AF545216

A Manual of DERMATOLOGY

A Manual of DERMATOLOGY

Second Edition

Zohra Zaidi MCPS
Former (Hon) Consultant
Jinnah Postgraduate Medical Centre
and
Dow Medical College and Civil Hospital
Karachi, Pakistan

Shernaz Walton MD FRCP (London)
Consultant Dermatologist
Hull and East Yorkshire, UK
and
Honorary Clinical Reader
Hull York Medical School, UK

Co-authors

Ijaz Hussain FCPS
Professor
Postgraduate Medical Institute
Lahore General Hospital
Lahore, Pakistan

Zarnaz Wahid FCPS
Professor and Head
Department of Dermatology
Dow University of Health Sciences and Civil Hospital
Karachi, Pakistan

Foreword

Hywel Williams

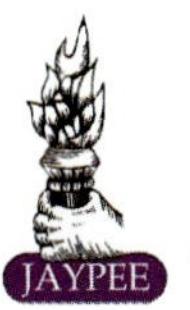

The Health Sciences Publisher
New Delhi | London | Philadelphia | Panama

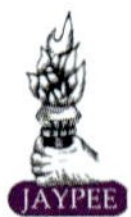

Jaypee Brothers Medical Publishers (P) Ltd

Headquarters

Jaypee Brothers Medical Publishers (P) Ltd
4838/24, Ansari Road, Daryaganj
New Delhi 110 002, India
Phone: +91-11-43574357
Fax: +91-11-43574314
Email: jaypee@jaypeebrothers.com

Overseas Offices

J.P. Medical Ltd
83, Victoria Street, London
SW1H 0HW (UK)
Phone: +44 20 3170 8910
Fax: +44 (0)20 3008 6180
Email: info@jpmedpub.com

Jaypee Medical Inc
The Bourse
111, South Independence Mall East
Suite 835, Philadelphia, PA 19106, USA
Phone: +1 267-519-9789
Email: jpmed.us@gmail.com

Jaypee Brothers Medical Publishers (P) Ltd
Bhotahity, Kathmandu, Nepal
Phone: +977-9741283608
Email: kathmandu@jaypeebrothers.com

Jaypee-Highlights Medical Publishers Inc
City of Knowledge, Bld. 237, Clayton
Panama City, Panama
Phone: +1 507-301-0496
Fax: +1 507-301-0499
Email: cservice@jphmedical.com

Jaypee Brothers Medical Publishers (P) Ltd
17/1-B, Babar Road, Block-B, Shaymali
Mohammadpur, Dhaka-1207
Bangladesh
Mobile: +08801912003485
Email: jaypeedhaka@gmail.com

Website: www.jaypeebrothers.com
Website: www.jaypeedigital.com

A Manual of Dermatology

First Edition: 2013
Second Edition: **2015**

ISBN 978-93-5152-792-3

Printed at: Ajanta Offset & Packagings Ltd., New Delhi

Dedicated to

The memory of my parents: my father, Syed Qadeer Hasan (Ex-Surveyor General of Pakistan) and my mother, Mrs Marzia Qadeer Hasan. Both my parents realized the importance of education and practically helped to promote it in many ways. This book is a small tribute to my loving and affectionate parents.

— Zohra Zaidi

My parents: my father, Dr Pesi Framroze Bilimoria (GP and Anesthetist) and my mother, Mrs Dinoo Pesi Bilimoria (English Scholar). They have always supported me in my quest for knowledge. Knowledge is a lifelong learning experience, and the book is a tribute to my dear parents.

— Shernaz Walton

Contributors

Anjum Kanjee MD FCPS CCFP
Skin Care Clinic
10171 Yonge Street
Richmond Hill
Ontario, Canada

Iain Foulds MBChB FRCP FFOM
Consultant Dermatologist and Senior Lecturer in Occupational Dermatology
Institute of Occupational and Environmental Health
University of Birmingham
Birmingham, UK

IS Nasr MRCP
Consultant Dermatologist
Queen's Hospital
Romford, UK

Khalid Hussain FCPS
Consultant Dermatologist
Lincoln County Hospital
Lincoln, UK

Major General Ashfaque Ahmed Khan MRCP
(Retd) Head of Dermatology and Advisor to Dermatology
Military Hospital
Rawalpindi, Pakistan

Mohammad Jafferany MD
Clinical Assistant Professor of Psychiatry
Michigan State University
Director
Psychodermatology Clinic
Saginaw, Michigan, USA

Ruqiya Shama Tareen MD
Associate Professor of Psychiatry
Psychosomatic Medicine
Director
Women Behavior Health Clinic
Michigan State University
Kalamazoo Center for Medical Studies
Kalamazoo, Michigan, USA

Sarwat Naseem FCPS
Associate Professor
Department of Dermatology
Ziauddin Medical University
Karachi, Pakistan

Shane Zaidi BSc (Hons) PhD MRCP FRCR
Academic Clinical Lecturer in Clinical Oncology
The Royal Marsden Hospital
Postdoctoral Training Fellow in Biological Sciences
Targeted Therapy Team
The Institute of Cancer Research
London, UK

Zarnaz Wahid FCPS
Professor of Dermatology
Dow University of Medical Health Sciences
Karachi, Pakistan

Foreword

No longer can a dermatology trainee working in Europe or the US say that he/she knows nothing about primary tuberculosis of the skin or leishmaniasis, as both conditions now crop up in skin clinics across the world—thanks to increased travel and the cosmopolitan nature of our societies. This book bridges the gap between the East and the West and is written by two busy clinical dermatologists having a vast experience of both the cultures. The book also bridges the gap between the introductory texts and the much larger definitive textbooks in dermatology. The book starts with a perfectly sized resume of the history of dermatology and then covers all of the main skin diseases and groups of diseases. Some of the chapters are arranged around common causes, such as ultraviolet light and the cold, which is helpful as patients rarely come into the clinic with their diagnosis. The chapters are supplemented with helpful summary tables and superb clinical photographs, as well as up-to-date treatment suggestions. The fact that two clinicians have written the entire book has helped its readability in terms of consistency and style. This book will be especially useful to trainee dermatologists, or any healthcare professional wishing to delve deeper into clinical dermatology than the introductory texts.

Hywel Williams
Director
Centre of Evidence-based Dermatology
University of Nottingham
Nottingham, UK

Preface to the First Edition

The book *A Manual of Dermatology* is written for residents and registrars of dermatology, physicians in internal medicine, general practitioners interested in dermatology, and for all doctors on rotation in dermatology. The book is simple-to-read, easy-to-understand and remember. The book should complement the textbooks of dermatology, and should serve as an introduction to the difficult and complex topics of dermatology.

Infectious and parasitic disorders that are prevalent in tropical countries are discussed in equal depth with the inflammatory and cutaneous malignancy due to ultraviolet radiation relatively common in the West. Today, in an outpatient clinic, patients from all over the globe are present in any metropolis city. It is, therefore, incumbent to know the diseases of the East and the West.

Poor economic conditions in developing countries preclude the use of expensive medicines and sophisticated diagnostic procedures. Therefore, time-tested inexpensive medications and simple laboratory techniques are mentioned. Majority of skin diseases are diagnosed on clinical examination, sometimes skin rashes become a conundrum. An appendix of differential diagnosis is included which should help the physicians in the diagnosis of cutaneous disorders.

A chapter on the history of dermatology is included. Our special thanks go to Professor LC Parish and Dr Nick Levell for their valuable suggestions on the subject. History of dermatology is a subject by itself; this chapter only gives a brief outline.

The book is an edited compilation of the lectures that we gave to the medical and postgraduate students of dermatology. The book could not be written without the support and help of innumerable friends and colleagues. We thank all our colleagues who allowed us to use their clinical photographs. Dr Rehan Alvi, Dr Naseema Kapadia, Dr Daulat Pinjani, Dr Badr Dhanani and Dr Aziz Khan are some of the consultants who have shared their photographs. We also thank Dr Shahbaz Janjua and Dr Ian McColl from the "Global Skin Atlas" for sharing their photographs. We are extremely grateful to our seniors and professors who taught us: Professor TS Haroon, Madam Naseem Zehra Jafri, Major General Ashfaque Ahmed Khan, Dr VR Metha, Dr Eustace J Desouza, Dr RJ Fernandez, Dr RG Valia from Mumbai, India, Late Dr K Keczkes, Dr EH Wyatt and Professor WJ Cunliffe from the UK. Whatever little we know is due to the hard work put by them. We also owe our thanks to Esen Rizvi for making all the illustrations for the book. Finally, we owe our sincere thanks to our family members for their extended support and help.

We would like to thank Shri Jitendar P Vij (Group Chairman), Mr Ankit Vij (Group President), and Mr Tarun Duneja (Director-Publishing) of M/s Jaypee Brothers Medical Publishers (P) Ltd, New Delhi, India, for publishing the book.

Zohra Zaidi
Shernaz Walton

Preface to the Second Edition

It is humbling indeed to write the preface for the second edition of our book *A Manual of Dermatology* within a short span of time. It gives us a sense of achievement and accomplishment. The former on account of its popularity with the trainee dermatologists, and the later due to a cause well served, as our younger colleagues found it useful in their clinical practice. It was unfortunate that due to some unavoidable circumstances the manual had some errors. This has been rectified; the manual has been extensively reviewed and updated. This edition is an easy to read, concise and up-to-date account of clinical dermatology to meet the needs of trainee dermatologists and general practitioners.

Finally, we owe our sincere thanks to our family members for their extended support and help.

We would like to thank Shri Jitendar P Vij (Group Chairman), Mr Ankit Vij (Group President), and Mr Tarun Duneja (Director-Publishing) of M/s Jaypee Brothers Medical Publishers (P) Ltd, New Delhi, India, for publishing the book.

Zohra Zaidi
Shernaz Walton

Contents

1. The History of Dermatology **1**

Ancient history 1
The middle ages 2
Modern age 3
Pioneer dermatologists 4

2. Skin: Structure, Function and Development **10**

Skin types 10
Structure of the skin 10
Epidermis 11
Desmosomes 15
Physiology of keratinisation 16
Characteristics of epidermal differentiation 16
The cell cycle 16
Control of the epidermal proliferation 17
The other cells of the epidermis 18
Basement membrane complex 20
Epidermal appendages 22
Hair 25
Nail 29
Dermis 32
Cellular components of the dermis 37
The cutaneous vasculature 37
Lymphatic circulation 38
Cutaneous nerves 38
Muscles of the dermis 39
Subcutaneous tissue 39
Skin lines 40
Occurrence of skin disease in relation to racial and ethnic characteristics 41
Development of skin 42
Investigations for hereditary disorders of the skin 45
Functions of the skin 46

3. Approach Towards a Dermatological Patient **49**

History taking 49
Examination 50
Some diagnostic hints 51
Special diagnostic procedures 51
Some clinical signs that help in diagnosis 52
Other laboratory investigations 52
Molecular diagnostics 53
Primary and secondary skin lesions 53
Commonly used descriptive terms in dermatopathology 56

4. Bacterial Infections **58**

Infections caused by *Staphylococcus aureus* and *Streptococcus haemolyticus* 59
Ecthyma 64
Infections caused by mycobacteria 70
Tuberculosis 70
Localized tuberculosis 72
Tuberculids 74
Diagnosis of tuberculosis 75
Diseases caused by atypical mycobacteria 77
Leprosy 79
Infections caused by other gram-positive bacteria 87
Corynebacteria 88
Actinomyces 90
Infections caused by gram-negative bacteria 92
Meningococcal infection 93
Glanders (Farcy) 95
Melioidosis (Whitmore's disease) 95
Tularemia (Ohara's disease) 95
Plague 96
Brucellosis (Undulant fever) 97
Rhinoscleroma 97
Rat-bite fever 97
Rickettsia 98
Spirochaetes 100
Chlamydia 104
Mycoplasma 104

5. Fungal Infections **106**

Superficial mycoses 107
Subcutaneous mycoses 128
Systemic mycoses 132
Opportunistic fungal infection 134

6. Viral Infections **136**

Herpes virus infections 137
Poxvirus 148
Human papillomavirus 152
Bowenoid papulosis 157
Picorna virus 158
Myxovirus and paramyxovirus 159
Erythema infectiosum (Fifth disease) 161
Other cutaneous disorders associated with virus infections 161

7. Parasitic Infestation, Diseases Caused by Arthropods and Other Venomous Animals **163**

Protozoal infestation 163
Trypanosomiasis 168
Toxoplasmosis 169

Helminthic infestations 170
Platyhelminths 175
Diseases caused by arthropods 176
Reptiles and other venomous animals 191
Dermatoses caused by aquatic animals 192

8. Sexually Transmitted Diseases 195

Syphilis 195
Latent syphilis 199
Tertiary syphilis 199
Congenital syphilis 202
Gonorrhoea 204
Non-gonococcal urethritis 205
Chancroid 206
Granuloma inguinale 206
Lymphogranuloma venereum 207
Human immunodeficiency virus infection 209

9. Eczema 216

Pathogenesis of eczema 216
Clinical and histological features of eczema 217
Special characteristic of eczema 218
(Secondary dissemination) 218
Treatment of eczema 219
Classification 219
Common contact eczemas 223
Infective eczema 230
Photosensitive eczema 230
Endogenous eczema 230
Seborrhoeic dermatitis 239
Nummular eczema 243
Hypostatic eczema 244
Pompholyx 245
Lichen simplex chronicus 247
Pityriasis alba 248
Asteatotic eczema 249
Juvenile plantar dermatosis 250
Eczematous drug eruptions 250
Hand eczema 251

10. Keratinising and Papulosquamous Disorders 255

Psoriasis 255
Lichen planus 274
Lichen nitidus 280
Lichen striatus 281
Callosity and corn 284
Acrokeratosis verruciformis 287
Follicular keratoses 288
Miscellaneous keratosquamous disorders 290

Porokeratosis 294
Congenital disorders of keratinisation 296

11. Connective Tissue Disorders **307**

Lupus erythematosus 307
Chronic discoid lupus erythematosus 308
Subacute lupus erythematosus 311
Systemic lupus erythematosus 311
Antiphospholipid syndrome 315
(Lupus anticoagulant syndrome) 315
Neonatal lupus erythematosus 316
Dermatomyositis 316
Scleroderma 319
Diffuse systemic sclerosis 321
Mixed connective tissue disease 324
Miscellaneous disorders of collagen tissue 325
Hereditary disorders of collagen and elastic tissue 328
Ehlers-Danlos syndrome 330
Marfran's syndrome 331
Juvenile hyaline fibromatosis 331

12. Bullous Disorders **334**

The pathogenic mechanisms of blister formation 334
Pemphigus 335
Other acantholytic bullous disorders 342
Pemphigoid 344
Dermatitis herpetiformis 348
Other subepidermal bullous disorders 352
Bullous disorders of children 354

13. Sarcoidosis **363**

Aetiology 363
Histopathology 364
Clinical features 364
Diagnosis 366
Treatment 367
Course and prognosis 367

14. Amyloidosis **368**

Aetiology 368
Histopathology 368
Clinical Features 369
Diagnosis 371
Treatment 371
Course and Prognosis 371

15. Diseases of Blood Vessels and Lymphatic System **373**

Vasculitis 373
Classification 373

According to the size of vessel involved 374
Cutaneous and systemic vasculitis 374
Neutrophilic vasculitis 374
Lymphocytic vasculitis 378
Granulomatous vasculitis 379
Vasculitis-miscellaneous 381
Erythemas of the skin 383
Other erythemas 387
Hypersensitivity syndromes (toxic erythemas) 392
Telangiectasia 393
Primary telangiectasia 393
Secondary telangiectasia 393
Disorders of the lymphatic system 396
Lymphoedema 396

16. Urticaria **399**

Aetiology 399
Pathogenesis 400
Classification 400
Differential diagnosis 403
Treatment 404
Angioedema (Quincke's oedema) 404
Mastocytosis 405
Papular urticaria 407

17. Purpura **408**

Aetiology 408
Investigations 409
Systemic causes of purpura 410
Purpura of dermatological interest 412
Miscellaneous purpuric disorders 415

18. Leg Ulcers **417**

Classification of leg ulcers 417
Venous ulcers 417
Arterial ulcer 421
Miscellaneous causes 422

19. Diseases of Pigmentation **425**

Physiology of pigmentation 426
Generalised Hyperpigmentation 426
Localised Hyperpigmentation 427
Reticular pigmentation 430
Generalised Hypopigmentation 432
Localised Hypopigmentation 435

20. Skin and Ultraviolet Radiation **441**

Sites of photosensitive eruption 442
Standard erythema dose 442
Ultraviolet radiation and its interaction with the skin 442

Effects of ultraviolet radiation on the skin at molecular level 443
Effects of solar radiation on the skin 445
Disorders of the skin caused by ultraviolet light 447
Classification 451
Treatment of porphyria 454
Photosensitisation due to abnormalities in DNA repair 457
Skin diseases aggravated by ultraviolet radiation 459
Protection and treatment of skin against UVR 459

21. Cutaneous Reactions to Cold **461**

Reaction of skin to cold—physiology 462
Dermatoses association with cold sensitivity 465

22. Pruritus **469**

Itch receptors 469
Central itch 469
Types of itch 469
Neural pathways of itching 470
Peripheral and central pharmacologic mediators of itch 470
Patterns of itching 472
Influence of skin temperature on itching 472
Causes of pruritus 472
Classification 473
Diagnosis and evaluation of the itching patient 477
Treatment 478

23. Disorders of the Sebaceous, Sweat and Apocrine Glands **480**

Acne vulgaris 480
Rosacea 491
Perioral dermatitis 494
Tumours of the sebaceous glands 495
Diseases of the sweat glands 495
Diseases of the eccrine glands 496
Hyperhidrosis 496
Intertrigo 498
Pitted keratolysis 498
Anhidrosis 499
Tumours of the sweat glands 500
Congenital disorders of the sweat glands 503
Diseases of the apocrine glands 504
Hidradenitis suppurativa (acne inversa) 504
Apocrine bromhidrosis 506
Apocrine chromhidrosis 506
Fox-Fordyce disease 506
Apocrine hidrocystoma 507

24. Hair Disorders **509**

Approach to a patient with hair disorders 509
Hypertrichosis 511
Hirsutism 512
Non-cicatricial alopecia 519
Alopecia areata 523
Cicatricial alopecia 528
Pseudopelade of Brocq 528
Folliculitis decalvans 529
Dissecting cellulitis of the scalp
(Perifolliculitis capitis abscedens et suffodiens) 529
Structural defects of the hair 531
Miscellaneous conditions of the scalp 535
Tumorus of the hair follicle 537
Hair cosmetics 539

25. Nail Disorders **544**

Nail changes in systemic disease 544
Nail changes due to cutaneous disorders 546
Discolouration (chromonychia) 549
Diseases of the nail fold 550
Abnormalities of the nail plate 552
Tumours adjacent to and under the nail 554
Congenital nail disorders 554

26. Diseases of the Subcutaneous Fat **557**

Panniculitis 558
Weber-Christian disease 560
Rothman-Makai syndrome 561
Panniculitis and pancreatic disease 561
(Nodular fat necrosis) 561
A1-antitrypsin deficiency-associated panniculitis 562
Sclerosing panniculitis 563
Dercums disease (Adiposis dolorosa) 563
Lipodystrophy 563
Cellulite 565

27. Tumours of the Skin **567**

Malignant tumours of the skin 567
Cutaneous T-cell lymphoma (Mycosis fungoides) 583
Primary cutaneous B-cell lymphomas 585
Premalignant dermatoses 588
Benign tumours of the skin 592
Tumours associated with congenital diseases 600

28. Naevi and Malformations **605**

Epidermal naevi 605
Epidermal keratinocytic naevi 606
Follicular naevi 609
Naevus sebaceous 610
Epidermal naevus syndrome 610

Vascular naevi 611
Venous malformation 616
Naevus anemicus 616
Blue rubber bleb naevus syndrome 617
Maffucci syndrome 617
Melanocytic naevi 617
Atypical naevus (Dysplastic naevus) 622
Dysplastic nevus syndrome 623
Spitz naevi (Juvenile melanoma) 624
Naevus achromicus 624
Lymphatic malformations 625
Connective tissue naevi 626
Angiokeratomas 627

29. Malnutrition and Skin **630**

Hypovitaminosis A 630
Hypervitaminosis A 631
Vitamin B complex 631
Vitamin D 634
Vitamin K 634
Vitamin E (α-tocopherol) 635
Vitamin C (Ascorbic acid) 635
Minerals 635
Essential fatty acids 637
Marasmus 638
Kwashiorkor 639
Plummer-Vinson syndrome 639
Obesity 640

30. Primary Cutaneous Immunodeficiency **641**

Innate immunity 641
Adaptive immunity 642
Humoral immunity 643
Classification of harmful allergic reaction 645
Cell-mediated immunity 646
Laboratory diagnosis and assessment of immunological disorders 647
When to suspect immunodeficiency 648
Disorders of phagocytosis 649
Disorders of the thymus and T lymphocytes 651
Diseases due to deficiency of antibodies 651
Combined antibody and T-cell deficiency 652
Severe combined immunodeficiency 653

31. Cutaneous Manifestations of Systemic Diseases **655**

Diabetes mellitus 655
Liver disease 657
Pancreatic disease 659
Cutaneous manifestations of malabsorption states 660

Miscellaneous disorders of gastrointestinal tract 660
Renal disease 661
Rheumatoid arthritis 663
Hyperthyroidism 664
Hypothyroidism 664
Cushing's syndrome 664
Addison's disease 665
Xanthomatosis (hyperlipidemias) 665
Disorders of lipid metabolism 667
Disorders of amino acid metabolism 669
Mucopolysaccharidosis 671
Calcinosis cutis 672
Angiokeratoma with systemic disease 673
Cutaneous manifestations of immunosuppression 674
Cutaneous manifestations of internal malignancy 675

32. Systemic Effects of Cutaneous Disease: Erythroderma 678

Causes of erythroderma 678
Manifestations cutaneous 679
Manifestations systemic 679
Treatment of erythroderma 680

33. Ages of Man and their Dermatoses 682

Neonatal dermatology 682
Transient neonatal dermatoses 683
Neonatal dermatoses 684
Specific neonatal dermatoses 685
Panniculitis in neonates 687
Oedema of the newborn 688
Cutaneous changes in pregnancy 688
Specific dermatoses of pregnancy 689
Cutaneous changes at menopause 691
Skin disorders of menopause 692
The ageing skin 692
Skin changes in the ageing skin 693
Histological features of the ageing skin 695
Dermatoses of the elderly 695
Premature ageing syndromes 695
Diagnosis of ageing syndromes 698
Methods of improving the skin in ageing 698

34. Skin and Sports 700

Skin diseases that prevent sports 700
Diseases transmitted to other players 701
Cutaneous injuries due to sport 701
Injuries due to mechanical trauma 701
Heat-induced injuries 704
Cold-induced injuries 705
Injuries due to the sun 705

Contact dermatitis 705
Miscellaneous 706
Skin diseases aggravated by sports 708

35. Skin and Psychiatry **710**

Classification of psychocutaneous disorders 710
Psychiatric disorders with dermatologic symptoms 710
Dermatologic disorders that are exacerbated by psychophysiological mechanisms 714
Approach to patients with psychocutaneous disorders 714

36. Diseases of the Oral Cavity **716**

Ulcers of the oral cavity 717
White lesions of the oral mucosa 723
Black/brown pigmented lesions of the oral mucosa 727
Red lesions of the oral mucosa 729
Tumours of the oral cavity 730
Cheilitis 732

37. Cutaneous Manifestation of Diseases of External Genitalia **736**

Specific disorders of female external genitalia 736
Specific disorders of male external genitalia 740

38. Miscellaneous Disorders **744**

Poikiloderma 744
Acanthosis nigricans 745
Pyoderma gangrenosum 747
Malignant atrophic papulosis 748
Sweet's syndrome (Acute febrile neutrophilic dermatosis) 749
Jessner's lymphocytic infiltration 751
Pseudolymphomas 751
Lymphomatoid papulosis 752
Gangrene of the skin 752
Treatment of gangrene 755
Histiocytosis 756
Mucinosis 759
Necrobiotic disorders 761
Perforating disorders 763
Piezogenic papules 766
Rieter's disease 767
Prurigo 771
Atrophy of the skin 772
Anetoderma 773
Cutis verticis gyrata 775
Pachydermoperiostosis 776
Ainhum 777
Pseudoainhum 777
Relapsing polychondritis 777
Cutaneous manifestations of drug abuse 778

39. Occupational Dermatoses **782**

Occupational hand dermatitis 782
Contact urticaria 783
Infections 783
Acne 784
Malignancy 785
Heat 785
Cold 785
Vibration syndrome 785
Connective tissue disorders 786
Importance of occupational skin diseases 786
Diagnosis of occupational skin disease 786
Treatment and prevention of occupational skin disease 787
Prognosis of occupational skin disease 788

40. Injuries Due to Burn **789**

Assessment of damage caused by burns 789
Clinical assessment of a burn injury 790
Factors to be considered in assessing burn injury 791
Special types of burn 791
Complication of burns 792
Treatment 792
Referral to a burn unit 794

41. Fundamentals of Topical Therapy and Some Common Dermatological Preparations **795**

Principles of topical therapy 795
Amount to be dispensed 795
Percutaneous absorption 796
Frequency of application 797
Ingredients in topical preparations 797
Topical preparations 797
Some common dermatological formulae 799

42. Systemic Therapy **804**

Corticosteroids 804
Antifungals 810
Retinoids 814
Psoralens 817
Immunosuppressive and cytotoxic drugs 819
Immunobiologics 824
Intravenous immunoglobulin 827
Topical immunomodulators 828
Antimalarials 830
Dapsone 832
Antiviral drugs 833
Ribavirin 837
Promise of the future: Gene therapy 837

43. Cutaneous Drug Reactions **840**

Classification of drug reactions 840
Approach to diagnosis of drug reactions 841
Skin lesions in drug reaction 841
Severe skin reactions 843
Uncommon reactions 845
Prevention 849

44. Physical Modalities in Cutaneous Therapy **850**

Biopsy 850
Curettage 852
Shave excision 852
Electrocautery 853
Electrolysis 853
Thermolysis 853
Iontophoresis 853
Mohs surgery 854
Cryosurgery 854
Lasers 857
Intense pulsed light 862
Photodynamic therapy 862
Cosmetic dermatology 863
Filling agents 866
Botox injections 867

45. Radiotherapy in Dermatology **869**

Types of ionising radiation used in dermatology 869
Treatment regimens 871
Postradiation changes in the skin 871
Indications for radiation 872
Side effects of radiotherapy and skin care 873

Appendices—Differential diagnosis

Appendix 1: Generalized Eruptions 875
Appendix 2: Hair Disorders 877
Appendix 3: Face 879
Appendix 4: Upper and Lower Limb 881
Appendix 5: Flexures 882
Appendix 6: Lesions Differentiated by Colour 883
Appendix 7: Lesions Differentiated by Appearance and Texture 884
Appendix 8: Vascular Reactions 885
Appendix 9: Nail Disorders 886
Appendix 10: Miscellaneous 888

Bibliography *891*

Index *895*

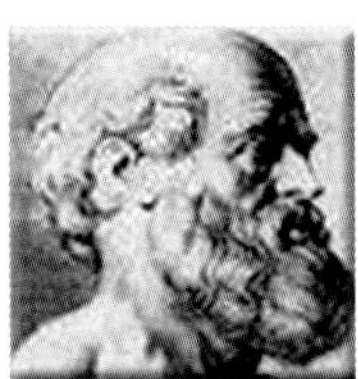
Hippocrates (460–370 BC)

Excerpt
from the
HIPPOCRATIC OATH

I swear to fulfil, to the best of my ability and judgment, this covenant:

I will respect the hard-won scientific gains of those physicians in whose steps I walk, and gladly share such knowledge as is mine with those who are to follow.

I will apply for the benefit of the sick, all measures that are required, avoiding those twin traps of overtreatment and ***therapeutic nihilism****.*

I will not be ashamed to say "I know not", nor will I fail to call in my colleagues when the skills of another are needed for a patient's recovery.

I will neither give a deadly drug to anybody if asked for it, nor will I make a suggestion to this effect. In purity and holiness I will guard my life and my art.

I will benefit the sick according to my ability and judgement; I will keep them from harm and injustice.

I will respect the privacy of my patients, for their problems are not disclosed to me that the world may know.

In every house where I come I will enter only for the good of my patients, keeping myself far from all intentional ill-doing and all seduction.

I will remember that I do not treat a fever chart, a cancerous growth, but a sick human being, whose illness may affect the person's family and economic stability. My responsibility includes these related problems, if I am to care adequately for the sick.

I will prevent disease whenever I can, for prevention is preferable to cure.

I will remember that I remain a member of society, with special obligations to all my fellow human beings, to those sound of mind and body, as well as the infirm.

If I do not violate this oath, may I enjoy life and art, respected while I live and remembered with affection after death.

Chapter 1

The History of Dermatology

INTRODUCTION

History of medicine forms an infrastructure on which modern dermatology is based. Evidence of disease is found in the earliest Egyptian literature, the Ebers Papyrus and then in Grecian, Roman and Arabic medicine. The history of dermatology can only be distinguished from the history of medicine at the beginning of the 19th century, when dermatology like the other specialities began to be recognised as a special branch of medicine.

ANCIENT HISTORY

Ebers Papyrus is the oldest and most important medical papyrus of ancient Egypt. It was written in about 1536 BCE, it is a compilation of medical lore going back to about 3000 BCE. The Papyrus devotes a considerable amount of space to skin diseases, leprosy is frequently mentioned. Healing was an art addressed on many levels. Turmeric powder and henna were used to treat open wounds. Acacia and aloe vera were employed for skin ailments. Remedy was evolved for removal of guinea worm by wrapping it round a stick and then slowly pulling it out, this method was still used as a standard treatment till recent times. The magicians and priests would drive away the evil demons. Cleanliness, bathing, shaving hair from the scalp were as significant for treating disease as were dietary restrictions such as eating raw fish unclean animals.

Other early writings from Mesopotamia come from the clay tablets, which have description of disease of ears, eyes, skin, heart and various venereal diseases. Mention is made of a child born with a birthmark was called 'spotted evil' which predicted a misfortune or even the death of a king.

Hippocrates (460–370 BCE) is said to have freed medicine from the shackles of magic, superstitions and supernatural phenomenon. He initiated the theory of four humors, but actually this concept is found in Cretan and Mycenaean medicine. According to this theory the body consists of four humours: blood yellow bile, black bile and phlegm. An imbalance of the humours caused disease and the physician's role was to restore health by correcting the imbalance and restoring harmony to the humours. Skin being a vehicle for the excretion of humours. The equilibrium could be disturbed by climate, environment and nutrition.

Hippocratic writings contained a number of passages which refer to cutaneous disorders. He divided skin diseases into two types: local (those with an independent existence) and constitutional (those that occur due to elimination of disease). Hippocrates made an astute observation "Eunuchs are not subject to gout, nor do they suffer from baldness", wisely reflecting on his own alopecia.

Aristotle (384–322 BCE) too was aware of the hormonal association of baldness. He noticed that neither normal women nor eunuchs went bald and that both were unable to grow hair on their chest. Aristotle mentions "*akari*" a kind of a tiny animal that may be applied to the mite of scabies-acarus. Aristotle also described lice, nits and bed bug. The cautery was effectively used by the Greeks to treat infection, wounds and tumors.

Cornelius Celsus (25 BCE–50 CE) of Rome, although a layman, he wrote books on agriculture, law, military science, philosophy and medicine. Only eight books comprising his "De Medicine" have survived. The sixth book is devoted chiefly to skin diseases. He called attention to the dangers of a carbuncle on the face. He also described patterns of alopecia, "Area Celsi" perhaps was alopecia areata, cradle cap was called mothers crust, thought to be due to the disturbance of humours by the mother's milk. Celsus recognised the common wart as "thymion" and "myrmecia" was another term used by Celsus for the deeper and broader variety of warts of the palms and soles. He is best known for the four signs of inflammation—calor, rubor, tumor and dalor.

Pedanius Dioscorides (40–90CE) was a celebrated Greek physician, pharmacist and botanist wrote "De Materia Medica", a precursor of all modern pharmacopeias. He found that the fig could be used for a number of skin diseases its juice could bleach freckles, while an unripe fig was used for treating warts, and when mixed with honey and salt it was used to treat oozing sores. Radish in a decoction with honey could remove the black and blue marks around the eyes.

Claudius Galen of Pergamon (131–201CE) was an eminent physician, he was born in Greece and later settled in Alexandria. His writings acquired a canonical status during the Middles Ages, but fell into dispute during the renaissance, as Galen's writing were based on animal anatomy, human dissection was legalised later. Galen distinguished skin diseases into those of the hairy parts of the body and those of the non-hairy parts, a classification that existed until the 18th century. Galen also advanced the theory of humours to linking them with the temperaments of the human body, sanguine, choleric, phlegmatic and melancholic.

Methods of prevention of disease have also been used since ancient times. Long before Jenner introduced the vaccination against smallpox, some tribes in Africa protected themselves against smallpox by inserting the fluid of smallpox blisters under the skin. In some parts of Asia, smallpox swabs were moistened in water and then pricked under the skin. Chinese were known to blow powdered scabs of smallpox into the nostrils. Wooden patens were worn in Sudan to prevent against guinea worm infection.

THE MIDDLE AGES

Al-Razi (865–925CE) was a Persian physician and philosopher. He wrote a number of books on medicine. The most popular one was "The Comprehensive Book on Medicine" (Kitab Al-Hawi Al-Tibb). In his treatise, he described smallpox and measles, diseases not described by Hippocrates. Al Razi's interest was exanthemata. Al Razi was also the first physician to relate hay fever with the smell of roses.

Ibn-Sina (Avicenna 980–1037CE), was also a Persian scholar, well versed in philosophy, medicine, music and mathematics. His book "The Canon of Medicine" became the leading medical encyclopedia for centuries. It was the first book which dealt with experimental medicine and evidence-based medicine. Avicenna stressed on testing of drugs before its use on the human body. Avicenna's medical philosophy was based on the theory of four humours similar to that of Hippocrates and Galen. Avicenna laid stress on the pores of the skin as a route to eliminate the excess of humours for cure of disease. He mentioned that exercise clears the pores of the skin and bathing dilates the pores, which help in the maturation of abscesses. Avicenna also wrote good descriptions of anthrax, carbuncle, and lesions on the head and neck. Avicenna was an authority on skin diseases in the Middle Ages.

Moses Ben Maimon (1135–1204) better known as Maimonides was a Jewish philosopher of the 12th century. He was born in Spain and eventually settled in Egypt. He was an outstanding Talmudic scholar and the first person to write a systematic code for all Jewish law. Maimonides also achieved fame as a physician, writing a number of medical treatises. His work on medical ethics has great depth.

Many contagious diseases were introduced into Europe by the returning crusaders. Epidemics of typhus, leprosy, smallpox and other diseases can be directly traced to the returning crusaders, but the most notorious epidemic to be imported from the East was that of Black Death or bubonic plague, which killed about 25 million people in the 14th century. Nostradamus, the famous French astrologer had studied at the medical school in Montpellier, he later settled as a practitioner at Agen. His healing powers soon spread throughout France and to neighbouring countries, where he was called to treat plague. Nostradamus is also famous for his prophecies.

After the crusade wars (1095–1291), new nursing and hospital orders were developed. The order of Lazarus, which was devoted to the care of the lepers, was found at the beginning of the 12th century. Leprosy was endemic in Europe, but with the return of the crusaders, the number of lepers increased considerably.

Leprosy patients were subjected to total ostracism from society, which was strictly enforced by the government. Leprosy was considered as a punishment of sin from God, the people considered that even a touch of a leper would result in death. Distinctive clothing was mandatory, as was segregation in places of public assembly and even worship. However, the order of Lazarus was so sympathetic to the care of the lepers that thousands of leprosoria were soon built throughout Europe.

MODERN AGE

Girolamo Fracastoro (1478–1553) was an Italian physician, a scholar in mathematics and geography, a poet and an astronomer. Fracastoro proposed the scientific germ theory of disease, more than 300 years before Louis Pasteur and Robert Koch. His book "De Contagione" also gives the description of typhus.

The name for syphilis is derived from Fracastoro's epic poem, written in three books. Syphilis was the name of a shepherd boy, who insulted a Sun god. He was punished by the god with a terrible disease, which had the features of the disease syphilis. The poem suggests its cure by mercury and guaiaco.

Girolamo Mercuriale (1530–1606) born in Italy and educated in Bologna, Padua and Venice. Mercuriale wrote many books on medicine, including one on skin diseases, "De Morbis Cutaneis et Omnibus Corporis Humani Excrementis Tractatus", this was published in 1572. In 1585, he published "De Decoratione", which deals what may be called cosmetic dermatology including plastic surgery.

Bernardino Ramazinni (1633–1714), an Italian physician is known as the "Father of Occupational Medicine". While still a medical student his attention was drawn towards the disease of working places. He would visit workplaces, observe workers activities and discuss their illness. His writings include "De Morbis Artificum Diatriba" (Disease of workers). Ramazinni described cutaneous ulcers in men working with mercury and contact dermatitis in men working with animal hides. Perhaps this was the beginning of the awareness towards industrial dermatology.

Percival Pott (1714–1788) reported that chimney sweepers had ragged sores on their scrotum. Most of the other doctors of the time thought it was some venereal diseases. But Pott was astute and said that it was skin cancer, caused by the lodging of soot in the rugae of the scrotum. The observation was a clinical milestone. It was the first cancer described caused by an external agent. The cancer was called the "chimney sweepers cancer", a classic in industrial medicine.

John Hunter (1728–1793) was a Scottish surgeon, who moved to London at an early age of 20 years. He inoculated himself with the secretion from a case of gonorrhoea. As the patient was suffering from both gonorrhoea and syphilis, Hunter developed syphilis and he thought that both the diseases had a common origin. He died 20 years later of syphilitic heart diseases. Philippe Record (1799–1889) later established the independent existence of syphilis and gonorrhoea.

James Currie (1758–1805) a Scottish physician, sparkled a renewal of interest in hydrotherapy. He used cold water to treat some contagious fevers in Liverpool. In 1777, he made public his views on experience in hydrotherapy. The spas of England were popular for the sufferers of gout and other metabolic diseases. Psoriasis is treated today at the Dead Sea Clinic in Israel, Swiss Alps and in the North Sea Islands

PIONEER DERMATOLOGISTS

Austria

Joseph Plenck (1735–1807), the Viennese protodermatologist is considered to be the forerunner of modern European dermatology. Plenck introduced the systematisation of dermatovenereological diseases, based on their paradigmatic differences. He wrote many treatises including dermatology and venereology. He also compiled a book which enlisted 800 plants with medicinal uses.

Ferdinand Ritter von Hebra (1816–1880) (Fig. 1), the "Father of the New Vienna School of Dermatology" was the first to specialise entirely in skin diseases. He established in the Vienna School of Medicine, a centre of dermatological training and research. He trained scholars from Europe and America.

He began his career working with Joseph Skoda who was the head of the department of chest diseases; Skoda saw Hebra's interest in skin diseases and supported him in opening a division of dermatology in the hospital. Hebra experimented on himself with the scabies mite. He transferred the mite on his skin and then observed the primary and secondary lesions of scabies. He also experimented on various chemicals on the skin and saw that it produced contact dermatitis.

These findings led him to prove that cutaneous diseases were due to agents acting on the skin itself. Skin was not only a mirror for the manifestation of internal disorders or a route for the excretion of humours. He discarded the theory of four humours. Von Hebra classified skin diseases in 12 categories based on their morphological and microscopic appearance. These were hyperaemia, anaemia, anomalies of secretion, exudations, haemorrhage, atrophy, hypertrophy, benign new growths, malignant new growths, ulcers, neurosis and parasitic disorders. His treatment was therefore directed at the local problems, rather than the abnormalities of the humours, which were still considered the primary source of disease.

Dermatology lends itself as a playground for artists, because skin diseases are visible to the naked eye. In Hebras atlas a whole spectrum of dermatological diseases are covered.

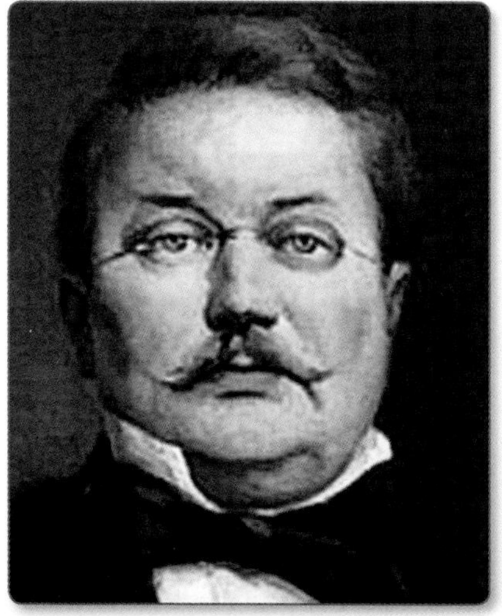

Fig. 1: Ferdinand Ritter von Hebra (1816–1880)

Hebra trained several men who rose to eminence; some of them were Kaposi, Kobner, Neumann, Pick, Duhrling and Auspitz. His students were not only from Austria, but also from other countries in Europe and America.

In his 40 years of service as a dermatologist, he had endeared to him the entire population of Vienna. On his death in 1880, his funeral was attended by the royalty, the nobility and the citizenry. Such a concourse had never before been witnessed in Vienna.

After the great Hebra were Kaposi, Austipz, Kobner, Hansen and Unna.

Moritz Kaposi (1837–1902) was the son-in-law and successor of Hebra, he married his daughter Martha Hebra. Kaposi was credited with the description of xeroderma pigmentosum. His atlas on skin diseases was extensive and most valuable at his time. Kaposi's name entered in history when he described Kaposi's sarcoma of the skin. The sarcoma was discovered in five elderly patients and Kaposi initially called it "idiopathic multiple pigmented sarcoma". More than a century later it was seen in gay men of New York.

France

French dermatology has been represented by so many brilliant minds, to name a few: Alibert, Lorry, Bazin, Virchow, Hallopeau, Brocq and Darier. Most of them were trained at the Hospital Saint Louis.

J L Alibert (1768–1837) (Fig. 2) laid the foundation of dermatology at the Hospital Saint Louis. Alibert first wanted to be a priest, but later took medicine as a career. He is called the "Father of French Dermatology". He classified skin diseases in 12 categories and likened his classification to a tree. An imaginary tree was drawn an on its branches were his classification. He is said to have taught dermatology to his students under a lime tree in the hospital, till his department was established.

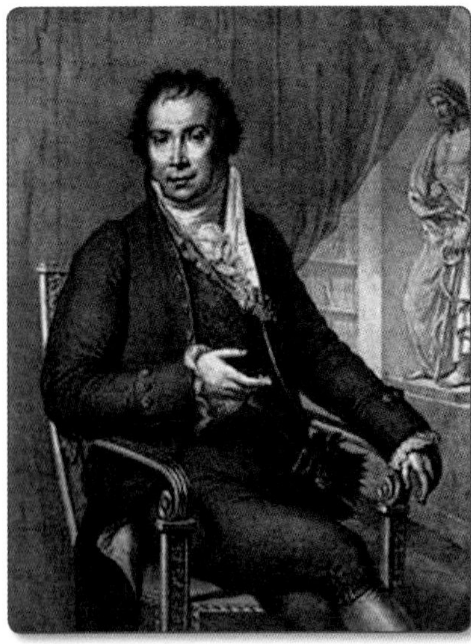

Fig. 2: J L Alibert (1768–1837)

Anne Charles Lorry was called the first French dermatologist; he had two special fields of interests, dermatology and mental diseases. He conceived the idea that the skin was an organ with its own blood vessels, nerves and lymphatics, but after being appointed as a physician to Louis XVI, he had to leave his interest in skin diseases. Similar was the case with Jean Louis Alibert.

Ernest Bazin (1807–1878) recognized the important role that parasites play in skin diseases. His revolutionary work in the treatment of scabies and fungal infections established him the chief at St Louis School.

United Kingdom

The pioneer English dermatologists were Daniel Turner, Robert Willan, Sir Erasmus Wilson, Tilbury Fox, Sir Jonathan Hutchinson and John James Pringle.

Daniel Turner (1667–1740) came into medicine as a Barber –Surgeon, but he was dissatisfied with it because of the lack of glamour in the profession. He then moved on to medicine, he was accepted as a licentiate of the College of Physicians in London. Turner showed a considerable practical knowledge of dermatology and had a considerable concern for the welfare of skin patients. He wrote the first dermatological text in English entitled "A treatise on Diseases Incident on the Skin". The book was translated into both German and French. He also wrote a book on syphilis. Turner should be regarded in a minor way as the founder of British Dermatology.

Robert Willan (1757–1812) (Fig. 3) a Yorkshire born physician practiced at the Public Dispensary in London. He is the accepted founder of British Dermatology. Willan was a general practitioner, but had a special interest in dermatology; his greatest achievement was the modified Plenk's classification of skin disease. He grouped skin disorders in eight categories, based on the morphology of skin lesions. Willan described the morphology of skin disease in detail, such as type of lesion, the shape and size, presence or absence of umbilication, redness, colour, consistency, pattern of distribution, etc. Willan elected to publish his findings in sections, four of which appeared between

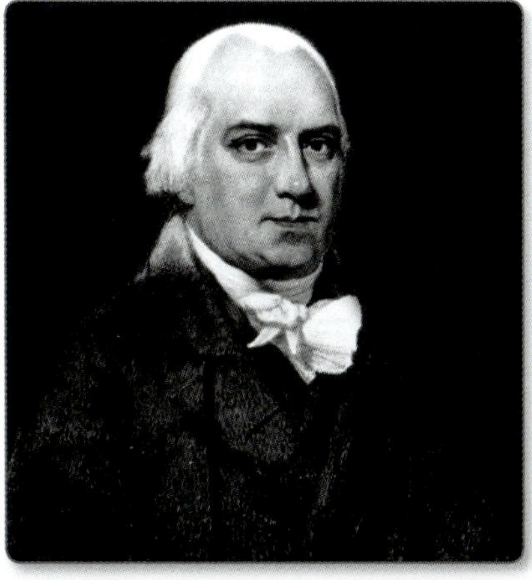

Fig. 3: Robert Willan (1757–1812)

1798 and 1808. The four sections were under the title "On Cutaneous Diseases". This work was completed later by Thomas Bateman, his student.

Thomas Bateman (1778–1821) completed Willans classification, later published his book "Practical Synopsis of Cutaneous Diseases". The book was a very successful work, it went through eight editions in 20 years. Bateman generously described his work to be merely an extension of Willan's work. Bateman died at the age of 43 after an illness associated with partial blindness. Had he not died prematurely, he would have added much more to the knowledge of dermatology.

Sir Erasmus Wilson (1809–1884) was one of the greatest dermatologists of his time. His book "Diseases of the Skin" ran through six volumes. Sir Erasmus Wilson was also known for his philanthropy. An extensive traveler and Egyptologist, he brought back from Egypt the monument known as the "Cleopatra's Needle" and set it on the Thames Embankment, at a cost of then £10,000. Altogether, his contributions towards arts and sciences were about £30,000. It is indeed a unique accomplishment among medical men. Erasmus Wilson was knighted in 1881.

United States

Dermatology in the United States began with two men who studied skin diseases briefly in the clinics of Paris in Europe. Henry Daggett Bulkley (1804–1872) a Yale graduate on return from Paris, established the first dispensary for the treatment of skin and venereal diseases, the Broome Street Infirmary for Skin diseases, and a year later delivered a series of lectures on dermatology, the first ever in North America.

Noah Worcester (1812–1847) a Dartmouth graduate after studying in the Parisian clinics joined the faculty of the newly founded Medical School of Ohio. Dr Noah Worcester published the first American textbook on skin diseases in 1845, "A Synopsis of the Symptoms, Diagnosis and Treatment of the More Common and Important Diseases of the Skin". Dr Worcester's early death from tuberculosis was a setback for American dermatology.

Most of the early American dermatologists travelled to Europe for postgraduate training, Vienna was the favourite place for most of them. James Clark White after postgraduate studies in Europe became the first professor of dermatology at Harvard in 1871. Other early American dermatologists were Louis A Duhring, Henry Granger Piffard, George Henry Fox, John T Bowen and William Allen Pusey. Duhring was a student of Hebra, his article on dermatitis herpetiformis ran through 18 papers. Duhring acquired large fortune and was second only to Erasmus Wilson in his benefactions.

This chapter is only a small tribute to the pioneers of medicine and dermatology great doctors and scientists have contributed to the history of dermatology, only a few have been listed above. We are living today in an age of great development and progress, but our past should not be forgotten. Winston Churchill addressing the Royal College of Physicians in March 1944 said, "The further you look back, the further you can look forward".

Wisdom lies in remembering past experiences and drawing benefits from them

FURTHER READING

1. Aliotta G, Capasso G, Strumia S, et al. Joseph Jacob Plenck. (1735–1807). Am J Nephrol. 1994;14(4-6):377-82.
2. Crissey JT, Parish LC. Two hundred years of dermatology. J Am Acad Dermatol. 1998;39(6):1002-6.
3. Holubar K, Frankl J. Joseph Plenck (1735–1807). A forerunner of modern dermatology. J Am Acad Dermatol. 1984;10(2):326-32.
4. Jackson R. Historical outline of attempts to classify skin disease. Can Med Assoc J. 1977;116:1165-8.
5. King JM. Historical review of early dermatology. South Med J. 1983;76(4):426-36.
6. Lyell A. Daniel Turner, and the first controlled therapeutic trial in dermatology. Clin and Exp Dermatol. 1986;11:191-4.
7. McCaw IH. A Synopsis of the history of dermatology. Ulster Med J. 1944;13(2):109-22.
8. O'Malley CD. Dermatological origins. Arch Dermatol. 1961;83(2):204-13.
9. Parish LC, Parish JL, Parish DH. Bibliography of secondary sources on the history of dermatology: 1. Journal articles in English supplemented through 2010. Clin Dermatol. 2011;29(4):469-74.
10. Potter BS. Bibliographic landmarks in the history of dermatology. J Am Acad Dermatol. 2003;48(6):919-32.
11. Sutton RL. Diseases of the skin: Mercurialis. Arch Dermatol. 1966;94 (6):763-72.
12. Zaidi Z, Wahid Z, Kapadia N. The History of Dermatology. Specialist. 1999;15(1):157-64.

Chapter 2

Skin: Structure, Function and Development

INTRODUCTION

Skin is the largest organ of the body. In the average adult man, it weighs 15% of the body weight and has a surface area of 1.7 m^2. The thickness of the skin varies from 1 mm over the eyelid and prepuce to about 2–3 mm on the palms and soles. The epidermis is only about 0.1 mm thick, but over the palms and soles it is much thicker. Skin is a tough elastic outer covering of the body; including the external auditory meatus and the lateral aspect of the tympanic membrane. It is continuous with the mucosae of the alimentary, respiratory and urogenital tracts at their respective orifices, where the specialised skin of the mucocutaneous junction occurs; it also fuses with the conjunctiva at the margins of the eyelids and with the lining of the lacrimal canaliculi at the lacrimal puncta. Skin is a complex sensitive organ necessary for the well-being and maintenance of life. It is not merely icing on an anatomical cake.

SKIN TYPES

Skin may be hairy or nonhairy (glabrous skin), such as on the palms and soles. Alternating ridges and sulci mark the nonhairy skin, these are arranged in unique individual configuration called dermatoglyphics.

Glabrous skin is characterized by thick epidermis, including a compact stratum corneum and by the presence of encapsulated sense organs in the dermis. There are no hair follicles and sebaceous glands in the glabrous skin.

The hairy skin on the other hand has both hair follicles and sebaceous glands, but lack the encapsulated sense organs. There is a wide variation in the structure of the skin in different regions of the body, e.g. in its distribution of hair, glands, its color, etc. Hairy skin constitutes the great majority of the body's covering.

Minor areas of the skin have special features that do not fall in the two types of skin described. Mucocutaneous junctions of the lips, outer rim of the anal canal, urethral opening, glans penis and glans clitoris have a characteristic histology; they have a thin epidermis lacking glands or hair.

STRUCTURE OF THE SKIN

The skin (Fig. 1) consists of epidermis and dermis, beneath which is the subcutaneous tissue. The epidermis and its appendages (nails, hair, eccrine, apocrine and sebaceous glands) are derived from the embryonic ectoderm. The dermis and the subcutaneous tissue are of mesodermal origin. The epidermis is

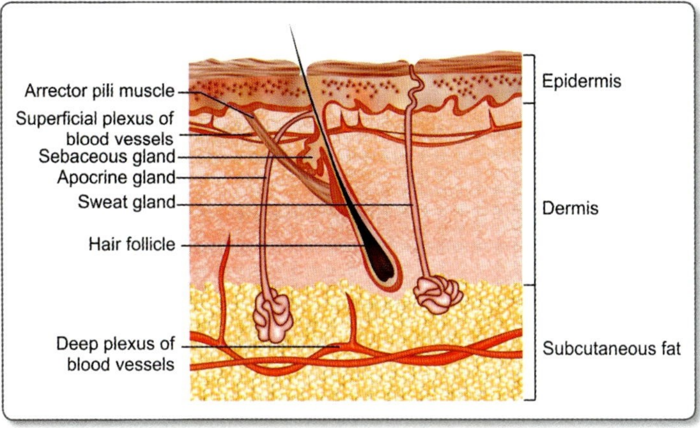

Fig. 1: Structure of the skin
Source: Ziadi Z, Lanigan S. Dermatology in Clinical Practice. Skin structure and function. London: Springer; 2010. pp. 1-15. With kind permission of Springer Science + Business Media.

multilayered that renews itself continuously by the cell division in its deepest layer, the basal layer. The epidermis is devoid of blood vessels and lymphatics; it derives its nutrition from the dermis. The lower surface of the epidermis is folded, in cross section, it appears wavy and these downward projections are the rete ridges, which interdigitate with the dermal papillae. The epidermis is attached with the dermis through the basement membrane.

EPIDERMIS

Epidermis is the major protective layer derived from the fetal ectoderm, it is mainly formed by cells called keratinocytes, these constitute about 95% of the epidermal cells. The basic function of these cells is to form keratin. The basic component of the cytoplasm of the keratinocytes are tonofilaments, these are intermediate filaments composed of fibrous protein arranged in an alpha helical pattern. The tonofilaments are fashioned into bundles; these converge upon and terminate at the plasma membrane, and where they end in specialised attachments called desmosomes. These filaments belong to the class of intermediate filaments of 100 Armstrong (Å) diameters.

Keratin

Keratin is a tough insoluble protein that forms the epidermal stratum corneum, hair and nail of humans, horn and hooves of animals. It consists of polypeptide chains linked by disulphide bonds, hydrogen bonds and salt linkages.

Keratins are a family of proteins with more than 50 individual members; each product is of a distinct and separate gene. The molecular weight of keratin varies from 40,000 to 67,000 Dalton (Da). The genes coding the individual keratins fall into two families, acidic and basic. The acidic keratins (Type I) range from 40–65 kDa and cover a pH range 4.5–6. The neutral-basic keratin (Type II) are larger 50–70 kDa covering a pH range 6.5–8.5. Type I keratin is encoded in chromosome 17q, type II keratin is encoded in chromosome 12q. These occur in pairs an acidic and basic pair in a cell. Basal keratins are K5/K14 and suprabasal keratins are K1/K10. Basal keratinocytes of the epidermis synthesises keratin 5 and 14. The suprabasal keratinocytes synthesise keratins 1 and 10. Abnormalities in the genetic coding for the keratins can result in diseases, such as epidermolysis bullosa and bullous ichthyosiform erythroderma.

Keratin may be soft or hard. Keratin of the skin is soft, while that of the nails and hair is hard. Hard keratin lacks keratohyalin granules; the tonofilaments harden through incorporation of disulphide bonds. Soft keratin desquamates due to the action of enzymes; hard keratin does not shed, but has to be cut. Soft keratin contains more glycine and hard keratin is rich in sulphur containing amino acids.

Layers of the Epidermis

The epidermis is composed of several distinct layers (Fig. 2), from the inner to the outer surface. These layers are:

- Stratum germinativum (Basal cell layer)
- Stratum malpighii (Prickle cell layer)
- Stratum granulosum
- Stratum corneum
- Stratum lucidum.

Stratum germinativum: The basal layer is the deepest layer of the epidermis; it rests on a basement membrane, which attaches it to the dermis. These cells are the only keratinocytes in the normal epidermis, which undergo cell division. It consists of a single layer of columnar cells, but it may be 2–3 cells

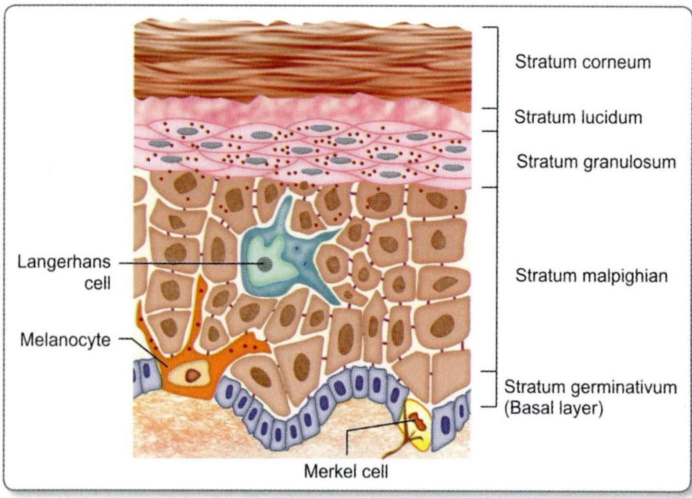

Fig. 2: Epidermis
Source: Ziadi Z, Lanigan S. Dermatology in Clinical Practice. Skin structure and function. London: Springer; 2010. pp. 1-15. With kind permission of Springer Science + Business Media.

thick in the glabrous skin (nonhairy skin) and hyperproliferative epidermis. Basal cells are small columnar cells with large dark staining nucleus, their long axis is perpendicular to the skin surface, and each cell is positioned next to the other in a pallisading pattern. The basic component of the cytoplasm is tonofilament. The basal cells are anchored to a basement membrane, this lies between the epidermis and the dermis. Present amongst the basal cells are the melanocytes and Merkel cells.

Basal cells contain a full range of intracellular organelles, such as Golgi apparatus, mitochondria, endoplasmic reticulum, ribosomes, etc. Hemidesmosomes are attachments present between the basal layer keratinocytes and underlying basement membrane. Desmosomes are attachments between two keratinocytes.

Basal cells contain keratin filaments (tonofilaments) organised into fine bundles around the nucleus and connecting to hemidesmosomes and desmosomes. Basal cells contain only low-molecular-weight keratins (46,000–58,000 Da). K5 and K14 are expressed in the basal layer of the epidermis. Other keratins expressed in small sub-population of basal keratinocytes include K15 and K19, which are associated with putative stem cells. Other cytoskeletal elements in the basal cells are microfilaments, such as actin, myosin and α-actinin; these assist in the upward movement of the cells as they differentiate.

The basal cells are the primary location of active mitotic cells in the epidermis. Three types co-exist in this layer: stem cells, transient amplifying cells and postmitotic cells. These cells are difficult to differentiate on morphology or protein expression. Only 30% of basal cells prepare for cell division. Stem cells reside amongst the basal cells and are also present amongst the cells of the external root sheath at the level of attachment of arrector pili muscle. These cells divide infrequently, but can generate new cells in the epidermis and hair follicles in response to damage.

Stratum malpighii (Stratum Spinosum, Malpigian Layer): This layer is the thickest and the strongest epidermal layer. It consists of 4–10 layers of polygonal cells placed in a mosaic-like pattern. The cells become flattened as they move towards the surface. The cells have a central oval nucleus and a cytoplasm packed with tonofilaments. Intercellular bridges called desmosomes connect the cells to one another. Desmosomes contain desmoplakins, desmogleins and desmocollins. Autoantibodies to these proteins are found in pemphigus. Tonofilaments radiate from the interior of the cell to the desmosomes, but do not pass to the adjacent cell.

New synthesis of K1/K10 occurs in the spinous cell, these keratins are characteristic of an epidermal-type pattern of differentiation or keratinisation. These filaments have both the high- and the low-molecular-weight keratins (55,000–65,000 Da).

This layer is also known as the prickle cell layer. These cells are closely packed and interdigitate by means of numerous projections and indentations on their surface, which are linked by many desmosomes. It acquires its name from the spiky appearance produced by the desmosomes. There are differences in the upper and lower part of the spinous layer that correlate to the progressive stage of keratinisation. The suprabasal spinous cells are polyhedral in shape and have a round nucleus. Those of the upper spinous layer are larger and more flattened. These cells also contain a full range of intracellular organelles. In the upper part of the stratum spinosum, lamellar granules appear which are called the Odland bodies; these consist of phospholipids, glycoproteins and acid phosphates. The contents discharge into the intercellular spaces between the cells of the granular layer and stratum corneum.

Marcello Malpighi (1628–1694) of Bologna discovered the lymphatic channels while examining a frog's lung. Malpighi was also the first to describe layers of the skin and glomeruli of the kidneys

Stratum granulosum: This layer is characterised by changes required for formation of superficial water-impermeable layer, the stratum corneum. This is the zone where the epidermal nuclei disintegrate. It consists of 1–4 layers of elongated diamond-shaped cells. It is named because the cells in this layer contain basophilic granules called the keratohyalin granules in the cytoplasm. Keratohyalin granules are composed of proteins, these include, profilaggrin, involucrin and loricrin, and keratin intermediate filaments. Loricrin is a protein of cornified cell envelope, variations of loricrin are found in Vohwinkel's syndrome. Profilaggrin is a high-molecular-weight protein, conversion of profilaggrin to filaggrin by specific phosphatases occurs during the transition of granular cell to a cornified cell. This is important for regulation of epidermal osmolarity and flexibility. It is a histidine rich electron dense precursor form of protein filaggrin, this is deposited in the interstices of the keratin filament network. Filaggrin in the cornified cell is said to function as the matrix protein that embeds and possibly promotes the aggregation of keratin filaments.

Processing of high-molecular-weight proteins also takes place in the granular layer. Keratin K1 is modified to K2 and K10 to K11. Keratin filaments have a high-molecular-weight (63,000–67,000 Da). Involucrin, a sulphur-rich protein of the cornified cell envelope. This is synthesised in the spinous layer, concentrated in the granular layer and organised as a dense layer beneath the plasma membrane in the cornified cell.

Other protein markers of keratinisation are the calcium requiring transglutaminases, these are present in all stratified epithelium. There are three glutaminases in the epidermis. Type I is present in the basal cells, but enzyme activity is prevalent in the granular layer and accounts for most of the differentiation of keratinocytes. Type II is present in fetal epidermis and in the basal cells and appears to play a role in apoptosis. Type 3 is expressed after early differentiation markers such as K1 and K10.

Stratum corneum: This layer consists of 20–25 layers of thin flattened dead anuclear, completely keratinised cells that overlap at their margins. Complete transition from a granular layer to a cornified cell is accompanied by 45–86% loss in dry weight. The stratum corneum barrier is made of lipid-depleted, protein-enriched corneocytes, surrounded by continuous extracellular lipid matrix. The three key lipids are cholesterol, ceramides and free fatty acids. The cells of the deeper layers of stratum corneum are called stratum compactum; here the cells are thicker and more compactly packed. The middle layer is called stratum dysjunctum; the cells here have the highest concentration of free amino acids, and are able to bind water with greater efficiency. The superficial cells are the outer dead cells that are inconspicuously shed. The desmosomes undergo proteolytic degradation in the outermost stratum corneum, which is one of the factors which allows the individual corneocytes to shed. Stratum corneum varies in thickness in different parts of the body, being thickest on the palms and soles.

This locking of the cells together with the intercellular lipid forms a very strong barrier. The corneocyte has an insoluble cornified envelope within the plasma membrane, this is formed by the cross-linking of the soluble protein precursor involucrin. These cells are made of plates of keratin that are shed from the free surface of the skin in the form of microscopic scales. The process of desquamation involves degradation of lamellated lipid in the intercellular spaces and loss of residual intercellular desmosomal interconnections.

The stratum corneum is not an inert covering as it was previously thought it can initiate skin diseases. It is not just the end result of processes in the subjacent cell layers.

Stratum lucidum: In the palms and soles, the skin has an additional layer called stratum lucidum, between the stratum granulosum and stratum corneum. The cells are nucleated unlike the cells of the stratum corneum, but have opaque membrane and dense cytoplasm.

DESMOSOMES

There are several types of cell junctions in the epidermis, which play a part in holding the cells together and allowing them to communicate. Some of these are: desmosomes, gap junctions (These allow the free movement of ions and small molecules between cells) and adherent junctions (These connect the actin filaments between two cells; they help in signalling and adherence of cells).

Desmosomes (Fig. 3) are the main junction between the two adjacent keratinocytes; they also provide resistance to mechanical stresses. Within each cell there is a desmosomal plaque, associated with the internal surface of the

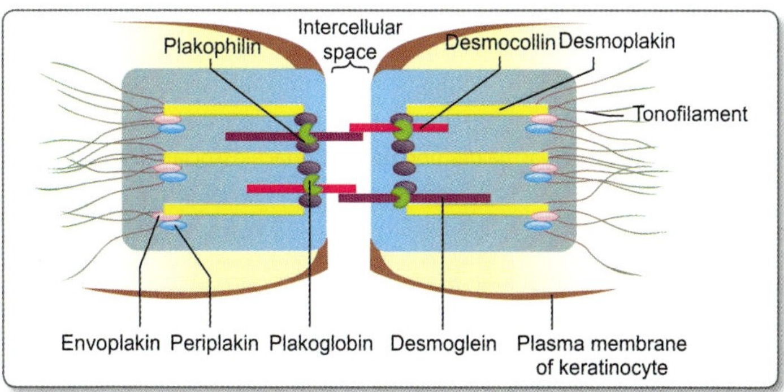

Fig. 3: Desmosome

plasma membrane. It is composed of a number of transmembrane adhesion proteins and cytoplasmic plaque proteins. Transmembrane glycoproteins are desmoglein 1 and 3, and desmocollin 1 and 2. These are calcium-dependent adhesion molecules (cadherins). The cytoplasmic plaque proteins are desmoplakin, plakophilin, plakoglobin, envoplakin and periplakin.

These plaque proteins link to tonofilaments of the cell, which in turn are linked to the nucleus. The whole network is stable and signals can be transmitted from the external surface of the cells through the desmosome to the nucleus. Autoantibodies to desmoglein proteins are responsible for pemphigus, and staphylococcal scalded skin syndrome (SSSS) is caused by a bacterial toxin damaging desmoglein.

PHYSIOLOGY OF KERATINISATION

The main function of the keratinocytes is to produce keratin. New cells are produced by mitosis in the basal layer of the epidermis. Each dividing cell produces two cells, one remains a basal cell, the other after a period of about 12 days becomes detached from the basal membrane and ascends towards the skin surface making its transit through the Malpighian layer in about 26–42 days. Various chemical changes take place in the cell during this period, so that when the cell reaches the stratum corneum it is an anucleated flat plate of keratin. After another 13–14 days, it is shed. Total transit time is 52–75 days. In psoriasis, it is reduced to 8–10 days.

CHARACTERISTICS OF EPIDERMAL DIFFERENTIATION

As the epidermal cells differentiate from the basal cells to the cells of the stratum corneum, a series of biochemical and structural changes occur in the postmitotic keratinocyte. These events involve the following changes:

- Synthesis of new structural proteins and modification of the existing ones
- Appearance of new cellular organelles, structural organisation of those present; and eventual loss of cell organelles from the cell
- Increase in the cell size and flattening of shape
- A progressive change from a generalised cellular metabolism to a more focused metabolism
- Alterations in the properties of the plasma membrane, cell surface antigens and receptors
- The end point of keratinisation is the production of a dead terminally differentiated keratinocyte that contains only tonofilaments; matrix proteins, protein reinforced plasma membrane and surface-associated lipids.

THE CELL CYCLE

Cell cycle (Fig. 4) is the period between two successive mitoses or the time taken for the individual cells to divide. Cell production must balance the rate of cell loss from the surface of stratum corneum. Epidermal homeostasis consists of a balance of stimulating and inhibitory signals. The normal cell cycle time is 163 hours.

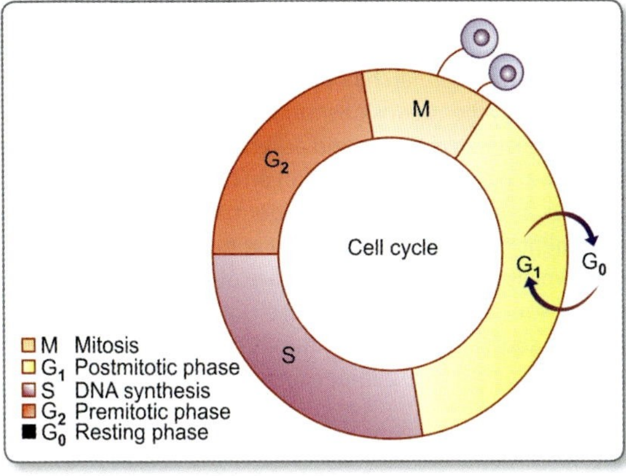

Fig. 4:
The cell cycle

The cell cycle begins at mitosis (M) this is followed by a prolonged period of growth (G_1), after this the cell has three options:

1. It may leave the cell cycle and undergo metabolic changes leading to differentiation and death, as occurs when cells reach the stratum corneum from stratum basale.
2. It may temporarily leave the cell cycle and enter a resting phase (G_0), perhaps analogous to hibernation, during which it neither proliferates nor differentiates, but can re-enter the cell cycle following suitable stimulation.
3. The cell may enter a period of active DNA synthesis (S) by the nucleus. This is followed by a short resting phase (G_2) prior to mitosis and start of another cycle.

CONTROL OF THE EPIDERMAL PROLIFERATION

Repeated rubbing of the skin produces a callosity, and stripping of superficial layers from the epidermis by repeated applications of adhesive tape, produces a burst of mitotic activity in the epidermal cells. These observations suggest that there must be a local mechanism, which controls the rate of cell division in the epidermis. Rate of cell production must balance the rate of cell loss from the surface of stratum corneum. Various intrinsic and extrinsic physiological and pathological factors regulate the proliferation, growth and differentiation of keratinocytes. Amongst the extrinsic regulating substances is the epidermal growth factor, oestrogens, progesterone, adrenaline, vitamin A and its derivatives. Important intrinsic factors that regulate proliferation are the epidermal cytokines, integrins, chalones and the level of cyclic nucleotides.

Calcium also plays a role in epidermal proliferation. It has been shown that keratinocytes grown in a medium with low calcium failed to stratify and differentiate. There is a calcium gradient in the epidermis, increasing from the basal cells to the granular layer. Calcium is required for desmosome formation and activation of glutaminase. Calcium homeostasis plays an important role in Darier and Hailey-Hailey disease.

Epidermal proliferation is due to the release of mitotic stimulators, but it is more likely that it is kept in control by an inhibitor of mitosis called a chalone.

Different tissues produce different chalones. Chalones are tissue-specific but not species-specific.

The exact nature of human epidermal chalone is unknown, but there is some evidence to suggest that the cyclic adenosine monophosphate (AMP) cascade may act as a chalone. Both hydrocortisone and adrenaline inhibit epidermal mitosis, this action can be explained by their action on the cyclic AMP system.

The dermis also plays a role in regulating epidermal proliferation, such as seen in the involvement of dermal papilla regulating the hair cycle. It is observed in studies in which tissue recombinants are prepared by removing the epidermis from one source and evaluating the outcome after attached to the dermis of another source. The new epidermis has the characteristics of the person in relation to age, species, regions, etc. These experiments are performed with embryonic tissue.

The terminal differentiation of the basal cell into the anucleated cornified cell is due to a modified apoptosis, which is gene-regulated.

THE OTHER CELLS OF THE EPIDERMIS

Following are the other cells of the epidermis:
- Melanocytes
- Langerhans cells
- Granstein cells
- Merkel cells
- Indeterminate cells.

Melanocytes

These are dendritic, pigment producing cells found in the basal layer with a clear halo around them because of the absence of desmosomes. They are derived from the neural crest. The melanocytes reside in the basal layer; the numbers differ at different sites. On the face, they may be one for every five basal cells, in the lower back there may be 1 to every 20 basal keratinocytes. On an average, they occur at a frequency of 1 to every 10 basal keratinocytes. The number of melanocytes in the epidermis is the same regardless of race or colour.

Melanocytes synthesise the pigment melanin. Melanosomes are melanin granules, these are small electron dense intracytoplasmic structures seen under an electron microscope. Melanosomes that are involved in the synthesis of brown/black pigment (eumelanin) are elliptical and those that are involved in the synthesis of the red pigment (pheomelanin) are spheroidal in shape. The size of the melanosomes is determined genetically; black skin typically contains large melanosomes than the more lightly pigmented skin.

Melanin is formed from tyrosine via dehydroxyphenylalanine (DOPA), which is catalysed by the enzyme tyrosinase to form melanin. Once melanin is formed, it is distributed along the dendrites of the cell to the surrounding keratinocytes. The combination of one pigment-producing melanocyte and about 36 surrounding keratinocytes forms the "epidermal melanin unit".

Melanocytes are also found in the hair bulb, eye and brain, and in very small amounts in the other organs. In the skin, they provide protection against ultraviolet radiation (UVR). Neuromelanin, the pigment found in substantia nigra and chromaffin system is different from eumelanin and phaeomelanin, it is derived from a different enzyme, tyrosine hydroxylase instead of tyrosinase. This is enzyme is not found is the melanocytes of the epidermis (Fig. 5).

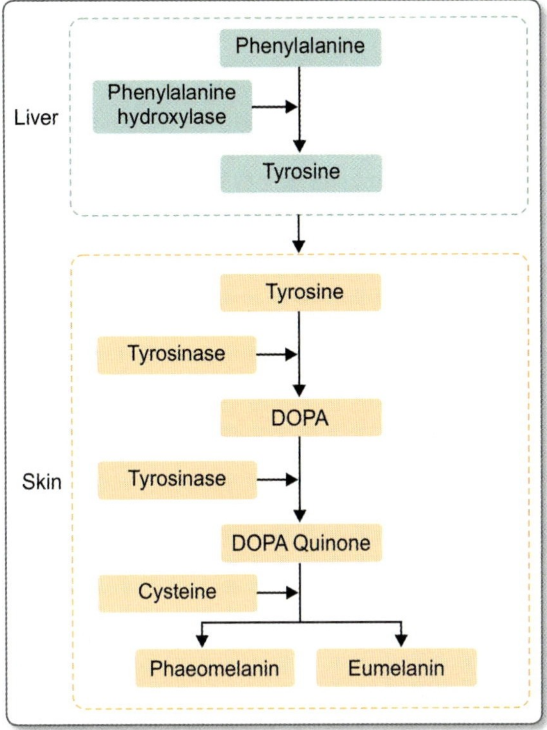

Fig. 5: Synthesis of melanin

Langerhans Cells

Paul Langerhans discovered these cells when he was a medical student in 1860. These are also dendritic cells scattered amongst the cells of the malpigian layer. These cells are slightly larger than the keratinocytes; they have a clear halo around them, probably because of the lack of desmosomes. On electron microscope, Langerhans cells are recognised by the presence of highly specific granules known as the Birbeck granules. They look like tennis or squash racquets, their function is not fully understood. Langerhans cells are also found in other squamous epithelia, including the oral cavity, oesophagus and vagina. They are also found in lymphoid tissue, such as the spleen, thymus and lymph nodes, they are also present in the dermis.

Langerhans cells are of monocytic-macrophage lineage of bone marrow origin. These cells present antigen to the helper T-cells. They are immunologically competent cells and play a role in graft rejection, primary contact sensitisation and immuno-surveillance. They also produce interleukin 1. These cells are the first line of immunological defence against environmental antigens. Abnormal Langerhans cells proliferate in the rare disease such as histiocytosis.

Granstein Cells

These are the most recently discovered and least understood of the epidermal cells. Granstein cells interact with the suppresser T-cells, probably acting as a "brake" on the skin activated immune response. Langerhans cells are more susceptible to damage by UVR than Granstein cells.

Merkel Cells

These cells are also found in the basal layer, they are present in the glabrous skin of the digits, lips, regions of the oral cavity and outer root sheath of the hair follicle. There are two hypotheses about its embryonic source. According to one hypothesis, they are derived from the neural crest and according to the other; they arise in situ from the epithelial cells. These cells require an electron microscope to be identified. They are found in large numbers in the touch sensitive sites, such as fingertips and around the lips. They are associated with mechanoreceptive cutaneous nerve endings. The cells are elliptical in shape, packed with granules; these contain large quantities of catecholamines. The cytoplasm is plain staining like other non-keratinocytic cells. Their exact function is not known, they are thought to be related to cutaneous sensation of touch.

Indeterminate Cells

These are dendritic cells; morphologically resembling the Langerhans cell, but characterised by the absence of Birbeck granules. These cells are related to the Langerhans cell and are Ia antigen positive.

BASEMENT MEMBRANE COMPLEX

The basement membrane zone (Fig. 6) forms the junction of the epidermis and dermis [dermal-epidermal junction (DEJ)]; it is the largest epithelial-mesenchymal junction in the body. It is about 80 nm thick. The main function of the basement membrane is to attach the epidermis to dermis and to provide resistance against shearing forces. This zone also supports the epidermis, directs the organisation of the cytoskeleton in the basal cells and helps in the transmission of nutrients, oxygen, antibodies, complement and trafficking immune cells to the epidermis, it acts as a semipermeable membrane.

The basement membrane is formed by the epidermis from the basal cells, with minor contributions from the dermal fibroblasts. The basement membrane zone can be divided into three components: the hemidesmosome-anchoring filament complex, the basement membrane (lamina lucida and lamina densa) and the lamina fibroreticulosa, which consists of the anchoring fibrils.

- The hemidesmosome anchoring filament complex, binds the basal keratinocytes to the basement membrane. The hemidesmosome consists of a cytoplasmic and transmembranous component. Intermediate filaments of the basal cells insert into the cytoplasmic component, which consists of bullous pemphigoid antigen 230 (BP 230) and plectin. The transmembrane component consists of integrin and bullous pemphigoid antigen 180 (BP 180). Integrins are adhesion molecules, which also transduce signals from the extracellular matrix to the interior of the cell.

- The lamina lucida is the primary location of several noncollagenous glycoproteins, such as laminin, entactin/nidogen and fibronectin. The anchoring filaments originate at the hemidesmosome and inserts into the lamina densa. The major component of this filament is laminin 5. Throughout the lamina lucida the anchoring filaments are oriented vertically. Laminins are the most abundant noncollagenous glycoproteins present in the basement membrane. They are multidomain molecules, consisting of a family of more than 50 members. Laminin 5 and 10 are specific to the basal lamina. They form a network throughout the basement membrane to which are attached other collagen glycoproteins and proteoglycans (PGs). Moreover they are signalling molecules, providing the adjacent cells with diverse information by interacting with cell surface molecules. Nidogen is a glycoprotein that interacts with several other components of basement membrane and may play a role in cell interactions with the extracellular matrix. The lamina lucida is the weakest zone of the basement membrane. It separates easily with heat and treatment with salt solutions and proteolytic enzymes.

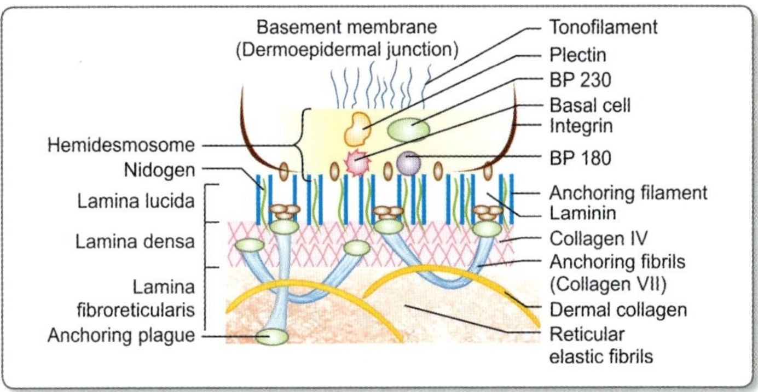

Fig. 6: Basement membrane

- Lamina densa accounts for 40–60% of total basement membrane proteins. The major protein is collagen type IV, synthesised by the epidermis. Nidogen is a glycoprotein, which is attached to the short arm of laminin; laminin-nidogen complex is then attached to collagen IV. Lamina densa gives support and flexibility to the basement membrane complex.
- Lamina fibroreticulosa consists mainly of the anchoring fibrils, elastic microfibril bundles. Anchoring fibrils are broad, elongated structures that originate in the lamina densa and extend into the papillary dermis, where they insert into amorphous bodies, known as the anchoring plaques or they curve backward to be inserted in the lamina densa. Anchoring fibrils are composed of Type VII collagen. Anchoring fibrils are also connected to the hemidesmosomes via laminin 5. Elastic microfibril bundles consist of many microfibrils, which extend into the dermis and enmesh with the microfibrillar system of dermal elastic tissue.

Basement membrane is multilayered and different bullous disorders result from the separation of dermal epidermal junction, e.g. bullous pemphigoid is due to antibodies acting against BP 230 and BP 180, linear IgA disease of childhood is due to the fragmentation of BP 180, epidermolysis bullosa aquisita is due to antibodies acting against the anchoring fibrils. Mutation in plectins of the hemidesmosome results in epidermolysis bullosa simplex. Mutations in anchoring filaments are responsible for junctional epidermolysis bullosa. Mutations in type VII collagen are responsible for epiderolysis bullosa dystrophica.

EPIDERMAL APPENDAGES

Eccrine glands, apocrine glands, sebaceous glands and the pilosebaceous units, nails and hair constitute the epidermal appendages (skin adnexa). Embryologically they originate as downgrowths from the epidermis and are therefore ectodermal in origin. While the adnexa serve special function, they can also serve as reserve function.

Eccrine Glands

The eccrine glands are seen on almost all parts of the body, there are about 2–4 million eccrine sweat glands distributed over the entire body surface. The glands are most profuse on the palm, sole, axilla and forehead while the surface of the limbs generally have the fewest. They are absent from the tympanic membrane, margins of the lips, nail bed, nipple, inner preputial surface, labia majora, labia minora, glans penis and glans clitoris. The number of sweat glands ranges from 80 to over 600/cm^2. These glands are anatomically independent of the other appendages. Sweat decreases the body temperature by evaporation, it also helps to maintain the pliability of the keratin, and it decreases friction on the palm and soles.

Sweat glands consist of three parts:

- Spiral intraepidermal part
- Straight intradermal part
- Coiled secretary part.

Sweat is formed by a process of active secretion, (the sodium pump) in the coiled secretary portion of the sweat duct; its electrolyte composition is modified as it travels up the intradermal portion of the sweat duct. The process is somewhat similar to the formation of urine in the nephron. Some drugs such as aldosterone and antidiuretic hormone (ADH), which act on the renal tubules, also act on the sweat ducts. The intraepidermal part of the duct helps to maintain its patency during changes in epidermal hydration.

Sweat contains sodium, potassium, chloride, lactate, urea and ammonia. Increased concentration is found in fibrocystic disease, sweat chloride estimation is a helpful diagnostic test. Metal handed by such workers rusts quickly; these workers are therefore often called rusters.

Sweat production is regulated by the sympathetic nervous system. The fibres to the sweat gland are unusual in secreting acetylcholine instead of adrenaline, they are cholinergic sympathetic fibres. The sweat glands can secrete from 300 mL to 12 litres of fluid each day, a further 200 mL diffuses directly through the horny layer of epidermis called the transepidermal water loss. The daily water loss under basal conditions is about 500 mL. There are three types of stimuli for sweating:

(1) Thermal
(2) Mental or emotional
(3) Gustatory

Thermal sweating: It is controlled by the heat-regulating centre of the hypothalamus, sweating follows when there is a rise in the central core temperature or a rise in the ambient temperature.

Mental sweating: The centre for mental sweating is not fully known. Sweating follows any type of mental stress; it is seen commonly on the palms, soles and axilla.

Gustatory sweating: The central connections of this type of sweating is not fully understood. Certain spicy foods will provoke sweating on the face. Gustatory sweating also occurs in pathological conditions involving the autonomic nervous system or a lesion in the central nervous system.

Histology

A thin fibrous dermal sheath and an investing basal lamina surround the whole length of the gland. The secretory portion consists of a psuedostratified epithelium enclosing a wide lumen. There are three types of cells: clear cells, from which most of the secretion is obtained, dark (mucoid) cells and myoepitheliocytes. The clear cells are located in the more basal or peripheral portion of gland and are rich in glycogen, the dark cells are located along the luminal surface and contain round mucoid granules. The clear and dark cells are pyramidal in shape. The clear cells are responsible for the production of water and electrolytes. The function of the dark cells is unknown; the myoepithelial cells are contractile with a smooth muscle like characteristics. The myothelial cells respond to cholinergic stimulation, they provide structural support to the secretary epithelium, especially when there is a stagnation to sweat flow due to ductal blockage. The myoepitheliocytes cells are numerous, they are elongated cells and lie among the foot processes of the other cells, just within the basal lamina of the gland. There is a rich plexus of nerves surrounding the gland.

Eccrine sweat ducts are lined by two layers of basophilic cuboidal epitheliocytes, the inner layer has short microvilli bordering the duct lumen. It seems that the proximal coiled duct is more active than the distal straight portion, it is here where most of the sodium, potassium and ATPase activity take place, and they also have a higher number of mitochondria.

Apoeccrine Glands

The apoeccrine glands are a family of the eccrine glands, present in the adult axillae. Their density is higher in persons who have axillary hyperhidrosis. Like the eccrine glands they have a large duct which opens independently on the skin surface. The secretary tubule consists of a segment of small diameter (80 μm) like that of the eccrine gland, and a segment similar to that of the apocrine gland, which can dilate up to 500 μg in diameter. These glands develop at puberty; they are larger than the eccrine glands, but smaller than the apocrine glands. The secretary rate is 10 times that of the eccrine glands, mainly because of its larger size. The gland responds to both epinephrine and methacholine. It can be said that apoeccrine glands are eccrine glands that have undergone apocrinisation.

Apocrine Gland

These epidermal appendages develop as a part of the pilosebaceous follicle. In the embryo, they are present throughout the skin surface, but most of the glands subsequently disappear. In adults they are found in the axilla, periareola, periumbilical and the anogenital region. The mammary glands are modified apocrine glands. Ectopic glands are found in the eyelids (Moll) and ear (Ceruminous).

These glands are larger than the eccrine glands; located at the junction of the dermis and the subcutaneous fat, they open in the hair follicles above the opening of the sebaceous glands. The secretion is proteinaceous, thick milky fluid which is at first sterile and odourless, but then undergoes bacterial metabolism to generate potent odorous compounds, such as short chain fatty acids, it is musky in smell. Their role in humans is uncertain, but it is responsible for the body odour. Their secretion is produced by breaking off the tip of the secretory cell cytoplasm, a process called decapitation. These glands become active at puberty, they are androgen dependent. Denervation does not stop the response to emotional stimuli, which suggests that the gland can be stimulated by hormones, such as circulating epinephrine and norepinephrine.

Histology

A single layer of cuboidal epithelium lines the walls of the apocrine glands; these have microvillus apices, which tend to protrude in the lumen. Among the bases of these cells lie the numerous epitheliocytes, the whole complex of cells rests on a thick basement membrane. Outside this is a connective tissue capsule rich in capillaries. The apocrine duct like the eccrine duct is lined by two layers of cubiodal cells, but has a much larger lumen than the eccrine glands; it has different set of enzymes.

Sebaceous Gland

Sebaceous glands are small saccular structures formed as an outgrowth from the upper portion of the hair follicle. It is composed of a cluster of usually two to five (occasionally up to 20) secretory acini opening by a short duct in the apical portion of the hair follicle. The acini consist of pale staining cells with abundant lipid in their cytoplasm. Sebaceous glands are found in great abundance in the face, scalp, chest and upper trunk. The number of sebaceous glands ranges from an average of 100/cm^2 over most of the body to 400–900/cm^2 on the face and scalp. They are distributed on all the body sites except the palms and soles. They are always associated with the hair follicles. In some areas of thin skin lacking hair follicles, the sebaceous ducts open directly on the skin surface, e.g. on the eyelids (Meibomian glands), buccal mucosa and vermillion border of the lips (Fordyce spots), prepuce (Tyson glands) and female areola (Montgomery glands).

Secretions of the sebaceous glands (sebum) is produced by a holocrine process, cells at the periphery of the gland break down and are completely converted into lipid secretion as they move to the gland centre, from where they are secreted through the sebaceous duct into the hair follicle. The secretion is activated by androgens. They may show glandular activity at neonatal period due to the effect of maternal hormones, the glands then shrink and become vestigial until puberty, when they respond to their body's own androgens. This overactivity is the main cause of acne vulgaris. Other hormones, such as thyroid and growth hormones also stimulate sebum production, oestrogens decrease sebum production. Another condition that can cause seborrhoea (increased sebum production) is Parkinsonism and this can be decreased by L-Dopa therapy.

Sebum is a complex mixture of which 50% is di- and triglycerides, with smaller proportions of wax esters, squalene, cholesterol esters and cholesterol. As sebum moves along its ducts, its triglycerides are partly hydrolysed by bacterial action to free fatty acids.

Sebum serves little useful purpose as children with virtually no sebum production have attractive skin and hair. It has mild fungistatic effect, which explains why children are more susceptible than adults to fungal infections. Sebum protects the loss of moisture from the skin, discourages blood-sucking ectoparasites, it may also contribute to body odour. In a newborn child, it could possibly play a part in the relationship between the mother and child.

Histology

The glandular acini are invested by a basal lamina supported by a thin dermal capsule and a rich capillary network. Within this is a single layer of flat polygonal epithelial cells, which lines each acinus. Functionally they are the active stem cells whose offsprings move towards the centre of the acinus, increasing in volume and accumulating swollen lipid vacuoles. Their nuclei become pyknotic as the cells mature and finally the large distended cells disintegrate, filling the central cavity and its effluent duct with a mass of fatty cellular debris. This mode of secretion is described as holocrine. The secretory products pass through the wide duct of the sebaceous glands lined by stratified squamous epithelium into the apical part of the hair follicle.

HAIR

Hair (Pili) are filamentous, keratinised structures present all over the body surface; they are absent in a few areas of the body, including the palms, soles, umbilicus, nipples, glans penis, clitoris, labia minora and inner aspects of the labia majora and prepuce. They vary from 600/cm^2 on the face to 60/cm^2 on the rest of the body. The length of the hair ranges from less than a millimetre to more than a meter. In width it ranges from 0.005 mm to 0.6 mm. The hair may be straight, coiled or wavy and the colour depends upon the type of pigment present.

Hair follicles (Figs 7A and B) are formed by the invagination of the epidermis into the dermis, which encloses at its base a small vascular dermal papilla. A small cluster of elastic fibres in the neck of the papilla is called the Arao-Perkins

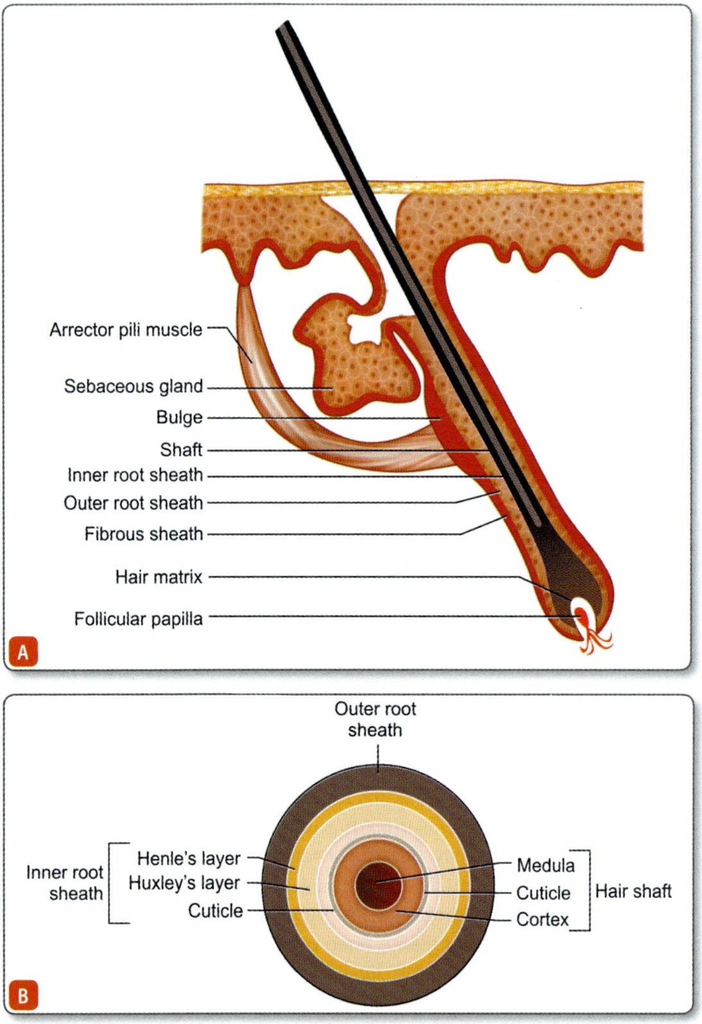

Arrector pili muscle
Sebaceous gland
Bulge
Shaft
Inner root sheath
Outer root sheath
Fibrous sheath
Hair matrix
Follicular papilla
A

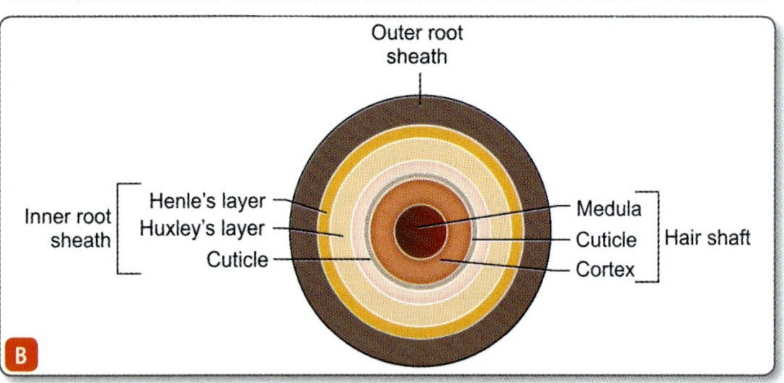

Figs 7A and B: (A) Hair follicle-longitudinal section; (B) Hair follicle-transverse section
Source: Ziadi Z, Lanigan S. Dermatology in Clinical Practice. Skin structure and function. London: Springer; 2010. pp. 1-15. With kind permission of Springer Science + Business Media.

body. These fibres are clumped in catagen and stay behind at the lowest point to which the papillae extend in anagen. Sebaceous glands open into the hair follicle and together they form the pilosebaceous unit. The region above the opening of the sebaceous ducts is the infundibulum and below as far as the attachment of the arrector pili muscle is the isthmus. The bulge is the site of attachment of the arrector pili muscle. Below the isthmus is the inferior segment of the hair follicle. Area of the follicle surrounding the hair bulb is called the fundus.

The isthmus is the site where the inner and outer root sheaths ascend in catagen, while the entire portion below disintegrates. It is the site of the lower end of the permanent follicle. At the isthmus, the inner and outer root sheaths disintegrate, either at or below the opening of the sebaceous duct. At this site the outer root sheath keratinises without the formation of keratohyalin granules. Above the opening of the sebaceous ducts, the follicular epithelium produces regular keratohyalin granules, which are different from epidermal keratohyalin granules; these are known as trichohyalin granules.

A thick perifollicular dermal coat containing collagen fibres, elastic fibres, blood vessels and nerves surrounds the follicle. Marking the interface with the dermis and follicular epithelium is a broad PAS positive basal lamina, the glassy membrane. Within this are arranged the epithelial outer and inner root sheath surrounding the hair shaft.

The outer root sheath (trichilemma) is an invagination of the epidermis. Above the level of the inferior segment its surface cells undergo keratinisation. In the deeper regions it is unkeratinised, forming a sheath of a few cells.

The inner root sheath is formed from the hair bulb, it occurs mainly in the inferior segment. It is a three layered structure, from outwards in they are: Henle's layer which is a single layer of keratinising cells, Huxley's layer made up of two layers of partially keratinised cells, and finally a single layer of flattened squames; this is the cuticle of the inner root sheath, facing and interlocking with the cells of the hair shaft cuticle.

The hair consists of a shaft and root; it lies within the hair follicle. At the proximal end of the root, the hair is expanded to form the hair bulb. The bulb is deeply indented on its deep surface by a conical vascular dermal papilla. The shaft has three concentric zones, the cuticle, cortex and the medulla. The cuticle forms the hair surface and is made of overlapping keratinised squames. The cortex contains numerous closely packed elongated cells, filled with keratin and melanosomes. The central medulla is composed of discoid cells containing keratin filaments, vacuoles, melanosomes and granular material. Medulla is absent in thin hair.

The hair bulb has at its base the germinative matrix, which generates the hair and the inner root sheath. The germinative matrix is composed of pluripotent polygonal cells capping the dermal papilla. Cells arising from the germinative matrix differentiate along several different routes, depending upon their position of origin. The cells from the centre of the base form the medulla; those from further out will transform into the cortex and cuticle of the hair and from further outside from the inner root sheath. Interspersed among the germinative matrix are the melanocytes. The largest portion of the matrix is used in producing the hair cortex.

The follicular papilla is a group of specialised mesenchymal cells that play a central role in follicular development and hair cycle. These cells are distinct from the dermal fibroblasts, for they send out signals that control the development of the hair follicle. Follicular papillary cells produce a number of growth factors, such as keratinocyte growth factor, cytokines and transcription factors that play a role in regulating the hair cycle.

Huxley in 1845, when still a medical student and only 20 years of age; described the layer of the inner root sheath of the hair follicle, which bears his name.

Types of Hair

There are three types of hair:

(1) Lanugo hair

(2) Vellus hair

(3) Terminal hair

Lanugo hair: These are long soft hair which covers the body of the foetus; it sheds into the amniotic fluid at about 7 months. Lanugo hair is not normally seen after birth except in very premature babies. These hairs are nonmedullated and nonpigmented.

Vellus hair: These are postnatal hairs, they are soft short unmedullated and occasionally pigmented. They cover most of the body surface.

Terminal hair: These hairs are medullated and pigmented.

Many hair of the body may be of an intermediate type.

Cyclic Activity of the Hair

Each hair follicle shows intermittent activity; hair grows to a maximum length, the growth then ceases, it is shed and then replaced. Hair growth and loss is not seasonal as in some mammals. The cyclic activity is random; it is not uniform throughout the scalp. This cyclic activity is studied under three phases:

- Anagen (period of active growth)
- Catagen (period of programmed cell death and apoptosis)
- Telogen (period of rest)

Anagen: About 85–90% of scalp hair is in the anagen phase. Scalp hair remains in the anagen phase for 2–6 years, 19–26 weeks on the legs, 6–12 weeks on the arms and 4–14 weeks on the upper lips (moustache). The anagen phase begins when mitotic activity is initiated in the hair bulb and dermal papilla. The follicle which has ascended at the isthmus in catagen, grows down and meets the dermal papilla, recapitulating the events of embryonic development of the hair follicle. This downward growth is regulated by the activation of cells in the bulge, or by the cells of the external root sheath, which in turn is activated by signals from the dermal papilla. Once the hair follicle reaches the original site of the dermal papilla, the matrix cells of the hair bulb take over the proliferation of the hair follicle, and the signals from the dermal papilla stop, thereby stopping the activation of the bulge cells, or the cells of the external root sheath. During anagen the hair grows at the rate of 0.4 mm/day (scalp hair), the rate diminishes with age. The growing phase is shorter and the resting phase longer in the hair of the other parts of the body, thereby explaining why these hair remain short.

Catagen: About 1% of hair in the scalp are in the catagen phase at one time. The duration is 2–3 weeks. In this phase, the cell division stops in the hair matrix. The lower follicle shrinks away from the connective tissue dermal papilla and ascends to the level of insertion of arrector pili muscle. The outer root sheath degenerates and retracts around the widened lower portion of the hair shaft to become a club hair.

Telogen: About 10–15% of scalp hair are in telogen phase. The duration is about 3 months in the scalp; it is longer in other parts of the body. This inactive dead hair (club hair), has a solid white base due to the lack of melanin. The club hair is firmly held in place and is later ejected. About 100 hairs are shed each day in the scalp; this is the hair that we see when we comb our hair.

Exogen: Some authors have recently focused attention to the mechanism of hair shedding known as exogen. Since hair can be retained for more than one cycle, the shedding phase is therefore more likely to be independent of anagen and telogen. Very little is known what controls exogen, perhaps proteolytic pathways have been implicated in club hair formation and removal.

In man, the activity of the follicles is independent of each other. Occasionally in a systemic upset, such as pyrexia, parturition or severe emotional stress many scalp follicles enter telogen phase simultaneously, causing a sudden thinning of the scalp hair. The dermatological term for moulting process is called telogen effluvium.

During anagen, the cells of the hair bulb have a high mitotic index and cytotoxic drugs therefore affect hair growth.

The hair follicles are metabolically very active and can convert testosterone into the more active form as 5-dihydrotestosterone. This increase in tissue androgenicity is thought to be important in the pathogenesis of male pattern alopecia and idiopathic hirsutism. Several factors regulate hair growth, such as androgens, oestrogens, glucocorticoids, thyroid hormones and growth hormones.

Hair Pluck Evaluation

In a trichogram, the anagen hair appears to have an equal diameter throughout its length; the root is largest at the base, which is pigmented. The inner root sheath is present and firm. The plucked root may show an angle of 20° or more with the shaft. This is presumably artefactual.

The telogen hair is club-shaped with smooth contours and it is colourless, due to the absence of melanin, there is no angulation, and telogen hair does not have the inner root sheath.

NAIL

Nails (Ungues) (Figs 8A and B) are highly modified skin appendages, formed by invaginations of the embryonic epidermis at about 9 weeks of gestation and the nails are completely formed by 12 weeks. Each nail consists of a plate of hard keratin, and four specialised epithelia, these are: the proximal nailfold, nail matrix, nail bed and the hyponychium. The nail lies immediately above the proximal phalanx, because the dermis is devoid of connective tissue; this is responsible for the disorders of the phalanx with nail disease. The fingernails present a major longitudinal axis and the toe nails a major transverse axis.

Nails are important aesthetically, they are used for scratching; protect the distal phalanx and tip of the fingers and toes. They are also important for picking small objects due to its enhanced tactile discrimination.

Nail Plate

The nail plate is produced by cell division in the matrix; it is firmly attached to the nail bed. It is surrounded by the nailfolds laterally and proximally. At the distal end of the digit, the nail plate separates from the nail bed at the hyponychium. Pink colour of the nail plate is due to the blood vessels in the nail bed. Pale halo at the proximal end of the nail is called the lunula. In this area the nail plate attachment to the underlying epithelium is loose and the keratin is not very mature. In the matrix the capillaries are thicker than that of the nailbed; this may also contribute to the white colour of the lunula. The onychocorneal

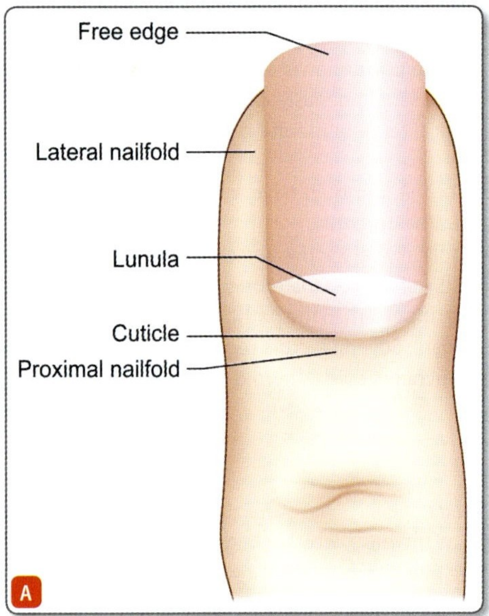

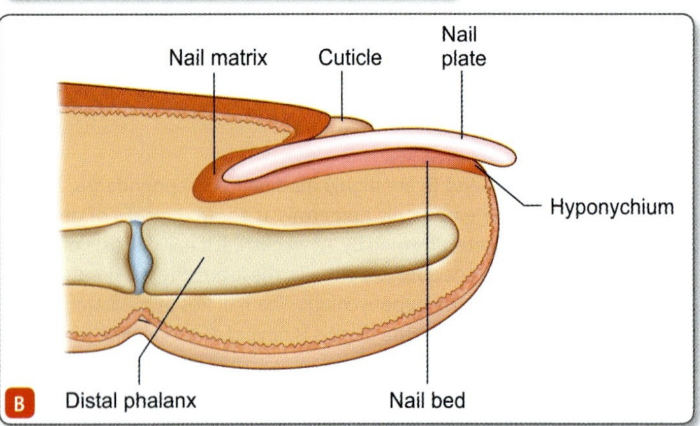

Figs 8A and B: (A) Nail-dorsal view; (B) Nail- lateral view
Source: **Ziadi** Z, Lanigan S. Dermatology in Clinical Practice. Skin structure and function. London: Springer; 2010. pp. 1-15. With kind permission of Springer Science + Business Media.

band is a thin transverse white band, which marks the most distal portion of the attachment of the nail plate with the nail bed. The onychocorneal band is separated from the free edge of the nail by a narrow pink band, 0.5–1.5 mm in diameter, called the onychodermal band, beyond which is the white free edge of the nail. The exact anatomical basis for this band is not known, but it appears that it has a separate blood supply from the main body of the nailbed. If the tip of the finger is pressed firmly, the band and an area just proximal to it blanch, and if the pressure is repeated, several times the band reddens.

In a transverse section the nail plate consists of three zones, the dorsal, intermediate and ventral. The dorsal and intermediate portions are formed by the nail matrix and the ventral by the nail bed. The nail thickens as it progresses towards the distal end. Thinning is a sign of nail matrix disorders, whereas nail thickness represents disorders of the nail bed.

Proximal Nailfold

The proximal nailfold consists of a dorsal and ventral surface. The dorsal nailfold is similar in appearance to the skin of the dorsum of the digit, but it is devoid of dermatoglyphic markings, hair and pilosebaceous glands. The ventral portion cannot be seen from the exterior, it is continuous with the nail matrix. The cuticle is an extension of the stratum corneum of the proximal nailfold; it prevents the separation of the nail plate from the proximal nailfold. It protects the nail from the injurious effects of the external environment. The dermis of the proximal nailfold contains numerous capillaries, which can be visualised by a dermatoscope. This is of help in diagnosing cutaneous disorders such as connective tissue diseases.

Nail Matrix

This is specialised structure from which most of the nail plate is formed. It lies above the middle part of the distal nail phalanx. In transverse section the matrix consists of a dorsal and ventral portion. The nail matrix keratinises in the absence of a granular layer. White spots may occasionally be seen in the nail plate if nuclear fragments persist in the intermediate layer of the nail plate; these often disappear before reaching the free edge of the nail.

The nail matrix can synthesise both hard and soft keratin. The dorsal nail matrix produces soft keratin and the ventral nail matrix produces hard keratin. The matrix cells are larger than the epidermal keratinocytes. Nail matrix melanocytes are usually quiescent, they can produce both DOPA-positive and DOPA-negative melanocytes. The melanocytes can be activated in Negroids, which is represented by longitudinal band of pigmentation on the nail plate. The Caucasians do not contain mature melanosomes.

Nail Bed

The nail bed extends from the lunula to the onychocorneal band. It is closely attached to the nail plate. This tight coupling prevents the invasion of microbes and impaction of debris under the nail. Beneath the epidermis is the rich vascularised dermis, anchored to the periosteum of the distal phalanx. Because of this, the infections of the nail bed cause severe pain. The rich blood supply of the dermis gives pink colour to the nail plate.

Nail bed epithelium produces the ventral surface of the nail plate, it represents one-fifth of the nail plate thickness. On histology the ventral nail plate is easily distinguished by its eosinophilic appearance. Nail bed keratinisation is not associated with the formation of granular layer.

Hyponychium

This is the area between the nail bed and the distal nail groove. The proximal part of the hyponychium is modified as the sole horn. Beyond the sole horn the hyponychium terminates at the distal groove, the tip of the digit beyond this ridge assumes the structure of the epidermis elsewhere. The hyponychium is normally covered by the nail plate, but may be visible in nail biters.

The nail apparatus does not contain subcutaneous tissue; it is also devoid of pilosebaceous units. Infection from the nail can easily spread to the distal phalangeal bone. The blood vessels in the nail bed are arranged longitudinally, which explains the linear pattern of nail bed haemorrhage. The nail bed dermis contains numerous glomus bodies. These are encapsulated neurovascular bodies, consisting of arteriovenous anastomosis and nerve endings. These help in the supply of blood to the digits in cold weather.

The fingernails grow more rapidly than the toe nails. The time taken for the fingernail to grow out completely from the base to the outer edge is approximately 6 months. For the toe nails is about 18 months or even longer. Fingernails grow at the rate of 1 cm in 3 months, toe nails at one-third of this rate. Nails grow rapidly in diseases due to increased cellular proliferation, the rate of nail growth maybe decreased by severe systemic illness. The nail matrix requires a rich blood supply; digital ischaemia predisposes to nail dystrophy. Nail disorders can provide a valuable clue to many systemic disorders. Even Sherlock Holmes has made use of these clues to solve his mysteries.

Nails consist of 80–90% of hard keratin, and 10–20% of soft keratin. Nails are rich in calcium; concentration is 10 times greater than the hair. Water content of the nail is 18%, most of it is in the intermediate nail plate. When the water content falls below 18% the nail becomes brittle, and when the water content rises above 30% the nails become opaque and soft. Nails are hard, strong and flexible. The strength is due to the hard keratin and flexibility due to its water content. Nails are more permeable to water than the skin; it behaves like a hydrophilic gel membrane. The nail plate is more prone to transverse fractures than vertical ones. This is due to the arrangement of keratin filaments which are oriented parallel and perpendicular in the ventral and dorsal nail plate; the orientation of keratin in the intermediate nail plate is perpendicular to the nail plate axis. Nail clippings can be used for DNA analysis and determination of blood groups.

DERMIS

The dermis or the corium is a thick layer located beneath the epidermis and above the subcutaneous layer. The constituents of the dermis are mesodermal in origin except the nerves, which like the melanocytes are derived from the neural crest. The dermis constitutes about 15–20% of the weight of the human body. It varies in thickness from 1 mm on the face to about 4 mm on the back and thigh. It is tough and resilient, provides nutrition to the epidermis and cutaneous appendages and cushions the body against mechanical injury. Two layers can roughly be distinguished in the dermis (papillary and reticular dermis), although there is no sharp boundary between them.

The outermost thinner layer is called pars papillaris, it is composed of relatively fine fibres, and the upper surface of this layer has numerous tiny projections called dermal papillae, which fit between the corresponding downward projections of the epidermis called rete pegs. Each papilla carries a vascular loop and some have specialised nerve end organs. The papillary dermis consists of small diameter collagen fibres and oxytalin. Mature elastic fibres are not found in the papillary dermis, but are present in the ageing skin and some disorders, such as Ehlers-Danlos syndrome. The papillary dermis also has a high density of fibroelastic cells, these proliferate more rapidly, have a higher rate of metabolic activity and synthesise special proteoglycans (PGs). The papillary dermis has influence over the epidermis through its soluble and diffusible characteristics. It consists mainly of type III collagen.

The bottom or the thicker layer of the dermis is called pars reticularis; it is composed of coarser interlacing bundles of fibrous tissue and mature elastic fibres (elastin). The elastic and collagen fibres increase in size as they progress towards the hypodermis. Subdivision of the reticular dermis into an upper intermediate and deep zone can be seen due to difference in the size of the fibres. The intermediate zone is more prone to trauma when compared with the deeper zone. The intermediate zone is also rich in fibroblasts and other connective tissue and inflammatory cells.

The dermis like other connective tissues consists of insoluble fibres, and soluble polymers. The insoluble fibres are the collagen and elastic fibres, and the soluble macromolecules are PGs (consist of protein core to which is bound one or more glucosaminoglycan chains) and hyaluran. These bind large volumes of water and thus occupy a large volume.

Fibronectin is an insoluble, filamentous glycoprotein synthesised in the skin by mesenchymal and epithelial cells, it ensheaths the collagen and elastic fibres. Fibronectin also binds platelets to collagen; it is found in fibrinogen-fibrin complexes and plays a role in organising the extracellular matrix. Vitronectin is another glycoprotein present in the dermis, it is widely distributed, but is absent from the oxytalin fibres in the papillary dermis. Tenascin surrounds the smooth muscles of the blood vessels, arrector pili muscle and sweat glands; it is strongly upregulated in conditions of epidermal proliferation.

Collagen

Collagen fibres constitute about 75% of the dry weight of the skin. It gives tensile strength and elasticity. Collagen is the most important structural protein in the body. The basic collagen molecule consists of three polypeptide chains known as the α-chains, which are coiled around each other to form a triple helix. These polypeptide chains consist of about 1,000 amino acids. The three main amino acids are glycine, proline and hydroxyproline and lysine. Every third amino acid is a glycine. The three polypeptide chains are held together by hydrogen bonds and intermolecular cross-links.

Collagen is produced by the fibroblasts; there are about 21 different types of collagen each with different amino acid sequences, present in various tissues. Collagen IV and VII are predominant in the basement membrane, and collagen I and III in the dermis.

Biosynthesis of Collagen

Collagen molecules are synthesised as precursor procollagen molecules, this is secreted by the fibroblast into the extracellular space where collagen molecules are then formed (Fig. 9). The synthesis of collagen can be studies in two stages:
(1) The intracellular stage
(2) The extracellular stage

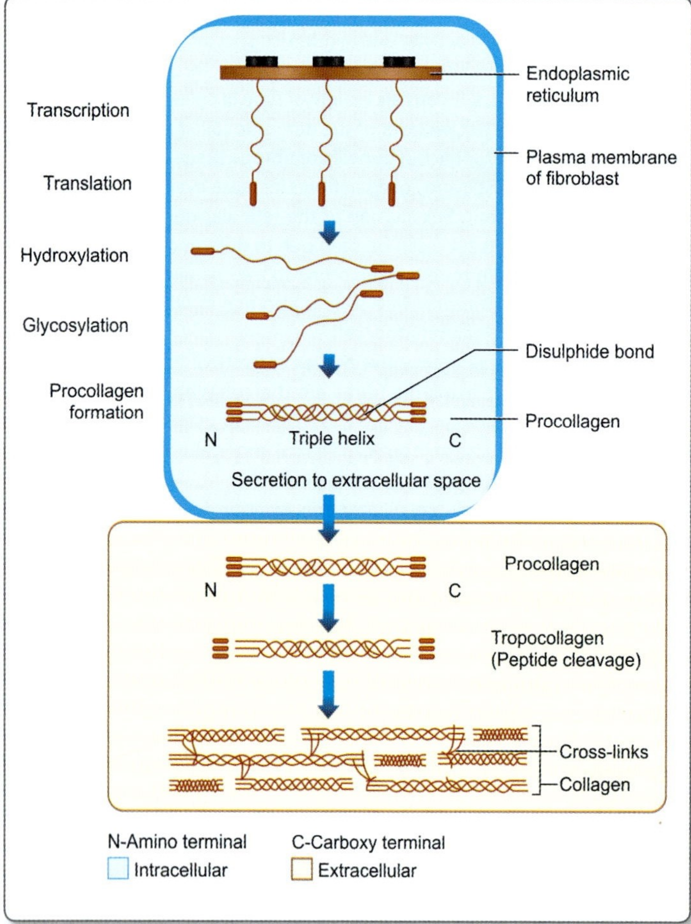

Fig. 9: Synthesis of collagen

Intracellular Stage

The procollagen molecules are formed in the ribosomes of the rough endoplasmic reticulum of the fibroblast. The initial polypeptide chains, consists of an amino-terminal signal. It serves as a signal for the attachment of ribosomes on the rough endoplasmic reticulum and release of polypeptides into the cisternae of the rough endoplasmic reticulum. The polypeptides released into the lumen of the rough endoplasmic reticulum are termed as pro-α chain. These chains are longer than the collagen chains, because they contain the extension peptides at both ends: the amino-terminal (N) and the carboxy-terminal (C).

After the assembly of α-chains, several modifications occur before the completed procollagen molecule is deposited into the extracellular space. Most of these reactions are catalysed by enzymes. Some of the proline and lysine residues become hydroxylated to form hydroxyproline and hydroxy lysine. A critical amount of hydroxyproline is necessary to stabilise the triple helix. Vitamin C is a necessary cofactor for the propyl hydroxylase enzyme. Patients of scurvy have poor wound healing.

Other modifications include attachment of carbohydrates galactose and glucosylgalactose onto certain hydroxyl lysyl residues, chain association, disulphide bonding and triple helix formation. Collagen produced by the fibroblast, is the larger precursor molecule called procollagen.

The procollagen chains are different from the collagen chains, they do not have a glycine as a third amino acid, they are poor in proline and hydroxyproline, but are rich in acidic amino acids. The extension peptides also contain cysteine and tryptophan, which are not present in type I and type II collagen.

The procollagen molecule is soluble under normal physiological conditions. The collagen molecule is insoluble. The procollagen levels are stable in the serum and can be estimated by a variety of methods. A well-known example is the use of serum level of amino-terminal polypeptide of type III procollagen, which is a marker for hepatic fibrosis. This investigation is used to assess the hepatic fibrosis, which can be induced by the use of methotrexate in the treatment of chronic psoriasis.

Proteolytic conversion of procollagen to collagen by the removal of the peptide extensions and cross-linking takes place extracelluarly.

Extracellular Stage

After secretion from the fibroblast the procollagen molecules are converted to tropocollagen by peptidase enzymes, which remove the peptide extensions at each end of the triple helix. These enzymes are procollagen N-proteinase and procollagen C-proteinase. Lack of peptidases can result in a type of Ehlers-Danlos syndrome. The collagen molecules develop full tensile strength by forming cross-links to stabilise. The first step in the formation of cross-links is the formation of aldehydes from the lysyl and hydroxylysyl residues. This requires the enzyme lysyl oxidase. Lysyl oxidase levels are low in some patients of Ehlers-Danlos syndrome. Cross-links are essential for the maturation and stability of collagen, this action can be prevented by the drug penicillamine.

Elastin

The elastic fibres form a continuous network throughout the dermis, and it extends into the connective tissue of the hypodermis. Elastic fibres return the skin to its original shape when stretched. Elastic fibres consist of elastin (85%), oxytalin and elaunin fibres. The oxytalin fibres are situated in the papillary dermis, they extend perpendicularly from the DEJ and merge into the horizontal network of elaunin fibres of the reticular dermis. The elaunin fibres evolve into the mature elastin fibres that extend throughout the reticular dermis. Elastic fibres are positioned between the bundles of collagen fibres.

The basic molecular unit of elastin is a linear polypeptide, which consists of about 800 amino acids, with a molecular mass of 70 KDa. About one-third of the amino acids are glycine, but these are not regularly placed as in collagen. The other rich amino acids are proline, alanine, and hydroxyproline. A characteristic feature of elastic fibres is the cross-links that bind elastin polypeptide chains into a fibre network. The two major cross-link compounds are desmosine and its isomer isodesmosine. These are unique to elastic fibres, an assay of desmosine and isodesmosine, can provide a quantitative measure of elastin content in the skin and other tissues.

Elastin comprises only about 4% of the dry skin weight. Its chemical composition and structure differs from the collagen. Elastic fibres of the papillary dermis are fine, directed vertically, while those of the reticular dermis are directed horizontally, they are coarse in texture. Elastic fibres are responsible for the resilience of the skin. With increasing age, the elastic tissue degenerates and the skin tend to sag and wrinkle.

Elastic fibres consist of two distinct components. The major component is a well-characterised connective tissue protein, elastin which is the electron-lucent core of the fibre; it is surrounded by electron dense microfibrils.

The Ground Substance of the Dermis

The PGs and glycosaminoglycans (GAGs) are molecules of the ground substance that embeds the fibrous components of the dermis. It also regulates the transmission of hormones and nutrients from the blood vessels to the cells. These account for 0.2% of the weight of the dermis. The PGs and GAGs can absorb up to 1,000 times their own volume of water; they also bind growth factors and link cells with fibrillar and filamentous matrix, thereby helping in repair, differentiation and proliferation. They are also components of the basement membranes and are present on the surfaces of mesenchymal and epidermal cells.

The major components of PGs are chondroitin sulphate/dermatan sulphate, heparan/heparan sulphate, and chondroitin-6-sulphate. Hyaluronic acid (HA) exists in the dermis as a free component of GAG and as a component of PGs. HA is much more abundant in fetal dermis, where it is associated with more watery and less stable dermis. As the dermis matures, the matrix is stabilised by a greater predominance of GAGs. With ageing the amount of dermatan sulphate increases, but there is a decrease in chondoitin-6-sulphate. Proteoglycans can be extracellular, intracellular or form part of the pericellular envelope.

Skin is the largest water storage. One-third of the total body fluid is contained in the skin

CELLULAR COMPONENTS OF THE DERMIS

The main cells of the dermis are the fibroblasts, macrophages, dentritic cells and mast cells. Fibroblasts are the main cells of the dermis; they form the collagen and elastic fibres. These cells are found in greatest concentration in the papillary dermis and in the sub-papillary region.

The fibroblasts are the key resident cells of the dermis. They are responsible for the synthesis and degradation of the fibrous and nonfibrous connective tissue proteins, and a number of soluble factors, that help in the transportation of substances to the epidermis. The origin of the fibroblast is unclear; they probably arise from the hair follicle connective tissue sheath.

Macrophages are derived from the bone marrow; they differentiate into monocytes in the blood and as macrophages in the dermis. These cells are morphologically identical to the fibroblasts, but can be differentiated from them by the antigen and enzymatic markers. Macrophages are microbicidal, tumoricidal, they process and present antigens to the immunocompetent lymphoid cells, they secrete growth factors, cytokines and other immunomodulatory molecules. Macrophages are also involved with coagulation, angiogenesis, wound healing and tissue re-modelling.

The dermal dendroctye is a stellate, dendritic cell, these probably represent a subset of antigen-representing macrophages, they represent a sub-population of Langerhans cells or perhaps originate from the bone marrow with a separate lineage. They are immunologically competent cells, they are highly phagocytic. They are likely to be the cell of origin of a number of disorders such as dermatofibroma and fibroxanthoma.

Mast cells are special secretory cells distributed throughout the connective tissue of the body, especially at sites where there is an interaction between the environment and an organ. These cells are recognised histologically by a round or oval nucleus and abundant darkly staining cytoplasmic granules. Mast cells originate in the bone marrow from stem cells. Mast cells synthesise histamine, heparin, tryptase, carboxypeptase, neutrophil chemotactic factor and eosinophilic chemotactic factor. These cells are responsible for immediate hypersensitivity reactions; they are also involved in subacute and chronic inflammatory disease. Mast cells become hyperplastic in mastocytosis.

The mast cells and macrophages are intimately involved in regulating fibroblasts and thus participate in dermal remodelling under physiological and pathological conditions.

THE CUTANEOUS VASCULATURE

The rich blood supply of the dermis originates from the numerous arterial branches that enter the skin from an intricate plexus in the subcutaneous tissue. At about the level of the base of the papillary layer these arteries further subdivide to form a secondary arteriolar plexus, capillary loops arise from this plexus and extend upwards into the papillae. The collecting veins and venules are distributed in the same fashion. The venous elements are larger in diameter and their walls are thinner than their arterial counterparts. Cutaneous vasculature not only supplies nutrition to the skin, but also involved in temperature regulation, blood pressure, wound repair and numerous immunological events. In comparison with the vasculature of other organs, the cutaneous blood vessels have thick walls supported by connective tissue and smooth muscle cells. This is of advantage because the skin is subjected to shearing forces.

In the dermis of the hands and feet there are multiple small arteriovenous (AV) shunts called the glomus bodies. In cases of extreme cold, they shunt the blood away from the skin surface and decrease the heat loss from the body. Rarely these become hyperplastic to form the painful glomus tumors.

All blood vessels of the cutaneous microcirculation are surrounded by veil cells. These cells are not a part of the vessel wall, but appear to define a domain for the vessel within the dermis.

LYMPHATIC CIRCULATION

Lymphatic vessels are also very abundant in the dermis. They are not normally seen in biopsy specimen, as they are extremely thin-walled channels that collapse when the block is dehydrated. The lymphatic capillary is a blind tube beginning in the sub-papillary region, but occasionally also in the dermal papillae. Near the surface the lymphatics are mere excavations in the ground tissue, but deeper in the corium there are distinct lymph channels lined with endothelium, outside the endothelium is a network of reticulum and elastic fibers. The lymph originates from fluid passed through the capillary walls into the tissue spaces.

CUTANEOUS NERVES

The skin has a rich supply of nerves; both free nerve endings and specialised receptors are seen in the dermis (Fig. 10). Receptors are particularly dense in the hairless areas, such as areola, labia and glans penis. Pattern of nerve fibers in the skin are similar to the vascular pattern. Nerve endings are best seen on light microscopy with a silver stain.

Nonmedullated nerve fibres extend into and through the epidermis up to the granular layer; they supply the epithelium of the hair follicles, arrector pili muscles and sweat glands. The other nonmedullated nerve fibres supply innervation to the blood vessels.

Medullated nerve fibers terminate in specialised end organs. There are several types of these end organs, the largest and most deeply situated are the Pacinian corpuscles; these are receptors for pressure sensation. Wagner-Meissner corpuscle are clubbed-shaped found in the dermal papillae, these are receptors of touch, Ruffini bodies found deep in the dermis and subcutaneous

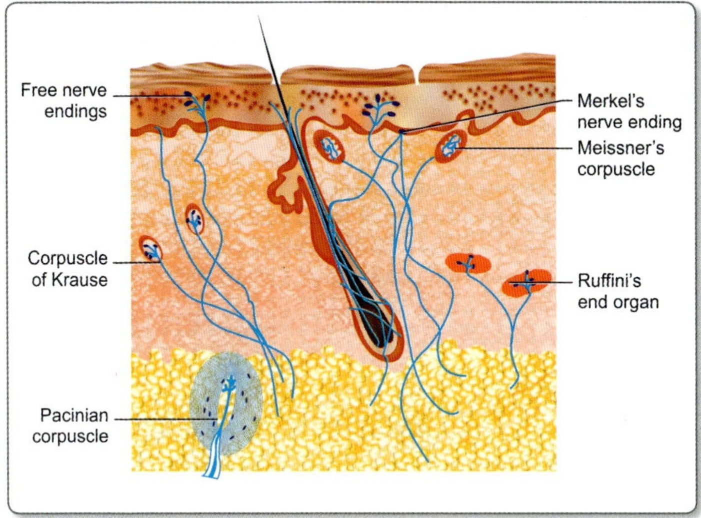

Fig. 10: Sensory nerve receptors

tissue are the heat receptors, and corpuscle of Krause found beneath the dermal papillae mediate cold sensations.

Sympathetic motor fibres are co-distributed with the sensory nerves in the dermis until they branch to innervate the sweat glands, vasculature, smooth muscle, the arrector pili muscle of hair follicles and sebaceous glands.

MUSCLES OF THE DERMIS

In man striated muscle fibres are found in the skin of the face and neck extending from the subcutaneous tissue into the dermis. They are responsible for the expression of emotions. Smooth muscle fibres in the skin are the arrectores pilorum, the dartos muscles of the scrotum and muscles around the areola and nipple. The arrectores pilorum is attached to the hair follicles at the bulge, below the sebaceous glands and extend upward into the papillary portion of the corium. On contracting, they pull the hair follicles upward producing goose flesh-like skin. Arrector pili muscles are absent from the face, axilla, eyelashes, eyebrows and hair around the nostrils and external ear canals.

SUBCUTANEOUS TISSUE

The subcutaneous tissue (hypodermis) lies immediately below the dermis and blends in it in an ill-defined border. The dermis and the hypodermis are structurally and functionally well-integrated through neural and vascular networks and continuity of the skin appendages. Hair follicles in anagen stage of the hair cycle extend into the hypodermis; the eccrine and apocrine glands are normally confined to this depth in the skin. Like the dermis, it is derived from the mesoderm.

The subcutaneous fat consists of lobules of fat cells or lipocytes separated by fibrous tissue septa. The collagen in the septa is continuous with the collagen in the dermis. The predominant cell is the lipocyte, which manufactures large amounts of lipids, mainly triglycerides. As a result, the nucleus is pushed and flattened against the periphery of the cell. The subcutaneous tissue contains nerves, vessels and lymphatics. It acts as a heat insulator, a cushion against trauma and it is storage of nutritional energy. The hypodermis also allows for the mobility of the skin over underlying structures. It also has a cosmetic effect in moulding body contours. The hormone leptin secreted by adipocytes, appears to provide a long-term feeding back signal regulating fat mass.

Skin constitutes a major energy reserve. Skin fat can provide energy for up to 40 days

SKIN LINES

The surface of the skin and its deeper structures show various skin lines. There are over 35 such lines, some visible to the naked eye, others recognisable after some sort of intervention, yet some are debatable postulates. Some of these are:

- Externally visible skin lines: these include the tension lines, flexure lines, dermatoglyphics, intrinsic scarring and Voigt lines of pigmentation.
- Lines detectable after manipulation or incision: these are the lines of Langer and Kraissl, and Blaschko.

Visible Skin Lines

Tension Lines

A simple lattice of skin creases or folds occurs on all the major areas of the hairy skin. The pattern is usually polygonal, this is divided by secondary creases into triangular areas, which are further subdivided by tertiary creases limited to the stratum corneum of the epidermis, and finally at a microscopic level to quaternary creases which are simply the outlines of the individual corneocytes. Apart from the quaternary creases, all the other tension lines increase the surface area of the skin, permitting considerable stretching, recoil and distributing stresses more evenly.

Flexure Lines (Skin Joints)

These are the major markings found near the synovial joints, where the skin is attached strongly to the underlying deep fascia. These are also conspicuous on the palms, soles and digits, these in combination with the associated skin folds, facilitate joint movement.

Dermatoglyphics

Dermatoglyphics (Papillary ridges, Friction ridges, Fingerprints) are impressions of the papillary ridges on the palmar aspect of the distal phalanx. These ridges contain the opening of the sweat ducts. The pattern is persistent throughout life and no two fingerprints are alike. It is therefore used for the identification of individuals. It can be used to identify criminals, identification in public offices, for passports, etc. There are four main configurations, whorl, loop, arch and composite. The most common are the loops and whorls.

Intrinsic Scarring

If the mechanical demands on the skin are greater than what the skin can accommodate, the reticular layer of the skin can rupture and it is then replaced by highly collagenous, poorly vascularised scar tissue. Sites of rupture are visible externally as striae or "stretch marks", e.g. striae gravidarum.

Lines of Pigmentation

Variations in pigmentation can also produce visible lines as "Voigt lines". Voigt lines mark the difference in pigmentation between the darker extensor and paler flexor surfaces of the arm.

Lines Detectable after Manipulation

Lines of Langer

Langer's lines reflect the systematic directional variation in the mechanical behaviour of the skin. There are two basic phenomenons, which are responsible for Langer's line. These are:

- Under passive resting conditions the skin has a series of built-in internal tension, this is because the skin acts as a container for its contents
- The skin also appears to be mechanically anisotropic

If the skin is mechanically punctured by a sharp circular instrument, the wound gapes open, it is oval rather than circular in shape. This is because of the relationship between the biomechanical behaviour of the skin and the built-in tension within the rhomboidal network of collagen fibres. Incisions made along the long axis of the oval, is in the direction of minimum skin extensibility. This direction along the line of least tension is called the Langer's line. The surgical significance of these lines was first proposed by Kocher, who advised that surgical incisions should be made parallel to Langer's line to minimise postoperative scarring. Langer made these observations on cadavers. Kraissl made observations on the living. The direction of these lines varies in different parts of the body.

Blaschko's Lines

These refer to the way in which patterns of naevi and related dermatological pathologies are distributed or developed. These do not correspond to vascular or neural elements, they may be related to early developmental boundaries of a "mosaic" nature. Blaschko's lines represent the migratory path taken by the embryonic skin cells, e.g. the migratory path of melanoblast clones are revealed in the whorled and linear melanosis of incontinentia pigmenti.

OCCURRENCE OF SKIN DISEASE IN RELATION TO RACIAL AND ETHNIC CHARACTERISTICS

Racial and cultural diversity are very complex. The main racial groups are based on division of human species on the grounds of physical characteristics. Ethnic group relates to human groups having racial, religious, linguistic and other cultural characteristics.

The main racial groups are:

- Caucasoid: Aryans, Semites and Hamites

- Congoid/Negroid: Africans, Hottentots, Melanesians, Papuans, Australian Aborigines, Dravidians and Sinhalese
- Mongoloid: North Mongolians, Chinese, Indo-Chinese, Japanese, Koreans, Tibetans, Malayans, Polynesians, Micronesians, Eskimos and American Indians.

Racial characteristics which predispose to skin disease are closely interwoven with cultural and socioeconomic factors. Genetic factors also play an important role.

The main characteristics of the Congoid skin are low incidence of solar keratosis and skin cancer in relation to UVR. But it has a tendency to develop keloids and pseudofolliculitis barbae. Tuberculoid leprosy predominates in black Africans, while psoriasis is rare. The hair is often spiral in Congoids.

Caucasoid skin has scanty melanin production it is susceptible to solar keratosis and skin cancer due to UVR. They are more prone to develop lepromatous leprosy. The hair may be straight, wavy or helical in Caucasoid.

Mongoloid skin has a tendency towards lichenification. The Mongoloids occupy an intermediate position between Caucasoid and Congoid with regards to the incidence of skin disease. The hair is straight in Mongoloids.

Vitiligo has a similar incidence in all races, but it is more conspicuous in the dark coloured people.

Other conditions that predispose to skin disease are the socioeconomic conditions, clothing, cultural characteristics, climate, etc. Malnutrition is common in developing countries. Overcrowding and poor hygienic conditions predispose to person-to-person contagion ranging from pyoderma to leprosy. Cultural factors such as tight braiding in Afro-Caribbeans result in alopecia. The use of oils and herbs can result in contact dermatitis. Humid conditions in hot countries predispose to fungal and bacterial infections, intertrigo and miliaria. Workers in fields are exposed to UVR. Bare foot individuals develop traumatic injuries leading to diseases, such as madura foot, creeping eruption, such as larva migrans. While those individuals who wear shoes and socks most of the time are prone to tinea pedis. Parasitic disorders, such as scabies is common throughout the tropics.

DEVELOPMENT OF SKIN

Development of the skin can be described into three distinct but overlapping stages:

(1) Embryonic development (specification): 0–60 days
(2) Early fetal development (morphogenesis): 2–5 months
(3) Late fetal development (differentiation): 5–9 months

Development of the Epidermis

During the third week of fertilization the three primary embryonic germ layers are formed: ectoderm, endoderm and the mesoderm. In the embryonic phase the epidermis develops from the ectoderm lateral to the neural plate. In a 4–6-week-old fetus, the epithelium divides and a layer of flattened cells, the periderm is laid down. By the end of 8 weeks the hematopoiesis shifts from the extraembryonic yolk sac to the bone marrow. With further proliferation of cells in the basal layer, a third intermediate layer is formed. Finally, at the end of 4th month the epidermis acquires its definite arrangement of four layers: the stratum basale, stratum spinosum, stratum granulosum and the stratum corneum. The formation of the cornified envelope is a late feature of differentiation.

The cells of the periderm are larger and flatter than the basal cells; they are usually cast off by 24 weeks. Together with shed lanugo hair, sebum and other materials they form the vernix caseosa. The periderm is a protective layer for the fetus before keratinisation of the epidermis. The periderm may also be concerned with the uptake of carbohydrates from the amniotic fluid.

Special cells of the epidermis: melanocytes, Langerhans and Merkel cells can be detected by the late embryonic period.

Melanocytes are derived from the neural crest. They are seen in the epidermis by 50 days of embryonic gestational age. During the first 3 months of development, the epidermis is invaded by cells of the neural crest. These cells synthesise melanin pigment, and are known as the melanocytes. The migratory path of melanoblast clones are revealed as "Blaschko's lines". Each melanoblast originates at distinct points along the dorsal midline, they migrate ventrally and distally to reach the epidermis.

Langerhans cells are derived from the monocyte-macrophage-histiocyte lineage. These cells are detectable in the epidermis by 40 days of embryonic gestational age. By the third trimester most of the adult number of Langerhans cells, are seen in the epidermis.

Merkel cells appear in the glabrous skin of the fingertips, lips, gingivae and nail bed at around 11–12 weeks of embryonic gestational age. The embryonic derivation of these cells is controversial. They either develop from in situ differentiation from fetal ectoderm or are derived from the neural crest.

Development of the Dermis and Subcutaneous Tissue

The formation of the dermis and subcutaneous tissue is more diverse than the epidermis, which is solely derived from the ectoderm. The embryonic tissue that forms the dermis depends upon the body site. Dermal mesenchyme of the face and anterior scalp is derived from neural crest ectoderm. The limbs and ventral body wall is derived from lateral plate mesoderm. The dorsal body wall mesenchyme is derived from dermatomyotomes of the embryonic somite. The protein components of the future elastin and collagen are synthesised in the embryonic period, but it is not assembled. The superficial mesenchyme becomes distinct from the underlying tissue at the embryonic-fetal transition. At 3rd–4th months of gestational age, the corium forms many irregular papillary structures: the dermal papillae that project upwards into the epidermis. Collagen bundles are seen by the end of 3rd month, later the papillary and the reticular fibres become distinct. Elastic fibers are first seen at 22 weeks. The dermal papillae contain a small capillary and sensory end organ. At the end of the second trimester the dermis changes from a non-scarring tissue to a scarring one.

The dermis is separated from the subcutaneous tissue by a thin plate of blood vessels by the 50–60 days of the embryonic stage. By the end of the first trimester of pregnancy the subcutaneous tissue can be differentiated from the dermis. By the second trimester adipocytes begin to appear, by the third trimester the subcutaneous tissue becomes organized into fat lobules and septa.

Development of the Blood Vessels, Nerves and Lymphatics

The blood vessels are derived from the endothelial cells at the endoderm-mesoderm interface. By 45–50 days of embryonic stage the horizontal plexuses are formed within the subpapillary and deep reticular dermis, which are interconnected by the vertical vessels. By the 3rd month of intrauterine life distinct networks of horizontal and vertical blood vessels have formed. Cutaneous vessels and nerves begin to form early in gestation, do not fully evolve into the adult until a few months after birth.

Lymphatics probably originate from the endothelial cells that bud off from veins. The development of the lymphatics therefore parallels to that of the blood vessels.

The development of nerves from the neural crest also parallels to that of the blood vessels in terms of patterning, maturation and organization. Early in development the nerves are predominantly small and unmyelinated. With development the nerves become myelinated, this process continues till puberty.

Development of the Basement Membrane

The basement membrane can be seen as early as 8 weeks of the embryonic stage. It contains all the major proteins common to all basement membranes. Components of the specific cutaneous basement proteins appear at the embryonic-fetal transition. By the end of the first trimester all the basement proteins are in place.

Development of Skin Appendages

All skin appendages contain two components: an epidermal component which produces the skin appendage, and a dermal component that regulates the differentiation of the appendage. Dermal-epidermal interactions are essential for induction and differentiation of these appendages.

Hair

Formation of hair is initiated by signals from the dermis, it instructs the basal cells to crowd at regularly spaced intervals. The process begins first on the scalp at 75–80 days of gestation. From the scalp the process spreads caudally to other parts of the body. Formation of the dermal papillae is thought to be initiated by the epidermal signals that are transmitted from follicle epithelium to the underlying mesenchyme.

The hair appears as solid epidermal proliferations (hair germ), penetrating the underlying dermis obliquely. At their terminal ends the hair buds invaginate, these are the hair pegs, they are rapidly filled with mesoderm in which blood vessels and nerve endings develop (hair papillae). At the bulbous hair peg, two epithelial swellings appear on the posterior wall of the follicle. At the lower bulge the arrector pili muscle becomes attached and the upper end is the rudiment of the sebaceous gland.

The center of the hair bud becomes keratinised and forms the hair shaft, while the peripheral cells become cuboidal forming the epidermal hair sheath. The dermal root sheath is formed by the surrounding mesenchyme. A small smooth muscle also derived from the mesenchyme is attached to the dermal root sheath; this is the arrector pili muscle.

Cutaneous proliferation of the epithelial cells at the base of the shaft pushes the hair upwards. By the end of the 3rd month the first hair appear on the surface in the region of the eyebrows and the upper lips. The lanugo hair (intrauterine hair) is shed at about the time of birth and is later replaced by the vellus hair.

Sebaceous Glands

The sebaceous glands appear as solid protuberances on the posterior surface of the hair peg. The sebaceous glands become differentiated at 13–15 weeks. The sebum forms a part of the vernix caseosa. At the end of fetal life, the sebaceous glands are well developed. After birth their size decreases to become functional again only after puberty.

Eccrine and Apocrine Glands

Eccrine glands first develop on the palms and soles at about 55–60 days of the embryonic stage. They like the hair begin as solid downgrowths of the epidermis into the dermis.

The interfollicular eccrine glands and the apocrine glands in contrast do not develop until the 5th month of gestation. Apocrine glands arise from the superficial parts of the hair follicle above the opening of the sebaceous glands. By the 7th month of gestation the cells of the apocrine gland become distinguishable.

Nails

Nails are demonstrable in the 3rd month of intrauterine life; they appear as primary nail folds of proliferative ectoderm, on the tips of the terminal segments of the digit. Fetal growth of the nail is gradual and they reach the tip of the digits at birth, the growth of the fingernails is more advanced than that of the toes.

INVESTIGATIONS FOR HEREDITARY DISORDERS OF THE SKIN

Abnormal development of the skin can give rise to various congenital anomalies, such as ichthyosis, naevi, absence of eccrine glands, congenital absence of the dermis, pseudoxanthoma elasticum, cutis laxa, etc. The techniques for detecting congenital skin disorders include invasive and noninvasive methods.

Noninvasive techniques include examination of the uterus through ultrasonography and maternal serum screen tests such as for alpha-fetoprotein. Blood tests for selected trisomies based on detecting fetal DNA present in maternal blood have become available. This can be done as early as 9 weeks of pregnancy. If an elevated risk of chromosomal or genetic abnormality is indicated by a noninvasive screening test, a more invasive technique may be employed to gather more information.

Invasive methods like chorionic villous sampling, taken at 8–10 weeks, amniocentesis at 16–18 weeks of gestation, fetal skin biopsy taken at 19–22 weeks of gestation. These can be associated with risks to the fetus.

FUNCTIONS OF THE SKIN

Skin is an organ of multiple functions and plays an important role in the normal activities of the body. The skin helps in protection, heat regulation, sensation, secretion, excretion, formation of vitamin D, respiration and immunological functions of the body.

Protection

All the layers of the skin participate in providing protection to the body. The tough elastic nature of the skin protects against mechanical injury. The cornified layer of the epidermis imbibed with lipids protects against the penetration of water and loss of fluids from the body. The skin thus acts as a two-way barrier to prevent the inward or outward passage of water and electrolytes. The keratinous and keratinising layers are poor conductors of heat and electricity, together with the melanin pigment in the deeper layers of the epidermis; these layers tend to screen out injurious UVR. The relatively impervious nature of the outer layers of the epidermis and their acid reaction protects against invasion of microorganisms and parasites. Sebum also protects the skin against fungi and bacteria.

Sensory Functions

The skin with its rich nerve supply can discriminate differences in weight of as little as 0.005 g, it can react to temperatures between −18°C and +44°C. They can send nerve impulses with a velocity of 2 m/s to the spinal cord and brain.

The skin perceives a number of sensations, such as touch, pressure, warmth and pain, by the help of these sensations the skin prevents the body against injuries such as due to heat and cold. Sensory nerve endings are unevenly distributed in a mosaic pattern and vary in density in different parts of the body. A number of cutaneous injuries are inflicted when sensations are lost as seen in leprosy and diabetes.

Heat Regulation

Temperature is regulated through the skin with the help of its physical properties, vascular responses and sweat secretion. On heating the blood vessels dilate, this increases the skin temperature. Heat is also lost through radiation, conduction and convection; sweating increases the heat loss by evaporation of sweat from the surface of the skin. Moisture also increases the skin conductivity of heat and favors heat loss. On exposure to cold blood vessels, constrict, sweat secretion decreases leading to dry skin that serves as a good insulator of heat and tends to conserve body heat. The blood vessels of the skin thus not only provide nutrition, but also help in maintaining a constant body temperature.

Secretory and Excretory Function

The sebaceous and sweat glands carry out the secretory and excretory functions of the skin. The oily secretion of the sebaceous glands keeps the hair and the surface of the epidermis soft. Sweat secretion helps to emulsify the sebum and thus prevents the occlusion of the sebaceous ducts.

Sweat secretion besides temperature regulation also serves as an excretory organ; it helps in the excretion of toxic products such as urea.

Synthesis of Vitamin D

Vitamin D is synthesised in the skin as a result of exposure of the skin to UVR. Vitamin D is formed principally in the stratum malpighii and stratum germinativum from the precursor 7-dehydrocholestrol.

Immunological Function

The skin is the front line for defence of the body. It prevents the entry of foreign antigens into the body. In the epidermis, the antigen presenting cells are the Langerhans cells, which present the antigen to the lymphocytes. The lymphocytes interact with the corresponding antigen, through adaptive immunity. Langerhans cells play an important role in contact sensitisation, immunosurveillance against viral infection and neoplasm. The indeterminate dendritic cells may also be concerned in immune responses. The keratinocytes secrete cytokines that regulate immunological and inflammatory response.

Respiration

The skin performs respiratory function of the body, but it is relatively insignificant. The skin gives off 1/220 as much of carbon dioxide as by the lungs and absorbs only 1/135 as much as oxygen. This is probably due to the passive diffusion of these gases through the skin.

Absorption

Gases and lipid soluble substances are better absorbed than electrolytes and water. Fat solubility increases penetration as it mixes with the normal lipids covering the skin. Some absorption occurs through the hair follicles, but apparently little through the sweat glands. Moisturizers, medicines such as corticosteroids, nitrates, antiseptics can be absorbed by the skin when applied with a proper vehicle; this property has been used as a therapeutic modality.

Skin is a wonderful thing,
Keeps the outside out and the inside in.

FURTHER READING

1. Burradori L, Sonnenberg A. Hemidesmosomes: role, adhesion, signalling and human disease. Curr Open Cell Biol. 1996;8:647-56.
2. Drake DR, Brogden KA, Dawson DV, et al. Antimicrobial lipids at the skin surface. J Lipid Research. 2008;49:4-10.
3. Egelrud T. Desquamation of the stratum corneum. Acta Derm Venereol. 2000;208:45-6.
4. Ekholm E, Sondell B, Dyberg P, et al. Expression of stratum corneum dystryptic enzymes in normal human sebaceous follicles. Acta Derm Venereol (Stockh). 1998;78:343-7.
5. Holbrook K. Ultrastructure of the epidermis. In: Leigh IM, Watt FM, Lane EB (Eds). Keratinocyte Handbook. Oxford: Oxford University Press; 1994. pp. 3-43.
6. Jungersted JM, Hellgren LI, Jemec GB, et al. Lipids and skin barrier function—a clinical perspective. Cont Dermatitis. 2008;58:255-62.
7. Maccari FM, Gheduzzi D, Volpi N. Anomalous structure of urinary glycosaminoglycans in patients with pseudoxanthoma elasticum. Clin Chem. 2003;49:380-8.
8. Marks R. The stratum corneum barrier: the final frontier. J Nuit. 2004.134(8 Suppl):20175-215.
9. Porter AM. Why do we have apocrine and sebaceous glands? J Royal Soc Med. 2001;94(5):236-7.
10. Prockop DJ, Kivirrko KI. Collagens: molecular biology, diseases and potential for therapy. Ann Rev Biochem. 1995:64:604-34.

Chapter 3

Approach Towards a Dermatological Patient

INTRODUCTION

Patients coming for dermatological problems are mostly treated in the outpatient clinic, very few need admission. It is therefore very important to take a detail history of the patient in an orderly and logical framework. Questions forgotten cannot be answered until the next visit. Although many diseases can be diagnosed immediately, but even then the history should not be omitted, as appearances can be misleading and serious mistakes can be made in the diagnosis if the patient's previous medical history and medication is ignored.

Examination of the skin is similar to that of other systems. History taking, family history, social history and drug history should all be taken into account as in other systems of the body. Skin lesions are exposed, so there is a tendency to examine these omitting the history taking. This is a gross mistake, as the history of the patient can unearth the true nature of the disease in a number of cases; this prevents the unnecessary diagnostic problems which can arise later. A systemic examination may be required on some patients, such as those with systemic lupus erythematosus, chronic erythroderma, porphyrias, chronic urticaria and pruritus.

Skin should be examined in sufficient light, be it sunlight or a fluorescent light in an examination room. A magnifying glass should be used to examine the minute details of a lesion. At the conclusion of the examination, one should come to a provisional diagnosis in most cases. When the patient is examined for the first time, the whole body should be examined. Some patients avoid telling about lesions on the genital organs, or one may miss lesions on the back, which cannot be seen by the patient.

HISTORY TAKING

Some important points to remember in dermatological history taking include:

- Duration of skin lesions.
- Are there any symptoms?
- Do the symptoms come and go?
- How did the initial lesion/rash start?
- The site of distribution of the rash leads to further questions, e.g. rash on the photosensitive areas should be questioned about the effects of sunlight and a rash on the foot should be questioned about shoe allergy.
- History of previous skin disease.
- History of previous systemic illness.
- History of drug allergy and medicines used in the last 6 months, including "over the counter" medicines.

The patients are often embarrassed by skin disease. Take the patient into confidence; treat the patient with understanding and sympathy. Very few skin diseases are infectious so do not make the patient feel untouchable by not examining them properly. The patients should remember their visit to the doctor with gratitude even if a cure cannot be provided.

EXAMINATION

Examine the patient in good light, preferably daylight. A torch is essential for examination in wards and for examination of the mouth. A magnifying lens is a useful means of detecting diagnostic minute. A better image is obtained by applying a drop of mineral oil over the lesion. This is especially useful in the diagnosis of Wickham's striae in lichen planus and follicular plugging in lupus erythematosus. Try to examine all the possible signs of a disease although many a times the patient will deny any lesion on the covered parts of the body. The following points should be noted in each examination:

- Site of the lesion: The skin differs in anatomy and physiology in various parts of the body that helps to locate certain diseases, e.g. acne vulgaris occurs on the face, chest and back.
- Size of the lesion.
- Colour of the lesion.
- Type of the lesion, is it primary or secondary?
- Distribution of eruption, whether localised or generalised, symmetrical or asymmetrical.
- Determine the pattern of eruption whether on the extensor or the flexor surface of the limbs, on the sun-exposed surface, profuse or scanty, grouped or scattered, along the lines of cleavage, etc.
- Determine the configuration of the lesion, whether it is annular, linear, serpiginous, circinate, polycyclic, zosteriform, target lesion, etc.
- Note any special features: Some diseases have a characteristic hallmark, which suggests the diagnosis, e.g. axillary freckling in neurofibromatosis, moon face of Cushing syndrome, ash leaf macule and periungual fibromas of adenoma sebaceum.
- Remember to examine the scalp, hair, nails and oral cavity as a part of the skin examination.

Then examine the patient closely. If necessary, use a magnifying glass for detailed examination.

- Determine the primary lesion
- Determine the secondary lesion
- Palpate to find out the degree of infiltration
- Examine the mouth, nails, scalp and whenever required the genitocrural area.

A complete physical examination is required in some cases, e.g. malignancies, collagen disorders, lymphomas, etc.

Always try to determine the anatomical location of the lesion, whether it is epidermal, dermal or subcutaneous. Are the hair, nails and other appendages involved?

SOME DIAGNOSTIC HINTS

- Depend more on what you see than on what you hear
- In all infective cases, palpate the regional lymph nodes
- In all pruritic cases, suspect parasitic infestations such as scabies and pediculosis
- In all patients with decreased sensitivity suspect leprosy
- In atypical or bizarre lesions suspect drug eruption.

SPECIAL DIAGNOSTIC PROCEDURES

- *Diascopy:* This is the blanching of skin on pressure with a glass slide. Diascopy differentiates erythema from purpura, naevus anaemicus from naevus depigmentosus and helps to see the apple jelly nodules of lupus vulgaris.
- *Wood's light examination:* This is a small lamp in which all ultraviolet light except UVA is filtered by a glass containing nickel oxide. Some fungal, bacterial, metabolic, genetic, pigmentary and parasitic disorders can be diagnosed by this method.
- *Immunofluorescence:* This test should be done when available; it helps in diagnosing autoimmune disorders, such as autoimmune bullous disorders, lupus erythematosus, collagen vascular disorders and vasculitis.
- *Dermatoscopy:* This is a noninvasive technique for diagnosing pigmented lesions in vivo, in particular malignant melanoma. The lesion is covered with mineral oil, illuminated and examined with a hand dermatoscope under 10x magnification. The oil makes the horny layer translucent and the pigmented lesions become more apparent. The newer polarised-light dermatoscopes may not require liquid interface or direct contact. Dermatoscope can also be used to examine scabies mites in the burrows. The pigmented lesion can be photographed with a digital camera for future references.
- *Tzanck test:* This test is useful for viral infections and acantholytic disorders such as pemphigus. The specimen is collected from the base of the blister. The material is placed on a glass slide, dried and fixed. The specimen is then stained with Giemsa or Wright's stain. Multinucleated giant cells are seen in herpes simplex and varicella zoster infections. In pemphigus, acantholytic cells are found. These are rounded cells with large basophilic nucleus and a rim of mildly eosinophilic cytoplasm.
- *Scraping of a burrow for scabies:* The finding of a scabies mite under a microscope confirms the diagnosis of scabies. Scraping of a burrow will show the mite, its faeces or eggs. The burrow can be made more visible by outlining them with black ink. The scraping is done with a number 15 scalpel blade moistened with oil, so that the contents of the burrow adhere to the blade. The contents are transferred to a glass slide, add a drop of oil on it and examine under a microscope. The key to a positive result is vigorous scraping.

  Scabies mite can also be examined on the skin with a dermatoscope.
- *Mycological examination for dermatophytes:* Direct examination of the skin, nail and hair is an essential step for confirming the clinical diagnosis

of a cutaneous fungal infection. These fungi can be examined by direct microscopy, with or without staining, or by fluorescence microscopy using specific fluorochromes for the fungal cell constituents.

Direct examination without staining is usually done in the ward to confirm the diagnosis of a dermatophyte infection. The specimen for fungus is taken from the edge of the skin lesion, which is the site where fungi are most likely to be found. The skin can be scraped with a sterile scalpel or curette; hair should be epilated with a tweezer. Nail specimen is best taken with a dental drill from the most proximal end of the infected nail. The specimen is placed on a glass slide, treated with potassium hydroxide (KOH), which destroys all non-fungal cells, and makes it easier to see if there is any dermatophyte present. The specimen is then examined under a microscope. It takes about 5–15 minutes to dissolve the keratin. A rapid clearing can be obtained by heating the slide gently over a low flame; overheating can destroy the specimen. To enhance clearing dimethyl sulfoxide can be added to the slide. To make the dermatophytes more prominent lactophenol cotton blue can be added.

SOME CLINICAL SIGNS THAT HELP IN DIAGNOSIS

Nikolsky's sign: When a gentle traction is applied to the skin, it peels due to the loss of adhesion in epidermal cells, e.g. pemphigus. It is also present in toxic epidermal necrolysis.

Bulla spreading sign: A slight pressure applied on a bulla, the bulla spreads due to the weakness in epidermal cell adhesions, e.g. pemphigus.

Auspitz sign: On forceful removal of a scale in psoriasis, pin-point bleeding spots are seen; this is due to the rupture of capillaries in the dermal papillae which are found underneath a thin epidermis. It is positive in psoriasis.

Dimple sign: This helps in differentiating dermatofibroma and malignant melanoma. Application of lateral pressure with the index finger and thumb over the nodule, results in the formation of a dimple in dermatofibroma.

Burns that form a blister but do not cause pain think of leprosy or neuropathic ulcers.

OTHER LABORATORY INVESTIGATIONS

These are advisable in some diseases and indispensable in others. They are indicated in persistent cutaneous disorders or to confirm a diagnosis. Common diagnostic procedures are:

- Skin biopsy
- Mycological studies
- Bacteriological studies
- Patch test for allergic contact dermatitis (test detects Type IV hypersensitivity)
- Prick test, radioallergosorbent test (test detects Type 1 hypersensitivity)
- Blood count, urine examination and blood chemistry
- Serological tests

- Search for parasitic organisms, e.g. scabies mite, Leishman-Donovan bodies.
- For hair shaft evaluations: hair pull test, trichogram, trichoscan, amino acid evaluations, hair window, electrophoretic characteristic of proteins and polariscopic examination.

MOLECULAR DIAGNOSTICS

Molecular diagnostic methods have increased the sensitivity and specificity in the diagnosis of infectious diseases, tumours, autoimmune disorders and genodermatoses. Some of these methods are:

Polymerase chain reaction (PCR): This provides rapid amplification of specific DNA sequences, leading to identification of foreign nucleic acids present in small amounts.

In situ hybridisation: The purpose is to analyse the intracellular distribution, transcription or other characteristics of nucleic acids.

Detection of immunoglobulins and T-cell receptor rearrangements: The test helps in assessing the clonality of B-cell or T-cell proliferation.

DNA microassays: This helps in analysing thousands of genes simultaneously.

False positive results are common the use of appropriate control measure is essential.

PRIMARY AND SECONDARY SKIN LESIONS

While examining the skin one should have a clear picture of the different kind of skin lesions. These give a clue to the diagnosis and prevent unnecessary investigations. The skin lesions can be primary or secondary.

Primary Lesions

The primary lesions are those, which are not affected by trauma, manipulations as scratching, scrubbing, etc. or regression over time. They arise on normal skin. The common primary lesions are:

Macule: It is a flat circumscribed discolouration of the skin; it lacks elevation or depression. These may be round, oval, angular or irregular in shape. These may be due to transient dilatation of the blood vessels (erythema), permanent dilatation of the blood vessels (capillary naevi), escape of blood in the skin (purpura), it may be due to deposition of melanin as in freckles, lentigines, macules may be hypochromic as in leprosy or achromic as in vitiligo.

Papule: This is an elevated solid lesion less than 5 mm in diameter. The lesions may be round, oval, polygonal, flat or angular in shape. The colour may be red, pink, purple or pigmented. The surface may be smooth, scaly or verrucous, e.g. pruritic purple papules of lichen planus.

Plaque: This is an elevated lesion more than 5 mm in diameter often formed by confluence of papules. It lacks a deep component, e.g. psoriasis, tinea corporis.

Nodule: Nodules are circumscribed solid, palpable, deep and indurated lesions. It is larger than 1 cm in diameter. When above the skin it is round or dome-shaped, e.g. erythema nodosum, nodules below the skin are better palpated than visible, e.g. fibroma.

Cyst: This is a cavity containing fluid, which is more than 5 mm in diameter; it may contain pus, blood, sebaceous secretion, mucous, etc.

Vesicle: This is a circumscribed accumulation of fluid that it is less than 5 mm in diameter. The content is usually serous, seropurulent or haemorrhagic. They often develop on inflamed skin. Vesicles are intraepidermal and heal without scarring.

Bulla: It is a vesicle of larger than 5 mm in diameter; it may be tense or flaccid. Bullae located in the epidermis are flaccid and rupture easily, e.g. pemphigus, those situated in the dermis are tense and remain intact for a longer time, e.g. pemphigoid.

Pustule: This is a localised collection of pus. It may appear as such or develop from a vesicle. They may be isolated or grouped. Large groups form a lake of pus. Pustules may be caused by infection or may be aseptic as in pustular psoriasis.

Wheal: It is a firm transient edematous elevation of the skin varying in shape and size, pale pink in colour. It is caused by oedema of the dermis and capillary dilatation. By coalescence large plateau like elevations is formed. Wheals are characteristic of urticaria and urticarial reactions.

Tumour: It is a circumscribed swelling larger than 2.5 cm in diameter. Tumours are located within or beneath the dermis or are attached to it by a pedicle, e.g. neuroma, fibroma, lipoma, etc.

Secondary Lesions

Secondary lesions are those that are superimposed on an existing skin lesion. These are:

Scales: These are desquamated horny flakes produced due to abnormal keratinisation. Under normal condition the stratum corneum is desquamated; this loss normally occurs imperceptibly. The desquamated scales when perceptible are due to increased proliferation or increased cohesion of the keratinocytes. Scales may be dry and silvery in psoriasis, greasy in seborrhoeic dermatitis, pityriasiform scales are branny, they are fine and loose as in pityriasis versicolor (furfuracious), scales of discoid lupus erythematosus are studded with a keratinous plug at their bottom. In pityriasis rosea, they form a centripetal collarette, ichthyotic scales are large and polygonal. Large scales of desquamated epidermis are seen in toxic epidermal necrosis and staphylococcal scalded skin syndrome.

Crust: This is a dry accumulation of exudate or secretion upon the skin. Crusts may be serous (yellow or honey coloured), purulent (yellowish-green), bloody (reddish-black) or a mixture of these.

Fissure: It is a small vertical crack of the epidermis, which is usually painful. Fissures are normally found in inflamed, inelastic, thickened skin such as the palms and soles, over the joints, mucocutaneous junctions, rhagades at the angle of the mouth and anal fissures.

Erosions: Is a partial loss of the epidermis. It may result from breaking down of a vesicle, bulla or a pustule. It could be due to trauma or chemicals. Erosions heal without scarring.

Excoriation: These linear erosions result from scratching and are often covered with bloody crusts. Excoriations are usually found in linear, parallel or punctate patterns.

Ulcer: This is a full thickness focal loss of the epidermis and dermis, it heals with scarring. Its location, size, configuration (round, oval, angular, annular or circinate), borders (flat, undermined, punched out, rolled), base (soft, infiltrated, membranous, washed leather), discharge (serous, sero-purulent, bloody), colour (bright red, livid), surrounding (oedema, erythema, fibrosis, pigmentation), symptoms (burning, painful, painless), and regional lymph node involvement should be noted.

Scar: This is the formation of new connective tissue. Scars may be hypertrophic or atrophic. Scars of certain diseases have a diagnostic value, e.g. scars of lupus erythematosus are shiny thin, telangiectatic, and minutely pitted. Scars are persistent, they become noticeable with time. Some scars become thick and tough such as hypertrophic scars and keloids. These hypertrophic scars are thick and elevated with increased growth of fibrous tissue. Atrophic scars are thin and wrinkled such as syphilitic scars. In some individuals, certain areas of the body are especially prone to scarring such as the anterior chest region.

Atrophy: This is thinning of the skin, it may be epidermal, dermal or of the subcutaneous tissue. Atrophy is characterised by loss of normal skin markings. Epidermal thinning is manifested by depression of the skin. Atrophy may occur with aging, healing of disease or drugs such as steroid therapy.

Sclerosis: Localised or diffuse induration of the dermis and subcutaneous tissue gives the skin a hard rigid feel when palpated. The overlying skin is pale, smooth and shiny as in scleroderma, but it may be rough and shows keratotic plugs as in lichen sclerosus et atrophicus.

Special Lesions

Burrow: These are short linear dark elevations of the horny layer characteristic of scabies, due to the presence of the mite in the stratum corneum. Long pink burrows forming bizarre patterns are diagnostic of larva migrans.

Comedone: This is a horny plug filling the orifice of the pilosebaceous duct. It may be closed (white head), or open (black head), comedones are characteristic of acne vulgaris and acneiform eruptions.

Telangiectasia: This is a thin red linear lesion caused by the dilatation of the blood vessels. It may be idiopathic or caused by diseases such as collagen disorders (scleroderma), vasculitis, etc.

Target lesion: The target lesion consists of typically three zones. The innermost zone is dark or contains a blister that is surrounded by a second pale zone. The third zone consists of a ring of erythema. These are characteristic of erythema multiforme.

Koebner's phenomenon: This is a linear lesion of a disease produced at the site of injury, when the disease is in its active form with a tendency to early relapse even with therapy. It is seen in some diseases such as psoriasis, lichen planus, molluscum contagiosum and verruca vulgaris.

Koebner's phenomenon occurs 7–14 days after injury. In a given patient all or none phenomenon occurs at all sites of injury. Clearing of existing psoriasis has also been observed in reverse Koebner phenomenon; this also observes the all or none phenomenon. Koebner's phenomenon is a marker for a subgroup of patients with a tendency to early onset and early relapse after various forms of therapy. The observations suggest the presence of a circulatory element controlling the expression of the disease throughout the skin. Serum from patients recovering from psoriasis inhibits Koebner's phenomenon.

COMMONLY USED DESCRIPTIVE TERMS IN DERMATOPATHOLOGY

Hyperkeratosis: This refers to an increase in thickness of the stratum corneum. Hyperkeratosis may be *orthokeratotic*; this consists of an increase in morphologically normal cells in the stratum corneum as seen in corns, ichthyosis, keratodermas and chronic discoid lupus erythematosus (CDLE).

Parakeratosis: This is retention of keratinocyte nuclei in the horny layer. It is due to disturbance of keratinisation, and is normally associated with absence or reduction in thickness of the granular layer. It is commonly seen in disease, such as psoriasis, subacute eczema, actinic keratosis, Bowen's disease and cutaneous horn.

Epidermolytic hyperkeratosis: Epidermolytic hyperkeratosis is an abnormality of epidermal maturation characterised by compact hyperkeratosis, accompanied by granular and vacuolar degeneration of the cells of the spinous and granular layers. It may be a congenital or an acquired. The change is characteristic of bullous ichthyosiform erythroderma.

Dyskeratosis: This is an abnormality of individual cell keratinisation as seen in Darier's disease, here the cells get separated by acantholysis and then proceed to keratinise as corps ronds and grains (benign dyskeratosis). It is also seen in premalignant and malignant tumours (malignant dyskeratosis).

Acanthosis: This denotes an increase in thickness of the malpighian layer. In *pseudoacanthosis,* there is an increase in the size of the cells; in *true acanthosis,* the number of keratinocytes is increased. This is often accompanied by hyperkeratosis as seen in epidermal naevi, molluscum contagiosum and psoriasis.

Acantholysis: This denotes a loss of cohesion between the keratinocytes, due to break down of the intercellular bridges. This results in the formation of bullae and vesicles. Primary acantholysis is seen in pemphigus, Darier's disease. Secondary acantholysis occurs when first there is damage to epithelial cells as seen in bullous impetigo.

Spongiosis: This is so called because of the spongy appearance of the epidermis. It is due to the intercellular edema of the malpighian layer. Increase in edema results in the formation of vesicles and bullae, these changes are characteristic of eczema.

Lichenification: This is thickening of the skin due to chronic rubbing, with exaggerated skin markings, as seen in lichen simplex chronicus.

Necrobiosis: Literary means life and death. It exhibits a localised damage to the dermis that affects the cells more than the fibers and is accompanied by deposits of abnormal substances. The dermal connective tissue becomes homogenised, resulting in mucinous, fibrinoid or sclerotic alteration. Changes of necrobiosis are normally surrounded by a palisading histiocytic granuloma. It is seen in necrobiosis lipoidica, granuloma annulare, rheumatoid nodule, granuloma multiforme and acne agminata.

The language of derrmatology is unique; it encompasses terms that are rarely used in other specialties. The use of correct dermatological terms is important; we can accurately describe diseases by looking at its morphological characteristics. Papules of lichen planus are violaceous, polygonal, flat, pruritic with Wickham's striae; these are located on the flexural surface of the wrist and ankles. It is therefore important to know the lesions, their distribution, the symptoms they produce to come to a diagnosis by simple examination of the skin; investigations should be done when necessary.

FURTHER READING

1. Bolognia JL, Orlow SJ, Glick SA. Lines of Blaschko. J Am Acad Dermatol. 1994;31:157-90.
2. Chren MM. Quality of care in dermatology: the state of measuring the art. Arch Dermatol. 1997;133(11):1349-57.
3. Gilchrest BA, Fitzpatrick TB, Anderson RR, et al. Localization of melanin pigment on the skin with Wood's lamp. Br J Dermatol. 1977;96:245-8.
4. Javkson R. The importance of being visually literate: Observation on the art and science of making a morphological diagnosis. Int J Dermatol. 1975;111:632-6.
5. Mysore V. Invisible dermatoses. Indian J Dermatol, Venereol and Leprol. 2010;76(3):239-48.

Chapter

4 Bacterial Infections

INTRODUCTION

The skin surface harbours saprophytic flora, such as *Staphylococcus (S.) epidermidis*, Micrococci, Corynebacteria and Yeast. The number of organisms varies in different parts of the body; it depends upon the age of the individual, the environment and climate. Besides harmless organisms some pathogenic bacteria also grow in certain areas of the body especially the body folds. When the barrier horny layer is broken these organisms proliferate and cause disease.

The skin's own defences such as unsaturated fatty acids and sebum keep the flora in check. In hot and humid climate, the body defences are lowered and minor trauma or abrasions often result in infection. Bacterial infections can be primary or secondary. Infections may be secondary to scabies, fungal infections, eczema, etc. The severity of the disease depends upon the following factors:

- The causative bacteria and its severity of toxicity
- The target tissue
- The immunological status of the patient.

Normal Bacterial Flora

The skin is sterile at birth, but only for a short period. *S. aureus* colonisation of the umbilicus begins during the first day of life in 25% of neonates. This figure increases steadily, perhaps due to the fall in the pH of the skin from 7.0 to 5.5.

The normal skin flora can be transient or resident. Organisms capable of multiplying as well as survival are classified as resident flora; these are found almost all over the skin. The transient flora, are deposited in the skin from the mucous membrane drop out or from the environment.

Opportunistic organisms are the nonpathogenic members of the resident or transient flora that produce infection in debilitated or immunocompromised patients.

Resident Flora

Propionibacterium acnes: This is an anaerobic diphtheroid present in the sebaceous follicles of the skin. Its presence in acne does not indicate a causative role, but the acne lesions are due to the physiological changes in the underlying disease.

Aerobic diphtheroids: These organisms are usually present in the intertriginous areas; *Corynebacterium* (C.) *tenuis* causes trichomycosis axillaris. *C. minutissimum* causes erythrasma.

Staphylococcus epidermidis: This organism is uniformly present on the normal skin; it exerts a suppressive action on the colonisation of the skin by other organisms. It is an important pathogen in prosthetic valve endocarditis and indwelling venous catheters.

Micrococci: These are not increased in number in dermatological diseases.

Gram-negative bacilli: These are present in the intertriginous areas; these include *Escherichia (E.) coli, Proteus, Pseudomonas, Enterobacter alcaligenes.* They often give rise to bacteraemia in patients with indwelling venous catheters.

Transient Flora

Aerobic spore forming organisms, such as Streptococci of various groups and Neisseria, are present on the skin surface for short periods. *S. aureus* is present in about 20% of individuals, their presence is associated with nasal or perineal discharge. Rifampicin is said to eradicate *S. aureus* from chronic nasal carriers. At times Streptococci can also colonise deeper in the skin and may become a part of the resident flora. Atypical mycobacteria occur as transient bacilli in the intertriginous areas.

INFECTIONS CAUSED BY *STAPHYLOCOCCUS AUREUS* AND *STREPTOCOCCUS HAEMOLYTICUS*

Staphylococcus and Streptococcus are the two common pathogens that infect skin. Most of the skin infections are caused by coagulase positive Staphylococcus, such as *S. aureus* producing invasive and toxin-mediated infection. *S. epidermidis* which is coagulase negative causes most of hospital infection. About 20% of individuals carry *S. aureus* in the nasal cavity and perineum; they act as carriers of infection. It is often the cause of recurrent furunculosis and wound infections.

Methicillin-resistant *Staphylococcus aureus* (MRSA) is becoming increasingly common because of the excessive use of antibiotics. The patient should be isolated to prevent spread of infection. Vancomycin is effective against MRSA, but resistance to this is also reported.

About 90% of streptococcal infection is caused by *S. pyogenes,* which belongs to β-haemolytic Streptococcus of group A, *S. viridans* (α-haemolytic Streptococci) and *S. pneumoniae* are also important members of streptococci. Subacute bacterial endocarditis and glomerulonephritis are complications of streptococcal infection; the patients should have a close follow-up after treatment. Patients should be monitored for anti-streptolysin O (ASO) and antistreptodornase titres till they normalise.

Impetigo

Impetigo is a contagious superficial skin infection caused by *S. aureus* or β-haemolytic streptococci. In some cases both the organisms are responsible for the lesion. It is the most common bacterial skin infection in children, but can occur at any age. The disease is common in the summer

Clinical Features

There are two clinical types of impetigo:

- Non-bullous impetigo (Impetigo contagiosa) (Fig. 1)
- Bullous impetigo (Fig. 2).

***Non-bullous impetigo*:** This is more common, it is responsible for about 70% cases of impetigo. The disease is characterised by the formation of thin walled vesicles, these occur predominantly on exposed parts of the body. The lesions are the most common on the face, especially around the mouth and nose. The vesicles rupture readily to form golden, yellow or brown crusts. There is gradual peripheral extension. Healing occurs without scarring.

***Bullous impetigo*:** The initial lesions are vesicles, which rapidly progress to form flaccid bullae. Bullae develop due to the action of an epidermolytic toxin on the granular layer, if the toxin becomes widely disseminated it results in staphylococcal scalded skin syndrome (SSSS). The bullae are at first clear, but later become purulent. The bullae rupture in a day or two. After rupture a brownish crust is formed. The lesions are more common on the trunk and extremities.

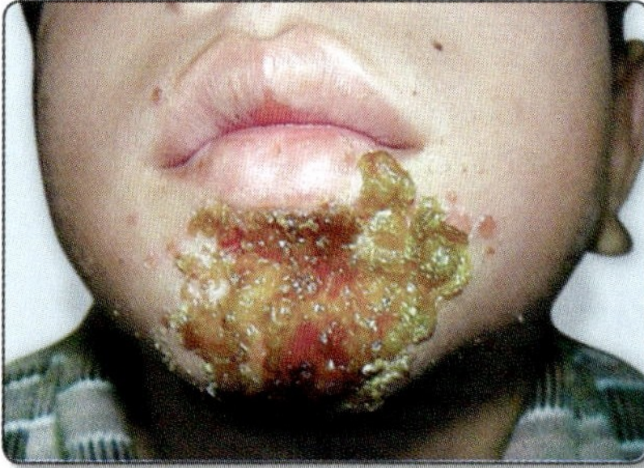

Fig. 1: Impetigo-non bullous

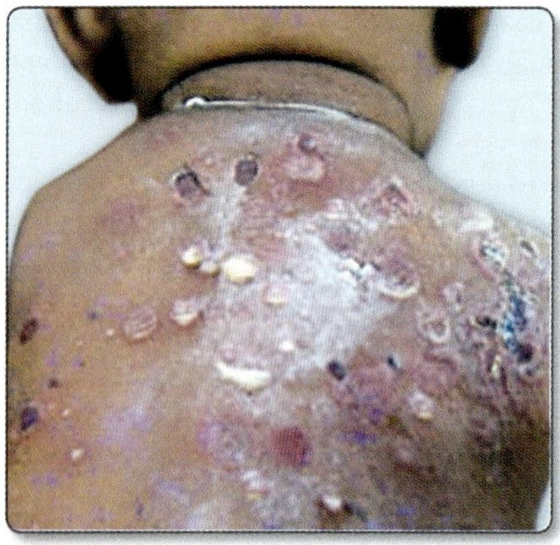

Fig. 2: Impetigo-bullous

Complications

Nephritogenic strains of streptococci that are sometimes responsible for impetigo can cause acute glomerulonephritis. The nephritis occurs 18–21 days after the infection, as compared to 10 days after the throat infection.

Scarlet fever, urticaria and erythema multiforme may follow streptococcal impetigo. Rheumatic fever is not a complication.

Complications following staphylococcal impetigo are cellulitis, lymphangitis, SSSS and bacteraemia.

months; prevalence is highest in tropical regions. Overcrowded and unhygienic conditions are important predisposing factors; it may complicate a pre-existing skin disease, such as scabies, pediculosis, atopic dermatitis and miliaria. Impetigo is contagious; infection can easily spread to other parts of the body and to close contacts.

Differential Diagnosis

The disease should be differentiated from herpes simplex in which the base is more erythematous and oedema more pronounced. In Tinea circinata the annular lesions have active vesiculations at the periphery, scraping with potassium hydroxide examination will show the fungus.

Treatment

Topical antiseptic creams, soaps or lotions containing hexachlorophene, triclosan, and chlorhexidine and povidone-iodine are effective for cleaning the lesion. Topical antibiotics are effective in most of the cases. The effective agents include bacitracin, gentamicin, mupirocin and fusidic acid.

Impetigo caused by erythromycin-resistant *S. aureus* is common in children. Amoxicillin plus clavulanic acid 25 mg/kg of body weight per day is given tid for 7–10 days. In extensive impetigo, penicillinase-resistant penicillin is initiated. Flucloxacillin or Cloxacillin is the antibiotic of choice and is given in a dose of 250–500 mg 6 hourly. Azithromycin 500 mg on the first day, followed by 250 mg for the next 4 days, is effective alternative therapy.

If impetigo appears resistant to treatment or is recurrent, then nasal swabs are taken for culture. Nasal mupirocin is useful to eradicate nasal carriage.

Tilbury Fox (1836–1879)

Tilbury Fox was an able and eminent English dermatologist. He was the first to describe dyshidrosis and impetigo. He described urticaria pigmentosa, lymphangioma circumscriptum, and epidermolysis bullosa but did not name these conditions.

Folliculitis

Folliculitis is an inflammation of the skin that is confined to the follicular ostium or slightly below it. Healing takes place without scar formation.

Aetiology

Infective: The offending agents include bacteria such as *S. aureus*, some gram-negative organisms, fungi such as *Pityrosporum ovale* and *Trichophyton rubrum*.

Chemicals: Oil folliculitis follows occupational exposure to mineral oil. Tar folliculitis is due to occupational or therapeutic exposure to tar.

Drugs: Topical steroids under occlusion.

Physical: Waxing, threading, plucking, occlusive dressings, etc.

Clinical Features

The lesions present as multiple, small follicular papules or pinhead-sized pustules. There is no pain. Tiny pustules with a central hair and an erythematous halo manifest Bockhart's impetigo. As the lesions dry, small yellow-brown crusts form. Folliculitis heals without scarring. The common sites are the scalp, beard region and the limbs.

Tropical folliculitis of the legs is common in Negroes and in other tropical races, its chronicity and atrophic sequelae characterise it. Clinically it resembles the Bockhart's type, but these are deep-seated nodules, as they heal they leave behind deep-seated atrophic depressions (Fig. 3).

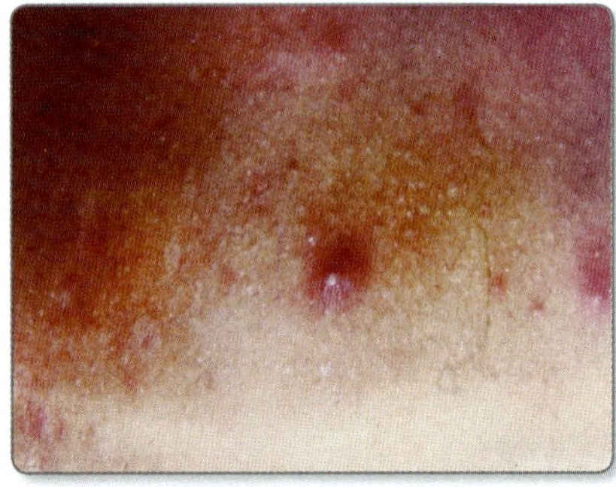

Fig. 3: Folliculitis

Treatment

- Remove the cause such as the physical and chemical agents
- One percent gentian violet or brilliant-green paint is a cheap and effective remedy
- Topical antibacterial agents: Fusidic acid, gentamicin cream, etc.
- Nasal and perineal carriage should be looked for and treated in chronic and resistant cases
- With availability of effective antibacterial agents, the need for systemic antibiotics is reduced
- Antimicrobial soaps are effective in treatment of folliculitis because they reduce the growth of Gram-negative, as well as Gram-positive bacteria. Soaps containing triclosan, chlorhexidine, hexachlorophene or povidone-iodine are beneficial. Systemic antibiotics should be used to treat tropical folliculitis of the legs.

Folliculitis in adults can be due to Ofugi's disease (Eosinophilic pustular folliculitis). The disease is seen mostly in Japan, the incidence is in the 3rd decade, most commonly on the scalp. It is often associated with AIDS. There is no effective treatment, topical and systemic and corticosteroids, topical tacrolimus, dapsone, colchicines and ultraviolet B (UVB) therapy have been used for treatment. Aetiology is unknown.

Furunculosis (Boils) and Carbuncles

Boil is an acute infection of the deeper part of the hair follicle, *S. aureus* is the most common pathogen. A carbuncle is a mass of boils that usually indicates an underlying debility.

Clinical Features

The initial lesion is a tender, hard red papule that rapidly develops into a nodule: this points and then discharges greenish-yellow pus. The sites of predilection are the face, neck, axillae and buttocks. The lesion should not be squeezed because this can lead to serious complications like osteomyelitis, cavernous sinus thrombosis or septicemia (Fig. 4).

A number of boils coalesce to form a carbuncle; it is often secondary to malnutrition, diabetes mellitus, prolonged steroid therapy, generalised debilitating diseases, etc. It presents as a red tender hard plaque, with a number of follicular orifices that discharge pus. Constitutional symptoms like fever may be present (Fig. 5).

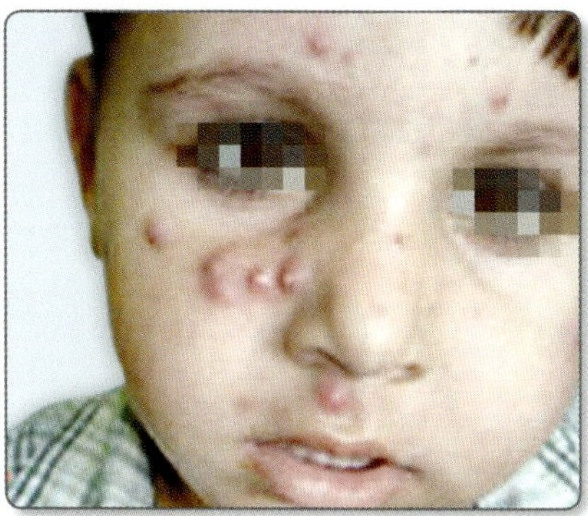

Fig. 4: Furuncles

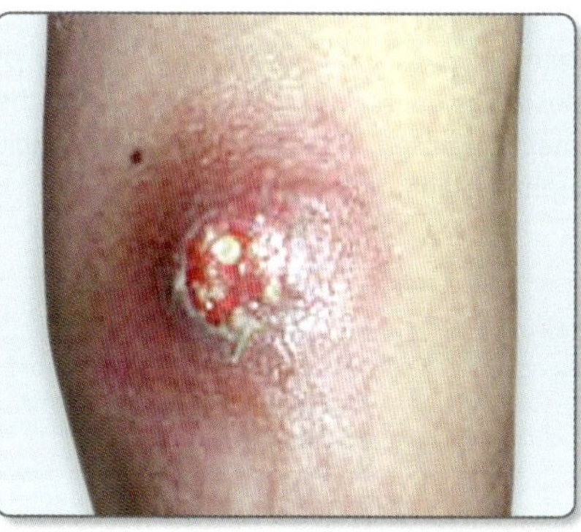

Fig. 5: Carbuncle

Treatment

Local heat relieves discomfort and aids in localization of the infection. If the boil is large and fluctuant; it should be incised and drained. Carbuncles usually require surgical treatment. Predisposing factors that cause carbuncles should be treated, such as malnutrition, diabetes mellitus, and general debilitating diseases.

Systemic antibiotics are effective in treating boils; local antibiotics do not penetrate deep into the dermis. The effectiveness of erythromycin and tetracycline is limited owing to emergence of resistant strains of ***S. aureus***. Flucloxacillin is effective in most cases. Unresponsive cases can be controlled by ciprofloxacin or low-dose clindamycin.

If methicillin-resistant strain of ***S. aureus*** is suspected vancomycin 1.0–2.0 g IV once in 12 hours is indicated. The infusion should be given slowly. Linezolid oral or intravenous may also be used.

Recurrent furunculosis: Recurrent furunculosis is common if patients harbour ***S. aureus*** in the skin or anterior nares. Diabetes mellitus can also lead to recurring attacks of furunculosis. Both topical and systemic medication is required for recurrent furunculosis.

Topical agents: Fusidic acid 2% cream or ointment is used three times daily. Mupirocin is effective against MRSA. In recurrent furunculosis, mupirocin is applied to anterior nares two or three times daily for 1 week each month; this effectively eradicates the nasal organisms.

Systemic therapy: Rifampicin is effective against recurrent furunculosis. The recommended dose is 600 mg daily for 1 week each month for 3 months. Ciprofloxacin and minocycline have also been used for recurrent furunculosis.

Systemic isotretinoin may clear many types of folliculitis, presumably by changing the microenvironment of the pilosebaceous units. It is used in doses of 1 mg/kg of body weight per day for 3–5 months. Isotretinoin should be reserved for patients who have failed other therapies.

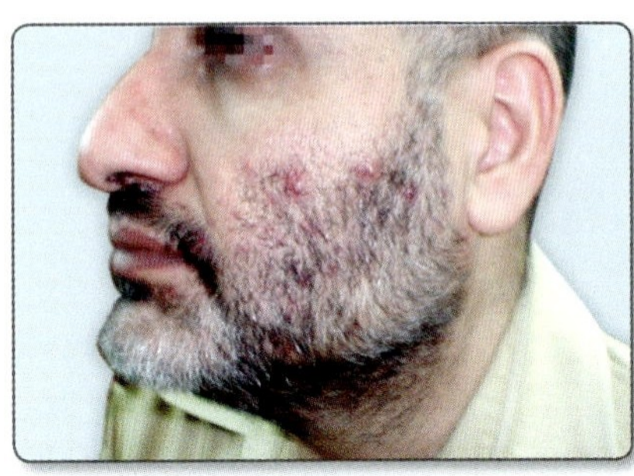

Fig. 6: Sycosis barbae

Sycosis Barbae

This is a subacute or chronic pyogenic infection involving the whole depth of the follicle. Sycosis appears in males after puberty and commonly involves the region of the beard and upper lip near the nose. Many patients are seborrhoeic they often suffer from chronic blepharitis and have a greasy skin.

Clinical Features

The essential lesion is an edematous red follicular papule or pustule around the hair, usually the follicles are discrete, but sometimes they may coalesce to form a plaque with studded pustules. The pustules rupture after shaving, leaving an erythematous red spot that is later a site of fresh eruption of pustules. The disease is chronic with attacks of varying duration, occurring at irregular intervals (Fig. 6).

Treatment

Subacute forms are treated relatively easily with antibiotics both topical and systemic. If the nasal swabs show a chronic carrier state, then the topical antibiotic should be applied to the nasal vestibule. The chronic form does not respond well to antibiotics and a steroid antibiotic combination is preferred. The treatment should be continued for a long time.

ECTHYMA

It is a pyogenic infection of skin characterized by the formation of adherent crusts beneath which ulceration occurs. The causative organisms are similar to that of impetigo, i.e. *S. pyogenes* or *S. aureus*. Some authors consider ecthyma as a subtype or ulcerated form of impetigo. In ecthyma, the infection spreads in depth while in impetigo it spreads on the surface.

Clinical Features

The infection begins as a vesicle or a pustule with a red halo, this rapidly turns into a bulla that breaks down to form punched out ulcer covered with a dark-brown bloody crust. Removal of the crust shows an irregular crateriform ulcer. The ulcer heals in 6–8 weeks often with scar formation. The lesions are few or numerous. The sites of predilection are lower extremities, buttocks and thighs. It is especially common in children and the elderly. There is a potential for developing post-streptococcal glomerulonephritis (Fig. 7).

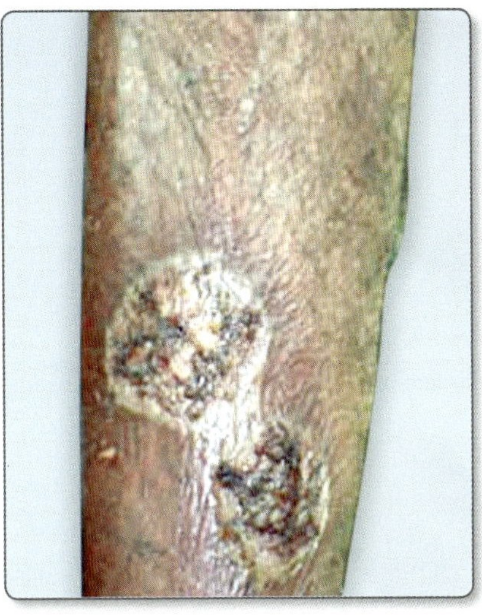

Fig. 7: Ecthyma

Treatment

- Removal of crusts by starch poultice
- Topical antibacterials, e.g. mupirocin or fusidic acid ointment
- Systemic antibacterial: The antibiotic chosen should be effective against both Staphylococcus and Streptococcus. The antibiotics used are similar to that of impetigo, but the treatment should continue for 3 weeks.

Erysipelas and Cellulitis

Erysipelas is the infection of dermis and upper subcutaneous tissue due to *S. pyogenes* or occasionally *S. aureus*. Cellulitis is the infection of the loose subcutaneous tissue. The two conditions may often coexit. The association of erysipelas/cellulitis is more common than each disease alone.

Clinical Features

Erysipelas: The onset of erysipelas is abrupt with fever, chills and pronounced malaise. The disease produces a sharply marginated red tender edematous plaque, which spreads peripherally, the borders are raised, the surface is shiny, bullae and vesicles may occur. It commonly affects the face, lower limbs and the feet may also be involved. There may be red streaks of lymphangitis with regional lymphadenopathy. Impairment of the lymphatic damage occurs in recurring erysipelas. The infection subsides in 1–3 weeks followed by slight pigmentation and desquamation. When located on the legs the swelling becomes covered with verrucous and papillomatous growths (Fig. 8).

Cellulitis: Cellulitis is characterized by red, hot, tender swelling around an ulcer or wound, the infection spreads into the surrounding tissue. The edge of the lesion is not well-defined. Cellulitis may be accompanied by fever and regional lymphadenopathy. It differs from erysipelas in being deeper and without a distinct edge (Fig. 9).

Cellulitis can occur on the face following sinus infection, otitis media, tooth extraction and trauma. In immunocompromised persons cellulitis can cause gangrene and

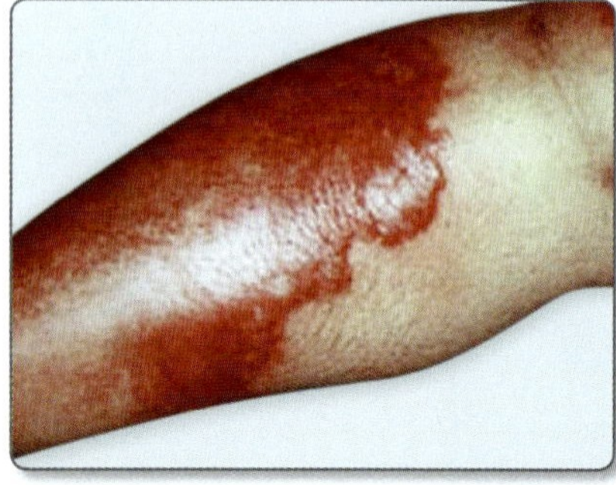

Fig. 8: Erysipelas- border raised

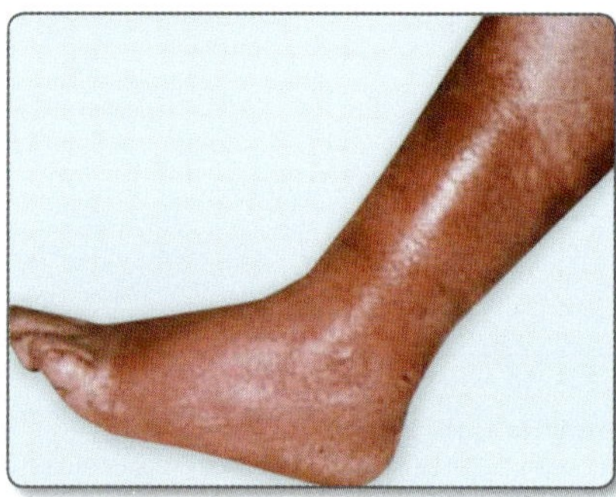

Fig. 9: Cellulitis

ecthyma gangrenosum. Other complications include fasciitis, myositis, subcutaneous abscess, septicemia and streptococcal nephritis.

Laboratory studies are usually not required for erysipelas/cellulitis; but they are required when the patient is immunocompromised. Successful identity of pathogens is difficult from the site of lesion, although injection of saline in the advancing border and then aspirating the fluid is tried, when the lesion is not open. Blood culture is a vital part of search for identifying the etiological agent. Magnetic resonance imaging (MRI) has gained favor in diagnosing soft-tissue infections.

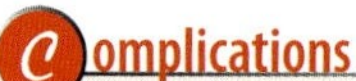

- Deep cellulitis
- Septicemia and metastatic abscess
- Glomerulonephritis, endocarditis
- Lymphedema in recurrent cases.

Treatment

Elevate the limb and use cool compresses locally.

Systemic antibiotics are required for treatment. A single injection of procaine penicillin will arrest the process. Penicillin should be given for 10–20 days. If no improvement occurs in a day, penicillin-resistant Staphylococcus should be suspected and flucloxacillin should be initiated. Macrolide antibiotics are used as an alternate, such as erythromycin, azithromycin or clindamycin.

In recurrent cases penicillin V daily for 5–7 days, benzathine penicillin G 2.4 million units once a month or erythromycin 1 g daily for 5 days every month for 4–6 months can prevent attacks. Vigorous treatment of any local skin damage is required. Some patients may require longer-term or life-long prophylaxis.

Lymphangitis

Lymphangitis is inflammation of the lymph vessels, often following an acute streptococcal infection of the skin, less often by staphylococci. Lymphangitis may be a sign that the skin infection is getting worse. It should raise concerns that bacteria may spread into the bloodstream, which can cause life-threatening problems.

Clinical Features

Lymphangitis is associated with constitutional symptoms, such as fever, malaise, headache, arthralgia, myalgia and loss of appetite. Painful, red streaks are visible along the course of the lymphatic vessels, which may be faint or obvious. The pain is throbbing in nature; the regional lymph nodes may be enlarged.

Complications

Abscess, cellulitis and septicaemia.

Diagnosis

A biopsy and culture of the affected area may reveal the cause of the inflammation. Blood cultures may be done to see if the infection has spread to the bloodstream.

Treatment

Lymphangitis may spread within hours. Treatment should begin promptly. Parenteral antibiotics may be required for a patient with signs of systemic illness; this should be started immediately without waiting for a culture report. Coverage should be provided for Group A Streptococci and ***S. aureus.*** These include penicillinase-resistant synthetic penicillin, cephalosporin or a second or third generation cephalosporin, such as cefuroxime, ceftriaxone. When erythema, warmth and edema are markedly reduced, antibiotics can be changed to the oral route.

Analgesics can help control pain, and anti-inflammatory medications can help reduce inflammation and swelling. Warm moist compressions may reduce inflammation and pain. Surgery may be needed to drain an abscess.

Necrotising Fasciitis

This is a dangerous, rapidly progressive and destructive inflammation of the dermis and underlying tissues including the deep fascia. It can be a polymicrobial infection following surgery, especially in a diabetic or immunocompromised patient; or it may be caused by *S. pyogenes* leading to streptococcal gangrene. The toxic bacterial products and necrotic debris trigger a massive destructive inflammatory reaction. Necrotising fasciitis is associated with profound toxaemia and multisystem failure (Fig. 10).

The condition often arises suddenly after a minor skin trauma. The legs are the most common site of

Investigation

Aspiration or Incision for culture and sensitivity, exclude clostridial infection with wound smear. Infections with clostridia and bacteriodes may lead to gas formation, which can then be diagnosed radiographically.

Magnetic resonance imaging scans are also helpful in diagnosing necrotising fasciitis or subcutaneous abscess. In patients with muscle damage or subcutaneous abscess, well-defined areas of high signal intensity are found.

Baseline laboratory tests should be performed, and then monitored for leucopenia, hypocalcaemia (fat necrosis), and elevated creatine phosphokinase (muscle necrosis).

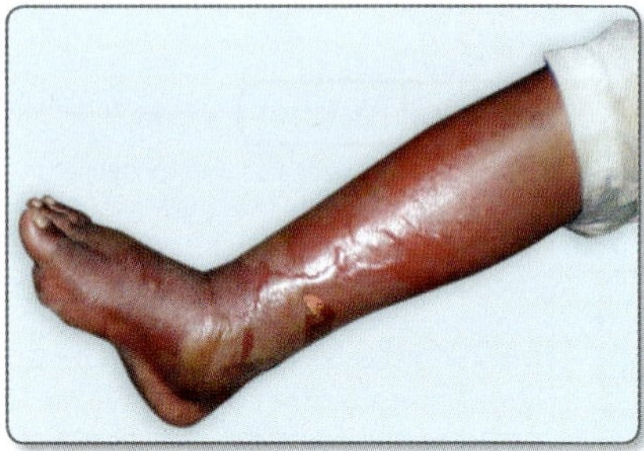

Fig. 10: Necrotizng fasciitis

infection. The clue to the presence of this infection is a rapidly spreading cellulitis in a very toxic patient, despite antibiotic therapy. Necrotising fasciitis is initially manifested as erythema and edema, the lesion progresses to brawny induration and cyanosis. Blister formation and gangrene rapidly follow. The central area of the lesion is anesthetic due to cutaneous nerve damage; the surrounding area is extremely tender and erythematous. In polymicrobial necrotising fasciitis subcutaneous gas may be present.

Necrotising fasciitis due to *Vibrio vulnificus* is found in tropical region, this is associated with liver disease and contact with shelfish.

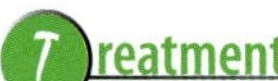

reatment

Necrotising fasciitis requires immediate treatment with generous surgical debridement. An appropriate antibiotic cover should be started immediately, without waiting for culture and sensitivity results; as the mortality rate is very high. Usually intravenous benzyl penicillin, a quinolone, and clindamycin or metronidazole for anaerobic Gram-negative organisms is started immediately. Even with prompt treatment mortality rate is high; in some cases amputation of the limb may be required.

Other adjunctive therapies include intravenous gamma-globulins; patients with poor granulocyte production may be helped by granulocyte stimulating factor. Recent literature recommends that nonsteroidal anti-inflammatory drugs (NSAIDs) should be avoided as they may interfere with leukocyte chemotaxis, decrease inflammatory response and therefore blur the cardinal signs of inflammation.

Eosinophilic fasciitis is a scleroderma-like disorder, seen in children and adults, although it is rare in children. It has a sudden onset, following strenuous exercise. The sites commonly affected are the arms and legs. The condition is characterized by pain, swelling, erythema and induration. The surface of the skin has a cobblestone appearance. The condition is associated with transient eosinophilia and elevation of sedimentation rate. The condition resolves spontaneously. Glucocorticosteroids, methotrexate and cimetidine are helpful.

Staphylococcal Scalded Skin Syndrome

Staphylococcal scalded skin syndrome (Ritter's disease) is characterized by epidermolysis and desquamation. The skin exfoliates below the granular layer. The disease is usually linked to infections with Group 2 *S. aureus*, phage type 71. Ritter von Ritterschein, who was a director of an orphanage in Prague; first described the disease. The focus of infection is not in the skin; the cutaneous lesions are due to the action of an epidermolytic toxin, elaborated by an infection at a remote site usually nasopharynx. The disease usually occurs in children under 5 years of age. Most patients are newborns or infants; the condition is primarily explained by a lack of immunity to the toxins and to renal immaturity that leads to a poor excretion of toxins. Epidermolytic toxin antibodies are present in 75% of normal people over the age of 10 years; this fact explains the rarity of SSSS in adults.

Histopathology

Intraepidermal cleavage occurs beneath and within the stratum granulosum. The remainder of the epidermis and the dermis contains no inflammatory cells.

Clinical Features

Initially a faint erythematous rash develops; cutaneous tenderness develops at this stage. Within 24–48 hours the rash progresses from a scarlatiniform eruption to spontaneous wrinkling of the skin, followed by the appearance of large flaccid bullae in the axillae, groins and around the body orifices, later spreading all over the body, but sparing the mucous membrane. As sheets of epidermis are shed, a moist erythematous base is revealed. The lesion dries quickly and healing is complete in 5–7 days.

The rare adult type of SSSS in adults is associated with underlying diseases related to immunosuppression, abnormal immunity and renal insufficiency.

Diagnosis

Examining the roof of the blister can make rapid diagnosis. The epidermis is cleaved below the stratum granulosum. Nikolski's sign is positive.

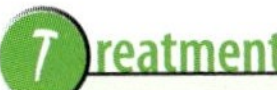

Treatment

Topical antiseptics or fusidic acid are used for local treatment. The body should be covered with nonadhesive covering. Intake-output chart should be maintained, fluid therapy and general supportive measures should be taken. Systemic antibiotic such as penicillinase-resistant penicillin or first generation cephalosporin is initiated as soon as possible. Erythromycin is also effective. The prognosis is good. Corticosteroids are contraindicated.

Toxic Shock Syndrome (TSS)

The condition is characterised by widespread erythema, and "circulatory shock". It is a multisystem disorder.

Aetiology

The syndrome is caused by the toxin of *S. aureus*. The organism is in most cases isolated from the vagina during menstruation, most women using tampons. The role of tampons remains uncertain; it probably provides a suitable condition for bacterial growth and injury to the vagina, which facilitates absorption of the toxin. TSS can occur after staphylococcal infection from any site, at any age and in either sex.

Clinical Features

The onset is sudden with fever and rash. The rash is erythematous and widespread usually clearing within 3 days. Edema of the hands and feet may occur. Conjunctiva is red. Desquamation occurs after 1–2 weeks, it may be localized on the fingers or it may be widespread.

Systemic manifestations: Diarrhea and vomiting occur due to gastrointestinal involvement. Liver, kidney, central nervous system (CNS) and cardiovascular system (CVS) may also be affected. Circulatory shock may be very severe.

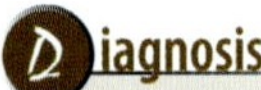

A history of fever, rash and shock help in the diagnosis of TSS. It should be differentiated from septicemic shock and other staphylococcal infections.

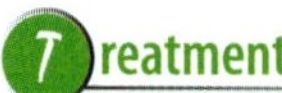

Appropriate antibiotic therapy should be given and general supportive measures are essential.

INFECTIONS CAUSED BY MYCOBACTERIA

Mycobacteria (M.) are acid-fast, aerobic, weakly Gram-positive, nonspore-bearing and nonmotile organisms. Mycobacteria have a lipid coating that makes them resistant to most stains. Once stained, they are difficult to decolorize (acid-fast). Because of the lipophilic coat, the mycobacteria are resistant to many antibacterial agents. Mycobacteria may be pathogens, facultative pathogens or some may even be nonpathogens. The most important human pathogens are *M. tuberculosis* and *M. leprae*. Mycobacteria are classified as follows:

Classification of Mycobacteria

- Slow growing mycobacteria
  - Obligate human pathogens
    - *M. tuberculosis*
  - Facultative human pathogens
    - *M. kansasii*
    - *M. marinum*
    - *M. scrofulaceum*
    - *M. ulcerans*
    - *M. xenopi*
    - *M. simiae*
  - Nonpathogens
    - *M. gastri*
    - *M. gordonae*
    - *M. terrae complex*
- Rapidly growing mycobacteria
    - *M. chelonei*
    - *M. fortuitum*
  - Nonpathogens
    - *M. phlei*
    - *M. smegmatis*
- Nonculturable mycobacteria
    - *M. leprae*

TUBERCULOSIS

Tuberculosis is an acute or chronic granulomatous disease that principally involves the lung, but may affect any other organ or tissue of the body, such as lymph nodes, bones, intestines, kidney, fallopian tubes, epididymis, meninges and skin. The people who are at a higher risk of tuberculosis are the elderly, infants and those who are immunosuppressed. The disease which was well under control in the West has a rebound after the increased incidence of AIDS. The poor, malnourished and people living in overcrowded, unsanitary conditions are very susceptible to tuberculosis.

The primary infection is usually in the lungs, following a droplet infection. The gastrointestinal tract may be the site of primary infection in undeveloped countries by drinking unpasteurised milk. The infection spreads to the regional lymph nodes; this is the primary or Ghon complex. After 2–4 weeks cell-mediated immunity develops, and the host is able to bring the infection under control. Healing occurs with fibrosis and calcification. Later when the host immunity diminishes, activation of a prior Ghon complex can spread the infection to another pulmonary site or to extrapulmonary sites such as the skin. The delayed hypersensitivity is marked by a positive tuberculin test, which is present in both primary and secondary infection.

The disease can be confirmed by a biopsy which shows the typical tuberculoid granuloma. The granuloma of tuberculosis is characterized by central caseation and Langhans giant cells. Langhans giant cells are formed by the fusion of epithelioid cells, which form an arc of nuclei at the periphery of the cell. Lymphocytes are found at the periphery of the granuloma.

Tuberculosis of the skin may be divided into the localized forms and the exanthematous or hematogenous forms.

Localized progressive forms are primary inoculation complex-tuberculous chancre, lupus vulgaris, tuberculosis verrucosa cutis, scrofuloderma and tuberculosis cutis orificialis.

The widespread exanthematous forms are tuberculosis miliaris, papulonecrotic tuberculides, lichen scrofulosorum. Some cases of erythema induratum meet the criteria of a tuberculid.

Classification

- Exogenous infection
  - Primary tuberculosis complex
  - Tuberculosis verrucossa cutis.
- Endogenous infection
  - Lupus vulgaris
  - Scrofuloderma
  - Tuberculosis cutis—orificialis
  - Acute miliary tuberculosis.
- Tuberculids
  - Papulonecrotic tuberculid
  - Lichen scrofulosorum
  - Erythema nodosum
  - Erythema induratum.

The following common types will be discussed in this chapter.

- Lupus vulgaris
- Scrofuloderma
- Warty tuberculosis
- Tuberculosis cutis orificialis
- Tuberculous gumma
- Tuberculous chancre

LOCALIZED TUBERCULOSIS

Lupus Vulgaris

It is an extremely chronic and progressive form of cutaneous tuberculosis. Lupus vulgaris is a post-primary form of skin tuberculosis, arising in previously sensitized individuals with only moderate immunity. Lupus vulgaris originates from tuberculosis elsewhere in the body by hematogenous, lymphatic or contiguous spread; rarely it may follow primary inoculation tuberculosis or Bacille Calmette–Guérin (BCG) vaccination.

Clinical Features

The initial lesions are the lupus papules, about the size of a pinhead, they are arranged in groups or irregular circles. Gradually the papules develop into nodules, which coalesce to form a plaque. The nodules are reddish-brown in color, soft and translucent resembling apple jelly. On diascopy the characteristic apple jelly nodules are seen, surrounded by a pale border. The plaques of lupus vulgaris tend to heal slowly in one area with scarring and progressing in another area. Lupus nodules are seen at the periphery of the plaque. Scarring is a prominent feature of lupus vulgaris. Atrophic scars occur subsequent to or independent of ulceration and new "apple jelly" nodules may develop within the cicatricial areas. The lesion is asymptomatic; the site of predilection is the face and the neck (Fig. 11).

The course of lupus vulgaris is very slow; a patch of the disease may be limited to a small area for several decades. A lupus patch may start in childhood and persist throughout life.

Histopathology

Tuberculoid granulomas are present in the upper dermis; the histology may be difficult to recognize as tuberculosis, the acid-fast bacilli are almost never found, epithelioid cells and Langhans giant cells are embedded in a shell of lymphocytes. Only slight caseation necrosis is seen.

Complications

- Cicatricial ectropion
- Cicatricial alopecia
- Lymphedema
- Infection
- Malignant change to squamous cell carcinoma or basal cell carcinoma.
- Microstomia
- Contractures causing reduced joint mobility
- Severe mutilation from destruction of cartilaginous structures of face

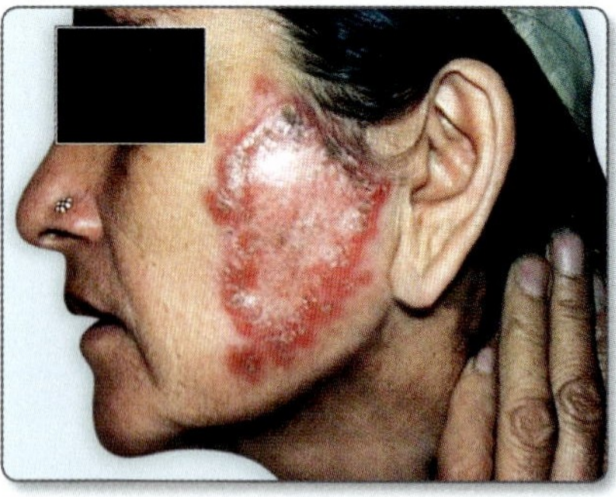

Fig. 11: Lupus vulgaris

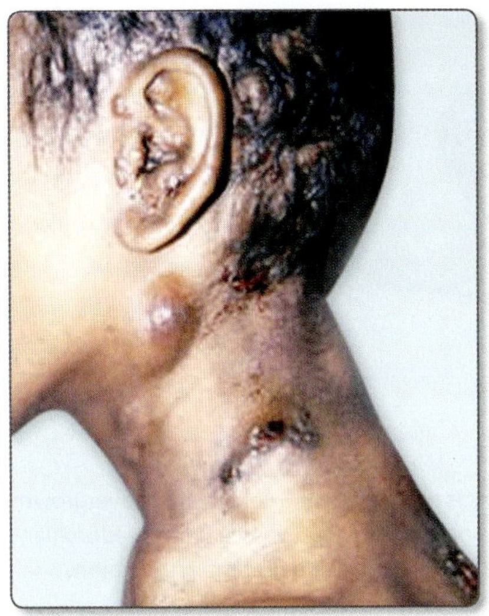

Fig. 12: Scrofuloderma

Scrofuloderma

This form of cutaneous tuberculosis spreads to the skin, from underlying foci of tuberculosis. The tuberculous foci may be in the lymph nodes, bones, joints, epididymis, intestines, parotid glands, etc.

Clinical Features

Scrofuloderma commonly involves the sides of neck, parotid, submandibular and supraclavicular areas due to the spread of tuberculosis from underlying lymph nodes. The skin lesions are first present as firm, subcutaneous nodules that breakdown to form undermined ulcers and discharging sinuses. Healing results in characteristic puckered scarring (Fig. 12).

Histopathology

The inflammation begins deep in the dermis with caseation necrosis and the formation of a cavity filled with liquefied debris, the walls of which are formed by tuberculoid granulomas. Tubercle bacilli are found in the lesion.

Warty Tuberculosis (Tuberculosis Verrucosa Cutis)

This is an indolent, warty form of tuberculosis that results from introduction of tubercle bacilli into the skin of a previously infected patient, with intact specific immune response. The organisms are introduced through minor abrasions or wounds. Occupational groups who handle the contagious material are particularly vulnerable like pathologists, butchers, farmers, and veterinary surgeons.

Clinical Features

The tuberculous lesions are present at sites exposed to trauma. The sites of predilection are hand, buttocks, ankles and feet. The lesion presents as reddish or brown verrucous plaque, it is asymptomatic and may be solitary or multiple. Regional lymph nodes are not enlarged. The extension is extremely slow. It does not penetrate deeply and even after many years does not lead to serious sequelae as lupus vulgaris (Fig. 13).

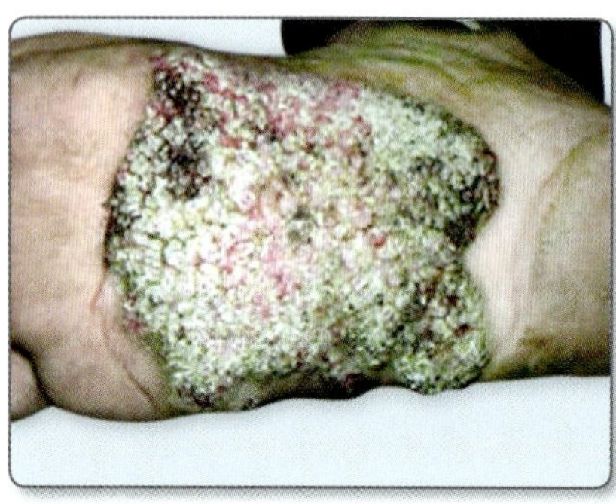

Fig. 13: Tuberculosis verrucosa cutis

Histopathology

In addition to the usual tuberculous nodule, there is considerable overgrowth of granulation tissue and formation of new blood vessels, with predominant acanthosis and hyperkeratosis. Tubercle bacilli are present in the lesion.

Tuberculosis Cutis Orificialis

Ulcerative lesions often occur in patients with advanced visceral tuberculosis. These are ragged, painful, shallow ulcers with a necrotic and purulent base. There is no tendency to spontaneous healing. Classical lesions are found around the orifices such as the lips, tongue, anus and the urethral meatus.

Tuberculous Gumma

This is due to hematogenous spread of mycobacteria, with formation of cold abscesses in the skin. It presents as hard deep-seated nodule not attached to the skin; it then slowly softens and breaks down. Nodules may be few or multiple. They heal with a depressed and keloidal scar. It should be differentiated from the gumma of syphilis.

Tuberculous Chancre

This primary cutaneous complex appears at the site of an abrasion usually on the lower extremities or the face. A nodule develops at the site of inoculation of the tubercle bacilli; this break down to form an indolent ulcer with undermined borders. A regional suppurative lymphandenitis occurs in 2–3 weeks. The ulcer heals spontaneously leaving a scar.

TUBERCULIDS

Tuberculid is an allergic reaction seen in an individual sensitized to a previous exposure to tuberculous bacilli. They are characterized by their self-limiting course, absence of bacilli in the lesion, a strong response to tuberculin test and its response to anti-tuberculous therapy. These are:

- Papulo-necrotic tuberculid

- Lichen scrofulosorum
- Erythema induratum
- Erythema nodosum

Papulo-Necrotic Tuberculid

The lesions are often seen on the extensor surface of the limbs in young adults, especially women. Successive crops of reddish-purple papules and nodules occur that undergo necrosis forming black adherent crusts. The lesions heal within a few weeks leaving a white scar, with a hyperpigmented halo.

Lichen Scrofulosorum

This is a rare condition seen in children with a recurrent history of tuberculous infection. The lesion consists of crops of tiny flat-topped skin colored or brownish papules, rough to touch. The eruption is symmetrically distributed, on the trunk and the limbs; they tend to heal spontaneously.

Eythema nodosum and erythema induratum are described in chapter 26.

DIAGNOSIS OF TUBERCULOSIS

Tuberculosis bacilli are difficult to see microscopically, because most of the cases are paucibacillary. The test is positive when large numbers of organisms are present. Mantoux test does not differentiate between an active infection, previous infection or due to vaccination. Therefore the criteria of diagnosis are:

Absolute criteria:

- Positive culture of tubercle bacilli from the lesion Lowenstein-Jensen medium or Bactec media
- Successful guinea pig inoculation
- Positive polymerase chain reaction (PCR).

Relative criteria:

- Demonstration of tuberculosis focus elsewhere in the body
  - X-ray chest
  - X-ray bones and joints if indicated.
- Presence of acid-fast bacilli in the lesion as demonstrated by Ziehl-Neelsen staining
- Characteristic histopathology; presence of caseating granulomas with Langhan's giant cells
- Tuberculin test (Mantoux test)
  - In the Mantoux test, the old tuberculin or purified protein derivative is injected intradermally into the flexor aspect of the forearm and results are read after 48–72 hours. The reaction is interpreted as positive if the diameter of skin thickening (due to edema and accumulation of lymphocytes) and erythema is 10 mm or more
  - The BCG vaccination and exposure to other mycobacteria blur the diagnostic value of Mantoux test.

Treatment

General

- Search for an underlying focus of tuberculosis
- Improve nutrition and general health of the patient.

Drug Therapy

Treatment of cutaneous tuberculosis is the same as that of tuberculosis anywhere else in the body. Directly observed therapy (DOT) is recommended for patients who are unlikely to comply with the treatment. Drugs commonly used are:

Isoniazid

- Adults: 300 mg daily
- Children: 10 mg/kg of body weight

Side Effects

- Peripheral neuropathy, pyridoxine 10 mg daily is given to prevent this side effect.
- Hypersensitivity
- Hepatotoxicity.

Rifampicin

- If under 50 kg: 450 mg daily
- If over 50 kg: 600 mg daily.
- In children: 10–20 mg/kg of body weight.

The drug is taken half an hour before breakfast.

Side effects

- Hypersensitivity reactions
- Induction of hepatic enzymes therefore oral contraceptives, oral anticoagulants, oral hypoglycemic and digoxin should be avoided
- Hepatitis
- Orange-red discoloration of urine, saliva, sweat and tears which causes undue alarm to patient.

Pyrazinamide

- Adults below 50 kg: 1.5 g daily; above 50 kg: 2 g daily
- Children:35 mg/kg of body weight.

Side effects

- Hypersensitivity
- Hepatotoxicity
- Gout.

Ethambutol

- Adults: 25 mg/kg of body weight
- Children: 15 mg/kg of body weight.

Side effects

Optic neuritis, which leads to decreased visual acuity and loss of red and green color perception. The drug should be avoided in children, as they are unable to detect the change in vision.

Streptomycin (the drug is best avoided because of ototoxcity)

Dose

- Adults over 45 kg: 1 g/daily
- Adults less than 45 kg: 0.75 g/ daily.

Side effects

- Hypersensitivity with pyrexia and erythematous skin eruption
- Vestibular disturbances with tinnitus and vertigo
- Deafness.

The drug should be prescribed with caution in elderly patients who find difficulties in compensating for vestibular disturbances and in patients with impaired renal function.

- Therapeutic test: In suspected cases, a trial of antituberculosis therapy may be given. A tuberculous lesion responds to treatment. Other mycobacterial disease either respond poorly or there is no response at all.

Regimen of Antituberculous Therapy

Short course: Six months regimen.
Four drugs are given in the initial stage.

Initial phase (*2 months*) with four drugs pyrazinamide, isoniazid, rifampicin and ethambutol.

Continuation phase (*4 months*) with three drugs isoniazid, rifampicin and pyrazinamide.

The continuation phase may be extended for 7 or more months if the patient has associated HIV infection.

Previously a long course (9 months) of treatment was used, with three drugs in the initial phase and two drugs in the continuation phase.

The other drugs used in the treatment of tuberculosis are para-aminosalicylic acid, cycloserine, kanamycin, capreomycin and interferon-α. These drugs are potentially ototoxic and nephrotoxic.

Langhans giant cells are also found in other granulomatous disorders, such as leprosy, syphilis, sarcoidosis and deep fungal infections.

Robert Koch (1834–1910)

Koch received the Nobel Prize for medicine in 1905. He qualified from Gottingen and worked with Virchow in Berlin. In his amateur laboratory, he proved that anthrax was due to a transmitted bacillus. Ten years later in 1882 he discovered the tubercle bacillus and in the next year the cholera vibrio. In 1885, he became the professor of Hygiene in Berlin. He also described the old and new tuberculin. He traveled widely and discovered a number of infectious diseases in India and Africa. Rokitansky and Virchow described the histopathology of tuberculosis.

DISEASES CAUSED BY ATYPICAL MYCOBACTERIA

A large number of atypical mycobacteria have been described. These may produce a variety of inflammatory, purulent or granulomatous tissue reactions, depending upon the antigenicity and individual immune reactions of the host. These atypical mycobacteria differ from Mycobacterium tuberculosis in the following ways:

- Less tendency to disseminate
- Not transmitted from person to person
- Acquired from environmental sources
- The infection runs a benign and limited course
- Less responsive to antituberculous drugs
- Larger and broader than mycobacterium tuberculosis bacilli
- Histological findings are nonspecific, dermal infiltration consists of lymphocytes, histiocytes and neutrophils. Tuberculous epithelial granulomas are seen in the older lesions, fibrinoid necrosis is present rather than caseation.

Classification of Atypical Mycobacteria

- Group I. This group contains photochromogens. A yellowish pigment is produced when exposed to light. This group includes *M. kanasasii*, *M. ulcerans*, *M. marinum*.
- Group II. These are scotochromogens; it produces a yellowish-orange pigmentation even when cultured in darkness. The main pathogen in this group is *M. scrofulaceum*.
- Group III. These are nonphotochromogens, they do not produce any pigment, e.g. *M. avium*
- Group IV. These do not produce pigment, but are rapid growers, e.g. *M. fortuitum* and *M. chelonae.*

Skin Infections with Atypical Mycobacteria

Fishing Pool Granuloma

Mycobacterium marinum is found in swimming pools, fresh and salt water and fish tanks.

Clinical Features

The disease begins as a violaceous papule at the site of trauma, which develops about 2–3 weeks after inoculation. The initial lesion is a pustule or a nodule that breaks down to form a crusted ulcer. It may become verrucous or psoriasiform. Nodules develop along the line of lymphatic drainage; the regional lymph nodes may enlarge, but do not break down. There is a tendency to spontaneous healing in 1–3 years.

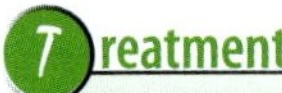

Treatment

There is no specific therapy, rifampicin, ethambutol, clotrimoxazole, tetracyclines especially minocycline may be effective. The drugs should be given for at least 6 weeks. Excision of the lesion when feasible is effective.

Buruli's Ulcer

This is caused by *M. ulcerans*. This atypical mycobacteria has several unusual features. It grows at a restricted temperature range from 24°–31°C, it is biochemically unreactive, and it can produce lethal disease in the mouse.

Clinical Features

The disease is found mainly in children and young adults. After an incubation period of about 3 months, a solitary, painless, hard, subcutaneous nodule forms that subsequently ulcerates, becomes undermined, necrotic fat is discharged from the lesion. ***M. ulcerans*** produces a toxin that is responsible for extensive necrosis and ulceration. The ulcer may reach a diameter of several centimeters in a few months. There are little or no constitutional symptoms. Healing occurs in 6–9 months. Fibrosis and calcification accompany the healing, which leads to contractures and deformity.

Treatment

Effective treatment is not available. Wide and deep excision of the ulcer is perhaps the best form of treatment. Heating of the limb beyond the viability of the organism seems logical.

Injection Abscess

This is caused by *M. chelonei*. The organism is found in water and soil. A sporotrichoid spread is occasionally seen. Disseminated nodules are rare. Localized cellulitis and osteomyelitis may also occur.

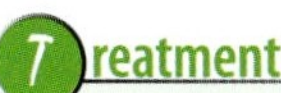

The organism is resistant to antituberculous treatment; kanamycin perhaps is an exception. Surgical excision of the abscess is the best method of treatment.

LEPROSY

Leprosy is a chronic, contagious disease that primarily involves the peripheral nerves and secondarily affects skin and other tissues, e.g. nasal mucous membrane, eyes, bones, lymph nodes, testes and small blood vessels. Leprosy does not affect the central nervous system. The disease is especially important because it is a social stigma, which is more troublesome for the patient than the disease itself.

Aetiology

Leprosy is caused by *M. leprae*, an acid-fast bacillus that was discovered, by Hansen in 1873. *M. leprae* grows at 30^0–32^0 C with a doubling time of 12 days. It remains viable in the environment for up to 10 days. It has a complex antigenic cell wall, comprising protein, lipids and carbohydrates. The disease is transmitted by droplet infection from oronasal mucosa of patients suffering from untreated lepromatous leprosy. Infection is most probably acquired in childhood, but because of long incubation period (2–5 years or longer); the disease usually manifests in adult life.

Types of Leprosy

Currently, two classification systems exist in the medical literature: the Ridley-Jopling system, and the World Health Organization (WHO) system. Comparative study of different types of leprosy is given in Table 1.

1. The Ridley-Jopling system is composed of six types of leprosy, depending upon the host's immunity against *M. leprae*, these are:
   - Lepromatous
   - Tuberculoid
   - Borderline lepromatous
   - Mid-borderline
   - Borderline tuberculoid
   - Indeterminate

   Lepromatous Leprosy (*LL*): The patient is unable to resist the infection and the bacilli are free to multiply. The organisms are found in highest number in skin and nerves. The disease is highly contagious unlike tuberculoid leprosy which is not infectious. Lepromin test is negative in this type of leprosy, due to the loss of cell-mediated immunity to *M. leprae*.

   The skin lesions are multiple, bilateral and symmetrically distributed. They present as slightly hypopigmented or erythematous macules, papules, plaques and nodules. Involvement of the ear is almost constant, leading

Table 1: Shows the differentiation between lepromatous, borderline and tuberculoid leprosy

Lepromatous leprosy	*Borderline leprosy*	*Tuberculoid leprosy*
Immunity to lepra bacillus None Abundant bacilli in lesion Lepromin test: negative	 Unstable Depends upon the spectrum of disease Lepromin test: negative or positive	 Well-developed immunity Few or no bacilli Lepromin test: positive
Early signs Edema of the hands and feet, nasal discharge *Lesions* Multiple, bilateral, symmetrical, nodules most common, those of the ear lobes are characteristic. Sensory changes occur late in the lesion	 Extensive severe neuropathy Multiple, bilateral, asymmetrical, annular or bizarre-shaped lesions, not sharply marginated Skin lesions hyperesthetic or paresthetic—early in disease	 Loss of sensation in the lesion One or few, usually annular, sharply marginated Skin lesions: hairless, hypopigmented, hypohidrotic and anesthetic—early in the disease
Nerve involvement Late with multiple nerves involved *Eye involvement* Positive: due to direct involvement by lepra bacillus	 Early with multiple nerves involved. Neuropathy most severe Positive: usually neural, depends upon the spectrum of disease	 Early—often limited to a single nerve or localized to a part of skin Positive: due to neural involvement
Leonine face due to cellular infiltration and involvement of the dermis. Loss of outer-third of eyebrows, eyelashes	Absent	Absent
Systemic signs Present in late stages- trophic and visceral changes. CNS Not affected	 May be present in BL Not affected	 Absent Not affected
Histopathology Diffuse involvement of the dermis, histiocytes prominent, contains lepra bacilli, Grenz zone present	 Depends upon the lepra immunological spectrum. Granulomas and epithelioid cells in BTL, histiocytes in BLL	 Granulomas predominate, epithelioid cells prominent, few or no lepra bacilli, Grenz zone absent
Lepra reaction Type 1 Absent Type 2 Positive in all cases	 Present in all borderline leprosy Positive only in BL	 Absent Absent

Abbreviations: BLL—Borderline lepromatous leprosy; BTL—Borderline tuberculoid leprosy

to elongation of the ear lobes. There is loss of eyebrows (especially outer one-third) and eyelashes. Acrocyanosis, edema of the hands and feet are common; it is often the earliest manifestation of lepromatous leprosy. The sites of predilection are face, legs, buttocks and arms. The sensations remain intact and there is no hair loss from the lesions in the early stages of lepromatous leprosy (Fig. 14).

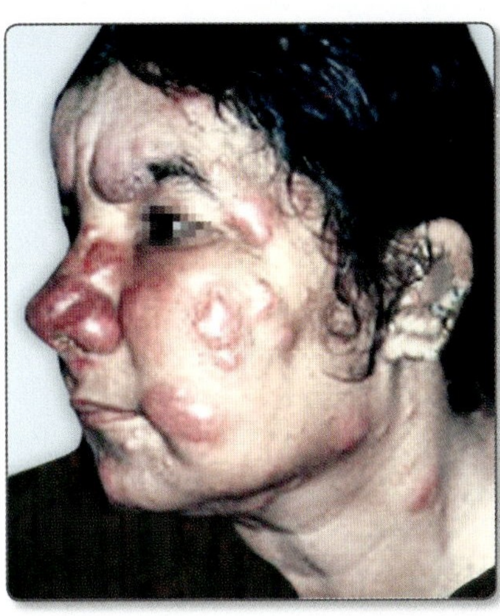

Fig. 14: Lepromatous leprosy

Later changes include ulceration of nasal and oral mucosa, diffuse thickening of skin of face (leonine face). Dryness of the skin and ichthyosis of the limbs are findings of late lepromatous leprosy. Peripheral nerve damage is a very late complication.

Variants of lepromatous leprosy: Diffuse lepromatous leprosy (Lucio-Latapi type). This type of LL does not have multiple lesions. It is characterized by shiny, waxy infiltration resembling myxoedema; there is alopecia of the eyebrows and eyelashes.

Histoid leprosy: The lesions are round or oval firm cutaneous or subcutaneous nodules.

Tuberculoid leprosy (TL): The only tissues clinically affected are nerves and skin. The lepromin test is positive due to the well-developed cell-mediated immunity to *M. leprae*. Few or no bacilli are seen in the lesion. The skin lesions are single or few and asymmetrical. Tuberculoid leprosy (TL) is limited to a single nerve or to a localized part of the skin. The lesions consist of macules or plaques which are erythematous, pigmented or hypopigmented, dry, scaly, anesthetic with hair loss. Infiltrated lesions are well-outlined; the margins are infiltrated and end abruptly. Annular lesions show a less infiltrated center.

Nerves are thickened with associated sensory loss and muscle weakness. The nerves commonly involved are facial, trigeminal, greater auricular, median, ulnar, radial, tibial and common peroneal. The eyes may be secondarily damaged due to involvement of facial and trigeminal nerves (Fig. 15).

Borderline leprosy: Borderline leprosy includes patients with intermediate grades of resistance to *M. leprae.* Depending upon the degree of immunity, it can be further subdivided into borderline tuberculoid (BT), mid-borderline (MB),and borderline lepromatous (BL). Lepromin test is positive in BT and negative in BL. Untreated they resolve towards the lepromatous type, and treated towards the tuberculoid type. Clinically there is an early extensive

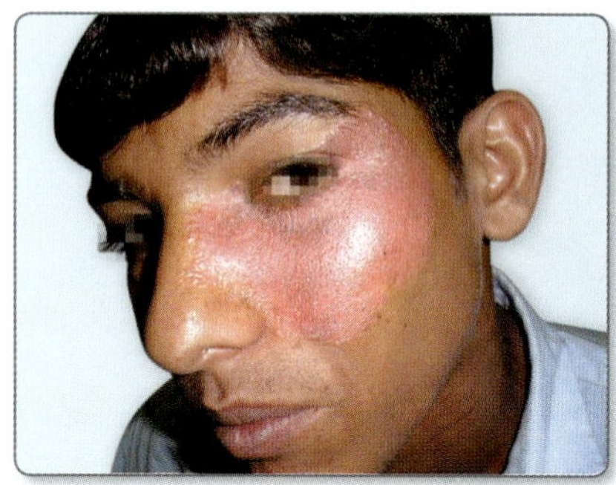

Fig. 15: Tuberculoid leprosy

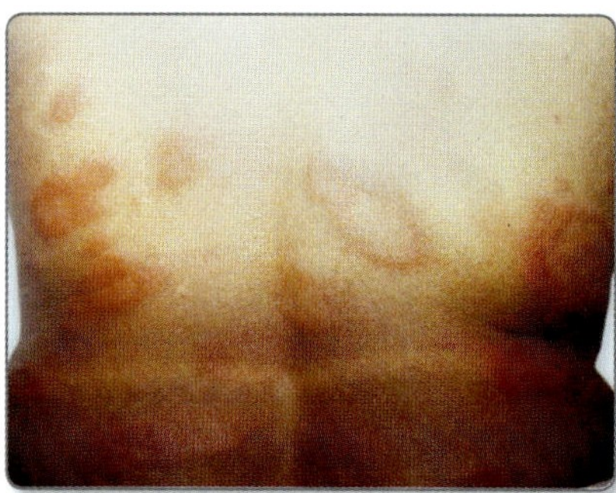

Fig. 16: Borderline leprosy

neuropathy several nerves are affected asymmetrically. These changes may develop months or years before the skin lesions appear. Skin lesions depend upon the location of the disease in the spectrum. In BL the skin lesions are usually multiple, but not as abundant as in LL. Neuropathy is most severe in this form of leprosy (Fig. 16).

Often a single lesion is present surrounded by several smaller ones. Skin and nerves are the only directly affected tissues in BL. The skin lesions consist of erythematous macules or plaques. Inverted saucer-shaped annular lesions are characteristic.

Characteristic features of BL are:

- Bizarre-shaped asymmetrical lesions in the form of bands or geographical pattern
- Large plaques are present with ill-defined margins and sharply outlined clean central spaces
- Asymmetrical distribution of lesions
- Extensive asymmetrical neuropathy.

Indeterminate leprosy: This is the type of leprosy with transitional immune status. The skin lesions comprise of single or few erythematous or hypopigmented macules. The lesions may show slight anesthesia. The lesions are always macular; if they become palpable, they are no longer in the indeterminate group. The condition resolves spontaneously in over 50% cases without treatment.

2. The 2009 WHO classification is simply based on the number of skin lesions as follows:
   - Paucibacillary leprosy: skin lesions with no or few bacilli (*M. leprae*) seen in a skin smear. Number of lesions less than or equal to 5.
   - Multibacillary leprosy: skin lesions with many bacilli (*M. leprae*) seen in a skin smear. Number of lesions more than 6.

The WHO classification is now universally used for the treatment of leprosy.

Neurological Manifestations of Leprosy

Peripheral nerves are the first site of attack of the lepra bacillus. The peripheral nerves are involved in all patients and in all forms of disease. The large peripheral nerves that lie just below the skin are mainly affected, as these are cooler. Nerves commonly involved are ulnar (at the epitrochlear groove), common peroneal nerve (at the head of the tibia), greater auricular nerve (at the side of the neck), superficial radial (above the wrist) and posterior tibial (behind the medial malleolus). The nerves are enlarged and can be felt as thick cords. They become tender during a lepra reaction.

Alterations of sensations are present at the onset, these may be hyperesthetic or paresthetic, but later the characteristic change is decreased sensation. First to disappear is the sensitivity to temperature, then to pain and finally to touch. Muscle atrophy is secondary to the nerve damage.

Trophic Changes

These are secondary to neural involvement; they range from dry, glossy, anhidrotic skin to blisters, ulcers, muscle atrophy and bone changes.

Palpation of the nerves will detect thickening, tenderness or even areas of softening. Leprosy should be suspected in any patient showing enlargement of the peripheral nerves. In TL, nerve enlargement occurs early and improves with treatment. In LL, it occurs late, often associated with trophic and motor damage and it is always bilateral.

Motor alterations result from nerve involvement; it causes paralysis and atrophy of the muscles. Varied manifestations may be found. On the face there may be inability to close the eyes; the patients may have a mask like face. On the limbs "claw hand" and "drop foot" may be found.

Other Manifestations

Nasal Changes

These are common in lepromatous leprosy. Bloody nasal discharge and nasal obstruction are amongst the earliest manifestations of leprosy. Later destruction of the nasal cartilage leads to saddle-shaped deformity of the nose.

Eye Changes

The eyes may be affected by the direct presence of *M. leprae* in the eye or indirectly by the involvement of trigemminal or facial nerve. Eye changes are seen in all forms of leprosy. Common ocular changes are superficial punctate keratitis, interstitial keratitis, miliary leproma or iris pearls. Iris pearls are yellowish-white round spots that appear stuck on the iris near the pupillary margin, and these are pathognomonic of leprosy. Cataracts and acute and chronic diffuse iridocyclitis are the other ocular changes.

Bone Changes

These changes are seen in the late, neglected and untreated cases of leprosy. The changes are due to trauma, defective nerve and blood supply. There is absorption and atrophy of the distal phalanges. On the feet, the metatarsal and the tarsal bones are affected, but in the upper extremities, the metacarpal and the carpal bones are not affected.

Visceral Changes

In lepromatous leprosy the liver, spleen and the lymph nodes are often enlarged, testicular atrophy can occur. Renal involvement is a common cause of death in lepromatous leprosy.

Histopathology

The histology depends upon the immune status of the host to the lepra bacilli. The changes are either simple inflammatory or granulomatous. In indeterminate leprosy the acute inflammatory reaction is predominant. In the tuberculoid type the granulomatous reaction is predominant.

The first evidence of infection is seen in the peripheral nervous system, *M. leprae* has a predilection for the neural tissue. The bacilli enter the nerves via the blood vessels. The target cell is the Schwann cell. The degree and type of cellular infiltrate depends upon the degree of cell-mediated immunity.

Indeterminate Leprosy

The histological features are nonspecific. There is mild lymphocytic infiltration around the blood vessels, skin appendages and the nerves. If the nerves are affected a few acid-fast bacilli may be seen within the cutaneous nerve.

Lepromatous Leprosy

The histological findings are diagnostic. There is proliferation of histiocytes, which at the onset of disease are found around the blood vessels and nerves. Later the infiltrate becomes diffuse and involves most of the dermis, but is separated from the epidermis by a band of normal connective tissue called the "clear zone" or the "Grenz zone". The papillary dermis appears as a clear band. In the reticular dermis, the infiltrate consists of "lepra cells"; these are histiocytes filled with lepra bacilli. Virchow's cells are old foamy histiocytes abundant in lipids, containing a few lepra bacilli; these are found in the later stages of LL.

In LL there is an asymptomatic proliferation of lepra bacilli in the Schwann cells, despite the large number of organisms present in the nerve the inflammatory response is mild. In late stages without treatment there is destruction of the axis cylinder and later Wallerian degeneration occurs.

Histoid variety is characterized by abundant histiocytes arranged in bands or whorls. Bacilli are numerous but foamy histiocytes are absent.

Diffuse lepromatous leprosy (Lucio-Latapi) shows an infiltration of foamy histiocytes around the dermal blood vessels and hair follicles, without node formation.

Tuberculoid Leprosy

The histological picture shows evidence of host resistance, as manifested by abundant epithelioid cells. These are present with or without the presence of Langhans cells. The cellular infiltrate extends up to the epidermis; there is no clear zone as in LL. Lymphocytes are present in the periphery of the granuloma. The granulomas are seen around the neuro-vascular elements. The nerves are surrounded, infiltrated or even destroyed by the tuberculoid granuloma. Bacilli are few or absent. No fat is found in the epithelioid cells or elsewhere. Tuberculoid granuloma is not diagnostic of leprosy; nerve involvement is the reliable feature.

Cutaneous nerves appear greatly swollen by the epithelioid cell granulomas, these granulomas are surrounded by a zone of lymphocytes, caseation may occasionally occur.

Borderline Leprosy

The histological picture varies with the position of the leprosy immunological spectrum. In BT, a thin clear Grenz zone is present that shows predominance of epithelioid cells. There are few vacuolated cells, few bacilli, some lipid may be found.

In BL, there is predominance of histiocytes and the clear zone becomes evident. Lipids are abundant.

Mid-borderline (MB) leprosy occupies an intermediate position, there is a clear zone and a diffuse infiltration of epithelioid cells, there are no giant cells, bacilli are numerous and some lipid is present in fat stained sections.

Nerve damage in boderline leprosy results from a combination of bacilli in the nerves and a granulomatous reaction resulting in widespread nerve damage.

Lepra Reactions

There are two main immunological reactions, involved in leprosy; the cell-mediated and the humoral antibody response.

The cell-mediated mechanisms are stable in the polar forms of leprosy and variable in the intermediate forms of leprosy. Patients with LL are unable to develop cell-mediated immunity; patients with TL have vigorous cell mediated immunity. In BL, the immunological status is affected favorably by treatment and unfavorably by intercurrent infection and other factors leading to downgrading reactions.

Leprosy patients often develop acute, subacute or protracted inflammatory reactions called the lepra reactions. These reactions result from an abrupt change in the clinical stability of the disease. There are two main types of lepra reactions:

- Type 1: Acute exacerbations
- Type 2: Erythema nodosum leprosum (ENL).

Type 1: Lepra Reactions

This result from alteration of cell-mediated immunity of the patient. It is present in all borderline patients, sub-polar form of leprosy; the polar forms of leprosy are exempt. The reaction may be upgrading (in patients under treatment), or downgrading (in untreated patients), often associated with pregnancy, infection, malnutrition. In this type of reaction, the existing lesions become swollen, erythematous, warm and shiny; the nerves may be enlarged and tender.

Type 2: ENL Reactions

This reaction is caused by an immune complex syndrome of humoral antibody response. It occurs in half of the cases of lepromatous leprosy. It may be triggered by a number of factors such as intercurrent infections, stress, surgical operations and aggressive anti-leprous treatment. Clinically it presents as appearance of new nodules while the pre-existing ones remain unchanged.

Treatment of Lepra Reactions

When lepra reactions occur, the treatment should not be stopped. It can be controlled by prednisolone 20–40 mg/day; clofazamine is also effective but slower in response. Type 2 reactions can also be controlled by antihistamines, antimalarials, thalidomide, 400 mg/day is given initially, the dose is then gradually reduced.

Early Signs of Leprosy

- Bilateral edema of the legs and ankles
- Burns that form a blister but do not cause pain
- Development of ENL in pregnancy
- Numbness and clumsiness of the fingers.

Cardinal Signs of Leprosy

- Anesthetic skin lesions
- Enlarged peripheral nerves
- Presence of acid-fast bacilli in skin or nasal mucous membrane.

Diagnostic Tests

- Skin smears for *M. leprae*
- Skin biopsy
- Nerve biopsy.

Results of Therapy

All forms of therapy lead to slow and progressive improvement. In lepromatous and borderline leprosy the first to improve are the ulcerative and the mucosal lesions.

Treatment

Objectives

Following are the objectives of treatment.

- Diagnose early to prevent complications
- Open cases of lepromatous leprosy should be isolated. The others should be treated as outpatients
- Reassurance and education. Almost all patients have feelings of guilt about the disease and fear they will spread leprosy to their families. These problems can be helped with reassurance and education.

Paucibacillary leprosy (TL and BT)

- Lepromin test positive
- Acid-fast bacilli absent or scant
- Number of lesions < 5

Rifampicin: 600 mg once monthly supervised.

Dapsone: 100 mg daily self-administered.

Duration of therapy: 6 months.

Multibacillary leprosy (LL, BL and BB)

- Lepromin test is negative
- Acid-fast bacilli numerous in skin smears
- Number of lesions > 5

Rifampicin: 600 mg once monthly supervised.

Dapsone: 100 mg daily self-administered.

Clofazimine. 50 mg daily self-administered.

300 mg once monthly supervised.

Duration of therapy: 1 year or until the patients become smear negative.

Several new bactericidal drugs for ***M. leprae*** have been identified, such as fluoroquinolones, minocycline and clarithromycin. The WHO is conducting multicenter trials of daily rifampicin/ofloxacin; this may lead to a shortening of duration of multiple drug therapy.

The improvement of the bacteriological index (count of dead and viable bacilli) is very slow. Morphological index (count for viable bacilli) decreases in a few weeks and disappears in a few months, rendering the patient noninfectious.

Prevention

- Improve living standards
- BCG vaccination based on the possible cross immunity with tuberculosis.
- Dapsone should be given to individuals exposed to open cases of leprosy

Gerhard Armauer Hansen (1841–1912)

Hansen was a Norwegian bacteriologist and leprologist, he discovered the lepra bacillus, Mycobacterium leprae; 14 years before Kock's discovery of the closely related Tubercle bacillus. 14th century writings refer to chalmoongra oil obtained from the seeds of an Indian tree as a specific cure for leprosy. This oil remained the principal anti-leprous drug even in the West for decades.

Leprosy is only contagious till the smears contain lepra bacilli. Once the treatment is started bacilli disappear, and the patient becomes noninfectious. Even lepromatous leprosy becomes noninfectious shortly after treatment.

Mahatma Gandhi

Leprosy work is not merely medical relief; it is transforming frustration of life into dedication, personal ambition with selfless service into joy.

INFECTIONS CAUSED BY OTHER GRAM-POSITIVE BACTERIA

Anthrax

Anthrax is primary disease of domestic and wild animals, humans become accidentally involved. The acute cutaneous lesion is called "malignant pustule". The patient is invariably employed in an animal product industry handling wool, hides, bones, etc. The disease is caused

Clinical Features

These may be cutaneous or systemic.

Cutaneous lesions: The first clinical manifestation is an inflammatory papule, which appears in a few hours or days of infection. The papule develops into a bulla; surrounded by intense edema and infiltration, the bulla often becomes hemorrhagic. Within a short time the bulla ruptures, contents are purulent or serosanguineous. A brown crust then forms; surrounded by vesicles and pustules upon a red-hot indurated area. The regional lymph nodes enlarge and suppurate. In severe cases there is high fever and prostration, often terminating in death in a few days or weeks.

In mild cases the constitutional symptoms are slight, the gangrenous skin sloughs and the ulcer heals. The lesion is neither tender nor painful.

Systemic manifestations: The disease can affect the lungs (woolsorter's disease) or the gastrointestinal tract. Inhalation anthrax is manifested by necrotizing hemorrhagic mediastinal infection. Bacteremia may follow with hemorrhagic meningitis.

Gastrointestinal anthrax results when the spores are ingested and they multiply in the intestinal submucosa. A necrotic ulceration in the terminal ileum or caecum may lead to haemorrhage.

Treatment

For mild lesions below the head and neck, ciprofloxacillin 500 mg b.i.d. or doxycycline 100 mg b.i.d for 7 days. If lesions are on the on the head and neck and in all severe cases medication by IV injection is recommended. Alternately a high dose of IV penicillin can be given. For prophylaxis routine vaccination is indicated for factory and laboratory workers.

(The above doses are when the lesions are only on the skin, but if the exposure is due to aerosol, then the treatment should be extended to 60 days)

by *Bacillus anthracis*. This is a large Gram-positive rod with square ends; it forms spores in the external environment and on culture but not in the tissues.

Erysipeloid of Rosenbach

This is an acute infection of traumatized skin caused by a slender Gram-positive rod: *Erysipelothrix* (E.) *rhusiopathiae* (*insidiosa*). The disease is seen in fishermen, butchers, people handling meat products and poultry.

E. rhusiopathiae is a Gram-positive bacillus, which tends to form filaments in culture. The organism is microaerophilic and nonmotile.

Clinical Features

The first symptom is pain at the site of inoculation; this is usually on a finger or palm. After an incubation period of 2–7 days, a violaceous raised swelling appears, this slowly spreads to produce a well-defined border. Central portion fades away without desquamation or ulceration. Brownish discoloration develops as the lesion resolves.

A diffuse or generalized eruption in regions remote from the site of inoculation may occur with fever and arthritis. Septicemia may occur; this may cause endocarditis, arthritis, prolonged fever and constitutional symptoms. The lesions consist of multiple serpiginous plaques with raised borders.

Treatment

Penicillin G, 1.2 million units given by IM injection daily or b.i.d. for 7–10 days is the treatment of choice. In patients who are allergic to penicillin, erythromycin 250 mg every 6 hours, for 7–10 days is an alternative. Ciprofloxacin and tetracycline are other alternatives.

In case of dissemination the dose of penicillin is increased to 2.4 million units given every 4 hours by IV route.

CORYNEBACTERIA

Corynebacteria (Diphtheroids) are Gram-positive nonspore-bearing rods, commonly referred to as diphtheroids. Corynebacteria (C.) appear club-shaped (tapered at one end) and are arranged in palisades or in V or L shaped formation. The rods have a beaded appearance. The beads consist of granules of highly polymerised phosphate, a storage mechanism for high-energy phosphate bonds. The granules stain metachromatically. The bacteria are widely distributed in nature; propionibacterium is the anaerobic variety of the organism. These may primarily affect the throat (*C. diphtheriae*), the skin (*C. minutissimum, C. pyogenes, C. hofmannii*).

The anaerobic variety affects the hair follicles (*P. acnes*).

The following are some of the diseases caused by the coryneform bacteria.

Erythrasma

Erythrasma (Greek, "red spot") is a common superficial skin infection caused by *C. minutissimum*. This is a Gram-positive rod with sub-terminal granules. It affects the intertriginous

Clinical Features

The disease may occur at any age, it is more common in adults. In the early stages red patches occur, which are irregular in shape and sharply demarcated. Later the lesions become brown in color and scaly. In the tropics, in diabetics and those with chronic disability, the disease may become generalized covering extensive areas of the body. The lesions appear as reddish-brown plaques.

Rarely erythrasma has been associated with systemic disease such as endocarditis (Fig. 17).

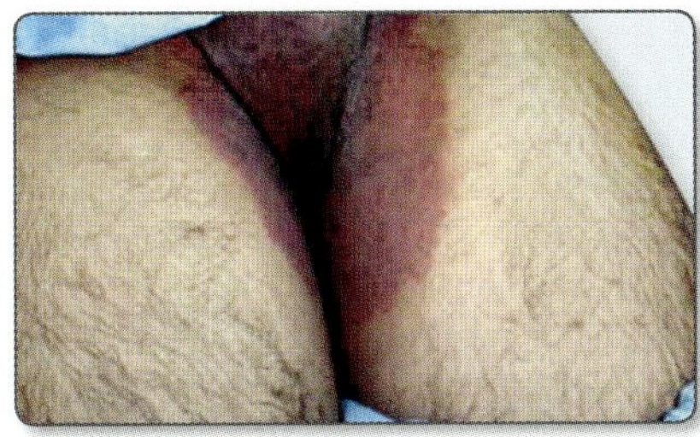

Fig. 17: Erythrasma

areas of the toes, groins, axillae, intergluteal and submammary regions. The organism is found in the horny layers of the skin. A warm humid climate is the predisposing factor.

Diagnosis

- Gram staining: This reveals rod like Gram-positive organism.
- Wood's lamp examination: Fluorescence with Wood's lamp gives a coral-red color due to the presence of porphyrins

Pathogenesis

The organism invades the upper-third of the stratum corneum, under favorable conditions such as heat and moisture. The stratum corneum is thickened. The organism is seen in the intercellular spaces and in the cells dissolving keratin fibrils. Coral-red fluorescence is due to the production of porphyrin by these bacteria.

Differential Diagnosis

The disease should be differentiated from tinea cruris, candida, inverse psoriasis, seborrhoeic dermatitis and contact dermatitis. Tinea is characterized by a pale center and active margins. Candidiasis has the peripheral papules. Fluorescence under Wood's lamp is diagnostic of erythrasma.

Treatment

Erythrasma responds well to topical azole antifungal agents. Duration of therapy is usually 2 weeks, relapses are frequent. For extensive lesions erythromycin 250 mg is given four times a day for one week.

In case of frequent relapses topical antibacterial soaps such as povidone iodine soaps, benzoyl peroxide bar is recommended. Topical erythromycin or clindamycin are also effective. Loose clothing should be worn and drying agents such as powders should be used in the affected areas.

Trichomycosis Axillaris

Despite its name, the condition is not a fungal infection. This is a superficial infection of the axillary and pubic hair; with the formation of adherent granular nodules, yellow, black or red in color on the hair shaft. The concretions consist of tightly packed bacteria. These grow within the cuticular cells of the hair and may invade the cortex. The disease is caused by *C. tenuis*.

Clinical Features

Yellow, red or black concretions are present on the hair shaft; these may be hard or soft. The hair may be brittle and easily broken. The underlying skin is normal. The axillary sweat may be yellow, red or black according to the color of the concretions. Yellow concretions are the most common and black the rarest.

Diagnosis

Potassium hydroxide mounts show the bacilli in the concretions.

Differential Diagnosis

The disease should be differentiated from pediculosis and piedra. Microscopic examination of the concretions is diagnostic.

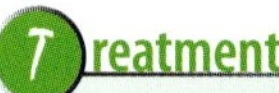

Treatment

Clipping of the affected hair and application of an antimicrobial ointment is effective. Antiperspirants should also be used.

Diphtheria

Diphtheria caused by *C. diphtheriae,* it primarily involves the pharynx and mucous membrane of the upper respiratory tract. It may produce membranous obstruction of the airway or affect the myocardium and peripheral nervous system, by the action of a potent cytotoxin. Very rarely the primary lesion is in the skin; it may infect a pre-existing wound. The hallmark of the infection is a gray leathery membrane.

Other infections due to Corynebacteria are pitted keratolysis and acne. Anaerobic corynebacteria are called Propionibacteria (P.). The lesions are discussed in chapter 23.

Clinical Features

Skin may be involved primarily or secondary to cutaneous infections and eczema.

Primary cutaneous diphtheria: This often begins as acutely pustular tender lesions; that breaks down to form an ulcer, the ulcer is punched out, has hard rolled elevated edges with a pale blue tinge. The lesion is covered by a leathery grayish membrane. Regional lymph nodes may be involved. The lower legs are commonly affected.

Treatment

A diphtheric antitoxin 20,000–100,000 unit is given after a test dose. Penicillin G 1.2 million units daily for 3 weeks, or erythromycin 500 mg q.i.d daily for 3 weeks.

ACTINOMYCES

Actinomyces (A.) are anaerobic Gram-positive bacteria. They cause two important human infections: actinomycosis and norcardosis.

Actinomycosis

This was previously regarded as a fungal infection, perhaps because of its microscopic appearance; they are filamentous bacteria producing branching hyphae (Fig. 18). The most common human infection is caused by *A. israelii*.

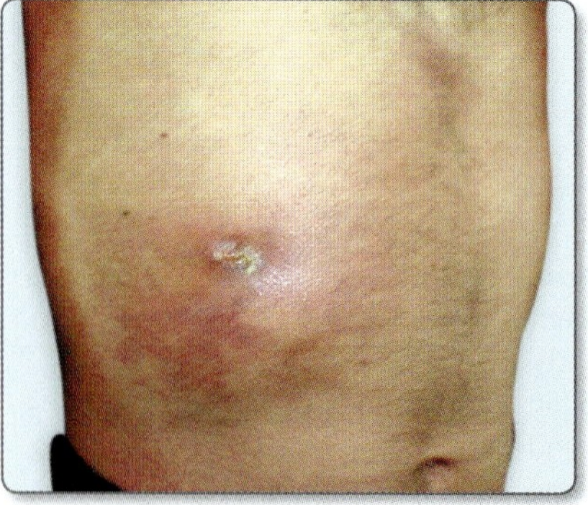

Fig. 18: Actinomycosis

Other pathogens are *A. bovis, A. naeslundii* and *A. viscosus*. Actinomycosis can affect all tissues and organs of the body. Five main clinical types can be recognized depending upon the primary site of infection: cervicofacial, thoracic, abdominal, pelvic and primary cutaneous.

Cervicofacial

The primary lesion is in the mandible or maxilla, which is infected from a periodontal abscess. The infection may spread to the orbital bones or outwards towards the skin. The skin lesion is characterized by a very hard induration, with nodules and sinuses. The nodules are dark-red in color; the sinuses discharge granules in the pus. These granules are yellowish in color and contain masses of microorganism.

Thoracic

The appendix or the caecum is the primary site of infection; stomach and gallbladder may also be affected. Extension to the abdominal wall produces draining sinuses in the skin. Infection may spread internally to the vertebrae, kidney, ovaries and the urinary bladder.

Abdominal

The lungs are the primary site of infection. The infection simulates pulmonary tuberculosis. Infection spreads inwards to the mediastinum and vertebrae, outwards to the chest wall and skin. The lesions in the skin are manifested by nodules and multiple draining sinuses.

Pelvic

This is often associated with the use of intrauterine contraceptive devices. The skin is usually not affected, only rarely tumor like masses, are seen in the skin.

Primary Cutaneous Actinomycosis

This is very uncommon, seen usually on the exposed skin. Subcutaneous nodules are found, they break down to form sinuses. Regional lymph nodes are enlarged. The pattern of infection is similar to mycetoma. The cutaneous variety may remain localized for years.

Mycetoma caused by actinomycetes is discussed in chapter 5.

Treatment

As actinomycosis is a chronic infection with marked fibrosis, quick response to treatment should not be expected. Mild cases can be treated by antibiotics, chronic cases require a combination of surgery and antibiotics. Actinomyces are sensitive to antibiotics effective against Gram-positive organisms such as penicillin, tetracyclines, rifampicin, erythromycin and sulphonamides.

High doses of penicillin, is the treatment of choice. 10–12 million units are given by IM injections for 30–45 days, this is followed by oral penicillin 4–6 g daily for 2–6 months or until the lesions have cleared.

Nocardiosis

This is an acute or subacute infection, caused by *Norcardia asteroides*. The bacteria are found in the soil, man is infected via the respiratory tract.

Clinical Features

The primary lesion is in the lung resembling pulmonary tuberculosis. Dissemination occurs via the bloodstream; in one third of cases dissemination occurs in the brain. Infection may also spread to the ribs, vertebra and pelvis. Multiple abscesses are found in the skin. ***N. asteriodes*** is often seen as an opportunistic infection in leukemia, and other debilitating diseases.

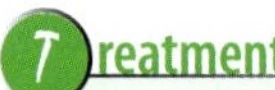

Trimethoprim-sulphamethoxazole is the treatment of choice, dapsone is also frequently used. Penicillin, tetracycline and chloramphenicol are alternatives.

INFECTIONS CAUSED BY GRAM-NEGATIVE BACTERIA

Pseudomonas

These are aerobic gram-negative rods seen as a transient member of the skin bacteria, present mainly in the intertriginous areas. Infection occurs in man when the general resistance to disease is lowered as seen in general debilitating diseases and immunosuppression. The following are the cutaneous manifestations of pseudomonal infection.

- Ecthyma gangrenosum
- Green nail syndrome
- Gram-negative toe web infection
- Pseudomonas folliculitis
- Otitis externa.

Ecthyma Gangrenosum

The lesion presents as grouped vesicles, surrounded by pink to violaceous halos. The vesicles become hemorrhagic; they rupture to form an ulcer with black necrotic center. It is treated with an aminoglycoside, and with antipseudomonal penicillin such as piperacillin.

Green Nail Syndrome

The condition is often seen in people who work with soap and water such as cooks, barmaids, nurses, etc. The lesion is characterized by distal onycholysis and green discoloration of the separated nails. Soaking the finger in 0.1% polymyxin B and 1% acetic acid solution twice daily has been said to be a successful treatment. Neosporin drops are also helpful.

Gram-Negative Toe Web Infection

Pseudomonal infection is often superimposed on a fungal infection of the toes. In later stages of the infection, there is purulent or serous discharge with edema and erythema of the surrounding tissues.

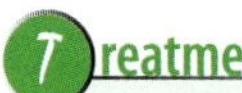

The underlying fungal infection should be treated with oral antifungals. Topically local antibiotics in acetic acid compresses are advisable. If the infection is severe, systemic antibiotics should be given. Quinolones are effective against pseudomonas.

Pseudomonas Folliculitis (Hot Tub Dermatitis)

This occurs 1–4 days after bathing in hot tubs or public baths. Pruritic follicular papules occur which become pustular. The lesions are seen on the trunk, axillae, buttocks and proximal extremities. Bacteremia is rarely reported. The folliculitis resolves without treatment in about 2 weeks. Acetic acid compresses are advised.

Otitis Externa

This is often seen secondary to swimming. A severe type referred to as malignant otitis externa, is associated with diabetes mellitus. Pain, swelling and erythema is pronounced, purulent foul smelling discharge from the ear occurs, necrosis of the cartilage may result. Appropriate systemic antibiotic such as ciprofloxacillin is the treatment of choice.

MENINGOCOCCAL INFECTION

Skin infection is often secondary to meningococcal bacteremia. Cutaneous lesions often provide a clue to the diagnosis. A purpuric eruption is characteristic, occurring mainly on the trunk or limbs. The purpuric lesions are in the form of petechiae, but in severe cases, ecchymosis may occur. Early lesions are not always hemorrhagic; they appear as macules or papules. Vasculitis may occur during the acute attacks. Intravenous benzyl penicillin is the treatment of choice. Cefotaxime can be used as an alternative. Rifampicin for 2 days is recommended as a prophylaxis for family contacts.

Bartonellosis

Bartonella are small Gram-negative bacteria, difficult to culture and classify. The human diseases associated with *Bartonella* (*B.*) are:

- Trench fever
- Cat scratch disease
- Oroya fever
- Bacillary angiomatosis

Trench Fever

This is caused by *Bartonella* (*B.*) *quintana*; it is transmitted to humans by the body louse. It spreads from person to person. The disease is characterizsed by recurrent febrile illness, widespread maculopapular eruption that fluctuates with fever. A myalgia that involves the lower part of the back and the legs (shin pain) is characteristic of the disease. The disease was seen only during the two world wars, hence the name "Trench Fever".

The illness is mild, spontaneous recovery occurs.

Cat Scratch Disease

The disease is worldwide; it affects both sexes of all ages. The causative organism is *B. henselae*. After an incubation period of about 5 days following the bite by a cat, a papule or a group of papules appears at the site of injury;

these become vesicular and later ulcerate. It takes several weeks for the ulcer to heal with a scar. The peripheral lymph modes are enlarged. The glands are painful and tender and occasionally progress to suppuration. Unilateral lymphadenitis is the usual presenting symptom. Constitutional symptoms are mild.

Systemic symptoms include low grade fever, malaise, hepatosplenomegaly, encephalopathy, lytic bone lesions, conjunctivitis and preauricular adenopathy (oculoglandular syndrome of Parinaud). It can cause endocarditis in patients with known valvular heart disease.

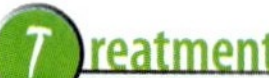

Most cases can be managed with conservative symptomatic treatment. The disease is self-limiting and resolves within 2–4 months. The fluctuant lymph nodes, should be aspirated, they should not be incised, to prevent chronic drainage.

Antibiotics are generally ineffective, despite the fact that they are used with success in bacillary angiomatosis. In some studies azithromycin for 5 days was demonstrated to reduce the lymph node volume during the first 30 days of observation.

Oroya Fever and Verruga Peruana

The causative organism for these diseases is *B. bacilliformis*. The disease is endemic in Peru, Equador and Colombia. The arthropod vector is a sandfly. The disease exhibits two characteristic forms; a severe febrile illness with hemolytic anemia known as Oroya fever and a benign nodular cutaneous form called verruga peruana or Peruvian warts.

Oroya fever is characterized by intermittent fever, myalgia, malaise, headache, gastrointestinal disturbances and severe hemolytic anemia. During the acute phase the patients are extremely susceptible to superinfection, either bacterial (Salmonella) or parasitic (Toxoplasmosis). During convalescence from Oraya fever, numerous cutaneous eruptions occur. The most common eruptions are miliary erythematous papules and macules on the face and extensor surface of the extremities. The lesions bleed easily and may ulcerate. Eruption heals without scarring.

Verruca peruana is characterized by chronic self-healing, soft verrucous vascular nodules. The lesions occur on the limbs and spare the trunk. Cutaneous lesions may occur without Oroya fever.

Treatment

Penicillin, chloramphenicol, tetracycline and streptomycin are all effective. Chloramphenicol is the treatment of choice, because of the frequent coexisting salmonella infection. Cutaneous lesions do not require any treatment, they resolve spontaneously within months or years.

Bacillary Angiomatosis

The disease is caused by *B. henselae* and *B. quintana*. This is found in AIDS and occasionally in patients with severe immunosuppression. The lesion is characterized by the development of friable angiomatous papules and nodules on any site of the body including the mucosa. Superficial lesions resemble pyogenic granuloma. The lesions

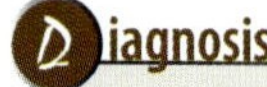

The skin shows a large number of organisms with Warthin-Starry stain. The diagnosis can be confirmed by PCR.

are due to vasculogenesis, there is a lobular proliferation of small blood vessels that contain swollen endothelial cells. Cyst-like inflammatory lesions may develop in the internal organs, such as the liver, spleen and bone marrow.

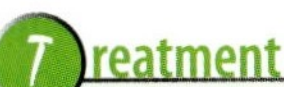

Treatment

Erythromycin 500 mg q.i.d. or other macrolides are the drugs of choice. It should be used for 8 weeks or longer. Doxycycline is also effective. Relapses are common; in these cases long-term prophylaxis is required. The nodules can also be destroyed by cryotherapy or laser.

GLANDERS (FARCY)

The disease occurs in people who handle horses and donkeys. The disease is rare in man; it is caused by *Burkholderia mallei*, previously known as *Pseudomonas mallei*, which is an aerobic, nonmotile Gram-negative bacillus.

Clinical Features

This may take one of the following two forms:

- Acute febrile illness, which may last for 10–30 days. Dissemination results in pneumonia, meningitis, arthritis and severe diarrhea. The disease may be fatal.
- Cutaneous variety: An inflammatory papule or vesicle arises at the site of inoculation; this may become nodular, pustular or ulcerative. In course of a few days other nodules (farcy buds) develop along the course of lymphatics, which subsequently breakdown to form ulcers. Repeated cycles of breakdown and healing occur for weeks or months.

Treatment

Prolonged therapy with a combination of antibiotics such as trimethoprim/sulfamethoxazole or amoxicillin/clavulanic acid have been used successfully for the treatment of glanders.

MELIOIDOSIS (WHITMORE'S DISEASE)

It is an infection caused by glander-like bacillus *Burkholderia pseudomallei*, previously known as *Pseudomonas pseudomallei*. The organism is isolated from the soil and water in the low-lying rice growing regions of the Far East.

The acute form of the disease often presents as acute pulmonary infection with multiple miliary abscesses in the viscera; it may result in early death. Severe urticara can result with pulmonary infection. The cutaneous lesion comprises subcutaneous abscesses.

Treatment

The majority of infections respond to tetracycline in a dose of 2–3 g daily for 30 days. Ceftazidime, piperacillin-tazobactam, imipenem, amoxicillin-clavulanic acid, trimethoprim and sulphamethoxazole are also effective.

TULAREMIA (OHARA'S DISEASE)

Tularemia is a febrile disease caused by *Francisella tularensis*, a Gram-negative coccobacillus that produces a powerful endotoxin. The organism resides in a wide range of animal species. In man, infection occurs by the bite of an infected

Clinical Features

The clinical manifestations depend upon the portal of entry; this may be the skin, gastrointestinal or respiratory tract.

Cutaneous form: This manifests as a punched out ulcer usually on the legs, this is firm and tender, and it heals in about 6 weeks with a scar. The regional lymph glands become painful, swollen and inflamed, similar to that of sporotrichosis. Other cutaneous lesions are nonspecific. These comprise of macules, papules, petechiael exanthema and erythema multiforme.

Gastrointestinal form: A typhoidal type of infection is seen when the portal of entry is through the gastrointestinal tract. The disease is characterized by fever, malaise and gastrointestinal symptoms.

Respiratory form: The pneumonial form is the most severe variety. This may give rise to a number of cutaneous lesions, such as macules, papules, vesicles, petechiae, erythema nodosum, etc.

Treatment

Streptomycin is the treatment of choice; 0.5 g IM is given every 12 hours. Clinical improvement is seen in 24–48 hours, but the treatment should be continued for 7–10 days. Other alternatives are gentamicin 5 mg/kg of body weight daily by IV or IM route, ciprofloxacin, tetracycline and chloramphenical. Lymph node drainage should be avoided until late in therapy.

tick or by direct contact with an infected rodent. The disease is usually seen in hunters.

PLAGUE

Yersinia pestis is a small-Gram-negative, nonspore bearing, nonmotile bacillus that causes plague. It is primarily an infection of rodents. The disease is transmitted to man by the bite of fleas, found on infected rats.

Clinical Features

The incubation period is 1-–6 days, followed by a sudden onset of malaise, headache, tachycardia and high fever. Infection can occur in three forms:

1. Bubonic Plague
2. Septicaemic Plague
3. Pneumonic Plague

Cutaneous form (Bubonic plague): The initial lesion is related to the flea bite. This is usually not visible, or occurs as an occasional papule or vesicopapule. Regional lymph nodes are enlarged and painful. The nodes become matted (buboes); with extensive erythema of the surrounding tissues, septicaemia may supervene with petechiae, due to disseminated intravascular coagulation.

Septicaemic plague: In septicaemic plague bacteria enter the blood from the lymphatic system, respiratory system or directly. The condition results in septicaemia with chills, fever, delirium hypotension, headache and vomiting. Septicaemic shock may occur.

Pneumonic plague: This is abrupt with fever, tachycardia and tachypnea. Signs of consolidation are seen in 24 hours. The patient is clinically ill with bloody sputum. Meningitis complicates all the three types of plague.

Treatment

Streptomycin is the drug of choice. Two gram daily is given in divided doses for 10 days. Side effect of ototoxicity should be kept in mind. Gentamycin, chloraphenicol, and tetracycline are alternatives. Gentamicin is the preferred alternative in pregnancy.

BRUCELLOSIS (UNDULANT FEVER)

Brucellosis is transmitted to humans by contact with animal or animal products such as raw milk or unpasteurized cheese. Brucellae are Gram-negative aerobic coccobacillus. These colonize in the reticuloendothelial system and induce a granuloma.

Clinical Features

After incubation period of 1–3 months, the disease is manifested by fever and headache, with involvement of the liver, joint or meninges. On the other hand, there may be an indolent disease with weakness, anorexia, low-grade fever that may persist for weeks or months. Rare forms of infection include suppuration, lymphadenitis and endocarditis.

Cutaneous Lesions

There are no typical skin lesions; a rash is reported in 5–10% of cases. Erythematous papules, urticarial and vesicular lesions may occur during the course of the illness. Rarely subcutaneous abscess or sinus tracts develop from an infected lymph node or bone infection. Sometimes a severe hypersensitivity reaction occurs in people directly exposed to infected material. Biopsy shows noncaseating granulomas.

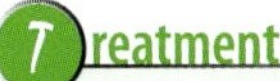

Treatment

Brucellosis is treated with doxycycline and rifampicin; both should be given for at least 6 weeks. Cotrimoxazole is an alternative drug.

RHINOSCLEROMA

This is a chronic inflammatory granulomatous disease of the upper respiratory tract, characterized by sclerosis and deformity. Death due to obstructive sequelae may occur. The infection is limited to the nose, pharynx and adjacent structures. The disease is caused by *Klebsiella rhinoscleromatis*, a Gram-negative, nonmotile rod, enclosed in a gelatinous capsule.

Clinical Features

The disease begins with nasal catarrh, increased nasal secretions and subsequent crusting. Gradually there are diffuse sclerotic enlargement of the nose, upper lip, palate and surrounding structures. The nodules are at first small, hard and movable, later they adhere to the underlying structures. Ulceration is frequent. The lesions have a distinctive stone hardness.

Advanced cases of rhinoscleroma produce extensive mutilation of the face, Eustachian tubes, middle ear cavity and the orbit.

Treatment

The disease is usually progressive and difficult to treat. A combination of surgery and antibiotics is required. Tetracycline 2 g daily for 6 months and then 1 g daily for another 6 months is the treatment of choice. In cases of recurrences, cephalexin may be helpful. The organism is also sensitive to streptomycin, kanamycin, rifampicin. Klebsiella rhinoscleromatis is insensitive to penicillin and sulphonamides. Surgery is needed to remove granulomatous tissue and scarring.

RAT-BITE FEVER

This is an acute infection, which is acquired from rodents. Fever, polyarthralgia or arthritis and a rash characterize the disease. It is caused by *Streptobacillus moniliformis*, a Gram-negative pleomorphic bacillus and *Spirillum minor*.

Clinical Features

There are two distinct forms of rat-bite fever: Sodoku caused by ***Spirillum minor*** and septicemia caused by ***Streptobacillus moniliformis***. After an incubation period of 10 days, a generalized morbilliform eruption occurs; palms and soles are also affected. The rash may become petechial, arthralgia and pleural effusion may occur.

Infection with ***Spirillum minor*** begins abruptly with fever and chills. Incubation period is from 1–4 weeks. The site of the rat bite is often inflamed, this may become ulcerated and lymphangitis occur. The eruption occurs as rose spots on the abdomen, which enlarge to form purplish and indurated plaques. Arthritis rarely occurs. Endocarditis, nephritis, meningitis and hepatitis are potential complications.

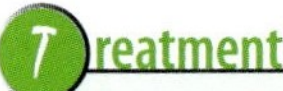

Treatment

Cauterization of the bite by nitric acid may prevent the disease. Penicillin is the drug of choice. Tetracycline and streptomycin are also effective.

RICKETTSIA

Rickettsiae are pleomorphic, coccobacilliary obligate intracellular parasites. They are Gram-negative bacteria, occurring as elementary bodies that multiply in the cells of the host. Rickettsial disease is transmitted to human by arthropods. Most of the infections result in vascular infarcts, extravasular fluid loss and disseminated intravascular coagulation. Rickettsia causes the following diseases:

- Epidemic typhus, endemic typhus and sporadic typhus
- Spotted fever group: These include Rocky Mountain spotted fever, tick typhus and rickettsial pox
- Scrub typhus
- Q. fever (has no exanthem)

Epidemic Typhus

Epidemic typhus is caused by *R. prowazekii*, it is the more severe form of typhus. It is associated with times of war and natural disasters. It has also been termed recrudescent or *sporadic typhus*, induced by poor living conditions or provocated by immunological stress.

Infection is transmitted to humans by the bite of the human body louse. After an incubation period of 7–10 days, there is fever, headache and malaise. A rash appears on the 4–7th day of fever; initially this appears as pink macules, first on the side of the trunk; it then spreads to the whole body, except the face, palms and soles.

During the second week, the rash becomes deeper red in colour and purpuric. Gangrene of the fingers, toes and genitals may result from vascular obstruction. Infection may involve the myocardium and central nervous system. Untreated about 40% of the cases are fatal.

Endemic Typhus

This is caused by *R. typhii*, it occurs worldwide. It is associated with fever, chills, nausea and vomiting. About 18% of patients exhibit an erythematous rash, petechiae may be present.

Spotted Fever Group

Rocky Mountain Spotted Fever

This is the most virulent of the rickettsial infections. The illness ranges from a virtually asymptomatic form to a fulminating disease with mortality rate ranging from 20% to 80%. The onset is abrupt with fever, chills, headache, myalgia and arthralgia. The rash is the most characteristic aspect of the disease. It generally appears on the 4th day of fever, the rash erupts on the ankles, wrist and forearms, it is pink and the macules fade on pressure, it increases in size with the rise of patient's temperature. After 6–18 hours the rash spreads to the body, it involves the palms and soles. A few days later the rash becomes papular and deep red in colour, it no longer fades on pressure. Small areas of gangrene may occur on the fingers, toes, ears and genitals. Involvement of the genitals often helps in the diagnosis.

In severe cases, there is diffuse vasculitis, resulting in the transudation of plasma. Fall of blood pressure, rising pulse, the patient appears toxic and ill, may even become comatosed.

Abdominal symptoms include enlarged spleen, abdominal distension and tenderness. Signs of neurological damage such as seizures and hemiplegia are associated with bad prognosis.

Rickettsial Pox

This is an acute influenza like febrile disorder, which presents for 4–5 days followed by the appearance of a rash resembling varicella. The lesions are firm papules; surmounted by a small vesicle which crusts and heals in a few days. Generalised lymphadenopathy may appear; illness is mild and recovery is complete in about 2 weeks.

Tick Borne Typhus (Mediterranean Fever)

The disease is endemic in North Africa and South Europe. It mostly affects children. The disease is characterised by fever, chills and headache. The tick bite produces a small indurated papule known as tache noir, which becomes a necrotic ulcer. A macular or maculopapular eruption later occurs which is generalised; palms and soles are also affected.

Scrub Typhus (Tsutsugamushi Fever)

After a prodormal illness of fever, malaise and headache, skin eruption appears. These are erythematous macules; lesions begin on the trunk and then spread peripherally. Deafness and tinnitus occur in one fifth of the cases.

An erythematous papule develops at the site of the bite, which becomes indurated; a multilocular vesicle rests on the top of the papule. Eventually a necrotic ulcer forms with regional lymphadenopathy.

Q. Fever

This is the only rickettsial disease, which does not produce skin rashes. Self-healing pneumonitis and hepatitis occurs in humans. It is now no more considered a rickettsial disease.

Treatment of Rickettsial Infections

Doxycycline is the drug of choice. Epidemic and scrub typhus respond to a single dose of 200 mg of doxycycline. Alternately a full dose of tetracycline can be used. In pregnant women, azithromycin or clarithromycin are alternative medications.

SPIROCHAETES

These are large flexible spiral, motile organisms. There are three genera important to humans, these are:

1. *Borrelia*
2. *Leptospira*
3. *Treponema* (*T.*)

Borreliosis

The spirochaete *Borrelia* causes relapsing fever, and Lyme disease. Lyme borreliosis is caused by three different species of *Borrelia* (B.): *B. burgdorferi*, *B. garinii*, *B. afzelii*. All three species are found in Europe, but only *B. burgdorferi* is found in USA. *B. afzelii* is more likely to cause neurological disease and acrodermatitis chronica atrophicans, perhaps explaining the paucity of these problems in USA.

Clinical Features

After an incubation period of a week, symptoms such as fever, malaise and headache, followed by jaundice, with hepatomegaly, splenomegaly and liver tenderness. Petechial or purpuric rash develops, especially on the trunk. A remission occurs for a few days, followed by relapse, which may continue for weeks. The cutaneous eruption does not occur after the initial episode.

Treatment

Tetracycline or erythromycin is the drug of choice.

Relapsing Fever

This is caused by the bite of a tick or louse. The louse borne relapsing fever is endemic in Ethiopia, Sudan and parts of Africa. Tick borne relapsing fever is worldwide.

Lyme Disease (Erythema Chronicum Migrans)

The disease is caused by *Borrelia burgdorferi*; it is transmitted to man by the bite of Ixodes ticks. The initial cases were found along the Lyme river in Connecticut, leading to the name of Lyme disease. The clinical symptoms can be described in three stages. Late Lyme borreliosis are those symptoms that are persistent or remitting after 12 months of initial infection.

Stage 1: Erythema chronicum migrans is the hallmark of Lyme disease. Red papule develops at the site of bite. The incubation period may be a few days to 3 months. Slowly a spreading annular erythema develops as the centre fades. The lesion is often pruritic. The diameter of the erythema ranges from a few centimeters to several centimeters. The peripheral reddish band may be 1–2 cm wide. Atypical variants, such as haemorrhage, scaling or blisters may be present. Erythema chronicum may pass unnoticed, or may be poorly visible or asymptomatic. The development of multiple erythema chronicum migrans like lesions may be due to hematogenous spread of the spirochaete. The lesion is associated with headache, malaise or joint pains. Resolution occurs in about 10 weeks with or without treatment.

Stage 2: Borrelial lymphocytoma. These develop after erythema chronicum migrans or in some cases may develop concomitantly. It develops as a solid bluish-red nodule, 1–5 cm in diameter, accompanied by regional lymphadenopathy. Tenderness and itching may be present. It is usually located on the ear lobe, nipple or cheeks. Microscopically it shows a proliferation of B cells.

Neurological manifestations include meningoencephalitis, peripheral paresis, such as facial palsy. About 50% of cases have peripheral neuropathy, which may be motor, sensory or combined. Emotional disturbances and personality changes are sometimes seen.

Cardiac lesions include myocarditis, pericarditis, artrioventricular block and heart failure. Occasionally complete heart block may occur.

Rheumatologic manifestations include arthralgia, myalgia and oligoarthritis, often of the knee, known as Lyme arthritis. The joint is swollen, pain often not severe. The arthritis may recur for months or years.

Other manifestations include lymphadenopathy, inflammatory ocular disease and renal disease.

Stage 3: Acrodermatitis chronica atrophicans. This is the development of a very atrophic skin over the distal extremities, first of the legs and then the upper extremity. Initially a dull vague erythema develops over the area, followed by atrophy and loss of subcutaneous tissue. The underlying vessels then become prominent. Involvement of the face and trunk is uncommon. Fibrous thickening of the skin may develop in some cases.

Juxtaarticular swellings are present around the elbows and knees. A fibrous band extending down the forearm is known the ulnar streak.

Systemic features include peripheral neuropathies, encephalomyelitis and chronic arthritis.

Serological diagnosis: The disease can be diagnosed by the presence of antibodies, detected by ELISA and Western Blot. In stage 1; 20–50% of cases show antibodies mainly Immunoglobulin M(IgM). In stage 2; 70–90% of cases are positive the antibodies are initially IgM and later IgG. In stage 3; 100% of cases are positive.

Complement levels are low, erythrocyte sedimentation rate is high and C-reactive proteins are positive. Neurological signs can be confirmed by a cerebrospinal fluid (CSF) examination, which shows increased lymphocytes and antibodies are detected in the CSF.

Histology can be conclusive for lymphocytoma and acrodermatitis chronica atrophicans.

Diagnosis

Cultivation of the spirochaete from skin biopsy using Kelly medium is the most reliable way of diagnosing Lyme disease. Successful cultivation can be seen in 60–70% cases with erythema chronicum migrans. Direct detection of *B. burgdorferi* (DNA) by cultivation or PCR can confirm the diagnosis.

Prognosis

Prognosis is good for patients who have been properly treated. But for those patients who have been treated inadequately morbidity is high. Morbidity from the disease is usually neurologic and rheumatic. Patients with neurologic disease who are not diagnosed and treated promptly can suffer from neurologic and cognitive dysfunction; that is difficult to treat. Some patients may have fixed neurologic defects that are unresponsive to antibiotics. Cranial nerve palsies usually resolve without treatment. Some genetically predisposed individuals with arthritis may have ongoing joint inflammation that is not responsive to further antibiotic therapy.

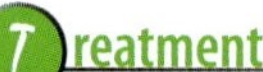

Adequate therapy is essential to avoid complications of the later stages. The treatment is dependent upon the stage of disease

Stage 1: Doxycycline 100 mg b.i.d. for 14–21 days. Tetracycline, ampicillin and cephalosporins can be given as alternative therapy.

Stage 2: Doxycycline 100 b.i.d. for 21 days. Penicillin G 5–10 million units IV t.i.d. for 21 days, ampicillin, amoxicillin and erythromycin can be given as alternative therapy.

Stage 3: Ceftriaxone 2 g IV for 14 days. Pencillin G 5–10 million units IV t.i.d. for 21 days can be given alternatively.

If symptoms persist after treatment, re-treatment with ceftriaxone should be considered.

Prevention

Avoid exposure to tick bite in endemic areas by the use of insect repellents. Check the body daily for ticks. Removal of ticks in the first 24 hours is the most important preventive measure to prevent infection.

A vaccine for Lyme arthritis was available for use in America. It was introduced in 1998, but withdrawn in 2002. The efficacy for the vaccine was about 76% after three injections, but a booster was required after 3 years. In Europe the situation is even more complicated because of the three species involved in the aetiology of the disease.

Leptospiral Infection

Infection from rodents, such as rats and dogs enters the human body from the urine and tissues of the infected animal, or indirectly from the soil or drinking water. Leptospira cause Weil's disease and pretibial fever.

Weil's Disease (Icteric Leptospirosis)

This is a systemic disease caused by many strains of genus Leptospira. The disease has an acute onset of chills, fever, intense jaundice, petechial and purpuric rashes in the skin and mucous membrane. Renal disease is manifested by proteinuria, haematuria and azotemia. Death may occur from renal failure in 5–10% of cases. Leucocytosis of 15,000–30,000 is usually present.

Pretibial Fever (Anicteric Leptospirosis)

The infection is got from domestic and wild animals. The disease is characterised by an acute exanthematous eruption most marked on the shin. The erythema may become generalised, erythema nodosum may appear.

High fever, conjunctival redness, nausea, vomiting and headache appear; these last for 1–3 days, followed by a relapse. The headache becomes intense, conjunctival redness increases; ocular pain and photophobia are prominent. Skin lesions resolve spontaneously in 4–7 days.

Treatment of leptospirosis: It is treated with penicillin or doxycycline. Doxycyline on a once weekly dose may be used as a prophylactic. Mortality is increased in icteric leptospirosis.

Endemic Treponematoses

The nonvenereal treponematoses are caused by spirochaetes that are identical to *T. pallidum*, both morphologically and serologically; but they differ in their mode of transmission, epidemiology and clinical presentation. Like syphilis they have a chronic relapsing course with prominent cutaneous manifestations. These disorders occur more common in children. Pinta is unique amongst nonvenereal treponematoses in having only cutaneous manifestations. It is the mildest of all treponematoses; discolouration of the skin is the most serious long-term sequela.

Yaws

This is a nonvenereal treponematosis, caused by *T. pallidum pertenue*. It is found in the hot humid regions around the equator. It is predominantly a disease of childhood. Seventy percent of cases occur before the age of 15.

Clinical Features

After an incubation period of 2–6 months, a primary lesion occurs at the site of inoculation, usually from an infected individual, flies or fomites. The primary lesion (mother yaw) begins as a nontender papule, which later becomes ulcerated. Regional lymph nodes are enlarged; they heal spontaneously leaving an atrophic scar. The secondary lesions are similar to the primary lesions but are smaller (daughter yaws). Lesions are prominent around the mouth and nose; there is hyperkeratosis of the palms and soles. The lesion disappears spontaneously within a month. Osteitis and periosteitis may occur. Later lesions called gumma are present predominantly on the lower limbs. Sabre tibia, saddle nose deformity and gangosa may occur.

Treatment

Penicillin is the treatment of choice. Doxycycline and erythromycin are alternatives.

Pinta

This is also a nonvenereal disease, caused by *T. carateum*. It is found mainly in South and Central America. It is a nonvenereal treponemal disease of underprivileged people, usually affecting people under 20 years of age.

Clinical Features

Clinical manifestations are confined to the skin. The primary stage is manifested by desquamating erythema on the exposed parts of the body. The lesions form multiple papules, which enlarge to form psoriasiform plaques. The lesions do not ulcerate as in yaws. In the secondary stage, the lesions become generalised and red scaly patches appear around the primary lesions. In the tertiary stage areas of depigmentation and hyperpigmentation appear. Dyschromia, hypochromia and achromia are seen in the same patient. Generalised lymphadenopathy is seen in the secondary and tertiary stages. Systemic symptoms are absent.

Begel (Endemic Syphilis)

Begel is a nonvenereal treponematosis, caused by *T. pallidum endemicum*, that closely resembles yaws, but with two exceptions. The primary lesion is often not identifiable and the lesions in the oral mucosa are frequent. The histological changes in the mucosa resemble those of venereal syphilis; the other clinical lesions resemble yaws.

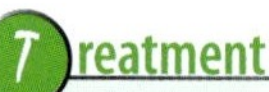

Treatment

Penicillin is the treatment of choice. Doxycycline or erythromycin can be used when the patient is allergic to penicillin.

CHLAMYDIA

These bacteria are intracellular parasites; they have a cell wall, contain both DNA and RNA, multiply by fission and are susceptible to antibiotics. They are seen under an electron microscope. Chlamydia produce cytoplasmic inclusions in susceptible host cells, these consist of a colony of small elementary bodies and large reticulate bodies in varying proportion. In man, chlamydia produces trachoma, conjunctivitis, pneumonia in newborns, psittacosis, Reiter's disease and lymphogranuloma venereum.

Psittacosis (Ornithosis)

The name psittacosis was introduced because infection was thought to be introduced in man by parrots only. It is now known that a number of domestic animals and some birds cause the disease. It is caused by *Chlamydia psittaci.*

Clinical Features

After an incubation period of 2 weeks there is severe pneumonitis, cyanosis and collapse. There is involvement of the liver, myocardium and central nervous system. In some case, the respiratory infection is mild.

Cutaneous signs include a morbilliform eruption, rose spots similar to typhoid fever. Erythema multiforme and erythema nodosum are also reported.

Treatment

Doxycycline is the treatment of choice, treatment is given for 2--3 weeks to prevent relapses.

MYCOPLASMA

These are a group of nonmotile microorganisms that lack a rigid cell wall and hence display a variety of forms. They can grow on cell free media. They are the smallest free-living organisms. These are about a dozen species known to be associated with human infection. The most important infection caused in man is pneumonia. Children and young adults are commonly affected. A number of cutaneous manifestations are seen during the infection. The most frequently reported is erythema multiforme, which may even present as Stevens-Johnson

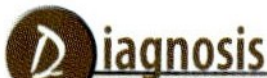

Diagnosis

Diagnosis of ***Mycoplasma pneumoniae*** is made either by culture of the organism or by a rise in the specific antibody titer.

Treatment

Macrolides are the active agents, and azithromycin is the most active macrolide, 500 mg PO once, then 250 mg once daily for 4 days. Erythromycin 500 mg t.i.d. for 6-10 days. Clarithromycin, and doxycycline are alternatives.

syndrome. Erythema nodosum, morbilliform, scarlatiniform uriticarial and vesiculo-papular lesions are also reported. Occasionally acrocyanosis may occur, secondary to the presence of cold agglutinins, which clears with antibiotic therapy.

Genital mycoplasma (M): In the genital region three species have been detected; *M. hominis*, *M. urealyticum* and *M. genitalium*. These are found in sexually active people without any manifestation of disease. The frequency of colonisation increases with sexual activity and change of partners. It has been associated with nongonococcal urethritis in men, but evidence in women is not confirmed. Mycoplasma is sensitive to tetracyclines and macrolides.

Reiter's disease described in chapter 38.

A mighty creature is the germ,
Though smaller than a pachyderm,
His customary dwelling place,
Is deep in the human race,
His childish pride he often pleases,
By giving people strange diseases.

FURTHER READING

1. Berger TG, Kaveh S, Becker D, et al. Cutaneous manifestations of Pseudomonas infection in AIDS. J Am Acad Dermatol. 1995;32:279-80.
2. Dale S and Shaw J. Eosinophilic pustular folliculitis. The Lancet. 2000;356:1235.
3. Hryniewicz W. Epidemiology of MRSA infection. 1999;27(Suppl):S 13-16.
4. Jakeman P, Smith WC. Thalidomide in leprosy reaction. Lancet. 1994;343:432-3.
5. Ji BH. Drug resistance in leprosy: a review. Lepr Rev. 1982;56:265-78.
6. Jopling WH. Reactions in leprosy. Lepr Rev. 1970;41:62-3.
7. Leppard BJ, Seal DV, Colman G. The value of bacteriology and serology in the diagnosis of cellulitis and erysipelas. Br J Dermatol. 1985;112:559-67.
8. Leyden JJ. Cellulitis. Arch Dermatol. 1989;125:823-4.
9. McCormick JK, Yarwoood JM, Schlievert PM. Toxic Shock Syndrome and bacterial antigens: an update. Ann Rev Microbiol. 2001;55:77-100.
10. Morse DC. Directly observed therapy for tuberculosis. BMJ. 1996;312:719-20.
11. Saiag P, Le Breton C, Pavlovic M, et al. Magnetic resonance imaging in adults presenting with severe acute cellulitis. Arch Dermatol. 1994;130:150-8.
12. Shetty VP, Mehta LN, Irani PF, et al. A study of the evolution of nerve damage in leprosy. Part 1-lesions of index damaged branch of radial cutaneous nerve in early leprosy. Lepr India. 1980;52:5-18.
13. Steere AC, Bartenhagen NH, Craft JE, et al. The early cutaneous lesion of Lyme disease. Ann Intern Med. 1983;99:76-82.
14. Swartz MM. Recognition and management of anthrax—an update. N Eng J Med. 2001;345:1621-6.
15. Torrelo A, Valverde E, Mediero IG, et al. Lichen Scrofulosorum. Pediatr Dermatol. 2000;17:373-6.
16. Wolfson JS, Sober AJ, Rubin RH. Dermatologic manifestations of infection in the compromised host. Ann Rev Med. 1983;34:205-17.

Chapter 5

Fungal Infections

INTRODUCTION

Fungi affect life of the common man in a number of ways. They destroy crops, they produce antibiotics; some fungi are used for brewing and baking. Fungi also cause disease. The fungi that infect skin are the dermatophytes, yeast and dimorphic fungi. These cause superficial fungal infections of the skin and they live on keratin. Other fungi invade living tissues to cause systemic disease, while some remain localised in the subcutaneous tissue.

The habitats of fungi are quite diverse. Most are terrestrial; living on soil or dead plant matter. A large number of fungi are parasitic on plants; a few fungi are parasitic on animals and humans. Some fungi are aquatic living primarily in fresh water, others are marine fungi.

Fungi exist in the form of saprophytes or parasites, as they are not capable of synthesising food from carbon dioxide and water. Fungi are morphologically more complex than bacteria. They possess a true nucleus unlike bacteria. Fungal cell wall resembles that of a plant architecturally, but not chemically. It contains large amounts of chitin or other glycosaminoglycans, 80–90% of the cell wall is made of polysaccharides. Fungi may exist in the unicellular form called yeast, or as multicellular organisms such as molds or hyphae, which consist of long filaments divided into cells by septa. Some fungi exist in both forms; these are called dimorphic fungi.

Fungi can reproduce sexually or asexually. Dermatophytes are anamorphic (asexual or imperfect) fungi, they multiply asexually through spores. Dermatophytes have the ability to form molecular attachment to keratin, which is used as a nutrient for dermatophytes to colonise keratinised tissues, such as the epidermis, hair and nails. Molds that produce sexual spores for reproduction are oospores, zygospores, ascospores and basidiospores.

Classification of Fungal Infection

- Superficial mycosis
  - Dermatophytosis
  - Candidiasis
  - Pityriasis versicolor
  - Pityrosporum folliculitis
  - Piedra
  - Tinea nigra

- Subcutaneaous mycosis
  - Sporotrichosis
  - Mycetoma
  - Chromomycosis
  - Subcutaneous zygomycosis
  - Lobomycosis
  - Phaeohyphomycosis
- Deep mycosis
  - Blastomycosis
  - Coccidioidomycosis
  - Histoplasmosis
  - Paracoccidioidomycosis
  - Zygomycosis
  - Penicilliosis
- Opportunistic fungi
  - Candidiasis
  - Aspergillosis
  - Cryptococcosis
  - Mucormycosis

SUPERFICIAL MYCOSES

Dermatophytoses

Dermatophytes invade dead keratinised tissues like hair, nail and stratum corneum. They cannot invade the deeper tissues because of the presence of an inhibitory factor in the serum. Their growth is considerably slowed at 37^0C. Mycosis caused by dermatophytes is called ringworm or tinea. Three genera of dermatophytes are recognised based on their macrospores (macroconidia).

- *Microsporum* (*M.*): The macrospores are spindle-shaped with a thick roughened wall and have 5–12 septa
- *Trichophyton* (*T.*): The macroconidium is spindle-shaped, thin-walled with 4–6 septa
- *Epidermophyton* (*E.*): The macrospore is pear-shaped, thick-walled with 4 septa.

Dermatophytes can also be classified by their habitat.

Geophilic: Geophilic organisms grow in the soil and occasionally infect humans; when they do the reaction is inflammatory, e.g. *M. gypseum*, *M. cookie*, *M. fulvum*. *M. gypseum* is the most common species; it produces a severe inflammatory reaction.

Zoophilic: Zoophilic species are found in animals, these can infect human beings via domestic pets or while slaughtering animals as seen in butchers, hunters, e.g. *M. canis* (dogs, cats); *M. nanum* (pigs), *T. equinum* (horses), *T. mentagrophytes* (cats, dogs, cattle and sheep), *T. verrucosum* (dogs, cattle, sheep, pigs and horses), *T. simii* (chickens and monkeys). Human infection with zoophilic species is usually suppurative. Infections can be clinically silent demonstrating the adaptation of the fungi to other animal hosts.

Anthrophilic: *Anthrophilic species* are transmitted from another human being, e.g. *T. rubrum*, *T. concentricum*, *T. schoenleinii*, *T. violaceum*, *T. tonsurans*, *M. audouinii* and *E. floccosum*. Infection can be inflammatory, such as kerion; or noninflammatory, representing the silent carrier state. This can delay the diagnosis and helps in spreading the infection to other human beings.

Diagnosis of Superficial Mycoses

On clinical examination, the characteristic ring shape of the infection is diagnostic, but the lesions should be differentiated from the other annular lesions, such as tuberculoid leprosy, granuloma annulare, annular erythemas, etc.

Wood's lamp examination: This is a lamp in which a light of 365 nm is produced, from ultraviolet (UV) radiation from a mercury vapour source. The radiation passes through a filter made of 9% nickel oxide and barium silicate. Some of fungi affecting hair produce a characteristic green fluorescence. Scales do not fluoresce. Dermatophytes which fluoresce are members of Microsporum species and *T. schoenleinii*. Other members of Trichophyton species do not fluorescence. *P. versicolor* produces a yellow fluorescence.

A number of other substances also fluoresce, such as salicylic acid, sebum and mineral oil. These should be excluded when using Wood's lamp for diagnosis of dermatophytes.

A negative Wood's lamp examination does not exclude a fungal infection

Microscopy: Scrapings from the affected skin are taken with a blunt scalpel. The affected hair should be plucked rather than cut. If the nails are involved, they should be clipped or scraped with a scalpel, the use of a dental drill is preferred for taking fungal nail samples. The material is collected on a glass slide or a piece of paper. Ten to thirty percent of potassium hydroxide (KOH) is added to the material on the glass slide, which should be heated gently to dissolve the keratin, this makes the examination of dermatophyte easier. Nail material can be kept for 24 hours in a weak (5%) KOH solution.

Dermatophytes are recognised by the presence of translucent hyphae and arthrospores.

Candida shows budding oval yeast with pseudo and true mycelium.

Silver impregnation techniques (Grocott, Gomori) can be used. Parker Quink is sometimes used to identify tinea versicolor.

Histology: Fungi are often conspicuous in histological preparation, but special stains may be necessary. Periodic-Acid Schiff (PAS) stain is usually used to identify fungi in tissue sections.

Culture: Sabouraud's medium is commonly used to grow the dermatophytes. It is an agar containing glucose and peptone. Chloramphenicol is added to inhibit bacteria and cycloheximide to inhibit saprophytic moulds. The growth is very slow; it is obtained in 4–6 weeks. Dermatophyte test medium is another medium used to culture the dermatophytes.

Dermatophytide

Dermatophytide are allergic reaction to a dermatophyte infection. These reactions should fulfill the following criteria:

- A proven focus of dermatophyte infection
- A positive reaction to a trichophytin antigen
- Absence of fungi in the dermatophytide lesions
- Clearing of the dermatophytide after the fungus has been eradicated.

These reactions can be in the form of follicular papules, eczematous lesions, vesicles on palms and soles, vesicles on sides of fingers, pompholyx, erythema multiforme, erythema nodosum like and pityriasis rosea like rash. A dermatophytide is more likely to develop in response to zoonotic infections.

Clinical Manifestations

Tinea corporis: This includes all superficial dermatophyte infections of the skin, other than those involving the scalp, beard, face, groins, hands and feet. It occurs in children and adults; both sexes are equally affected. All the three species of dermatophytes, i.e. Microsporum, Trichophyton and Epidermophyton can cause tinea corporis. *T. rubrum* is the predominant fungus in tinea corporis.

Clinical Features

Tinea corporis is characterised clinically by single or multiple patches with central clearing and a well-defined raised edge; this is the classical ring or annular infection of dermatophytes (Fig. 1). Itching is usually present in these lesions. In acute inflammatory tinea corporis caused by ***T. mentagrophytes*** and ***T. verrucosum***, there is no central clearing; severe pustular reaction may be present. Long standing cases may become very extensive and present as very large confluent areas or as a follicular pustular reaction on the hairy limbs (Figs 2A and B).

Variants of Tinea Corporis

Tinea imbricata: An anthropophilic fungus known as *T. concentricum* causes this infection; it perhaps has an autosomal recessive inheritance. Numerous concentric scaly rings, with severe pruritus and a prolonged course

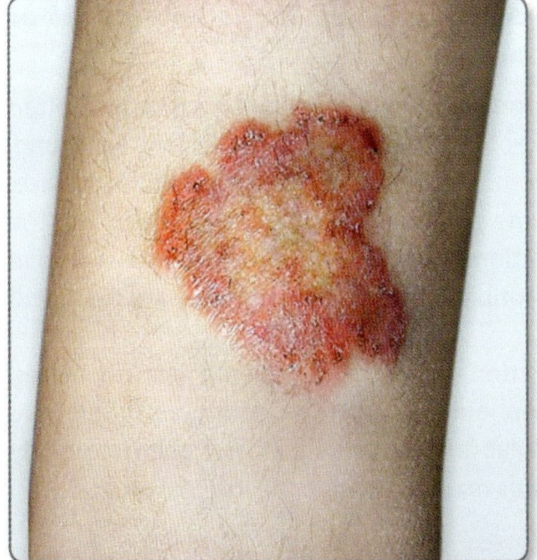

Fig. 1: Tinea corporis

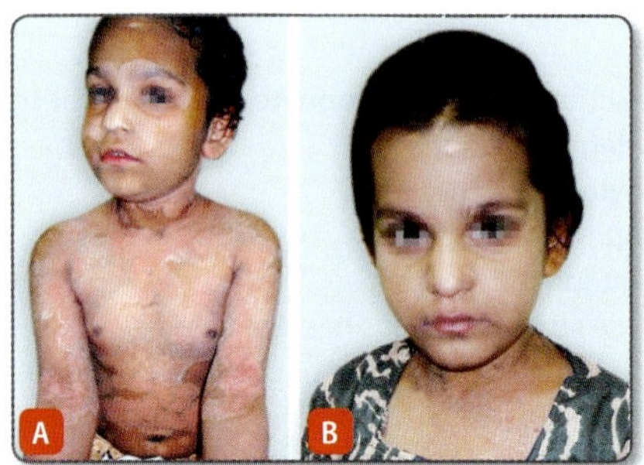

Figs 2A and B: (A) Tinea corporis generalised; (B) Same patient after treatment

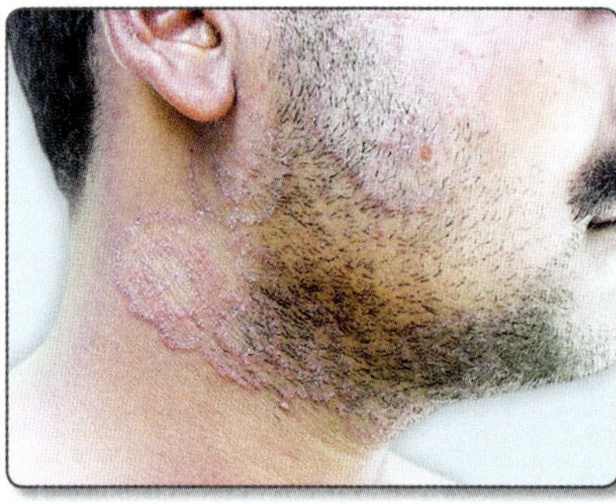

Fig. 3: Tinea imbricata

characterise *T. concentricum* (*Fig. 3*). Lichenification may develop secondary to pruritus.

Majocchi's granuloma: This is a superficial fungal infection caused by *T. rubrum*, which due to decreased immunity may penetrate the dermis and subcutaneous tissue to form a granuloma (Fig. 4). The site of predilection is the skin over the calf muscles. The primary lesion is a follicular papule, pustule or inflammatory nodule. Intracutaneous or subcutaneous granulomatous nodules arise from these lesions. Clinically these lesions are psoriasiform, lichenified plaques without central clearing. The lesions are not as inflammatory as that of *T. verrucosum*.

T. verrucosum can sometimes produce a deep inflammatory response, often seen in areas where cattle are kept in close quarters. The lesions are round, intensely inflamed, with a uniformly elevated red boggy pustular surface. The pustules are follicular with the penetration of the fungus deep into the follicle. Secondary bacterial infection can occur. These deeper lesions require 1–3 months of therapy. Topical antibiotics do not work as they are destroyed by the inflammatory response.

Invasive dermatophyte infection can occur in patients with depressed cellular immunity, such as in lymphomas or patients on immunosuppressive drugs. The lesions appear as nodular, firm or fluctuant masses; seen frequently on the extremities. Dermatophytes may also invade the internal organs.

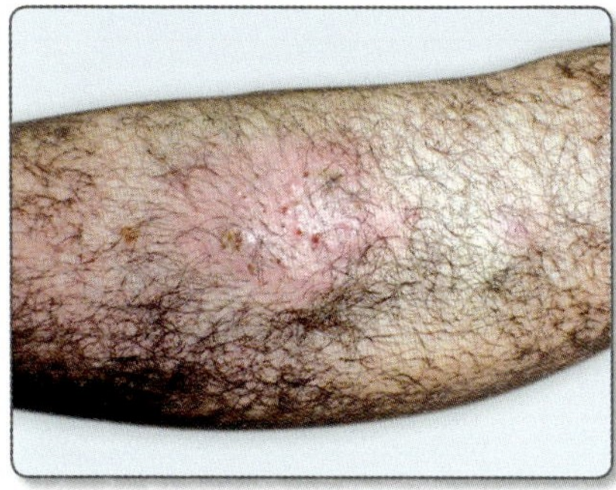

Fig. 4: Majocchi's granuloma

Differential Diagnosis

Seborrhoeic dermatitis, this infection can lead to confusion in some cases, but the condition is symmetrical with involvement of scalp, chest, back and body folds.

Psoriasis, this can cause diagnostic difficulty if present at atypical sites, however, lesions on scalp, elbows, knees and nail changes are helpful. Psoriasis has a characteristic morphological appearance of an erythematous plaque with silvery white scales.

Leprosy (tuberculoid) is often confused with tinea corporis, because of its annular lesions. Enlarged peripheral nerves and anaesthetic skin lesions are two cardinal signs of leprosy.

Nummular eczema may cause difficulty, but the lesions are symmetrically distributed on the limbs.

Pityriasis rosea: The presence of herald patch, typical arrangement and distribution of the lesions and collarette of scales allow the diagnosis of pityriasis rosea to be made. Pityriasis versicolor, candidiasis and tertiary syphilis must also be excluded.

Tinea Capitis

This is a fungal infection of the scalp in which the hair shaft is invaded by dermatophytes. It is a disease of children and is very rare after puberty. The infection is more common in males. Most dermatophytes can invade the hair shaft, however *E. floccosum*, *T. concentricum* and *T. interdigitale* does not cause tinea capitis. Depending on the pattern of hair invasion, tinea capitis is divided into ectothrix, endothrix and the favic type.

Ectothrix infection: This type of infection can be caused by small-spored ectothrix or large-spored ectothrix, in which the arthrospores are found on the external surface of hair shaft, e.g. *M. audouinii*, *M. canis*, *M. equinum*, *T. verrucosum* (small-spored ectothrix), *T. rubrum*, *T. mentographytes* (large-spored ectothrix).

Endothrix infection: In this type of infection the arthrospores are found within the hair shaft. Fluorescence is not seen with this type of hair invasion, e.g. *T. tonsurans*, *T. soudanese* and *T. violaceum*.

Favus: This infection is caused by *T. schoenleinii*. Hyphae and air spaces are seen in the hair shaft, but arthrospores are absent. This type gives a greenish fluorescence.

Clinical Features

The clinical pattern varies with the type of hair invasion and the response of the host. The following clinical types are recognised.

Common type (***Grey patches***): The most common clinical appearance is that of bald patches on the scalp. Closer examination reveals numerous short hair of varying length, but usually less than 0.5 cm. The scalp is slightly scaly; the affected patches are of varying sizes, inflammation is minimal. This clinical pattern is produced by small-spored ectothrix. School children are the most commonly affected (Fig. 5).

Black dot: In this type of infection, black dots are formed as the affected hair breaks at the surface of the scalp. This clinical pattern is produced by endothrix dermatophytes. The patches are usually multiple with minimal scaling (Fig. 6).

Kerion: This variety of tinea capitis is usually caused by zoophilic organism typically ***T. verrucosum*** or ***T. mentagrophytes***. There is a pronounced inflammation probably due to delayed hypersensitivity reaction to fungal elements. Clinically there is a boggy inflammatory mass with discharge of pus, crusting and matting of hair. Regional lymphadenopathy is common. Scarring alopecia may follow kerion (Fig. 7).

Favus: This infection is caused by ***T. schoenleinii***; it commonly affects the scalp, but may involve skin and nails. The condition is characterised by the presence of yellow cup-shaped crusts called scutula around the infected hair. There is a characteristic mousy odour. Later cicatricial alopecia and atrophy occur which is irreversible (Fig. 8).

Agminate folliculitis: This condition is caused by zoophilic organisms and is characterised by sharply defined plaques with follicular pustules.

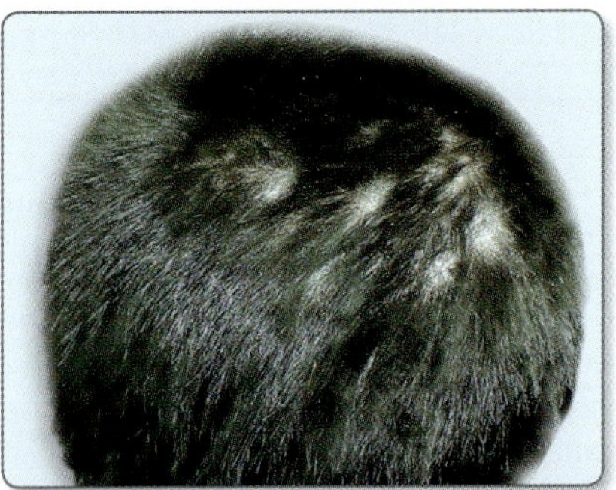

Fig. 5: Tinea capitis-grey patch

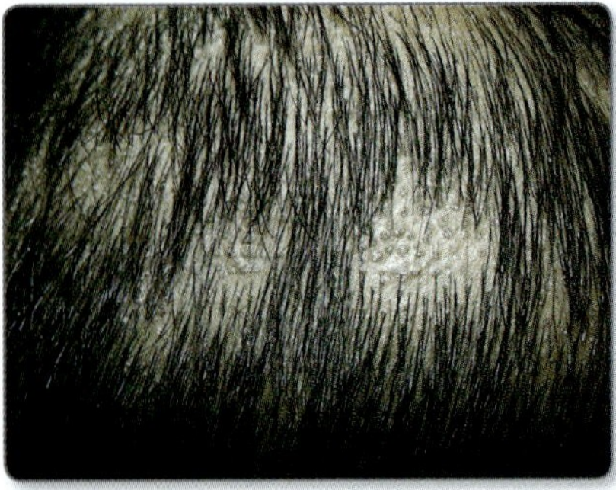

Fig. 6: Tinea capitis-black dot

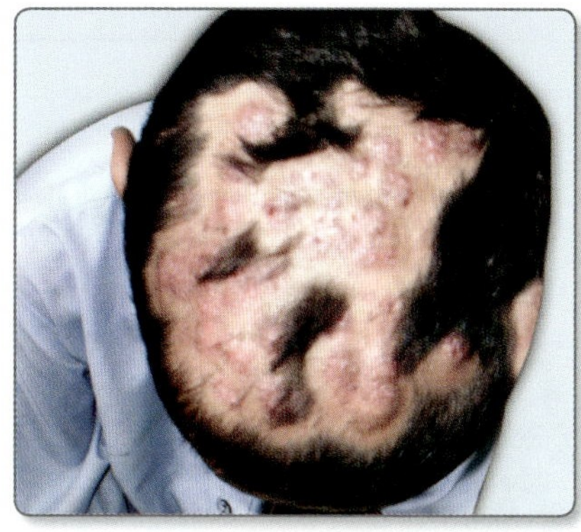

Fig. 7: Kerion

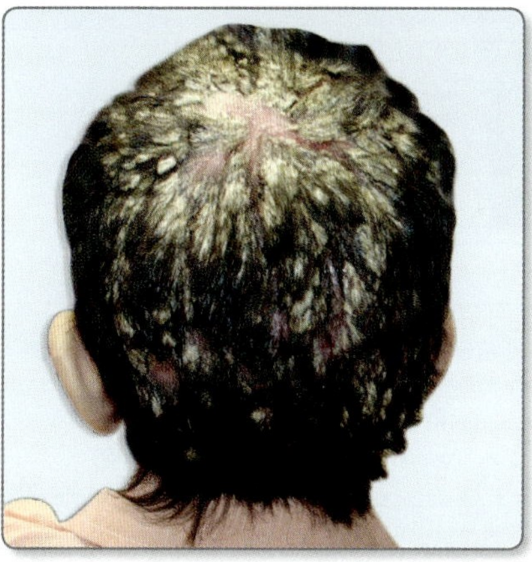

Fig. 8: Favus

Differential Diagnosis

In alopecia areata there is no scaling, the scalp is normal and exclamation mark hair are present at the edge of the lesion. Traumatic alopecia results from hair dressing procedures; there is a patchy hair loss without any signs of inflammation, alopecia occurs at the site of traction. Seborrhoeic dermatitis is more diffuse with adherent scales with usually no hair loss. Impetigo secondary to pediculosis must be differentiated from kerion. Psoriasis, lichen planus and discoid lupus erythematosus must be excluded in some cases; these conditions give rise to scarring alopecia and have other cutaneous lesions. Trichotillomania presents as irregular patchy hair loss, with no scaling; the patient is often tense or anxious.

E. floccosum, T. concentricum and T. interdigitale never cause tinea capitis

Tinea Cruris (Tinea Inguinalis)

This is an infection of the groins with dermatophytes; *E. floccosum* and *T. rubrum* are the main organisms causing tinea cruris; however, *T. interdigitale* is also responsible in some cases.

Clinical Features

This condition is more common in men. A number of cases are due to autoinfection from tinea pedis. Hot weather, excessive sweating, friction and obesity are important predisposing factors. It is characterised clinically by an erythematous, well-defined plaque with central clearing and variable scaling involving the groin. The lesion may extend down to the thighs or up to the buttocks, lower back and abdomen. Itching is a prominent feature (Fig. 9).

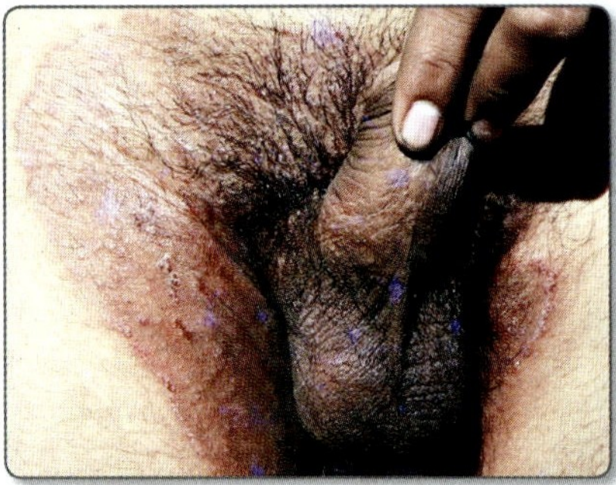

Fig. 9: Tinea cruris

Differential Diagnosis

Candidiasis: The presence of satellite papules and pustules, and absence of distinct raised margin help in differentiating the lesion from dermatophytosis.

Pityriasis versicolor: It may be localised to the groins, but the condition is asymptomatic, noninflammatory without central clearing. It gives yellow fluorescence with Wood's lamp examination.

Intertrigo: It is common in obese patients and needs to be differentiated from tinea cruris. In intertrigo there is maceration, and other body folds like submammary and axillary folds may be involved.

Contact dermatitis: Contact dermatitis from textiles and deodorants may be confused with tinea cruris. Erythrasma presents as reddish confluent plaque, there is no central clearing, Wood's light examination shows coral-red fluorescence.

Always check for tinea pedis or onychomycosis, if present they would require oral antifungal therapy

Tinea Pedis (Athletes Foot)

Tinea pedis is commonly called athletes foot, it is the infection of the feet or toes with dermatophytes. It is a disorder of young and middle-aged adults; the condition being more common in men than in women due to heavy and occlusive footwear used by males. *T. rubrum*, *T. interdigitale* and *E. floccosum* are the main dermatophytes causing the infection.

Clinical Features

In the interdigital form of tinea pedis, the skin between the toes is involved with scaling, maceration and sometimes fissuring. Occasionally the infection may spread to the dorsum of the foot or the soles. In the vesiculobullous variety, there are vesicles, pustules and sometimes bullae involving the soles. The hyperkeratotic or the moccasin type is characterized by erythema and scaling involving the soles and may extend to the dorsal aspect of the feet (Fig. 10). There may be associated nail infection.

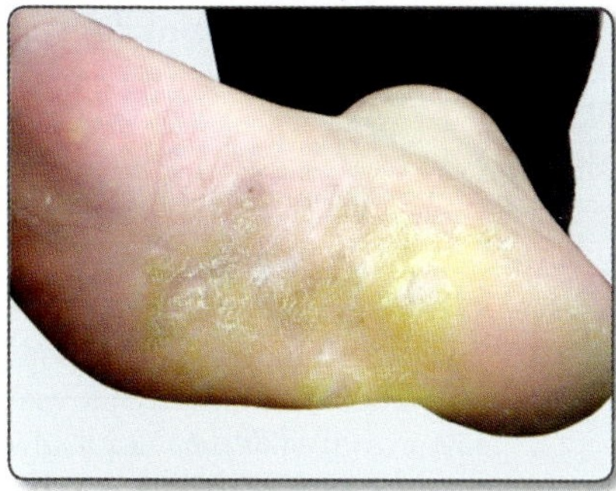

Fig. 10: Tinea pedis

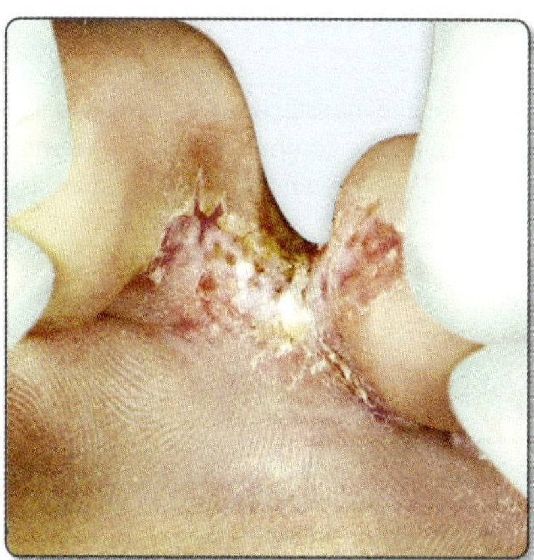

Fig. 11: Tinea pedis-interdigital

Interdigital tinea pedis often tends to be a persistent problem, it may be possible to clear the lesion, but the condition tends to recur. This may be due to re-infection and partly due to the failure to eradicate the fungus completely. The ideal conditions for growth of the fungus, are warmth and moisture which exist at this site (Fig. 11).

Differential Diagnosis

The interdigital form of tinea pedis must be differentiated from erythrasma, candidiasis, soft corns and infected eczemas. Tinea pedis involving the soles should be differentiated from psoriasis, tylosis, contact dermatitis and Reiter's disease. Fungal infection is usually unilateral, the infection is seen between the toes.

Tinea Manuum

Tinea manuum is infection of the palmar skin of hand with a dermatophyte fungus. *T. rubrum*, *E. floccosum* and *T. interdigitale* are the main organisms causing this infection. It is a disease of adults with no sex predilection.

Clinical Features

The condition is unilateral in about 50% of the cases. There is diffuse hyperkeratosis with fine scaling and accentuation of the flexural creases. There may be associated nail infection (Fig. 12).

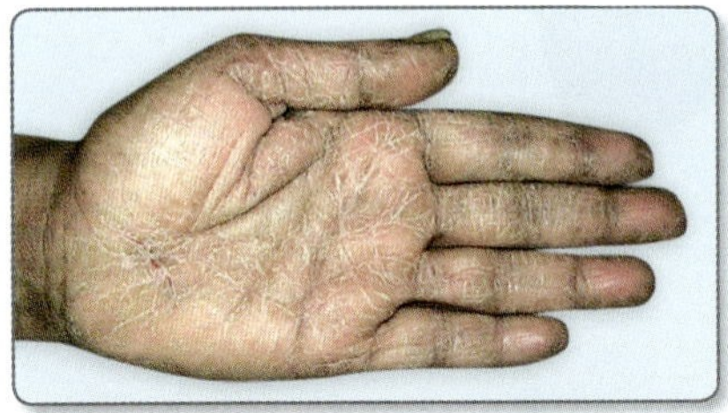

Fig. 12: Tinea manuum

Differential Diagnosis

Tinea manuum must be differentiated from psoriasis, contact eczema, tylosis and syphilis. Unilateral scaling and nail changes are suggestive of dermatophyte infection and should be confirmed by scrapings.

Tinea Barbae

This is the ringworm infection of the beard and moustache areas in adult males. The source of the infection is often animals; the common species concerned are *T. verrucosum* and *T. mentagrophytes*. *T. violaceum* and *T. rubrum* may also cause tinea barbae.

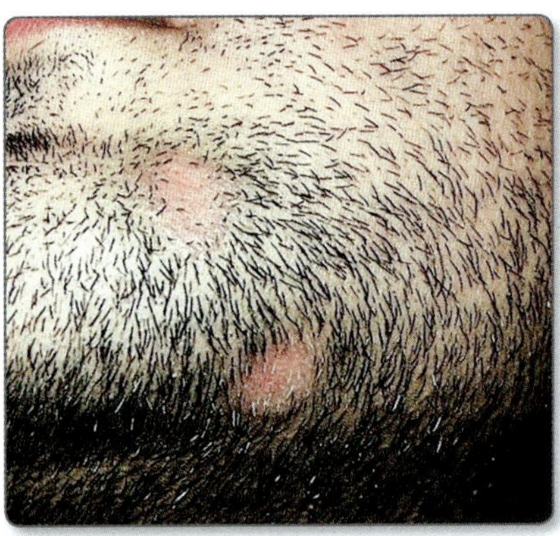

Fig. 13: Tinea barbae

Clinical Features

The lesion may be very inflammatory; it resembles a kerion, in which there is pronounced inflammation with pustular folliculitis, exudation, crusting and loss of hair. Some amount of irritation is usually present. In less severe infections, there are dry, circular, red and scaly lesions with broken hairs (Fig. 13).

Differential Diagnosis

Severe infections of tinea barbae must be differentiated from sycosis barbae in which there is no hair loss and the lesions are painful. Acne, rosacea and pseudofolliculitis must also be excluded from the mild infections of tinea barbae.

Tinea Faciei

This is an infection of the glabrous skin of the face excluding the beard and moustache area. *T. mentogrophytes* and *T. rubrum* are the main organisms causing tinea faciei. It may be caused by sleeping with pet animals or by spread from other sites to the face.

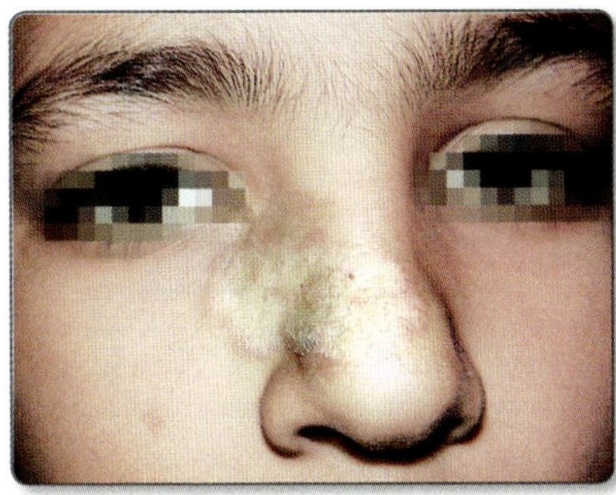

Fig. 14: Tinea faciei

Clinical Features

The clinical picture is often distorted because the patient has used a number of topical remedies before coming to the doctor. Sunlight causes burning and itching.

Some patients show annular lesions typical of ringworm infection (Fig. 14), others may present as simple papules, or as flat patches of erythema, a few vesicles or pustules may be found (T incognito).

Differential Diagnosis

Tinea faciei should be differentiated from lupus erythematosus, rosacea, polymorphic light eruption and seborrhoeic dermatitis, these are usually bilateral and skin scrapings would be negative for the fungus. Solar keratosis, Bowen's disease, impetigo and benign lymphocytic infiltrations should also be excluded.

If topical steroids have been used, it is better to stop the drug for a few days; typical lesions of tinea faciei may then appear making the diagnosis easy.

Onychomycosis (Tinea Unguium)

Onychomycosis is the fungal infection of nails. It can be caused by dermatophytes, yeasts or molds. The dermatophytes responsible for infection are *T. rubrum*, *T. mentagrophytes* and *E. floccosum*. Amongst the yeast, candida is a common cause of nail involvement. Moulds like Aspergillus and Scopulariopsis also infect nails.

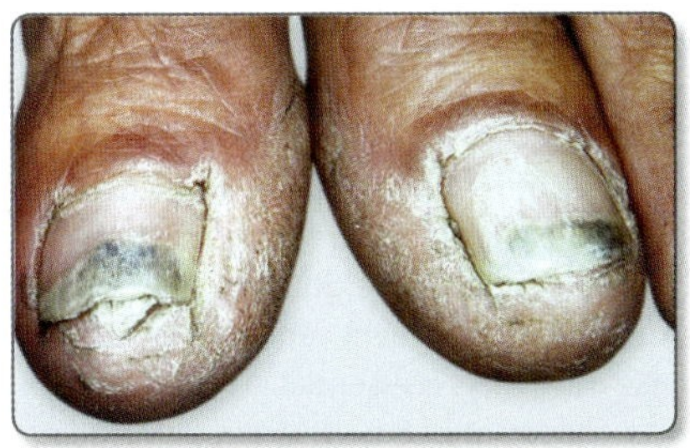

Fig. 15: Onychomycosis

Differential Diagnosis

Onychomycosis must be differentiated from nail involvement of psoriasis, bacterial paronychia, eczema and lichen planus. In psoriasis, pitting of nails is a prominent feature that is not seen in fungal infections. Asymmetrical nail involvement is another feature, which differentiates onychomycosis from psoriasis. In bacterial or candidal paronychia, proximal and lateral portion of the nail plate is affected, usually with the sparing of the free edge.

Clinical Features

Onychomycosis can be distal, superficial or proximal. Distal onychomycosis is the most common.

In distal onychomycosis, there is discolouration at the free or lateral edge of nail plate. The discolouration may be white or yellow; it may be brown or black from contamination, e.g. by pseudomonas. There is thickening of nail plate and separation of nail plate from underlying nail bed. The whole nail plate may be eventually affected. The nails are brittle, they can be broken easily, and white powdery keratinous debris is often found under the nails. Paronychia is rare in dermatophyte infection (Fig. 15).

A cinnamon like discoloration and thickening of nail plate characterize onychomycosis caused by Aspergillus or Scopulariopsis. In candidal infection, there is prominent paronychia. The nailfold is red swollen with pussy discharge and loss of cuticle. The proximal portion of the nail plate may be involved with discoloration and thickening.

Hendersonula (Scytalidium) also affects the palms and soles, the lesions resemble those of ***T. rubrum*** infection. Paronychia is often associated. The nails often show increased pigmentation. There is no effective treatment; Whitfield's ointment may be applied on the palms and soles. Terbinafine may be effective for the nails.

Nail clipping for diagnosis should be done by expert hands. The fungus is found at the growing edge as in dermatophyte infection of the skin. Nail clippings taken by a dental drill at the appropriate site yield the best results.

Management of Ringworm Infections

Topical Therapy

The topical agents commonly used in dermatophyte infections include:

- Benzoic acid compound (Whitfield's ointment) contains 3% salicylic acid, 6% benzoic acid and emulsifying ointment. It is a cheap remedy, but the ointment is irritant and greasy. It should be diluted to half strength for use in groins and flexures
- Castellani's paint is a brilliant green paint. It is cheap but stains the skin
- Undecenoic acid is also a cheap topical agent
- Tolnaftate is another cheap agent, available as cream, powder and lotion
- Imidazoles include miconazole, clotrimazole, econazole, sulconazole, ketoconazole, etc. These are effective, but more expensive
- Allylamines: Naftifine is available as a topical antifungal cream
- Amorolfine nail lacquer (2–5%) used once weekly for 6 months is said to be effective in a number of patients of onychomycosis.

Systemic Therapy

Griseofulvin: This is a fungistatic agent and due to its low cost and effectiveness, is still the drug of choice especially in undeveloped countries. It is given orally in a dose of 10 mg/kg of body weight. The drug should always be given after meals. The duration of treatment varies with the site of involvement, but a minimum course of 3 weeks is essential.

Griseofulvin has a very narrow spectrum being effective only against dermatophytes. It is not effective in candidiasis and pityriasis versicolor. Griseofulvin interacts with a number of drugs like phenobarbitone and anticoagulants. Side effects of major concern are rare, but it may cause headache, irritability and nightmares. Urticaria and photosensitive eruptions are also seen. The drug may exacerbate porphyrias and systemic lupus erythematosus (SLE).

Itraconazole: It is a triazole and a broad-spectrum antifungal agent. Side effects include nausea and headache. It is given in a dose of 100 mg daily for 2–4 weeks or as pulse therapy for nail involvement.

Fluconazole: It is a triazole and a broad-spectrum antifungal agent. It is given in a dose of 150 mg weekly for 2–6 weeks.

Terbinafine: It is an allylamine antifungal agent, which is fungicidal. It is effective against dermatophytes and some species of candida. It is not effective in *T. versicolor* except as topical cream. It is given orally in a dose of 250 mg daily for 2 weeks in ringworm infections of the skin.

Ketoconazole: This is an imidazole that is effective when given orally. It is given in a dose of 200–400 mg/day with food. Side effects include headache, nausea, hepatitis and gynecomastia. It is a broad-spectrum antifungal agent. Its use is limited because of hepatotoxicity.

Treatment Schedules

Tinea Capitis

There is very little place of topical therapy in the treatment of tinea capitis. When a child is diagnosed as suffering from tinea capitis, the other members of the family should also be examined. Sharing of combs and brushes should be discouraged. Cutting or shaving the child's hair has no added benefit.

Griseofulvin: It is given in a dose of 10–20 mg/kg of body weight daily after meals for 4–6 weeks.

Itraconazole: It appears to be as effective as griseofulvin, but is in the investigative phase for use in children. The dose is 5 mg/kg of body weight/day for 4–6 weeks.

Terbinafine: It is also recommended in children above the age of 2 years. In children, less than 20 kg, 62.5 mg/day is given for 2–4 weeks. In children between 20 Kg and 40 Kg, the dose is 125 mg/day for 2–4 weeks and in children above 40 kg, the dose is 250 mg/day for 2–4 weeks.

Ketoconazole: This drug can be used in those cases that are slow to respond or are resistant to other antifungal therapy. The dose is 3.3–6.6 mg /kg of body weight daily with breakfast for 6–8 weeks. It is not much used because of hepatotoxicity.

Shampoos: Selenium sulphide and ketoconazole shampoos are also useful in tinea capitis.

Tinea Corporis and Tinea Cruris

If the lesion is localised, then topical therapy is recommended applied twice daily for about a month. In more widespread or chronic infection, systemic antifungal agent is preferable. The newer broad-spectrum antifungal agents, such as itraconazole 100 mg daily, will achieve clinical clearance within 3 weeks or sooner. Terbibafine, 250 mg daily is given for 2–4 weeks. Griseofulvin usually produces remission in about 4 weeks.

Tinea Pedis

Preventive measures are a very important aspect of the treatment. The importance of keeping the feet dry should be explained to the patient. Cotton socks are preferable to nylon socks because of their ability to absorb moisture. The patient should use lightweight ventilated footwear and should remain barefoot when convenient. In mild interdigital involvement tolnaftate, powder or imidazole creams are effective. If there is inflammation of toe clefts, potassium permanganate solution or magenta paint is useful. If secondary bacterial infection is pronounced, then a systemic antibiotic is needed. Extensive or severe cases require systemic therapy.

Terbinafine is a fungicidal agent, which gives an excellent long-term remission. It is given in a dose of 250 mg twice daily for 4–6 weeks.

Itraconazole is a useful alternative. It is given in the dose of 100 mg daily for 30 days or 200 mg twice daily for 7 days.

Griseofulvin is effective in moccasin type of infection, but is not recommended in the interdigital infection. It is given in a dose of 500 mg twice daily for 2–3 months or longer if required.

Tinea pedis is a common infection, difficult to eradicate, re-infection is common

Tinea Unguium (Onychomycosis)

Recurrences after treatment are high, but with the advent of new broad-spectrum antifungal agents, the results are more encouraging.

Onychomycosis caused by Aspergillus or Scopulariopsis does not respond to griseofulvin or ketoconazole.

Fingernails respond better to treatment than toenails because of faster growth.

Terbinafine is given in a dose of 250 mg daily for 6 weeks and 3 months in fingernails and toenails respectively. It is most effective in dermatophyte infection.

Fluconazole is used for both dermatophytes and yeasts. Dose of 150 mg provided weekly for 3–6 months.

Itraconazole is an antifungal agent effective against dermatophytes and yeasts. Pulse therapy with this agent is now recommended in a dose of 200 mg twice daily for 1 week. This is repeated after a gap of 3 weeks. About 3–4 courses are required for cure.

Griseofulvin can be given 500 mg–1 g daily for 5–6 months for fingernail and 8–18 months for toenail. The treatment is discontinued when clinical and mycological clearance is achieved. There is a high chance of recurrence on stopping the therapy.

If the patient cannot tolerate systemic therapy, then the affected nail can be removed by chemical or surgical avulsion. Topical antifungals should be applied as soon as the nail starts to form.

Pityriasis Versicolor

Pityriasis versicolor is a mild chronic infection of skin caused by dimorphic yeast *Malassezia (M.) furfur*, (previously known as *Pityrosporum (P.) ovale* and *P.*

orbiculare). The infection may cause hypopigmentation, erythematous or hyperpigmented lesions, hence the name versicolor: meaning of various colours. Malassezia can be classified into three serovars A, B and C. Microscopically serovars A and B have round blastopore whereas serovar C has oval blastopores. It is generally seen in young and middle aged adults. *M. furfur* produces pteridin, which produces a pale yellow colour on fluorescence under Wood's lamp.

Malassezia furfur is frequently present in yeast form, it colonises normal skin. The scalp is the most abundant reservoir of the yeast. In case of infection, the spores proliferate in the outer layers of the stratum corneum, often beginning in the areas of follicular openings. When the spores are transformed to hyphae infection occurs. The hyphae do not penetrate the viable epidermis; they cause thickening and disruption of the stratum corneum, which is expressed as fine scales.

The hypopigmentation is due to fungal enzymes, which act on surface lipids to produce decarboxylic acid that diffuses into the epidermis. This acid inhibits tyrosinase; the enzyme responsible for pigment formation, it is also toxic to melanocytes. The infected thick stratum corneum acts as a sunscreen which prevents the ultraviolet light from reaching and stimulating underlying melanocytes. Mechanism of producing hyperpigmentation and erythematous lesions remains unclear; it may be due to hyperkeratosis or inflammation.

Clinical Features

The condition is common in hot humid environment. It mainly affects young adults. Increased sweating is an important factor in causing transition of the commensal yeast to its pathogenic form. There are two distinct presentations; the first is that of slightly scaly hypopigmented or brownish well-defined macules, which may coalesce to form irregular patches. The decarboxylic acid has the ability to inhibit melanin formation. The other presentation is that of reddish-brown scaly lesions, it should be differentiated from seborrhoeic dermatitis; the latter is confined to the center of the chest and back. In long-standing cases, the patches may coalese to form large confluent areas on the skin. The sites of predilection are upper trunk and upper arm, although it may spread to involve neck, face, scalp and abdomen. The condition is asymptomatic. The involved skin gives a pale-yellow fluorescence under Wood's light (Fig. 16).

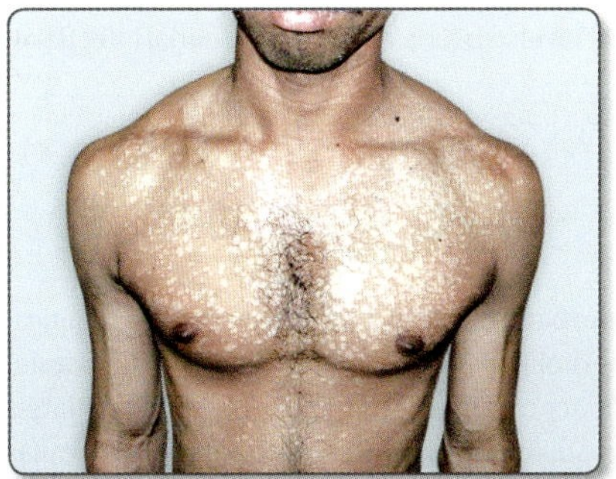

Fig. 16: Pityriasis versicolor

Differential Diagnosis

The macules of vitiligo are milky-white and there is no scaling. Other conditions that need to be differentiated from *P. versicolor* are seborrhoiec dermatitis, secondary syphilis, pityriasis rosea. Syphilis is characterised by lymphadenopathy; changes in the skin, mucous membrane and hair, the infection can be confirmed by a Venereal Disease Research Laboratory (VDRL) test. In pityriasis rosea, the lesions are present along the line of cleavage parallel to the ribs; the herald patch is also present.

Diagnosis

Diagnosis is usually clinical. In cases of doubt, a scraping for the yeast and a KOH examination reveals hyphae and spores with a characteristic spaghetti and meatball appearance.

Examination under a Wood's light shows the pale-yellow fluorescence.

Treatment

Treatment can be local or systemic. If the lesions are chronic and very extensive then the oral treatment is preferred. Griseofulvin is not effective in *P. versicolor*; the newer anti-fungal drugs are used such as the imidazole and fluconazole.

Local treatment: Topical preparations such as half strength Whitfield's ointment (benzoic acid 3% and salicylic acid 1.5%), imidazole creams such as clotrimazole, miconazole 20% sodium thiosulphate solution may also be used; it is cheap and effective. These preparations should be applied for at least a month. The pigment in hypopigmented areas may not return for a few months.

Shampoos containing selenium sulphide and zinc pyrithione are effective in *P. versicolor*.

Selenium sulphide 2.5% shampoo is applied to affected areas daily for 10 minutes for 7 days. Alternatively, it is applied to entire body and left overnight to be washed in the morning.

Zinc pyrithione 1% shampoo or 2% soap is applied to affected areas for 10 minutes daily for 2 weeks. Ketoconazole shampoo is also effective. As recurrences are frequent, the medicated shampoos can be used 1–2 times a week for an indefinite period.

Systemic treatment: Itraconazole 200 mg daily for 7 days. For prophylaxis, 200 mg b.i.d. a day, every month for 6 months.

Fluconazole, 300–400 mg once, repeat after 2 weeks.

Ketoconazole 200 mg for 10 days or 400 mg for two consecutive days.

For prophylactic purposes, it is given as 200 mg tablet for three consecutive days each month. Hepatotoxity limits its use.

Inverse Pityriasis Versicolor

The condition is similar to *P. versicolor*, but it is seen in flexures, it should be differentiated from other lesions of the flexures, such as seborrhoeic dermatitis, candidiasis, intertrigo, erythrasma, inverse psoriasis and other fungal infections.

Always treat the scalp, as it is a major site of the commensal yeast
Hypopigmentation persists for 1–2 months or longer after treatment

Malassezia Folliculitis

The lesions are typically seen on the back, chest and sometimes the extremities. The primary lesion is a pruritic, perifollicular, erythematous papule or pustule. The lesion can be confused with acne vulgaris, but should be differentiated by KOH examination; the face is usually not involved. The treatment is similar to *P. versicolor* (Fig. 17).

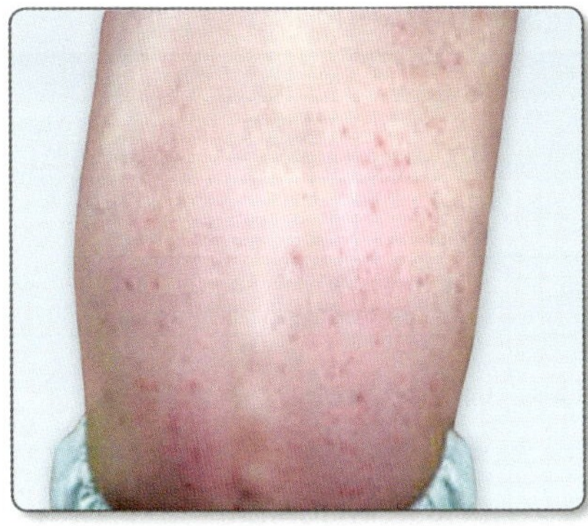

Fig. 17: 'Malassezia folliculitis

Tinea Nigra

This is a superficial asymptomatic fungal infection caused by exophytic nondermatophyte *Phaeoannellomyces werneckii ((Hortaea werneckii)*; it produces a melanin-like pigment. The lesions are usually present on the palms and soles. They appear as brown or black macules single or multiple that may coalesce to form patches, these resemble junctional naevus, melanoma or silver nitrate stains, from which it should be differentiated.

Potassium hydroxide examination reveals brown to olive coloured hyphae and spindle-shaped yeast cells occurring singly or in pairs.

Treatment is by Whitfield's ointment or 40% salicylic acid plaster. Topical imidazoles are also effective.

Piedra (Trichosporosis)

This is an asymptomatic fungal infection confined to hair shafts, resulting in the formation of superficial nodules on them. Two varieties exist, Black and White Piedra. Table 1 shows the difference between Black and White Piedra.

Black Piedra: This is caused by *Piedraia hortae*; it is characterised by the formation of dark gritty, hard nodules, composed of a mass of fungal cells, firmly adherent to the hair shaft. These nodules are gritty to touch. The hair of the scalp, moustache and the beard are commonly affected.

White piedra: This is caused by *Trichosporon beigelii (Trichosporon asahii)*; it is characterised by the formation of soft, white or light-brown nodules that can easily be detached from the hair. The nodules are carried outwards as the hair grows away from the surface of the scalp.

The disease is diagnosed by examining the asci and mycelium with KOH preparation. Cultures produce black colonies composed of hyphae and clamydospores.

Treatment is by cutting the hair, and using imidazole or ciclopirox olamine lotion.

Candidiasis

Candidiasis is the name given to a diverse group of infections caused by *Candida* (*C.*) *albicans* and other members of the genus Candidia; a group

Table 1: Showing the difference between black and white piedra

Black piedra	*White piedra*
Causative organism *Piedraia hortae*	*Trichosporon beigelii* *(Trichosporon asahii)*
Epidemiology Tropical climate	Temperate climate
Site Scalp hair	Facial, axillary and genital hair
Predisposing factors Infestation encouraged by religious and aesthetic factors	Unhygienic conditions
Symptoms Symptomless	Symptomless
Clinical manifestations Fungi firmly attached to the hair Dark nodules Gritty on palpation Can weaken and break the hair Other cutaneous manifestations absent	Fungi less adherent to the hair Beige colored nodules Not gritty on palpation Broken hair less common Cutaneous manifestations may be present, such as onychomycosis, papules, papulovesicles
KOH examination Nodules consist of well-aligned hyphae, packed with thick walled cells. Colonies dark brown or black in colour	Nodules less organised, hyphae arranged perpendicularly on the hair shaft, which can be easily fragmented. Colonies creamy in colour
Treatment Shaving and topical antifungal therapy	Shaving and topical antifungal therapy

which includes at least 150 yeast species. These organisms infect the skin, nails and mucous membranes; they can also infect the internal organs and cause systemic disease. *C. albicans* colonises in oral cavity and bowel especially the colon. Candidiasis is probably caused by infection of the host with its own commensal yeast following its transition to the mycelial form.

Pathogenicity in tissues is associated with the conversion of the organism from yeast to filamentous form. The most important local factor in conversion is moisture; skin folds are commonly involved, so are areas occluded by wet diapers. After the penetration into the stratum corneum the organism elicits a complement mediated acute inflammatory reaction that produces dermatitis and prevents deeper penetration. The increase in glycogen content, and changes in acidity, such as seen in vaginal epithelium, due to oral contraceptive pills and antibiotics predispose to candidiasis.

Candidiasis usually involves the skin, nails and mucous membranes. In case of immunodeficiency, the internal organs are also involved.

The primary lesion is a pustule; the contents of which dissect horizontally under the stratum corneum and peel it away. Clinically this process results in a red denuded glistening surface, with long cigarette paper like scaling and an advancing border. Accumulated scales and inflammatory cells form the characteristic yellowish -white curdy material.

Yeast grows in a warm and moist environment. It is usually confined to the skin, mucous membranes and intertriginous areas. The advancing border usually stops when it reaches the dry skin.

Conditions predisposing to candidiasis include diabetes mellitus, systemic corticosteroid therapy, cytotoxic drugs, prolonged use of antibiotics, AIDS, immune suppression, leukaemia and reticuloses. Excessive exposure to soap and water, warm, occluded and wet environment favours the development of candidiasis.

Clinical Forms of Candidiasis

Oral candidiasis

Thrush. This is a form of oral candidiasis, which is common in infancy, elderly and immunosuppressed patients. It is characterised clinically by bright erythematous lesions covered with a curd-like membrane. The lesions are easily scraped away to leave a red, raw bleeding base (Fig. 18).

Acute atrophic candidiasis. This is often painful, presents as flat eythematous areas usually on the tongue. It is secondary to long-term use of antibiotics.

Chronic hyperplastic candidiasis. This presents as thick white plaques, usually seen in men. It should be differentiated from leukoplakia.

Chronic atrophic candidiasis. This is seen in people wearing dentures. The lesion presents as dusky erythematous areas. The condition should be differentiated from allergic or irritant dermatitis.

Angular cheilitis. Presence of saliva at the angles of the mouth is the most important factor in producing candidiasis. This may occur as a result of mouth breathing, poor fitting dentures and compulsive lip licking. Aggressive use of dental floss may produce mechanical trauma to the angles of the mouth. Advancing age is another factor as excessive folds develop at the angle of the mouth due to the sagging of skin. Shortening of the lower-third of the face from loss of teeth and resultant absorption of the alveolar bone, results in the fluid being drawn into the angle of the mouth due to capillary action. Clinically, this results in maceration of the skin, erythema and secondary infection, both bacterial and due to candida.

Intertrigo or Flexural candidiasis. Any body fold may be involved; large skin folds like axilla, groins, submammary region and area between the buttocks

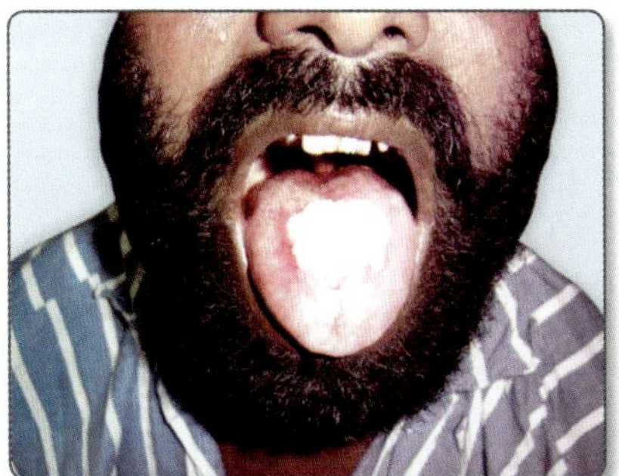

Fig. 18: Thrush

and smaller skin folds such as the web spaces and the angle of the mouth. Candidiasis is common in obese patients. It is characterised clinically by erythematous macerated lesions (pustules get macerated under the skin folds) with satellite papules and pustules. There is itching and soreness (Fig. 19).

Erosio interdigitalis blastomycetica. This is common in housewives who spend long hours working at wet tasks. Macerated white skin is seen on finger webs. The third web between ring and middle finger is the most commonly involved. Usually at the center of the lesion, there are one or more fissures with raw red base; as the condition progresses, the macerated skin peels off, leaving a painful raw denuded area, surrounded by a collar of overhanging white epidermis. The macerated white scale becomes thick and adherent. In this particular condition, candida and Gram-negative bacteria, blastomycetes are co-pathogens (Fig. 20).

Candidal paronychia. The characteristic feature of this disease is redness and swelling of the posterior nailfold, the cuticle is lost at an early stage of the illness and small quantity of pus may be expressed from underneath the nailfold. There is secondary involvement of the nail plate with ridging and

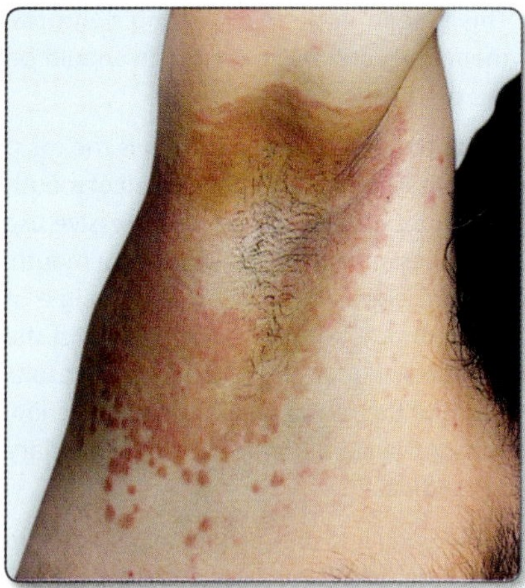

Fig. 19: Flexural candidiasis—note the peripheral papules

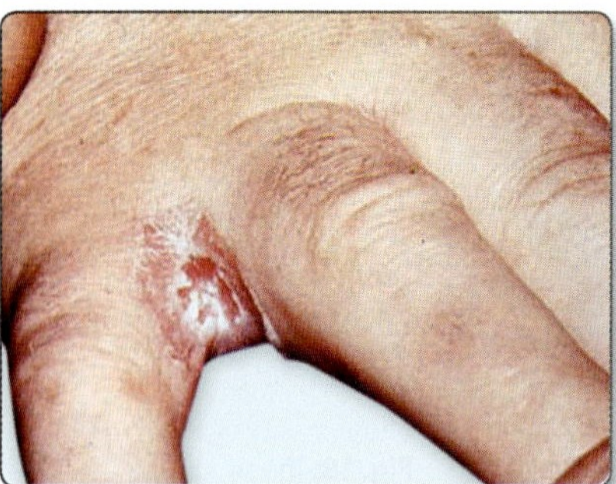

Fig. 20: Interdigital candidiasis

brownish-green discolouration. Initially one finger is infected, but eventually other fingers are involved. It is rare for all fingers to be involved. It should be differentiated from bacterial paronychia, which lacks chronicity and the infection shows all the signs of acute inflammation. Ringworm infection and psoriasis do not involve the nailfold.

It takes weeks or months for the paronychia to clear even with treatment and removal of the predisposing factors. Once the infection is cured, the patient should be instructed to wear gloves for housework and keep the hands dry.

Treatment

General treatment: Remove predisposing factors. In paronychia and flexural candidiasis the importance of keeping the skin dry should be explained to the patient. The patients suffering from paronychia should wear gloves when performing wet tasks. In vulvovaginitis, the use of cotton undergarments should be encouraged. The male partner should use a condom. Good oral hygiene and avoidance of trauma is important in patients suffering from thrush.

Topical therapy: The drugs commonly used in candidiasis include gentian violet, Burrow's solution, imidazole creams and nystatin ointment. Dr Scholls Lamb wool can be placed between the toe webs to separate them and to promote dryness.

Systemic therapy: These include itraconazole and fluconazole. Ketoconazole, can be used in resistant cases.

Vulvovaginitis. Candidal vulvovaginitis is common in pregnancy, diabetes mellitus and in patients on prolonged antibiotic therapy. It is characterised clinically by beefy-red erythema of vaginal mucous membrane and vulval skin, with curdy-white discharge.

Balanitis. There is involvement of glans penis in uncircumcised male. It is characterised clinically by erythematous lesions with papules and pustules. The female partner could be a carrier of infection.

Napkin candidiasis (Diaper candidiasis). This type of candidiasis is characterised by erythematous macerated lesions with satellite papules and pustules. It involves the napkin area excluding the folds.

Chronic mucocutaneous candidiasis. This is persistent candidal infection of the mouth, skin and the nails, which is resistant to ordinary therapy. It is associated with some endocrinological or immunological disorder; a deficiency of iron may also play a part. The clinical presentation may be divided into granulomatous or nongranulomatous. The granulomatous disease is found in children, sex distribution is equal. The lesion usually commences on the face or scalp, the lesion is localised, raised, has an irregular surface that is red and scaly. The lesion gradually enlarges; new lesions develop at the periphery. The nongranulomatous forms such as thrush, intertrigo and paronychia are widespread; paronychia may be present in all the fingers.

Specific Treatment

- Oral candidiasis: Nystatin suspension, imidazole or amphotericin lozenges can be given for oral thrush. Nystatin 100,000 IU/ml oral suspension, 4–6 ml. is held in mouth for a few minutes before swallowing four times a day. Miconazole oral gel can also be used.

Itraconazole 100 mg once daily for 15 days. Alternatively fluconazole 50 mg is given once daily for 2 weeks. In severe cases, ketoconazole 200 mg tablet given daily for 7–14 days.

Dentures if used should be cleaned, soaked overnight in a dilute 1:10 sodium hypochlorite solution and 0.12% chlorhexidine solution.

- Vulvovaginal candidiasis: Nystatin vaginal suppositories 100,000 units are inserted into the vagina twice daily for 10–14 days. Miconazole 2% cream is inserted intravaginally at bedtime for 7 days.

  Fluconazole is given as a single 150 mg dose. Itraconazole 200 mg is given twice for a single day only. Ketoconazole 200 mg can be given daily for 3 days.
- Intertriginous candidiasis: Drying the area is of paramount importance. Gentian violet is very effective, but it discolours the skin and clothes. Other drying solutions are methylrosaniline chloride and eosin solutions.

  Specific topical therapy with imidazoles or nystatin is applied for 2 weeks.

  If the disease is recurrent then oral itraconazole or fluconazole is recommended.
- Napkin candidiasis: The nappies should be changed frequently. The use of plastic panties should be discouraged. Topical anticandidal therapy with imidazoles or nystatin.
- Chronic paronychia requires prolonged treatment. Hands should be kept dry by the use of gloves while doing wet work. Topical nystatin or imidazoles are applied twice daily. Itraconazole pulse therapy is the treatment of choice. 200 mg b.i.d. for 7 days every month for 3 months.

  For prophylaxis:
  - Itraconazole 200 mg once a month
  - Fluconazole 150 mg once a month
  - Ketoconazole half of 200 mg tablet once a month for 6 months. The patient should be monitored for hepatoxicity.
- Chronic mucocutaneous candidiasis: Fluconazole 200–800 mg daily. In resistant cases voriconazole 200–400 mg daily has given promising results. Correct the predisposing factors.

Exclude immunosuppression, diabetes mellitus, hematological malignancies, long-term antibiotic therapy in patients with recurrent candidiasis

SUBCUTANEOUS MYCOSES

These fungi infect the skin and subcutaneous tissue; it rarely disseminates to produce systemic disease. The organisms are present in the soil, plants and decaying vegetable matter. They are inoculated into the skin through local trauma.

Mycetoma (Madura Foot)

It is a chronic localised infection of the skin, subcutaneous tissue and bones caused by various fungi or Actinomycetes. The condition is acquired by penetrating injuries, e.g. thorn prick in those who walk bare foot. It is common in tropical climate.

Aetiology

Mycetoma can be caused by a true fungus (eumycetoma), or by Actinomycetes (actinomycetoma). The causative organisms present in eumycetoma are *Madurella* (*M.*) *grisea, M. mycetomatis, Exophiala (E) jeanselmei, Acremonium recifei.*

The causative organisms in actinomycetoma are *Nocardia* (*N.*) *asteroides, N. brasiliensis*. *Streptomyces (S.) somaliensis*, and *Actinomadura madurae*.

Bacteria such as Staphylococci and Streptococci may also cause mycetoma.

Clinical Features

Mycetoma begins as a firm, painless, subcutaneous swelling on the foot usually the instep or the toe webs. This then forms a painless, nontender firm rubbery mass. The overlying skin is normal or attached to the underlying structures. The mature fully developed lesion is a tumefaction accompanied by the formation of nodules, tubercles or draining sinuses. These sinuses secrete micro-colonies or grains of the causative organism. The grains can be of three varieties: black, red or pearly-cream or yellow. There is no lymphadenitis. The further course depends upon the causative organism. In the black variety, spread is mainly subcutaneous. In the red and yellow varieties, deep penetration occurs early, the muscles and the underlying bones become infiltrated, but unexpectedly nerves and tendons are highly resistant to invasion. Neurological signs are conspicuous by their absence. Blood dissemination does not occur. In course of time, even the black variety involves the underlying fascia, muscles and bone. The lesion extends by local extension and the foot enlarges. Eventually secondary infection occurs. The leg atrophies from disuse (Fig. 21).

Investigation

The colour of the grains gives a clue to the type of the causative organism. Light coloured grains are due to ***A. madurae***, Nocardia, Cephalosporium, ***S. somaliensis***. Red grains are due to ***S. pelletieri***. Black or dark coloured grains are caused by ***M. grisea***, ***E. jeanselmei*** and ***M. mycetomatis***.

Periodic-Acid Schiff stain shows the presence of fungi, Grams stains are positive for Actinomyces species.

X-rays will show the bony involvement.

Diagnosis

Clinically the characteristic triad of tumefaction, sinuses and grains are suggestive of the diagnosis of mycetoma. The diagnosis is confirmed by culture of the organism.

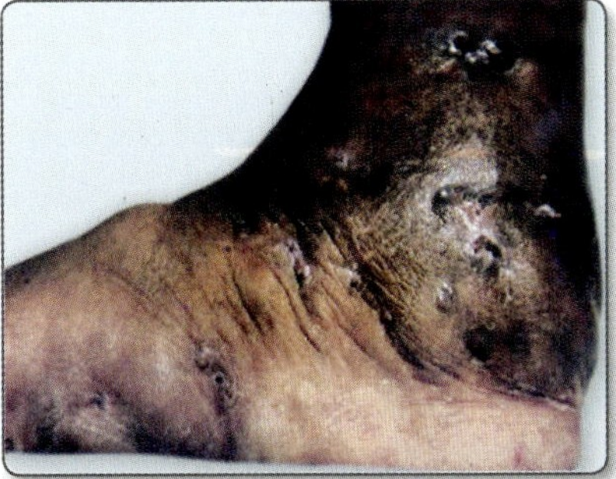

Fig. 21: Madura foot

Differential Diagnosis

The condition needs to be differentiated from chronic osteomyelitis caused by bacteria or tuberculosis. Direct microscopy of pus reveals the characteristic granules. The clinical features of mycetoma are the same whatever the causative organism may be (actinomyces or fungus). Black granules are due to fungus, light coloured grains due to actinomyces. The culture confirms the diagnosis.

Madura foot should also be differentiated from podoconiosis (Price's disease); this is an allergic reaction to silicates found in the red volcanic soil. The soil particles penetrate the skin when walking barefoot then pass to the lymph nodes, where they cause lymphadenopathy, lymph stasis and elephantiasis.

Treatment

Treatment is difficult. Localized lesions can be excised. The fungal mycetoma responds poorly to antifungal therapy. However, itraconazole, fluconazole griseofulvin and ketoconazole, are worth attempting. Amphotericin B has helped some cases. Mycetoma caused by actinomycetes gives a good respond to chemotherapeutic agents. The combination of dapsone with streptomycin or sulphamethoxazole-trimethoprim plus streptomycin gives good result. Alternatively rifampicin can be used.

A combination of systemic therapy and surgical excision of sinuses and tracts is the most effective treatment for madura foot.

Radical surgery should be considered in resistant cases.

Sporotrichosis

This is a granulomatous fungal disease caused by *Sporothrix (S.) schenckii*. It has a worldwide distribution, but is endemic in North and Central America. The fungus penetrates the skin through accidental abrasions or injuries. The incubation period is about 3 weeks.

Clinical Features

The earliest manifestation is a small nodule or an ulcer that may heal before the advent of other symptoms. In course of a few weeks, nodules develop along the lymphatics. These nodules may remain hard or soften and ulcerate. Cutaneous lesions last for months or years.

A chronic localised form "fixed variety" is found in about one third of the patients, this may sometimes present as a verrucous lesion. Subcutaneous abscesses and visceral form manifest a rare disseminated form of sporotrichosis. Histologically, the cutaneous forms show a tuberculoid granuloma.

Diagnosis

Sporothrix schenckii is often not found in histological tissue and it is difficult to stain. Sporothrix schenckii appear as small 3–5 μ, cigar-shaped budding organisms. On culture, a moist white colony develops in 7–10 days.

Differential Diagnosis

The cutaneolymphatic type should be differentiated from atypical mycobacterium infection, leishmaniasis, glanders and tuluremia. The fixed variety should be differentiated from other deep fungal infections and carcinoma.

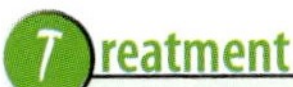

Sporotrichosis is treated by saturated solution of potassium iodide, starting with an initial dose of 5 drops three times a day in milk, increasing according to tolerance up to 30–40 drops at each dose. Signs of intolerance are gastric disturbances, lacrimation, swelling of the salivary glands and skin eruptions of iododerma. Amphotericin B is effective in relapsing or the disseminated variety. Other drugs such as terbinafine 250 mg and itraconazole 200 mg daily are well tolerated. Treatment should be continued for at least 4 weeks after clinical cure.

Chromomycosis (Chromoblastomycosis)

Chromomycosis (verrucous dermatitis) is a chronic cutaneous and subcutaneous infection that persists for years with minimal discomfort. The infection is most common on the lower extremity and 95% of cases occur in males. It is caused by a dematiaceous fungus. The typical patient is a rural agricultural worker of the tropics. At the site of inoculation, red papules develop that eventually coalesce to form a plaque. The plaque slowly enlarges to form a verrucous or warty surface. If not treated a cauliflower-like mass develops with lymphatic obstruction and elephantiasis.

Histopathology shows a foreign body granuloma with isolated areas of abscess formation. Potassium hydroxide preparations show deeply pigmented thick-walled "muriform" cells; culture shows dark velvety colonies. Medical therapy is disappointing;, intralesional amphotericin B, oral 5-flucytosine or itraconazole may help. Surgical excision is often required.

Lobomycosis

Jorge Lobo originally described Lobomycosis in 1931. The disease is reported in tropical countries. Any part of the body may be affected; usually it is the head and neck. The lesion is keloidal, purplish to brownish in color that may ulcerate. The lesions are painless, generally not associated with lymphadenopathy. There is no systemic dissemination. Histological examination shows granulomas with abundant giant cells.

The fungus is not found in nature, snake or arthropod bites may inoculate the fungus into the skin. The causative organism is Loboa loboi, a blastomyces-like organism. Surgical excision is the treatment of choice; this is often followed by recurrence. Chemotherapy is of no value.

Subcutaneous Zygomycosis (Phycomycosis)

Zygomycosis is caused by *Basidiobolus haptosporus* of the class Zygomycetes. Infection may be subcutaneous, visceral and disseminated. Subcutaneous zygomycosis is of two types involving different anatomic sites. Well-defined subcutaneous masses involving the nose, para-nasal tissue and upper lips are involved in one type. The second type has lesions on the extremities, buttocks and trunk. The lesions occur as indurated nodules, these are painless, firm, and freely mobile over the deeper structures, the overlying skin may be tense, edematous, hyperpigmented or normal. Ulceration does not occur and regional lymph nodes are not enlarged. Histology shows eosinophilic granuloma, lying deep in the subcutaneous tissue, largely replacing the fat. The systemic form usually affects the lungs and central nervous system; it is often associated with diabetes and leukaemia. Potassium iodide is the treatment of choice; surgical excision may be helpful. Amphotericin B and itraconazole may be used in some cases.

Phaeohyphomycosis

This is a rare generally localised cutaneous and subcutaneous infection, caused by a variety of brown pigmented (dematiaceous) fungi. Subcutaneous infection begins as a firm tender nodule that may develop into a large cyst up to several centimetres in diameter. The overlying epidermis is greatly thickened. There is no tendency to spread to the lymphoid tissue; systemic dissemination is very rare. Cutaneous disease is similar to that caused by dermatophyte infection. The disease may respond to topical antifungal agents. Other options include surgical excision of the nodule. Systemic Amphotericin B, itraconazole and fluconazole are also helpful.

SYSTEMIC MYCOSES

Deep fungal infections are widely distributed throughout the developing and tropical countries. These infections are slowly progressive; the diseases may eventually become incapacitating or cause death of the patient. The following general features are characteristic of most deep fungal infections.

- They have a chronic course
- Systemic symptoms are usually mild or absent. When the lesion disseminates from the primary focus constitutional symptoms become severe
- Each disease has its own geographic distribution
- The diagnosis is often made by finding the causative fungus in the lesion, exudate, sputum and by the histological examination of the tissue.

Some systemic respiratory fungal infections include blastomycosis, histoplasmosis, coccidioidomycosis and paracoccidioidomycosis. These diseases are similar in pathophysiology, but each has different clinical characteristics. The causative organisms are found in the soil and infection occurs with the inhalation of the organism. The primary infection is in the lungs, dissemination occurs via the lymphatics and blood vessels. Each fungus has a predilection for particular organ system.

Histoplasmosis (Darling's Disease)

This is an infectious disease caused by *Histoplasma* (*H.*) *capsulatum*. The disease begins as a primary acute pulmonary infection, at times erythema nodosum may be the presenting feature. Dissemination occurs to the liver, spleen, kidney, central nervous system, lymph nodes and mucous membrane of the mouth and genitals. The skin lesions may be ulcerated, granulomatous or verrucous.

Histoplasma is unique amongst pathogenic fungi in being predominantly intracellular, found within the cells of the reticuloendothelial system in the form of budding yeast. Potassium hydroxide stains reveal intracellular yeast in the sputum. Peripheral blood culture of *H. capsulatum* are exceedingly infectious, laboratory infections are frequent.

North American Blastomycosis

North American Blastomycosis is caused by Blastomyces dermatitidis; this is a diamorphic fungus producing yeast-like cells in tissues and mycelium in vitro. Potassium hydroxide mounts show thick round refractile spherical cells with broad-based buds. On culture, the colonies are white and cotton like.

The disease first affects the lungs, pulmonary changes resembles tuberculosis. Disseminated skin lesions are rare, these occur as nodules that become ulcerated and vegetating, often forming large masses with peripheral extension. Primary cutaneous form of North American Blastomycosis is similar to sporotrichosis with the formation of primary nodules and subsequent nodules along the draining lymphatics.

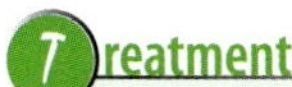

For mild cases itraconazole 200 mg three times daily for 3 days and then 200 mg once or twice daily for a total of 6–12 weeks is recommended. For severe cases lipid formulation of amphotericin B 3–5 mg/kg of body weight, by IV route is given for 1–2 weeks, followed by itraconazole 200 mg three times daily for 3 days, then 200 mg twice daily for a total of 12 weeks is recommended. Ketoconazole 400–800 mg/daily or fluconazole 400–800 mg/daily can be used as an alternative.

Although some patients may tolerate full intravenous doses of amphotericin B without difficulty, most will exhibit some intolerance, often at less than the full therapeutic dose. Tolerance may be improved by treatment with aspirin, antipyretics, such as acetaminophen, antihistamines, or antiemetic.

Amphotericin B is the drug of choice. Ketoconazole 400 mg/day with early reduction to 200 mg/day to be continued for 2–5 months is also helpful. Itraconazole and miconazole are alternative to amphotericin B.

Coccidioidomycosis

This is an infection caused by Coccidioides immitis, found in dry deserts like regions of North and South America. Human infection may be caused by very little exposure to the organism; so that travel cases of coccidioidomycosis are found in many parts of the world. Potassium hydroxide preparations show the characteristic arthrospores produced at intervals along the hyphae.

The primary infection is in the lungs, erythema nodosum and erythema multiforme are common cutaneous presentations. Dissemination occurs in the bones, joints, viscera and the skin. The skin lesions manifest as subcutaneous abscesses that remain localised for several years. Some lesions are like those of mycosis fungoides, in the form of nodules and plaques.

Ketoconazole and itraconazole are effective in patients without central nervous system involvement. Amphotericin B is the drug of choice in immunosuppressed and in patients with involvement of the central nervous system.

Paracoccidioidomycosis (South American Blastomycosis)

The disease is caused by *Paracoccidioides brasiliensis*; it is confined to hot and humid tropical and subtropical forests, especially in Brazil. The disease is more common in men, the male female ratio is 15:1, and it is presumed that the sex difference is due to the inhibitory action of estrogen on the mycelium to yeast transformation necessary for infectivity.

Histology shows a granulomatous and pyogenic inflammation, giant cells are frequent. Potassium hydroxide preparation shows round refractile cells. The fungus is diamorphic; mycelial phase is present only at room temperature.

The first manifestation of the disease occurs in the buccal, oral, pharyngeal or laryngeal mucosa, the lesions present as plaques that become ulcerated and show a characteristic yellowish-white granulation with hemorrhagic spots. Skin lesions are polymorphic, single, multiple, grouped or sparse. Regional lymph nodes enlarge and suppurate. Liver, spleen and central nervous system may be affected. The course is progressive; it may lead to death if untreated.

The treatment of choice is itraconazole; it can produce remission in 3–6 months. Amphotericin is used in more rapidly progressive and extensive infections. Long acting sulphonamides were previously used in the treatment of paracoccidioidomycosis.

Penicilliosis

Penicillium (*P.*) *marneffei* is a recently discovered fungal pathogen, which causes disseminated mycosis. Infection in humans is mainly confined to Southeast Asia. *P. marneffei* is yeast-like oval-shaped organism, about the size of H capsulatum, they reproduce by fission.

The primary site of infection is the lung with respiratory symptoms, such as fever, cough and chest pain. Signs of dissemination include anaemia, hepatosplenomegaly and skin lesions. Cutaneous signs are present in about 50% of cases. These are small papules, ulcers or molluscum-like lesions, scattered on the face and trunk. If untreated the infection is fatal.

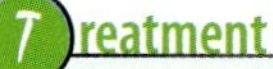

Itraconazole 200–400 mg/day is given for a long time to prevent relapse. Amphotericin B is recommended for severe cases.

OPPORTUNISTIC FUNGAL INFECTION

Opportunistic infections are caused by organisms that typically produce disease in a host with lowered resistance. Many opportunistic fungi involve the skin.

Cryptococcosis

The infection is caused by *Cryptococcus neoformans*; it is encapsulated yeast found in the soil, particularly which is contaminated by pigeon excreta. It is the leading cause of fungal meningitis.

Cryptococcosis unlike other systemic mycosis occurs throughout the world. Portal of entry is usually the lung, central nervous system manifestations predominantly present as meningitis or focal brain lesions simulating a tumour. In the disseminated form skin, liver, bone, prostate and the kidney are affected. Cutaneous lesions are more frequent on the head and neck. A variety of morphological lesions are reported, such as abscesses, tumour-like growths, molluscum contagiosum like lesions, sinuses, plaques, ulcers and cellulitis. Often the skin lesions provide the first evidence of dissemination.

Amphotericin B is the treatment of choice; flucytosine, itraconazole and fluconazole are effective in suppressing recurrences after induction of clinical remission.

Aspergillosis

Aspergillosis is the most frequently encountered fungus in the laboratory. It is second only to candida in the frequency of opportunistic fungal infections. Aspergillus fumigatus is the most common cause of disseminated aspergillosis.

Aspergillus species are primary respiratory pathogens with the lungs and sinuses as the major site of infection. Disseminated disease is seen in 30% of cases. Cutaneous lesions develop in 5%. Cutaneous lesions can be grouped in five categories, solitary necrotising dermal papules, subcutaneous granulomas or abscesses, persistent eruptive dermal papule with suppurative, vegetating or necrobiotic lesions and miscellaneous erythemas. Aspergillosis is a frequent contaminant from thick friable, dystrophic nails.

Amphotericin B is the drug of choice in invasive and cutaneous infection and in immunocompromised patients.

Mucormycosis

Mucormycosis is caused by several fungal genera of the class Zygomycetes. These fungi are present in decaying vegetable matter, fruit and bread. About one-third of the patients have diabetes. There are five major clinical sites of infection: pulmonary, cerebral, cutaneous, gastrointestinal and disseminated. They all share the common feature which includes the invasion of the blood vessel walls this leads to infarction and gangrene. Ulcers, cellulitis, ecthyma and necrotic abscesses comprise cutaneous lesions.

Treatment is by excision of the necrotic lesions and amphotericin B.

Candidiasis

Described earlier.

FURTHER READING

1. Ashben HR, Evans EG. Immunology of diseases associated with Malassezia species. Clin Microbiol. 2002;15:21-57.
2. Chastan MA, Reed RJ, Pankey GA. Deep dermatophytosis: report of two cases and review of literature. Cutis. 2000;67:457-62.
3. Farah CS, Ashman RB, Chailacombe SJ. Oral candidiasis. Clin Dermatol. 2000;18:553-62.
4. Ingham E, Cunningham AC. Malassezia furfur. J Med Mycol. 1993;31:265-88.
5. Kirkpatrich CH. Chronic Mucocutaneous candidiasis. Ped Infec Dis J. 2001;20:197-206.
6. Krowchuk DP, Lucky AW, Primmer SI, et al. Current status, identification and management of tinea capitis. Paediatrics. 1983;72:625-31.
7. Monod M, Baudraz-Rosselet F, Ramelet AA, et al. Direct mycological examination in dermatology and comparison of different methods. Dermatol. 1989;179:183-6.
8. Palestine RF, Rgers RS. Diagnosis and treatment of mycetoma. J Am Acad Dermatol. 1982;6:107-11.
9. Reinel D. Topical treatment of onychomycosis with amorolfine nail lacquer: comparative efficacy and tolerability of once and twice weekly use. Dermatology. 1992;182(Suppl):21-4.
10. Rinaldi MG. Dermatophytosis: epidemiological and microbial update. J Am Acad Dermatol. 2000;43(Suppl):S120-4.

Chapter

6 Viral Infections

INTRODUCTION

Viruses are ultramicroscopic living organisms that multiply in the living cells. They have a central core of nucleic acid either DNA or RNA, a protein coat (capsid) that surrounds the central core, with an outermost lipoprotein envelope. The genetic information is sufficient to encode the protein involved in viral replication, but requires host ribosomes for replication. Host specificity and tissue tropism are hallmarks for viral infection, e.g. polio virus infects neurons; human papillomavirus has a tropism for epithelial cells. As viruses proliferate within a cell, inclusion bodies develop, these can be in the cytoplasm, nucleus or in both. Viruses can be diagnosed by the growth of the virus in cell culture, examination under an electron microscope, detection of antiviral antibodies and immunofluorescence studies.

The following are the common cutaneous viral infections:

- DNA viruses

Herpes virus

- ➢ Herpes virus hominis (Type 1 and 2)
- ➢ Varicella-zoster virus
- ➢ Human cytomegalovirus
- ➢ Epstein-Barr virus
- ➢ Herpes virus 6, 7 and 8

Pox virus

- ➢ Variola, vaccinia virus
- ➢ Molluscum contagiosum virus
- ➢ Orf virus
- ➢ Milker's nodule virus

Papova virus

- ➢ Human papillomavirus

- RNA viruses

Picorna virus

- ➢ Coxsackie virus
- ➢ Echovirus

Myxovirus and Paramyxovirus

- ➢ Measles virus
- ➢ German measles virus
- ➢ Mumps virus

- Retro virus

HIV virus (Discussed in chapter 8).

HERPES VIRUS INFECTIONS

Herpes viruses are large DNA viruses, they multiply in the nucleus and produce typical intranuclear inclusions. A typical feature of all herpes viruses is that after clinical recovery the virus persists in patients as a latent infection. Under certain conditions the virus becomes reactivated to produce an acute infective episode with cellular damage.

Herpes Simplex

Herpes simplex virus (HSV) is a common viral disease distributed throughout the world. There are two types of herpes simplex infections:

1. Type 1 affects the face and trunk above the waist.
2. Type 2 causes genital lesions; this usually spreads by sexual contact.

Pathogenesis

Clinically, HSV infection can be divided into three stages: acute infection, a latent period and reactivation of the virus. In the primary or acute infection, the virus replicates at the site of primary inoculation, usually a mucocutaneous junction. It then travels by retrograde axonal route to regional sensory ganglia where further replication occurs. Here the viral DNA is incorporated in the host DNA and becomes inaccessible to immune mechanisms and chemotherapy before recurring as outbreaks of reactivation.

Reactivation occurs at frequent intervals. Reactivation of HSV 1 is frequently from trigeminal ganglia; and of HSV 2 from sacral ganglia. Some factors responsible for activation of HSV are sunlight, stress, fever, infection and menstruation. The viral particles then move down the anterograde axonal route to a peripheral site, usually near the original site of entry, and replicate in the epithelial cells of the skin, to produce an outburst of cold sores.

The recurrent infection is usually mild, of a shorter duration than the primary lesion. After many recurring attacks in the same location, telangiectasia, lymphoedema, depigmentation and scars may appear.

Histopathology

This is similar for HSV, varicella and zoster infections. Intraepidermal vesicles, ballooning degeneration of keratinocytes and large multinucleated giant cells are present in the epidermis. The nucleus of the affected cells shows specific intranuclear inclusions. The individual cells become greatly enlarged with pale vacuolated cytoplasm. Early in infection the inclusion bodies are basophilic, they rapidly become acidophilic. Giant cells are formed by the fusion of infected cells. Intranuclear inclusions and giant cells are not found in poxvirus infections.

Clinical Features

Herpes simplex is characterised by a group of vesicles on an erythematous base. In course of a few days, these vesicles rupture and the dried serum forms a flaky crust. The lesions heal without scarring in a few days. It usually occurs at or near the mucocutaneous junction; the common locations are around the mouth, eyes and the genitals.

Herpes Simplex 1

Orofacial herpes simplex: The infection is caused by HSV 1. The primary infection often occurs in the oral cavity (herpes gingivostomatitis); the disease is common in children. The primary lesion may be in the soft palate, hard palate, buccal mucosa or even the pharynx, this should be differentiated from streptococcal sore throat. It is accompanied by fever, myalgia and difficulty in swallowing. The lesion is manifested by swelling and redness of the mucous membrane; this bleeds easily and it is painful. After one or two days small vesicles in a group occur, these rupture to form shallow ulcers. There is regional enlargement of the lymph nodes. Lesions heal without scarring in 2–4 weeks.

Reactivation of the virus usually involves the lips. Most of these are on the vermilion border. The lesions appear as grouped vesicles on an erythematous base. These rapidly develop into pustules, often painful with dysesthesia and neuralgia. The lesion resolves in 10–15 days. It is not associated with systemic symptoms. Recurrences are usually at the same site or a few millimeters away. Herpes virus can spread by autoinoculation to other parts of the body such as the eyes and hands (Fig. 1).

Herpetic whitlow: Primary infection on the finger is called herpetic whitlow. This is commonly seen in dentists, doctors and nurses.

Herpes gladiatorum: This is a herpetic infection seen primarily in contact sport players such as wrestlers and rugby players. The players abrade their skin and come into contact with an active HSV infection of their opponent. The virus then becomes latent in the sensory nerve ganglia and recurrent attacks at ectopic sites are possible. The common sites affected are the head, then the extremities and trunk. The disease is often misdiagnosed because of its atypical position.

Herpes Simplex Virus 2

Genital herpes simplex: This is caused by herpes virus 2 and it is more common in women. The primary infection is similar to herpes virus 1 infection. The primary infection is associated with extensive genital lesions; these may be papules, vesicles, pustules or superficial painful ulcers, with associated bilateral lymphadenopathy. The lesions are present on the vulva, vagina or cervix in females and on the penis in males. The cervix is involved in 80%

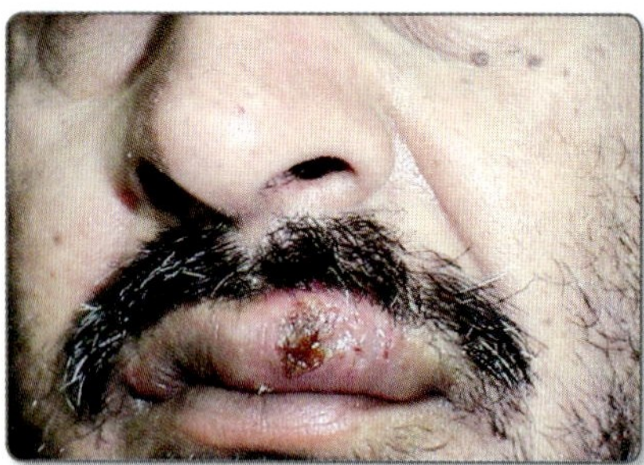

Fig. 1: Herpes simplex (Virus 1)

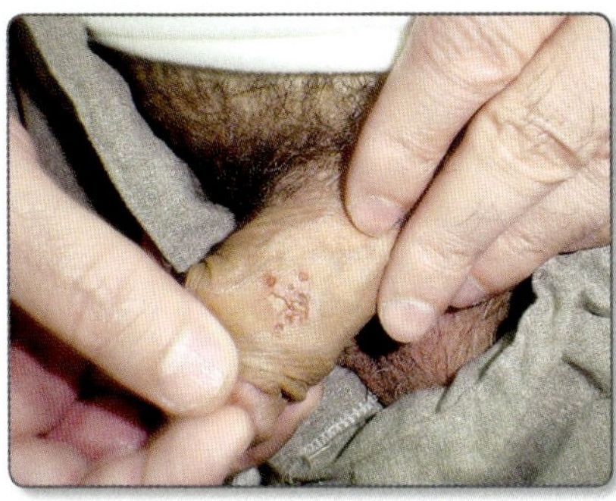

Fig. 2: Herpes simplex (Virus 2)

of cases. Symptoms include dysuria, pain, itching and urethral or vaginal discharge. Healing occurs after 2–3 weeks (Fig. 2).

Lesions reactivate more frequently in herpes 2 infections. The clinical manifestation is typical of herpes infection; grouped vesicular lesions on an erythematous base, with minimal symptoms. Burning, itching and pain may herald the recurrent lesion.

Genital infections can also occur with Herpes simplex virus 1, following oral-genital contact

Neonatal herpes simplex: Primary herpes can also occur in a newborn from herpes simplex infection in the mother through the vaginal secretions. The infection is seen 4–7 days after birth. Neonatal infection can occur without skin lesions, it may directly involve the central nervous system and visceral organs. This infection is devastating in a neonate. It should be diagnosed and treated promptly.

The infection occurs through maternal HSV 2 virus. The course in the newborn is severe because of incomplete immune response. Cesarean section should be performed in cases where the mother has HSV infection.

Associations and Complication

- Recurrent erythema multiforme: Herpes simplex acts as a trigger for erythema multiforme. Perhaps in these patients the serum contains immune complexes composed of antibodies and herpes simplex antigen. The erythema multiforme can be prevented by oral acyclovir.
- Eczema herpeticum (Kaposi's varicelliform eruption): This is a widespread infection, in a skin damaged by eczema usually atopic dermatitis. It can also be seen in other conditions, such as patients receiving immunosuppressive therapy, bullous disorders, Darier's disease, mycosis fungoides, etc. There is a generalised eruption of vesicles, which become pustular and umbilicated. There is high fever, lymphadenopathy, mortality rate is high (Fig. 3).
- Recurrent keratoconjunctivitis, corneal opacity and visual loss may occur, if the eye is affected.
- Herpes simplex virus 2 increases the risk of cervical cancer when associated with papillomavirus.

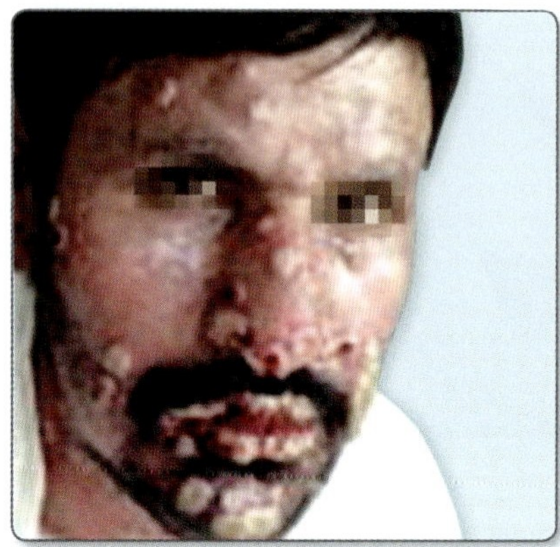

Fig. 3: Eczema herpeticum

Diagnosis

Clinical examination is usually sufficient for diagnosis. Specific tests for herpes simplex infection are:

- Viral culture: This is most specific but less sensitive on culture, there is 75% sensitivity in primary and 50% in recurrent infection.
- Tzanck test: A smear is made of the cells from the base of the vesicle. The cells are spread on a glass slide and stained with Giemsa's or Wright's stain. Multinucleated giant cells are seen
- Enzyme-linked immunosorbent assay (ELISA) for epidemiological studies
- Monoclonal antibodies: The use of specific monoclonal antibodies directed against HSV 1 and HSV 2 for rapid and precise diagnosis of HSV infection
- Nucleic acid hybridisation: This is used to detect viral nucleic acid in the infected tissues.

- After many recurring attacks of herpes simplex in the same location, telangiectasia, lymphoedema, depigmentation and scars may appear.
- Herpes simplex virus is a common cause of encephalitis in adults. Often there is no skin, or mucosal lesions. Lesions are found in the temporal lobe and the limbic system. Mortality is high.

Differential Diagnosis

Impetigo is commonly mistaken for secondary infected herpes simplex infections. Site of infection and the golden crust of impetigo should help in differentiating the two conditions. Contact eczema is associated with a history of irritation. Genital herpes should be differentiated from the syphilitic chancre, which is superficial and indurated. Other ulcers of the oral cavity should be differentiated such as aphthous ulcers, Behcet's disease, etc.

Treatment

Both the primary and recurrent attacks of herpes simplex are usually self-limiting and require only symptomatic treatment. Antiviral therapy reduces the time of healing in both cutaneous and genital herpes. Thus if required the treatment should be started within 48 hours of the onset of the rash. The paediatric dose of acyclovir is 15 mg/kg of acyclovir suspension, given five times a day for 7 days. The adult dose of acyclovir is 200 mg five times daily for 7 days. The antiviral treatment of primary herpes simplex does not decrease subsequent recurrences. For genital herpes, the sexual partners should also be investigated and treated.

Contd...

Contd...

For recurrent attacks the precipitating factors should be avoided. Protection from ultraviolet radiation (UVR) may help to reduce viral reactivation of herpes labialis. The treatment for recurrent attacks of herpes simplex is with topical acyclovir cream, which should start within the first 48 hours of the infection. Symptomatic treatment with calamine lotion, betadine paint, analgesics for pain; topical antibiotics are helpful if there is secondary infection. Steroids should not be applied. If a person has multiple attacks of herpes simplex, 200 mg of acyclovir may be given twice a day for several months. This may reduce the number of attacks.

Herpes simplex infection can be life-threatening in atopic individuals and immunosuppressed patients, in such case hospitalisation, systemic therapy with acyclovir, and supportive care is required. Acyclovir is given in a dose of 200 mg every 3 hours, or by IV route 5 mg/kg every 8 hours. Other antiviral drugs that can be used are famciclovir 250 mg three times a day for 7–10 days and valacyclovir 500 mg thrice daily for 7–10 days. Topical idoxuridine is also helpful.

For patients who are scheduled for surgery and have a history of herpes infection, should receive antiviral therapy 2 days before the surgery and for 5 days after surgery.

Neonatal HSV infection should be treated with immunoglobulin and IV acyclovir.

Suppressive therapy is required in patients who have recurrent attacks of herpes and who develop erythema multiforme after each recurrence. These patients should be started on long-term therapy with acyclovir 400 mg twice daily, valacyclovir 1 g once daily or famciclovir 250 mg twice daily. Once adequate suppression has been established, the dose should be tapered to the minimal effective dose.

Always exclude herpes simplex infection in recurrent erythema multiforme

Varicella (Chickenpox)

Varicella is an acute contagious disease, often seen in childhood, caused by Varicella-zoster virus; a member of herpes virus family.

Incubation period is from 14 to 21 days. The eruptions start as small macules that develop into vesicles within 24 hours. The rash begins on the face and scalp; then rapidly spreads on the trunk. The limbs are relatively less affected. The lesions are also seen on the mucous membrane of the mouth. The exanthem is polymorphous. In children, systemic symptoms are mild. Low-grade fever, malaise and headache are usually present. After recovery from infection, the virus may remain dormant in the sensory root ganglia; this may give rise to herpes zoster later in life (Fig. 4).

The infection is more virulent in adults. The rash is preceded by malaise, fever and headache 2–3 days before the rash. Systemic complications are often seen. Adults should be treated with acyclovir.

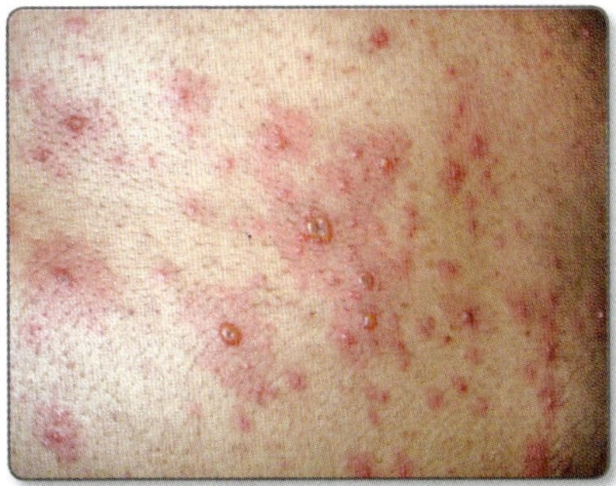

Fig. 4: Chickenpox

Complications

These are rare; encephalitis, pneumonia, glomerulonephritis are most frequently seen. Local infections, such as impetigo, furuncles, cellulitis and gangrene can occur. Most of the infections are due to secondary infection by *Staphylococcus* or *Streptococcus*. Thrombocytopenia with purpura and bleeding into the mucous membrane is a rare complication.

Maternal infection with varicella in the first 4 months of pregnancy may result in fetal malformations, such as central nervous system (CNS) disorders, ocular defects, limb hypoplasia and neonatal deaths. Infection in the second trimester results in undetected fetal chickenpox. The newborn child is at risk of developing herpes zoster. If the mother gets varicella infection a few days before or after birth of a child, the neonate has no antibodies and is at risk of severe varicella. Mortality of about 30% will occur in the absence of treatment. Infants should receive varicella-zoster immune globulin and IV acyclovir therapy.

Pregnant women with chickenpox should receive high doses of acyclovir in a dose of 18 mg/kg of body weight every 8 hours.

Reye's syndrome is acute noninflammatory encephalopathy associated with hepatitis or fatty metamorphosis of the liver. Twenty to thirty percent of Reye's syndrome is preceded by varicella. The fatality rate is 20%. Salicylates used during varicella infection may increase the risk of development of Reye's syndrome.

Diagnosis

This is usually clinical. Definite diagnosis is by viral culture. Immunofluorescent or immunoperoxidase staining of cellular material from fresh vesicles can detect varicella-zoster virus often faster than viral culture.

Treatment

In children only symptomatic treatment is required; calamine lotion is soothing and prevents itching. Local or systemic antibiotic may be required for secondary infection. Oral antihistamines help in relieving pruritus and providing sedation. In severe cases, acyclovir is given in a dose of 800 mg every 3 hours for 7 days. Adults should always be treated with oral acyclovir to prevent systemic complications.

Vaccination: Life attenuated varicella vaccine is available. Children in 12–18 months of age should receive one dose of the vaccine. Children over 13 years of age should receive two doses at 4–8 weeks interval. The effect lasts for 6 years.

Herpes Zoster (Shingles)

This eruption is usually confined to an area supplied by one sensory nerve ganglion and thus it is unilateral. The skin lesions are preceded by pain in the affected area, after 2 or 3 days the pain subsides and the skin lesions appear. These are red grouped vesicles on an erythematous base. After a few days, the vesicles may become pustular, dry up or rupture forming a crust. The scabs form after 7–10 days, these then eventually fall off. There may be some constitutional upset with the eruption; the regional lymph nodes may be enlarged. In severe cases, the vesicles may become haemorrhagic or necrotic. Peak age is 50–70 years.

Aetiology

After recovery from chickenpox the virus remains dormant in the sensory root ganglion. The reasons for the activation of the virus are not known, after activation the virus travels down the sensory nerve from the ganglion to the skin. Pain preceding the eruption is due to the involvement of the sensory nerve. Generalised herpes zoster may occur in persons with impaired immunity.

Clinical Features

There is usually a prodomal phase of pain or dysaesthesia before the eruption of the rash. The phase may last for about 7 days. Sometimes the pain is severe, and may be misdiagnosed as a myocardial infarction when present on the chest, or appendicitis in the abdomen.

The most common site of involvement is the thoracic region followed by the lumbar and the cervical dermatomes. This could possibly be due to the centripetal distribution of chickenpox; most of the lesions are on the trunk. The lesions appear as grouped vesicles on an erythematous base, which last for about 7 days. In some cases the lesions can become haemorrhagic or necrotic. Widespread lesions suggest immunosuppression (Fig. 5).

In the ophthalmic zoster, there is involvement of the ophthalmic division of the trigeminal nerve. Lesions appear on the side of the forehead that is affected and there may be a vesicle on the nose (Hutchinson's sign) if the nasociliary branch of the nerve is affected. The eye complications occur in about 50% of cases; these include keratitis, iridocyclitis and ulcers of the cornea and conjunctiva. Involvement of the ciliary ganglion may give rise to Argyrll-Robertson pupil. Involvement of maxillary division of the trigeminal nerve produces vesicles along the nerve, on the uvula and tonsillar region. Involvement of the mandibular division produces vesicles on the anterior part of the tongue, floor of the mouth and buccal mucosa.

Involvement of the geniculate ganglion results in the Ramsay Hunt syndrome with pain and vesicles on the pinna and external auditory canal. Lesions are present on the anterior two-thirds of the tongue, facial palsy and auditory symptoms may also occur.

If the virus affects the anterior horn cells of the corresponding sensory ganglion then paresis may occur, myelitis and encephalitis are rare complications of herpes zoster infection. Skin lesions may become generalised in persons with immune deficiency. The most common complications of herpes zoster are secondary infection and postherpetic neuralgia.

Postherpetic neuralgia is common in the elderly and may persist for months or years. It is persistence or recurrence of pain, which occurs a month after zoster, better considered after 3 months. Postherpetic neuralgia is more likely to develop if the acute attack of zoster pain was severe, and if zoster rash was prolonged.

An attack of herpes zoster does not confer lasting immunity. It is possible that a patient may have 2–3 episodes in a lifetime.

"Zoster Sine Herpete", is neuralgia without a rash. Varicella-zoster complement fixation tests are required to confirm the diagnosis.

Children and adults exposed to herpes zoster may get chickenpox if they did not have chickenpox earlier in life.

There is an increased incidence of herpes zoster with increasing age as T cell immunity for the virus wanes.

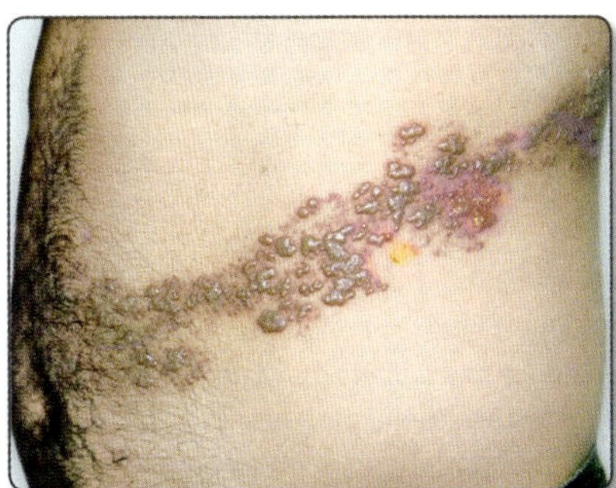

Fig. 5: Herpes zoster

Complications

Postherpetic neuralgia is the most common complication of herpes zoster and the most difficult to treat. It is unusual in children, it increases in severity with age. The pain can be continuous, burning, spasmodic or shooting. The pain is neuropathic; it results from injury to the peripheral nerves, and altered CNS signal processing.

After injury the peripheral neurons discharge spontaneously, have lower activation thresholds and display exaggerated response to stimuli. Axonal regrowth after injury produce nerve sprouts; which are prone to unprovoked discharge. The excessive peripheral activity is thought to lead to hyper-excitability of the dorsal nerve, resulting in exaggerated CNS response to all input. These changes may be so complex that no single therapeutic approach will ameliorate all the abnormalities.

In immunocompromised patients or patients with lymphomas, disseminated zoster develops, which may be haemorrhagic. Systemic involvement may occur that can be fatal.

In the elderly and undernourished, the local eruption often becomes necrotic; this may be followed by scarring.

Visceral involvement may lead to abdominal pain, pleural pain and temporary electrocardiography (ECG) abnormalities.

Motor involvement may occur in 5% of cases. This is due to the spread of infection from the dorsal to the anterior horn of the spinal cord. Motor neuropathies are usually transient and about 75% of cases recover.

Abdominal hernia may follow zoster of the 10th and 11th thoracic nerve root. Zoster of the anogenital area is associated with disturbances of defecation and urination. Facial palsies have occurred with herpes zoster oticus.

Secondary infection, eczematisation, scarring and keloid formation may follow herpes zoster. Scar sarcoidosis may occur.

In trigeminal zoster, ocular complications, such as uveitis, keratitis, conjunctivitis, ocular muscle palsies, proptosis, scleritis, retinal vascular occlusion, scarring and necrosis of the lid may occur. Involvement of the ciliary ganglion may result in Argyll-Robertson pupil.

Encephalitis and meningoencephalitis.

Granulomatous angiitis of cerebral arteries.

Anesthesia of the involved segment, this is especially troublesome, when it affects the area supplied by the ophthalmic nerve.

Superficial gangrene and delayed healing.

Acute retinal necrosis and Guillian- Barre syndrome are rare complications of herpes zoster

Differential Diagnosis

Ophthalmic zoster should be differentiated from erysipelas, in which eruptions are usually bilateral vesicles in erysipelas are present on the edge of the eruption and are not grouped.

Pre-eruptive zoster is easily confused with the pain of pleurisy, myocardial infarction, cholecystitis, appendicitis and renal colic depending upon the site of zoster.

Diagnosis

The clinical picture is characteristic, usually no investigations are required. Tzanck's smear, immunofluorescent staining of smear with monoclonal antibodies, may be needed in some cases.

Prophylaxis of Postherpetic Neuralgia

Systemic corticosteroids with antiviral therapy; and vitamin B12 have been used, but there is no satisfactory evidence that it alters the course of the disease and prevents postherpetic neuralgia in the elderly patients.

Low dose of nortriptyline 10–20 mg at night, as soon as herpes zoster is diagnosed may be helpful in patients above the age of 60 years.

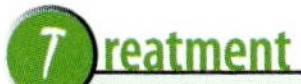

The patients are elderly and so, oral acyclovir should be initiated, to avoid complications. Oral acyclovir should be instituted within 48 hours of the rash. This is given in a dose of 800 mg given five times daily for 7–10 days. Symptomatic treatment is required in most cases for the pain, pruritus and paresthesia. Topical antiseptics for secondary infections, calamine lotion applied every 4–6 hours is soothing. Eye involvement should be treated by an ophthalmologist.

It is possible that early aggressive treatment may prevent the postherpetic neuralgia. Pain must be controlled. The dose and drug should be selected according to the needs of the individual. If less potent analgesics are inefficient, stronger agents should be prescribed until the pain is relieved.

Oral acyclovir with steroids is recommended for severe zoster especially if it involves the ophthalmic division of the trigeminal nerve. The steroid is then tapered over 21 days. The other antiviral drugs that can be used are famciclovir, valacyclovir and foscarnet.

In the treatment of herpes zoster oticus (Ramsay-Hunt syndrome), corticosteroids are usually given in order to reduce the inflammatory swelling and consequent compression of the facial nerve. It is given in a dose of 60 mg/day/for 2 weeks and then tapered off in the 3rd week.

Vitamin E 400 mg, one to three times daily has been used in the treatment of herpes zoster.

Treatment of Postherpetic Neuralgia

Postherpetic neuralgia is one of the most unrewarding conditions to treat. It is important to avoid analgesics that are addictive.

Lidocaine patches, eutectic mixture of local anaesthetics (EMLA) cream, aspirin tablets crushed in alcohol are easy to use. Capsaicin (0.025%) can be applied locally; it causes intense burning which may reduce patient compliance.

Simple analgesics such as nonsteroidal anti-inflammatory drugs (NSAIDs): a higher dose may be required, e.g. ibuprofen 600–1,200 mg daily, acetaminophen 1.5–4 g daily. Ibuprofen is ineffective in the normal dose.

Tricyclic antidepressant drugs are important components of therapy for postherpetic neuralgia. They block the reuptake of serotonin and norepinephrine. These drugs relieve pain by increasing the inhibition of spinal neurons involved in pain perception. Amitriptyline is better tolerated in older patients; it should be started at a low dose (12.5–25 mg) at bedtime, increased weekly until the pain subsides. Maprotiline or nortriptyline may be tried if amitriptyline is ineffective.

Anticonvulsant drugs, such as carbamazepine 400–1,200 mg daily, are used to reduce the lancinating component of neuropathic pain.

Gabapentin and pregabalin may also be used. Gabapentin is structurally related to neurotransmitter gamma-aminobutyric acid (GABA), the exact mechanism how it acts is not known. It is given in a dose of 300–600 mg tid. Start at 300 mg qd, gradually increase the dose.

If the pain does not improve, then a weak opium analgesic may be added such as tramadol 200–400 mg daily or codeine 120 mg daily. These are used keeping the risk of sedation and dependence in mind.

Intralesional injection of xylocaine may be injected at the most painful site. The injection may be repeated every 4–5 days. Nerve block may be tried in difficult cases. Patient should be referred to pain management centres, if required.

Prevention of Varicella-Zoster Infection

In 1995, the US Food and Drug Administration approved attenuated varicella vaccine. The recommended age for vaccination is 12–18 months. The vaccine is administered as 0.5 mL subcutaneous dose to children who have not had chickenpox. Those over the age of 12 should receive two 0.5 mL subcutaneous doses at 1-month interval.

Because the vaccine is a live attenuated virus, vaccine recipients are at a risk for developing herpes zoster in later life. It should not be given to immunocompromised patients, patients who have received blood transfusions within the last 5 months and those who have received varicella-zoster immune globulin within proceeding 5 months.

Varicella-zoster immunoglobulin (VZIG): It is used for passive immunisation of immunocompromised patients after exposure to chickenpox or herpes zoster. It is given within 96 hours after exposure.

Cytomegalovirus Infection

Cytomegalovirus (CMV) is a herpes virus, it occurs worldwide, 90% of the patients are asymptomatic. CMV is so named because it induces megalocytes (large cells) in cell culture. In the newborn, it is associated with cerebral and cerebellar atrophy, microcephalus, deafness and blindness due to optic atrophy. Cutaneous manifestations result from anaemia and thrombocytopenia. Primary infection is followed by lifelong carriage of the virus, with intermittent shedding in various secretions of the body. Systemic infection in infants can lead to sepsis, extramedullary haemopoiesis with cutaneous nodules; blueberry muffin baby.

Symptomatic infection in adults is unusual, except in the immunocompromised. In these patients the symptoms include pneumonia, chorioretinitis and hepatic dysfunction.

Cytomegalovirus mononucleosis: This presents as follicular, maculopapular or rubelliform eruptions, on the legs. Lymphocytic vasculitis manifests as papules and plaques in an annular configuration. Livido reticularis is also described.

Diagnosis

The disease is diagnosed by finding the typical intranuclear inclusions, surrounded by a clear halo in the large cells (owl eye cells). Congenital CMV can only be diagnosed by virus isolation or the presence of CMV IgM antibody within 3 weeks of birth.

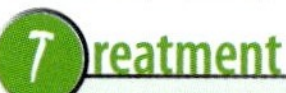

Cytomegalovirus does not require specific therapy. In severe infections two antiviral agents, ganciclovir and foscarnet have been found to be successful.

*Cytomegalovirus is transmitted via the placenta to the fetus. It is associated with the TORCH syndrome, which stands for: **T**oxoplasmosis, **O**thers, **R**ubella, **C**ytomegalovirus and Herpes simplex.*

Epstein-Barr Virus

This is an antigenetically distinct member of the herpes virus group. This virus was originally observed in Burkitt's lymphoma. Epstein-Barr virus (EBV) selectively infects the B lymphocytes and occasionally certain squamous epithelial cells. Primary infection may be asymtomatic or presents as infectious mononucleosis. Following infection, the virus persists for life in the B lymphocytes, 0.1–5% of these cells are infected per millimeter of blood. Under certain conditions, these cells are activated. EBV is associated with the following diseases:

- Infectious mononucleosis
- Burkitt's lymphoma
- B cell tumour
- Post-transplant lymphoproliferative disease.

Other diseases associated with EBV are:

- Oral hairy leukoplakia
- Gianotti-Crosti syndrome
- Lipschutz ulcer
- Erythema multiforme
- Erythema nodosum
- Erythema annulare centrifugum.

Infectious Mononucleosis (Glandular fever)

Epstein-Barr virus infects B cells and the epithelial cells of the oropharynx and nasopharynx. The infection is associated with fever, malaise and headache. Cutaneous and mucous membrane lesions are present in one-third of patients. Macular eruption is seen on the trunk and upper extremities. Lesions of the mucous membrane consist of pinhead-size lesions, 5–20 in number, present on the soft and hard palate. Patients have pharyngitis, and are often treated with ampicillin or amoxicillin; they then develop the characteristic morbilliform drug eruption.

Lymphadenopathy, splenomegaly, lymphocytosis and atypical lymphocytes in the peripheral blood characterise infectious mononucleosis. After an incubation period of a few days to several weeks, there is bilateral lymph node enlargement of the cervical glands. Axillary and inguinal glands may occasionally be infected.

The blood shows absolute lymphocytosis and monocytosis with abnormally large lymphocytes, these are basophilic and contain foamy cytoplasm and fenestrated nucleus. Atypical lymphocytes (Downey cells) are present in 1–10% of total lymphocyte count.

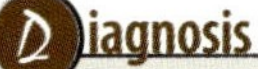

- Examination of blood for abnormal lymphocytes
- Test for hetrophilic antibodies, that agglutinate sheep or horse RBC, but not by guinea pig
- Paul-Bunnell test is positive
- During infection IgM antibody persists for a few months, IgG for life.

In small children EBV is one of the triggers of Gianotti-Crosti Syndrome. EBV is responsible for oral hairy leukoplakia in HIV patients. EBV is an important cofactor in Burkitt's lymphoma.

Human Herpesvirus (HHV) 6, 7 and 8

These viruses are newly recognised viruses; that share close genetic, biologic and immunologic features. They differ from the other human herpes viruses, in their primary T cell tropism and their inability to directly induce cellular transformation in vitro. They are present in normal population in a latent phase and have been implicated in various disorders. At birth most of the children have IgG antibodies to HV 6 and 7 because of their exposure to maternal immunoglobulin.

The most accurate method for the detection of these viruses is by the polymerase chain reaction. Other methods employed include immunohistochemistry and RNA in situ hybridisation.

Human Herpes Virus 6 (Roseola Infantum, Sixth Disease)

Salahuddin first described this infection in 1986. It was isolated from a lymphoproliferative disorder in the B lymphocytes. Serologically the virus differs from the HSV, it is closest to CMV, there is cross hybridisation between the CMV and herpes virus 6.

As seen with other HV infection; after primary infection HV 6 remains latent in the monocytes and macrophages, probably also in the salivary glands. The virus infects infants through saliva mainly from the mother.

Roseola infantum is a common cause of high fever in infants and young children. High-grade fever, convulsions and lymphadenopathy characterise the disease. Lymphadenopathy usually of the occipital region begins before the eruption of the rash and persists until after the rash has subsided. Suddenly on the 4th day the fever drops, the child sits up and commences to play. With the drop of fever, a morbilliform rash appears on the neck, trunk and buttocks. The rash may occasionally be seen on the face and extremities. In a few days complete resolution occurs, with no sequelae.

Herpes virus 6 is thought to play an important role in activation and propagation of HIV infection.

Only symptomatic treatment is required. Ganciclovir or foscarnet can be helpful in severe cases.

Human Herpes Virus 7

This is a new virus isolated from T lymphocytes. At present, it is not known if it causes any disease.

Human Herpes Virus 8 (Kaposi's Sarcoma Associated Herpes Virus)

In 1994, Chang et al. found two DNA fragments of HV 8 in AIDS-associated Kaposi's sarcoma. This virus is also associated with classic Kaposi's sarcoma.

POXVIRUS

The poxviruses are the largest animal viruses, being only slightly smaller than the smallest bacteria; they are just visible by the ordinary microscope. They replicate in the cytoplasm and form eosinophilic inclusion bodies (Guarnieri bodies). The virus is especially adapted to the epidermal cells. Poxvirus causes a number of diseases, such as smallpox, cowpox, orf, milker's nodule, tanapox and molluscum contagiosum. Smallpox is now eradicated globally.

Molluscum Contagiosum

This is a worldwide disease caused by a poxvirus. There are three types of molluscum contagiosum virus (MCV): MCV 1, MCV 2 and MCV 3. No clinical difference has been found in the different strains. MCV 1 is responsible for the majority of infections. The virus occurs throughout the world, the infection is rare before the age of one year, and peak incidence of infection is between 10 years and 12 years. In adults the condition is transmitted sexually.

Aetiology

Molluscum contagiosum virus is a poxvirus; it multiplies in the cytoplasm of the infected cells and induces hyperplasia. Unlike the other poxvirus, it has not been reproduced in tissue culture.

Pathogenesis

Viral growth is confined to the epidermis. The virus particles are synthesised in the malpighian and granular layers. The rate of cell division is much higher in the basal layer of lesional skin. The viral DNA synthesis causes cellular proliferation, this produces a lobulated epidermal growth that compresses the papilla, until they appear as fibrous septa between the lobules, which are pear-shaped with the apex upwards. The basal layer remains intact. The cells at the core of the lesion are distorted and are ultimately destroyed. These appear as hyaline bodies (molluscum bodies), containing cytoplasmic masses of viral material. These inclusion bodies increase in size and move towards the surface of the skin. In the horny layer the molluscum bodies are enmeshed in a fibrous network; that dissolves the centre of the lesion, forming the central core, which is composed primarily of molluscum bodies.

Inflammatory changes in the dermis are slight or absent. This may be due to:

- The production of a glutathione peroxidase homolog which protects the virus and infected cells from damage by peroxides
- The production of a major histocompatibility complex (MHC) Class 1 heavy chain homologue, which prevents presentation of molluscum contagiosum genomes
- The production of a chemokine homologue that inhibits inflammation.

Histopathology

The histology shows hypertrophic and hyperplastic epidermis. This is essentially an acanthoma, with a downward proliferation of the rete pegs and enveloped by the connective tissue to form a deep crater.

In the cytoplasm of the epidermal cells there are numerous small eosinophilic and later basophilic inclusion bodies develop, called the molluscum contagiosum bodies (Handerson-Patterson bodies). These bodies first develop as single, minute ovoid eosinophilic structures in the lower cells of the stratum malpighii; at a level, one or two layers above the basal cells. The molluscum bodies increase in size as the infected cells move towards the surface. The molluscum bodies in the upper layer of the stratum malpighii, compress the nucleus, so that it appears as a thin crescent at the periphery of the cell. At the level of the stratum granulosum, the staining reaction of the molluscum bodies changes from eosinophilic to basophilic. In the horny layer the molluscum bodies measure up to 35 µm in diameter, they are enmeshed in the network of tonofilaments. In the centre of the lesion the stratum corneum ultimately disintegrates, releasing the molluscum bodies. Thus a central crater forms, secondary infection and ulceration can occur.

Electron microscopy reveals that molluscum inclusion bodies consist of large number of molluscum contagiosum virus.

Clinical Features

The distribution of the lesion depends upon the mode of infection, type of clothing and by the climate. In temperate regions, the lesions are found on the trunk and neck, in the tropics they are mainly found on the limbs. Molluscum can also occur on the mucous membranes such as the tongue and buccal mucosa.

The disease is common in young children, lesions are commonly seen on the face, neck and trunk. The genital area may be involved in adults. Lesions may be single or multiple, 1–3 mm in diameter. The papules are first solid, firm and flesh-coloured, and on reaching maturity they become soft with an umbilicated centre, which is whitish or pearly in colour. The lesions spread by autoinoculation (Figs 6 and 7). Conjunctivitis and keratitis may complicate lesions around the eyes. Patients with atopic dermatitis may have extensive lesions. The incubation period varies from one to several weeks. The disease is self-limiting and spontaneous remission may occur within a year.

Large lesions of 3-5 cm in diameter (giant molluscum), are seen in HIV infection.

Diagnosis

The clinical picture is diagnostic. A skin biopsy will show the characteristic molluscum bodies.

Differential Diagnosis

A single molluscum contagiosum should be differentiated from a nodular cystic basal cell carcinoma. The latter appears at a late age, it has telangiectasia on the surface, the surface is uneven and there is no central depression.

Multiple lesions may be confused with chickenpox, milia, sebaceous hyperplasia and eruptive xanthoma.

Lymphangiomas are compressable and have no central punctum.

Treatment

The lesion can be easily removed by curettage, light electrodesiccation or cryotherapy. Other methods include expressing the contents of the papule and squeezing it by forceps, or piercing the papule by a sharpened orange stick dipped in 1% iodine solution. Topical EMLA is useful while removing molluscum in children. Salicylic acid plasters, 10% podophylin in alcohol are also effective.

Antiviral drug cidofovir has recently been found to be effective against molluscum contagiosum, used either topically as 1–3% ointment or by IV route in extensive lesions.

Five percent imiquimod cream can be applied overnight three times a week, in uncontrolled cases.

As the disease is infectious, the patient should avoid the use of public pools, communal baths and shared towels. Patients should avoid contact sports.

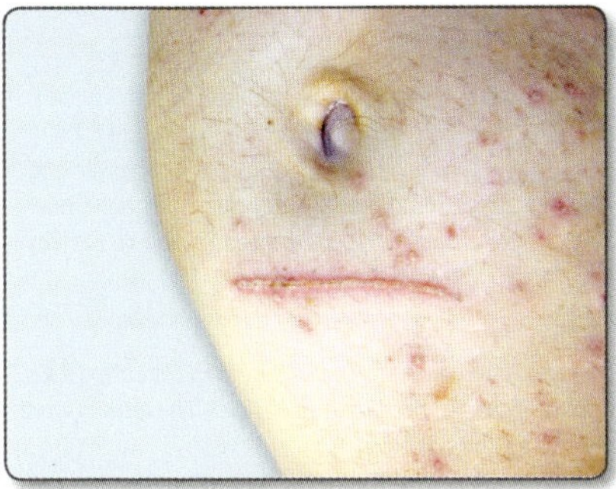

Fig. 6: Molluscum contagiosum with Koebner's phenomenon

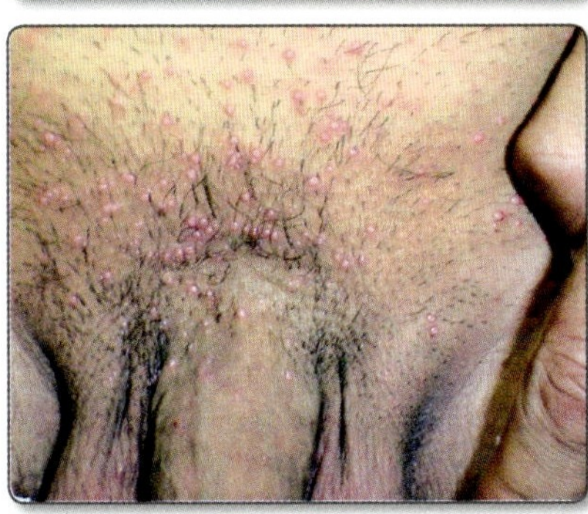

Fig. 7: Molluscum contagiosum

ORF (Sheep Pox)

This is a disease of the mouth and udder of lambs, goat and sheep. Man is infected through direct contact with the infected animals or through contaminated objects.

The lesion is usually single at times multiple, the common sites of infection are the hands, forearms and the face. A painless red papule appears at the site of inoculation, the red centre is surrounded by a white ring with a peripheral red halo, later the lesion oozes and becomes crusted. Lymphangitis due to secondary bacterial infection may develop. The lesion heals spontaneously in a few weeks. Transmission from man to man is not known. One attack gives lasting immunity.

Differential Diagnosis

The lesion should be differentiated from the milker's nodule, pyogenic granuloma, cowpox, anthrax and squamous cell carcinoma. Milker's nodules are usually multiple, infection is got from infected cows or calf muzzles, there is no grayish-white ring as seen in orf. Pyogenic granuloma bleeds easily and they do not heal spontaneously.

Milker's Nodule

Jenner first described this disease; it is contracted from the teeth and udder of cows. It is characterised by one or several red dome-shaped nodules on the hands and forearms. The lesions start as macules, this changes to a papule and then to a nodule, through a vesicular stage. It is surrounded by a red halo.

Differential Diagnosis

It should be differentiated from anthrax, which appears as a hemorrhagic bulla with a central brown crust, the surrounding tissue is oedematous and there is constitutional upset.

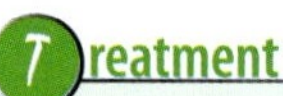

Treatment

No treatment is required, as the disease is self-limiting; it heals in 6–8 weeks. There is no scarring; one infection gives lifelong immunity. Milking machines have now largely replaced these traditional hazards of the dairy farmers.

Smallpox caused by pox virus is now eradicated. It was declared extinct by WHO in early 1980s. It was a severe infection, with an exanthem of macules, papules and vesicles. The lesions were monomorphic, and would leave disfiguring scars on healing.

HUMAN PAPILLOMAVIRUS

Human papillomaviruses (HPVs) are small viruses which infect the squamous epithelium. The most common lesion produced by the HPV is the common wart. The virus infects the basal cells, but viral replication takes place in the upper part of the stratum malpighii and stratum granulosum. There are different types of HPV; these are distinguished by their DNA sequence. These vary in different types of infection, and have different anatomical sites, e.g. HPV 1 infects the palms and soles, HPV 16 has a predilection for the genital areas, some may progress to dysplasia and malignancy. These viruses do not have a lipoprotein envelope surrounding the capsid.

Warts (Verrucae)

The papova virus causes warts; these are benign tumours that commonly infect the skin, less commonly the mucous membrane. Some of the viruses in the group are oncogenic; they are all ether resistant. DNA viruses are slow growing and replicate in the nucleus. Warts are also known as verruca vulgaris, there are a number of different varieties of warts depending upon their location on the skin. Incubation period ranges from a few weeks to more than a year.

Types of verruca virus

Type 1	Palmar and plantar warts
Type 2	Common warts
Type 3, 10	Flat warts
Type 4	Common warts
Type 6, 11	Anogenital warts
Type 16, 18	Bowenoid papulosis, cervical condylomata
Type 5, 8, 9, 12, 14, 15, 17, 19–24	EDV (Epidermal dysplasia verruciformis)

Human papillomavirus 16 and 18 have an oncogenic potential, these are the causative agents for cervical carcinoma. EDV has a high risk of developing cutaneous malignancy, the viruses responsible are HPV 5 and 8.

Pathology

The main histological feature is vacuolation of cells in and below the granular layer; the infected cells are called koilocytes. These are large keratinocytes with an eccentric nucleus, surrounded by a perinuclear halo; the cells contain basophilic inclusion bodies of the viral particles and eosinophilic inclusions of the keratohyalin granules. The other features of the infection are hyperkeratosis,

Clinical Features

Warts are rare in infancy, but are very common during the school years. The highest incidence is between the age of 9 to 16 years. Genital warts usually appear between the ages of 20 years to 50 years, the sexually active years.

Plane warts appear on the face and back of the hands. They are small, flat-topped skin coloured papules; often multiple which may cause cosmetic problems (Fig. 8). Regression of plane warts is often preceded by inflammation of the lesion, causing itching, erythema and swelling. Depigmented halos may appear around the lesion. Resolution occurs within a month. Plane warts should be differentiated from molluscum contagiosum, which are smooth pearly papules with central umbilication. It should also be differentiated from the papules of lichen planus; these occur in adults and involve other parts of the body.

Common warts are firm papules, which has a rough hyperkeratotic verrucous surface (Fig. 9). They resolve spontaneously within two years. Multiple clustered warts should be differentiated from tuberculosis verrucosa cutis.

Filliform warts are common in males, they are long, narrow, frond-like and flesh coloured growths that can occur singly or as clusters around the eyelids, face, neck, or lips (Fig. 10).

Plantar warts occur on the soles, usually on pressure points such as the heels or metatarsal heads (Fig. 11). They are often painful on walking. Planter warts should be differentiated from punctate keratodermas. They resemble corns, but gentle paring with a scalpel will reveal a well-defined margin with free bleeding points. Skin markings are absent in warts, but present in corns in the earlier stage of development, these later disappear as the corn thickens. Sometimes multiple shallow confluent warts are present over a wide area of the sole, these are called mosaic warts. Myrmecia is a term used for deep domed-shaped tender warts mostly present on the palms and soles, besides a nail or on the pulp of digits. A term first introduced by Celsus and later used by Lyell. Histologically they are characterised by eosinoplilic bodies, at first intracellular and later extracellular.

Genital warts (condylomata acuminata) resemble the common wart virus, but it is antigenically different. Viral warts 16 and 18 are oncogenic. Clinically it appears as soft pink verrucous growths around the anus, vulva and the penis (Fig. 12). As it is contagious; it is classified as a venereal disease. Genital warts are asymptomatic, but may cause pruritus, discharge and bleeding. Giant condylomata accuminata known as Buschke-Lowenstein tumour is rare and aggressive, it penetrates the dermis. Clinically it behaves like a carcinoma, but is benign histologically.

These warts should be differentiated from condylomata lata due to syphilis. Syphilitic condylomas are broad flat and pink in colour, the other signs of syphilis are present.

Treatment

Plane warts. Three to four percent salicylic acid ointment, topical retinoids, light cryotherapy, light electrocautery, imiquimod cream are usually effective. Treatment can cause lesions to spread; the treatment should therefore be slow and gentle.

Common warts. Common warts are best treated by wart paint containing salicylic acid and lactic acid in flexible collodion, 40% salicylic acid plaster can be used. Unresponsive warts will usually clear with carbon dioxide snow or liquid nitrogen. Application may have to be repeated at 3 weekly intervals. The treatment is painful and overenthusiastic freezing may produce blisters and even scars. Electrodessication and curettage of warts is widely used, but even in skilled hands may leave an unsightly atrophic scar. Trichloracetic acid (TCA) can be used for any type of warts.

Filliform warts. These are easily removed by clipping with scissors, under local anaesthesia, and electrodessication of the base if necessary.

Plantar warts. The treatment of plantar warts is similar to common warts; those resistant to treatment should be removed. Cryotherapy is more difficult in plantar warts, because of the difficulty in raising a blister.

Other treatments. 4% formalin soak is applied daily on the warts for 15 minutes and the skin around the warts is protected by petrolatum. Gluteraldehyde in 20% solution with aqueous ethanol in a gel base is also effective in plantar warts. It colours the skin brown , it is therefor not used in for the treatment in other areas. Mosaic warts are very resistant to treatment keeping the warts well pared down with the use of a pumice stone or file, may help in reducing the duration of treatment.

Genital warts. Genital warts are treated by 25% podophyllin in tincture benzoin; this is irritant to the surrounding skin, which should be protected by petrolatum or vaseline. The podophyllin solution is removed after 6 hours or else chemical burns may occur. This is repeated at weekly intervals. Podophyllin should not be used during pregnancy as it may damage the fetus.

Podophyllotoxin (condylox): This is used in a concentration of 0.5%; it is a purified derivative of podophyllin. It is available in solution and gel form, to be applied twice daily for three consecutive days per week to the genital warts, for 1–3 months. Side effects include burning, stinging and pain.

In pregnancy, podophyllin is not used, electrodessication of the warts is preferred. Carbon dioxide laser is quite useful in the treatment of condyloma.

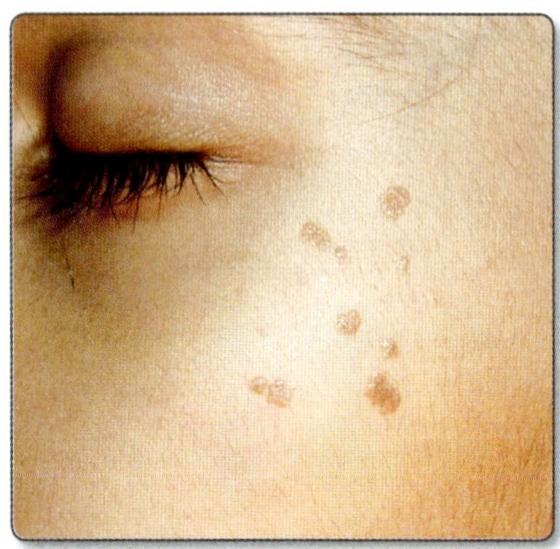

Fig. 8: Plane warts

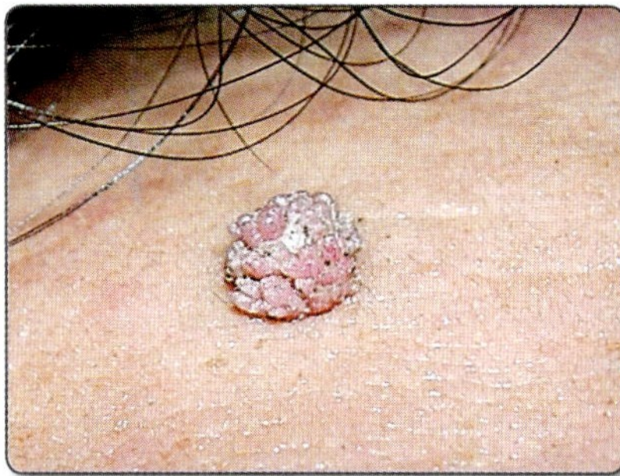

Fig. 9: Verruca vulgaris

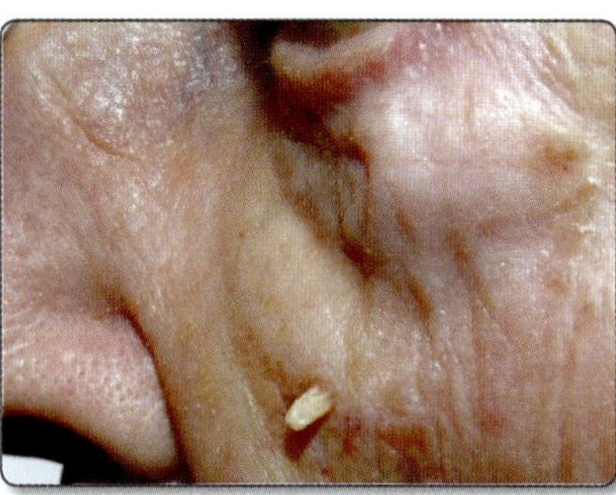

Fig. 10: Filiform wart

acanthosis and papillomatosis. The dermal capillary vessels are prominent and may be thrombosed.

Mucosal Warts (Extracutaneous)

These occur as pink or white papules in the oral cavity, lips, larynx and the cervix. In the cervix atypical warts may present as flat or slightly elevated lesions. Laryngeal warts present as hoarseness, it may cause respiratory distress in a newborn. Several studies have shown a correlation between condylomata

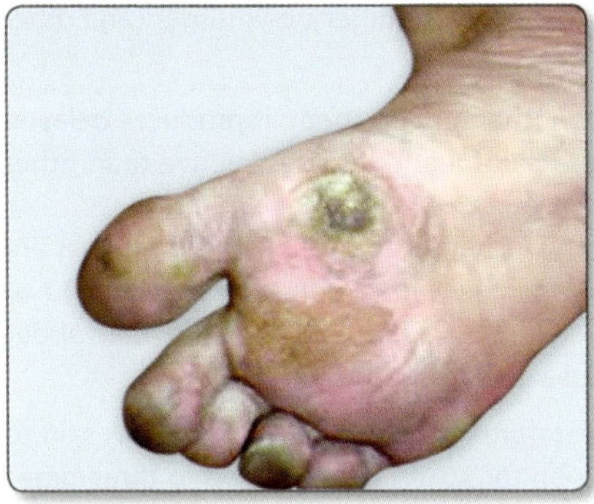

Fig. 11: Plantar wart

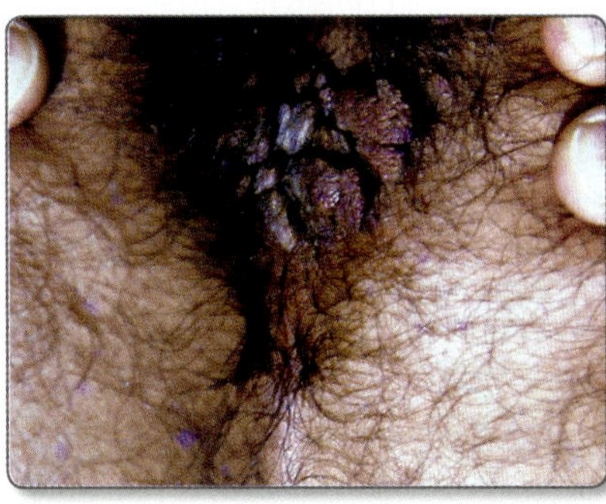

Fig. 12: Condylomata acuminata (Genital warts)

acuminata of the mother and laryngeal warts in a newborn baby. A cesarean section is indicated for women having genital warts.

Treatment of Resistant Warts

Retinoids. Acitretin is useful for extensive and hyperkeratotic warts in immunosupressed patients. It does not eradicate the warts, but the size is greatly reduced, the warts relapse once the treatment is stopped. Once the size is decreased, other treatments can be used.

Cimetidine. 30–40 mg/day when given for 3 months has shown complete resolution of the wart without recurrence after one year.

Intralesional bleomycin. 0.5 units/mL is injected into the warts, the treatment is effective if the warts blanch after injection. The injection is painful and local anaesthesia should be given before the injection. A haemorrhagic eschar develops after 2–3 weeks of injection, which separates along with the wart.

Psychological methods. Hypnosis is said to clear the warts. Children are said to have higher success rate than adults.

Antiviral therapy. Recent studies have shown that cidofovir applied locally as 1% gel can be effective in treating warts. A search for therapeutic vaccination is in progress.

Interferon. Different interferons have been used by different routes to treat warts. In many cases the reports of its effectiveness have been disappointing.

It has been used as an adjuvant therapy with surgery, cryosurgery and other topical measures.

Diphencyprone. This is an immunotherapeutic agent; it produces delayed type of hypersensitivity. It is less painful and less destructive than other modalities.

Squaric acid dibutylester (SADBE). SADBE is a topical allergen. Patients are sensitised with 2% SADBE in acetone; the warts are then treated with 0.1 or 0.01% SADBE once a week or every other week. In uncontrolled trials, about two-thirds of the patients showed a good response.

Local heat. Increasing the temperature of the skin to about 50°C is said to result in wart clearance. Immersion for 30–45 minutes, two to three times weekly for 16 weeks can be effective, as the wart virus is heat labile.

Laser. Carbon dioxide laser has been useful to treat cutaneous and mucosal warts. It is also useful in difficult warts such as the periungual and subungual warts. Local anaesthesia is required; it has a potential for scarring. Pulse dye laser is also used for removing warts, it targets the blood supply of the wart, and it is less painful and has a less potential for scarring. However, pulse dye laser may not be as effective as the carbon dioxide laser. Newer laser systems such as erbium-doped yttrium aluminum garnet (Er: YAG) laser may play a role in the treatment of warts by thermal damage.

Bleomycin. Bleomycin can be used when other treatments fail. The drug is expensive. One unit/mL of solution is used for treatment. The treatment is painful, local EMLA is applied to the wart, and then add 1-2 drops of bleomycin solution onto the wart. Prick till bleeding points appear. Cover the wart with plastic bandage for 24 hours. Repeat the procedure after 2 weeks. The method is contraindicated in pregnancy and lactation.

Imiquimod. Imiquimod (aldara) cream activates the host immune system. The cream is applied three times a week to the wart until it resolves it usually takes 1–3 months. This agent is used for genital warts where the efficacy rate is about 70%. For nongenital areas, it is not very effective.

Most warts resolve spontaneously, procedures that cause scarring and are painful should be avoided
All forms of therapy have a high recurrence rate
Always think of child abuse if children present with condylomata acuminata.

BOWENOID PAPULOSIS

Bowenoid papulosis (BP) affects young adults (Fig. 13). The disease histologically resembles Bowen's disease, but may regress. It is characterised by reddish-brown verrucous papules and plaques on the genitalia, they look like condylomata acuminata. It is caused by HPV 16, 18 and 33.

The course of BP is variable it may regress, or transform to Bowen's disease and invasive squamous cell carcinoma. The course resembles that of cervical dysplasia. Patients with BP and their sexual partners should be examined periodically, because of the risk of developing squamous cell carcinoma (SCC).

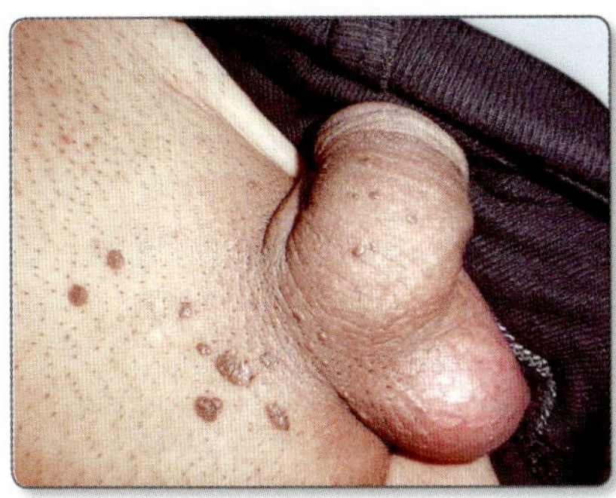

Fig. 13: Bowenoid papulosis

Bowenoid papulosis responds well to treatment with local destructive measures, such as electrodesiccation, cryotherapy and curettage.

Epidermodysplasia Verruciformis

Lewandowskey and Lutz first described epidermodysplasia verruciformis (EDV) in 1922. It is a rare familial disease characterised by widespread papillomavirus induced macules and papules, appearing in childhood. In 2–3 decades the sun-exposed lesions may change into bowenoid papulosis and carcinoma.

Aetiology

About 1–2% of cases of EDV are a product of consanguineous marriages and about 10% are familial with one or more siblings affected with the disease. The mode of inheritance appears to be autosomal recessive. Some cases are said to be X-linked recessive, others may be autosomal dominant. A number of papillomavirus are said to cause EDV. HPV 5 and 8 are found in malignancies caused by EDV. Ninety percent of the patients with EDV have depressed T cell function, humoral immunity is said to be intact. Sunlight acts as a cofactor in production of skin cancer.

Histopathology

This is similar to that of the papillomavirus. However, vacuolation is more extensive and may affect the upper half to three fourths of the stratum malpighii. Viral particles may be found not only in the malpighian layer, but also in the basal cells. There may be a gradual progression towards dysplasia.

Clinical Features

Macular scaly lesions are found in early childhood, most commonly seen on the trunk and upper extremities. The lesions may range in colour from tan to red, may be depigmented or brown in colour. Macules tend to become confluent with polycyclic borders. The eruption at times resembles tinea versicolor.

Lesions on the dorsum of the hands are like flat warts, while the lesions on the knees and elbow are psoriasiform. Bowenoid changes are seen on the sun-exposed areas, they appear as raised plaques that may metastasize to the regional lymph nodes. Local invasion is common to the orbit, sinuses and the brain.

About 10% of cases have mental retardation. Most of the patients have normal intelligence and behaviour.

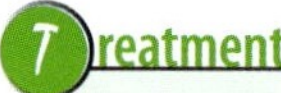

Lesions on the trunk resemble tinea versicolor, but the presence of plane wart like lesions on the hands and absence of fungus from the lesion helps in differentiation. Acrokeratosis verruciformis, lichen planus, simple plane warts should be differentiated from the lesions of the hands, biopsy and other cutaneous findings are important differentiating factors.

Treatment

There is no effective treatment for EDV. Patients should avoid sun-exposure and use sun blocks. Oral retinoids such as acitretin reduce the number of viral particles in benign lesions. It tends to reduce the scaling of macular lesions and flattens the raised papules. It is not proven whether retinoids reduce the incidence of carcinoma in EDV. Genetic counseling is useful for families who have a child with EDV. Prenatal diagnosis is not possible.

Course and Prognosis

The darker the complexion of the patient the better is the prognosis. Cancers appear to be slow to metastasize, death has occurred from invasion of the vital organs by direct spread or metastasis.

PICORNA VIRUS

These are small RNA containing virus, resistant to lipid solvents. They are widely distributed, they replicate in the gastrointestinal tract. Infection spreads by droplet infection or by fecal contamination. The infections are usually mild, but in some cases myocarditis and paralysis may occur, similar to the poliovirus. Poliovirus has no exanthem.

The viruses in this group include:

- Enterovirus

Poliovirus

Coxsackie virus

Echo virus

- Rhino virus

Foot and mouth virus

Influenza virus

Hepatitis A

Enterovirus

Coxsackie Virus

These viruses are divided into two groups A and B. Group A causes herpangina, and hand, foot and mouth disease. Group B viruses are associated with myalgias, myocarditis, etc. Relationship between Coxsackie group B virus and juvenile dermatomyositis has been suggested.

Herpangina

This is an infection caused by coxsackie group A virus. It usually affects children. The disease is manifested by fever, sore throat, and dysphagia. Vesicles are found in the pharynx, tonsils, pillars of the fauces and uvula. The vesicles are surrounded by a red areola. The vesicles rupture to form ulcers. Recovery occurs in 5–7 days.

Treatment is symptomatic.

Hand, Foot and Mouth Disease

It is a disease of young children, characterized by the formation of vesicles in the oral cavity. The vesicles are larger and fewer than that of herpangina.

Cutaneous lesions manifest as vesicles surrounded by a red areola. These vesicles are present on the dorsum of the hands and around the margins of the heel. Palms and soles may also be affected. The lesions are few and heal in 2–3 days. Relapses are rare.

Echo Virus

It was previously thought that the Echo virus does not cause human disease, hence the name Echo Virus (**E**ntero-**C**ytopathic **H**uman **O**rphan). It has now been found that there are about 34 different serological types of echo virus, they cause a wide variety of syndromes. It may cause encephalitis, aseptic meningitis, diarrhea, vomiting. It may also be associated with dermatomyositis like syndrome.

Rhino Virus

This virus is present in farm animals; children and adults are infected when they come in contact with the infected stocks. It causes foot and mouth disease and hepatitis A.

Foot and Mouth Disease

After incubation period of 7–10 days, vesicles occur in the oral cavity and soles; they then rupture to form ulcers, which are painful. The disease tends to be more severe in children than adults. The lesion often heal within a week.

Treatment is symptomatic.

MYXOVIRUS AND PARAMYXOVIRUS

These RNA viruses; cause measles, German measles, mumps, para influenza and respiratory syncytial disease. Measles causes the characteristic morbilliform eruption.

Measles

This is an acute contagious disease, seen mostly in children. It spreads by droplet infection. It is contagious from the 5th day of the incubation period to as long as the eruption clears. One attack confers permanent immunity.

Clinical Features

The incubation period is 10–12 days. Prodromal symptoms are fever, coryza and cough. The eyes are congested, photophobia is present. On the 2nd or 3rd day the diagnostic Koplik spots appear. These

Contd...

Contd...

are whitish spots, surrounded by reddish areola, found opposite to the molar teeth. On the 4th day the eruption appears, first behind the ears, it then spreads to the face, neck and then caudally downwards to the rest of the body.

The exanthem consists of small brick-red macules or a maculopapular eruption, which coalesce to form blotchy patches, the characteristic morbilliform eruption.

The rash lasts for 3–5 days; there may be slight pruritus. The rash fades in order of appearance. Hemorrhage in the rashes may occur in undernourished and debilitated individuals. Other complications include laryngitis, bronchopneumonia, otitis media and encephalitis.

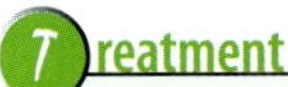

There is no specific therapy. Treatment is symptomatic. Prevention with live attenuated measles vaccine is effective. Those who are exposed to infection gamma globulin will prevent or attenuate measles vaccine if given within 6 days of exposure.

Rubella (German Measles, Three days Measles)

Rubella has a worldwide distribution; the disease runs a mild course in children, if acquired in pregnancy it results in the congenital rubella syndrome. The disease spreads by droplet infection, maximum infectivity occurs during the prodromal period, and during the time the rash is present.

Signs and Symptoms

The incubation period is usually 14–21 days during which the patient complains of fever, malaise, sore throat and conjunctivitis. On the mucous membrane, small petechial lesions are seen on the soft palate and uvula (Forchheimer's sign). The rash appears first on the forehead, then spreads on the face, and moves downwards on the trunk and extremities. On the second day, the facial exanthem fades, and on the 3rd day, the exanthem fades completely. The exanthem is reddish-pink, discrete and macular. The lymphadenopathy is characteristic; it involves the suboccipital, postauricular and posterior cervical group of lymph nodes.

Congenital rubella syndrome: If rubella is acquired in the first trimester of pregnancy, malformations are seen in 80% of fetuses. The malformations include patent ductus arteriosus, ventricular septal defects, cataracts, microphthalmia, hydrocephalus, microcephalus, mental retardation and deafness.

Treatment is symptomatic.

Prevention

Combined measles, mumps and rubella (MMR) vaccine provides good protection against rubella, it is given in infancy. The vaccine is contraindicated in pregnancy or if there is a likelihood of pregnancy within 3 months of immunization. Human immunoglobulin can decrease the symptoms of rubella, but cannot prevent the teratogenic effects.

ERYTHEMA INFECTIOSUM (FIFTH DISEASE)

This is an infection caused by parvovirus. The disease is common in children between the ages of 5 years and 10 years. The incubation period is 6–14 days. The virus has a special affinity for the erythropoietic cells of the bone marrow. The disease has two classic skin findings:

- Erythema of the cheeks (Slapped-cheek appearance)
- Reticulate erythema of the extensor surface of the proximal extremities.

Sometimes the above two classic signs are absent, and the patient may present only with a maculopapular rash. Associated findings include fever, pharyngitis, and lymphadenopathy. Infection in children can be associated with chronic anemia.

If the infection occurs in pregnancy it can lead to abortion, hydrops fetalis or transient aplastic anemia of the newborn.

The treatment is symptomatic.

OTHER CUTANEOUS DISORDERS ASSOCIATED WITH VIRUS INFECTIONS

Several cutaneous syndromes are associated with viral infections. These include the TORCH syndrome, erythema nodosum, erythema multiforme, histiocytic necrotizing lymphadenitis, etc. Torch syndrome is caused by toxoplasmosis, rubella, cytomegalic and herpes virus.

Erythema nodosum may occur in milker's nodule and infectious mononucleosis. Erythema multiforme is caused by herpes virus, it also occurs in mumps, milker's nodule and orf. Hepatitis A virus causes panniculitis.

Gianotti-Crosti Syndrome (Papular Acrodermatitis of Childhood)

This is usually a response to hepatitis B virus. Other viruses responsible are EBV, coxsackie and echovirus. The syndrome affects children between the ages of 6 months and 12 years.

Clinical Features

Dull-red papules occur on the thigh, buttocks, extensor aspect of the arms and the face. The papules are asymmetrical. Constitutional symptoms are usually mild.

In cases due to hepatitis B virus, liver involvement is mild and anicteric. Occasionally there may be jaundice.

Treatment

There is no specific treatment. Lesions fade in 2–8 weeks.

Table 1: Differentiating features of measles, mumps and rubella

Scarlet fever	*Measles*	*Rubella*
Causative organism Bacteria—Hemolytic *streptococcus*	Virus—Paramyxovirus	Virus—Togavirus
Incubation period 3–7 days	10–15 days	14–21 days

Contd...

Contd...

Scarlet fever	*Measles*	*Rubella*
Prodromal phase 1–2 days, fever and sore throat	3–5 days, moderate to severe coryza-like symptoms	1–2 days, mild coryza-like symptoms
Rash Generalized pinhead-sized yellow-red papules on erythematous skin, red tongue (strawberry), circumoral pallor present	Generalized red maculopapular rash , with marked coalescence on the face and thorax. No circumoral pallor	Scattered to generalized pinkish-red maculopapular rash, minimal coalescence on the thorax, small, deep, papular eruptions on soft palate. No circumoral pallor
Characteristic sign Schultz-Charlton sign +	Koplik spots +	Posterior cervical glands enlarged
Duration of rash Depends on treatment	3–5 days	1–3 days
Postexanthem desquamation Severe, most marked on the hands and feet	Common and branny	Occasional and branny

FURTHER READING

1. Brown ZA, Selke S, Zen J, et al. The acquisition of Herpes simplex virus during pregnancy. N Eng J Med. 1997;337(8):509-15.
2. Bryson YJ, Dillon M, Lovell M, et al. Treatment of first episode of genital herpes virus infection with oral acyclovir. N Eng J Med. 1983;308:916-21.
3. Dahl H, Fjaertoft G, Norsted T, et al. Reactivation of herpes virus 6 during pregnancy. J Infect Dis. 1999;180:2035-8.
4. Ewin DM. Hypnotherapy for warts (Verruca vulgaris): 41 consecutive cases with 33 cures. Am J Clin Hypn. 1992;35:1-10.
5. Fairris GM, Statham BN, Waigh MA. The investigation of patients with genital warts. Br J Dermatol. 1984;111:736-8.
6. Hengge UR, Esser S, Schultewother T, et al. Self-administered topical 5% imiquimod for the treatment of common warts and molluscum contagiosum. Br J Dermatol. 2000;143: 1026-31.
7. Huang CC, Chang YC, Liu CC, et al. Neurological complications in children with enterovirus 71 infection. New Eng J Med. 1999;341:136-42.
8. Kost RG, Straus SC. Postherpetic neuralgia: pathogenesis, treatment and prevention. N Eng J Med. 1996;335:32-42.
9. Lin L, Chen XC, Cui PG, et al. Topical application of penciclovir cream for the treatment of herpes simplex facialis/labialis: in a randomized double-blind multicentre, acyclovir controlled trial. J Dermatolog Treat. 2002;13:67-72.
10. McGregor JM, Yu CC, Lu QL, et al. Post-transplant cutaneous lymphoma. J Am Acad Dermatol. 1993;29(4):549-54.
11. Porter CD, Blake NW, Archard LC, et al. Molluscum contagiosum virus types in genital and non-genital lesions. Br J Dermatol. 1989;120:37-40.
12. Smith KJ, Skelton H. Molluscum contagiosum: recent advances in pathogenic mechanisms and new therapy. Am J Clin Dermatol. 2002;3:535-45.
13. Watson CPN, Evans RJJ, Watt VR. Postherpetic neuralgia and topical capsaicin. Pain. 1988;33:333-40.
14. White WB, Grant-Kels JM. Transmission of herpes simplex Type1 infection in rugby players. JAMA. 1984;252:533-5.
15. Whitley RJ, Yeager A, Kartus P, et al. Neonatal herpes virus simplex infections: follow-up evaluation with viderabine therapy. Pediatrics. 1983;72 (96):778-85.
16. Woolfson H. Oral acyclovir in eczema herpeticum. BMJ. 1984;288:531-2.

Chapter 7

Parasitic Infestation, Diseases Caused by Arthropods and Other Venomous Animals

INTRODUCTION

Animals can cause cutaneous disease, some are parasites, others act as vectors of disease. Skin damage can also be caused by bites, stings or injection of toxic substances. A number of these disorders are found in tropical countries, due to the ecological conditions which favour the habitat of animal parasites and vectors of disease. Scabies is the most common parasitic disease of tropical countries. It is found in endemic proportions in many areas, often becoming epidemic. Other parasitic diseases, such as trypanosomiasis, leishmaniasis and filariasis also prevail in the tropics. Insect bites are common in children, scratching leads to infection and pyoderma. The common cutaneous infestations caused by animals are listed below.

Common Infestations

Protozoal infestations
- Cutaneous amoebiasis
- Leishmaniasis
- Trypanosomiasis
- Toxoplasmosis

Helminthic infestations
- Nematodes
- Platyhelminths

Diseases transmitted by arthropods
- Class Hexapoda such as insects
- Class Arachnida such as scabies
- Class Chilopoda such a centipedes

Diseases caused by reptiles

Diseases caused by sea animals

PROTOZOAL INFESTATION

Cutaneous Amoebiasis

Amoebiasis is an intestinal disease that can infect the skin by a primary inoculation, or from an internal focus such as the intestines or a liver abscess. Dissemination is due to lymphatic or haematogenous spread.

Clinical Features

Perianal region or the genitals are commonly affected. Nodules appear that become rapidly ulcerated or vegetating lesions develop. Pain is a constant feature. Fully developed ulcers have three zones; a central area with granulation and necrotic tissue covered with dark purulent exudate, an undermined violaceous border with a wide red halo.

Differential Diagnosis

The ulcer should be differentiated from phagedenic tropical ulcer, deep mycosis, mycobacterial ulcer and venereal disease.

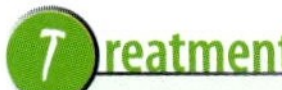

Treatment

The amoebic ulcer is treated with metronidazole 800 mg, 3 times daily for 10 days. Daily cleaning of the ulcer is necessary.

Leishmaniasis

These are a group of diseases caused by several species of the parasite of genus *leishmania*; different species cause infection of the skin, mucous membrane and viscera. Each species has a particular geographical distribution, they are morphologically identical, but can be differentiated by isoenzyme pattern, DNA analysis and monoclonal antibodies.

Cutaneous Leishmaniasis

Cutaneous leishmaniasis is caused by *Leishmania* (*L*) *tropica*, *L. major*, *L. aethopica*, and *L. infantum*. These are often referred to as Old World Leishmaniasis. Man is infected by the bite of a sandfly. Other diseases caused by the sandfly are sandfly or papatasi fever, harara fever and bartonellosis (Oroya fever).

The parasite can exist in two forms. In the humans, the amastigotes (Leishman-Donovan bodies) are found. These are small spherical bodies 2–6 μm long, 1–2 μm wide. They have an external membrane the periblast, a spherical nucleus and a pinpoint like kinetoplast, from which a thin element emerges, the flagellum. The other reservoirs of infection are rats, gerbils and dogs.

The flagellated form known as the promastigote is found in the insect vector (sandfly) and artificial media. These are about 15–20 μm long and 1.5–3.5 μm wide with a 15–20 μm flagellum. The flagellum consists of 8 firm filaments that surround a thick central one, it is responsible for mobility. The sandfly is infected by feeding on a lesion or from the blood of an animal infected with *Leishmania*. In the intestine of the insect, they become flagellated, multiply and migrate to the oropharynx in great numbers. When the infected sandfly bites the human skin, they enter the macrophages, loose the flagella and assume the amastigote form. The reticuloendothelial system appears to play a central role in leishmanial infection.

Cutaneous leishmaniasis due to *L. major* (wet or rural type) has an incubation period of less than 2 months. Clinically the lesion appears as a small bluish-red papule that slowly enlarges and develops into a nodule; this looks like a furuncle. The nodule then breaks down to form an ulcer that is covered by a crust. The lesion heals in about 6 months heals in about 6 with scarring. Multiple small secondary nodules may occur in the lymphatics (Fig. 1).

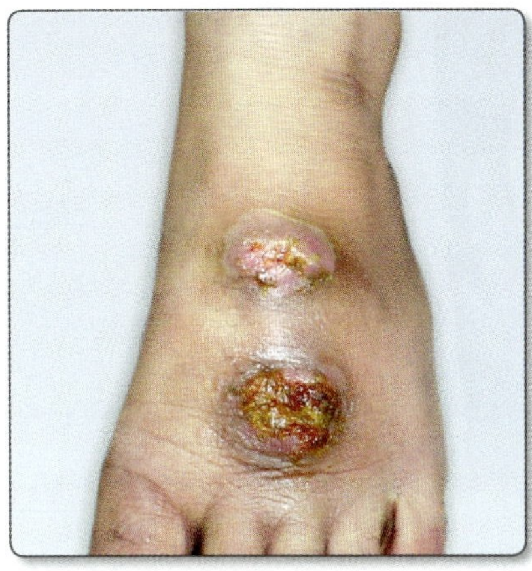

Fig. 1: Leishmaniasis major—note the secondary nodule

Cutaneous leishmaniasis due to *L. tropica* (dry or the urban type) occurs after an incubation period of 2 months or more. A small reddish-brown nodule appears which develops into a slowly extending plaque 1–2 cm in diameter. A shallow ulceration appears in the centre, a closely adherent crust develops on it. Secondary nodules occur less frequently than in the wet form, it heals spontaneously in 12 months with scarring. (Fig. 2).

Leishmaniasis recidivans (chronic leishmaniasis) is due to the result of a peculiar host reaction in which the cellular immunity fails to sterilise the lesion. Brownish-red or brown papules appear close to a scar of an old lesion of cutaneous leishmaniasis, these coalesce to form a plaque, closely resembling lupus vulgaris. After infection, the patients are normally immune to reinfection with the same species (Fig. 3).

Cutaneous leishmaniasis due to *L. aethiopica* does not ulcerate; lesions are seldom inflamed and heal in 2–5 years. This form of leishmaniasis is not sensitive to antimony. The disease may become widespread and can infect the mucous membrane.

Cutaneous leishmaniasis due to *L. infantum* is seen in infants; it may have visceral involvement, but if adults are infected only cutaneous lesions are seen. Evolution of the lesion is slow and mild.

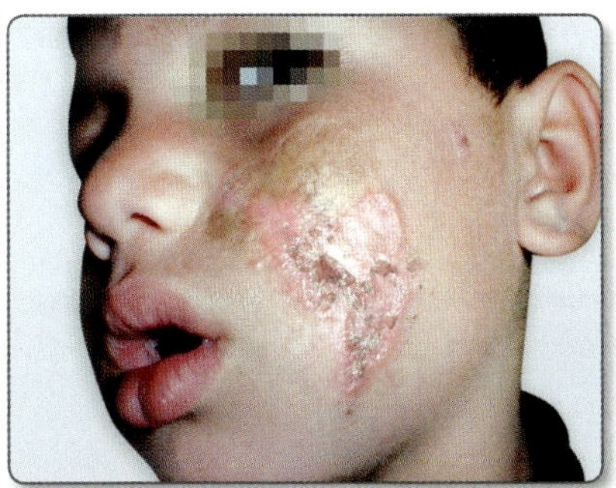

Fig. 2: Leishmaniasis tropica

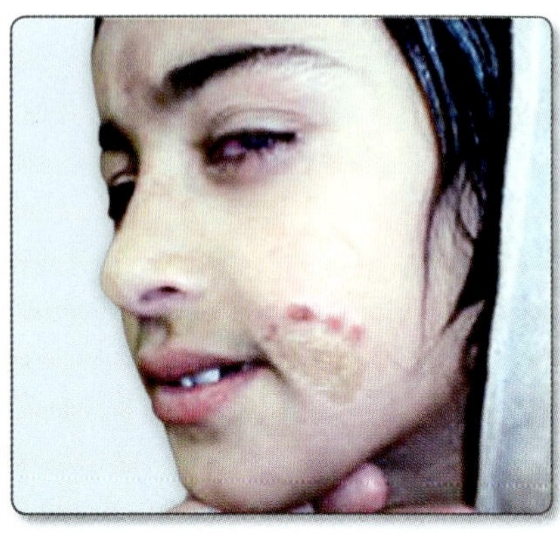

Fig. 3: Leishmaniasis recidivans

New world cutaneous leishmaniasis: Cutaneous leishmaniasis due to *L. mexicana* are multiple, ulcerative and destructive than Old World counterpart. It characteristically involves the pinna of the ear (chiclero ulcers).

Cutaneous leishmaniasis due to *L. braziliensis* is similar to Old World cutaneous leishmaniasis, but some cases may develop mucosal lesions.

Diffuse cutaneous leishmaniasis: In both Old and New World leishmaniasis *L. aethiopica* and *L. braziliensis* lesions can become disseminated. The disease presents initially as a single nodule, it then spreads locally through extension, and eventually the lesions become widespread through metastasis. The lesions bear a close resemblance to lepromatous leprosy. The disease runs a protracted course, but does not visceralise. Parasites are present in abundance in the skin lesions. The disease is not due to the virulence of the organism, but due to defects in the host immune response.

It responds poorly to treatment.

Differential Diagnosis

In the earlier stages before ulceration, leishmaniasis can be mistaken for a boil, sarcoidisis, keloid or leprosy. When ulceration appears, it should be distinguished from malignant neoplasms, tuberculosis and other infected granulomas. The recidvians lesion should be differentiated from lupus vulgaris, tertiary syphilis and psoriatic plaque.

Diagnosis

A smear should be taken from the edge of the lesion for the detection of ***Leishman-Donovan*** (LD) bodies. Biopsy will show a granulomatous lesion with numerous LD bodies in the macrophage in early stages. A culture on the Nickole-Novy-McNeal (NNN) medium will grow the organism and demonstrate the promastigotes. Intradermal test with heat-killed parasites gives a positive reaction in 48 hours.

Treatment

Pentavalent antimonials form the basis of treatment. Sodium stibogluconate (pentostam) or meglumine antimoniate (glucantime) are the drugs of choice. It is given in a dose of 20 mg/kg of body weight by intramuscular injections (IM) given daily for 15–21 days. The injections can be repeated after an interval of a week, if the response is not good. Antimonials should be given with great care, bradycardia, dysrhythmia and circulatory collapse may occur during the use of these drugs.

Treatment

Small sores can be treated by local injections of pentostam (1 mg/kg of body weight), curettage, photodymanic therapy or cryotherapy. Heat treatment using a novel and low-technology device named Hand-held Exothermic Crystallisation Thermotherapy for Cutaneous Leishmaniasis (HECT-CL) has been introduced recently. This device produces a stable thermal reaction ranging from 50° to 54°C which is considered therapeutic. It is cheap, simple to use, and well tolerated by patients. It can be used for small lesions less than 6 cm in diameter, in places where antimony is not available or it cannot be afforded by the patient.

The other drugs that can be used for leishmaniasis are dapsone 2 mg/kg of body weight for 3 weeks, rifampicin 600 mg bid for 4 weeks, itraconazole 7 mg/kg of body weight for 3 weeks, fluconaazole 200 mg daily for 6 weeks, ketoconazole 600 mg daily for 30 days, pentamidine 4 mg/kg of body weight by IM injections every other day for 3 doses, levamisole 300 mg weekly, paromomycin 11 mg/kg of body weight by IM injections for 21 days, and amphotericin B 1 mg/kg of body weight every other day for 30 days. Chloroquine and miltefosine have also been used in resistant cases.

Leishmaniasis recidivans is resistant to treatment; a combination of oral allopurinol (20 mg/kg of body weight for 30 days) and IM injection of meglumine antimoniate (50 mg/kg of body weight for 15 days) is helpful, with a follow-up for 2 years.

Mucocutaneous Leishmaniasis

Mucocutaneous leishmaniasis (American leishmaniasis) is a granulomatous disease caused by *L. braziliensis* in South America and by *L. aethiopica* in Africa. The disease first affects the skin and then mucous membrane of the upper respiratory tract. The disease is found in the tropical and subtropical regions of South and Central America and Africa. Cutaneous lesions are similar to that of cutaneous leishmaniasis, metastatic mucous membrane lesions occur several years later, usually 2–10 years. The anterior part of the nasal septum is first affected. Ulceration and vegetating lesion cause considerable destruction and deformity of the nose, upper lip and palate. The disease causes marked disfiguration called espundia. Bones are usually spared. An anergic-disseminated form is also seen.

The diagnosis is largely clinical, as it is difficult to isolate the parasite from the mucosa of the respiratory tract.

Visceral Leishmaniasis (Kala-azar)

Kala-azar means black fever; it acquires its name because of the dark macular pigmentation of the skin due to deposits of melanin. The deposits are most prominent on the forehead, temples, perioral region and the abdomen. Post kala-azar dermatosis develops 1–3 years after the treatment of systemic disease.

Kala-azar is a systemic disease, caused by *L. donovani* found in the tropical and subtropical parts of Asia and Africa. The earliest lesion is a cutaneous nodule, which develops at the site of sandfly inoculation. Endogenously the primary target for the parasite is the reticuloendothelial system; the liver, spleen, bone marrow and the lymph nodes. There is intermittent fever, hepatosplenomegaly, agranulocytosis, anaemia and thrombocytopenia. Purpura develops as the disease progresses. The pigmentation of the skin appears later, it is prominent on the face and abdomen. The disease is fatal if untreated.

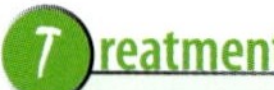

Local treatment is of no value. Pentavalent antimonials should be given in a high dose in repeated courses. Minocycline and methyluracil have also proved to be effective.

Post kala-azar dermal leishmaniasis develops 1–3 years after a course of therapy, in some cases it may be delayed for as long as 10 years. The lesions are hypopigmented, erythematous or nodular. Hypopigmented lesions are widespread and asymptomatic. Erythematous macules appear on the central part of the face and may later become yellowish pink. Nodular lesions are widespread and clinically resemble lepromatous leprosy. The lesions heal without scarring. The parasite can be demonstrated in the erythematous and nodular lesions, but seldom in the hypopigmented ones.

Leishmaniasis should be suspected in a person who has a nodule on the face, and has visited an endemic area of leishmaniasis

Sir William B Leishman (1865–1926)

Leishman was born and qualified in Glasgow at the Military Hospital. He worked with Sir Almroth Wright and discovered the stain by which he is known. The organism of Leishmaniasis was discovered in a soldier dying of 'dum dum fever'. With Wright, Leishman worked on typhoid vaccination, which was tried out first during the Boer war and was remarkably successful.

TRYPANOSOMIASIS

African Trypanosomiasis

African trpanosomiasis (Sleeping sickness) is caused by *Trypanosoma brucei* (*T b gambiense* and *T b rhodesiense*). It is transmitted to man by the bite of a tsetse fly. At the site of the bite, usually the forearm a chancre-like ulcer is formed. This is followed by secondary erythematous eruptions of an annular or circinate type. Erythema nodosum may also occur. Enlargement of the posterior cervical gland is characteristic (Winterbottom's sign). The tertiary stage is manifested by changes in the central nervous system, such as apathy, somnolence and finally coma and death.

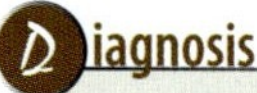

Both African and American trypanosomiasis is diagnosed by finding the trypanosomes in the chancre fluid, blood and the lymphatic fluid.

American Trypanosomiasis

American trypanosomiasis (Chagas disease) is caused by *Trypanosoma cruzi*; it is transmitted to man by the bite of a reduviid bug. The bug frequently bites at night at the mucocutaneous junction, where it deposits the infected faeces. When the sleeping person rubs the skin, the

Treatment

Suramin and pentamidine are effective in early stages of sleeping sickness. Once the central nervous system is affected, specific therapy consists of intravenous injections of melarsoprol or eflornithine.

Chagas disease should be treated with a trypanocidal drug, either nifurtimox or benznidazole. Allopurinol has recently been used.

infected faeces passes into the skin and the person becomes infected. If the bite is near the conjunctiva, an oculoglandular syndrome develops (Romana's sign). This consists of unilateral conjunctivitis, oedema of the eyelid and an ulceration of the area (chancre). Soon secondary cutaneous morbilliform eruptions occur. In the tertiary stage, the heart, thyroid and the spleen may be affected.

TOXOPLASMOSIS

Toxoplasmosis is a worldwide infection caused by *Toxoplasma gondii*. This is a crescent, round or oval protozoan. The organism invades the reticuloendothelial system and endothelium of the blood vessels forming granulomas and causing tissue necrosis. The disease is acquired through contact with animals especially cats. Meat used for human consumption may contain cysts serving as a source of infection or drinking contaminated water. The disease may be congenital or acquired.

Congenital Toxoplasmosis

Congenital toxoplasmosis affects the central nervous system, eyes, heart, lungs and the adrenals. If the infant survives, the parasite soon disappears from most organs except the central nervous system and retina.

Manifestations of congenital infection include hydrocephalus, microcephalus, convulsions, tremors and paralysis. Radiological examination shows patches of calcification in the brain.

Ophthalmic lesions include micro-ophthalmos, nystagmus and chorioretinitis. Other manifestations are enlarged liver, jaundice, thrombocytopenia and purpura. Congenital infection is usually fatal; those who survive are usually blind and disabled.

Cutaneous lesions are manifested by haemorrhagic eruptions; "blueberry muffin" lesions predominate reflecting erythropoiesis. Occasionally abnormal hair growth, exfoliative dermatitis has also been observed.

Acquired Toxoplasmosis

The acute form may be manifested by pneumonia, fever, cough, malaise, rarely jaundice and myocarditis. The cutaneous lesions consist of maculopapular eruption, subcutaneous nodules and haemorrhagic eruption, followed by scarlatiniforn desquamation.

Chronic infections are afebrile with enlargement of the lymph nodes with atypical mononuclear cells. Toxoplasmosis is a cause of chorioretinitis in adults.

Diagnosis

Serological tests are of value; antibodies detectable by fluorescence appear early in the disease and persist for years.

Smears taken from the tissues, body fluids and from lymph node biopsy show the protozoa, anti-toxoplasma antibodies are detected by the Sabin-Feldman dye test.

Toxoplasmosis and Pregnancy

A seronegative woman, who acquires toxoplasmosis during pregnancy, has a high risk of producing an abnormal fetus, and termination of pregnancy should be considered. Women who are seropositive before pregnancy do not carry the risk of fetal damage.

Pregnant women should avoid handling cat litter. Eating undercooked meat should be avoided.

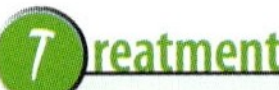

Treatment

Pyremethamine (daraprim) 25 mg every other day after a loading dose of 100 mg is given in two equal doses for 2 days. Sulphadiazine should be given in combination after a loading dose of 75 mg/kg of the body weight and then 100 mg/kg of body weight/day for 1 month. Side effects are due to interference in the folic acid metabolism, folinic acid is given concomitantly to the patient. Clindamycin is also effective.

Toxoplasmosis is one cause of the TORCH syndrome –Toxoplasmosis, Other agents, Rubella, Cytomegalovirus, Herpes simplex

HELMINTHIC INFESTATIONS

Helminthic diseases are divided into Nematodes or roundworms and Platyhelminths or flat worms. Nematodes can be intestinal roundworms or tissue roundworms such as filaria. Flat worms include tapeworms and flukes.

Larva Migrans

Larva migrans (Fig. 4) is caused by the larva of some nematodes that are parasitic to cats and dogs, usually *Ancylostoma* (*A*) *braziliense* and *A. canis*. Larva migrans is found throughout the hot and humid tropics. The larva penetrates the skin but remains unchanged, as man is not the natural host.

The feet, buttocks and trunk are frequently affected. Papules appear at the site of inoculation preceded by slight local itching. Pruritus is severe especially at night. Migration occurs in about 4 days after inoculation and progresses at the rate of 2 cm daily. Cord-like superficial burrows develop, these linear lesions may be interrupted by papules which mark the site of resting larvae. The larvae usually die in 2–8 weeks with resolution of the eruption. Secondary infection and lichenification may obscure the clinical picture.

Larva migrans may be accompanied by Loeffler's syndrome particularly in severe infection. Similar eruption can be caused by larva of flies such as *Gasterophilus*, the horse bot fly and cattle warble fly (*Hypoderma bovis*) and other nematodes.

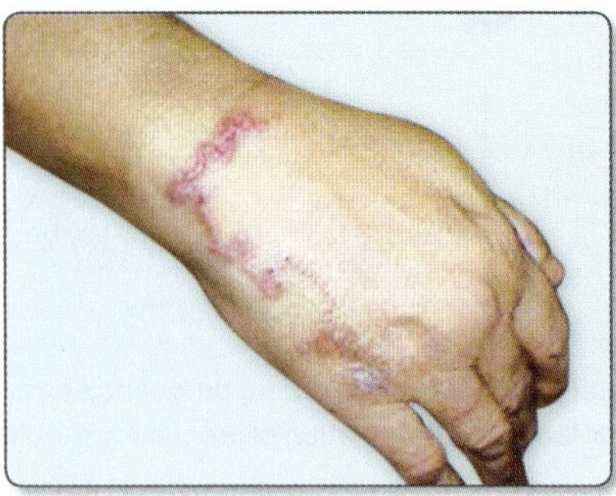

Fig. 4: Larva migrans

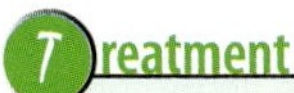

Larva migrans: Treatment of choice is topical application of 10% thiobendazole. Two tablets of 0.5 g of thiobendazole are triturated in 10 g of petrolatum and applied twice daily. 95% of cases clear within a week. Oral thiobendazole is toxic to use. Albendazole tablets 400 mg daily for 3 days, is safe and often effective. A single dose of 12 mg of oral ivermectin gives good response.

Larva Currens

Larva currens is due to the larva of *Strongyloides stercoralis*. There is rapid migration of larvae in the skin. Intense papular reaction develops at the site of penetration, often accompanied by urticaria, papulovesicular or a non-specific eruption. Often the eruption is associated with intestinal strongyloidiasis, cutaneous lesions are then seen around the anus. The skin of the abdomen is also affected, but the genitals are spared. The pruritus is intense, lesions spread at about 5–10 cm/hour. The larvae leave the skin enter the blood and settle in the intestinal mucosa. The disease is self-limiting, 80% of the lesions disappear in about 4 months, and some persist for many months.

Visceral Larva Migrans

Visceral larva migrans is caused by the roundworm of dogs. In humans the ingested eggs release larvae in the intestines. The larvae pass through the systemic circulation to the organs, such as the liver, heart, brain, spinal cord, eyes and muscles. Because the larvae cannot mature in humans they lie dormant or wander in the tissues for years. Most patients are asymptomatic. Occasionally a prolonged or debilitating illness occurs, symptoms relating to the organs affected.

Albendazole is the treatment of choice, alternate therapy is mebendazole.

Gnathostomiasis

This is a roundworm infestation caused by *Gnathostoma (G.) spinigerum*, less frequently by *G. hispidum* and *G. nipponicum*. The definite hosts are cats and dogs. The eggs are passed in the faeces of these animals, which are then hatched in water. The larvae are ingested by Cyclops, that are eaten by fish, frogs and snakes. Man becomes infected by eating undercooked fish. As man is not the definite host, the larvae wander in the human tissues or become encysted in them.

In man the ingested larvae penetrate the wall of the stomach, and migrate in tissues, causing inflammation, haemorrhage and necrosis. The parasite may reach any site of the body. Migration in the skin and subcutaneous tissue results in intermittent migratory swellings, which are erythematous and cause itching. These swellings remain at one site for 2–4 weeks. They then migrate to reappear at another site. Thighs and the trunk are the sites commonly affected. The infestation may continue for months or years. Facial migratory lesions may lead to involvement of the eye or the central nervous system.

The disease should be differentiated from onchocerciasis, loiasis, sparganosis, larva migrans and larva currens. The finding of the larva in the tissue confirms the diagnosis. Peripheral eosinophilia is high.

Surgical excision and albendazole is the treatment of choice.

Filariasis

Filariasis is an infestation with helminths of the class Nematodes and family filiarioidae. The adult filaria is a thread-like worm that inhabits the lymphatic vessels and connective tissue of man and some animals. Filariasis is transmitted by the bite of a mosquito. The following are some of the clinical varieties of filariasis:

- Bancroftian and Malayan filariasis
- Onchocerciasis
- Dracunculiasis
- Loiasis

Bancroftian Filariasis (Lymphatic filariasis)

Bancroftian filariasis (Lymphatic filariasis) is an infestation caused by *Wuchereria bancrofti*, *Brugia (B.) malayi* and *B. timori*. The adult filaria is a thread-like long worm that inhabits the lymphatic vessels and connective tissue of man and some animals. The disease is transmitted by many species of anthropophilic mosquitoes of the species *Culex*, *Aedes* and *Anopheles*. The disease is characterised by lymphoedema with resultant hypertrophy of the skin and subcutaneous tissue.

Man is infected by the bite of an infected mosquito; the larva passes through the peripheral lymphatics and migrates centrally where they eventually grow into adults. The adults mate in the lymphatics proximal to the lymph nodes; fertilised females discharge their microfilariae in the peripheral blood 12 months after the initial infection. The discharge is cyclical and occurs principally at night. The adults are found in the dilated lymphatics.

Clinical Features

The clinical features depend upon the lymphatics (usually lower extremity, scrotum and penis) affected, age of first exposure and the presence of immunity. Manifestation may be acute, chronic and recurrent.

The onset of filariasis is characterised by recurrent attacks of acute lymphangitis; this starts in the groin and then extends peripherally. The lymph nodes are enlarged and tender, associated with fever and chill that last for several days to several weeks. These episodes occur over a period of several months or years, there may be a dozen or more attacks in a year. Filarial orchitis and hydrocele are common.

In the later chronic obstructive stage, lymphatic varices and elephantiasis develop (Fig. 5). The latter is characterised by pronounced enlargement of the leg or scrotum with thickening of the skin, papillomatous and warty growths with fissuring. These changes cause considerable deformity and incapacitation. The course of the disease is slow and progressive.

The upper extremity, breasts and vulva are less commonly involved. Tropical pulmonary eosinophilia develops in some patients; this is associated with progressive restrictive pulmonary disease.

Diagnosis

Microfilariae can be found in the blood taken from the finger or ear, and then examined under a microscope. Specimens should be taken between 12 pm and 2 am at night, as the microfilariae enter the peripheral blood at that time. Micofilariae can also be seen in the peripheral blood after a single dose of 100 mg of diethylcarbamazine. The drug releases the microfilariae in the circulation.

Differential Diagnosis

Acute cases should be differentiated from bacterial lymphangitis. Verrucous enlarged legs may be found in chromomycosis, madura foot, leprosy and deep fungal infections.

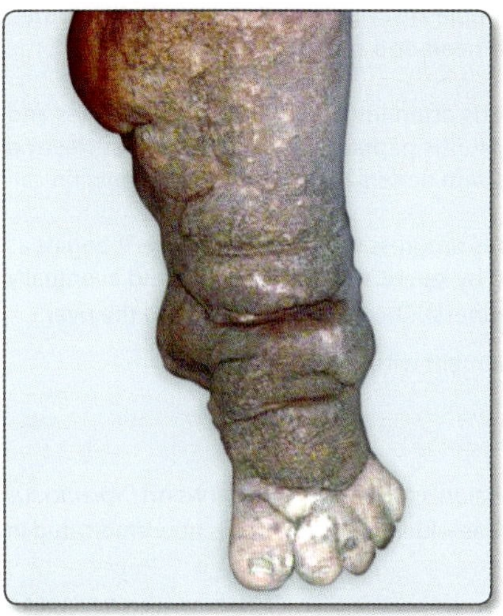

Fig. 5: Filariasis

Treatment

Treatment can be medical, conservative and surgical.

Medical-Ivermectin 200 µg/kg in a single dose. Diethylcarbamazine can also be used; it kills both microfilariae and the adult worm.

Conservative- to remove the lymph in the extravascular tissue by decongestive therapy with multilayered compression bandage bandage, skin care and exercise.

Surgery-surgical operations to remove oedematous subcutaneous tissue.

Prophylactic measures for adequate mosquito control

Onchocerciasis

Onchocerciasis (River blindness) is a filarial disease caused by *Onchocerca volvulus*. It is transmitted by the bite of a buffalo gnat. It is found in the tropical region of Africa and America, mainly along the fast flowing streams. After entering the skin the larvae mature into adults worms that are encapsulated in fibrous tissue as nodules. These are seen in the subcutaneous tissue and deep fascia.

The skin is affected first and then the eye. The disease commonly affects the legs; it presents as itchy papules which later become lichenoid and pigmented, followed by scarring.

Diagnosis

Onchocerciasis is diagnosed by finding the microfilariae in the skin, and the adult worm in the nodules. In heavily infected patients the microfilariae can be found in the blood.

Treatment

Ivermectin is the treatment of choice. It is given as a single dose of 100–200 µg/kg. It is nontoxic and does not trigger severe reactions as seen with diethylcarbamazine. Nodules may be removed surgically.

It may be necessary to repeat the dose after a few months if the disease reappears.

The disease can also present as erysipelas like eruption and marked oedema. This is often followed by speckled depigmentation of the skin (leopard skin), which later becomes dry and ichthyotic (lizard skin). Subcutaneous nodules appear at various parts of the body; these are pea sized or larger. These nodules (onchocercomas) contain a large number of microfilariae. In Africa, these nodules are widespread as the people are only partially covered with clothes. In America, they appear on the head and neck. The lesions later become fibrotic and calcified.

Acute papular onchodermatitis often involves the face, extremities and the trunk; the lesions consist of pruritic papules that progress to vesicles and pustules. This may be associated with oedema and erythema. Ivermectin can precipitate a similar rash.

Ocular involvement is a serious progressive disabling feature. It begins as a painless conjunctivitis followed by keratitis, iritis, choroiditis and eventually this leads to blindness (river blindness). The gnats breed close to the river.

Prevention: Mass population treatment with ivermectin.

Dracunculiasis

Dracunculiasis (Guinea worm infection) is caused by a filarial worm *Dracunculus medinensis*: the guinea worm. It was widely distributed; it is now eradicated in many parts of the world.

The disease is contracted by drinking water infected with crustacean cyclops, which is found in stagnant water. The adult worm migrates to the subcutaneous tissue of the legs. When the leg or the foot comes in contact with water, a blister forms that ulcerates, larvae come out of the wound, these are taken up by the cyclops, which become infected by engulfing these free-swimming larvae. The ulcer heals in 4–6 months.

Treatment

Niridazole in a dose of 25 mg/kg of body weight is given for 7–10 days. Metronidazole is also effective. The old traditional approach was to induce the worm to discharge the larva by applying ethyl chloride or hydrochloric acid and then removing the worm. The worm was wound around a matchstick, gradually more and more of the worm was wound as it came out until the whole of the worm was removed. The procedure must be done with great care, the worm should not be broken or else a severe reaction would occur at the site.

The disease is now under control in many parts of the world as the drinking water is well disinfected, which kills the larvae. Improved public health measures can help in the control of dracunculiasis.

Loiasis

Loiasis (Calabar swellings) is caused by Loa loa filarial worms and transmitted to man by the bite of a chrysops fly. It is found in the hot humid climate of equatorial Africa.

The larvae enter the body by the bite of a chrysops fly. The larva matures, into an adult worm in the subcutaneous tissue; it then migrates along fascial planes to different parts of the body. The adult worms produce microfilariae that enter the bloodstream during the day, and they reside in the lungs when not circulating.

Clinical symptoms: Then disease is characterised by painful itchy inflammatory swellings (calabar swellings) caused by the migration of the worm into the subcutaneous tissue. Any part of the body can be affected. The swelling later subsides leaving hyperpigmented areas. Infection of the eyes and joints can be incapacitating. When the eye is infected, unilateral palpebral oedema may develop; the worm may actually be seen crossing the eye. Generalised urticaria and oedema of the limbs can occur. The finding of microfilaria in the blood is diagnostic.

Diagnosis

Blood test for identification of the microfilariae during the day. Peripheral eosinophilia is common. Calcified worms may be seen on X-ray films.

Treatment

Diethylcarbamazine is the treatment of choice. Alternative treatment is with albendazole. Topical antipruritics and oral antihistamines are helpful.

PLATYHELMINTHS

Cestodes

Subcutaneous cysticercosis is due to the larva of *Taenia solium*, the pork tapeworm. Man gets infected by ingesting the eggs of the adult worm. The outer shell of the egg disintegrates in the small intestine; the embryos released enter the circulation. From here they are disseminated widely. It causes asymptomatic soft rubbery nodules; any part of the body may be affected. The disease should be differentiated from sebaceous cysts, lipomas and fibromas. The nodules should be removed surgically. Praziquantil in low doses as 10 mg/kg of body weight is said to cure almost every patient infected with *T. solium*. Treatment with albendazole, trivalent antimonial compounds such as niridazole is also effective.

Sparganosis

Sparganosis is a tapeworm larva of genus Spirometra (S). The species are *S. mansoni*, *S. erinaceri* and *S. mansoniodes*. The definite hosts for Spirometra are the cats and dogs. Two intermediate hosts are required; these are a copepod and a vertebrate. Humans are incidental hosts for the second stage larvae. Other vertebrates that can be infected are amphibians, reptiles and birds.

The skin can be infected by two routes, first by ingestion and secondly when infected flesh is applied to the skin.

The clinical signs depend upon the route of infection. When infected by ingestion, the larvae migrate to the muscles or subcutaneous tissue, where they provoke an inflammatory reaction. Resulting in the formation of a slow-growing subcutaneous nodule, that is occasionally migratory. The other organs which may be infected are the brain, eye, lungs, urethra and the epididymus.

When the infected flesh containing the larvae is applied to the skin, it results in pruritus, erythema, oedema and later nodules develop. These are painful on palpation.

The disease is diagnosed by finding the larvae in the tissue. There is peripheral blood eosinophilia.

Treatment is by excision of the nodule.

Trematodes

These are blood flukes that are parasitic to the skin or the internal organs. The viscera may be infected by *Schistosomia* (*S.*) *hematobium*, *S. masoni*, *S. japonicum*. The cercaria penetrates the skin, where it produces a local inflammatory response. They then enter the venules to reach the pulmonary capillaries. Worms mature in the hepatic sinusoids and then migrate to mesenteric vessels (*S. intercatum*, *S. japonicum*, *S. masoni*), in the rectovesical plexus (*S. hematobium*). The mature worm pairs and produces eggs 1–3 months after infection. Most of the eggs remain in the tissues or blood vessels, some reach the bowel or the bladder, from where they are excreted.

The cutaneous manifestations of schistosomiasis (bilharziasis) begin with mild itchy papular dermatitis of the feet and often other parts of the body. Swimming in polluted streams containing cercarie causes the infection. After an asymptomatic latent period, there may be a sudden illness with fever and chills, pneumonitis and eosinoplilia. Petechial haemorrhages may occur.

Praziquantel is effective in treating trematode infections.

A severe urticarial reaction occurs with *S. japonicum* this is known as Katayama fever. In addition to urticaria, fever, malaise, abdominal cramps, arthritis and involvement of the liver and spleen may occur.

S. hematobium is associated with dysuria, urinary frequency, renal calculi, haematuria, hydronephrosis and renal failure. Infection with *S. japanocum* and *S. masoni* results in hepatosplenomegaly, portal and pulmonary hypertension, intestinal polyps and strictures.

Schistosomal cercarial dermatitis (Swimmer's itch): This is caused by the penetration of a cercaria of non-human schistosomes. Man is infected by swimming in fresh water. After coming out of the water, the bather begins to itch, erythematous eruptions occur. Then after a quiescent period of 10–15 hours, the symptoms reappear. Erythematous macules and papules occur throughout the body. Cercarial dermatitis should be differentiated from sea bather's itch which is only restricted to the bathing costume area.

Treatment is by soothing lotions and corticosteroids.

DISEASES CAUSED BY ARTHROPODS

Arthropods are invertebrate animals having jointed limbs, a segmental body, and an exoskeleton made of chitin. In the tropics man is exposed to a large number of venomous arthropods. These may sting, bite or inject a toxin. These may elicit an allergic or toxic reaction. An individual never bitten by an arthropod reacts to the bite with a minimal pinpoint haemorrhagic spot; sensitization to the salivary antigen develops later, followed by a hypersensitivity reaction. In some cases repeated bites lead to a decreased sensitisation, the individual becomes immune to the particular arthropod.

Arthropods that cause dermatological diseases are:

- Class Hexapoda are insects, such as lice, fleas, bees, flies, mosquitoes and ants
- Class Arachnida are arthropods, such as mites, scorpions, spiders and ticks.
- Class Chilopoda arthropods, such as centipedes and millipedes

Class Hexapoda

True insects belong to the class hexapoda. Insects are small air breathing arthropods, having a body divided into head, thorax and abdomen, with three pairs of legs, some have wings. Insect bites cause an urticarial wheal with a central punctum, which may be followed by a papule. The following are the diseases of dermatological interest:

- Pediculosis
- Myiasis
- Papular urticaria

Pediculosis

Pediculosis (Phthiriasis) is caused by the infestation with lice. Lice are six-legged wingless insects 1-4 mm in length, grey in colour, reddish when engorged with blood. The body louse is the largest. The pubic louse is round and small with powerful claws, as they feed on the skin an irritating substance is injected causing itchy papules. Man is parasitised by two species of lice, *Pediculus humanis* and *Pediculus pubis*. There are two subspecies of *Pediculus humanus*, *Pediculus capitis* and *Pediculus corporis*. Each species of lice has predilection for different parts of the body and rarely migrates to other sites. The lice attach themselves on the skin and live on the blood they suck. In piercing the skin, the parasite exudes an antigenic salivary secretion; this together with the mechanical punctures produce pruritus and inflammation. The bite of a louse is painless.

Pediculosis capitis: This is a common infestation, found mainly in children, no class is exempt. It is transmitted by intimate personal contact through hats, brushes and combs.

Clinical Features

The infection usually begins with severe itching of the nape of the neck and behind the ears. Red papules with a central haemorrhagic dot may be found, but these papules are usually excoriated, by scratching. Neglected cases show secondary impetigo, furuncles, eczematization and cervical adenitis is common (Fig. 6).

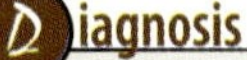

Diagnosis

Is made by finding nits attached to the hair, lice are often difficult to find unless heavily infected. The nits fluoresce with a greyish-white glow under the Wood's light. The lice attach the nits close to the base of the hair shaft at the scalp level. As hair grows, the nits are seen at some distance from the scalp. The presence of persistent impetigo of the scalp should suggest pediculosis capitis.

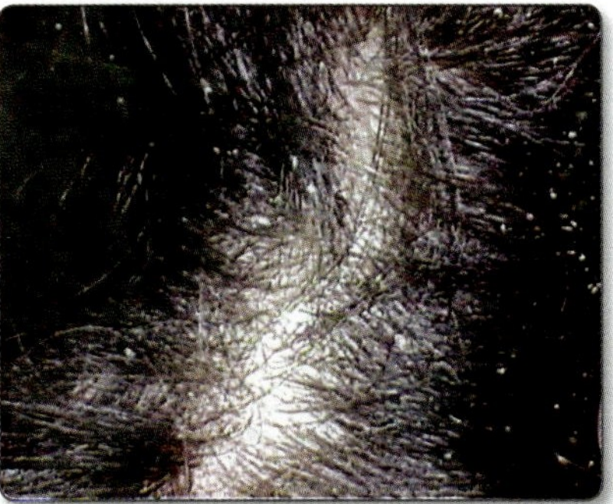

Fig. 6: Pediculosis capitis

Life cycle: Adult female head lice are 3–4 mm long; the male is slightly smaller. The colour varies from white to greyish black. The lice attach themselves to the host tissue by strong crab like claws and suck blood through a stylet. During the life cycle of about 40 days, the female is capable of laying about 300 eggs at the rate of 7–10 eggs per day. The eggs are firmly cemented to the base of the hair. The eggs are operculated and have a characteristic disc-like structure with holes for the entry of oxygen. The nymphs hatch in about 8 days following 3 moults the adult lice develops, in about 10 days.

Treatment

This should aim at destruction of the lice and ova. Permethrin 1% cream is applied to the scalp overnight and washed next morning. A repeat application after 7–10 days is necessary. After washing, the hair should be combed with a fine-tooth comb.

Gamma benzene hexachloride (Lindane) is available in the form of cream or shampoo. The shampoo may be thoroughly massaged into the scalp for 5–10 minutes and then rinsed out. The remaining nits may be removed with a fine-toothed comb. Lindane should not be used on infants, pregnant and nursing women.

Malathoin lotion is absorbed in the keratin, a process that takes about 6 hours; it also has a residual effect against reinfection for about 6 weeks. It should remain on the scalp for about 12 hours before being washed out. Malathoin and carbaryl are degraded by heat; therefore hot hair dryer should not be used after the use of these drugs. Treatment should be repeated after 10 days.

Crotamiton in a 10% cream or lotion is effective as a 24-hour application, followed by a shampoo. A fine comb removes nits.

Twenty-five percent benzyl bezoate lotion left for 24 hours is also effective. Nits can be removed with 5% acetic acid or white vinegar left for a few hours on the scalp and wrapping the head with a towel.

For mass delousing 2–5% DDT emulsion or 10% DDT powder are applied to the scalp overnight. The treatment should be repeated in 7–10 days.

Oral therapy with cotrimoxazole is reported to be effective in eradicating head lice. The antibiotic is ingested by the louse, this affects the symbiotic behaviour between the louse and the bacteria, these are essential for the synthesis of vitamins, without which the louse cannot survive. The minimal effective dose of co-trimoxazole for pediculosis is one tablet twice daily for 3 days. The course has to be repeated in 7–10 days.

Oral ivermectin 200 μg/kg of body weight may be used to treat resistant or widespread cases.

In treating lice infestation, other family members should also be examined and treated simultaneously or else reinfection will occur.

Pediculosis Corporis

This is generally found in persons with poor hygiene and in vagabonds. *Pediculus corporis* is about 30% larger than *Pediculus capitis*, but has essentially the same morphology. The body louse lives on the seams of clothing where it lays its eggs and attacks the body only to feed. The eggs are cemented to the clothing; seams are the favourite site for laying the eggs. The body louse does not survive at high temperature such as washing and ironing. It is therefore found in individuals who rarely change or wash their clothes.

Clinical Features

The clinical findings of a body louse are macula cerulae (blue macules), found in areas where the clothing comes in close contact with the skin, such as the waist, buttocks and thigh. The macule often has

Contd...

Contd...

a central punctum. The other sign of a body louse are excoriations often linear, primarily on the interscapular region, posterior aspect of the axillae, hips and thighs. These scratch marks are often diagnostic. Long-standing cases show patches of pigmentation, pyoderma, eczematization and lichenification.

Body lice are important because they are also carriers of infections caused by *Ricketsia prowazekii* (epidemic typhus), *Bartonella quintana* (trench fever) and relapsing fever caused by *Borrelia recurrentis.*

The disease is diagnosed by finding the eggs or lice on the seams of clothing.

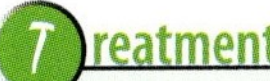

Topically soothing antipruritic lotions after baths usually suffice. If secondary bacterial infection is present, it is treated by topical or systemic antibiotics. The clothing should be sterilised by boiling followed by ironing of the seams. Dusting with 10% DDT powder, 1% malathion or gamma benzene hexachloride is effective.

Pediculosis corporis is also the vector of epidemic typhus, relapsing fever and trench fever

Pediculosis Pubis

Pediculosis pubis is caused through sexual contact. It may also be contracted via public toilets seats, bathing or contaminated bedding and towels. Pediculosis pubis frequently coexists with other sexually transmitted diseases. The diagnosis of pediculosis pubis should initiate a search for other sexually transmitted diseases.

It differs in appearance from the head louse. The body is somewhat rounded like that of a crab, with small claws on the front legs and larger claws on the hind legs, which allows the louse to grip the widely spaced pubic hair. It is mainly sedentary but becomes active

Clinical Features

Itching is the main symptom. Pruritic red papules, with a central punctum are found on the pubis, which soon becomes excoriated and eczematized. The hair of the axillae, thighs, chest, beard, eyebrows and eyelashes may also be involved. The scalp is spared, as the lice of pediculosis pubis are adapted to living in hair of a particular density, scalp hair is too dense for the habitation of the pubic louse. In neglected cases bluish or steel-grey asymptomatic macules may be found on the abdomen, these are called "maculae cerulae", similar to that found in pediculosis corporis.

Infants may be infected on the eyebrows and eyelashes from contact with infected persons (Fig. 7).

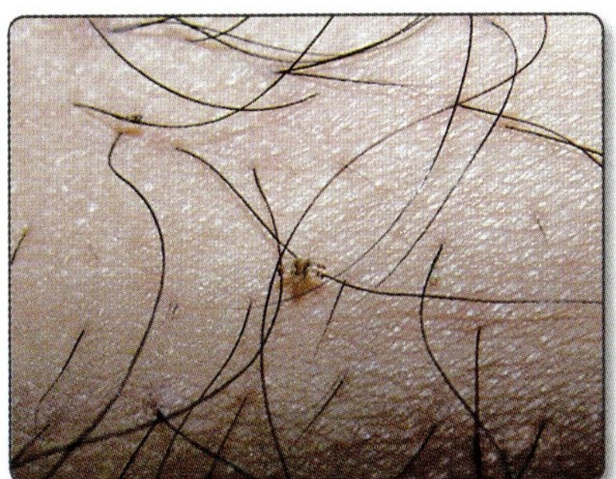

Fig. 7: Pediculosis pubis – note the thin density of hair

at night, when the host is sleeping. It moves by transferring its grip from one hair to another. The crab louse has difficulty moving when taken from its host, whereas the body and head louse are quite mobile. Pubic louse lives on pubic hair, eyebrows and eyelashes, where the density of hair is low. The pubic louse moves at a slow rate (10 cm/day) compared to the body and head louse (23 cm/min).

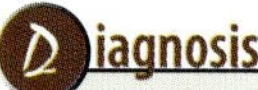

The diagnosis is made by finding the crab-like pediculi against the skin, often firmly attached to the hair by the claws or finding nits glued to the hair.

Treatment

The treatment is the same as for pediculosis capitis; sexual contacts should also be treated. Therapy for the eyelashes is the use of petrolatum applied thickly twice daily for 8 days, followed by removal of the nits mechanically. The ointment interferes with the respiratory function of the louse by blocking its spiracle. Clothing and fomites should be boiled or sprinkled with DDT powder.

Always think of pediculosis in a patient with recurring folliculitis of the scalp
In cases of pediculosis corporis look for lice and nits in clothing and not on the skin

Myiasis

Myiasis is infestation of any part of the body by the larva of diptera. The eggs are laid in neglected ulcers, which later crawl with maggots. In ancient times maggots were applied by doctors to treat necrotic tissue.

Clinical Features

Clinical manifestations may be:

- Myiasis of a wound in which eggs and larvae (maggots) are present. This is common in neglected ulcers and wounds in rural tropics. Abscess, lymphangitis, cellulitis and tetanus may develop
- Furunculoid lesions
- Subcutaneous tunnels such as larva migrans.

The nasal, ocular, auricular cavities and internal organs can be affected by the migration of the larva.

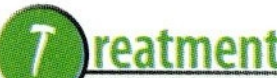

Wound myiasis is treated by surgical removal of the maggots and douching of the wound for 30 minutes with 15% chloroform, dissolved in light vegetable oil. Treatment of furuncular myiasis is by injections of local anaesthetics into the skin, which anaesthetize both the skin and the larva. Then incising the lesion or pushing the larva out with pressure from beneath removes the larva. The larva can be suffocated by topical application of thiobendazole. Albendazole can also be used.

Papular Urticaria

Papular urticaria is a common chronic pruritic papular eruption caused by an allergic skin reaction to insect bites. It is common in children from families of low socioeconomic status, adults develop the disease when they move to a new environment and are exposed to bites by different arthropods. In urban areas, the common causes are fleas and bedbugs. In rural areas mosquitoes, mites, fleas, chiggers are the common causative agents.

Clinical Features

The lesions pass through two stages; an urticarial wheal that fades in 1–2 days and is replaced by a firm papule. A vesicle often develops at the apex of the papule that becomes excoriated by scratching; each attack may last for 2–10 days. The lesions occur in crops usually at night, the lesions are few millimetres in diameter usually discrete but may occur in groups. Pruritus is severe; scratching causes lichenification and secondary infection.

The distribution of the eruption may offer a clue to the causative arthropod. Involvement of the exposed parts suggests a flying insect, infection on the ankles and legs are frequently caused by fleas, lesions on the trunk are often caused by bedbugs. A change in environment causes recovery, residual hyperpigmentation is common. Host sensitivity is probably important since only one member of the family is affected. The disease may gradually disappear due to desensitisation following repeated exposure to the bites. The course of the disease is chronic, the eruption prevails in warm and rainy weather, relapses may occur every summer. New lesions may activate the old ones.

Differential Diagnosis

The disease should be differentiated from scabies, in the latter burrows are found, family history is often positive for scabies. Atopic eczema particularly if lichenified and papular, may resemble papular urticaria. In atopic eczema, a family history is positive for atopy, the rash is common in the flexures.

Treatment

The treatment should begin with elimination of the insects; insecticidal powders, such as pyrethrin is effective in treating furniture and bedding. If the source cannot be isolated, insect repellents may be helpful. Oral antihistamines may reduce itching; antipruritic lotions may be applied topically. Corticosteroids may also be applied in severe cases.

Fleas

These are wingless arthropods, flat from side to side with highly developed legs for jumping. They are capable of jumping by approximately 2 feets. The body is armoured with chitin and the mouth is highly specialised for penetration and sucking. Fleas live on rugs and bodies of animals. They jump to the body of humans.

Fleas that infect man are the human, cat and the dog flea. They cause bubonic plague. Fleas usually bite around the legs and waist; they extract their blood meal from the superficial capillaries. Haemorrhagic puncta occur surrounded by an erythematous and urticarial patch. In some persons immediate or late hypersensitivity reaction develops.

Treatment

Flea control is essential by pyrethrin and malathion. Calamine lotion and corticosteroid creams give prompt relief.

Tungiasis

The sand flea causes this infection. The bite causes a pruritic swelling about the size of a pea. This usually occurs at the ankle and feet. The lesions are very painful and become secondarily infected. Although both male and female flea live on the skin, only the female burrows into the skin, the eggs are laid and then the female falls off to the ground. The egg develops into larvae and then into the insect in about 10 days.

Treatment

Curettage of the burrow is recommended. Thiobendazole 25 mg/kg of body weight/day is used in heavily infested individuals. Antibiotics should be used for secondary bacterial infections. Tetanus prophylaxis should be given. Insecticides should be used to disinfect infected playing grounds. Wearing of shoes will prevent infection.

A typical feature of flea bite is that when a new bite occurs, the previous ones also begin to itch.

Bees and Wasps

Bees are widely distributed, especially found in warm climate. Honey bee can sting only once, because the barbed stinger is left on the skin. Wasps can sting several times. The venom of bees has a haemolysing factor and histamine.

Bite reaction depends upon the degree of sensitivity, and the amount of venom injected. A reddish flare develops at the site of bite, with a whitish peripheral zone. Systemic reaction can range from simple urticaria, to generalised oedema and shock. Serum sickness like reaction can occur after 2 weeks.

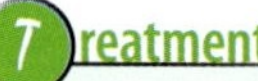

Remove the stinger with forceps. Elevate the limb, apply ice packs. Hydrocortisone skin ointment and IM antihistamine are indicated in mild cases. In severe systemic reaction subcutaneous injection of epinephrine (1:1000) 0.2–0.5 mL subcutaneously, repeated every 15 minutes. Injection of antihistamine and systemic steroids by IM route are helpful. Oxygen is indicated if there is cyanosis.

BedBugs

Bedbug (*Cimex lectularius*) is a smelly parasite with non-functioning wings; it is found all over the world. It lives in crevices during the day and feeds on human blood at night. The bedbug bite is painless; the saliva contains a protein that gives rise to a hypersensitive reaction about the punctum. Bites often follow a line or are grouped together. Papular urticaria and extensive erythema have been reported by the bite. The females must have a bloody meal to lay eggs; these are deposited in the corners of the wooden bed-stands and other crevices. The bedbug may survive starvation for many months and is readily transported in baggage and clothes. Hepatitis B virus has been demonstrated in the bug and it is thought that the bedbug may be responsible for transmitting hepatitis.

Itching is relieved by soothing antipruritic lotions. Bedbugs should be removed from the crevices in the furniture, floors and walls; these should be sprayed with 0.1% trichlorfon, pyrethrin, malathion, or lindane. An infected house should be treated with methyl bromide fumigation.

Cockroaches

These belong to the primitive order of insects such as crickets and the grasshoppers. They were originally adapted for the hot climates but are now also found in the cooler regions. The cockroaches are active nocturnally. Inhalation of cockroach allergens may play a part in allergic asthma, chronic rhinitis and conjunctivitis. Contact dermatitis has been reported in laboratory workers.

Flies

Black flies transmit onchocerciasis
Sandfly transmits leishmaniasis, bartonellosis and sandfly fever
Tsetse fly transmits African trypanosomiasis
The common fly causes myaisis

Mosquitoes

Mosquitoes transmit malaria, dengue fever, yellow fever and filariasis

Class Arachnida

All adults in this class of arthropods have four pairs of legs, two body parts the cephalothorax and an abdomen.

Scabies

Scabies is a contagious disease caused by a mite called *Sarcoptes scabiei*, it has a worldwide distribution, both sexes are affected, it is most common in infants, children and young adults. The mite has an ovoid body, having a head and abdomen, which has four pairs of short legs, and the dorsal surface is marked by bristles and spines. The mite appears to avoid areas with a large density of pilosebaceous glands. The average number of adult mite on an individual with scabies is about 12.

Incidence and epidemiology: Scabies is a worldwide infection and affects all races; it is more common in overcrowded environment. Incidence of scabies in developed countries shows cyclical variation, perhaps this is due to different ways of living in different times. During the world wars there was a high incidence of scabies, by the early 1950s there was a decline in the incidence of scabies and in mid-1960s there was again a rise, perhaps this was due to sexual promiscuity in this decade. Another explanation is the "herd immunity", after an epidemic of scabies there is a high degree of immunity in people so that another epidemic will not occur, until another new susceptible population has developed. Spread of scabies is dependent upon the customs and social factors, rather than inherent susceptibility.

In developing countries, overcrowding and poor hygiene are responsible for the high incidence of scabies. Scabies is transmitted by close physical contact. Fertilised female mite is mainly responsible for transmission. The mite survives for 24–36 hours at room temperature away from the host.

Life cycle: After copulation the male dies, the pregnant female burrows under the skin along the horny layer mainly at night, advancing 2–3 mm daily, 2–3 eggs are laid each day for 4–5 weeks and then the female mite dies. In 3–4 days the eggs hatch and a 6-legged larva appears which migrates from the burrow, by cutting through the roof on to the surface of the skin. They then dig small burrows in which they transform into nymphs. After further moults, adult male and female develop. The cycle from an egg to an adult takes about 15 days.

The adult female mite measures about 0.4 mm long and 0.3 mm broad; the male mite is smaller 0.2 mm long and 0.15 mm broad. The body is creamy-white marked by transverse corrugations, on its dorsal surface bristles and spines are present. There are four pairs of legs; the anterior two pairs end in elongated peduncles tipped with small suckers. In the female two hind legs end in long bristles, but in the male there are bristles in the third pair and elongated puduncles in the fourth.

Immunology: Immediate and delayed hypersensitivity reactions is involved in the development of lesions of scabies. Levels of IgE are variable, in some cases, there is an increased level of IgE and in others, it is normal. High levels of IgM and IgG and low levels of IgA are found during the infection. After the infection IgG and IgM levels fall, whereas IgA level rises. Involvement of delayed hypersensitivity reaction results in papules and nodules; this is suggested by the predominance of T lymphocytes in the cutaneous inflammation.

It takes 1–2 weeks for the stratum corneum to turn over and shed the foreign material and for the hypersensitivity reaction to subside.

Pathogenesis: Sensitisation begins 2–4 weeks after the onset of infection. During this time, the parasites may persist in the skin without causing any discomfort or pruritus. Severe itching begins with sensitisation of the host. In reinfection, this itching begins immediately and may be clinically more intense.

Clinical Features

The first symptoms appear in about 2 weeks after infestation. The main complaint is generalised irritation more severe at night. The pathognomonic lesion is a burrow, the typical burrow is greyish, scaly, tortuous or linear, up to 1 cm in length, and it may have a small vesicle at one end, which contains the mite. The burrows are found on the palms, interdigital folds, flexural aspects of the wrist, they are also seen on the head and neck region of babies, the head and neck is not affected in adults. Mites prefer areas that are not hairy and those with low sebum excretion.

The hypersensitivity pruritic papules are generalised, but occur predominantly over the axillae, around the areola, periumbilical area, genitals, buttocks and the thighs. The primary manifestations are present along an imaginary arch; intersecting points are axillae, elbows, wrists, hands and the crotch. This was known as the circle of Hebra. The papules are very itchy and may persist for weeks or months after the scabies infection has been treated. In addition to these primary manifestations, secondary lesions are due to infections, such as impetigo, eczematization and glomerulonephritis occur as complication of scabies. Patients who are clean and bathe frequently the eruption is seldom pronounced this makes the clinical diagnosis difficult (Figs 8A to D).

Scabies in infants: The clinical features of scabies in infants differ slightly from those of older children. There is more extensive distribution of burrows, vesicles and vesiculo-pustular lesions, lesions in the hands and feet are common. Bullous lesions are also found. Extensive eczematization, multiple crusted nodules are found on the trunk and limbs.

In the elderly pruritus is a problem because of the already dry skin; bullous lesions are also seen.

Scabies in patients with good hygiene is often difficult to diagnose, as the lesions are few, and the burrows are difficult to find.

Scabies incognito: This is seen in patients who are immunocompromised or on immunosuppressive drugs. The presentation of scabies is not typical. Presentation similar to crusted scabies, Darier's disease or even contact dermatitis. Scabies should be considered whenever severe widespread pruritus is present in an immunocompromised patient.

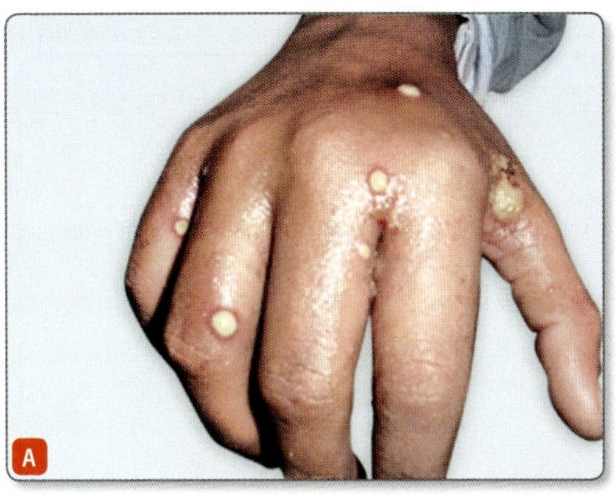

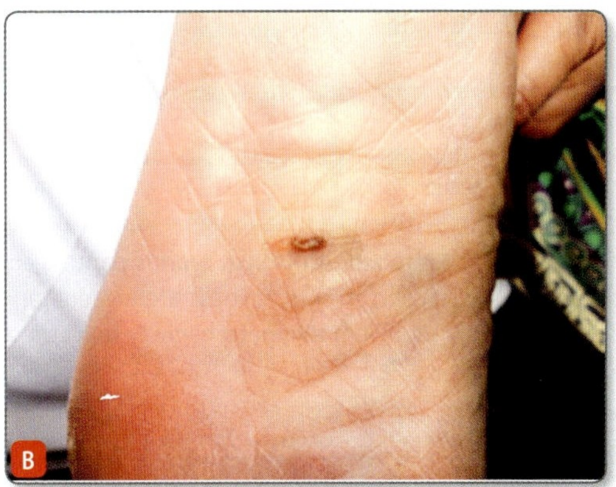

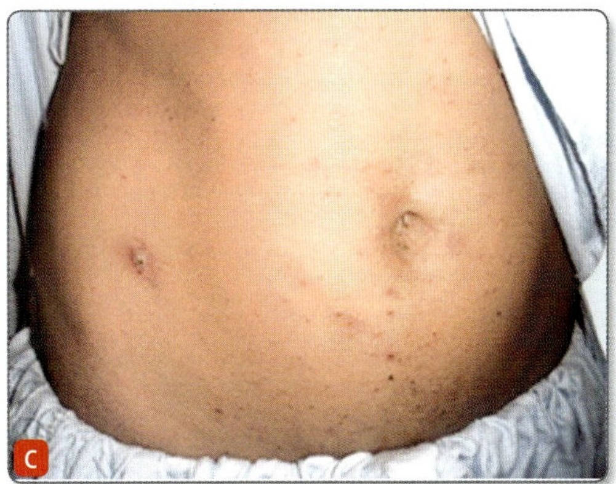

Contd...

Contd...

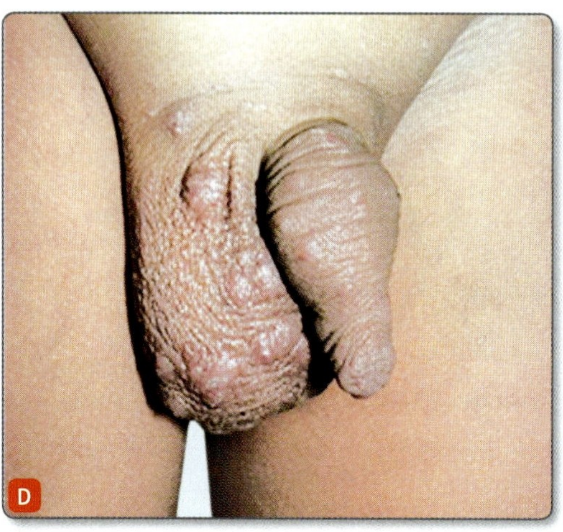

Figs 8A to D: (A) Infected scabies-note the finger web involvement; (B) Scabies burrow; (C) Scabies hypersensitivity—generalized involvement; (D) Scabies-nodules on the genitals

Nodular scabies: The lesions are reddish-brown pruritic papules and nodules on the male genitalia, axillae, and the groin. These are present long after the treatment. These probably represent a hypersensitivity reaction to retained parts of mite or antigens.

Diagnosis

The three diagnostic features of scabies are the burrow, nocturnal pruritus and the characteristic distribution of the eruption. Itching in other members of the family often helps in the diagnosis. Inflammatory papules and nodules on the male genitals are also characteristic of scabies. The presence of a female mite in the burrow confirms the diagnosis. The burrow is opened with the help of a scalpel (burrow can be outlined with black ink); the contents of the burrow are examined under a microscope. Potassium hydroxide is not used for examination as it dissolves the faeces, which may be the only sign of infestation.

Dermoscopy shows small, dark triangular structures, corresponding to the pigmented anterior segment of the mite, and a subtle linear segment containing air bubbles, which is thought to be a burrow, with eggs and fecal pellets.

Differential Diagnosis

Scabies should be differentiated from generalised pruritus in which there are no visible skin lesions, but there may be secondary changes due to scratching. The absence of burrows confirms the diagnosis.

Eczema should be differentiated from secondary eczematization due to scabies by the presence of burrows, demonstration of acarus, nocturnal itching and by a family history of scabies in the family.

Dermatitis herpetiformis is also another very pruritc condition; excoriated papules on the buttocks are similar to scabies. Herpetiform vesicles are also present in the elbows and knees. Biopsy shows neutrophilic microabscesses in the papillary dermis, with subepidermal blister formation.

Treatment

A number of drugs are used for the treatment of scabies. The pattern of treatment should be as follows in countries where scabies is endemic.

- A hot soap and water bath is taken preferably at night, scrubbing the affected areas where the burrows are found such as the wrist and finger webs, to open the burrows.
- Application from the neck down to the body with a thin layer of the medication, which is allowed to dry and kept overnight.
- Often a second application of the drug with a change of clothing, the following night without a bath.
- A bath on the 3rd day, followed by a change of clothing and bed linen.
- All family members should be treated.
- Repeat medication after 5 days, when the eggs have hatched.

Patient should be warned that it may take several days for the irritation to subside. The papular lesions on the genitals may persist for months, although the patients are no longer infectious

For adults 10% sulphur ointment in soft yellow paraffin is safe, effective and cheap. It can be used to treat a number of family members especially those of low income. 2.5% concentration may be applied to infants. Two applications are required as outlined above.

Twenty-five percent benzyl benzoate emulsion can also be used; it should also be applied once daily for 2 days.

0.5% malathion in aqueous base is also an effective scabicide, it is left on the skin for 24 hours; a second application is required after an interval of a few days.

Permethrin 5% cream is an effective scabicide it can be used as a single application, washed after 8–12 hours.

Gamma benzene hexachloride is used as a single application, washed after 12–24 hours is recommended, but a 6 hourly application is also effective. Adverse neurological effects especially seizures can occur in infants. Lindane should not be used in pregnant and lactating women.

Crotamiton has limited scabicidal activity and several applications on consecutive days are needed.

Oral ivermectin can be used in the treatment of scabies, pediculosis, onchocerciasis, filariasis, larva currens and strongyloidiasis. It is used in resistant, epidemic or crusted scabies in a single dose 200 µg/kg of body weight, and repeated after 2 weeks. The drug paralyses the parasite. Topical ivermectin has also been used for the treatment of pediculosis and scabies.

Albendazole and cotrimoxazole are other oral medications used to treat scabies.

Think of scabies when patients complain of pruritus worse at night and other family members are affected. Sulphur and benzyl benzoate are cheap and are mostly used when a number of family members are to be treated, where low socioeconomic conditions prevail.

Norwegian Scabies

Norwegian scabies is a rare clinical variant of scabies seen in mentally retarted, immunosuppressed patients, patients who are severely incapacitated as in severe arthropathy or neurological disorders with skin anaesthesia, in these conditions the patients are unable to scratch. A number of mites are present in the skin with gross hyperkeratosis of the palms, soles and elbows. Irritation is minimal or absent, generalised lymphandenopathy is present in some cases and blood eosinophilia is common. Treatment is like that of ordinary scabies, but both clothing and the surrounding are contaminated with live mites, which results in the spread of infection to the attendants and nursing staff, for which adequate measures should be taken. Ivermectin is used in resistant cases (Fig. 9).

There is a squeak of pure delight from a matey little mite,
As it tortuously tunnels in the skin,
Singing furrow, folly furrow, come join me in my burrow,
And we will view the epidermis from within.

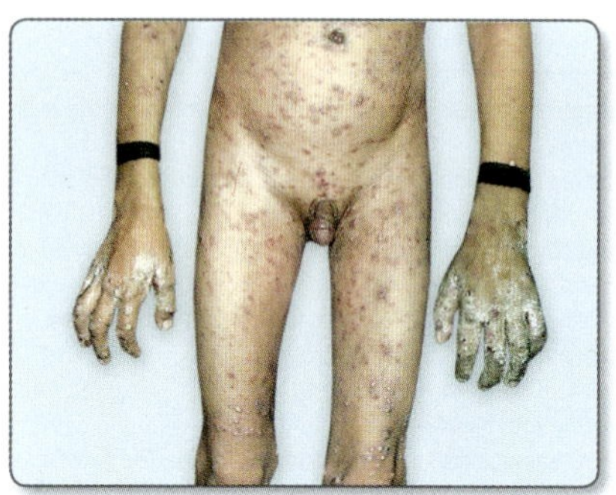

Fig. 9: Norwegian (crusted) scabies—note the crusts on the hand

Infections Caused by Other Mites

Animal scabies: A number of acari affect animals, when man comes in close contact with these animals, the parasite can be transferred to human beings. The parasite does not find the human skin a favourable habitat so that human cases generally run a mild form of the disease. The host specificity is not complete; the mite usually survives for a short period in another host. The disease in man is self-limited; there are no burrows. The common animals through which the infection can spread to the human beings are dogs, cats, poultry, birds and horse.

Demodiciosis: The Demodex mite is generally found in adults, the children rarely have them. The larval form of *Demodex folliculorum* inhabits the sebaceous glands of the nose, it may also be found on the forehead, chin and scalp. The larval form has a flattened head and an elongated abdomen, which gives it the appearance of a worm.

The pathogenesis of the *Demodex* has been a subject of controversy for many decades, as the *Demodex* is found in adults without any evidence of disease. On the other hand, rosacea and rosacea-like lesions are considered to be due to *Demodex*. When the number of mites in the follicle is large, the follicle ruptures and the mite comes in contact with the dermis, giving rise to the formation of inflammatory papules.

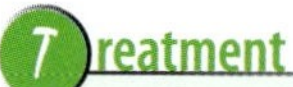

Treatment

Permethrin, benzyl benzoate emulsion is applied twice a day, usually after 3 days of the therapy the Demodex can no longer be demonstrated in the treated area. Other scabicides can also be used.

House dust mite (Dermatophagoides): This mite occurs worldwide. These mites are mainly found in houses that are damp and are inadequately heated. The main food of the house dust mite is the scales of human skin. There is increasing evidence of the role of the house dust mite in the production of atopic dermatitis and asthma. A number of patients have a positive intracutaneous test to house dust mite. A case of purpuric dermatitis is also reported to be due to house dust mite allergy.

Mites of stored food: These mites are found in flour, grains, cheese, dried fruits, etc. Skin lesions are produced in people who handle these foods. These mites are haematophagus, but irritation results from mite products, either faecal or secretory. The eruption is called 'grocer's itch'; the lesions consist of minute pruritic papules or papulovesicles on the exposed parts of the body. The eruptions on the face resemble that of acute contact dermatitis.

Pyemotes mites: These are primary parasites of insects or their larvae. The insects are found infesting grains, straw, hay or stored food. Dermatitis in found in persons who handle stored grains. The lesions are urticarial papules surmounted by a vesicle.

Cheyletiella mites: These are mites present in some mammals such as dogs, cats, rabbits, etc. their entire life cycle is completed in the host. The infected animals are usually symptomless or it may cause itchy papules. The most obvious sign is the presence of excessive dandruff on the back often called 'walking dandruff' by veterinary surgeons.

Harvest mites: Harvest mites (Trombiculidae) are found on low vegetations. Man is infected by walking on grass or through low vegetation. The lesions are due to the irritant effect of the mite's saliva, an acquired hypersensitivity reaction develops to the salivary antigen. Within a few hours of the bite erythematous macules occur, these develop into itchy papules and papulovesicles. Thrombiculid mites have provided evidence to suspects in murder investigations.

Birds, rodents and reptile mites (Dermanyssidae): These mites are haematophagus. Infection in man is manifested by profuse eruption of itchy wheals and papules. The lesions have a central punctum. There is intense pruritus excoriation is common. *Rickettsia akari* causes Rickettsial pox.

Trombidiasis (chiggers): The common chigger is also called scrub mite or red bug. It is prevalent in rural areas of the tropics especially in the rainy season. The chiggers attach themselves to the host to feed. They usually attack the ankles. The lesion consists of haemorrhagic puncta surrounded by red swelling, these later become papular, umbilicated and pruritic. The lesions can be secondarily infected and eczematized. Chiggers transmit scrub typhus (Tsutsugamushi fever).

Mites are responsible for the transfer of Rickettsial pox and Scrub typhus.

Scorpions

Scorpions have a crab-like shape, large frontal pincers and a stinger at the end of a long tail. A sting causes a severe painful local and systemic reaction. Lymphadenopathy, necrosis and death may occur, due to respiratory or cardiac failure. Ice packs and tourniquet should be applied at the site of the bite. Antivenom should be injected; calcium gluconate 10 mL of 10% solution IV is effective against muscle pain.

Spiders

Spiders differ from insects by having two body parts, five paired appendages, and by the absence of antennae. Some spiders are poisonous to man and may cause a severe reaction called arachindism; this usually develops in a few hours after the bite. The most dangerous spiders are of the genus *Loxoceles* and *Latrodectus*.

Loxoceles: This spider can be recognised by a dark violin-shaped band on the cephalothorax and three pairs of eyes. It is usually found in storage closets. Two types of reaction are seen by its bite. In the localised type a star-shaped necrotic area occurs (cutaneous loxoscelism), which heals with scarring in 2–3 weeks. In the generalised type, high fever, erythematous and purpuric rashes, haematuria are common. Death may occur in children.

Latrodectus mactans (Black widow spider): The black widow spider is found in the tropical and subtropical regions. It is found under stones, in dark buildings and huts. These spiders have a characteristic red hourglass or double triangle on the ventral surface of their abdomen. The bite of a female spider causes a pricking sensation followed by a severe muscular pain and rigidity. Within a few hours there may be chills, vomiting, violent cramps, delirium, partial paralysis, spasm and abdominal rigidity. The pain is very severe and is often mistaken for acute appendicitis. Death may occur in children and debilitated individuals.

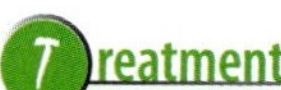

A tourniquet should be tied immediately, antivenom should be given IM, calcium gluconate 10% administered IV and muscle relaxants are indicated. Tetanus prophylaxis must be administered. Antibiotics are given to reduce the morbidity of secondary bacterial infection.

Immediate IM 80 mg of triamcinolone, followed by oral prednisolone 60 mg daily is given this is tapered over 2 weeks. Ice bags, antibiotics and analgesics are helpful. Dapsone has also been used with success.

Ticks

These are blood-sucking sac like arthropods, which are common parasites of domestic animals and often man. Ticks may be soft body ticks; these are found in the dry tropical and subtropical regions. The hard body ticks have a worldwide distribution. Ticks are vectors of relapsing fever, tuluremia, various rickettsial and viral infections, Lyme disease, Rocky Mountain spotted fever and typhus fever.

The female tick attaches itself to the skin by sticking its proboscis and then sucks the blood of the host from the superficial blood vessels. It remains attached to the skin until it is engorged and then falls off. This usually takes about 12 days. In a few hours at the site of puncture, an urticarial wheal is produced. During this period, the patient may have fever, abdominal pain and vomiting (tick bite pyrexia). The bite of a hard tick is painless, while that of a soft tick is painful. A pruritic urticarial swelling develops with a central necrosis. Tick paralysis may follow a hard tick bite.

Treatment

If the tick is attached to the skin, it should be removed by applying ether or petrol to the tick or by pulling it off gently. An attempt can also be made to pull the tick out of the skin by tying a thread around the neck of the tick and then pulling it off gently. Oral antihistamines relieve the symptoms. Rickettsial infections respond to tetracyclines. In children with sudden ascending paralysis, search should be made for the removal of a tick, often unnoticed in the scalp, may be life-saving.

Ticks are vectors of relapsing fever, tuluraemia, viral, and various rickettsial infections, such as Lyme disease, Rocky Mountain spotted fever, typhus fever.

Class Chilopoda

The arthropods in this class have elongated segmented bodies, with legs protruding from each segment. A flattened or rounded head, from which protrude the antennae.

Centipedes

Centipedes are nocturnal carnivores; they have numerous segments, each with a pair of legs. Some tropical species have strong claws that inject a poisonous substance in the bite. The bite is manifested by numerous haemorrhagic puncta surrounded by an erythematous swelling. This may lead to lymphangitis and lymphadenopathy. Locally there may be itching and pain. The venom of the centipede contains histamine and polypeptides, these may be neurotoxic. Rubbing with raw garlic, using a cut clove may rapidly relieve the pain. Injecting local anaesthesia is more helpful.

Millipedes

Millipedes are generally harmless, they have numerous segments; but each segment has two pair of legs. Most of these are harmless, but tropical species may cause injury to humans by their defensive secretions. They are found in decaying vegetable matter. Children often pick these up, contact with the human skin produces a burning sensation, and a brownish pigmentation develops over the next 24 hours. There is intense erythema and vesiculation. The colour is produced by the oxidation of quinone in the secretion.

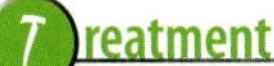

Treatment

The skin should be washed with plenty of water and the area cleaned with alcohol. Blisters should be treated with topical antiseptics.

REPTILES AND OTHER VENOMOUS ANIMALS

Snakes

Poisonous snakes fall into two families: elapidae and viperidae.

The elapidae are characterised by neurotoxic venom, these include the cobra, krait and mamba. The viperidae and crotalidae possess haemotoxic venom; these include the puff adder of Africa, the rattlesnake and copper head of the Americas.

Clinical Features

These vary with the type of snake, the amount of venom injected, the age and size of the patient. Elapidae snakes cause little local pain or swelling, but pronounced neurotoxic symptoms leading to paralysis and possibly death may occur. Viperidae snakes cause severe pain and pronounced local reactions. External and internal bleeding occurs, leading to shock and even death.

Treatment

Immediate application of tourniquet, incisions of fang marks, aspiration of the venom, ice packs and sedatives are recommended.

Treatment of shock and haemorhage, antivenom IM or IV should be administered, antibiotics, IV steroids and tetanus prophylaxis are recommended.

Lizard Bite

Venomous lizards are the Heloderma, the beaded lizard of Mexico. Bites from poisonous lizards may cause paralysis, dyspoea and convulsions. Local treatment is the same as that of snakebite.

Human Bite

Human bites are common, although man does not produce venom; its bite may produce bacterial infection as the saliva contains both aerobic and anaerobic bacteria. It may produce gangrene due the presence of fusospirochetal organism. Transmission of herpes virus 1 and 2, hepatitis B and C virus has been recorded. Rabies should be considered as possible sequelae to human bite.

DERMATOSES CAUSED BY AQUATIC ANIMALS

Venomous Fishes

These include stingray, catfish, stonefish and scorpion fish. They cause painful laceration, systemic symptoms and shock. Abscess, necrosis and gangrene may occur. Local infiltration with lidocaine and powerful analgesics are indicated. Antibiotics, tetanus prophylaxis and treatment for shock are required.

Portuguese man-of-war and Jelly fish dermatitis

Portuguese man-of-war and jellyfish are common on tropical shores. Portuguese man-of-war produces dermatitis due to the venom injected by stinging nematocysts, which break the skin. The venom of physalia is neurotoxic; it may produce marked cardiac changes. Systemic symptoms include severe dyspnoea, prostration, nausea, abdominal cramps, lacrimation and muscular pain. The cutaneous lesion is usually linear; but there may be urticaria, erythema and even hemorrhage. The lesions are painful. Bullae and necrosis may develop local ulcers are traumatic.

Treatment

The part of the body bitten should be immobilised, to prevent mobilisation of the venom. It is important to remove or inactivate the nemocyst as rapidly as possible. Nematocysts should be removed by rubbing with sand or papain from the meat tenderisers diluted in water. Dermatitis can be treated with cold compresses and topical corticosteroids.

The tentacles and toxins should be washed with sea water, vinegar or alcohol, which inactivates the nematocysts. The remaining tentacles should be removed with gloved hands by a paste made of baking powder or talc and sea water. The dried paste is scraped off with a knife.

If the area is washed with fresh water or dried with a towel, the unfired nematocysts become activated

Jellyfish Dermatitis

The lesions produced by jellyfish are similar to those of Portiguese man-of- war, but the lesions are not so linear.

Sea Urchins

Sea urchins are characterised by the presence of numerous brittle fragile spines that break off while piercing the skin. This causes local pain and swelling. The wound is often stained bluish black by the black spines. Infection and later granulomatous reaction may occur.

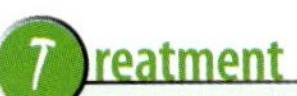

Visible spines should be removed. Hot water compresses and an antibiotic is helpful. Apply hot wax over the wound, when cool, scrape off the wax, spines come out with it.

Coral Cuts

These injuries are caused by the exoskeleton of corals. They become inflamed and infected easily. Cleaning of the wound as soon as possible after the injury is advisable.

Sponges

Tedania ignis (Bermuda fire sponge) can cause severe dermatitis. It may produce erythema multiforme like reaction on the face, palms and soles, 10 days after the contact.

Mollusca

The stings of molluscs are painful; they cause local ischemia, cyanosis and numbness, the reaction quickly spreads to involve the whole body. Sting of some species may be fatal. Some molluscs have venom that contains a vasoactive substance. Blue ringed octopus found mainly in the Australian coastal water is said to be the world's most deadly octopus, its bite causes severe systemic symptoms, death is due to respiratory failure.

Leeches

Blood sucking leeches are segmented worms that exist in salt water; they are also numerous in fresh water and on land. Leeches attach themselves to the skin causing distinct, painless triradiate wounds. They feed until engorged and then fall off the human body. The saliva of leech contains heparin-like substance, this prevents the blood from clotting and the wound may continue to bleed for hours, after the leech has detached. Secondary infection often develops.

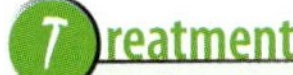

The leech may be detached from the skin touching it with a lighted cigarette, a match flame or sprinkling it with salt. Bleeding is controlled with a styptic pencil.

Seaweed Dermatitis

This is often seen in the shores that contain marine plant Lyngbya majuscula. The symptoms appear within a few minutes after leaving the ocean. There is severe itching and burning followed by dermatitis, blisters are formed and painful desquamation is seen in areas covered by the bathing suit. Scrotum, perianal and perineum are mainly involved. Prophylaxis is achieved by refraining from swimming in water, which is turbid with such algae. Patch tests are negative, as the algae are a potent irritant. A shower should be taken within 5 minutes of bathing. Active treatment in severe cases is the same as that for burns.

Dogger Bank Itch

This is an eczematous dermatitis caused by seaweed-like animal colony chervil *Alcyonidium hirsutum*. These seaweeds are found on the Dogger Bank, this is an immense elevation under the North Sea, between Scotland and Denmark.

Halecium Dermatitis

This dermatitis results from contact with a small marine hydroid *Halecium beani*. It grows as a thick coat of moss in the submerged portions of the ship or rafts in the sea. The lesions produced by the hydroid are extremely painful.

Some other cutaneous diseases caused by animals:
Orf by sheep and goats
Milker's nodule by cows
Anthrax by horses, sheep, goat and wild herbivores
Erysipeloid caused by fish, pig and poultry products
Tularaemia caused by tick or infected rodents
Psittacosis by parrots
Glanders by horses
Haverhill fever/rat bite fever (Streptobacillus moniliformis) by rats
Plague by rats
Leptospirosis by cattle, pigs, dogs, squirrels and rats

FURTHER READING

1. Amr ZS, Nusier MN. Pediculosis capitis in Northern Jordon. Int J Dermatol. 2000;39:919-21.
2. Barkwell R, Shields S. Death associated with ivermectin treatment of scabies. Lancet. 1997;349:1144-5.
3. Bennett CE, Keefe M, Reynolds JC. Perception of the incidence of scabies and efficacy of treatment in UK Hospitals. Br J Dermatol. 2000;143:1337-8.
4. Bhutani LK. Pediculosis capitis. Arch Dermatol. 1979;115:675.
5. Burgass I. Human lice and their management. Adv Parasitol.1995;36:271-342.
6. Burns DA. Action of co-trimoxazole on head lice. Br J Dermatol. 1987;117:399-400.
7. Chosidow O. Scabies and pediculosis. Lancet. 2000;355:819-26.
8. Curnie MA. Treatment of cutaneous leishmaniasis by curettage. BMJ. 1983;287:1053-6.
9. Davis RR. Filariasis. Dermatol Clin. 1989;7:313-21.
10. Downs AMR, Harvey I, Kennedy CTC. The Epidemiology of head lice and scabies in UK. Epidemiol Infec. 1999;122:471-7.
11. Fugita WH, Barr RJ, Cottschaulk HR. Cutaneous amebiasis. Arch Dermatol.1981:117:309-10.
12. Griffiths WA, Dutz W. Repeated tissue sampling with a dental broach. A trial in cutaneous leishmaniasis. Br J Dermatol. 1975;93:43-5.
13. Paul J, Bates J. Is infestation with common bed bug increasing? BMJ. 2000;320:1141.
14. Rausmussen JE. Lindane a prudent approach. Arch Dermatol. 1987;123:1008-10.
15. Valencia BM, Miller D, Witziq RS, et al. A novel low-cost thermotherapy for cutaneous leishmaniasis in Peru. Plos Negl Trop Dis. 2013;7(5): e 2196.
16. Wolf R, Krakowski A. Atypical crusted scabies. J Am Acad Dermatol. 1987;17:434-6.

Chapter 8

Sexually Transmitted Diseases

INTRODUCTION

Sexually transmitted diseases (STDs) are a diverse group of infections caused by multiple microbial pathogens. Cutaneous inoculation is the most common route for the five classical STDs (syphilis, gonorrhoea, chancroid, lymphogranuloma venereum and granuloma inguinale), as well as for herpes simplex. Blood-borne infections transferred are human immunodeficiency virus (HIV), hepatitis B, hepatitis C and cytomegalovirus. Scabies, candidiasis and molluscum contagiosum can also be sexually transmitted.

SYPHILIS

Syphilis (Lues) has been associated with dermatology because of the syphilitic rash. The rash in early European history was mentioned as the "great pox". From the 16th century until well into the 19th century most doctors assumed that gonorrhoea and syphilis were manifestations of the same disease. Mercurial ointment was used for treatment, which was also used to treat parasitic disease. In 1837, a French venereologist Philippe Record established the specificity of the two infections. Ricord was also amongst the first to differentiate primary, secondary and tertiary syphilis. In 1905, two German researchers Fritz Schaudinn a protozoologist and Erich Hoffman a syphilologist identified the spirochete *Treponema (T.) pallidum*. In 1909, Paul Ehrlich discovered Salvarsan an arsenal for the cure of syphilis. In 1944, the arsenal was replaced by penicillin of Fleming.

Syphilis is an STD caused by the spirochete *T. pallidum*. It is a spirochete with tapered ends, and 10–20 spirals. The width of the organism is very narrow (0.10–0.18 μm), and so it cannot be seen under an ordinary microscope without silver staining. Under dark ground examination, the spirochete shows its characteristic rotatory movements. *T. pallidum* replicates after every 30–33 hours by fission. Infection occurs by close contact, with the entry of *T. pallidum* through minor abrasions in the skin or mucous membrane.

The course of syphilis can be divided into three stages:

- Primary syphilis (primary and secondary stage)
- Latent syphilis
- Tertiary syphilis

In the primary stage, there is localised infection at the site of entry of the *Treponema* with regional adenitis. In the secondary stage, there is dissemination of the infection via the blood, this results in multiple lesions on the skin, mucous membrane and other organs. Between the secondary and the tertiary stage is the latent stage. In this stage, the *Treponema* are dormant and inactive. There are no clinical symptoms, but the serological tests are positive. In the tertiary stage, any organ may be involved with specific changes in the skin, cardiovascular and central nervous system (CNS).

Clinical Features

PRIMARY SYPHILIS

Primary Stage: After an incubation period of 3–4 weeks, the primary lesion called the chancre appears at the site of inoculation. This is usually on the genitals, but it may also occur on the lips, nipples, fingers and buccal mucosa. The initial lesion is a dark-red nodule, which breaks down to form an ulcer (chancre) (Fig. 1). The ulcer is painless, usually single, round or oval, about 1 cm in diameter, with sharply defined raised indurated border. Multiple chancres can occur. The ulcer base is smooth, brownish-red, or covered with yellowish or greyish slough. A narrow red border about 1–2 millimeters wide surrounds the ulcer. The adenopathy develops within a week of the onset of the chancre; it is unilateral initially later becoming bilateral. The lymph nodes are small, multiple, discrete, firm, mobile and painless. The overlying skin is normal and the nodes do not suppurate. The chancre heals spontaneously in 3–8 weeks leaving an atrophic scar.

In women the chancre occurs on the labia, fourchette, cervix and uretha. Chancres in women are more oedematous than indurated.

Diagnosis

A dark field examination for the *Treponema* is helpful in differentiating syphilitic ulcer from the other genital ulcers. Alternative to the dark ground microscopy is the direct fluorescent antibody test (DFAT).

Differential Diagnosis

Chancre has an incubation period of about 3 weeks, it has a very narrow erythematous margin, it is painless, single, round or oval, and the surface is smooth. Chancre has a dark velvety-red lacquered appearance, it is cartilage hard on palpation and lymphadenopathy is usually bilateral. Chanchroid (soft sore) has an incubation period of 1–3 days, the ulcer is acutely inflamed, it is very painful, has a large surrounding inflammatory zone. The lesions are usually multiple and merge into one another. The edge of the ulcer is undermined, it is yellowish-red in colour, the base of the ulcer is covered with a membrane and the ulcer is soft to touch. Lymphadenopathy is usually unilateral and the glands ulcerate. Granuloma inguinale begins as an indurated nodule that later becomes hypertrophic and vegetative. It is soft beefy-red in colour and bleeds easily. Lymphogranuloma venereum is a small painless vesicle or superficial nonindurated ulcer. The lesion is transient, primary lesion is followed in 7–30 days by adenopathy of the regional lymph nodes. Herpes simplex begins with grouped vesicles often accompanied by burning pain; after rupture of the vesicles, lobulated irregular soft erosions form. Only rarely are the lymph nodes involved.

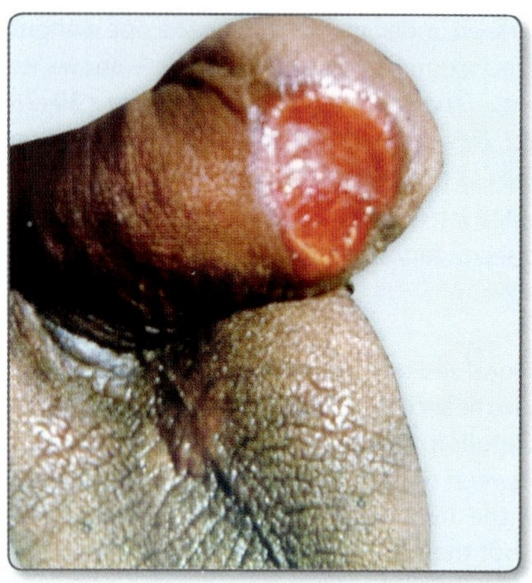

Fig. 1: Primary syphilis—chancre

Secondary Stage

The secondary stage occurs about 8 weeks after the infecting exposure. This stage is manifested by lesions on the skin, the mucous membrane and other organs. The rashes of secondary syphilis do not itch.

Clinical Features and Cutaneous Manifestations

Early secondary syphilis is characterised by macular lesions (roseola); these are more or less generalised, superficial, nondestructive and transient. The colour varies from light pink to rose; the lesions may disappear spontaneously after a few days or weeks without any trace or may leave postinflammatory hyperpigmentation. Syphilitic leukoderma (collar of Venus) is a peculiar round or oval depigmented syphilid on the neck and shoulders, more commonly seen in coloured races.

Cutaneous lesions appear later in successive crops, lesions in different stages of development are present at the same time, giving it a polymorphic appearance. Lesions are prominent on the face, palms and soles, genitalia and the perianal region. On the genitalia, the affected papules become hypertrophic, they are broad, moist and pink in colour, these are known as condylomata lata. Maculopapular lesions around the forehead, is called "corona veneris". The lesions on the palms and soles are characteristic. Always suspect syphilis when a patient is confronted with acute palmoplantar rash. If the patients also have HIV infection; or is immunosuppressed, larger lesions ulcerate (malignant syphild). The crusted lesions are called rupial syphilis (Figs 2A to C).

Painless erosions on the oral mucous membrane (mucous patch) form circinate pattern or arcs (snail track ulcers). These lesions contain a large number of spirochetes and are highly infectious.

There is generalised lymphadenopathy; the lymph nodes frequently affected are the inguinal, posterior cervical, postauricular and the epitrochlear. The nodes are firm, slightly enlarged, nontender and discrete.

In the late stages of secondary syphilis, the lesions tend to be more localised. Variants of secondary syphilis are follicular, pustular and corymbose (large papule surrounded by smaller ones).

Nail changes: The nails are brittle, they break easily. Other changes include onycholysis, pitting and dystrophy. Amber coloured nails are said to be characteristic of secondary syphilis. Cyanotic painful toes are sometimes seen.

Hair changes: Alopecia occurs in 3–7% of cases. The hair loss may be diffuse, patchy or both. Small irregular patches of nonscarring alopecia are commonly seen in the scalp in occipital and parietal areas (moth-eaten appearance).

Malignant syphilis (Lues maligna) is characterised by widespread papulopustules, or nodules, that become necrotic and breakdown to form ulcers. The eruption is associated with toxicity, fever, malaise, arthralgia and occasionally hepatitis. Most patients have an abnormal immune system or are in poor health.

Systemic manifestations: Acute membranous glomerulonephritis, proctitis, hepatitis, acute meningitis, sensorineural hearing loss, iritis, anterior

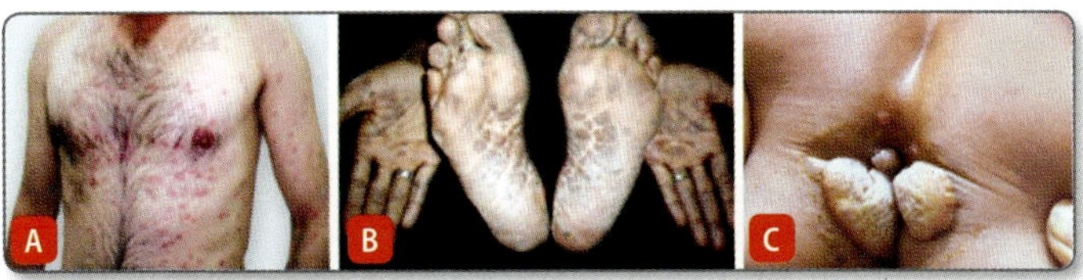

Figs 2A to C: Secondary syphilis. (A) Generalised maculopapular eruption; (B) Palmoplantar keratosis; (C) Condylomata lata

uvietis, optic neuritis, Bell's palsy, pneumonitis, periostitis, polyarthritis, glomerulonephritis, hepatitis may occur in secondary syphilis. Spleen is enlarged in almost all cases.

Histopathology: Syphilitic lesions show superficial and deep involvement of the blood vessels. There is swelling of the endothelial cells of the vessel walls with marked perivascular infiltrate. The infiltrate consists chiefly of lymphocytes and plasma cells. In the late secondary eruptions, multinucleated giant cells and degenerative changes in the vessel walls may be seen.

Diagnosis

A triad of oral ulcers, lymphadenopathy and non-itchy symmetrically distributed skin lesions are almost pathognomonic of secondary syphilis. A history of genital ulcer is an additionally highly suggestive feature. However, diagnosis should always be confirmed by serological tests. These are non-treponemal tests which identify antibodies against phospholipids such as lecithin and cardiolipin. Treponemal tests are those that identify antibodies against ***T. pallidum***.

Venereal disease research laboratory (VDRL) is positive in all cases of secondary syphilis. It is a flocculation test which detects antibodies that react with cardiolipin and ***T. pallidum*** cell wall phospholipids. The patient's serum is mixed with a colloidal solution of cholesterol, lecithin and cardiolipin. If antibodies to ***T. pallidum*** are present in the patient's serum a flocculation occurs. VDRL is a useful test for screening purposes. It is cheap and sensitive.

Biological false positive cases are found in a very small number of normal individuals, it is positive in diseases, such as malaria, collagen diseases, rheumatoid arthritis, genital herpes, leprosy, pregnancy, etc. It is therefore important to carefully evaluate a person before diagnosing syphilis. VDRL test normally decreases by at least two dilutions within several months of adequate treatment. A rise of serum titre indicates re-infection or a relapse.

False Negative test could result due to very high titres of antibody (prozone phenomenon). The prozone phenomenon is said to be present when dilution of a previously negative sample leads to a positive test. High levels of antigen or antibody may prevent the formation of antigen-antibody complexes.

Rapid plasma reaginic test (RPR) is a modified VDRL test. In this test the antigen contains carbon particles that is mixed with the unheated serum and is then put on a plastic card. Because of the inclusion of carbon particles, the flocculation can be determined by the naked eye. For screening purposes, RPR test is technically easier.

Test specific for syphilis is the fluorescent treponema antibody absorption test (FTA-ABS). In this test the non-specific group antibodies are first removed from the patients serum and then the fluorescent treponema test (FTA) is performed.

Treponema pallidum hemagglutination test (TPHA-Test). In this test sheep's erythrocytes are coated with T. pallidum antigens, it is mixed with the patient's serum. If the patient's serum contains antibodies to ***T. pallidum***, the sheeps red blood cells (RBC) get agglutinated.

Differential Diagnosis

Syphilis has long been known to be a great imitator of many cutaneous disorders. It should be considered in the differential of any unusual rash or atypical presentation of papulosquamous diseases. Pityriasis rosea begins on the trunk, characterised by the herald patch; oval patches along the line of cleavage, absence of lymphadenopathy and mucous membrane lesions differentiate it from syphilis. Drug eruptions produce a picture similar to syphilis, but the lesions are scarlatiniform or morbilliform, history of drug intake is present. Lichen planus is differentiated by the presence of Wickham's striae, typical characteristic appearance, severe pruritus, typical sites and mucous membrane involvement in the form of white reticulate striae. Other dermatoses to be differentiated from syphilis are guttate psoriasis, pityriasis lichenoides chronica, urticaria pigmentosa. Lesions of the mucous membranes should be differentiated from aphthous stomatitis and geographical tongue.

Course and prognosis: The early lesions of syphilis involute either spontaneously or by treatment, but relapses occur in approximately 25% of cases. Cutaneous recurrences may be generalised; the lesions are larger and separated by a wider area of healthy skin.

LATENT SYPHILIS

This is the period after the lesions of secondary syphilis have disappeared and the patient is asymptomatic. The serological tests are positive, but the patient is noninfective. Early latent syphilis is of less than 1 year duration, and late when the duration is more than 1 year. This stage may last for a few months or may continue for the rest of the patient's life. Always have a cerebrospinal fluid (CSF) examination, neurological evaluation, ultrasonography for assessment of the aorta and an eye examination in all cases of latent syphilis.

TERTIARY SYPHILIS

This stage may occur as early as 1 year after infection, but most cases occur after 3–5 years. Some cases are seen after many years of contracting the disease, it can occur as long as after 30 years. Tertiary syphilis affects the skin, nervous system and the cardiovascular system.

The cutaneous lesions are more localised; these occur in groups and are destructive. The skin lesions are of two types:

- Superficial and nodular
- Deep or gummatous.

Nodular lesions: These firm coppery-red nodules appear in groups with a tendency to form circinate arrangement. The lesions heal centrally and extend peripherally. The eruption may appear on any part of the body, but favours the face, arms and the back. The lesions are symptomless; they heal forming a soft fine wrinkled scar (cigarette paper scar). In the early stages the scar is pink later it becomes white.

Gumma is a mass of syphilitic granulation tissue that may originate in the subcutis, muscle or the bone. It tends to grow in all directions; superficially it ulcerates in the skin. Gummas are usually single, they may be multiple, and there is no regional lymphadenopathy. Gummas are painless, the central necrotic tissue may turn into a shiny adherent mass and this gives it the name "gumma". Gumma may vary in size from a few to several centimetres in diameter. The sites of predilection are the scalp, face, chest, palate and the legs. The lesions may progress in one area while healing proceeds in another. Gummas are locally destructive and may lead to perforation of the hard palate. They heal leaving a thin "tissue paper" scar.

Lesions of the mucous membrane are present in all stages of syphilis. On the tongue, the lesions may be localised or diffuse. Gumma of the tongue usually involves the edge towards the back; it rapidly breaks down to form a punched out ulcer with irregular soft edge. The lesion can become malignant. It is often said that if there is a patch of leucoplakia on the tongue look forwards to malignancy and backwards to syphilis.

Osseous lesions: Skeletal syphilis occurs most commonly on the face, head and tibia. Late manifestations of syphilis are periostitis, osteomyelitis and gummatous osteoarthritis. Bone pain occurs often at night. Charcot's joint is the most prevalent manifestation; knees and ankles are most commonly affected. There is loss of contours of the joint and the joints are painless.

Neurosyphilis: This may be meningovascular or parenchymatous. Parenchymatous neurosyphilis manifests as general paresis of insane or tabes dorsalis.

General paresis of insane: The damage is in the grey matter of the anterior lobe of the cerebral hemisphere, causing widespread neurological and psychiatric manifestations.

Meningovascular syphilis manifests as meningitis, cranial nerve disorders convulsions and delirium.

Tabes dorsalis is as common as general paresis of insane. The posterior column of the spinal cord and dorsal nerve roots are involved. Tabes dorsalis is characterised by neurotropic ulcers on the feet, severe abdominal pain and changes in the pupil. The movements are uncoordinated, Romberg's sign is positive (patient is unable to stand when the eyes are closed). Signs and symptoms of paresis may be present.

Optic atrophy may occur independently or in association with other forms of neurosyphilis. Examination of the visual fields is essential in all cases of late syphilis. Argyll Robertson pupil is that which responds to accommodation but not to light.

Cardiovascular syphilis: Aortitis is the basic lesion in cardiovascular syphilis. This may lead to aortic insufficiency and coronary disease, ultimately aortic aneurysm occurs. It is said that Christopher Columbus died of syphilitic aortic disease.

Diagnosis of tertiary syphilis: CSF examination should be done in all cases of tertiary syphilis, this shows an increase cell count (lymphocytes) of 5 or more cells, increase in total proteins and the serological tests for syphilis are positive. Blood serology is reactive, but the titre is low. The treponemal tests become positive early and remain so. Thus in late or latent syphilis these tests are most sensitive.

Differential Diagnosis

Skin lesions of late syphilis should be differentiated from granulomatous diseases and tumours. Lupus vulgaris is slow growing, has the characteristic apple jelly nodules. There may be a recurrence of lupus vulgaris in its scars but not in syphilis. Histoid leprosy does not ulcerate; the other signs of leprosy are present. Iododerma and bromoderma present as red oozing nodules or plaques, mostly on the face or the limbs, there is a history of prolonged administration of iodides or bromides. In endemic area leishmaniasis, rhinoscleroma and South American blastomycosis should be differentiated. Tumours such as basal cell carcinoma, squamous cell carcinoma, mycosis fungoides and other lymphomas resemble gummas.

Treatment of Syphilis

Penicillin is the drug of choice in the treatment of all forms of syphilis. Patients allergic to penicillin should be treated with erythromycin or tetracyclines. Dose of medication depends upon the stage of syphilis. All sexual contacts should be traced and treated simultaneously.

- Treatment of early syphilis (primary, secondary and latent syphilis of less than 1 year duration).
  Benzathine penicillin G 2.4 million units, IM at a single session (1.2 million units distributed in each buttock).
  Aqueous procaine penicillin G 600,000 units IM for 8 days.
- Treatment of late syphilis (latent syphilis of more than 1 year duration and tertiary syphilis).
  Benzathine penicillin G, a total dose of 7.2 million units is given as 2.4 units IM weekly for 3 weeks.
  Aqueous procaine penicillin G 600,000 units daily for 15 days.

Treatment of neurosyphilis: As benzathine penicillin G has low concentrations in the CSF, crystalline penicillin G is used in the treatment of neurosyphilis. Crystalline penicillin G 20 million units IV are given every 4 hours for 15 days. Also recommended is procaine penicillin G 600,000 units IM for 15 days.

Patients allergic to penicillin should receive erythromycin or tetracycline 500 mg four times daily for 15 days in early syphilis and for 30 days in late syphilis. Azithromycin and ceftriaxone have also been used for cases resistant to penicillin therapy.

Reactions to Penicillin

Jarisch-Herxheimer reaction: The reaction is due to the result of rapid killing of *Treponema*, it occurs in more than half of the patients with early syphilis, 2–3 hours after the first injection of penicillin. Patients have fever and there is an exacerbation of syphilitic lesions. The patient should be warned of the complication, the treatment should be discontinued.

The importance of Jarisch-Herxheimer's reaction is that it may result in a flare-up of infection in a vital structure, such as aortic aneurysm or iritis, leading to serious consequences. When the CNS is involved, special importance is attached to avoid Jarisch-Herxheimer reaction, even though the paralysis may be temporary. Gumma of the brain is first treated surgically, followed by the medical treatment. It is advisable to use concomitant treatment with corticosteroids in treating neurosyphilis.

Other reactions: Anaphylactic shock is a rare but serious complication; this requires immediate administration of epinephrine 0.5 ml subcutaneously with other emergency measures. Erythematous or urticarial eruptions may also develop. Penicillin should be discontinued.

Follow-Up

Adequate therapy should lead to a fourfold drop of serological titres. Until this is reached monthly tests should be carried out. Then the tests should be done at 3 months interval for 2 years. A fourfold rise in titre indicates relapse or reinfection and is an indication for retreatment. FTA-ABS remains reactive even after adequate treatment.

Table 1 showing the differentiating points between condylomata lata and condylomata acuminata

The rashes of secondary syphilis usually do not itch
The rashes of secondary syphilis are usually not bullous
Suspect syphilis when a patient develops acute palmoplantar rashes
Suspect tabes dorsalis when a patient has Argyll Robertson pupil

CONGENITAL SYPHILIS

Congenital syphilis is transmission of infection from the mother to the fetus. Infection through the placenta does not occur before the 4th month of pregnancy, so treatment of the mother before this period will almost prevent the infection in the fetus. If prenatal infection occurs soon after this, then fetal death and miscarriage will result. During the remainder of pregnancy, infection is likely to produce characteristic developmental stigmata of syphilis, if infection occurs after 8 months of pregnancy active infection of secondary syphilis is seen. In utero infection of the fetus is rare when the pregnant mother has had syphilis for more than 2–3 years.

Prenatal syphilis can present as early and late congenital syphilis.

Early Congenital Syphilis

This develops before the age of 2 years. It has the similarities of secondary syphilis but is more severe and is highly contagious. The infant is underweight, anaemic and shrunken. There is a generalised maculopapular

Table 1: Differentiating points between condylomata lata and condylomata acuminata

Condylomata lata	*Condylomata acuminata*
Causative organism *Treponema pallidum*	*Human Papilloma virus*
Clinical appearance Multiple broad, smooth, dome-shaped papules, pinkish in appearance	Multiple verrucous papules, brownish or skin coloured
Lesions at other sites Skin, palms, soles, oral mucosa, lymph nodes	Other sites not involved
Histopathology Superficial and deep involvement of blood vessels, plasma cells present	Hyperkeratosis and acanthosis
Lesions do not become malignant	HPV 16 and 18 are oncogenic
Diagnosis Serological tests Dark field examination	Punctate haemorrhage on paring, Histopathology PCR, serotyping
Treatment Penicillin	Podophyllin tincture
Note: Keep in mind sometimes condylomata lata can become verrucous	

or papulosquamous eruption that may become eczematised or secondarily infected. Vesiculobullous eruption (syphilitic pemphigus) occurs on the palms and soles. Mucous patches occur on the oral mucosa and nose causing a characteristic mucoid haemorrhagic discharge (snuffles). Perioral lesions cause radiating furrows that heal with scars. Patchy alopecia and paronychia may be found.

Osteochondritis of the long bones with painful swelling of the epiphysis occurs; this may interfere with the movements of the limbs (syphilitic psuedoparalysis). There may be periostitis of the phalanges (syphilitic dactylitis).

Late Congenital Syphilis

The eruptions of the skin and mucous membrane are like those of tertiary syphilis (nodular and gummatous lesions), cardiac involvement is uncommon. Interstitial keratitis develops at puberty; antisyphilitic treatment does not alter the course of the disease, which may lead to blindness. Early and intense treatment with corticosteroids may be helpful. Hydroarthrosis of both the knee joints begins between the ages of 10–20 years; the condition is painless (Clutton's joint). Eighth nerve deafness begins at about the age of 10 years; it is often associated with interstitial keratitis. This is often bilateral and progressive, it does not respond to antisyphilitic treatment; systemic steroids may be helpful. Bone changes include perforation of the palate, destruction of the nasal septum, saber tibia, bony masses of the skull (Parrots nodes) and frontal bossing.

The stigmata of congenital syphilis:

- Saddle nose is caused by defective bone growth following rhinitis (snuffles)
- Hutchinson's teeth, the upper incisors are widely spaced, pegged with a central notching (screwdriver nails). The Hutchinson's triad is an association of Hutchinson's teeth, interstitial keratitis and the 8th nerve deafness
- Mulberry molars are characterised by small extra cusps of the first molar resembling mulberries
- Rhagades; these are the radiating scars found about the mouth and the anus
- Parrot's node on the skull, frontal bossing
- Pepper and salt fundus due to scarring choroiditis and optic atrophy
- Higoumenakis sign; this is a unilateral thickening of the inner end of one of the clavicles, due to hyperostosis resulting from syphilitic osteitis.

Treatment of Congenital Syphilis

Infants with congenital syphilis should be given a single injection of 50,000 units/kg of benzathine penicillin G. If the patient has neurosyphilis, then aqueous crystalline penicillin G 50,000 units/kg of body weight IM or IV is given for at least 10 days or penicillin G procaine 50,000 units IM for at least 10 days should be administered.

It is often said that syphilis was imported to Europe from Hispaniola (Haiti), by the crews of Christopher Columbus. Syphilitic bone changes have been found in the skeletons of Australians, Africans and American aborigines.

An Italian pathologist Giro Lamo Fracastoro gave a complete description of syphilis in 1530, in a poem entitled "Syphilis Sivi Morbus Gallicus". In this poem, he describes a mythical shepherd named Syphilis, who was affected by a sexually transmitted disease as a punishment for blasphemy to the Sun god.

Shaudinn and Hoffman in 1905, discovered the causative organism of syphilis: Treponema pallidum. Wasserman, Neisser and Bruck in 1906, detected the lipoidal antibodies in the serum of infected individuals.

Sir Jonathen Hutchinson (1828–1913)

Hutchinson qualified from the medical school at York and then studied under Sir James Paget at the St. Bartholomew's Hospital. He became the surgeon to the London Hospital and is said to have treated a million cases of syphilis. He was an outstanding clinician of the 19th century.

GONORRHOEA

Gonorrhoea is an acute or chronic STD caused by *Neisseria gonorrhoeae*, a Gram-negative diplococcus. Urethritis and various lesions of the genital tract manifest the disease. It may cause ophthalmic lesions in the adult and the newborn. As no immunity develops after the infection, re-infection is common. Most of the cases are seen in young adults; about 50% of cases are seen in people less than 25 years of age.

Clinical Features

Gonoccocal infection may be local or disseminated. There may be associated local complications.

Primary lesion: After an incubation period of 2–5 days, there is a slight burning sensation in the urethra that is more pronounced after urination. Soon afterwards a characteristic spontaneous urethral discharge develops, at first scanty and later profuse. The urethra shows multiple erosions, these are red in colour, 0.2–2 centimetres in diameter, round or oval in shape, with a nonindurated areola. Anterior urethra is involved first and later the posterior urethra. In chronic cases, strictures develop in the urethra making urination difficult, leading to urinary retention. In men, infection spreads to the surrounding glands resulting in the involvement of the Tyson's gland, Littre's gland, prostate, seminal vesicles and the epididymis (Fig. 3).

In women the incubation period is more than 2 weeks, symptoms are absent in more than one third of the cases. Cervicitis is the most frequent manifestation followed by urethritis. Involvement of the cervix results in low backache and low abdominal pain. There may be a profuse yellowish vaginal discharge; the vaginal mucosa is resistant to infection by gonococcal infection. The infection may spread to the vulva, Bartholin's gland, Skene's glands and fallopian tubes that may lead to infertility in females.

Extragenital dissemination occurs in 1% of males and 3% of females. Disseminated gonococcal arthritis develops in 3–4 weeks of infection, mainly in women. The knee, ankle, hip and wrist joints are frequently infected. The joints are red, hot and swollen containing a purulent exudate rich in gonococcus or it may be a tenosynovitis in which the synovial cultures are negative.

Skin lesions in disseminated gonorrhoea are rare; these manifest on the extensor surface of the extremities as macules, papules or small vesicles with a red halo, these soon develop into pustules or bullae that may become haemorrhagic or necrotic. They heal after a few days leaving small superficial scars.

Gonorrhoea in neonates is caused by the spread of infection through the birth canal. The disease is manifest by erythema and swelling of the eyelids, conjunctivitis associated with purulent discharge. Corneal ulceration can occur.

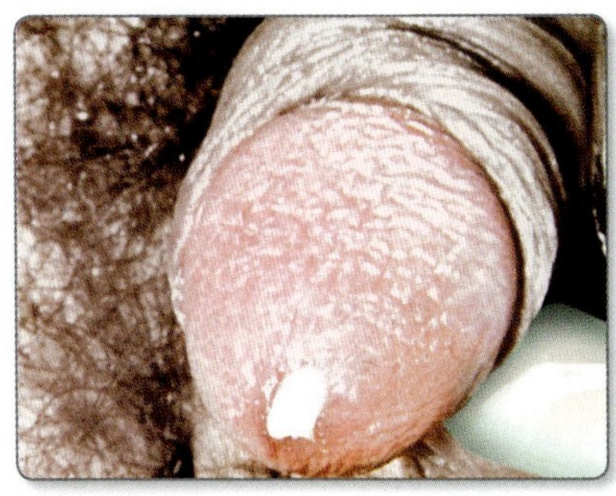

Fig. 3: Gonorrhoea

Diagnosis

Acute gonococcal urethritis is easily diagnosed by the microscopic examination of the urethral smears. Typical intracellular diplococci are diagnostic. Chronic cases should be cultured.

Differential Diagnosis

Gonococcal urethritis should be differentiated from non-gonococcal urethritis, intraurethral chancre and Reiter's disease. Examination of the urethral smear helps in differentiating these conditions. Intracellular diplococci are diagnostic of gonorrhoea.

Treatment

Previously gonorrhoea was treated with penicillin or tetracycline; but now these are no longer used due to resistance of the organism.

As resistance to penicillin is worldwide, the current recommendation for the treatment of gonorrhoea is injection of ceftriaxone 250 mg IM as a single injection; this is then followed by doxycycline 100 mg daily for 7 days, to treat concurrent chlamydial infection. (ceftriaxone also treats syphilitic infection, but the dose is higher and of longer duration).

Alternative therapy includes cefixime 400 mg once orally; azithromycin1 gm in a single dose, ciprofloxacin 500 mg orally in a single dose, and ofloxacin 400 mg in single dose. Spectinomycin hydrochlorides 2 gm by IM single injection, can also be used.

John Hunter (1728–1793)

The Hunter brothers (William and John) were dominating figures in the study of anatomy in England. John Hunter was a brilliant surgeon and experimentalist, who has left a great impression in the history of medical sciences. After becoming an expert anatomist, John studied surgery under Percivall Pott and William Cheseldon.

It was previously thought that gonorrhoea and syphilis were caused by a single organism. John inoculated himself with the secretion from a case of gonorrhoea. Hunter developed syphilis, as the patient was suffering from both syphilis and gonorrhoea. Hunter thought that both the diseases had a common origin. John Hunter died 27 years later of syphilitic heart disease. Philip Record cleared the confusion half a century later.

NON-GONOCOCCAL URETHRITIS

Many cases of urethritis are non-gonococcal. Typically, non-gonococcal urethritis (NGU) predominates in the higher socioeconomic group. *Chlamydia trachomatis* causes 30–40% of NGU; other cases are due to *Ureaplasma urealyticum* and *Trichomonas vaginalis*.

Clinical Features

Nongonococcal urethritis is less contagious than gonorrhoea. Incubation period is 7–14 days. Patient complains of itching, urethral discharge and dysuria. The discharge is not spontaneous, but becomes apparent after milking the urethra in the morning. The mucopurulent discharge is thin and cloudy. *T. vaginalis* has a typical scanty discharge.

Diagnosis

Gonococcal urethritis is ruled out by preparing Gram smears of the exudate (intracellular Gram-negative diplococci are positive for gonorrhea). When interpretation of the Gram stain is not clear then culture on Thayer-Martin medium is appropriate. Urethral smears in chlamydial infection stained with methylene blue show large blast-like cells with deeply staining nuclei. Inclusion bodies may be found in Giemsa's stain. Smears of *T. vaginalis* show the protozoan with 4–5 flagellae. Culture of *T. vaginalis* is diagnostic.

Treatment

Tetracycline is the drug of choice for chlamydial infection; 500 mg is given orally four times daily for 3 weeks. Doxycycline 100 mg twice a day may also be given as an alternative. If tetracycline is contraindicated then erythromycin is given in the same dose. Azithromycin given as a single oral dose of 1 gm is highly effective and is associated with increased compliance.

Metronidazole is the therapy of choice in *T. vaginalis*, 250 mg three times daily for 7 days.

(Reiter's disease is discussed in chapter 38)

CHANCROID

Chancroid (Soft chancre) is a localised STD caused by *Haemophilus ducreyi*; it is a Gram-negative rod with rounded edges. It is nonmotile and nonspore-bearing organism.

Clinical Features

The incubation period is 2–4 days. The first lesion is a papule within 24 hours it becomes pustular and soon ulcerates. The ulcer is extremely painful, it is irregular with undermined edges and the base is covered with a yellowish-grey exudate. The base of the ulcer is granulomatous and bleeds easily. The lesions are usually multiple but may be single. Inguinal lymphadenopathy often unilateral is found in about half of the cases. The lymph nodes enlarge become tender and suppurate without treatment. The adenitis is unilateral in most cases.

Haemophilus ducreyi possesses agglutination properties that accounts for the clumping of the organism, when the colonies are dispersed in saline. Agglutination is responsible for the "school of fish pattern" seen on Gram staining. Exudate for the smear is taken from the base of the ulcer with a cotton swab or flat surface of a tooth pick.

Treatment

Local treatment includes soaks with potassium permanganate; fluctuating lymph nodes should be aspirated. Chancroid is usually treated with erythromycin 500 mg 6 hourly for 7 days. Ceftriaxone is an alternative given as a single dose of IM injection of 250 mg. Azithromycin 1 gm orally in a single dose and ciprofloxacin 500 mg orally in a single dose can also be used.

The sexual partners should be examined and treated.

GRANULOMA INGUINALE

Granuloma inguinale (Fig. 4) is a mildly contagious disease caused by *Calymatobacterium granulomatis (Klebsiella granulomatis)*. It is locally destructive, characterised by progressive indolent serpiginous ulcerations of the groin, pubis, genitalia and the anus. The lesions enlarge by autoinoculation and peripheral extension with satellite lesions. A membranous exudate

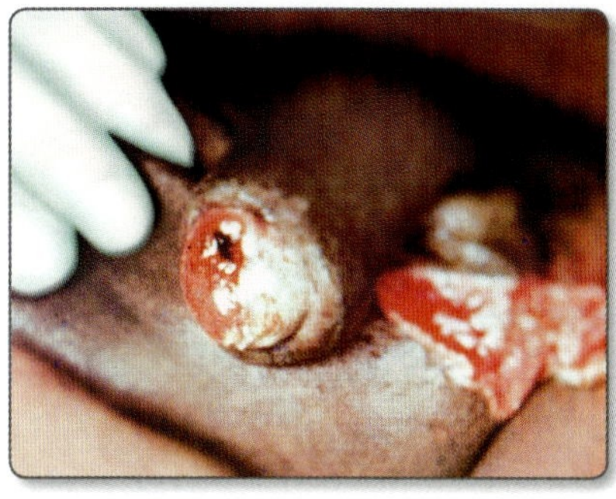

Fig. 4: Granuloma inguinale

covers the floor of the lesions, which are moderately painful. In later stages vegetations, ulceration and scarring occur, carcinomatous changes may develop. Due to cicatrisation, the lymphatic channels are sometimes blocked and pseudo-elephantiasis of the genitals may result. The course is chronic and progressive. Regional lymph nodes are not enlarged.

Diagnosis

The diagnosis is confirmed by finding of the Donovan bodies in the smears, these are found in macrophages, presenting as a characteristic bipolar (closed safety-pin) appearance.

Treatment

Cotrimoxazole, tetracycline or erythromycin 500 mg given four times a day is effective. Streptomycin and gentamicin, ciprofloxacin are also the drugs of choice. Relapses are common, bimonthly examination for 1 year is indicated.

Donovan in 1905, first described the bipolar staining, intracellular inclusions in macrophages from exudates in granuloma inguinale.

LYMPHOGRANULOMA VENEREUM

Lymphogranuloma venereum (LGV) also known as Durand-Nicolas-Favre-disease is caused by *Chlamydia trachomatis*, which is an obligate intracellular pathogen. It is found in all races, affecting people between the ages of 20–40 years. It is more common in men.

Clinical Features

After an incubation period of 1–3 weeks a transient primary lesion appears at the site of contact, this is usually on the genitals. It consists of small herpetiform vesicles or a tiny papule that heals spontaneously in a few days. In about 2 weeks after the appearance of the primary lesion enlargement of the regional glands occur, these are usually unilateral, some cases may be bilateral. The lymph nodes fuse together to form a large mass, the overlying skin becomes violaceous; the mass is tender and may break down with multiple fistulous openings. When both the inguinal and the femoral glands are involved, a groove is seen between these two groups of glands corresponding to the inguinal ligament, this groove is considered pathognomonic for LGV. Women have a low incidence of involvement of the inguinal glands, their bubo is typically pararectal, and this may later lead to rectal strictures. The iliac nodes may also be involved. Women may also develop elephantiasis of the genitals with chronic ulceration and scarring of the vulva.

There may be systemic symptoms such as fever, malaise, joint pains and loss of appetite. Patients may even develop hepatitis or aseptic meningitis. Erythema nodosum, photosensitivity and exanthems represent cutaneous lesions due to systemic involvement.

Late complications include destruction of lymphatics with elephantiasis of the penis, scrotum or the vulva, accompanied by fistula formation.

Diagnosis

Presence of purplish wrinkled adenopathy is characteristic. Laboratory diagnosis is made by a positive intradermal test to a specific antigen (Frei's test). The albumin globulin ratio is 1:1 or it is reversed.

Treatment

Tetracycline 500 mg four times a day for 3 weeks is adequate, it will also treat syphilis. Erythromycin can also be used in a dose of 500 mg four times daily. The fluctuant nodes should be aspirated to prevent rupture. Alternatively doxycycline 100 mg bid for 3 weeks may be used.

Sulphonomides are also effective, but these do not mask a syphilitic infection. Sulfisoxazole in a first dose of 4 gm, then 1 gm four times a day. Trimethoprim-sulphamethoxazole two tablets twice a day is also effective.

Follow-Up

The patient should be examined periodically for at least a year. A persistent high titre of complement fixation test for LGV is an indication for retreatment.

Table 2 showing the differential features of syphilis, chancroid, lymphogranuloma venereum, granuloma inguinale and herpes simplex.

HUMAN IMMUNODEFICIENCY VIRUS INFECTION

Human immunodeficiency virus (HIV) is responsible for the acquired immunodeficiency syndrome (AIDS). HIV is a member of the lentivirus group of Retroviridae. Viruses in this group are characterised by life-long persistence in their host, after seroconversion there is a long asymptomatic phase before the appearance of the clinical manifestation.

Retroviruses are RNA viruses that replicate via DNA intermediary made by the viral reverse transcriptase enzymes. The virus has a special affinity for T cells, which exerts cytopathic and cytolytic effects. During viral replication structural proteins are produced, antibodies against these proteins are used for the diagnosis of HIV infection. In the course of infection, new mutations of HIV appear. There are three types of HIV virus:

1. HIV-1 was the first HIV virus discovered in 1983 as a causative agent for AIDS. During the 1980s and 1990s, the HIV-1 spread widely and became a worldwide pandemic. It has a specific core protein p-24 and an envelope glycoprotein gp-41; these are used for its diagnosis.
2. HIV-2 virus was isolated in 1985; it is less aggressive with a longer latent period than HIV-1 virus. Although HIV-2 virus shares many biological and genetic characteristics with HIV-1 virus, each of the two viruses has regulatory and structural genes that are unique. Core protein p-24 is the same but the glycoprotein is specific, it is gp-36. It is found predominantly in West Africa.
3. HIV-0 virus identified in 1994 as a new human variant appears to be confined geographically to the Southern parts of Cameroon and the surrounding areas.

Throughout this chapter, the term HIV for HIV-1 virus is used, as this is the virus, which is found worldwide.

Table 2: Differential features of syphilis, chancrpoid, lymphogranuloma venereum, granuloma inguinale and herpes simplex

Syphilis	*Chancroid*	*Lymphogranuloma venereum*	*Granuloma inguinale*	*Genital herpes*
Causative organism *Treponema pallidum*	*Haemophilus ducreyi*	*Chlamydia trachomatis*	*Calymma-tobacterium granulomatis*	*Herpes simplex virus*
Incubation period 3–4 weeks	2–4 days	1–3 weeks	3–6 weeks	3–10 days
Site Genitals, peri-anal	Genitals, peri-anal	Genitals, perianal	Genital, perianal, inguinal	Genital, perianal
Ulcer Oval or Round, shallow, indu-rated, narrow rim of erythema, dark, velvety-red lacquered appearance	Shallow inflamed ulcer, soft, yellowish-red in colour	Transitory lesion appears as herpetic vesicles or papule	Progressive indolent, serpigi-nous ulceration	Grouped vesicles on ery-thematous base, erosions have a yellowish-white surface
Painless	Painful	Painless, slight irritation	Painless	Painful
Duration 3–6 weeks	Undetermined usually months	2–6 days	Undetermined maybe years	Primary 2–6 weeks Recurrent,7–10 days
Lymph nodes Bilateral, firm, movable, do not suppurate or break down	Unilateral or Bilateral, break down and ulcerate, matted	Inguinal or femoral-unilateral or bilateral, break down and ulcerate	Lymph nodes not involved, lymphoedema may be present	Bilateral tender lymphadenopa-thy in primary herpes, not in recurrent herpes
Diagnosis Treponema in smears positive, serological tests	Gram stain shows Haemo-philus	LGV complement test positive	Smear shows Donovan bodies in mononuclear cells	Tzanck test shows multinu-cleated cells
Treatment Penicillin	Azithromycin, ceftriaxone	Doxycycline, eryth-romycin	Azithromycin, erythromycin	Acyclovir

Pathogenesis

Progressive immune dysfunction is the hallmark of HIV infection. HIV has a tropism for cells expressing CD4 molecules on their surface. Soon after the patient becomes infected, the number of CD4 lymphocytes begins to fall from its normal value of about 1,000 cells per mm^3, at a variable loss of 40–80 cells/mm^3 per year. This progressive deterioration of the immune system is initially manifested as generalised lymphadenopathy, diarrhoea and weight loss. AIDS develops when the count of CD4 falls below 200 cells/mm^3.

Kaposi's sarcoma is felt to be due to concurrent infection with herpes virus 8. This virus is present in normal adults, but is commonly expressed in an immunocompromised person.

Transmission

Human immunodeficiency virus survives poorly outside the human body; it is transmitted by blood, semen and the breast milk. Thus the main routes of transmission are sexual, administration of blood or blood products, injection with blood contaminated equipment (seen in drug abusers) and from the mother to the child. Transmission can also occur by organ transplantation (risk is small), saliva (risk is small), no transmission occurs by close personal contact or by insects.

Clinical Manifestation

The clinical manifestation of HIV infection with its acquired immunodeficiency depends upon the loss of functional integrity of the T helper cells. This in turn leads to impairment of other immune responses. Depressed T helper cell function impairs T suppressor cells, T cytotoxic cells, macrophages, killer cells and the B cells. HIV infection can be studied in four phases:

1. The acute infection. This is commonly seen as flu-like illness, with fever, malaise, chills, myalgia and arthalgia. In several cases there is erythematous macular, nonpruritic eruption of the trunk and face that lasts for 3–7 days.
2. A prolonged asymptomatic period that lasts from a few months to many years.
3. A phase of generalised lymphadenopathy, there are no other signs or symptoms of infection. The nodes are rubbery, mobile and intermittently tender. Virions are present in large numbers in the follicular dendritic cells of the germinal centres of the lymph nodes and the spleen, which undergo intense hyperplasia. As the HIV disease progresses over the years, the architecture of the lymphoid tissue is disrupted and plasma viraemia intensifies.
4. Symptomatic disease. This phase may be subdivided according to the clinical manifestation into groups A–E. The majority of the patients have decreased number of CD4 lymphocytes usually below 100/mm^3.

A—Constitutional disease (AIDS-related complex)
B—Neurological disease
C—Secondary infections
D—Malignancy secondary to HIV disease
E—Other conditions

Cutaneous Manifestations of AIDS

Cutaneous manifestations of AIDS are more widespread, have an unusual character, have a more prolonged course and the condition is more resistant to therapy than the original infection. Infection with unusual organisms and neoplasms also occur.

Kaposi's sarcoma: In a patient under 60 years of age this should prompt an investigation into HIV infection. The initial lesions of the sarcoma appear as purple or hyperpigmented patches, papules, nodules or tumours on any part of the body. Common sites affected are the tip of the nose and the hard palate. Lesions may develop at the site of trauma (Koebner's phenomenon). Kaposi's sarcoma may be the presenting sign of HIV disease. Surgery is advised for large tumours. Small tumours can be treated by intralesional injection of vinblastine, cryotherapy or irradiation. For widespread lesions ABV (Adriamycin, bleomycin, vinblastine) chemotherapy is advised. Treatment is more or less successful.

Other malignancies: AIDS-related lymphomas are not uncommon; they are usually of high grade and of the immunoblastic type. Extranodal sites are frequently involved.

Seborrhoeic eczema: This may have an abrupt onset and is often severe. It is believed to be associated with an overgrowth or abnormal activity of pityrosporum yeasts.

Psoriasis and Reiter's syndrome: Psoriasis becomes worse in HIV patients. Pustular, erythrodermic, flexural and palmoplantar forms are common. Rieter's syndrome is often severe and refractory to treatment. Sometimes both psoriasis and Rieter's syndrome occur simultaneously with HIV infection; the immune changes caused by HIV are believed to be responsible for the association.

Eosinophilic pustular folliculitis: This is also called the itchy bump disease; it is characterised by itchy-red papules on the head, neck, trunk and the limbs, pustules and excoriations occur. Individual lesions may coalesce to form plaques. Ultraviolet B (UVB) can relieve the symptoms, the condition responds to a short course of oral retinoids.

Pruritic papular eruption (itchy folliculitis): This is an extremely itchy eruption that consists of skin coloured papules situated on the head, neck and the trunk. Histology shows a non-specific perifollicular mixed cell infiltrate. Antihistamines, PUVA (psoralen + UVA) and UVB have helped many patients.

Xeroderma: This is common in AIDS especially in patients who have chronic diarrhoea; it may be related to malabsorption.

Viral infections: Infections like herpes simplex, herpes zoster, warts and molluscum contagiosum may be severe and widespread, necrotic lesions may be present. Herpes zoster may involve more than one dermatome.

Oral hairy leukoplakia: This is an asymptomatic, vertically corrugated whitish plaque on one or both sides of the lateral borders of the tongue. Epstein-Barr virus (EBV) seems to be responsible. Treatment is indicated if there is severe discomfort, with systemic acyclovir in a dose of 400 mg five times a day.

Fungal infections: Infection with dermatophytes and *Candida* is extremely common in all stages of HIV disease, affecting the mouth, genitals and the intertriginous sites. Angular stomatitis (also involves *Staphylococcus aureus*) is common. In severe cases of HIV, one-third of HIV patients have ringworm infections. Nail involvement is common, it causes white diffuse thickening.

Deep fungal infections, such as cryptococcosis, coccidioidomycosis, histoplasmosis and blastomycosis can produce cutaneous lesions in HIV infection due to dissemination.

Bacterial infections: Staphylococcal infections are common, folliculitis, furunculosis and even staphylococcal scalded skin syndrome (SSSS) have been reported. Syphilis may coexist with HIV infection, mycobacterial infection usually causes systemic lesions, but cutaneous lesions may also occur.

Bacilliary angiomatosis: These angioma like lesions may affect the skin, mucosa and the internal organs. Cutaneous lesions begin as tiny pinpoint papules resembling Campbell de Morgan spots; they appear in large numbers and are very widespread. As they enlarge, they have the appearance of pyogenic granulomas. It is caused by *Bartonella henselae*. The condition responds to erythromycin 1–2 gm daily given for several weeks, doxycycline is also effective.

Infestations: Amoebiasis, scabies and demodicidosis are common pathogens; these manifest with severity. Amoebiasis can lead to progressive encephalitis, skin lesions present as pustules, nodules and ulcers on the face and limbs. Scabies presents as Norwegian scabies. Treatment must be meticulous; it should be prolonged and may involve more than one scabicide. Demodicidosis due to Demodex folliculorum causes itchy eruptions on the head, neck trunk and arms. There is a rapid response to treatment with insecticides such as γ-benzene hexachloride.

Drug eruptions are common in AIDS especially with sulphonamides. The cause of these eruptions in immunocompromised individuals is not fully understood. Altered drug metabolism and increased basophilic reactivity have been suggested as possible factors.

Itching: Itching is an important symptom in HIV infection. It may be associated with systemic disease, such as hepatic or kidney failure, cutaneous disease, such as seborrhoeic dermatitis and scabies. Pruritus is also a presenting feature of adverse drug reactions in HIV positive patients. Patients with intense pruritus tend to have high IgE levels. Thalidomide can be useful in the treatment of intractable pruritus in HIV positive patients. Other treatments reported to be effective include dapsone, pentoxyphylline, UVB phototherapy and PUVA.

Systemic Manifestations of AIDS

Nervous system: HIV is neurotrophic and infection of the CNS is found in all cases of AIDS. This may be in the form of encephalitis, behavioural disorders, opportunistic fungal infections, such as cryptococcosis, toxoplasmosis. AIDS-related B cell lymphomas frequently involve the CNS. Cerebral involvement with syphilis and herpes zoster is more common than in normal persons.

Lungs: Pneumocystis carinii (P. jiroveci) pneumonia affects 85% of patients with AIDS; it is a major cause of death. Treatment is usually with cotrimoxazole, although it causes a high incidence of cutaneous and other reactions. Other organisms affecting the lungs are cytomegalovirus (CMV) and tuberculosis.

Gastrointestinal tract: Candida may affect the oral mucosa, perianal region and the oesophagus. The other organisms affecting the gastrointestinal tract are CMV, salmonella, shigella, and some protozoa such as *Giardia lamblia* and amoeba. Diarrhoea, weight loss and malabsorption result.

Renal disease: These include AIDS-associated nephropathy, ischemic injury and drug-associated nephropathy.

Arthritis: A seronegative oligoarthritis or polyarthritis is reported for which no definite cause is found; its response to non-steroidal anti-inflammatory drugs (NSAIDs) is poor.

HIV in Children

Failure to thrive, delay of milestones, chronic parotid swelling and hepatosplenomegaly are common in HIV-infected infants, in addition to the lymphadenopathy and chronic diarrhoea of adults. There is frequency of major bacterial infections, such as septicemia, pneumonia, otitis media and SSSS. The infections are severe and prolonged; Kaposi's sarcoma is seen in only 5% of cases. HIV is not an established cause of congenital malformations.

Criteria of Diagnosing AIDS in Underdeveloped Countries

In underdeveloped countries, World Health Organisation (WHO) has recommended the following criteria for AIDS, as expensive investigations are not easily available. Two major and one minor criteria of the following should be present for the diagnosis of AIDS.
Major signs

- Weight loss of more than 10% of body weight
- Chronic diarrhoea for more than 1 month
- Fever for more than 1 month (intermittent or continuous).

Diagnosis

CD4 absolute counts and CD4/CD8 ratios will indicate the severity of infection. CD4 counts below 200 indicate severe infection. Complete blood picture, hepatic and renal function tests, antibodies for hepatitis A, B and C, VDRL should also be done to find out the extent of disease and presence of any coexisting STD.

Human immunodeficiency virus infection is diagnosed by the detection of serum antibody to HIV by the enzyme-linked immunosorbent assay (ELISA); it is confirmed by the Western blot. Individuals who are recently infected are antibody negative, for these individuals re-testing should be done at 6 weeks, 3 months and at 6 months.

The major disadvantage of the ELISA test is the high incidence of the false positive reactions. All positive ELISA tests should be repeated, if the repeat test is also positive, then it should be confirmed by the Western blot. Western blot is expensive; it is specific for the HIV core protein p24 and envelope glycoprotein gp41.

Enzyme-linked immunosorbent assay test and the Western blot are only positive after the appearance of the antibodies to HIV infection. In majority of individuals, the antibodies develop within 5 months of the infection. Within this period, detection of the virus is necessary for the diagnosis of the HIV infection. A latex agglutination test has been developed to detect the core protein of the virus. Another very sensitive test for the detection of the virus is the polymerase chain reaction (PCR), which detects the HIV DNA present at very low levels in the infected cell. However, most of these tests are unreliable and not well standardized; they are therefore not in routine use. Viral culture remains the ultimate test for diagnosing the HIV infection in the early phases of infection, the test is however technically difficult and expensive.

Minor signs

- Persistent cough of more than 1 month
- General pruritic dermatitis
- Recurrent herpes zoster
- Oropharyngeal candidiasis
- Chronic progressive disseminated herpes simplex
- Generalised lymphadenopathy.

Treatment

Antiretroviral therapy: These drugs block the translation of viral RNA into DNA. A large number of drugs are continually appearing in the market against HIV, they reduce the circulating virus titre before the mutations in the virus render it resistant to the antiviral drug. At present, the best results are obtained by using two reverse transcriptase inhibitors (RTI) and a protease inhibitor.

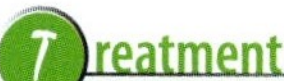

There are four basic principles for the treatment of HIV infection. These are:

1. Antiretroviral therapy
2. Immunorestorative therapy
3. General management
4. Treatment of opportunistic infection

The drugs that inhibit HIV reverse transcriptase are the nucleoside reverse transcriptase inhibitors (NTRI), such as zidovudine (AZT), didanosine (DDI), zalcitabine (DDC), stavudine (D4T) and lamivudine (3TC).

The nonnucleoside reverse transcriptase inhibitors (NNRTI) are nevirapine, efavirenz and delavirdine.

Protease inhibitors (PI) block the maturation and discharge of new viral particles. The drugs that inhibit HIV protease are saquinavir, indinavir, ritonavir, nelfinavir and amprenavir.

The fusion inhibitors block the entry of HIV into the cells; such as enfuvirtide.

Monotherapy with one of the RTI inhibitors causes a less than tenfold decrease in plasma viral load (PVL); monotherapy with the more potent protease inhibitors causes a 100 fold decrease in PVL. Greater decrease in PVL (up to 1,000 fold) can be achieved by a combination of a protease inhibitor and one or more RTIs (e.g. indinavir/zidovidine/lamivudine).

Treatment is usually started with 2NRTI combined with a NNRTI or a PI. A combination of antiretroviral therapy known as highly active antiretroviral therapy (HAART), has been instituted by WHO for the treatment of AIDS; which reduces the chances of infection with common and opportunistic infections, reduces the chances of malignancy and improves constitutional symptoms, but has serious side effects. The regime requires careful monitoring.

The drugs should be well monitored; they tend to cause a bone marrow depression with anaemia and leucopenia. It also causes a distinct pigmentation of the neck especially in dark coloured persons.

Immunorestorative therapy: the drugs used for immunorestorative therapy, are interferons, interleukin-2, bone marrow transplantation and infusion of histocompatable lymphocytes.

Prevention

As the disease is spread through sexual contact, the guiding principle is to avoid contact between infected secretions, mucosal surfaces and broken skin. The practice of "safe sex" includes monogamous relationship, reduction in the number of partners, avoidance of high-risk partners, such as drug abusers, prostitutes and those with evidence of genital infection. Use of a latex condom is important in preventing transmission.

No satisfactory vaccine has been developed against HIV. Prevention of transmission of infection is therefore of paramount importance.

FURTHER READING

1. Bagovac J, Lukas D. Condylomata of secondary syphilis. New Eng J Med. 2005;352:708.
2. Finkelstein M, Berman B. HIV and AIDS in inpatient dermatology. Approach to the consultation. Dermatol Clin. 2000;18:509-20.
3. Hoorer WD, Lang PG. Pruritus in HIV Infection. J Am Acad Dermatol. 1991;24:1021-1.
4. Jensen BL, Weisman K, Sindrip JH, et al. Incidence and prognostic significance of skin disease in patients with HIV/AIDS; A 5 year observational study. Acta Derm Venereol (Stockh). 2000;80:140-3.
5. Koff AB, Rosen T. Nonvenereal treponematoses: Yaws, Endemic Syphilis, Pinta. J Am Acad Dermatol. 1993;29:519-35.
6. Parish JL. Treponemal infection in the pediatric population. Clin Dermatol. 2000;18:687-700.
7. Welch J. Antenatal screening for syphilis (Editorial). BMJ. 1998;317:1605-6.

Chapter

9 Eczema

INTRODUCTION

The word eczema is derived from a Greek word meaning to boil out. The word was first used by Aetius Amidenus, a Greek physician to the Byzantine court in the 6th century. He was referring to a phlyctenular condition the Greeks called "eczemata". It is not known whether he was referring to a boil, eczema or something else. Any vesicular or bullous disorders are suggestive of bubbling. Even today, there is no clear-cut definition of eczema. It is often said that eczema is like jazz; one assumes that everyone recognises it and that this makes it unnecessary to define it.

Eczema is an epidermal reaction to injurious agents; it is induced by external or internal factors; acting singularly or in combination. It is characterised histologically by spongiosis (epidermal oedema), varying degrees of acanthosis and a superficial perivascular lymphohistiocytic infiltrate. The dermal reaction is secondary and rather non-characteristic except that it involves the blood vessels of the superficial plexus. Clinically, it is characterised in the acute stage by papules, vesicles and oozing, in the subacute stage by mild erythema and scaling, and in chronic stage by scaling and lichenification.

The word dermatitis should not be used, as dermatitis is any inflammation of the skin, perhaps eczematous dermatitis would be a better terminology.

PATHOGENESIS OF ECZEMA

General Concept

Different types of eczema represent a common type of inflammatory response of the epidermal cells to damage resulting in secretion of proinflammatory cytokines. These cytokines cause dilatation of dermal blood vessels, which explain the redness of eczematous rashes. The dilatation of blood vessels results in exudation of fluid, this leads to intercellular oedema (spongiosis) and sometimes discrete collections of fluid resulting in vesicle formation. The action of these mediators on nerve endings causes itching. As the process becomes subacute or chronic, the keratinisation process in the damaged epidermal cells becomes affected, resulting in disturbed formation of horny layer, which clinically manifests as scales and lichenification.

Eczema can be studied under two headings:

- Clinical features of eczema, these are the same in every type of eczema and so is the treatment of eczema in general
- Aetiology of eczema, here the pattern, morphology, age, distribution, specific treatment and prognosis differ.

CLINICAL AND HISTOLOGICAL FEATURES OF ECZEMA

Clinically eczema can be acute, subacute or chronic. This simple clinical classification is a useful guide to the treatment of eczema, but is of little value in assessing the factors responsible for eczema.

The appearance of the eczema depends upon its severity, duration and the site. The main symptom in eczema is pruritus.

Acute Eczema

This affects the epidermis and the papillary dermis. It is characterised clinically by erythema, papules, vesicles, oozing and crusting (Figs 1A and B). Histologically the eczema is characterised by the development of spongiosis, starting irregularly in the mid-epidermal region, but as the eczema becomes severe, the oedematous areas coalesce to form clinical vesicles. As the pressure increases, the fluid leaks on to the surface and the skin weeps. There is usually a dermal infiltrate composed mainly of lymphocytes, but in some cases, polymorphs and red blood cells also accumulate.

Subacute Eczema

As the eczema becomes more chronic, the oedema diminishes and acanthosis develops. Due to the disturbances of keratinisation, parakeratosis (retention of nuclei in the horny layer) and hyperkeratosis develop. Clinically there is redness, swelling, scaling and crusting (Fig. 2).

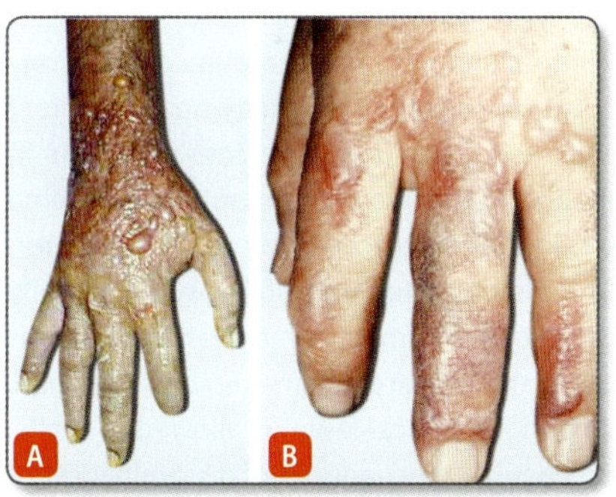

Figs 1A and B: (A) Acute eczema-erythema, vesicles and bullae; (B) Acute eczema

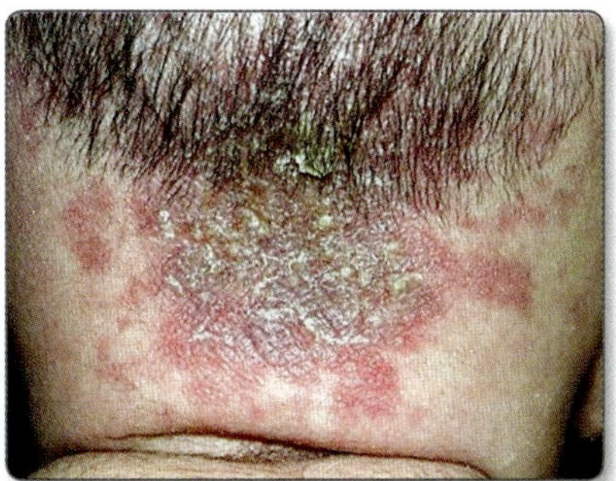

Fig. 2: Subacute eczema-erythema and scaling

Chronic Eczema

In chronic eczema the vascular dilatation decreases and gradually becomes less marked, the lymphocytic infiltrate persists particularly around the blood vessels. The increased thickness of the epidermis, produces areas of the skin in which the normal skin lines become exaggerated, this change is called lichenification. Chronic eczema is associated with severe itching.

Chronic eczema is characterised clinically by thickening, lichenification, fissuring and pigmentation of the skin (Fig. 3).

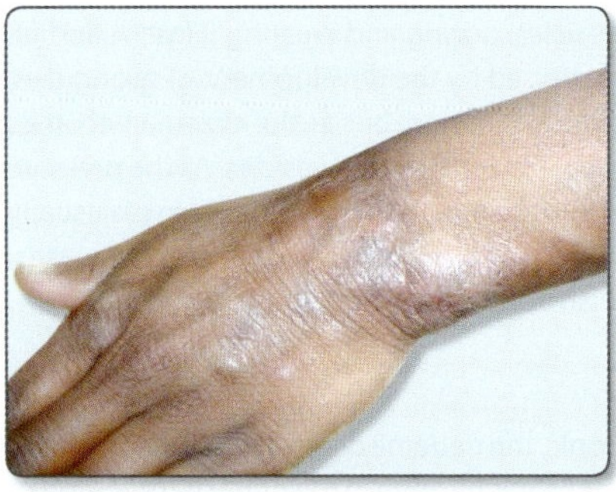

Fig. 3: Chronic eczema—thickening and lichenification

SPECIAL CHARACTERISTIC OF ECZEMA (SECONDARY DISSEMINATION)

A very characteristic feature of all forms of eczema regardless of aetiology is a tendency to spread far from its point of origin. This may occur by direct extension of the eczema from the affected area or new patches may occur in a completely new area. Dissemination occurs more commonly with eczema present over the legs. The dissemination is preceded by an exacerbation of eczema at the primary site. The disseminated eruption is symmetrically distributed over the body consisting of erythematous macules, eczematous papulovesicles or utricarial lesions. If the primary eczema remains inflamed, the eruption increases in severity and if the local lesion is allowed to settle, the secondary eruption subsides. Possible mechanisms of dissemination of eczema are:

- Direct spread of the allergen: Lesions are not spread by the rupture of the contents of the blister or vesicle, as the fluid does not contain the offending agent
- Spread by contact with a foreign antigen
- Spread by ingestion of the antigen
- Conditioned hyperirritability. An area of eczema on one part of the body is associated with hyperirritability of the skin at distant sites making these sites more vulnerable to eczema. This may be immune-mediated
- Bacterial hypersensitivity. Heavily infected eczema can disseminate probably as a result of allergy to bacterial products.

TREATMENT OF ECZEMA

Removal of the irritant is the most important part of the treatment. If this is impossible, minimise the contact by wearing protective gloves and washing the skin after contact with the irritant. Emollients serve as a protective layer for the skin and also prevent its dryness. In acute eczema, wet dressings such as potassium permanganate are applied, until a subacute stage is reached. Topical steroids are the mainstay of treatment.

- Low potency steroids should be used on the face and groins
- Medium potency steroids should be used on the body and extremities
- Strong steroids are used in severely affected areas.

In persistent cases, it may be advisable to resort to systemic steroids rather than to continue with potent topical steroids for a prolonged period.

Acute Eczema

This is a moist weeping eczema, which should be treated several times daily with potassium permanganate soaks, normal saline or Burrow's solution. Potassium permanganate is a soothing lotion; it also prevents secondary infection due to its antibacterial properties. These solutions tend to reduce the weeping, but will cause dryness and cracking when used for a long time. A topical steroid should be applied later if these are ineffective. Oral steroids may be used in acute severe eczema. Antihistamines relieve itching due to sedation. If secondary bacterial infection is present, it should be treated with an appropriate antibiotic.

Subacute and Chronic Eczema

Here it is advisable to use a less water-soluble preparation. In patients with dry skin, simple emollients will often relieve pruritus. Lubrication is an essential part of treatment; chronic eczema will quickly relapse back in to subacute eczema if lubrication is neglected. Lubricants are best applied a few hours after the steroid application and these should be continued for days/weeks after the inflammation has subsided. Frequent bathing causes removal of the skin lipids with subsequent dehydration of the keratin and this makes the eczema worse.

Topical steroids are mainstay of suppressive treatment of eczema. Patients should be warned of the possible side effects, the weakest preparation effective for a particular patient should be used. Patients who have failed to respond to treatment will often improve when hospitalised.

Intralesional steroids can be used in thickened patches of eczema; steroids can also be used under occlusion.

Steroids become less effective on long-term treatment, various tar preparations are effective alternatives. Tar can also be used on long-term or between short courses of steroids. PUVA (psoralen + UVA) has been used to treat chronic hand eczema.

CLASSIFICATION

Classification of eczema is not easy as many pathogenic factors are involved; most of these are poorly understood. There are two important groups of eczema, the exogenous and the endogenous. The differentiation is important to the patient, as removing the cause can prevent exogenous eczema.

Exogenous eczema

- Contact dermatitis (CD)
  - Irritant
  - Allergic
- Infective eczema
- Photosensitive eczema

Endogenous eczema

- Atopic dermatitis (AD)
- Seborrhoeic dermatitis
- Discoid or Nummular eczema
- Hypostatic eczema
- Pompholyx
- Asteatotic eczema
- Lichen simplex chronicus
- Pityriasis alba
- Juvenile plantar dermatosis.

Exogenous Eczema

Irritant Contact Dermatitis

This is a nonallergic exposure of the skin to irritating substances. It accounts for 80% cases of occupational dermatitis. Irritant eczema occurs in all ages and in both the sexes. Most irritant eczemas occur on the hands as these are most exposed to irritants; both the palms and the back of the hands are affected. It can be acute or it may occur after a delayed response, this is known as the cumulative insult dermatitis.

Pathogenesis: Little is known about the pathogenesis of irritant CD. Penetration of the irritant is primarily via the sweat ducts and the hair follicles; the reaction is reduced in the absence of sweating. Irritants can also cause damage by degreasing the skin, the irritants gain access to the epidermal cells, causing separation of the cells and they also cause damage to the cell membrane and cytoplasm, which may lead to its death. The influx of inflammatory cells; release cytokines causing oedema and inflammation. The reaction also involves the stimulation of sensory nerve endings.

The weak irritants predominantly affect the horny layer, causing dryness and scaling by destroying the lysozomal enzymes in the horny layer. The irritants denature the keratin, and remove the stratum corneum lipids and alter the water-holding capacity of the skin. This eventually leads to the damage of the living cells of the epidermis.

Weak irritants, such as bleaches, soaps, solvents, weak acids and alkalis, plants and cutting oils cause primary irritant eczema, after prolonged exposure to the irritant. Irritant CD is sharply localised to the site of contact of the irritant. The eczema is dry, scaly, and often lichenified.

A primary irritant when strong can produce an eczematous reaction in all individuals following a single exposure such as strong acids and strong alkalis. Strong irritants damage the keratinocytes and blood vessels resulting in hyperaemia, formation of vesicles and bullae.

Allergic Contact Dermatitis

Allergic CD is a manifestation of delayed hypersensitivity. Contact allergy is rare before the age of 15 years and in the extreme old age, due to the diminished cell-mediated immunity in the young and the very old. Irritant CD is independent of age. Sex incidence depends upon the allergen, e.g. nickel sensitivity is more frequent in women, chromate and cement sensitivity in men.

Allergic CD develops in susceptible individuals after weeks or years of exposure to a sensitising agent. Once the individual is sensitised, further exposure will cause dermatitis within 48 hours. Certain elements and compounds have the ability to act as contact allergens, these then cause allergic CD. Common sensitisers are nickel, paraphenylenediamine (found in hair dyes), rubber, cosmetics, medications, plants and wood. Allergic CD is not sharply demarcated to the site of contact of the allergen, it spreads to the adjacent sites, e.g. from back of the hands to the wrist.

Pathogenesis: Allergic CD is a Type IV delayed cell-mediated hypersensitivity reaction. Initially a low-molecular-weight antigen (hapten) contacts the skin and forms a hapten-carrier protein complex. This complex associates itself with epidermal Langerhans cells; this presents the complete antigen to the helper T cells causing a release of various mediators. Subsequently T cell expansion occurs in the regional lymph nodes producing specific memory T effector lymphocytes, which circulate in the general blood stream. The whole process of sensitisation takes about 5–21 days.

On re-exposure of the antigen within minutes a sensitisation reaction occurs, this is localised to the area of maximal contact. Absorption of the allergens is promoted by moisture, such as sweating, and thin skin as that of the eyelid. Similarly degreased and chapped or broken skin is more liable to sensitisation.

Clinical Features of Contact Dermatitis

Primary irritant dermatitis causes an inelastic feeling of the skin, there is discomfort related to dryness, pruritus secondary to inflammation, pain related to fissures, blisters and ulcers.

Chronic exposure to mild irritants results in dry, thick and fissured skin. Strong irritants cause blisters, erosions and ulcers. Mild irritants sometimes produce erythema, microvesiculation and oozing that may be indistinguishable from allergic CD. This may be associated with AD or when the skin is broken due to injury.

Mild allergic CD is similar in appearance to irritant eruptions. A more typical allergic reaction will consist of grouped or linear vesicles and blisters. If the involvement is severe, there may be marked oedema, particularly on the face, periorbital and genital areas. The allergy is frequently transferred from the hands and to other areas of the body, where the allergic rash appears. Palms, soles and scalp are more resistant to allergic CD, because of the thicker stratum corneum and greater barrier function.

Non-eczematous variants of allergic CD: These include lichenoid CD (metals, paraphenylenediamine derivatives, photographic colour developers, aminoglycosides, fragrances), erythema multiforme (exotic woods, drugs, dyes, epoxy resins, paraphenylenediamine), contact purpura (phenylenediamine, textile resins, epoxy resins, quinidine, oxyquinolone), contact leukoderma (paraphenylenediamine), cellulitis like CD, and erythema dyschromicum perstans. Patch testing is the means for accurate diagnosis.

Morphological Pattern of Contact Dermatitis

The eczema may be acute, subacute or chronic. Irritant contact eczema is localised to the site of contact, whereas allergic dermatitis is not sharply demarcated to the site of the allergen, there is a spread to the adjacent sites, e.g. from the back of the hands to the wrists. Distant sites may be involved such as the eyes and the antecubital fossae; severe allergic contact eczema may become generalised.

The distribution of the eczema corresponds to the site of exposure to the allergen, e.g. wrist in watch allergy, back of the hands and wrist in rubber glove dermatitis. Nail varnish allergy does not affect the nails, but areas touched by the fingers such as the eyelids. Clothing eczema due to dye and fibre finishes, commences in the moist and occluded areas, such as the popliteal and antecubital fossae, the vault being commonly spared. Airborne allergens affect the face and the neck. Shoes and socks affect the feet. Scalp is affected by the hair dyes. Buttocks are involved in napkin dermatitis.

The palms, soles and scalp are more resistant to allergic CD because of the greater thickness of the stratum corneum and greater barrier function.

Irritant and allergic CD may coexist, making the diagnosis difficult.

Factors Affecting Contact Dermatitis

A number of factors affect the development of CD. These include the concentration of the active ingredient in the offending substance, its physical and chemical properties, the vehicle used, the duration of exposure, the genetic make-up of the patient, the site of exposure and the age of patient. Environmental factors, such as humidity and temperature, also play a role in the pathogenesis of contact eczema.

Differential Diagnosis

Contact eczema should be differentiated from other eczemas as nummular eczema, AD and seborrheic eczema. Nummular eczema affects the extensor surface of the limbs, hands and feet, particularly on the dorsal surface. The lesions are bilateral and symmetrical; they are well-defined coin like in shape. Atopic dermatitis is seen in individuals who are potentially atopic; they have a predisposition to asthma, allergic rhinitis and urticaria. It has special sites of predilection as the face and neck in infants, flexures in the children and adults. Atopic eczema is associated with intense pruritus. Seborrhoeic eczema is often associated with greasy scales, areas rich in sebaceous glands and intertrigenous areas are most often affected.

Contact eczema, should also be differentiated from other diseases, e.g. hand eczema should be differentiated from palmar psoriasis, fungal infection, palmar lichen planus, congenital palmoplantar keratosis. A proper history, examination of other parts of the body, scraping for fungi, and examination of the nails, and biopsy will help in diagnosis. Similarly, clothing eczema in the axilla should be differentiated from other intertriginous disorders.

Allergic contact eczema can be confirmed by the patch test. Once a substance is suspected to cause allergic CD, it may be tested by applying the offending agent (preferably in solution), to the back of the patient under a small patch of adhesive tape. The patch is removed after 48 hours or earlier if severe irritation develops. A positive reaction consists of erythema and papules, if the reaction is severe there may be vesiculations and oedema.

Patch test should be avoided when the eczema is acute. A positive test may cause a severe exacerbation of the eczema and it may become generalised.

A biopsy helps to distinguish allergic CD from other eczemas. Allergic CD is charcterised by the presence of hyperplasia of Langerhans cells or nesting of antigen presenting cells. Eosinophilic spongiosis or eosinophils distributed individually within an oedematous epidermis and the presence of eosinophils in the dermal inflammatory infiltrate.

Table 1 shows the difference between irritant and allergic contact dermatitis.

Table 1: Difference between irritant contact dermatitis and allergic contact dermatitis

Irritant contact dermatitis	*Allergic contact dermatitis*
• Common • All persons susceptible • Does not extend beyond the site of contact • Concentration of the substance to produce the reaction should be high. • The reaction is immediate in acute dermatitis, and late in chronic irritant dermatitis • No hypersensitivity involved, reaction it is due to the direct toxic effect of the substance • Patch test not diagnostic	• Less common • Some people susceptible • Extends beyond the site of contact • Minute amount of substance required to elicit the reaction • Sensitisation requires 2–3 weeks • Type IV hypersensitivity reaction • Patch test diagnostic

COMMON CONTACT ECZEMAS

Footwear Dermatitis

It usually starts on the dorsal surface of the big toe, and then spreads on the dorsum of the other toes and feet. Eczema does not involve the insteps, skin between the toes and the flexural areas of the foot, as these areas are not in contact with the offending agent.

Shoe dermatitis (Fig. 4) may be caused by dichromates of leather, rubber accelerators, gum, tar, formaldehyde, felt, cork, asphalt, dyes and nickel. Patch testing may be done to find out the allergen; this helps in making footwear without the sensitizing substances. A simple method to establish a diagnosis is to cut out a piece of the area of the shoe that is in direct contact with the eczematous skin and applying this piece as a patch test. The sensitisation is common in people with hyperhidrosis of the feet. Those who have shoe dermatitis should change shoes frequently as chromate is gradually liberated from the leather by the action of hydroxy acids in the sweat.

Rubber Dermatitis

Rubber dermatitis may be caused by rubber gloves, shields, girdles, panties in infants, rubber sheets, condoms, pessaries, etc. Natural rubber does not cause sensitisation, but it is the chemicals added to it in the manufacturing processes, make it sensitive. The main chemicals added are the antioxidants and the accelerators.

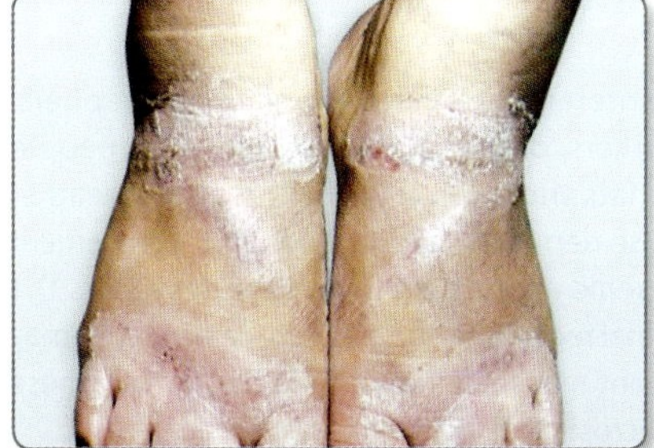

Fig. 4: Shoe dermatitis

- Accelerators: These are substances used to increase the vulcanisation of rubber. The common chemicals included are:
  - Mercaptobenzothiazole (MBT)
  - Tetramethylthiuram disulphide
  - Diphenylguanidine.
- Antioxidants: In order to preserve rubber, antioxidants are used. These include phenyl-alpha-naphthylamine. Hydroquinone antioxidants can cause depigmentation of the skin and allergic reactions. A frequent antioxidant sensitiser is propyl-paraphenylenediamine; this is also used for hair dyes, cross sensitivity may occur.

Nickel Dermatitis

Nickel sensitisation (Fig. 5) is one of the most common causes of sensitisation, especially in women. Nickel occurs everywhere from the cooking utensils and military armament to ornaments and work of art. Nickel produces more cases of allergic CD than all the metals combined together. Nickel is present in artificial jewellery, in wrist watches, spectacle frames, buttons, handle of doors, handbags, etc. Cobalt and nickel often occur together, as cobalt is a contaminant of nickel.

The diagnosis is established by a positive reaction to 5% nickel sulphate solution used as a patch test. Fisher's sensitivity test to detect articles containing nickel is by applying freshly prepared 1% alcoholic solution of dimethylglyoxime and a freshly prepared solution of 10% ammonia in equal amounts, to the test object. If nickel is present in the article, it will turn orange pink in colour.

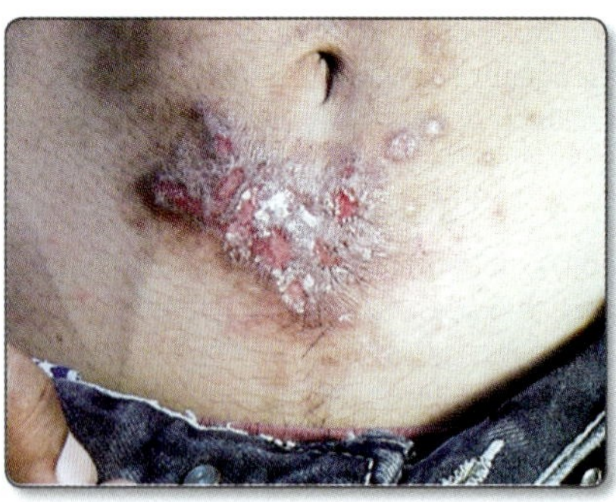

Fig. 5: Nickel dermatitis

Chromium Dermatitis

Chromium dermatitis is encountered in tanners, dyers, photographers, polishers, welders, aircraft workers, diesel engine workers, and people concerned with the bleaching of fats and oils. Traces of dichromate in leather in the shoes and gloves may cause dermatitis of the hands and feet. Cement contains dichromate, nickel, arsenic and cobalt. In cement dermatitis the elbows, knees, flexures and inguinal region may be affected, cement dust may affect the face. Alkalinity of cement may lead to caustic burns. Initially these burns are asymptomatic, later necrosis and ulceration may occur.

Heavy exposure to industrial workers can cause chrome ulcers on the back of the hands and forearms usually beginning around the hair follicles, creases of the knuckles and finger webs. It begins as a small abrasion in the skin that deepens and widens, edges grow thick, eventually forming conical indolent ulcers. Chrome ulcers may also perforate the nasal septum. Patch testing is done with 0.5% potassium dichromate.

Paraphenylenediamine Dermatitis

Paraphenylenediamine (PPDA) dermatitis is found in hairdressers, photographers, rubber vulcanising industrial workers, etc. In industrial workers sensitisation is seen on the back of the hands, wrists, forearms, eyelids and the nose. In those who use hair dyes, sensitivity is manifested by itching, redness and puffiness of the upper eyelids, top of the ears, temples and back of the neck. Patch test is done with 2% PPDA in petrolatum.

Persons sensitive to PPDA hair dye should use semipermanent dyes or vegetable dyes such as henna.

Fibreglass Dermatitis

Small spicules of fibreglass can penetrate the skin and cause severe irritation. Tiny erythematous papules are formed; itching is severe resembling scabies or an insect bite. Fibreglass dermatitis may be occupational or it may occur in persons whose clothes have been washed with fibreglass curtains. Occupations that deal with fibreglass are automobile factories, furniture industries, manufacture of fibreglass curtains, draperies, thermal installations, gasoline tanks and aircraft.

Washing of clothes after handling fibreglass is helpful in preventing fibreglass dermatitis. Talcum powder dusted on the flexural surfaces of the arms makes the fibre slide off the skin.

Clothing Dermatitis

Clothing dermatitis occurs in persons who perspire freely, who are obese and wear tight-fitted clothing. Axillary folds are commonly affected while the vault is spared; intertriginous areas will leach dyes from the clothing to cause dermatitis. Pure cotton, silk and wool do not sensitise. Synthetic fibres, such as nylon, acrylics, rayon, polyesters cause sensitisations, this is due to the dyes and finishes in the clothing such as antiwrinkling chemicals make it prone to sensitisation. Formaldehyde is added to make it less vulnerable to the effects of perspiration and to make it water repellent. Some clothing provoke a purpuric reaction such as khaki dermatitis.

Clothing dermatitis should be differentiated from seborrhoeic dermatitis, AD and neurodermatitis.

Fisher recommends that the test fibre be soaked in 1 mL of water and a drop or two of vinegar for 24 hours. The solution is applied as a patch test for 24 hours. In testing for axillary dermatitis, the suspected fibre is soaked in 250 ml of water to which a drop of 20% of sodium hydroxide has been added and then applied to the skin for 48 hours.

Dermatitis due to Heavy Metals

Mercury Poisoning (Arodynia)

Also called calomel disease or pink disease, it is caused by the ingestion of mercury usually in infancy. The skin changes are characteristic and pathognomonic. It consists of painful swelling of the hands and feet, sometimes associated with considerable itching. The hands and feet are cold and clammy, pink or dusky red. Erythema is usually blotchy, but it may be diffuse. Haemorrhagic puncta are frequently evident, stomatitis and loss of teeth may occur. Constitutional symptoms, such as fever, irritability, tendency to cry most of the time and increased perspiration may be present. There is often associated respiratory infection and sore throat.

The diagnosis of acrodynia is made by the urine examination. Finding over 0.001 mg of mercury in one litre of urine is diagnostic. Albuminuria and haematuria are usually present.

Arsenism

Arsenic was used in the past for the treatment of psoriasis, AD, asthma and syphilis. Arsenic poisoning may be acute or chronic.

Acute arsenic dermatitis: Cutaneous manifestations are generalised erythematous papules, pustules, bullae, erythema multiforme and even exfoliative dermatitis may occur. The systemic manifestations are abdominal pain, diarrhoea, painful extremities, fever and oedema of the eyelids, feet and hands.

Chronic arsenism: This is seen when arsenic is used for a long time, such as in Fowler's solution in the treatment of syphilis. This may be in the form of arsenic keratosis and arsenic melanosis.

Arsenic keratosis: This is chiefly seen in the palms and soles. Basal or squamous cell carcinoma may develop on arsenic keratosis. The keratosis is especially prominent about the sweat pores, small pegs of keratin are mounted on the pores and when these are removed, pits are seen. Multiple basal cell carcinomas develop on the trunk in arsenic poisoning. Carcinoma may also be found in the gastrointestinal tract, larynx and genitourinary system.

Arsenical melanosis: This is characterised by generalised black pigmentation confined to the trunk and depigmented macules (raindrops) scattered in it. The hyperpigmentation is due to arsenic combining with sulphydryl groups in the epidermis that stimulates the oxidation of tyrosine to DOPA. Transverse white striations on the fingernails may appear (Mee's lines).

Chronic arsenic poisoning also occurs in several parts of the world. Water and soil contain large quantities of arsenic in Cordobe in Argentina and South coast of Taiwan. Normal excretion of arsenic in the urine is 0.005–0.04 mg/day. In acute arsenic poisoning, it may be 0.1 mg/day. The hair and nail tend to store arsenic. In the hair, normal amount is 0.008–0.025 mg/100 g, in arsenic poisoning it is 0.1 mg/100 g of hair.

Dermatitis due to Plants

This was previously called dermatitis venenata. Dermatitis may be due to trees, shrubs, flowers, fruits, leaves, weeds, pollen or any other part of a plant. The plant poison ivy causes rhus dermatitis. This is an acute phytodermatitis characterised by linear vesicular bullous eruptions. Common plants causing dermatitis are money plant (philodendron); chrysanthemum and primrose Eruption is usually vesicular often accompanied by marked oedema. Apart from the hands the eyelids are commonly involved.

Plant-Associated Dermatitis

Some plants will produce a phototoxic reaction in certain individuals. The ultraviolet A (UVA) of the sun is mainly responsible. It is known as phytophotodermatitis. Plants that produce phytophotodermatitis are psoralens, dil, parsely, celery, lime, bergamot, mustard, etc. Plants of the Umbelliferae family are frequent causes of this eruption.

Insecticides

Many insecticides on the plants also produce dermatitis. This is especially true of arsenic and malathion containing sprays. Herbicides such as randox are reported to cause large bullae on the feet of farmers.

Mechanical Irritants

Barbs, spines, thorns, cactus needles are some of the mechanical accessories of the plants, they may produce dermatitis.

Sabra Dermatitis

This is an occupational dermatitis resembling scabies. It is seen amongst the pickers of prickly pear cactus plant and in persons handling Indian figs. It is caused by the penetration of invisible thorns in the skin.

Dermatitis due to Plant Derivatives

The sensitising substances derived from the plants are found in the oleoresin fraction, which contains camphors, essential oils, phenols, resin and turpentine. The chief sensitisers are the essential oils. These may be localised in certain parts of a plant such as peel of citrus fruit, leaves of eucalyptus tree and bark of cinnamon.

Testing for Plant Allergies

The method of testing for plant hypersensitivity is by the application of the plant leaf or substance as a cover patch test. A 1 cm square leaf is left on the skin for 48 hours. A test should be done on several controls to make sure that the leaf is not irritant.

Many plants are also photosensitizers. Tests should be done in duplicate, one set covered and the other exposed to light for the detection of photosensitivity.

Cosmetics

Cutaneous reactions to cosmetics may be allergic, irritant or photosensitive. The leading causes of allergic CD are the fragrances, preservatives, lanolin and wool wax.

Amongst the axillary antiperspirants least irritant is aluminum chlorohydrate, zirconium preparation produce a generalised granulomatous reaction. Axillary deodorants rarely produce allergic sensitization, addition of antibacterials drugs such as neomycin and bithionol cause allergic CD.

Hair Dyes

Permanent hair dyes such as paraphenylenediamine (PPDA) are potent sensitisers and may cross-react with other chemicals such as sulphonamides and local anaesthetics. Azo dyes can cross-react with PPDA. Currently popular metallic hair dyes contain nickel, cobalt, chromium or lead.

Hair Bleaches

These contain peroxides, persulphates and ammonia. These may act as local irritants.

Permanent Waves

These rarely sensitize, but may cause hair breakage. In cold type of hair waving thioglycolates are used, in the hot type alkaline sulphides are used.

Hair Straighteners

Greases and gums are not sensitisers; however, the perfumes added to it can cause sensitisation.

Hair Sprays

These contain gum and synthetic resins; they act as sensitisers and frequently cause allergic reactions.

Depilatories

Calcium thioglycolate and sulphides are used for removing the hair. These may cause primary irritant dermatitis. Mechanical hair removers such as wax may cause allergic CD.

Nail Lacquers

These contain sulphonamides and formaldehyde resins. These are frequent causes of eyelid and neck dermatitis.

Lipstick

Dibromofluorescein and tetrabromofluorescein in the indelible dyes and perfumes of the lipsticks, cause sensitisation reactions. The reactions may be enhanced if allantoin compounds are also included.

Eye Makeup

These consist of mascara, eye shadow and eyeliners. The preservatives and perfumes are the components that may cause sensitisation but it is rare.

Sunscreens

Para-aminobenzoic acid and its esters, cinnamates and benzophenones are photosensitisers. Hydroquinone is not only used as a sunscreen, but also as a bleaching agent can sensitise occasionally.

Depigmenting Creams

These contain hydroquinone, which can sensitise occasionally. Previously ammoniated mercury was used which was a sensitising agent.

Perfumes

Almost all cosmetics contain perfumes. Photoallergy is frequently reported. Almond oil may produce rhinitis and dermatitis. Other perfumes that cause sensitisation are coriander, lemon, jasmine, lavender, lemon grass, oil of clove, peppermint, spearmint and winter grass.

Use Test for Cosmetics

The strategy is to use a small amount of the suspect cosmetic on a normal area of skin; the forearm is used for testing. If a rash appears at the site, the cosmetic should be discontinued.

Diaper Dermatitis

This primary irritant dermatitis occurs in infants due to prolonged exposure with urine and faeces because of ammonia produced by the bacteria. Ammonia is formed in the wet diaper by splitting of urea by ammonia forming bacillus in the faeces. Conditions that favour development of napkin dermatitis are delay in napkin changing, frequent loose stools, inadequate cleaning of buttocks or nappies, and occlusive rubber or plastic pants. In napkin dermatitis the skin folds are usually spared, dermatitis is limited to the areas covered by the napkin.

Most cases respond to improved hygiene, frequent changing of nappies and application of emollients. In severe cases, mild steroids may be prescribed. Disposable nappies should be used.

Treatment of Contact Dematitis

The successful treatment of CD requires identification of substances causing CD, its avoidance, appropriate barrier creams, wearing heavy vinyl gloves while working, emollients after use and appropriate occupational advice.

Acute reactions require wet soaks and application of soothing creams and lotions. After vesiculation subsides, a topical corticosteroid cream or lotion should be applied. Occasionally a severe episode of acute CD may require oral corticosteroids.

Subacute and chronic dermatitis responds to topical steroids and systemic antihistamines. Steroid under occlusion and intralesional steroids can be used in localised resistant cases of CD. Tar preparations are a useful adjunct in chronic eczema. Bacterial infections are usually common, which should be treated with topical and systemic antibiotics.

In persistent cases UVR can be tried such as hand UVB or bath PUVA for localised hand or foot dermatitis, and oral PUVA for generalised lesions. Systemic immunosuppressive agents, such as azathioprine, cyclosporin, and methotrexate can also be considered. Topical tacrolimus and pimecrolimus can be used as an alternative to topical steroids.

Hyposensitisation may be required in patients who cannot avoid exposure to the substance causing CD, dangerous adverse effects may occur with hyposensitisation.

Hand eczema is discussed separately later in the chapter.

INFECTIVE ECZEMA

Infective eczema is an eczema, which is caused by microorganisms or their products, and which clears once the organisms is eradicated. This should be differentiated from infected eczema in which eczema is superimposed by bacterial invasion.

Infective eczema is common in the tropics, especially in the hot humid areas; it develops in susceptible individuals by an unknown mechanism. The organisms commonly found are coagulase positive staphylococci, β-haemolytic streptococci or both. Infective eczema presents as an area of advancing erythema with microvesicles seen around discharging wounds and ulcers. Predisposing factors are poor hygiene, seborrhoeic diathesis, malnutrition or excessive perspiration. It often follows insect bites, parasitic infestations, miliaria, infected wounds and ulcers.

Clinical Features

Eczamatous patches develop over another lesion such as abrasion fungal infection or scabies. The lesions are erythematous oozing and crusting. The borders are sharply demarcated, the eruption spreads with vesicles and pustules at the periphery. Large areas may be affected often in a polycyclic pattern. Itching is minimal except when the eczema is secondary to parasitic infections such as scabies and pediculosis.

Common sites are behind the ears, groin, axilla and dorsum of the feet. Eczema due to scabies is often on the genitals and nipples. In pediculosis it is found in the nape of the neck, in pinworm infection the perineum is involved. The course is subacute and chronic with a tendency to relapse.

Treatment

The source of infection should be treated. Systemic antibiotics are needed to control the infection. Oral corticosteroids are often needed. Treatment should be prolonged as relapses are common.

PHOTOSENSITIVE ECZEMA

This is generally seen in middle aged or older patients, in whom photosensitivity develops after many years. Histology is consistent with chronic lichenoid dermatitis. The most common photosensitivity is due to UVA.

Treatment

The identification and withdrawal of the photoactive agent is the most important factor. Topical steroids are helpful in those who are mildly affected. Severely affected persons may require a course of systemic steroids. Patients with chronic actinic dermatitis may require azathioprine, PUVA or cyclosporin. Broad-spectrum sunscreens, wearing of tightly woven cotton clothing, and a hat with broad brim must be recommended for such patients.

ENDOGENOUS ECZEMA

Atopic Dermatitis

Atopic dermatitis is a chronic inflammatory skin disease, affecting about 10–20% of infants and 1–3% of adults globally. The incidence is increasing dramatically. The reason is not clear; it may be due to the reduced exposure to infections, thereby preventing the normal immunological maturation. Early infection may lower the incidence of allergy by boosting the production of y-interferon.

The word atopy was coined by Coca in 1923, it means "out of place", or different. It is often associated with asthma, hay fever and urticaria. The predisposition to these diseases is called atopic diathesis. Atopic dermatitis is often the first clinical manifestation of atopic disease.

Atopic dermatitis is characterised by intense itching, dry skin, inflammation, exudation, and lichenification in chronic cases. The dry skin is mainly due to increased transepidermal water loss.

Pathogenesis

The exact cause of AD is unknown. There is evidence that a combination of factors are responsible for the development of AD. The disease seems to be a result of genetic susceptibility, epidermal barrier dysfunction and immune dysfunction.

Heredity

A family history is obtained in 70% of patients. Atopic parents do not in all cases have atopic children; this excludes a simple autosomal dominant inheritance. The inheritance may be polygenic, influenced by environmental factors. There is no constant influence of human leukocyte antigen (HLA) system in AD.

The Inherited Barrier Defect

Inflammation in AD results primarily from inherited abnormalities in the skin, the skin "barrier defect". Defects are found in filaggrin, fatty acid metabolism and stratum corneum chymotryptic enzymes.

Filaggrin. An inherited abnormality in filaggrin expression is now considered as a primary cause of disordered barrier function. The gene for filaggrin is present on chromosome 1. This gene was first identified in ichthyosis vulgaris. The loss of filaggrin results in:

- Corneocyte deformation, which disrupts the organisation of extracellular lipid.
- An increase in the skin pH encourages serine proteases activity. These are enzymes that digest lipid processing enzymes and proteins that hold epidermal cells together. Serine proteases also activate IL 2, which promotes inflammation.
- A reduction in natural moisturising factors which include metabolites of profilaggrin.

Abnormalities in the essential fatty acid metabolism. Abnormalities are found in the arachidonic acid metabolism and the release of mediators from it. There are decreased amounts of ceramides in both the lesional and nonlesional skin of AD. There is decreased amount of lipids in the intercellular spaces, decrease in the hydrolysis of sphingomyelin. Metabolites of linoleic acid are decreased. Evening primrose oil which contains linoleic acid is used in the treatment of AD. Topical treatment with primrose oil is not effective, as this does not penetrate the skin.

Stratum corneum chymotryptic enzyme (SCCE). There is a genetic predis-position in patients of AD to synthesise elevated levels of SCCE; this results in early degradation of corneodesmosomes, thereby damaging the epidermal barrier.

Loss of barrier function leads to increased water loss, irritants and allergens can easily penetrate the skin.

The Immune System

Immunoglobulin E levels: Increased levels of immunoglobulin E (IgE) are found in a large number of patients of AD. These are highest in patients with asthma and hay fever. Its level corresponds to the severity of AD. It may remain elevated or decrease in patients with remission. However, not all patients of AD have elevated levels of IgE. Some patients with agammaglobulinemia have AD. Patients of AD may be IgE-dependent or IgE-independent.

Increased levels of IgE are found in patients allergic to food and other allergens, they are also found in patients harbouring *Staphylococcus (S.) aureus*.

It has been postulated that AD should be subdivided into two broad categories. In the first category, allergy plays a role in provoking pruritus by interacting with IgE on the cell surface of the mast cells and macrophages. The second category might be independent of allergens; these patients have low levels of IgE and are nonallergic. Both groups are characterised by intrinsic skin hypersensitivity, resulting in a lowered itch threshold to mechanical or chemical stimulus.

T cells: The immune system develops in the 6th month of life. There is generally an equilibrium in the two main types of T helper cells, Th1 and Th2. In AD there is often an imbalance with far more Th2 cells and their associated chemical messengers.

Patients with AD have diminished cell-mediated immunity as shown by the increased incidence of viral, bacterial and fungal infections. Atopic dermatitis is associated with impaired function of Th2 cells, in response to environmental and bacterial stimuli. Th2 cells secreting IL4 are found in early lesions of AD, and a mixed Th1 and Th2 cells dominance in chronic cases of AD producing IFN-γ.

Mucosal IgA deficiency: According to this hypothesis there is a transient decrease in mucosal IgA during the first few months of life. The absence of IgA in the intestinal mucosa and lumen allows allergens in the food to enter the blood stream; these then stimulate IgE antibodies and other immune mechanisms. In normal infants, intestinal IgA neutralises these antigens. The mechanism by which eczema is produced is unknown. It has been postulated that breast-feeding at this time eliminates the allergens and lowers the incidence of atopy. However, a few cases of AD have occurred inspite of breast-feeding this could be due to allergens in the mother's milk or it may be caused by inhalation allergens.

Keratinocytes: A number of cytokines and chemokines are produced by the keratinocytes of AD patients such as RANTES, GM-CSF and thymic stromal lymphopoietin (TSLP). These promote and maintain skin inflammation.

Allergens and Colonisation with *Staphylococcus*

Allergens in atopic dermatitis: Food as an allergen has received a great deal of attention. Many studies have been carried out with milk, egg and wheat being used as a challenge for producing AD; no positive result has been postulated. So is the case with other allergens, such as house dust mite, pollens and animal dander.

Allergens differ in the different age group in AD as shown by the radioallergosorbent test (RAST). In infants, RAST levels are found against foods usually egg, dairy products and fish. After about a year IgE is directed against house dust mite, animal hair and dander.

Colonisation with Staphylococcus aureas: S. aureas is present in both acute and chronic AD in a large number of patients. Treatment with an appropriate antibiotic has resulted in improvement of the eczema. This suggests that patients with AD may be sensitised not only to common allergens, but also to pathogenic bacteria colonising the skin.

Other Factors Associated with Atopic Dermatitis

Vascular reactions: Disturbances in vascular reactivity have been well-documented in AD. The best-known abnormality is white dermographism; this is development of a white line on the skin instead of a red response as normally seen in the triple response of Lewis. Nicotinic acid esters produce erythema in normal skin; a blanching reaction is seen in patients of AD. Intracutaneous injection of cholinergic agents produces blanching around the wheal instead of a normal red reaction.

Atopic individuals are prone to cold, they often have periocular pallor (headlight sign), perinasal and even generalised pallor.

The increased sensitivity of vascular smooth muscles to α-adrenergic stimulation, and increased sensitivity of sweat glands and basophils to cholinergic stimulation are consistent with impaired β-adrenergic stimulation.

Studies have shown that the skin of AD has failed to show inhibition of DNA synthesis following exposure to β-adrenergic agonists. Blood leukocytes of patients with AD show decreased cyclic adenosine monophosphate (AMP) production following stimulation of with β-agonists, histamine and prostaglandin. This could be due to a deficit in multiple receptors or decrease in the binding affinity of β-agonists. Antibodies against β-adrenergic receptors have been detected in the sera of some patients with AD.

Sebum production: There is a deficiency of lipids in the sebum (wax esters and squalene); which contributes to the dryness of skin.

Phosphodiesterase and phospholipase C-activation: In AD both the second messenger systems of the cell are affected, resulting in the alteration of both cyclic AMP and inositol triphosphate. Decrease in the levels of cAMP, leads to increased release of histamine from the mast cells.

Neuropeptides: Neuropeptides mediate vasodilatation, oedema, axon reflex flare, sweat gland secretion, itch, pain and ability to regulate T-cell activation. The neuropeptides could play a significant role in the vascular changes, leukocyte infiltration and itch of AD. Some of the neuropeptides are substance P, calcitonin, gene-related peptides, somatostatin, and vasoactive intestinal polypeptides. In AD, there are increased amounts of vasoactive polypeptides and reduced amounts of substance P.

Changes in leukocytes other than lymphocytes: Eosinophils are increased and the number correlates to the disease severity. Basophils show increased release of histamine. Langerhans cells show increased expression of IgE receptors.

Clinical Features

Atopic eczema is a chronic pruritic skin disease with a characteristic clinical picture and course. Both sexes are equally affected; the patients are often highly-strung, tense individuals. Atopic eczema has a natural course that is divided into three distinct stages:

- Infantile phase
- Childhood phase
- Adult phase

Personality traits: A characteristic personality is seen in most cases of AD. Many patients have a suppressed feeling of resentment; they are sensitive, easily depressed, tense, intolerant and overactive. Aggressive and hypochondriac nature is often seen, the cause of this personality is unknown.

Clinical Features

Infantile phase: The skin lesions are never present at birth; they develop between 4 and 6 months of age. Scalp, face and the trunk are commonly affected (Fig. 6). The infant is irritable, restless and wakeful at night due to severe pruritus. Dietary allergens particularly cows milk may play a part in provoking eczema, such patients should be breastfed for at least 3 months to reduce the risk of eczema. This eczema may be triggered by teething, upper respiratory tract infections, etc. In about 40% of the cases, AD clears spontaneously by the age of 2–5 years.

Childhood phase: The disease tends to be localised to the flexural aspect of the elbows, knees, wrists, ankles and the neck (Fig. 7). Hand lesions may be exudative; a prurigo-like eruption is common on the extensor aspect of the limbs in tropical races. Prominent infraorbital folds are common (Dennie-Morgans fold); these give a weary and prematurely aged appearance to the child. Firm stroking of erythematous skin produces a white line possibly due to vasoconstriction; this is known as white dermographism. Thinning of the lateral part of the eyebrows (Hertoghe's sign) is frequently present due to continued rubbing. The atopic patients tend to have a generalized dry skin. A mild degree of ichthyosis and keratosis pilaris may also be present. In childhood, allergens provoking eczema are found in dust, pollen and animal dander; rather than food as seen in the infantile phase. In most cases the eczema remits by the age of 10 years.

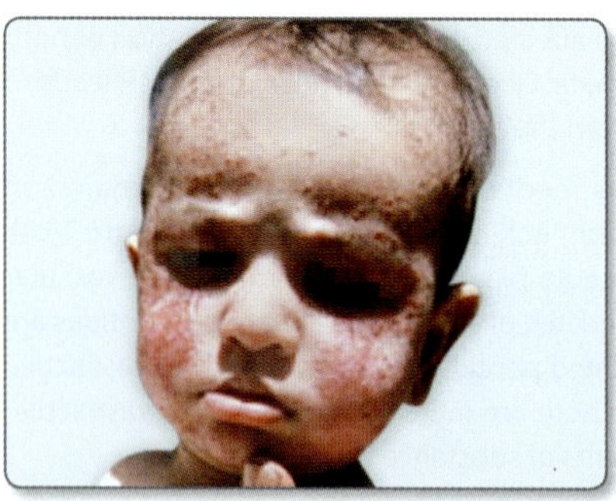

Fig. 6: Atopic dermatitis

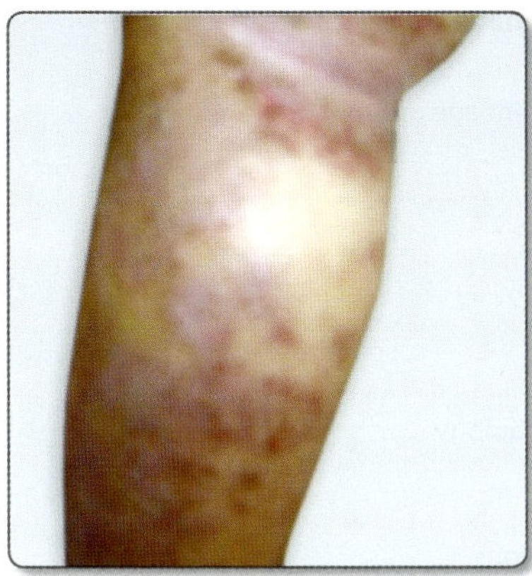

Fig. 7: Atopic dermatitis—flexural involvement

Adult phase: This shows a persistence of the flexural involvement. The lesions are hyperpigmented, pruritus is severe, and excoriations and lichenification are common. As the disease tends to disappear, the eruption may retreat to one or more patches on the hands, wrist and ankles. In severe cases, large areas of the face and trunk are involved with diffuse itchy plaques. Adults are more liable to develop erythroderma.

Kaposi's varicelliform eruption: This is a dramatic and uncommon complication of atopic dermatitis. If patients of AD develop herpes simplex, a widespread dermatitis may occur with umbilicated vesicles (eczema herpeticum), similar reactions may be seen after threats of bioterrorism with smallpox and other vaccinations (eczema vaccinatum), and following coxsackie infection (eczema coxsackium).

Factors Aggravating Atopic Dermatitis

- Excessive washing of the skin without using lubricants
- Irritants such as wool, synthetic fibres, mineral oil, sand, etc.
- Airborne allergens, such as animal dander, smoke, tobacco and house dust mite
- Secondary infections
- Increased perspiration.

Physical Findings in Atopic Dermatitis

- Dry skin
- Pruritus
- Characteristic morphology in the different age groups
- Accentuation of palmar creases
- Keratosis pilaris
- Dennie-Morgan fold
- Pityriasis alba
- Increased susceptibility to infections
- Pallor around the nose, mouth and eyes
- Early onset of posterior subcapsular cataract
- White dermographism
- Keratoconus
- Scaling scalp.

Major Diagnostic Criteria (Must have three)

- Pruritus
- Typical morphology in the different age groups
- Family history of atopy
- Chronic relapsing dermatitis

Minor Diagnostic Criteria

- Related to subclinical eczema
- Related to dry skin
- Related extra skin folds
- Related to ophthalmological pathology
- Raised serum IgE
- White dermographism
- Increased susceptibility to infections
- Susceptibility to skin infections

Cause of Pruritus in Atopic Dermatitis

- Increased transepidermal water loss (TEWL)
- Increased levels of histamine and prostaglandins
- Low threshold for pruritus
- Decreases production of lipids in sebum
- Scratching aggravates the itch-scratch cycle
- Stress

Associations of Atopic Dermatitis

Immunodeficiency disorders

- Wiskott-Aldrich syndrome
- Ataxa telangiectasia
- Agammaglobulinemia
- Ichthyosis vulgaris
- Netherton's syndrome

Metabolic/Miscellaneous disorders

- Phenylketonuria
- Hurler's syndrome
- Cystic fibrosis
- Coeliac disease
- Anhidrotic ectodermal dysplasia
- Nephrotic syndrome.

Differential Diagnosis

Atopic dermatitis is easy to diagnose because of its typical morphology, excessive pruritus and family history. It should be differentiated from seborrheic dermatitis especially in infants. In adults AD should be differentiated from lesions that involve the flexures, such as fungal infections, flexural psoriasis, candidiasis, intertrigo, seborrhoeic dermatitis and clothing dermatitis.

Complications

There is a tendency to develop bacterial and viral infections. The eczema may be secondarily infected. Children have a slightly higher incidence of viral warts and molluscum contagiosum. Kaposi's varicelliform eruption is a serious complication secondary to vaccinia virus or herpes infection. Patients with AD are more prone to develop cataract and keratoconus.

Treatment

General principles: There is yet no definite cure for AD. The goal of treatment is to reduce inflammation, itching, to help in skin hydration, prevent or reduce recurrences and to provide long-term management by preventing exacerbations.

General Guidelines for Treatment are as follows:

Atopics should avoid extremes of heat and cold. Xerotic skin tends to be worse in winter; it should be hydrated, by avoiding soaps and using hydrophilic creams and lotions. Moisturisers reduce dryness by trapping in moisture.

The patient should not wear wool, as its fibres are irritating. Stress should be minimised, it is an important factor in causing exacerbations of AD, an appropriate antibiotic should be prescribed, as Staphylococcus is often a secondary invader. The nails should be kept short to avoid scratching the skin. There should be a close cooperation between the doctor, patient and the family members.

Reduction of triggering factors: Following triggering factors need to be reduced.

Irritants: Soaps and detergents can irritate the skin. A dispersible cream can be used as a soap substitute to clean the skin. Avoid hot baths. Avoid occlusive clothing and direct contact with wool. Try to avoid extremes of heat and cold. Avoid activities causing increased sweating.

Food: In children where food appears to be a precipitating factor substitutes can be used. Wheat can be substituted with oats, rice, barley, corn, soya bean and rye. Soya bean emulsions can substitute cow's milk. Other dietary elements like seafood, dairy products, eggs may have to be avoided if necessary.

In cases where food does not appear to be a factor in the pathogenesis of AD restricted diets should be discouraged.

Airborne allergens: Airborne allergens like house dust mite, dander and pollens are aggravating factors and should be avoided by regular hovering and dusting, pets should be discouraged. Spray the entire house and soft furniture with methoprene spray. House dust mite cannot live at altitudes above 1,500 m, explaining remissions during vacations in high altitudes. Carpets should be removed from the house, because they serve as a reservoir for house dust mite and animal dander.

Vaccination/Drugs: As most vaccines contain egg protein, so caution should be taken in vaccination and it should be supervised in an environment where resuscitation facilities are available. Care should be taken while giving penicillin and sera.

Herpes simplex infection: Avoid contact with patients infected with active cold sores, as it can lead to eczema herpeticum.

Stress: The doctors should explain the condition to the patient and the family. They should show empathy to their patients. Try and eliminate any stressful situation. Psychological counselling may be required in some cases.

Prevent scratching: Avoid scratching as it prolongs and complicates the disease.

Active treatment:

- Topical steroids are the mainstay of treatment
- Low potency steroids should be used on the face and groins
- Medium potency steroids should be used on the body and extremities
- Strong steroids are used in severely affected areas
- Oral corticosteroids have a definite role in the management of severe exacerbation of AD.

Antihistamines: These help in controlling the itching. The commonly used drugs are hydroxyzine and diphenhydramine.

Antibiotics: S. aureus has long been known to be a frequent resident of both normal and involved skin in AD; an appropriate antibiotic should be prescribed when needed.

Immunomodulators: Pimecrolimus and tacrolimus inhibit inflammatory cytokine transcription in activated T-cells and other inflammatory cells through inhibition of calcineurin.

Tacrolimus ointment 0.03% in a bid application is used in children from 2 to 15 years of age. Tacrolimus ointment 0.1% is used in adults and children over 15 years. Side effects are burning and itching. These immunomodulators are safe in long-term use and do not have the side effects seen in topical steroids.

Pimecrolimus 1% cream can be used in infants, children and adults. Low dose cyclosporin therapy is said to be effective in the treatment of severe refractory AD. The dose recommended is 2–5 mg/kg of body weight/day

Phototherapy: Narrow band UVB is very helpful in chronic cases of AD. UVA 1 is helpful in acute flares of the disease.

Other modalities: In adults, evening primrose oil is said to reduce itching and scaling. This contains gamma linolenic acid; it can also be given to children in a reduced dose. The other drugs that can be tried in resistant cases of AD are papaverine, sodium chromoglycate, psoralens followed by UVA therapy.

Desensitisation plays a limited role in AD; it is more effective in asthma and allergic rhinitis.

Atopics have an imbalance of T cell function and poor production of gamma interferon. Daily injections of interferon 50 μg/m^2/day for 12 weeks have shown some benefit. Thymopentin an extract of thymic hormone has shown some improvement in patients of AD.

Sedatives/Psychotherapy/Hypnosis. These can be helpful in certain cases.

Mast cell stabilisers like oral sodium cromoglycate in high doses are helpful in some patients. Its topical use has been found helpful in children.

The use of probiotics, such as *Lactobacillus fermentum,* in AD is in the experimental phase, some studies have shown promising results. These are given to mothers who are predisposed of having an atopic child during pregnancy and for 6 months after birth of the child.

Desensitisation: It has a very limited role in the management of AD even when an allergic factor has been fully established clinically. It may be effective in house dust mite allergy.

Course and Prognosis

Almost half of the infantile cases clear by the age of 18 months. Many show spontaneous healing by the age of 2–4 years. Generally speaking, extensive and early onset of the rash; worse is the prognosis. Not all patients pass through all the phases; a few may begin in adult life. The eruption usually disappears by the age of 25–30 years. Severe cases persist longer; often flare-ups are related to nervous tension or climatic factors.

The UK Working Party's Diagnostic criterion for Atopic Dermatitis are that the patients should have an itchy skin condition plus three or more of the following: a history of asthma/hay fever, a history of generalised dry skin, onset of rash under two years of age or visible flexural dermatitis.

Robert Willan first described atopic dermatitis in 1808 as a prurigo-like eruption. In 1844 Hebra noted the flexural distribution of the pruritic rash.

SEBORRHOEIC DERMATITIS

This is a common eczema, areas rich in sebaceous glands or the intertriginous areas are most affected. The greatest incidence of seborrhoeic dermatitis is between adolescence and middle age. It occurs in infancy, but is rare in children and old age. In developing countries, it is easily infected. The eruption may be triggered by upper respiratory tract infections and is easily irritated by external agents. Obesity, debilitating diseases, a diet rich in carbohydrates and fats are predisposing factors. Seborrhoeic dermatitis is common in patients with acne, rosacea and psoriasis.

Aetiology

Many hypotheses have been put forward, but the exact cause of seborrhoeic dermatitis is still not known. It is a dermatitis that affects areas rich in sebaceous glands, but hypersecretion of the sebum is not always present. A hormonal influence could be postulated, as the disease is not seen before puberty. The two main factors responsible for seborrhoeic dermatitis are: increase in epidermal lipids and colonisation by *Malassezia (M.) furfur*, at least transiently in adults. In infants colonisation by *Candida albicans* is often found. Immune responses also play a role; the disease tends to be more severe in AIDS. Some authors view an overlap of seborrhoeic dermatitis with psoriasis, and consider it may be a mild form of the disorder. The term sebopsoriasis is sometimes used for this overlapping condition.

Presence of lipophilic, pleomorphic fungus, *M. furfur* in the scalp is seen in most cases, the use of ketoconazole cream and shampoo is often effective. Recently *M. restricta* and *M. globosa* have also been found.

It is worse in conditions that increase perspiration. Emotional stress, neuroleptic drugs, such as haloperidol that may induce parkinsonism, also cause seborrhoeic dermatitis.

Seborrhoeic dermatitis may be associated with or accentuated by several internal diseases such as diabetes mellitus, sprue, malabsorption, and epilepsy. Reaction to arsenic and gold can also produce seborrhoeic dermatitis. Parkinsonism is often associated with severe seborrhoeic dermatitis, involving the face and the scalp with waxy profuse scaling and little erythema. In AIDS seborrhoeic dermatitis may be an early marker of the disease in the risk population. It may have an abrupt onset and is often severe.

Seborrhoeic dermatitis is also seen in patients with facial palsy, and in patients with paralysis of the trunk. This could be due to increased pool of sebum in the immobile areas.

There is an increased incidence of bacterial and viral infections in seborrhoeic dermatitis. Seborrhoeic dermatitis is one of the established manifestations of HIV infection.

Drugs that cause seborrheic dermatitis like infections are methyldopa, cimetidine, chlorpromazine and PUVA therapy.

Low temperature and low humidity are known to worsen seborrhoeic dermatitis.

Seborrhoeic dermatitis in infancy may have a different pathogenesis. It may be associated with acrodermatitis enteropathica and improves with therapy. In adults, zinc deficiency plays no role in the pathogenesis of seborrhoeic dermatitis. Biotin deficiency, whether secondary to holocarboxylase deficiency or a biotinase deficiency, and abnormal metabolism of essential fatty acids have been proposed as probable mechanism for the aetiology of seborrhoeic dermatitis in infants.

Clinical Features

The sites mainly affected by seborrhoeic dermatitis are the scalp, face, trunk and the intertriginous areas.

Scalp

The scalp is almost always affected; there is redness and diffuse scaling of the scalp, which may be mild or severe. The mild form is known as pityriasis capitis (dandruff). This is manifested by dry flaky branny desquamation with fine powdery scale, beginning in small patches and rapidly involving the entire scalp. The oily type (pityriasis steatoides) is accompanied by erythema and an accumulation of thick greasy scales, the disease may spread to the upper border of the forehead as red scaly band with festooned borders called "corona seborrhoeica".

Face

On the face, there is involvement of the supraorbital margin, edges of the eyelid, glabella, ears, cheeks and the nasolabial folds. Persistent erythema of the ala-malar angle is called dyssebacea; it is almost specific for seborrhoeic dermatitis (Fig. 8).

Trunk

There are three main patterns of the rash that may occur in any combination. The lesions start with follicular and perifollicular redness, these spread until

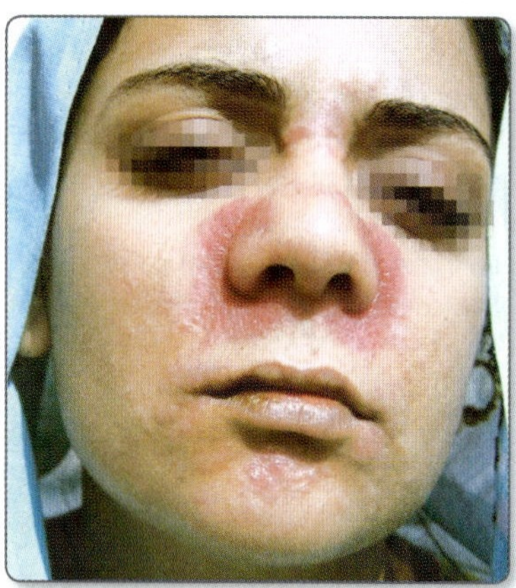

Fig. 8: Seborrhoeic dermatitis

they form clearly outlined circinate lesions (petaloid type). In the pityriasiform type, there are generalised erythemato-squamous lesions, similar to but more extensive than pityriasiform rosea. In some patients, the lesions may be psoriasiform.

On the trunk, lesions are commonly seen on the areola of the breast, inframammary folds, presternal area, interscapular region, umbilicus, groin and gluteal folds. The lesions may be generalised or localised to one area. Seborrhoeic dermatitis may progress to exfoliative dermatitis. The lesions are characterised by a yellowish colour, mild to severe erythema, thick oily scales and crusts.

Body folds

The body folds (axillae, groins, submammary areas) are affected particularly in the middle aged and the elderly. Obese women are chiefly affected and the condition should be differentiated from candida and fungal infections. The body folds are bright-red, moist and macerated, the edge is ill-defined and it is often very itchy. There is a rare follicular form with tiny perifollicular pustules. Swabs for bacteria and candida should exclude secondary infection of the intertriginous areas; scrapings should be examined for fungus.

Seborrhoeic Dermatitis in Infants

In infants pronounced crusting and oozing of the scalp (cradle cap), appears shortly after birth, it may be the sole manifestation of the disease or seborrhoeic dermatitis may affect the body folds, napkin area, buttocks and the neck. Eczema in the napkin area is due to the irritant effect of urine and faeces on the skin. The pronounced scaly rash in the napkin area is termed psoriasiform. Secondary infection of the napkin area is very common.

Erythroderma Desquamatum (Leiner's Disease)

This is a severe form of seborrhoeic dermatitis seen in nursing infants. There is generalised exfoliative dermatitis, the infants are in poor general condition, there is severe diarrhoea, wasting and intercurrent infections. It may be associated with the dysfunction of the fifth component of the complement, with decreased opsonin activity. The disease appears to have an autosomal dominant inheritance. The disease may be ameliorated by the infusion of fresh frozen plasma.

Differential Diagnosis

This varies from site to site. On the scalp, it should be differentiated from psoriasis, impetigo, dermatophyte/ringworm infection and pediculosis. In pediculosis nits are seen, pruritus is common; often, the cervical lymph nodes are enlarged due to secondary infection. On the face, in infants seborrhoeic dermatitis should be differentiated from AD, this is seen at the age of 3 months, the nasolabial folds, eyebrows and eyelids are not involved, there is a positive family history and the condition is very itchy. The other facial conditions from which seborrhoeic dermatitis should be differentiated are rosacea, CD and systemic lupus erythematosus. In the intertriginous areas inverse psoriasis, candidiasis and dermatophyte infections should be differentiated. On the trunk, the lesions should be differentiated from pityriasis rosea, psoriasis and tinea corporis.

Table 2 shows the difference between infantile AD and infantile seborrhoeic dermatitis

Table 2: Difference between infantile atopic dermatitis and infantile seborrhoeic dermatitis

Infantile atopic dermatitis	*Infantile seborhoeic dermatitis*
• Begins three months after birth • Markedly pruritic • Presents as erythema, papules and vesicles • Prominent on the cheeks and extensor surfaces of the limbs	• Begins shortly after birth • Asymptomatic • Presents as greasy scales on an erythematous base • Prominent on the scalp, cheeks, eyebrows, nasolabial folds and proximal flexures

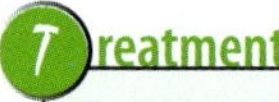

Treatment

Treatment of the Skin

Application of topical antipityrosporal agents, such as clotrimazole, itraconazole, miconazole are commonly prescribed. These are often prescribed with low potency corticosteroids for the trunk, and 1% hydrocortisone for the face and flexures. If there is no response then 5% lithium succinate cream, metronidazole 1% gel have shown a significant improvement of seborrhoeic dermatitis when used against a placebo.

In refractory cases topical immunomodulators such as tacrolimus or pimecrolimus can be used. The anti-inflammatory properties of vitamin D3 analogues (calcipotriol) are also useful in selected cases.

Unresponsive cases should be treated with oral itraconazole 100 mg daily for 21 days, followed by 100 mg for 2 days a month for 9–11 months.

Prednisolone 30 mg daily is helpful in erythroderma due to seborrhoeic dermatitis. Narrow band UVB has also been used successfully in erythrodermic form of seborrhoeic dermatitis. Isotretinoin is also helpful.

Treatment of the Scalp

The scalp seborrhoeic dermatitis is helped by topical antipityrosporal creams/gel and shampoos. Antifungal ketoconazole shampoo is the most widely used shampoo; it eradicates the fungus Malassezia furfur. Other shampoos used are ciclopirox, zinc pyrithione and selenium sulphide. These should alternate with a regular shampoo. Frequent shampooing should be encouraged. Thick greasy-yellowish scales have a high incidence of the fungus. Corticosteroid gels can also be used with antipityrosporal agents.

If there is increased crusting of the scalp then application of 2% sulphur and 2% salicylic acid ointment applied overnight is helpful. Resistant cases may require 5% sulphur, 5% salicylic acid and 30% coconut oil in emulsifying ointment. This should be applied 2–3 times a week.

Treatment of resistant or unresponsive cases is similar to that described above with oral intraconazole.

Treatment in Children

Management of mild cradle cap is simple by rinsing the scalp with warm olive oil, which is left for few minutes, and the area is then combed gently, scales are easily removed. The scalp later is washed with mild shampoo.

In children the cradle cap is best treated with 1% sulphur and 1% salicylic acid ointment. It should be applied overnight and the scalp is shampooed the next day. Salicylic acid ointment should not be applied to newborns and infants. Difficult cases can be treated by itraconazole cream.

Psoriasiform diaper dermatitis is treated with topical 1% hydrocortisone and an antifungal ointment twice a day. Secondary infection with candida is often present which should be appropriately treated. A barrier ointment should be applied after each diaper change.

Leiner's disease: Hospitalisation is necessary with correction of fluid and electrolyte balance. These patients respond to antibiotics and infusions of fresh frozen plasma or whole blood.

Course and Prognosis

Seborrhoeic eczema in infants has a very good prognosis. In most children the disease clears by the age of 18 months. It does not predispose to adult seborrhoeic eczema. Seborrhoeic eczema in adults runs a very chronic course, often persisting indefinitely. There are periods of relapses and remissions. Different areas may be affected at different times.

NUMMULAR ECZEMA

Nummular eczema (Discoid eczema) presents with characteristic round or nummular lesions distributed commonly on the extensor surface of the extremities, especially on the hands and forearms. The trunk is also involved in some cases. The lesions are sharply demarcated.

Aetiology

In most cases, the cause is unknown. Infection, trauma, emotional stress, drugs, xerosis have been stressed as possible aetiological factors. Drugs such as isoniazid, aminosalicyclic acid, gold, methyldopa have also been implicated as a cause for nummular eczema. It is often associated with dry skin. Nummular eczema occurs in all age groups, peak incidence is between the ages of 55 and 65 years; another peak is seen at the age of 15–25 years. It is uncommon in children.

The cutaneous sensory nerves contain increased amount of substance P, vasoactive polypeptide, and calcitonin gene-related peptide. These vasoactive neuropeptides act as a potential mechanism for mast cell degranulation.

Clinical Features

Acute lesions of nummular eczema are coin-shaped, studded with vesicles on an erythematous base. As the disease progresses, the lesions become less vesicular and more scaly, often with a central clearing, forming ring-shaped annular lesions. Finally the plaque fades, leaving dry scaly patches. The eruption is worse during the winter months.

Discoid eczema recurs at intervals, many cases are worse in winter. Some cases of discoid eczema are dry from the beginning; they present as dry scaly round patches with scattered microvesicles on an erythematous base. Itching is minimal in this form of eczema and is more resistant to treatment (Figs 9A and B).

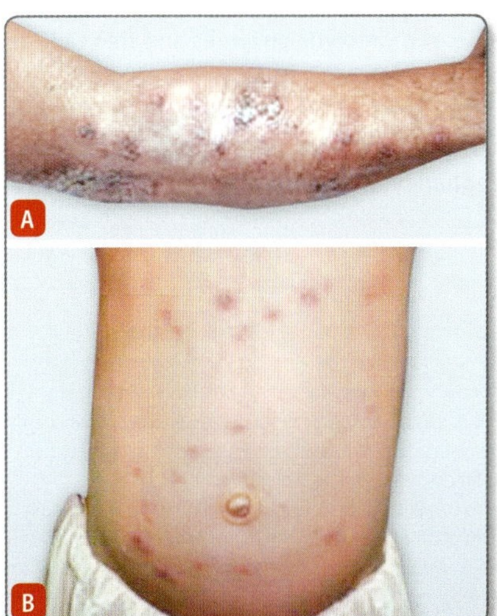

Figs 9A and B: Discoid eczema

Differential Diagnosis

The disease should be differentiated from ringworm infection, especially when the eczema clears from the centre. The edge is broader and vesicular in eczema, scraping should be done in doubtful cases. The other annular lesion which should be considered in the differential diagnosis is annular psoriasis. Contact dermatitis should also be differentiated, when the lesions are few and of an unusual configuration.

The histological features are a cross between psoriasis and eczematous dermatitis. The epidermis is regularly acanthotic. Focal collections of neutrophils are seen within the overlying parakeratotic scale. In addition spongiosis is found in the epidermis.

Treatment

Topical steroids are the mainstay of treatment. A combination of tar and corticosteroids is effective in long-term management. Skin should be kept hydrated. As the condition is often persistent in winter, bathing oils and emollients should be applied frequently. Irritants should be avoided as in other forms of eczema. Pruritus can be treated with H1 antihistamines.

Other anti-inflammatory agents such as tacrolimus and pimecrolimus are also effective.

If there is no response a course of systemic antibiotics such as penicillinase-resistant penicillin or cephalosporins should be tried.

HYPOSTATIC ECZEMA

Hypostatic eczema (Varicose eczema) occurs on the lower legs because of underlying insufficient venous drainage. It is common in middle-aged women. Pregnancy, obesity and thrombophlebitis are predisposing factors.

Aetiology

Venous insufficiency leads to increased hydrostatic pressure in the leg veins, which is transmitted to the capillaries in the lower leg skin. This distends the local capillary bed and widens the capillary pores allowing the fibrinogen to leak out forming a fibrin coating around the capillary. This fibrin forms a barrier to diffusion of oxygen and nutrients leading to decreased vitality of the skin making it more damage prone. In addition the sequestration of white blood cells in the venules leads to release of proteolytic enzymes and free radicals leading to tissue damage and inflammation.

The cause of varicose ulcer is not clear, an inherited tendency may play a part, long periods of standing, any condition causing prolonged intra-abdominal pressure such as pregnancy and thrombophlebitis may cause incompetence of the veins.

Clinical Features

Onset is gradual with oedema at the end of the day. Later brown pigmentation develops on the inner aspect of the ankle and gradually extends to the rest of the leg. Varicose veins are often present, chronic pruritic dermatitis develops with periods of exacerbations; the dermatitis may be weepy or dry, scaly or lichenified. The pigmentation is due to melanin and hemosiderin. Leakage of fibrinogen is believed to eventually coat the capillaries with a layer of fibrin that inhibits the passage of oxygen and thus causes anoxia; this sets the stage for dermatitis and ulceration.

Secondary bacterial infection may lead to cellulitis and lymphangitis. Irritation of the eczematous patches may trigger an autoeczematous eruption of the upper extremities and the trunk. Venous ulcers, with sharp borders surrounded by inflamed skin are a common and persistent complication. It often occurs on the inner side of the lower leg (Fig. 10).

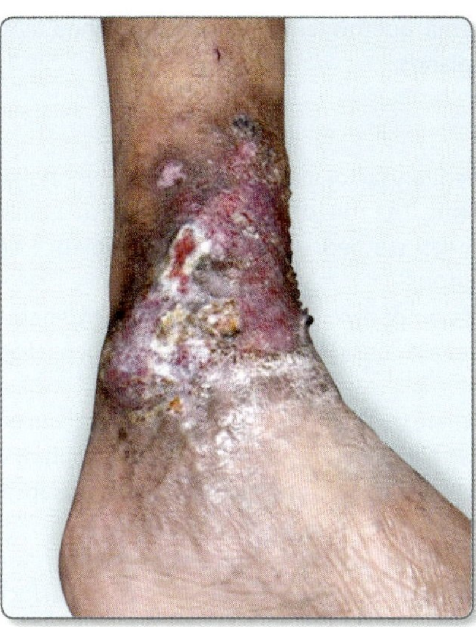

Fig. 10: Hypostatic eczema

Complications

Ulcers are the most common complication of hypostatic eczema. The thin skin due to the poor blood flow and high back pressure is easily damaged, which results in the formation of an ulcer. This ulcer heals slowly. The other complications include allergic and irritant CD, often due to local medicaments. Varicose eczema of long duration may become generalised.

Treatment

The only effective way of treating venous hypertension is by external compression of the leg by bandaging or support stockings. This compresses the superficial veins so that the blood can flow to the deeper veins. The patient should use their calf muscles, so they need to be mobile and walking. When sitting, the feet should be raised on a stool and dorsiflexed frequently.

Weak topical steroids should be applied twice daily, once before applying the bandage or stocking and once before going to bed. Any potent sensitiser should be avoided; local antiseptics are preferable to topical antibiotics for secondary infection.

Course and Prognosis

The prognosis is poor unless the cause of hypostasis is removed. Varicose ulcers require a cooperative and motivated patient if permanent healing is to be acquired.

POMPHOLYX

Pompholyx (Vesicular palmoplantar eczema) is a chronic relapsing vesicular eruption of unknown cause, which mainly affects the palms (cheiropompholyx) and at times the soles (podopompholyx). Pompholyx is common in young adults; it is rare in children and old age. Both sexes are equally affected. Emotional stress is a common predisposing factor. Chronic pompholyx characterised by small vesicles on the inner aspect of the fingers, it was previously called dyshidrotic eczema, but this term should be abolished, as it has no relationship to the sweat glands.

Aetiology

The exact cause is unknown. A hereditary factor may be involved as pompholyx has occurred in monozygotic twins. The role of atopy is difficult to assess because not many cases have been studied; although the prevalence of pompholyx is slightly higher in atopics.

Contact dermatitis may cause pompholyx; soluble oils, paraphenylenediamine, dichromates, and perfumes are considered as potential allergens that cause pompholyx.

Fungal infections found elsewhere on the body could produce eczema of the palms (id reaction); this is known as pompholyx dermatophytid. Pompholyx disappears when the fungal infection is treated and reappears with a relapse of the infection.

In some cases, an allergic reaction to contact dermatitis of the foot can produce palmar pompholyx as a sympathetic eruption. Similarly, bacterial foci can also produce palmar pompholyx.

Pompholyx has also been related to stress; it may follow a drug eruption, e.g. aspirin, oral contraceptives.

Clinical Features

In acute pompholyx there is an explosive outbreak of deep seated, sago like vesicles on the palms, the lateral aspect of the fingers and sometimes the soles (Fig. 11). The distribution is bilateral and symmetrical. Vesicles appear in crops, which last for a few days, these either rupture or dry forming a crust that slowly desquamates. Each attack lasts for a few weeks, recurrences are common, secondary infection and lymphangitis are common in the tropics. Larger blisters should be drained to avoid discomfort, but should not be unroofed. Sometimes there is discomfort and itching before the eruption of blisters. The blisters heal in 2–3 week; there is a tendency to recur. Secondary bacterial infection should be avoided; it can lead to cellulitis and lymphangitis.

Repeated attacks present as small vesicles on the lateral aspect of the fingers, palms and soles. As the condition becomes more chronic the eczema becomes hyperkeratotic, and fissured, this is usually on the centre of the palms. Spongiosis is manifest on histology.

After recurrent attacks the nails may become dystrophic, they are irregular with transverse ridging, pitting, thickening and discolouration. In some cases, it may be the presenting complaint.

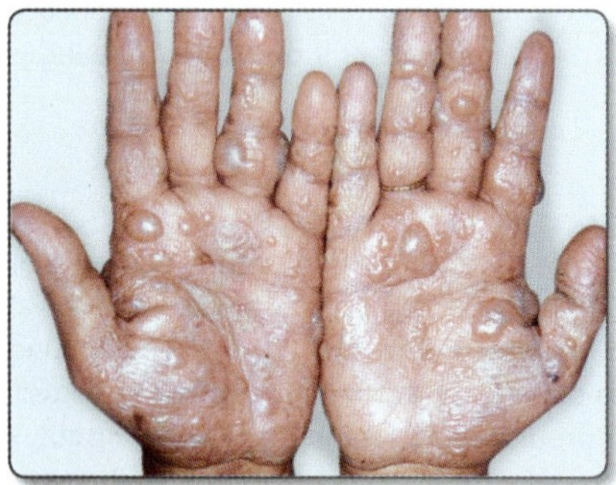

Fig. 11: Pompholyx

Differential Diagnosis

The vesicles should not be confused with acute fungal infections or the pustules of psoriasis. The chronic stage resembles irritant CD, atopic eczema, psoriasis or fungal infections. Fungal infection and psoriasis are less itchy, psoriasis is found in other parts of the body. Fungal scrapings exclude dermatophyte infections. Contact allergic dermatitis usually involves the back of the hand. Chronic irritant dermatitis usually presents as thickening and hyperkeratosis of the palms with fissuring.

Treatment

Any obvious cause of eruption should be eliminated. Acute pompholyx should be treated by soaking the hands and feet in potassium permanganate solution (1:5,000) three to four times a day, followed by the application of high potency corticosteroids. A sterile syringe should aspirate large bullae. Systemic corticosteroids are required in severe cases. Antihistamines are given for pruritus.

Tacrolimus and pimecrolimus are also effective. The more chronic forms of pompholyx are difficult to treat. Intralesional corticosteroids, retinoids or keratolytics may provide benefit. Severe cases and those resistant to therapy can be treated by UVB, PUVA, cyclosporin, methotrexate or mycophenolate mofetil.

Course and Prognosis

Pompholyx is a very variable condition. Its severity ranges from an isolated attack every few years to months of recurrent attacks or a severe persistent incapacitating condition. In some patients it is lifelong.

LICHEN SIMPLEX CHRONICUS

The term lichen simplex is used when there is no preceding skin disorder and the skin is lichenified due to scratching. Lichenification can also be secondary to other dermatoses, such as atopic eczema, chronic fungal infections, etc.

Clinical Features

Lichen simplex chronicus (LSC) usually develops at a localised site such as the ankles or nape of the neck, which is easy to reach and can be scratched without thinking. Itching occurs in paroxysms and the scratching continues until the skin is sore; relief is then obtained until the next paroxysm, which occurs some hours later.

During the early stages, the skin is red and slightly oedematous; the normal markings of the skin are exaggerated. As the disease progresses the redness and oedema subside, the skin becomes thickened, dry and pigmented. Surrounding the central plaque is a zone of lichenified papules. Chronic cases often show hyperpigmented and hypopigmented spots on the lichenified plaque.

Lichen simplex chronicus is rare in children and the elderly, commonly seen between the ages of 30 years and 50 years. It is more frequent in tense and nervous individuals.

Differential Diagnosis

Nummular eczema causes pruritic eczematous plaques, but lichenification is absent. The purple colour of the plaque and the presence of Wickham's striae are characteristic of lichem planus. Lichen amyloidosis on the lower limbs is very itchy, its symmetrical distribution and rippled appearance differentiate it from LSC. Prurigo nodularis is also associated with pruritus, lesions involve comparatively large areas of the body, usually the legs and arms. The lesions are nodular and very itchy.

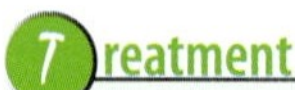

Treatment

This should be aimed to break the itch-scratch-itch cycle. The treatment consists of antihistamines to reduce pruritus, topical steroids to reduce inflammation and tar/salicyclic acid preparations for the antipruritic/keratolytic effect. Occlusive dressings help to prevent scratching and can produce dramatic improvement. In some cases, where lichenification is intense, intralesional injection of steroids is very helpful.

Other therapeutic modalities include doxepin cream, capsaicin cream, PUVA, and narrow band UVB therapy.

Course and Prognosis

Lichen simplex may resolve with treatment, but recurrence at the same place or at a different site is common.

PITYRIASIS ALBA

Pityriasis alba is a nonspecific dermatitis of common occurrence. It was first described by Fox and named by O'Farrell. Erythematous scaly patches are present on the face; this subsides to leave behind areas of hypopigmentation. Hypopigmentation is probably postinflammatory.

Aetiology

The exact aetiology is unknown. It is said to be an eczematous dermatitis, some regard it as a manifestation of AD. Excessive dryness followed by exposure to strong sunlight may be a contributory factor. All races are affected; it is more obvious in the black people.

Histopathology

There is hyperkeratosis, parakeratosis, acanthosis and mild spongiosis. The number of melanocytes is decreased and the size of the melanasomes is small. There is moderate dilatation of the superficial dermal blood vessels and slight oedema of the papillary dermis.

Clinical Features

Over 90% of cases are seen between the ages of 6 and 12 years. The typical lesion is a pink scaly macule with indistinct margins. The erythema fades to a whitish macule with powdery scales. The face particularly the areas around the mouth and malar ridges are commonly involved. The lesions are 0.5–2 cm in diameter, but may be larger. Most cases persist for months. The lesions may sometimes become generalised. The condition is asymptomatic or slightly pruritic (Fig. 12).

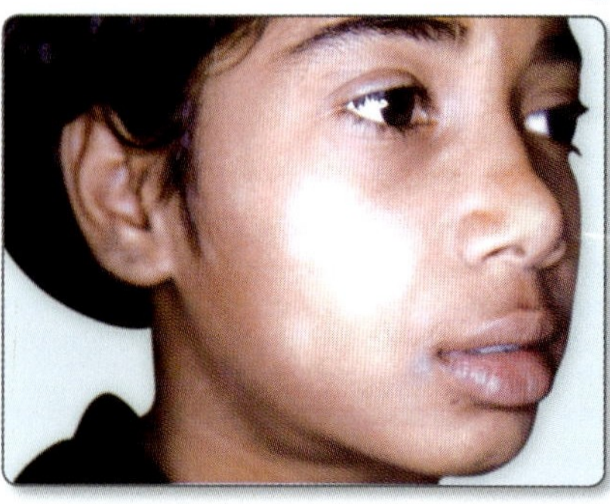

Fig. 12: Pityriasis alba

Differential Diagnosis

The age, distribution and color of the lesions help in the easy diagnosis of pityriasis alba. The condition should be differentiated from other hypopigmented lesions, such as pityriasis versicolor, vitiligo, leprosy, postinflammatory hypopigmentation and hypopigmented naevi. Pityriasis alba is tan coloured with indistinct margins, vitiligo on the other hand is milky-white in colour and the margins are sharp.

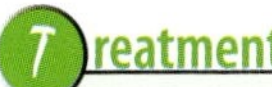

Treatment

Response to treatment is often disappointing. Emollient creams, mild tar preparations, 1% hydrocortisone ointment may be helpful. Spontaneous healing is seen within several months to a few years.

ASTEATOTIC ECZEMA

It is an eczematous eruption common in the elderly, but can be seen in any age group. Asteatotic eczema is characterised by dry, cracked and fissured patches on the limbs. It is common in winter. Sun, wind and low humidity are predisposing factors. Asteatotic eczema is seen secondary to epidermal lipid depletion.

Aetiology

Following factors cause decrease in skin surface lipids and lead to asteatotic eczema: naturally dry skin, old age, malnutrition, low environmental humidity, dry cold environment, degreasing of the skin by excessive use of soaps and by industrial solvents, drugs like diuretics, cimetidine, topical steroids, myxoedema and zinc deficiency.

Clinical Features

The eczema commonly affects the legs, arms and the hands, the surface of the skin is marked by dryness and crackling in a criss-cross fashion (Fig. 13). On the legs, the pattern of superficial marking is more marked and the lesions are deeper. In some patients fissures develop. The condition may remain in this state for months or recurs every winter. Irritation of the skin is often intense, particularly with change of temperature and on undressing at night. Frank eczematous changes finally develop. Extensive or generalised eczema craquele, should increase the suspicion of internal malignancy.

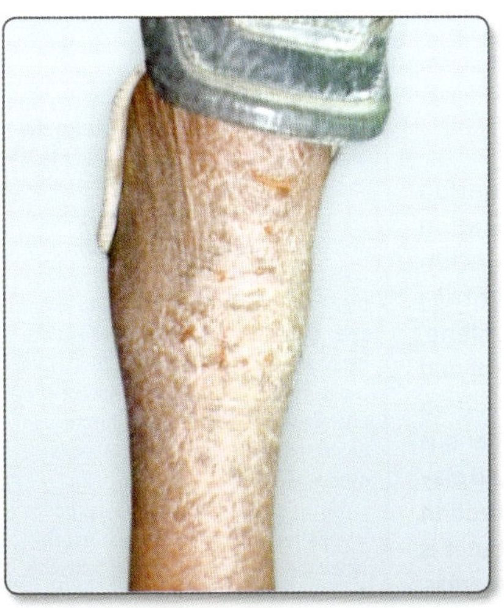

Fig. 13: Asteatotic eczema

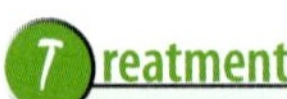

Treatment

Any precipitating factor should be recognised and removed. Environment should be humidified and irritants should be avoided. Baths should be restricted and should not be hot. Soaps should be avoided and use of bath oils should be encouraged. Emollients should be used after bathing and several times in a day. Urea-based weak corticosteroids are also helpful. Topical steroids should be avoided in the elderly, as the skin is already thin and fragile.

Course and Prognosis

Healing of the skin is rapidly achieved; continuous use of greasing agents usually prevents recurrences.

JUVENILE PLANTAR DERMATOSIS

This is a type of endogenous eczema characterised by dry fissured lesions on the plantar surface of the forefoot.

Aetiology

The exact aetiology of this condition is not known but it has been postulated that wearing of less porous socks and occlusive footwear for long hours by children, and friction from sports lead to retention of sweat and maceration, which aggravates the condition. Atopy may be present.

Clinical Features

This condition, which is strikingly symmetrical, occurs exclusively in children aged 3–14 years. There is redness and pain on the forefoot, which appears, glazed and cracked. The condition spares the non-weight bearing areas. Most cases clear with passage of time.

Treatment

Topical preparations including urea, tars, emollients and Lassar's paste may be helpful. Change to cotton socks and change of footwear may be helpful.

ECZEMATOUS DRUG ERUPTIONS

Eczematous eruptions secondary to drugs are due to gold, bleomycin, penicillin, quinine, β-blockers, methyldopa, clonidine, pyrazolone compounds and chloramphenicol.

Tropical Eczema (Unclassified Eczema)

This peculiar eczematous eruption does not fit into any classification of eczemas. The eruption is often seen in underdeveloped countries where malnutrition, poor hygiene, secondary bacterial infection, hot and humid climate could play a role in producing tropical eczema. Exogenous or endogenous factors both could play a role in its production. The eruption is seen in adults of either sex, but it is more common in men from rural areas.

Clinical Features

The lower limbs are usually first affected, the eruption then spreads to the trunk and neck. The lesions are not well defined; they are erythematous oozing and crusted plaques. These may coalesce to form circinate or polycyclic patterns. Pruritus is severe. When the lesions become infected pustules appear, these are more pronounced at the periphery of the plaque. Chronic lesions are papillomatous and verrucous. Adenopathy often develops secondary to infection. In neglected cases, the lesions resemble a pyoderma.

Nutritional deficiency may produce lesions resembling nummular eczema, seborrhoeic dermatitis and neurodermatitis.

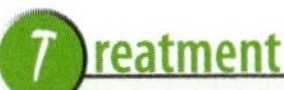

The treatment is similar to that of acute infected eczema, with antibiotics and corticosteroids. Chronic cases should be treated with keratolytics and tar preparations. Recovery is slow.

HAND ECZEMA

Hand eczema is one of the most common eczema; it is a burden to the patient and a challenge to the physician. It is due to a variety of causes; most of these have already been mentioned. Hand eczema is the result of several factors including an atopic tendency, dry skin, repeated exposure to mild irritants, repeated trauma, secondary infections, etc. It can be difficult in medicolegal cases to apportion blame. Hand eczema can occur alone or it can occur in association with other diseases such as fungal infections of the feet in pompholyx. All parts of the body should be examined in hand eczema particularly the feet. Many diseases such as psoriasis, lichen planus and fungal infections may mimic hand eczema.

Pruritus is the primary symptom, but dryness, fissuring, inelasticity and superinfection often lead to inability to work with the hands (Fig. 14). This dermatitis is a cause of social, personal and financial grief.

Aetiology

Hand eczema may be due to both irritant and allergic CD. Hand eczema is a very common manifestation of occupational dermatoses. It is seen in food handlers, dentists, nurses, bartenders, surgeons, cooks, housemaids, hairdressers, farmers, construction workers, etc.

Common causative agents causing housemaids eczema are foodstuff handled in the kitchen such as garlic, onion, carrot, tomatoes, spinach, radish, fig, parsnip, cheese, soaps and detergents. Doctors and nurses may be sensitive to rubber gloves, antiseptics, surgical instruments, soap and detergents. Other common sensitisers are nickel, hair dyes, cement, dichromates and plants. Hand dermatitis is 4–10 times more common in people with AD.

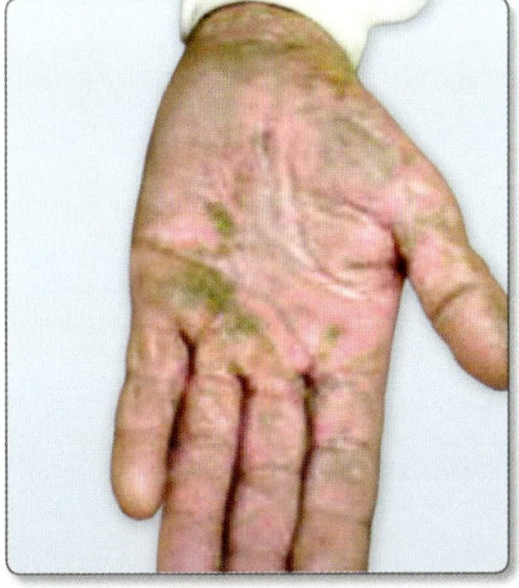

Fig. 14: Chronic hand eczema

Secondary candidiasis can develop in the finger webs and secondary bacterial infection especially with *Staphylococcus aureus* may occur in the fissured areas.

Atopic patients have an increased risk of hand eczema, and it is most difficult to treat.

Morphological Varieties of Hand Eczema

- Diffuse and patchy, dorsal and palmar
- Particular patterns:
  - Ring eczema
  - Fingertip eczema
  - Apron eczema
  - Discoid hand eczema
  - Hyperkeratotic hand eczema
  - Palmar eczema
  - Pompholyx
  - Keratolysis exfoliativa.

Clinical Features

Diffuse and Patchy, Dorsal and Palmar

Most cases of hand eczema are patchy, vesiculosquamous in nature and without any particular morphological features. These in most cases are due to allergic or irritant CD. Exceptions are finger web dermatitis which is an indication of irritant dermatitis due to liquids. Id reactions and the effect of ingested allergens affect the palmar surface of the hand.

Particular Pattern

Only about one-third of cases of hand eczema present with a particular pattern. Some of these are:

Ring eczema: The frequent site is under the ring, but it may spread to the adjacent fingers and palms. It is more common in women wearing cheap artificial rings. Pure gold is less likely to sensitise. Irritant contact eczema is often associated due to soaps and detergents accumulating under the ring.

Fingertip eczema: This is known as "pulpite" in France, because it affects the pulp of the fingers. The fingertip is dry and scaly, thickened and fissured. The fissures are painful, which is the cause of referral to the doctor. Fingertip eczema is more common in women, due to cutting of vegetables, fruits, garlic, ginger, etc. It may be traumatic, as seen in people who count currency as bankers and shopkeepers. In some cases, the finger pulps may become acutely eczematous. Patch tests and 20 minute contact tests are indicated.

Apron eczema: This is so called because of its appearance like apron. It involves the proximal palmar aspect of two or more adjacent fingers and the continuous palmar skin over the metacarpophalyngeal joints in a semicircular pattern. It is an endogenous eczema.

Discoid hand eczema: This pattern is similar to discoid eczema elsewhere. It is localised to the hands and fingers, usually the dorsal surface. The patches are resistant to treatment, and tend to recur at the same site.

Hyperkeratotic hand eczema: This type of eczema is more common in men, usually seen between 40 years and 60 years. The cause is not known, it is not associated with allergic CD. Only one-third of patients were associated with manual labour. The eczema tends to run a stable chronic course; few patients have reported spontaneous recovery. It should be differentiated from psoriasis.

Palmar eczema: Most cases are associated with CD. It can be dry or vesicular.

The dry palmar type is called the "wear and tear" dermatitis of housewives. The palms are dry, with a criss-crossing of fractured horny layer, without deep fissuring. It affects the palmar surface of the fingers and palms. It may be unilateral or bilateral. The dominant hand is more affected. The common offending agents are soaps, detergents, washing and cleaning agents. It may be an extension of fingertip or ring eczema.

The recurrent vesicular type should not be confused with pompholyx. This eczema has longer duration of recurrent attacks and the vesicles rupture. After a time, the condition becomes chronic and there is no healing between the attacks. The cause is not known in majority of cases.

Recurrent focal palmar peeling (***Keratolysis exfoliativa***): This is probably a mild form of pompholyx. Small areas of superficial desquamation of the palms and soles are sometimes seen. It is asymptomatic; some patients may progress to pompholyx.

Pompholyx is described earlier.

Severity of Hand Eczema

The severity of hand eczema can be estimated by some parameters such as duration, symptoms, extent of hand involvement, need for medical consultation, if it causes cessation of work, or in some cases change of occupation. Irritant CD is the mildest form of hand eczema, while atopic hand eczema is more widespread and debilitating.

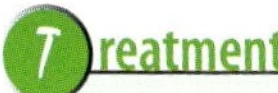

The treatment of hand eczema is the same as that of eczema in general. The following principles should be observed:

- Avoidance of irritants
- Frequent application of emollients
- Sparing use of steroids
- Protection of the hands by gloves
- Avoid abrasive soaps
- Use of barrier protective creams

In all cases of hand dermatitis look at the soles to exclude any fungal infection
Exclude atopic dermatitis
Nail changes indicate chronic disease
If pustules are present, exclude pustular psoriasis
Moisturisers should be continued even after the hand heals

Ferdinand von Ritter Hebra (1816–1880)

Hebra was the founder of modern dermatology. His discoveries and teachings, together with his successor Kaposi, laid the foundations for modern day dermatology. He was the first to prove that skin diseases were due to agents acting on the skin. He experimented with local irritants and found that it produced eczema. He also experimented with the scabies mite. Hebra discarded the theory of four humours and classified skin diseases on the morphological and microscopic appearance. He opened the department of dermatology in the Vienna school of medicine, taught dermatology to people not only from Vienna, but also to people from all over Europe and America. His motto was "never abandon a case as hopeless, but continue to study it on the basis of knowledge, its pathology and aetiology, until you find some way to help".

FURTHER READING

1. Bandmann HJ, Clnan CD, Cronin E. Dermatitis from applied medicaments. Arch Dermatol. 1972;106:335-7.
2. Bos JD, Leent EJ, Smitt JH. The millennium criteria for the diagnosis of atopic dermatitis. Exp Dermatol. 1998;7:132-8.
3. Dattner AM. Breastfeeding and atopic dermatitis: preventive or harmful? Facts and controversies. Clinical Dermatol. 2010;28:34-7.
4. De-Groot AC, Frosch PJ. Adverse reaction to fragrance. A clinical review. Contact Dermatitis. 1997;36:57-86.
5. Flohr C, England K, Radulovic S, et al. Filaggrin loss-of-function mutations are associated with early-onset eczema, eczema severity and transepidermal water loss at 3 months of age. Br J Dermatol. 2010;163:1333-6.
6. Hanifan MJ, Rajka G. Diagnostic features of atopic dermatitis. Acta Dermatol Venereol (Stockholm)Suppl. 1980;92:44-7.
7. Li FL, Liu G, Wang J. Prognosis of Unclassified eczema. A follow-up study. Arch Dermatol. 2008;144(2):160-4.
8. Sehra S, Tuana MB, Holbreich M, et al. Clinical correlations of recent developments in the pathogenesis of atopic dermatitis. An Bras Dermatol. 2008;83(1):57-73.

9. Sugarman JL, Parish LC. Efficacy of a lipid-based barrier repair formulation in moderate-to -severe pediatric atopic dermatitis. J Drug Dermatol. 2009;8(12):1106-11.
10. Wickens K, Black NP, Stanley VT, et al. A differential effect of 2 probiotics in the prevention of eczema and atopy: A double-blind, randomized, placebo-controlled trial. J Am Acad of Allergy Clin Immunol. 2008;122(4):788-94.
11. Williams CH, Burney GJP, Pembroke CA, et al. The UK Working Party's Diagnostic Criteria for Atopic dermatitis. Independent hospital validation. Br J Dermatol. 1994;131:406-16.

Chapter

10

Keratinising and Papulosquamous Disorders

PSORIASIS

Psoriasis is a genetically determined chronic papulosquamous disorder with relapses and remission, characterised by the presence of sharply demarcated dull-red plaques covered with silvery scales, particularly on the scalp and extensor surfaces of the body, such as knees and elbows.

Incidence and Prevalence

Psoriasis has a universal distribution. The overall prevalence is about 1–3% of the population. The highest incidence is in Faroes Island, Denmark and Sweden. Mongoloids have a much lower incidence (0.3%) as compared to others.

The peak age of onset is 2nd or 3rd decade. The onset of psoriasis is earlier in females than in males. However, the incidence of psoriasis is equal in both sexes.

Aetiology

Genetics

Psoriasis has an autosomal dominant inheritance with incomplete penetrance. A positive family history is obtained in about 35% of patients; identical twin studies show a concordance of 75%. Various studies have revealed an association of psoriasis with HLA B 13, HLA B 17, HLA CW 6, HLA DR 7, HLA B 27 and HLA B 37.

At least nine total or partial gene loci have been reported in psoriasis (PSOR 1–9). The putative gene at PSORS 1 is undoubtedly the major genetic determinant for psoriasis.

Some authors have classified psoriasis into the following two types:

Type I: Onset under 40 years of age, with a positive family history.

Type II: Onset over 40 years of age, sporadic and with no family history of psoriasis.

Immunological Aspects

It has been known since the mid-1980s that psoriasis is an immune disorder and that abnormal T cell activity plays an important part in the pathogenesis of psoriasis. Three lines of evidence implicate that T cells are responsible for the pathogenesis of psoriasis. First T lymphocytes are present in the plaques of psoriasis. Second it has been demonstrated that the initiation and maintenance of lesions require activated T cells. Finally drugs that suppress T cell activity such as cyclosporin have led to the improvement of psoriasis.

Current hypothesis is that hyperproliferation and inflammation in psoriasis are due to release of mediators from activated T lymphocytes, which are triggered by an unidentified antigen.

An unknown antigen causes the antigen processing cells (APCs) to be activated in the epidermis. The activated APCs then travel to the lymph nodes and activate naïve T cells. This is due to recognition of intercellular adhesion molecule-1 (ICAM 1) on the surface of the APC by lymphocytes functioning antigen-1(LFA-1) on the surface of T cell. The activated T lymphocytes roll along the microvasculature then traffic into the dermis and then to the epidermis by the binding between T cell LFA 1 and endothelial ICAM 1.

Once in the skin activated T lymphocytes undergo a second activation similar to the previous encounter with APCs in the lymph node. This is due to the expression of ICAM 1 and HLA DR on keratinocytes, which causes release of inflammatory mediators, such as IL 2, IFN-γ, IL 8 TNF-α and granulocyte macrophage colony-stimulating factor(GM-CSF). These cytokines are characteristic of Th1 cells.

Endocrine Factors

The peak incidence of psoriasis is at puberty and menopause. Pregnancy can improve or deteriorate psoriasis.

Provoking Factors

Several factors provoke or exacerbate psoriasis. These include:

Trauma: Psoriatic lesions appear at the site of injury; this is known as Koebner's phenomenon.

Infection: It has long been recognised that streptococcal pharyngitis may provoke guttate psoriasis. AIDS is associated with severe and recalcitrant psoriasis.

Drugs: Certain drugs may precipitate or exacerbate psoriasis, such as antimalarials, β-blocking agents, lithium, nonsteroidal anti-inflammatory agents, interferons and withdrawal of systemic corticosteroids.

Stress: The role of emotional stress in psoriasis is not well understood. Possibly stress deteriorates psoriasis by decreasing the capacity to cope with treatment.

Sunlight: Although sunlight is usually beneficial, it may provoke psoriasis in a few patients.

Metabolic factors: Dialysis and hypocalcaemia precipitate psoriasis.

Other factors: Alcohol and smoking may aggravate psoriasis.

Whatever the provocation, the result is an increased number of cycling cells recruited from the normal resting cell proportion. This leads to an increased number of dividing cells. Cellular turnover is increased sevenfold, and the transit time from the basal layer to the stratum corneum is reduced to 8–10 days from 52–75 days. Growth factors, especially transforming growth factor-α seem to mediate these events. The cell cycle time is not reduced.

Pathogenesis

The abnormalities found in psoriatic skin are increased epidermal cell proliferation, dilatation and proliferation of dermal blood vessels, and an inflammatory cell infiltrate in which neutrophils and T helper lymphocytes proliferate. The increased epidermal proliferation in psoriasis is caused by an excessive number of germinative cells entering the cell cycle rather than by a decrease in cell cycle time. This leads to increased epidermal cell turnover with decreased shedding, this results in the accumulation of dead cells, which appear as silvery white. The trapping of air between the scales also contributes to the silvery white aspect of the clinical lesion.

Various in vivo models of angiogenesis demonstrated that epidermal keratinocytes are the primary source of angiogenetic activity. These cells produce an array of soluble mediators with angiogenetic activity, such as interleukin 8 (IL 8), tumour necrosis factor-α (TNF-α), thymidine phosphorylase, endothelial cell-stimulating angiogenesis factor and more importantly vascular endothelial growth factor (VEGF).

Other mediator systems involved in excess cellular proliferation and inflammation are arachidonic acid and its products. There is an increased level of phospholipase A2 that acts on phospholipids in cell membrane. This releases arachidonic acid, which is a precursor of prostaglandin, hydroxyeicosatetraenoic acid and leukotrienes, these mediate inflammation and proliferation in psoriasis. Indomethacin potentiates psoriasis due to an increase in the production of leukotrienes. Benoxaprofen decreases leukotrienes and ameliorates psoriasis.

Arachidonic acid is present in red meat, green leafy vegetables, corn and safflower oils.

Other factors increased in psoriasis are proto-oncogenes, cyclic guanosine monophosphate (cGMP), polyamines, cyclic nucleotides, phosphoinositol, calmodulin and proteinases. Perhaps the underlying abnormality in psoriasis is a genetic defect in the control of keratinocyte growth. Interferon-γ inhibits growth and promotes the differentiation of normal keratinocytes. In psoriasis, interferon-γ fails to inhibit growth of keratinocytes and they proliferate out of control.

Others think that psoriasis is caused by a genetic defect of retinoid signaling, that is why it improves with retinoid therapy.

Whether the initiating factor responsible for psoriasis is epidermal or dermal is debated. The following factors are indicative of epidermal origin for psoriasis:

- Koebner's phenomenon
- Retinoid receptors in the epidermis
- Release of proteases that provoke epidermal proliferation
- Presence of antibodies against the stratum corneum
- The initial response may be due to an intrinsic reaction of the keratinocytes with increased cytokine production, this in turns leads to epidermal proliferation, accumulation of T cells in the papillary dermis, proliferation of blood vessels, and migration of neutrophils into the epidermis
- Various in vivo models of angiogenesis demonstrated that epidermal keratinocytes are the primary source of angiogenetic activity.

Histopathology

The histology of psoriasis is usually diagnostic. Psoriasis is the main disease giving rise to the psoriasiform tissue reaction. The two principal features of which include, the suprapapillary exudate and focal parakeratosis related to it.

Of great importance is its intermittent character, which is expressed as the "squirting papilla". The earliest change of the psoriasiform tissue reaction is the oedematous dermal papillae with engorged capillaries. This gives rise to increased mitosis of the basal cells and corresponding acanthosis. Mitosis may appear one or two layers above the basal layer. The focal parakeratosis is due to the damage to the suprapapillary cells. The epidermis over the epidermal papillae is thinned thus explaining the Auspitz sign. Parakeratosis may alternate with orthokeratosis, reflecting the episodic nature of the disease. In areas of parakeratosis the granular layer is thinned or absent. A fully developed plaque shows extensive hyperkeratosis and confluent parakeratosis.

Collections of neutrophils extend from the tip of dermal papillae into the epidermis. The neutrophils present in the stratum corneum are known as Munro's microabscess. These are present in about 75% of cases. This migration of neutrophils from the dermal papillae into the overlying epidermis is known as the squirting papillae. More marked in pustular psoriasis, neutrophils are present in the stratum malpighii (Kogoj's pustules). The dermal papillae are prominent and contain ectatic vessels. There is perivascular mononuclear infiltrate. These dermal changes precede the epidermal changes. When the papillary oedema subsides, the papillae become inconspicuous.

Histological characteristics are:

- Hyperkeratosis
- Parakeratosis
- Absence of granular layer
- Acanthosis
- Elongation of rete pegs
- Long-edematous club-shaped papillae
- Thinning of supra-papillary plate
- Munro's microabscess in stratum corneum
- Kogoj's pustule in stratum malpighii (pustular psoriasis).

Clinical Features

Lesions of psoriasis show four prominent features: they are sharply demarcated, the surface is covered with silvery-white scales, under the scale the skin is glossy, homogenous and erythematous and finally Auspitz sign is positive. Auspitz sign is a special feature of erythrosquamous psoriasis; it is not present in inverse and pustular psoriasis. The different morphological presentations are related to the activity of the disease process, due to factors not fully understood. In children guttate, erythrodermic and pustular forms are more common; these eventuate into chronic plaque psoriasis.

Psoriasis Vulgaris

The classic lesion is a salmon pink plaque covered with silvery scales. On removal of psoriatic scales, small-bleeding points may be seen; this is called the Auspitz sign. The lesions are well-defined and may be single or multiple. The sites of predilection are scalp, extensor aspect of elbows and knees, sacrum, palms and soles. Although it is said that psoriasis is not itchy, it is often seen that patients complain of some itching. In fact Greek word "psora" actually means itch. Guttate psoriasis is more prone to irritation than chronic plaque psoriasis.

Woronoff's ring is a concentric blanching of erythematous skin at or near the periphery of a healing psoriatic plaque. It does not turn red with ultraviolet-induced erythema or with anthralin therapy. It has been suggested that the ring is mediated via an endogenous inhibitor of prostaglandin synthesis (Figs 1A to C).

Koebner's phenomenon is seen in an active lesion of psoriasis.

Guttate Psoriasis

There is a sudden onset of multiple small lesions mainly on the trunk and proximal extremities. It is common in children and young adults and may be preceded by streptococcal sore throat. An episode of guttate psoriasis may be the first indication of the patient's propensity for psoriasis. In children silvery scale is only minimally expressed and the lesions may appear quite red (Fig. 2).

Flexural or Inverse Psoriasis

This involves the groins, axillae, submammary folds, vulva, gluteal cleft and other body folds. Typical scaling is absent but edges of the lesions are well defined and the characteristic colour is retained.

Erythrodermic Psoriasis

Erythroderma in psoriasis is characterised by extensive erythema and scaling that involves more than 90% of the body surface area. Erythema is the most prominent feature and scaling usually is less severe. This may be the initial manifestation of psoriasis, or chronic and pustular psoriasis may gradually evolve into erythrodermic phase.

Unstable Psoriasis

This is a term used when the disease activity is marked and the course and immediate outcome is unpredictable

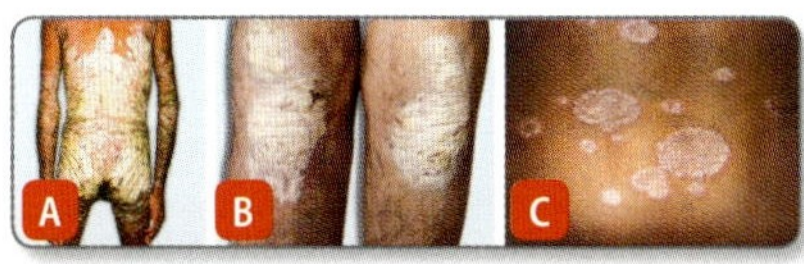

Figs 1A to C: (A) Psoriasis—note the silvery white scales; (B) Psoriasis knee-common site; (C) Annular psoriasis

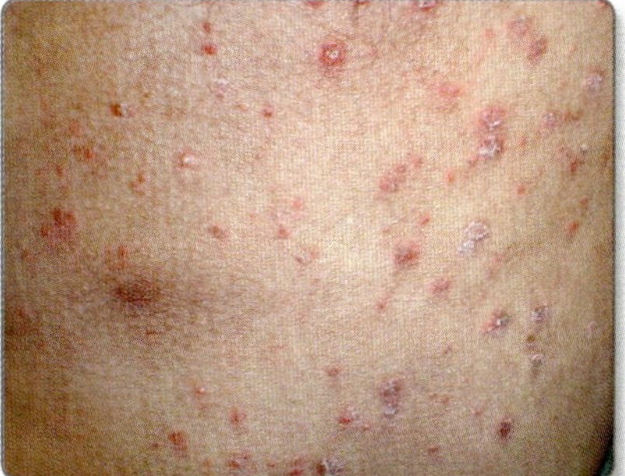

Fig. 2: Guttate psoriasis

Psoriasis of the Scalp

Psoriasis may affect the scalp associated with cutaneous lesions elsewhere on the body, or it may be the only part of the skin affected. There may be only one or a few plaques or it may affect the entire scalp. The plaques are raised and the scales frequently become adherent to the hair, these are heaped up upon one another. The surface of the psoriatic lesion is often irregular because of the thick scales and the lesions are easily palpable (Fig. 3).

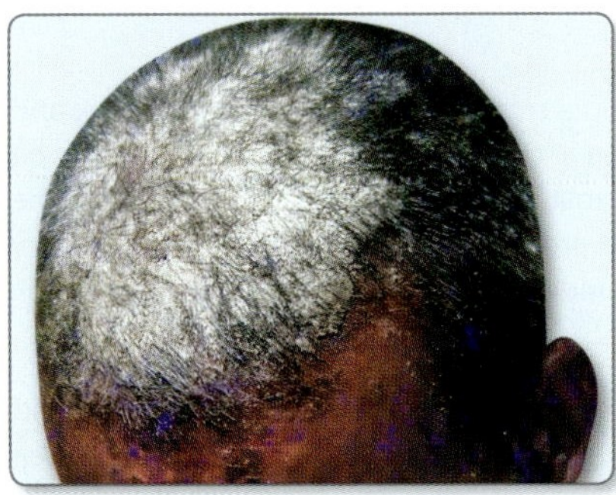

Fig. 3: Psoriasis—scalp

Nail Involvement

Nail changes occur in 25–50% of all cases. This is seen in all types of psoriasis, but is especially common in patients with joint involvement. Nails may be involved in the absence of psoriasis elsewhere. Pitting is the most frequent change, due to parakeratosis. The other changes include yellow discolouration, onycholysis (this is caused by a plaque of psoriasis in the distal nail bed, with accumulation of scales that lifts the nail plate from its bed), subungual hyperkeratosis and splinter haemorrhages. The yellow colour is due to the presence of glycoproteins. The nail may lose its structural integrity, resulting in fragmentation and crumbling (Fig. 4).

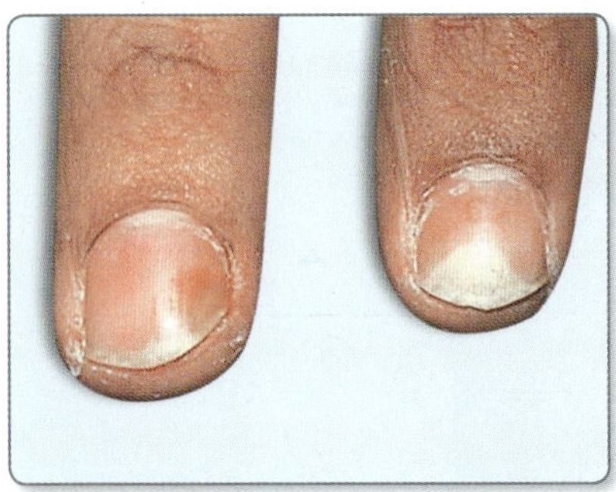

Fig. 4: Nail psoriasis—pitting and onycholysis

Psoriatic Arthritis

Skin lesions usually precede arthritis, but arthritis can precede skin lesions or both may be involved simultaneously. There is an increased incidence of HLA B 27 in patients with psoriatic arthritis. Nail changes are more frequent in patients with arthritis especially in distal and mutilating types. Raised erythrocyte sedimentation rate (ESR) is the best guide to disease activity.

The arthritis is inflammatory in nature. It may affect any peripheral joint, as well as the axial skeleton and the sacroiliac joints. Patients have pain associated with stiffness, which is more in the morning and improves with activity. Joints in psoriatic arthritis are less tender than in rheumatoid arthritis. The inflamed joints in psoriatic arthritis are purplish-red in colour, which is not often seen in rheumatoid arthritis. Women tend to have small joints and upper limb involvement, while men tend to have axial involvement. Psoriatic arthritis is asymmetrical in distribution.

A typical feature of psoriatic arthritis is the development of dactylitis, which presents as a swelling of the whole digit, the exact cause of dactylitis is unclear. It may be related to extensive inflammation and effusion in all joints of a particular digit, with an associated tenosynovitis, or to soft tissue inflammation in the whole digit. Tenosynovitis is also a feature of psoriatic arthritis. The more advanced imaging techniques help to delineate the pathogenesis of "sausage digits" (Figs 5 and 6).

The spondyloarthritis of psoriasis is more common in males, the symptoms improve with time and their spinal mobility is generally good. Enthesitis or inflammation of tendons at the site of their insertion is frequent in psoriatic arthritis, seen particularly at the Achilles tendon. The cervical spine has received attention in recent literature. High prevalence of atlantoaxial subluxation was found in some cases of psoriasis. Osteolysis and ankylosis is more common in psoriatic arthritis as compared to rheumatoid arthritis. Erosions and joint space

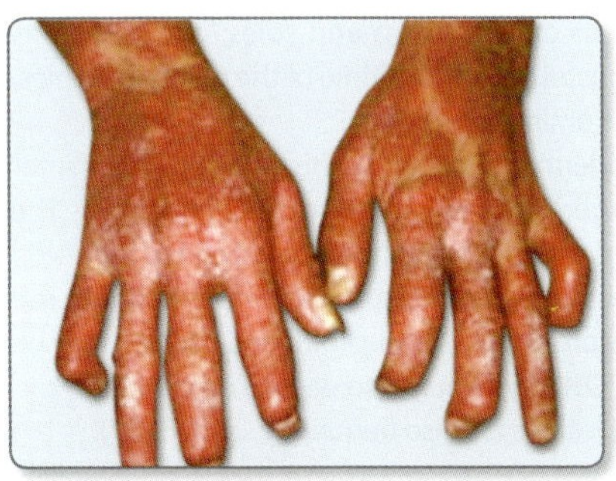

Fig. 5: Psoriatic arthritis—note the sausage-shaped digits

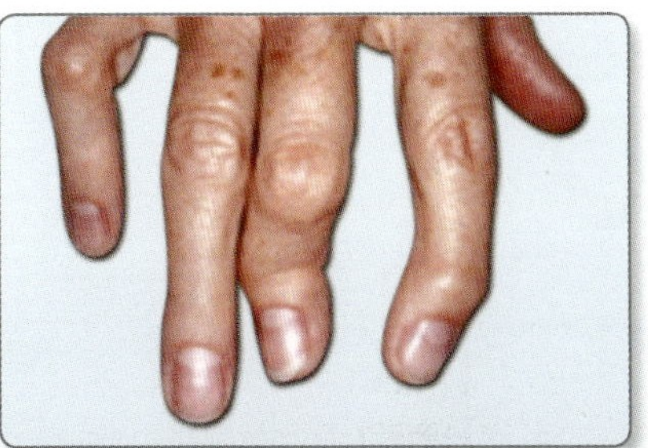

Fig. 6: Psoriatic arthritis—note the involvement of distal interphalangeal joints and showing rheumatoid arthritis like changes

narrowing is seen on X-ray. Psoriatic arthritis is not associated with vasculitis and autoantibodies, which are associated with rheumatoid arthritis.

The different types of psoriatic arthritis are:

- *Monoarthritis or Oligoarthritis*: This is the most common form with swelling and tenosynovitis of one or a few joints of the fingers and toes. Usually one or more proximal interphalangeal joint (PIP), distal interphalangeal (DIP), metatarsophalangeal or metacarpophalangeal joints are involved
- *Distal interphalangeal arthritis*: This is the classic form but is less common. There is a sausage swelling and flexion deformity of the digits, which is asymmetrical. The nails may be involved and dystrophic
- *Arthritis mutilans*: This is a deforming arthritis involving hands, feet and spine. There is destruction of bone (osteolysis) and ankylosis. Osteolysis may cause complete dissolution of phalanges and digital shortening
- *Rheumatoid-like polyarthritis*: This is a symmetrical, seronegative arthritis and is not accompanied by rheumatoid nodules
- *Axial arthritis*: This is spondylitis and/or sacroiliitis, with or without peripheral arthritis.

Pustular Psoriasis

Pustular psoriasis is a condition in which macroscopic pustules are associated with psoriasis. The condition can be localised or generalised; these may be acute or chronic.

Localised pustular psoriasis: Its relationship with psoriasis is controversial. It is not associated with HLA B 13 and HLA B 17, and it is not provoked by factors that precipitate psoriasis. There is no seasonal variation and it tends to start at a later age. The typical lesions are seen on the palms and soles.

There are two types of lesions on the palms and soles; one is seen as psoriatic plaques studded with pustules on the middle of the palms and soles, or on the thenar and hypothenar eminences.

The other type of lesion is acrodermatitis continua; this type of palmoplantar psoriasis affects the tip of the fingers or toes. It is a disease of middle life. The disease begins as patches studded with pustules, the proximal end of the lesion is bordered by a line of vesiculo-pustules that later exfoliate, leaving a bright-red surface. The lesions extend slowly proximally. The nailfolds and nail bed may be involved leading to nail atrophy. Osteolysis may also occur. The condition can lead to generalised psoriasis; oral lesions are also frequently seen (Fig. 7).

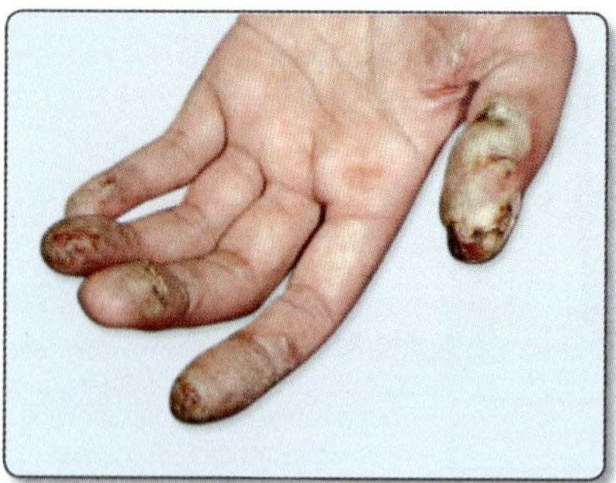

Fig. 7: Acrodermatitis continua

Generalised pustular psoriasis: This may be acute, subacute or chronic, it is an extreme form of psoriasis in which all the pathological features of psoriasis are exaggerated.

Acute generalised pustular psoriasis (Von Zumbusch): This form of psoriasis usually develops from typical psoriatic lesions that have not been adequately controlled; it is often seen on steroid withdrawal.

There may be a prodromal phase of burning sensation in the skin; the skin lesions become dry and tender, the lesions become red and pustules develop. Waves of pustulation are seen, the oral cavity is often involved, the nails may become thick or they may shed. Systemic symptoms such as fever and malaise are present. The condition is serious; patients may die of exhaustion, toxicity or infection.

Complications of acute generalised pustular psoriasis. These include hypoalbuminaemia, oliguria, renal tubular necrosis, hepatic damage, deep venous thrombosis, pulmonary embolism, polyarthritis, hypocalcaemia and septicaemia (Fig. 8).

Generalised pustular psoriasis of pregnancy (Impetigo herpetiformis): The onset is usually in the last trimester of pregnancy; the disease is similar to that of acute generalised pustular psoriasis with a flexural onset, constitutional symptoms are severe. The oral cavity and even the oesophagus may be involved. Placental insufficiency may lead to stillbirth, neonatal death or fetal abnormalities. The disease may recur in subsequent pregnancies and even after oral contraceptives.

Psoriasis in children: This may manifest as guttate psoriasis, inter-digital psoriasis napkin and scalp psoriasis. Psoriasis of the face is more common than in adults. It can occur on the eyelids, cheeks and angle of the mouth.

Concomitant Diseases

Epidemiological studies reveal a number of diseases associated with psoriasis. These are arthritis, diabetes, ischaemic heart disease, Crohn's disease, atopy, urticaria and atopic dermatitis.

Complications

Complications are rare; these are mostly seen in erythrodermic psoriasis. These include infection, hypocalcemia, renal failure, amyloidosis and apical pulmonary fibrosis. Apical pulmonary fibrosis is a nonarticular complication of ankylosing spondylitis.

Hypocalcaemia and low folic acid levels are due to enhanced epidermopoiesis.

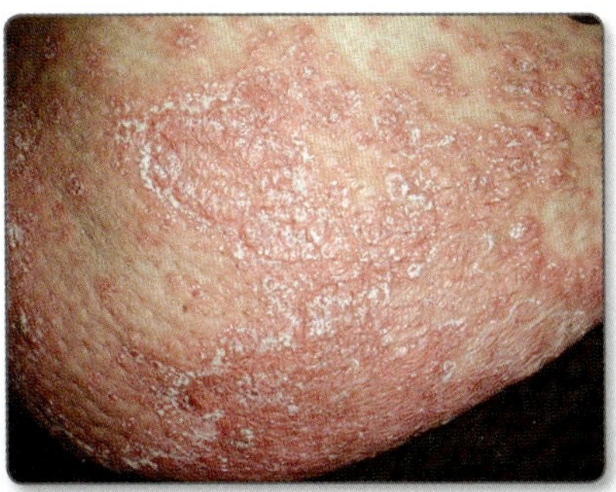

Fig. 8: Pustular psoriasis

Laboratory Findings

There are no consistent laboratory findings in psoriasis. The ESR is normal, but it may be raised in pustular psoriasis. Anaemia may be found due to deficiency of iron or folic acid. Mild hyperuricemia may be present due to increased epidermopoiesis. Hypoalbuminemia is due to excessive scaling and hypocalcaemia is seen in some cases.

Diagnostic Features of Psoriasis

- Erythematous sharply defined plaques, covered with silvery-white scales
- Extensor surface primarily involved as the knees and elbows
- Auspitz's sign positive
- Koebner's phenomenon present in active phase of the disease
- Woronoff's ring often present in the healing phase of the disease
- Characteristic histopathology.

Method of Measuring the Severity of Psoriasis

Psoriatic area and severity index (PASI). PASI is used to measure the severity of psoriasis. The following parameters are measured in relation to the site and surface area affected.

Sites: The body is divided into four segments: head (H), trunk (T), upper extremities (U), and lower extremities (L).

Surface area: The surface area of body segments are represented as: H = 0.1, T = 0.3, U = 0.2, L = 0.4.

Parameters

Area involved in each segment: 0 = none, 1 = ≤ 10%, 2 = 10–30%, 3 = 30–50%, 4 > 50–70%, 5 = 70–90% 6 = 90–100%.

Severity of disease: 0 = Nil , 1 = Mild, 2 = Moderate, 3 = Marked, 4 = Severe.

The points to be noted are–erythema (E), induration (I) and scaling (S).

Calculations of PASI score

PASI= $0.1(E_H + I_H + S_H)$ AH + $0.3(E_T + I_T + S_T)$ AT + $0.2(E_U + I_U + S_U)$ AU + $0.4(E_L + I_L + S_L)$AL

The PASI score can this range from 0 to 72.

Differential Diagnosis

This depends upon the type and location of psoriasis.

Seborrhoeic dermatitis: The lesions of seborrheic dermatitis have a lighter colour with less sharply delineated edge and covered with yellowish greasy adherent scales.

Eczema: Hyperkeratotic eczema of palms is often difficult to differentiate from psoriasis clinically. However, the colour and silvery scales are suggestive of psoriasis.

Lichen planus: The lesions of lichen planus are differentiated by its violaceous colour, pruritus, scantiness of scales and by the presence of oral lesions.

Pityriasis rosea: The presence of herald patch, typical arrangement and distribution of the lesions and collarette of scales are characteristic of pityriasis rosea.

Pityriasis lichenoides chronica: This resembles guttate psoriasis, but lesions are brownish-red with mica-like scales.

Candidiasis: This can cause confusion with flexural psoriasis, but scaling is confined to the edge and satellite papules and pustules are seen in candidiasis.

Tinea cruris: This has a well-defined edge. Scraping for dematophytes confirms the diagnosis.

Psoriasiform syphilid: This may cause difficulty but condylomata and other signs of disease are usually present.

Pityriasis rubra pilaris: This may closely resemble psoriasis, but follicular lesions are present and hyperkeratosis of the palms and soles have a yellowish hue.

Lichen simplex chronicus: In lichen simplex chronicus, the skin markings are exaggerated, the edge is ill defined and there is marked itching.

Treatment

Each patient must be assessed individually before commencing treatment. It should be made clear to the patient that there is no cure for psoriasis and the disease can only be controled. Treatment depends upon age, sex, occupation and resources; as well as on the site, extent, type, duration and previous treatment. The goal of therapy is to decrease the epidermal proliferation and decrease the underlying dermal inflammation.

If the disease is minimal, stable (no new lesions are developing), and the lesions are on the covered parts of the body then perhaps no treatment is required or simple emollients are applied to remove the scales. All treatments topical or systemic have potential side effects, which must be remembered before treatment is undertaken.

If the disease is very active (new lesions appearing and the disease is extensive), treatment is difficult and there is a high tendency to relapse, some form of maintenance therapy will be required. If the lesions are chronic and stable, the treatment is usually effective.

Treatment of psoriasis can be studied under the following headings:
- Topical treatment
- Treatment by ultraviolet light
- Systemic treatment.

The treatment has to be adjusted for the skin, scalp, nails, joints and for pustular psoriasis.

Topical Treatment

Topical corticosteroids: The potent corticosteroids are effective in psoriasis. As a rule, weak topical steroids such as 1% hydrocortisone skin ointment are not effective in clearing the lesion. For lesions on the trunk and limbs ointments are better than creams, these should be applied once or twice daily; the lesions can be occluded if very thick. The potent steroids should be effective within 3 weeks, if not discontinue the treatment. Topical steroids become less effective on continual use, short intermittent courses are a better approach. If psoriasis involves the face and the intertriginous areas then low strength corticosteroids are used to avoid the side effects of potent steroids.

Intralesional steroids may be used in persistent, hypertrophied, localised patch of psoriasis in a concentration of 5 mg/ml, usually one injection produces clearing at the site of injection. Intralesional steroids may cause atrophy of the skin, which disappears in a few months.

Foam delivery system of betamethasone helps in rapid absorption.

Topical vitamin D_3 derivatives (Calciprotriol 50 µg/g cream, ointment or lotion, calcitriol 3 µg/g, and tacalcitol 4 µg/g): These drugs induce differentiation and suppress proliferation of keratinocytes. Calcipotriol is applied once or twice daily, and tacalcitol once daily, for about 6 weeks. It can cause irritation, erythema and allergic contact dermatitis. Tachyphylaxis does not occur and there is no risk of cutaneous atrophy. Excessive use may elevate the serum calcium levels. Calcipotriol can be used up to 100 g/week (40% of the body surface on a twice daily basis), and tacalcitol ointment up to 35 g/week (20% of the body surface on a once daily dose).

Calcipotriene should not be given with salicylic acid, as it is rapidly inactivated in an acid environment.

Tazarotene: Tazarotene 0.1% cream is a topical vitamin A derivative, also available as a gel 0.05%. Like calcipotriol, it is steroid sparing, but it is more irritating than calcipotriol. Tazarotene is not inactivated by ultraviolet B (UVB); it thins the stratum corneum allowing the skin to burn easily with UVB. UVB doses can be reduced by one third, if tazarotene is added to a course of phototherapy.

A combination of potent corticosteroids and calcipotriol or tazarotene is often effective, when monotherapy does not work. New ointments combine both corticosteroids and calcipotriol; these are effective and also reduce the irritability of vitamin D analogs. These are effective topical preparations.

Tacrolimus: Tacrolimus 0.1%, 0.03% ointment, and pimecrolimus 1% cream are topical immunomodulators, they inhibit calcineurin. They are ineffective in chronic plaque psoriasis as they do not penetrate the thick stratum corneum; but it is used for inverse psoriasis. Tacrolimus is more effective for atopic dermatitis.

Ultraviolet Light

It has long been known that ultraviolet light (UVL) clears psoriasis. Dead Sea has been a resort in the past for the treatment of psoriasis, due to the beneficial effects of UVL. Dead Sea is 400 meters below sea level; here UVB is absorbed, so the UVL is dominated by UVA, which helps to clear psoriasis.

More recently, "solarium lamps" have been used in the treatment of psoriasis. If carefully monitored the patients do not burn; it clears psoriasis in about 6 weeks. Both Goekerman's and Ingram's regimen use UVB for treatment.

Tar: Coal tar is a keratolytic and an antimitotic agent. It is a mixture of thousands of substances produced by destructive distillation of coal. Tar has a propensity to stain the skin and is messy to use. It may also photosensitise the skin, exacerbate acne and cause folliculitis. Tar is contraindicated in pustular or erythrodermic psoriasis, unstable psoriasis and psoriasis on the face, genitalia and flexures. Allergic contact dermatitis is rare. There are few reports of carcinoma at the site of local tar therapy especially when tar is combined with UVB therapy.

Geokerman regime: Crude coal tar is generally used in a concentration of 2–5%. It can be used up to a concentration of 10%. After a tar bath, crude coal tar 2–5% is applied to all affected areas and is left for about 7 hours each day. The tar is then removed by bathing and this is followed by a minimal erythema dose of UV radiation. Regular treatment over 2–3 weeks is required for a therapeutic response. However this treatment is for inpatients; or can be used in psoriatic outpatient centers where present. Goekerman's regimen produces long-term remissions.

Dithranol (Anthralin): It is the treatment of choice for plaque psoriasis. It has irritating and staining properties, staining is due to the oxidation of dithranol to a purplish-brown dye. Dithranol paste is not suitable in unstable psoriasis and on face, flexures and genitalia. It is unstable and is stabilised by addition of salicylic acid. For best effects, the paste should be stiff to prevent spread to the normal skin; Lassar's paste forms a good vehicle.

Ingram's regimen was introduced in 1916 and is effective in dealing with extensive and resistant psoriasis. After a tar bath and UVB therapy in suberythemal dose, diathranol is applied to all involved areas in a concentration of 0.1–0.8%. This treatment is repeated daily and clearing of psoriatic lesions is achieved within 3 weeks. Discolouration of treated skin is reversible, but the staining of linen is permanent.

Routine anthralin therapy: 0.1% anthralin is applied to all psoriatic plaques daily at bedtime. The therapy is continued until the lesions clear and then taper the application.

Short contact therapy: 0.5–3% dithranol is applied to the psoriatic plaques. After 30–60 minutes, dithranol is removed by bathing or washing. This therapy is based on the principle that when dithranol is applied to psoriatic skin, considerable amount is retained in scaly plaques even after washing. Treatment is repeated daily until the lesions clear.

Narrowband UVB: Long wavelength of UVB have good penetration, they are anti-inflammatory and antiproliferative. The more carcinogenic shorter waves are avoided. Narrowband UVB suppresses the production of interferon (IFN)-γ, and interleukin (IL) 2, and increases the production of IL 4 and IL 10, which together could account for the shift of the immune response in the direction of T helper (Th) 2 like responses. The shift from an IFN-γ-dominated Th 1 to an IL 4-dominated Th 2 response appears to be one of the major factors determining the therapeutic efficacy of narrowband UVB phototherapy.

Narrowband UVB is a popular method of treating psoriasis; it is used to treat all forms of psoriasis except pustular psoriasis.

Psoralen plus UVA (PUVA) radiation: PUVA is most often used with oral 8 methoxypsoralen (MOP), topical 8 MOP can also be used. Standard oral dose of 8 MOP is 0.6 mg/kg of body weight and this is followed after 2 hours by UVA irradiation. The dosage of UVA radiation is calculated according to patient's skin type (I to VI). Alternatively, treatment is started with 1J/cm^2 and increments of 0.5–1.5 J/cm^2 are made at intervals of not less than a week, depending on the patient's response. This treatment is given 2–4 times weekly. When the lesions have cleared, the patient is kept on maintenance therapy; the frequency of treatment is gradually reduced to once every 1–4 weeks. Prior to the therapy, routine laboratory tests and the eye examination should be done. Eye protection with UVA opaque goggles is necessary during therapy and UVA blocking glasses should be worn during the rest of the day as psoralens are deposited in the lens of the eye.

After the initial clearing phase of psoriasis, patients require a minimum of 30 treatments/ year for the first one and half years.

PUVA is indicated in extensive psoriasis vulgaris, in patients over 50 years that are not responding to the conventional topical therapy. For pustular and erthrodermic forms of disease, methotrexate and retinoids are considered to be better than PUVA therapy.

Contraindications to the use of PUVA include pregnancy, children, photosensitivity, cataract or aphakia, cardiovascular, renal and hepatic disease. In addition, any previous cutaneous malignancy and history of exposure to arsenic or radiotherapy contraindicate this form of therapy. The common side effects include erythema, sunburn, pruritus, pigmentation, hypertrichosis, hepatotoxicity, gastrointestinal disturbances, premature cataract formation and carcinogenic hazard. There are reports of increased incidence of Bowen's disease, keratoacanthoma, and squamous cell carcinoma in patients on long-term PUVA therapy.

PUVA therapy can also be used with topical psoralens. Both 8 methoxy-psoralen and trimethylpsoralen have been used topically in baths or in a cream base.

A combination of PUVA with retiniods (RE-PUVA) reduces the duration of treatment and the total UVA dose. Acitretin is given in a dose of 0.6–1 mg/kg of body weight about 2 weeks before starting the PUVA therapy. Treatment is continued for 4–8 weeks, and then the dose of acitretin is decreased to 0.3 mg/kg of body weight and PUVA is then either stopped or used alone. The duration of the remissions is prolonged if retinoids were given as maintenance therapy.

Growing evidence of the increased risk of nonmelanoma skin cancer associated with a high dose of long-term PUVA, means that a maintenance therapy is now not recommended. Upper life time limit of UVA is 1000 J/cm^2. A combination of retinoids with PUVA, reduces the number of treatments, improves the efficacy of PUVA and decreases the long-term risk of malignancy of PUVA.

Balneophototherapy: This is a combination of selective UVL therapy with a prior bath with 5–10% table salt, or a solution simulating ocean water. The method is based on treatment of psoriasis at Dead Sea and other health spas.

Tar and dithranol should not be used in unstable psoriasis and psoriasis of the face, genitalia and the flexures.
UVL is not used for treatment of scalp psoriasis, as UVL does not penetrate through the scalp hair
UVL treatments should not be used on the face, because of photoageing
PUVA is used to treat severe forms of psoriasis
In young patients PUVA can cause increased photodamage and increase the lifetime risk of skin cancer
Goeckerman's and Ingram's regimen are good for long-term remissions

Lasers: Excimer and pulsed dye lasers can also be used for localised plaque psoriasis.

Systemic Therapy

While topical therapy will control a great majority of psoriatic patients, a small proportion will require systemic treatment. The choice generally lies between methotrexate, retinoids, fumaric acid esters and PUVA. These drugs should only be considered after a trial of topical therapy has failed. None of the systemic drugs is safe for women in the childbearing age without adequate oral contraception. The aim of systemic therapy is to control the disease rather than to achieve complete clearance. After this is achieved, appropriate topical therapy should be continued. To minimise long-term toxicity of drugs a rotational therapy of drugs may be effective and treatment continued for many years.

Biologics are used to treat difficult and recalcitrant cases of psoriasis.

Methotrexate: Methotrexate is a folic acid antagonist; it is also an immunosuppressive drug that inhibits the chemotaxis of polymorphonuclear leukocytes. Methotrexate is indicated in extensive and resistant plaque psoriasis, erythrodermic psoriasis, pustular psoriasis and psoriatic arthritis. Contraindications to the use of methotrexate include disease of renal, hepatic, haematopoietic system, pregnancy, lactation, alcoholism, gastric ulcers and unreliable patients. Before starting methotrexate renal, haematologic and hepatic functions must be assessed. These investigations should also be performed periodically during the therapy. Liver biopsy is mandatory after a cumulative dose of 1.5 g. Serum level of amino-terminal polypeptide of type III procollagen is a marker for hepatic fibrosis.

Methotrexate is given in a dose of 0.2–0.4 mg/kg of body weight every 7–14 days. The total dose is divided into three parts and is given at 12 hours interval. Clinical response is obtained in 1–2 weeks. The maximal response may take up to 8 weeks. Do not exceed the maximum dose of 30 mg/week. The common side effects include bone marrow suppression, hepatic fibrosis and cirrhosis, oligospermia, teratogenicity, anagen alopecia, pulmonary fibrosis, gastrointestinal irritation, depression and psychosis. Long-term toxicity is manifested by cough and shortness of breath.

Folic acid supplements are given to patients on methotrexate therapy. Increase in mean corpuscular volume of RBCs is a useful indicator of folate deficiency and impending toxicity.

Acitretin: Acitretin is the active carboxylated metabolite of etretinate. It is rapidly eliminated from the body and is 50 times less lipophilic than etretinate. Some of acitretin gets re-esterified into etretinate. This necessitates that pregnancy should be avoided in women up to 2 years after stoppage of acitretin.

Acitretin is given in a dosage of 0.25–1 mg/kg body weight. A therapeutic effect occurs after 2–4 weeks and maximum benefit after 6 weeks. It is indicated in extensive and resistant psoriasis vulgaris, generalised pustular psoriasis and erythrodermic psoriasis.

Contraindications to the use of acitretin include pregnancy, children, hyperlipidemia, and active liver disease. The most serious side effects is the teratogenic potential of retinoids and contraceptive precautions should be taken 1 month prior to and during therapy, for 2 years after discontinuing treatment. Acitretin also causes hyperlipidemia, generalised pruritus, diffuse alopecia, cheilitis, skeletal changes, and dryness of skin and mucosae. It can be used along with PUVA, and UVB.

Concomitant therapy with tetracyclines and corticosteroids increases the risk of intracranial pressure. Caution should be taken when prescribing other drugs that raise serum lipids such as thiazide diuretics and corticosteroids. It increases methotrexate plasma concentrations and the risk of hepatotoxicity. Acitretin probably antagonises the action of warfarin.

Cyclosporin: Cyclosporin is the T helper cell suppressant. It is given in a dose of 3–5 mg/kg daily in two divided doses. Maintenance doses should be reduced to the minimum, which allows adequate control. Do not exceed the maximum dose of 5 mg/kg. The major side effects associated with cyclosporin are dose-dependent hypertension and nephrotoxicity. Cyclosporin affects the renal blood flow and is toxic to renal cells. It is indicated only as a crisis therapy or when other drugs have failed. Regular monitoring is important during the therapy especially of blood pressure, serum creatinine and liver function tests. Contraindications to the use of cyclosporin include pregnancy, lactation, renal dysfunction, hepatic diseases, past or present malignancy, history of epilepsy, acute infection, hypertension, alcoholism and unreliable patients. PUVA and UVB therapy should not be used with cyclosporin because of immunosuppression and chances of malignancy are high.

Cyclosporin is used for rapid control of psoriasis, followed by transition to other methods. Numerous drug interactions occur with concomitant use of NSAIDs, cimetidine, macrolide antibiotics, ketoconazole; rhabdomyolysis occurs with HMG-Co A reductase inhibitors. The drug is safe to use in pregnancy.

Systemic corticosteroids: These are not indicated for routine cases of psoriasis. The most serious side effects associated with the withdrawal of steroid therapy is the rebound phenomenon, which takes the form of widespread and eruptive psoriasis. Steroids are only indicated in uncontroled erythrodermic psoriasis with metabolic complications, pustular psoriasis of pregnancy and acute episodes of psoriasis arthropathy, for a short-term period.

Fumaric acid esters: These are popular in Germany; they can be used for all forms of psoriasis, including inverse psoriasis, pustular psoriasis and psoriatic arthritis. The drug is anti-inflammatory. The clinical response is slow; it comes as the dose is gradually increased. There is no cumulative toxicity. The initial dose of fumaderm (containing 30 mg of dimethyl fumarate), is one tablet at night, gradually building it up to one tablet three times a day, and then to two tablets three times a day. Then fumaderm tablets (containing 120 mg of dimethyl fumarate) are introduced, starting with one tablet at night and then slowly increasing the dose to three times a day.

Side effects of the fumarates are diarrhaea, flushing, leucopenia, lymphopenia, proteinurea and renal toxicity.

The white blood cells (WBCs) count falls in almost all cases, but there is no risk of increased infection. The drug should be monitored for WBC counts, lymphocytes, creatinine, eosinophils and proteinurea. Liver and renal functions should also be monitored. If the WBC count falls below 4,000/μL, lymphocytes below 500/ μL, creatinine more than 30% of initial value and eosinophils more than 25% for more than 6 weeks; then the dose should be reduced to the tolerant level. If problems persist then the medication should be stopped.

Mycophenolate mofetil (MMF): MMF is the ester of mycophenolic acid. It inhibits purine synthesis by inhibiting the enzyme inosine monophospahte dehydrogenase. It induces apoptosis of activated T cells; it also decreases the recruitment of lymphocytes and induces immune tolerance. MMF is best suited for individuals in whom other systemic immune-therapies are contraindicated because of hypertension, impaired renal functions and liver disease.

Dose is 1 g twice daily.

Neutrophil counts should be done frequently, as severe neutropenia is seen in 2% of patients.

Lefluonomide: Lefluonomide inhibits pyrimidine synthesis; it inhibits T cell proliferation and production of autoantibodies by B cells. The drug is contraindicated in patients with liver disease.

Dose 100 mg once daily for 3 days and continued with 10–25 mg daily.

Biologic Therapy for Psoriasis

Psoriasis is driven by activated T memory cells; many biological agents are available to selectively target the immune system. Biological agents are proteins that can be synthesised by using recombinant DNA techniques (genetic engineering). Biological agents bind to specific cells, and modulate cytokine production. They do not have multiple adverse effects as seen with other drugs. The potential for interaction with other drugs is also very low. The risk of immunosuppression is unlikely to be worse than other commonly used dermatological drugs. Long-term effects of immunosuppression are yet to be studied; malignancies of the lymphatic system are reported with some.

T cell inhibitors: Alefacept is a fusion protein that binds to T cells expressing CD2. It inhibits T cell activation and induces apoptosis of memory T cells. Alefacept reduces the population of these cells in the circulation. Patients remain in remission for weeks or months after treatment.

Dose: 10–15 mg IM or IV injection weekly for 12 weeks.
The other biological agents that act against T cells are daclizumab and basiliximab.

Efalizumab which was approved by FDA in 2003 was withdrawn in 2009 due to adverse effects such as leukoencephalopathy caused by a fatal viral infection.

Tumour necrosis factor-α inhibitors: Etanercept is a fusion protein that acts against TNF-α and β

Etanercept is given by subcutaneous injection 25 mg twice weekly.

Infliximab is a chimeric monoclonal antibody that acts against TNF-α.

Dose: 5 mg/kg given intravenously. Three doses are given over 6 weeks, and every 8 weeks for maintenance.

The other TNF-α inhibitors are adalimumab and golimumab.

Inhibitors of leukotrienes. IL12, IL17 and IL 23: Ustekinumab was approved by the US Food and Drug Administration (FDA) for the treatment of psoriasis in 2009. It blocks IL 12 and IL 23, immune system proteins linked to inflammation. It is given by subcutaneous injection (45 mg) twice in the first month; and then 45 mg every 12 weeks. This results in approximately five treatments in 1 year. The dose may have to be increased to 90 mg for patients who weigh above 100 kg. Secukinumab targets IL17A and Apremilast, a phosphodiesterase 4 inhibitor, is a new oral agent for the treatment of moderate severe plaque psoriasis. It reduces production of multiple cytokines involved in the pathogenesis of psoriasis.

Janus Kinase inhibitors are promising potential therapeutic options for psoriasis.

No biologics are currently approved for use in children.

The other drugs that may be used in psoriasis are hydroxyurea, sulphasalazine, dapsone, liarozole, colchicine and somatostatin. Photodynamic therapy and excimer lasers have also been used in the treatment of psoriasis.

Treatment of Scalp Psoriasis

Many of the topical preparations are not suitable mainly because it is difficult to wash them out of the scalp or it may irritate the surrounding skin. Tar containing shampoos should be used daily or two or three times a week, depending upon the severity of psoriasis. Tar lotions may be rubbed at night and washed the following morning.

As the scales are thick and heaped up, it is preferable to use a coconut oil based tar and salicylic acid pomade overnight for 2–3 days; this will soften the scale to allow a corticosteroid scalp lotion or gel to be substituted. Salicylic acid mixed with steroid ointment can also be used. Steroid lotion mixed with equal parts of liquid petrolatum is used for milder cases. Baker's solution (phenol, sodium chloride and liquid paraffin) can also be used for removal of scales. This is applied at night and washed in the morning. A shower cap enhances penetration. Diffuse thick psoriatic scalp can also be treated by short-term anthralin therapy.

Once the scales are removed potent topical steroid gels, lotion or foam preparations are applied.

Treatment of Psoriatic Arthropathy

The treatment of psoriatic arthropathy is the same as that of rheumatoid arthritis. In mild form salicylates should be given, nonsteroidal anti-inflammatory agents such as ibuprofen, indomethacin and phenylbutazone may be given in severe cases. Methotrexate or cyclosporin can be used when other methods have failed. In fulminating arthritis, systemic steroids in small doses of less than 7.5 mg daily are given. Some of the newer biologic agents can be used as in rheumatoid arthritis in resistant cases.

Treatment of Pustular Psoriasis

Treatment of acute generalised pustular psoriasis needs admission, removal of provocative factors and general supportive measures. Tar and dithranol should be withdrawn immediately. Initial treatment should be conservative with bed rest, mild sedation and bland applications (potassium permanganate, 1% gentian violet), protein and fluid replacement. In many cases this promotes spontaneous reversion to erythrodermic psoriasis or even psoriasis vulgaris. If no improvement occurs then systemic treatment with IV methotrexate is regarded as the first choice. Oral therapy is less predictable because of variable absorption. Treatment of localised pustular psoriasis is often frustrating for both the physician and the patient. Tar, diathranol and steroids are generally disappointing, PUVA using psoralen lotion or gel is the most effective treatment. Acitretin is another drug of choice in localised pustular psoriasis.

Treatment of Nail Psoriasis

Nail psoriasis is difficult to treat. These may show improvement when systemic therapy is used to treat psoriasis. Systemic therapies are seldom a first-line therapy for nail psoriasis. If systemic therapy does not show any response in nail disease or when nails are only affected in psoriasis then topical therapy is used as follows:

Topical treatment with high-potency corticosteroid solution or ointment under occlusion with cellophane wrap at bedtime can improve nail psoriasis. Prolonged occlusion (not to exceed 2 weeks) should be avoided. A combination of high-potency corticosteroid and calcipotriol may benefit some patients.

Topical 1% 5-fluorouracil solution or 5% cream applied twice daily to the matrix area for 6 months without occlusion improves pitting and subungual hyperkeratosis.

Intralesional triamcinolone acetonide suspension of 2.5 mg/ml into the proximal nailfold is very helpful for nail matrix psoriasis (pitting, ridging, and leukonychia). This medication may be administered every 4–6 weeks. The proximal nailfold is sprayed first with a refrigerant spray for anaesthesia, and the injection is given with a 30-gauge needle.

Systemic therapy with acitretin, methotrexate, cyclosporin and PUVA may be used if topical therapy fails. Both oral and topical PUVA therapies have improved nail psoriasis in 3–6 months. A possible adverse effect of PUVA may be nail discolouration.

Avulsion therapy by chemical or surgical means can be used as an alternative therapy for psoriatic nail disease. Chemical avulsion therapy includes the use of urea ointment to the affected nail under occlusion for 7 days, the nail becomes soft and it is removed atraumatically. Chemical avulsion therapy is painless, involves no blood loss, and is less expensive than surgical avulsion.

Surgical avulsion therapy can be performed for psoriatic nail disease when other treatments have failed.

Rotation of Treatment

Rotational therapy minimises risk to the patient with severe psoriasis requiring systemic treatment. Changing between different compounds, with respect to individual risk factors, such as cumulative dose of methotrexate, exposures to UVL in PUVA therapy, kidney function in cyclosporine, etc. should be kept in mind while prescribing systemic drugs. Rotation of treatment reduces these risk factors.

Course and Prognosis

The course of psoriasis is unpredictable as it was 150 years ago. There is a tendency of disease to persist and recur. Rarely the patient may remain completely free of the disease, for many years. Guttate psoriasis has a better prognosis than the other types. Erythrodermic and pustular psoriasis carry a greater mortality and psoriasis arthritis has a considerable morbidity.

Earliest description of psoriasis is found in "Corpus Hippocratum". Hippocrates used the terms psora and lepra for the condition he recognised as psoriasis.
Heinrich Auspitz (1835–1886): was a brilliant pupil of Hebra. The terms parakeratosis and acanthosis were introduced into pathology by Auspitz. He also called attention to the bleeding points in psoriasis, which is named after him.

LICHEN PLANUS

Lichen planus is a papulosquamous disorder, which involves the skin and mucous membranes. It is characterised by the appearance of papules that are polygonal, plane topped, purplish coloured and usually highly pruritic. The appearance of lichen planus is similar to that of a scurfy, finely furrowed, dry excrescence of symbiotic vegetation known as lichen.

Lichen planus is a relatively common disorder with a worldwide distribution. It is most common between the ages of 30 years and 60 years. The incidence varies considerably; generally, it is present in about 0.1–1.2% of the population. Lichen planus has also been reported in families and in monozygotic twins.

Aetiology and Pathogenesis

The exact cause is unknown. The disease is probably immunologically mediated. Cell-mediated immunity is involved, T cells are found in the lesional skin of lichen planus. The basic process is thought to be an immunological attack on the basal layer. The presence of inflammatory cells and other changes in the epidermis are believed to be secondary events. However, the nature of the antigen remains obscure; it could be a metal, bacteria, fungi, virus or drugs. Langerhans cells are increased in early lesions and are probably involved in processing and presentation of the antigen to the lymphocytes. The dermis is largely infiltrated by T lymphocytes. Both CD4 and CD8 cells are found in the lesional skin of lichen planus. Progression of the disease may lead to the accumulation of CD8 cells. These cells are said to be responsible for the most characteristic change in lichenoid reactions namely apoptosis. The epithelial lymphocyte interaction can be divided in to three major stages: antigen recognition, lymphocyte activation and keratinocyte apoptosis.

Immunofluorescence shows a dense ragged band of fibrin and fibrinogen at the dermo-epidermal junction with clumps of IgM, IgA, IgG and complement deposits.

A genetic predisposition is suggested by the occurrence of lichen planus in families. There is also an increased frequency of HLA B7 in patients of lichen planus.

Histopathology

The two basic histological features of lichen planus are damage to the basal cells and lichenoid-interface lymphocytic reaction. Damage to the basal cells is manifested in several ways:

- Normal columnar cells are rarely seen, the lowest cells of the epidermis often look like prickle cells and lymphocytes are present between them.
- Round and oval acidophilic bodies about the size of a basal cell are present within or below the epidermis (Civatte bodies, apoptotic cells).
- Occasionally the impression is gained that most of the rete ridges have been transformed into colloid bodies, leaving only a pointed saw-tooth appearance.
- Melanocytes are more or less absent or degenerating. Melanin granules are engulfed by the melanophages in the subepidermal region.

Because of the damage to the basal cells, the rate of mitosis is low; this leads to long retention of cells, leading to pseudoacanthosis (hypertrophy of the prickle cells), focal hypergranulosis and cohesiveness in the stratum corneum.

A band-like lymphocytic infiltrate of lymphocytes is seen in the papillary dermis that abuts the epidermis. Many histiocytes and a few plasma cells are also seen. Plasma cells are more prominent in the mucous membranes. Interspersed melanophages are also present. Focal separation of the dermis and the epidermis occurs; these form the Max Joseph spaces, which is a prominent feature in bullous lichen planus.

Clinico-Histological Correlation

- Lichen planus does not have an exfoliating scale, but an adherent horny layer
- Wickham's striae are due to varying thickness of the granular layer
- Keratohyalin granules reflect and diffuse light; they also influence the transmission of the colour of blood, causing a bluish tinge. This and deposition of melanin below the epidermis give rise to the violaceous hue of the disease
- Scraping of a lesion of lichen planus produces subepidermal haemorrhage known as Brocq's phenomenon; this is analogous to the Auspitz sign in psoriasis. It is due to the increased vascularity in the subepidermal layer
- Scratching produces pain in lichen planus; so scratch marks are seldom seen inspite of the intense pruritus. This is because the free nerve endings are in the very layer that is affected by the inflammatory process.

Clinical Features

Lichen planus is characterised by shiny violaceous, polygonal flat papules varying in size from pinpoint to a centimeter or more across. The onset of the disease is usually insidious, but may be acute. White lines may be seen on the surface of these papules, known as Wickham's Striae. These striae are more prominent after applying oil or water and then examining the lesion with magnifying lens. In the active phase of the disease, linear lesions may be seen along the scratch marks due to Koebner's phenomenon. The sites of predilection are flexor aspects of wrist and forearm, back of hands, ankles, shins and lower back. Prutitus is also a consistent feature of LP, but may be absent. It is generally related to the extent of involvement. Pruritus is more intense in generalised lichen planus. Spontaneous resolution of lichen planus is common in about 18 months. Chronicity is seen in hypertrophic LP and ulcerative oral lesions (Fig. 9).

Involvement of the mucous membrane is seen in 30–70% cases and can occur without skin lesions. Oral mucosa is most commonly affected, but lesions may be found on genitalia, anus, larynx, bladder, conjunctiva, gastrointestinal tract and nasal mucous membrane. Reticulate white streaks on the buccal mucosa are very characteristic, but ulcerative lesions can also occur in the oral cavity. There is a risk of developing carcinoma with the ulcerative form of LP. On the tongue, the lesions appear as a fixed white plaque (Figs 10A and B).

Nail involvement is seen in 10% cases. The nail changes include thinning, longitudinal ridging, pterygium, distal splitting of the nail plate (onychoschizia), partial or complete destruction of nails (Fig. 11).

Lichen planus of the scalp: Lichen planopilaris or follicular lichen planus may affect the scalp. Individual papules of lichen planus coalesce on the scalp to form plaques and patches of atrophy. Perifollicular erythema and acuminate keratotic plugs are commonly seen. Lesions of the skin, nails and mucous membrane may also be present, helping in the diagnosis. The end stage of the disease is scarring alopecia.

The typical papules of LP on the skin may be associated with patches of cicatricial alopecia on the scalp known as pseudopelade.

Palmoplantar lichen planus: This presents as very pruritic, erythematous plaques on the soles, the lesions are usually seen on the internal plantar arch. Yellowish keratotic papules or nodules are seen on the lateral margins of the fingers, and surface of the palms. The lesions appear like callosities, but have an erythematous halo. The lesions are less likely to affect the fingertips. The ulcerative form of lichen planus on the palms and soles is very painful and difficult to heal; the nails may be lost permanently (Figs 12A and B).

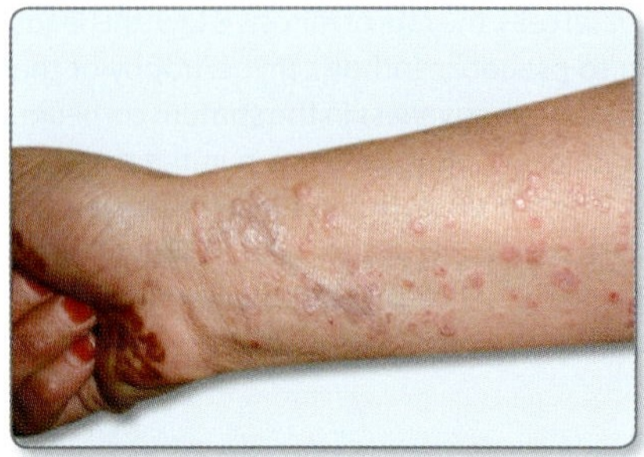

Fig. 9: Lichen planus

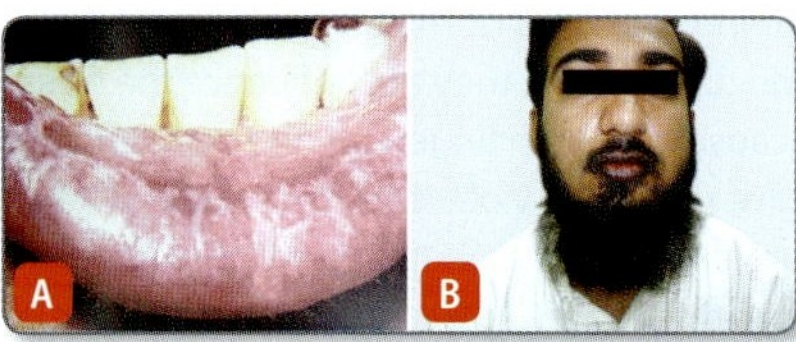

Figs 10A and B: (A) Lichen planus of the lips—reticulate white streaks; (B) Lichen planus of the lips—plaque form

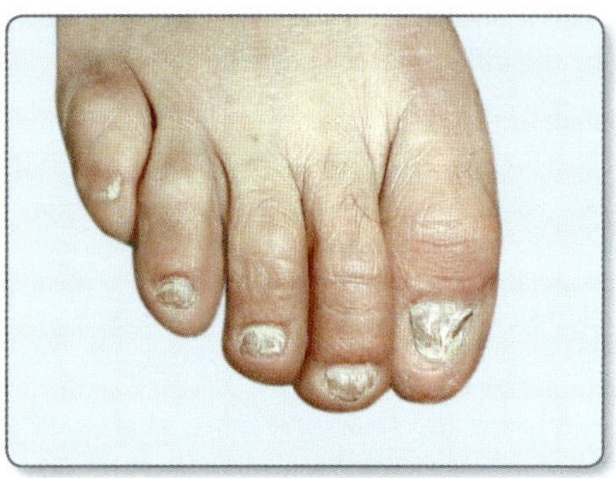

Fig. 11: Lichen panus—nails

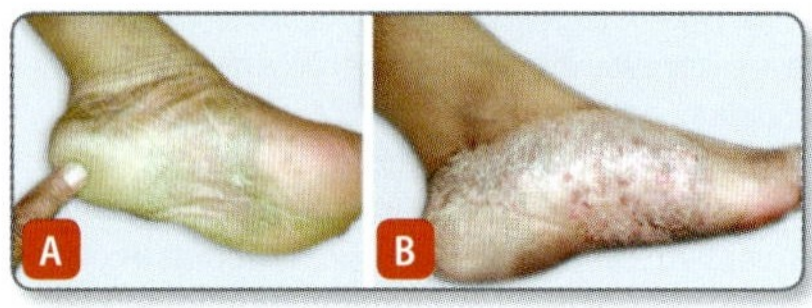

Figs 12A and B: (A) Plantar lichen planus; (B) Lichen planus—erosive

Variants of Lichen Planus

Hypertrophic Lichen Planus

This is characterised by firm, rough, verrucous, highly pruritic plaques which may be single or multiple. The sites of predilection are shins and ankles. The lesions may be symmetrical and lichenified. This type of LP has a chronic course and heals with scarring or pigmentation (Fig. 13).

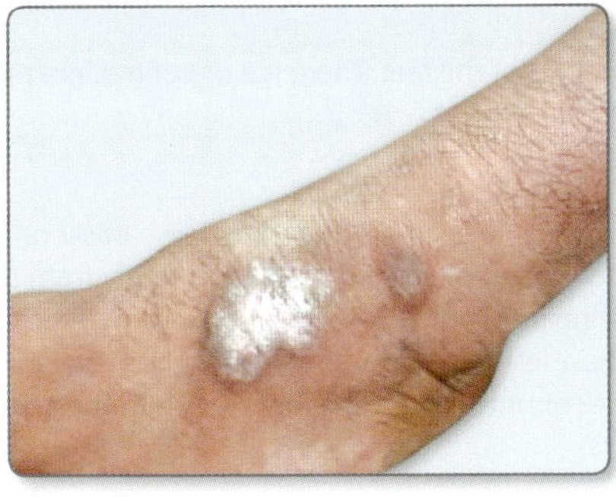

Fig. 13: Hypertrophic lichen planus

Lichen Planopilaris (Follicular Lichen Planus)

Spiny follicular papules are seen usually with typical lesions of LP. The common sites are the abdomen and medial aspect of the proximal extremities. Follicular lesions on the scalp lead to scarring alopecia. The triad of follicular lichen planus of the skin, cicatricial alopecia of the scalp and nonscarring alopecia of the axillary and pubic area is known as Graham-Little-Picardi syndrome. Lichen planopilaris should be differentiated from lichen spinulosus, Darier's disease, follicular mucinosis and lichen scrofulosorum.

Lichen Planus Actinicus

This is common in tropical and subtropical areas. Lesions occur on the exposed areas of the skin, creating patches of hyperpigmentation surrounded by a striking hypopigmented zone (Fig. 14).

Annular LP

These lesions have a narrow rim of activity with slightly atrophic centre. Annular lesions are characteristically found on the penis in the males. This type of LP must be distinguished from granuloma annulare.

Atrophic LP

The lesions are few in number and may result from resolved hypertrophic or annular lesions. The histology at this stage is not specific. The lesions resemble lichen sclerosus, however the histology is characteristic.

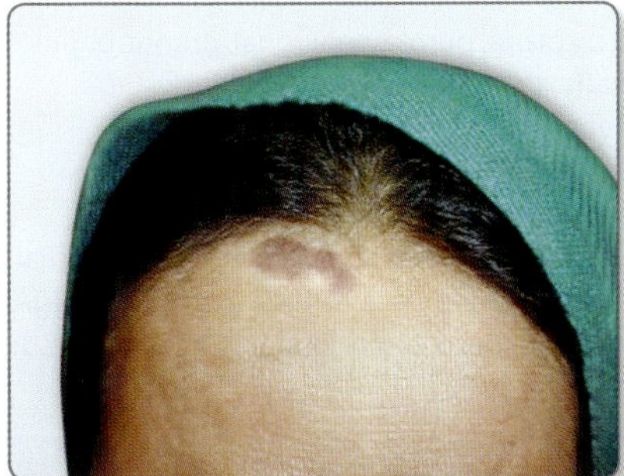

Fig. 14: Actinic lichen planus

Ulcerative (Erosive) LP

This may involve vulva, mouth or soles of the feet. There is a risk of malignant transformation in this type of LP.

Bullous LP

This type of LP is usually seen on lower legs and is due to extreme basal cell vacuolation. The bullae arise from the papules of lichen planus, rarely from a normal appearing skin. Bullae arising from normal skin are more characteristic of lichen planus pemphigoides. These lesions can be differentiated from bullous lichen planus by direct and indirect immunofluorescence. Bulllae in the oral cavity can lead to painful erosions.

Lichen Planus Pigmentosus

This variant is characterised by macular hyperpigmentation of the sun-exposed areas and the flexures. It spares the mucous membranes, palms and soles. This variant of lichen planus bears striking resemblance to ashy dermatosis or erythema dyschromicum perstans. It is common in Latin Americans and dark-skinned people.

Invisible LP

In this rare entity lesions of lichen planus cannot be seen by the naked eye under visible light, but become apparent under Wood's lamp examination. The only symptom is pruritus and the biopsy will show lichenoid histology.

Lichen Planus-Like Eruptions

Lichenoid eruption may be caused by a number of drugs or other chemical agents, such as thiazide diuretics, heavy metals (gold, bismuth), chloroquine, mepacrine, methyldopa, streptomycin, phenothiazine, β-blockers, para-aminosalicylic acid, quinidine and photocolour developers. In treating a case of lichen planus, a drug history should always be taken. Lichenoid stomatitis has been reported from lithium carbonate. Lichenoid eruption is also seen in graft-versus-host disease. Lichenoid drug eruptions are usually larger and scaly, it fails to exhibit classic Wickham's striae. Mucous membrane involvement is rare. The eruptions usually appear symmetrically on the trunk and extremities, unlike the flexural distribution of lichen planus. The latency for the appearance of the rash after drug intake varies from months to a year.

Diagnostic Features of Lichen Planus

- Lichen planus is characterised by plane, purple, polygonal, pruritic papules
- These are chiefly found on the flexors of the wrist and ankles
- Wickham's striae may be present
- Oral mucosa involved in 50% of cases
- Koebner's phenomenon present in active disease
- Direct immunofluorescence shows numerous apoptotic cells at the dermal-epidermal junction, staining with IgM and occasionally with IgG and IgA. Deposition of fibrinogen at the dermal-epidermal junction is characteristic of lichen planus

- Characteristic histological features are:
  - Hyperkeratosis
  - Focal hypergranulosis
  - Irregular pseudoacanthosis
  - Liquefactive degeneration of the basal layer
  - Band like upper dermal lymphocytic infiltrate
  - Incontinence of melanin
  - Colloid bodies present
  - Small separations between the epidermis and the dermis (Max-Joseph's Spaces)

Differential Diagnosis

Hypertrophic lichen planus must be differentiated from lichenified eczema on the legs, unless there are features of lichen planus elsewhere, it may be difficult to distinguish the two disorders. The papules of lichen planus may be found around the lichenified patch. Lichenoid drug eruption has a similar appearance; in these cases a drug history is very important. Lichenoid drug eruption displays the following features: parakeratosis, a normal granular layer, eosinophils and plasma cells in the inflammatory infiltrate. Inflammation is also more likely to be perivascular in contrast to band like in lichen planus, the inflammation is around middle and deep vascular plexus. Lichenoid drug reactions are often larger and scaly, Wickham's striae are usually absent, and mucous membrane involvement is less common, sun-exposed areas are more commonly involved. Guttate psoriasis may mimic widespread lichen planus, psoriasis is more erythematous and silvery scales are present. The papulosquamous lesions of secondary syphilis are not itchy and show a predilection for the palms and soles, there is generalised micro-lymphadenopathy especially of the posterior cervical and epitrochlear lymph nodes, condylomas on the genital areas may be present. A serological test for syphilis may be required. The white streaks on the buccal mucosa should be distinguished from candidiasis and leukoplakia; severe erosions in the oral cavity may mimic pemphigus.

Treatment

The treatment of LP is mainly symptomatic. Pruritus can be relieved by menthol, phenol, and camphor preparations, doxepin hydrochloride or lidocaine cream. Sedating antihistamines are helpful at bedtime.

Corticosteriods are the most effective agents in the treatment of LP. Potent fluorinated topical steroids are beneficial in most cases. Short-term occlusion is recommended for persistent or hypertrophic lesions. Intralesional triamcinolone is effective for localised hypertrophic LP.

Systemic corticosteriods are indicated for erosive mucosal lesions, progressive nail destruction, and hair involvement causing cicatricial alopecia and generalised lichen planus. Prednisolone 15–30 mg daily for 6 weeks clears the lesions, which is then gradually tapered. However, the recurrence rate after the withdrawal is very high and a maintenance dose may be required until the disease goes into remission.

Isotretinoin 10 mg orally bid, acitretin 30 mg daily for 2 months can be used when steroids are ineffective.

Chloroquine 250 mg 2–3 times a week can be used in the treatment of actinic lichen planus.

Other therapies for generalised LP are PUVA, narrow band UVB, cyclosporin 2–5mg/kg of body weight daily, azathioprine 1–3 mg/kg of body weight daily, griseofulvin 125 mg twice a day for 3–6 weeks. Levamisole 150 mg daily for two consecutive days per week, for 6 weeks.

In recalcitrant cases of lichen planus, methotrexate, cyclophosphamide and dapsone can be tried. Thalidomide has been used for erosive lichen planus.

Oral metronidazole 500 mg bid. for 1–2 months has shown good results in some patients with generalised LP.

Based on the benefit in bullous pemphigoid, combination therapy with tetracycline or doxycycline and nicotinamide, have been reported to be useful in the treatment of lichen planus pemphigoides.

Recent trials have shown the efficacy of pioglitazone hydrochloride in the treatment of lichen planus planopilaris. Primary cicatricial alopecia is said to be irreversible, but recent studies have found that the initial trigger of inflammation in the cause of these alopecia is abnormal functioning of peroxisome proliferator-activated receptor -γ (PPAR-γ). This leads to aberrant lipid metabolism in the sebaceous glands, a toxic build up of lipids, and a subsequent inflammatory response. Oral PPAR-γ agonist pioglitazone hydrochloride 15 mg/daily can inhibit the inflammatory process in lichen planopilaris. More studies are required to confirm these findings.

Oral Lichen Planus

Provocative factors such as spicy food, tobacco and alcohol should be avoided. Bland food should be substituted. Dental prosthesis should be tested, if found to be allergenic it should be removed. Intercurrent candidiasis should always be treated.

Triamcinolone in orabase should be applied 3–4 times a day for 2–4 weeks. Other topical preparations used are cyclosporin mouth washes and tacrolimus 0.1%. Intralesional corticosteroids can also be used.

In severe cases prednisolone 40–60 mg daily tapered over 3–6 weeks. Acitretin 25–50 mg daily is also effective. Treatment of oral lichen planus with 308 nm excimer laser has also shown clinical improvement.

If the eyes and other mucosal sires such as the oesophagus are involved cyclosporin, azathioprine or mycophenolate mofetil can be helpful.

Course and Prognosis

In most cases, the rash clears spontaneously leaving residual postinflammatory hyperpigmentation, which may take months to disappear. Scarring alopecia of the scalp is permanent.

Sir Erasmus Wilson first described lichen planus in 1869. Wickham described the characteristic striae in 1895 and Graham Little described the scalp involvement. The histological features were defined by Darier in 1909.
Sir Erasmus Wilson (1809–1884), was a pupil of Hebra. He described trichorrhexis nodosa, erythema nodosum, and assembled the various forms of lichen planus in one group.
He made a large fortune by his successful practice and by skilful investments, and since he had no family he devoted a great deal of his money to charitable and educational purposes.
Sir Erasmus Wilson is said to have brought the Egyptian obelisk called Cleopatra's Needle from Alexandria to London, where it was erected on the Thames Embankment.

LICHEN NITIDUS

This is a chronic inflammatory disorder characterised by pinpoint to pinhead sized, flesh coloured asymptomatic papules. The condition is usually seen on the penis, forearms, lower abdomen and inner side of the thighs. Pinkus first described lichen nitidus in 1901.

Aetiology

The exact cause of lichen nitidus is unknown. It is often said to be a variant of lichen planus and it often co-exists with the lesions of lichen planus. The lesions of lichen planus are very pruritic, they are purplish in colour, their distribution differs and there is absence of immunofluorescence in lichen nitidus. Others consider it an inflammatory granulomatous disease.

Histopathology

The histology is characteristic. The solitary dermal papillae are widened; these contain a dense infiltrate of lymphocytes, histiocytes, some Langhans giant cells and melanophages. The overlying epidermis is flattened, with liquefactive degeneration of the basal layer. A central area of parakeratosis is characteristic.

The rete ridges at the margins of the dermal papillae are elongated and tend to encircle it in a claw-like manner. The collagen and elastic fibres may be destroyed in the centre of the lesion.

Clinical Features

Lichen nitidus may be localised and discrete or generalised and confluent. In the discrete form the papules of lichen nitidus are flat topped, pinhead size and asymptomatic. They are flesh-coloured and shiny. The sites of predilection are the penis, wrists, forearms, lower abdomen and inner sides of the thigh. It often co-exists with lichen planus. It is a disease of children and young adults (Fig. 15).

In the generalised variety, lichen nitidus loses its papular appearance; it appears as reddish-yellow or brownish plaques, covered by fine scales. Primary papules may be seen at the periphery of the plaque. The palms and soles may be thickened, nails may show pitting, ridging or may be thickened. Minute grayish, flat papules are seen in the buccal mucous membrane.

The course is very unpredictable, spontaneous healing is seen in some cases, without any residual pigmentation. In some cases it persists for a long time.

Differential Diagnosis

The disease should be differentiated from lichen planus, lichen scrofulosorum and flat warts. Lichen planus is purplish in colour, it is very pruritic, its distribution and histology differentiates it. Lichen scrofulosorum is perifollicular; it is darker in colour and it is scalier. Warts are brownish in colour, their distribution is different and so is the histology.

Treatment

The disease is self-limiting and asymptomatic, usually no treatment is required. Some resistant cases can be treated with fluorinated steroids. The generalised variety can be treated with PUVA or acitretin. H_1 antihistamines have helped a few cases.

LICHEN STRIATUS

This is a unilateral linear eruption that appears suddenly on the extremities or the sides of the neck. The lesions are grouped papules that coalesce to form linear plaques. The lesions are said to develop along the lines of Blaschko. The condition is usually seen in children. Female to male ratio is 2:1. The papules are flat topped, lichenoid, purple or skin coloured, covered with greyish scales. The lesions often run for months, before spontaneous involution occurs.

The histology is like lichen planus; band like inflammation of lymphocytes in the dermis with overlying epidermal changes. The earliest epidermal change is intercellular oedema. Dyskeratotic keratinocytes are seen in 50% of cases. There

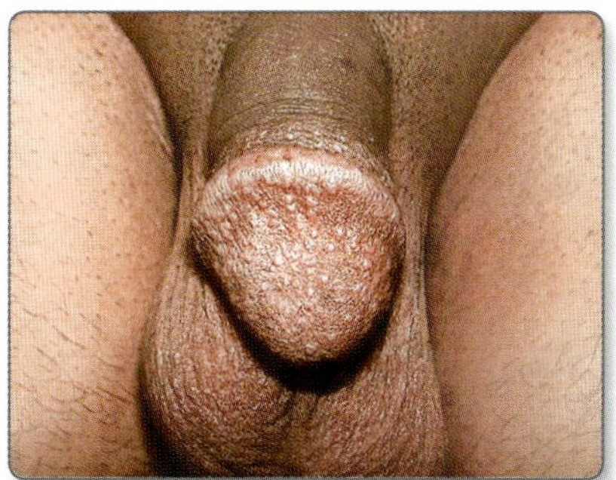

Fig. 15: Lichen nitidus

is focal liquefactive degeneration of the basal layer. The dermis is edematous with infiltration of lymphocytes and histiocytes around the blood vessels and appendages.

The condition should be differentiated from linear lichen planus, linear psoriasis, and linear epidermal nevus. No treatment is required as the lesion involutes spontaneously.

Nekam's Disease (Keratosis Lichenoides Chronica)

Papulonodular violaceous lesions on the extremities and buttocks characterise the disease, with seborrhoeic dermatitis like eruptions on the face. Lesions are often linear or reticulate. Mucous membrane, genitalia and nails may also be affected. The course is chronic and resistant to treatment. PUVA and calcipotriene have shown some benefit.

Localised Hyperkeratosis

Hyperkeratosis of the Palms and Soles

Palmoplantar keratoderma is characterised by excessive formation of keratin on the palms and soles. This may be congenital or acquired; it may accompany other diseases or may be a part of a syndrome.

Congenital palmoplantar keratodermas: The hereditary palmoplantar keratodermas have an early onset, it is usually present by infancy, and most have an autosomal dominant inheritance.

The Unna-Thost is the most common type of palmoplantar keratosis, there is a generalized thickening of the palms and soles, and epidermis is thick, yellow, viscous and horny. The uniform thickening may form a rigid plate; it ends abruptly at the periphery of the palms and soles. Hyperhidrosis is frequent that causes a sodden appearance. Occasionally there are associated changes; nails may become thick, opaque and malformed (Fig. 16).

Howell-Evans reported a diffuse keratoderma of the palms and soles occurring as an autosomal dominant trait, associated with carcinoma of the oesophagus. Skin lesions appear between the ages of 5 and 15 and carcinoma appeared between the 4 and 5th decade.

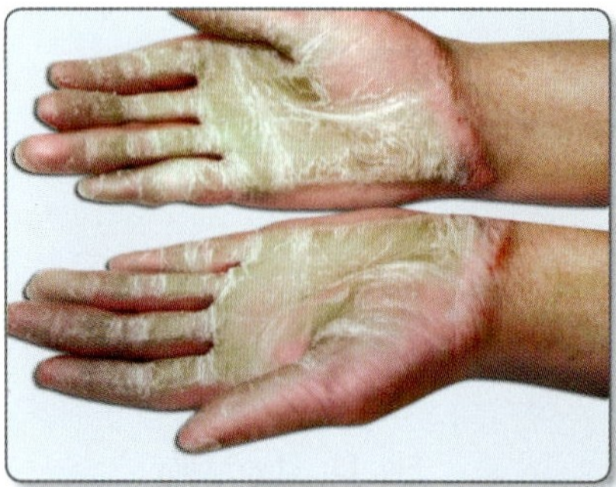

Fig. 16: Palmar keratoderma

Progressive type: These are other congenital types of palmoplantar keratodermas, some may spread over the dorsum of the hands and feet, as well as the elbows and knees it may be mutilating (Vohwinkel), with pseudoainhum formation.

Punctate keratosis: The keratosis is present as discrete firm, elevated papules on the palms and soles.

Striate palmoplantar keratoderma is characterised by linear hyperkeratotic plaques, which run through the length of the fingers onto the palms, it can be very disabling.

Papillon-Lefevre syndrome has an autosomal recessive inheritance; it is associated with mutation in cathepsin C gene, which is essential for neutrophil function. There is severe periodontosis affecting both the deciduous and the permanent teeth, resulting in the loss of both the deciduous and permanent teeth. Psoraisiform plaques are seen on the knees and elbows (Fig. 17).

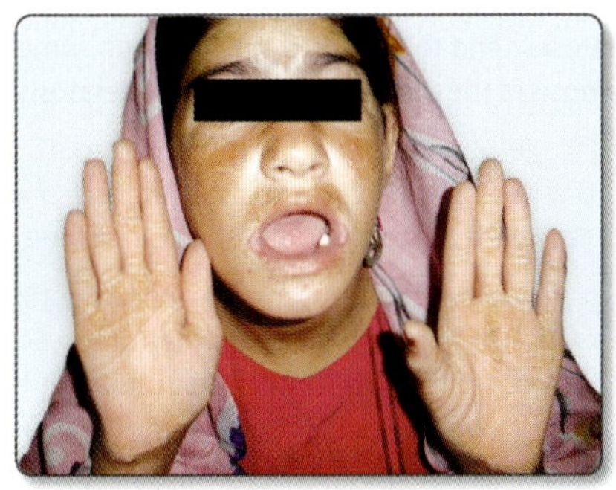

Fig. 17: Papillon-Lefevre syndrome

Mal de Meleda is an autosomal recessive skin disorder, with an onset in infancy. Clinical features include diffuse, thick keratoderma with a prominent erythematous border. Lesions spread onto the dorsum of the hands and the feet. Constricting bands are present around the digits and can result in spontaneous amputation. Well-circumscribed psoriasis like plaques or lichenoid patches may be present on the knees and the elbows. Patients may have hyperhidrosis, possibly accompanied by malodor. Secondary bacterial and fungal infections are common.

The congenital palmoplantar keratodermas should also be differentiated from other genodermatosis associated with palmoplantar keratosis, such as basal cell nevus syndrome, pachyonychia congenita, pityriasis rubra pilaris, ichthyosis, Darier's disease and dyskeratosis congenita.

Acquired palmoplantar keratodermas: The acquired palmoplantar keratodermas appear later in life, these may be due to psoriasis, eczema, fungal infections, lichen planus, Reiter's disease, arsenic keratosis, syphilis, yaws, etc. These keratoses can be diagnosed by the history and lesions at other sites.

Keratoelastoidosis marginalis: Linear plaques located symmetrically on the medial and lateral aspect of the fingers and thumbs. These are probably due to actinic damage, seen in people with repeated mechanical trauma.

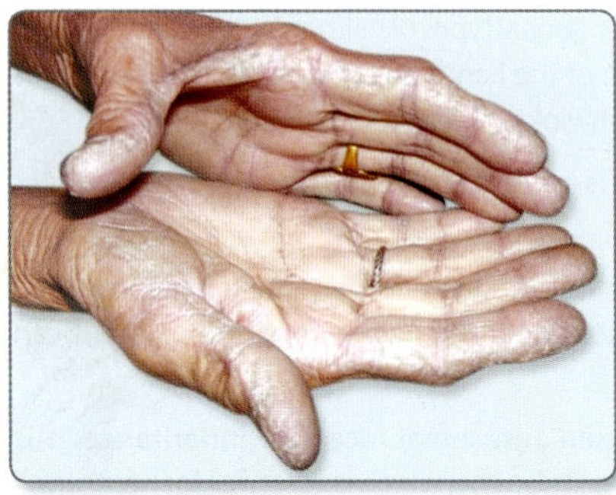

Fig. 18: Keratoelastoidosis marginalis
Source: Global Skin Atlas, Dr S Janjua

Histological examination shows degeneration of collagen, solar elastosis, calcification is characteristic and the epidermis is hyperkeratotic (Fig. 18).

Prognosis

The hereditary palmoplantar keratoses tend to be persistent, although some may improve later in life. The prognosis of the acquired palmoplantar keratosis depends upon the primary disease.

Treatment

Keratolytics are the only treatment. On the palms and soles the concentration of keratin is greater than elsewhere, and so the concentration of the keratolytic agents used locally on the palms and soles is higher. Salicylic acid up to 15% may be necessary or urea up to 20% may be used. Benzoic acid compound ointments are mild kerolytic and are useful in reducing fungal and bacterial growths and the resulting bad odour. In extreme cases, systemic treatment by acitretin may be considered. Long-term treatment with an antifungal agent such as itraconazole 100 mg daily is beneficial, when dermatophyte infection co-exists.

Emollients should be applied regularly

Treat the cause in acquired keratodermas.

Table 1 shows the difference between the common palmoplantar keratosis.

CALLOSITY AND CORN

The earliest known discussions of corns and callosities can be found in the writings of Cleopatra, who authored a textbook on cosmetics. Corns and calluses occur in response to chronic and mechanical or frictional forces applied to the skin, leading to thickening of the stratum corneum. Corns are formed when the mechanical forces are applied to a focal location. Calluses are formed when the frictional forces are applied over a wide area.

Heredity does not determine frictional dermatoses. Heredity does play a role in configuring the skeletal architecture. If there is a family history of abnormal bony architecture, it can be a site of corns or calluses.

Callosity

Callosity is a nonpenetrating area of greatly thickened skin, which occurs as a protective measure when intermittent pressure is distributed over a comparatively large area of the skin. At the periphery, cornified skin ceases abruptly, where it is continuous with the normal skin. Callosities appear

Table 1: Differential diagnosis of palmoplantar keratoses

Psoriasis	*Lichen planus*	*Hereditary palmoplantar keratoses*	*Contact dermatitis*	*Tinea manuum/Tinea pedis*
Lesions Sharply demarcated plaques with silvery-white scales or may be pustular in pustular psoriasis	Rough firm plaques with a yellowish hue, may be localized or diffuse	Generalised thickening of the palms and soles, with a yellowish hue; or may be punctate or glove stocking type	Erythema and scaling, generalised, localized or at the tip of the fingers	Interdigital, localised or maybe generalized
Age of onset Young adults	Young and middle age	Infancy	Adults usually housewives	Adults
Lesions at other sites Knees, elbows, lumbosacral areas	Wrist, ankle, oral cavity and penis	Absent, except in the progressive variety	Absent	Absent
Itching Usually absent	Very itchy	Absent	Itchy	Itching may be present
Histopathology Hyperkeratosis, parakeratosis, absence of granular layer, dilated dermal papillary blood vessels	Hyperkeratosis, liquefaction of the basal layer, band like infiltration of the dermo-epidermal junction with T cell lymphocytes	Hyperkeratosis	Hyperkeratosis and spongiosis	Hyphae present on microscopy
Nail changes Pitting, onycholysis, subungual hyperkeratosis	Thinning, pterygium formation	Thickening, yellowish in colour	Usually not affected, longitudinal striations and ridging when eczema is present near the nails	Usually not infected in tinea pedis, in onychomycosis the nails are yellowish thickened and friable

where the skin is normally thick, most frequently on the soles, beneath the heads of one or more of the metatarsal bones around the heels and along the beneath the inferomedial side of the great toe. Callosities appear as a yellowish thickening over which the dermatoglyphic markings are absent.

It is often seen due to ill-fitting shoes, abnormal gait or some anatomical abnormality of the foot. Prayer nodules may appear on the knees and ankles in Muslims, due to the squatting position adapted for worship. It may appear on the forehead, when it is touched on a prayer stone. On the hand, calluses mostly occur due to occupational reasons.

Corn

A hard corn occurs when intermittent pressure occurs over a very limited area. It consists of a conical wedge of hyperkeratosis that penetrates in the dermis, impinges on the nerve endings and causes pain. It is characterised by a central core of whitish appearance, this is composed of degenerated cells and cholesterol encircled by a narrow area of keratosis, this disappears gradually at the periphery. Palpation reveals a bony projection beneath the corn. Corns occur chiefly where the normal skin is thin, it is found particularly over the lateral surface of the fifth toe.

Interdigital corns are soft when it occurs deep between the fourth and the fifth toes. The softness is due to maceration of keratotic tissue. Interdigital corns can be hard when they are adjacent to the interdigital joints. Soft corns should be differentiated from interdigital candidiasis.

Due to the close proximity to joints and bone, septic arthritis and osteomyelitis can occur as a complication of corns and callosities. Mechanical forces that cause corns and calluses can also rupture the subcutaneous vessels, leading to haemorrhage in the hyperkeratotic tissue (Fig. 19).

Histopathology

Corns and callosities demonstrate changes in the epidermis, dermis and the subcutaneous tissue. There is epidermal hyperplasia, the stratum corneum is

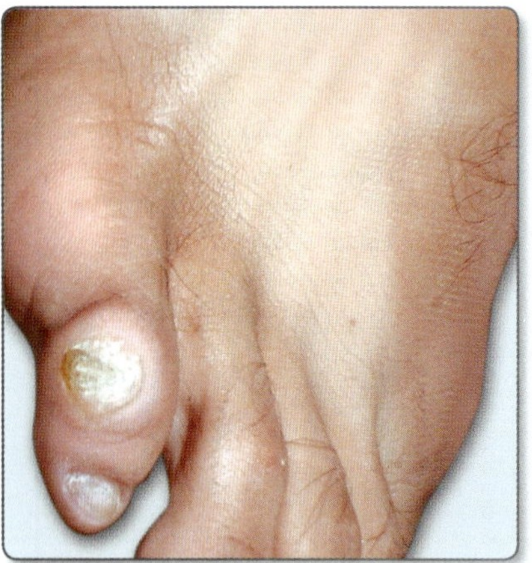

Fig. 19: Corn

thickened and parakeratotic over the dermal papillae, relative loss of stratum granulosum, atrophy of the malpighian layer. There is significant fibrosis in the dermis, with dilated eccrine glands and blood vessels, hypertrophied nerves and scar tissue replacement of subcutaneous tissue.

Treatment

Callosities require symptomatic relief by careful and regular paring. Salicylic acid 10–20% can be of some help. Footwear and the gait of the patient should be corrected. Any anatomical abnormalities if present should be treated.

Corns require a 40% salicylic acid plaster, this is applied for 48 hours, the plaster is then removed, the skin is cleaned and scraped and a new plaster is then applied. This procedure is repeated until the corn is cleared. Salicylic acid 16.7% and lactic acid 16.7% in a collodion base can also be applied; this is especially useful for soft corns. Soft corns also respond to biweekly infiltrations of a sclerosing solution of 4% alcohol mixed with a local anaesthetic. Table 2 shows the difference between corn and warts.

ACROKERATOSIS VERRUCIFORMIS

This is inherited as an autosomal dominant condition; the lesion may be present at birth or appears in early childhood, it may be delayed until the 5th decade.

Skin-coloured warty papules are present on the dorsum of the hands, feet, knees, elbows and the forearms. The palms may be diffusely thickened or show small keratoses. Transformation to squamous cell carcinoma has been reported. The nails may be thickened and white. Acrokeratosis verruciformis may be associated with basal cell carcinoma, congenital poikiloderma, steatocystoma multiplex and hypertrophic lichen planus.

Other frictional dermatoses are described in chapter 34.

Table 2: Difference between corn and warts

Warts	*Corns*
Site Anywhere on the palm or sole	Only on pressure points
Aetiology Viral	Due to abnormal intermittent pressure over a bony prominence
Painless, unless at pressure points	Painful
Infectious, usually in clusters	Not infectious, usually single
Histopathology Hyperkeratosis, koilocytes, acanthosis, prominent dermal capillary vessels which may be thrombosed	Hyperkeratosis, parakeratosis, increase in collagen fibres around neurovascular bundles. Absence of koilocyte
Gentle paring shows the bleeding points of thrombosed vessels	Thrombosed vessels absent
Usually resolves spontaneously within 6 months to a year	Does not resolve spontaneously unless the abnormal pressure is removed

Retinoids have been successful in the treatment of acrokeratosis verruciformis.

FOLLICULAR KERATOSES

These are a group of disorders in which abnormality of keratinisation involves the pilosebaceous follicles. Variable degrees of hyperkeratosis fill the follicular ostia; rupture of the follicular wall may result. Follicular keratosis is found in lupus erythematosus, follicular lichen planus, follicular psoriasis, follicular ichthyosis, pityriasis rubra pilaris, Darier's disease, keratosis pilaris, Kyrle's disease, lichen spinulosus, phrynoderma and keratosis cirumscripta.

Phrynoderma (Hypovitaminosis A)

The condition is due to deficiency of vitamin A; skin and eyes are mainly affected.

Cutaneous changes: Phrynoderma is characterised by hyperkeratosis of the hair follicle. The lesions consist of dry, firm, pigmented papules containing a central intrafollicular keratin plug. These are present on the anterolateral aspect of the thighs and posterolateral aspect of the upper arms. As the condition progresses, it spreads to other parts of the body. The skin is dry and scaly.

Ocular changes: These include night blindness xerophthalmia and keratomalacia. Dryness of the cornea produces well-defined white spots (Bitot's spots).

The condition is treated by 50,000 IU of vitamin A daily.

Lichen Spinulosus

The disease is commonly seen in children. It is characterised by formation of minute, filiform, horny spines, which protrude from follicular openings. These appear as grouped lesions that are present on the trunk, limbs, neck, buttocks and abdomen. The lesions are usually symptomless. Histologically there are inflammatory changes and mild follicular hyperkeratosis (Figs 20 and 21).

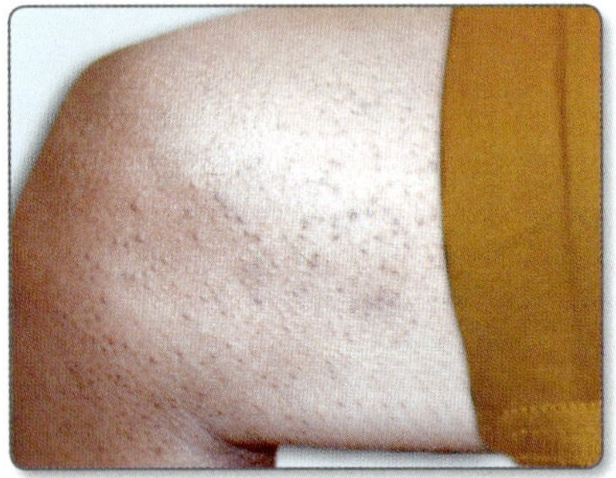

Fig. 20: Lichen spinulosis—knee

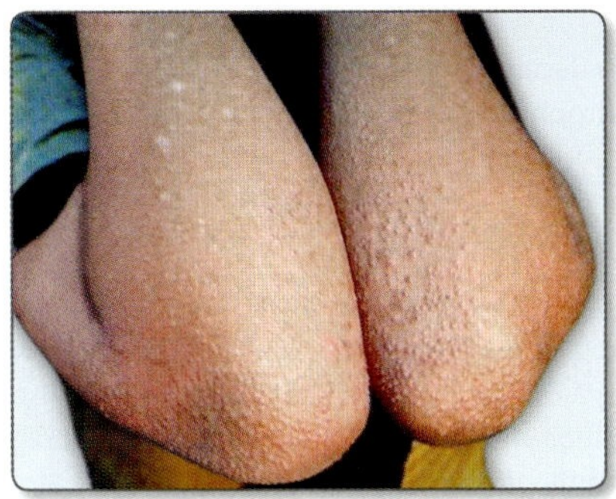

Fig. 21: Lichen spinulosus—elbow
Source: Global Skin Atlas, Dr S Janjua

Keratosis Pilaris

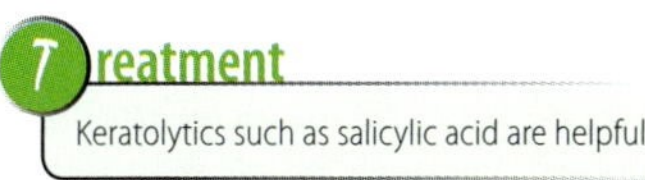

Treatment

Keratolytics such as salicylic acid are helpful.

The disease usually is common; it is seen in almost everyone at some stage in life. The lesions are present on the upper arm and thigh. In severe cases the disease is widespread. The lesions comprise small follicular papules. They may be erythematous or appear greyish because of the superimposed keratotic cone. Occasionally inflammatory papules and pustules may occur. The lesions are arranged in poorly defined groups.

Keratosis pilaris is often seen in xerotic and atopic patients. It is also associated with Netherton's, KID and Fairbanks syndromes. It is treated with topical tretinoin; lactic acid is also helpful (Fig. 22).

Keratosis Circumscripta

This condition has an autosomal recessive inheritance. The onset is at 3–5 years of age. The lesions consist of diamond-shaped plaques and follicular hyperkeratosis over the knees and elbows. The palms and soles may be thickened; back of the hands may also be involved. The hip and lower sacrum show discoid areas of follicular keratosis. The lesions do not progress.

Keratosis Pilaris Atrophicans

These are a group of syndromes in which follicular keratoses is followed by atrophy. There are variations in the distribution, severity of inflammation and genetic heterogeneity in the different syndromes.

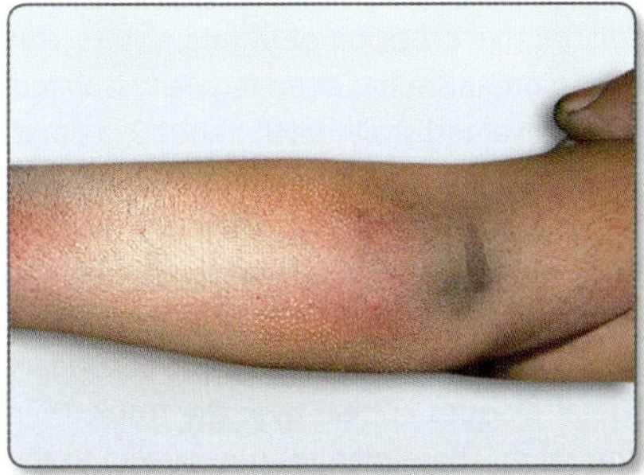

Fig. 22: Keratosis pilaris

These syndromes include:

- Keratosis follicularis spinulosa decalvans
- Keratosis rubra pilaris faciei atrophicans
- Ulerythema ophryogenes
- Atrophoderma vermiculatum
- Folliculitis decalvans (Discussed in chapter 24).

Keratosis follicularis spinulosa decalvans: This is an X-linked recessive disorder. Keratotic follicular papules develop on the scalp in the first few years of life, progressive scarring alopecia follows. Similar papules may also be found in eyebrows. The condition may be associated with cutix laxa, big pinnae, Noonan's syndrome and aminoaciduria.

Treatment is unsatisfactory; retinoids topically or systemically produce little improvement.

Keratosis rubra pilaris faciei atrophicans: In this condition, the face is mainly involved, keratosis pilaris may also be seen on the extensor surface of the arms. The condition is inherited as autosomal dominant.

Ulerythema ophryogenes: The condition affects the eyebrows and scalp. It may be associated with Noonan's syndrome. Erythematous or skin-coloured horny papules are formed in the eyebrows followed by cicatricial alopecia.

Atrophoderma vermiculatum: The cheeks and preauricular regions are primarily involved, giving rise to an atrophic worm-eaten appearance. The condition is very rare.

Inverted Follicular Keratosis (Basosquamous Cell Acanthoma)

Inverted follicular keratosis is a benign epithelial tumour of the infundibulum of the hair follicle. Some consider it an irritated seborrhoeic keratosis.

The benign tumours are seen on the face and scalp of elderly persons, these appear as skin coloured papules 2–10 mm in diameter. It closely resembles seborrhoeic keratosis. The papules have a sharply marginated edge.

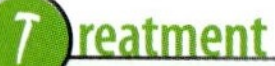

The condition responds to shallow shave biopsy with subsequent haemostasis.

MISCELLANEOUS KERATOSQUAMOUS DISORDERS

Pityriasis Rosea

This is a common self-limiting distinctive eruption of young adults. It is presumed to be due to a virus, but no organism has been regularly isolated. The first sign is the appearance of an oval red scaly patch about 2–5 cm in diameter; the patch may at times be discoid or annular. It is usually situated on the trunk, sometimes on the neck or extremities. This is the herald patch: this is usually larger than the succeeding lesions and persists for a week before the other lesions appear. The centre of the lesion clears and assumes a wrinkled atrophic appearance, with a collarette of scales at periphery. The secondary smaller, discrete, dull-red centripetal plaques appear over the trunk, then spreads to the upper arms and the thigh. These plaques run parallel to the lines of cleavage, forming a "Christmas tree" pattern. The interval between the primary and secondary eruptions is between 2 days and 2 months. The rash fades in about 6 weeks, there is mild pruritus and occasionally malaise and lymphadenopathy occur.

Recurrences are unusual, suggesting lasting immunity after an attack of Pityriasis rosea (PR). If recurrences occur, the primary plaque may develop at the same location or at another site (Fig. 23).

Drug-induced PR is due to drugs such as arsenic, barbiturates, captopril, isotretinoin, ketotifen, metronidazole, omeprazole, and terbinafine. Drug-induced PR may be of the classic type, or may show atypical features such as large lesions, protracted course, resistant to therapy and residual hyperpigmentation.

Atypical forms of Pityriasis Rosea

Pityriasis circinata et marginalis of Vidal. This is regarded as a special form of pityriasis rosea in adults. The lesions are few and large, often localised to one region of the body, especially axillae and groins. The lesions tend to be confluent and persist for several months.

In some cases the primary plaque may be missing or present as double or multiple lesions. The primary plaque may also be the sole manifestation of the disease.

Unilateral distribution, or flexural involvement (PR inversa), facial involvement in children are other atypical presentations of pityriasis rosea.

Enanthem may appear in the oral mucosa, the lesions resemble aphthous ulcers. Nail dystrophy has also been reported.

A purely vesicular form is seen in children and young adults, it is said to be common in Africa.

Differential Diagnosis

Pityriasis rosea should be differentiated from drug eruptions, secondary syphilis, seborrhoeic dermatitis and viral exanthems. Seborrhoeic dermatitis has a characteristic distribution and the scales are greasy. In secondary syphilis, the lesions are generalised, papules are present on the palms and soles, and there is generalised lymph node enlargement. A VDRL test should exclude syphilis. Drug eruptions have a rapid and generalised onset.

Treatment

No treatment is required as the lesions heal spontaneously in about 6 weeks. Soothing lotions, such as calamine, may be given for pruritus. Erythromycin has recently been shown to clear PR in 2 weeks.

Dapsone is used in severe vesicular PR.

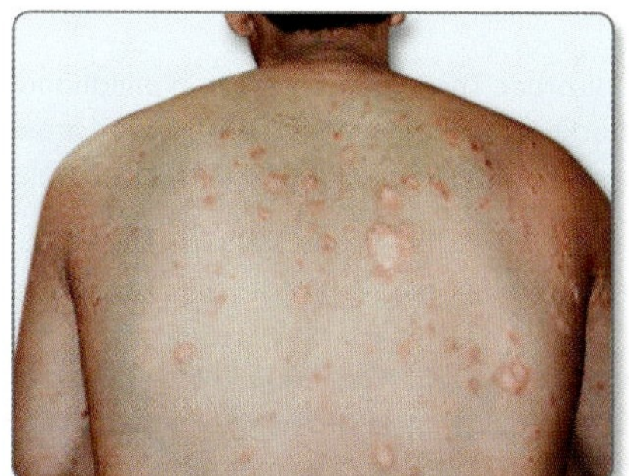

Fig. 23: Pityriasis rosea—note the herald patch

Pityriasis Rotunda

A variety of acquired ichthyosis that manifests as persistent, sharply defined circular patches of ichthyosiform scaling without inflammation. The lesions may be single or multiple; they appear mostly on the trunk or extremities. Some cases are a manifestation of internal malignancy.

Peeling Skin Syndrome (Erythrokeratolysis)

Peeling skin syndrome is an autosomal recessive disorder. Peeling of the skin occurs above the granular layer. The syndrome is associated with pruritus, short stature, easily removable anagen hair, moderate aminoaciduria and low plasma tryptophan levels. Areas of 2–5 cm of the skin often exfoliate leaving polycyclic denuded red areas. The stratum corneum can be pulled off in a sheet. Palms and soles are red and dry. There is no effective treatment, the condition is lifelong.

Erythrokeratoderma Variabilis

Two types of lesions characterise the condition; erythematous scaly patches that vary in colour and extend over short periods and the fixed lesions. The following are the two types of erythrokeratoderma variabilis:

1. Mendes de Costa syndrome
2. Degos syndrome

Mendes de Costa syndrome: This is a rare autosomal recessive disorder, it usually presents at birth or during the first year of life. There are two kinds of skin lesions. There may be localised sharply demarcated hyperkeratotic plaques, which vary in colour and extend over short periods of time; lesions may reappear at different sites. The other type consists of generalised, hyperkeratotic plaques with accentuated skin markings, these lesions are more persistent. Keratoderma of the palms and soles may sometimes occur. Hair, nails and mucous membranes are normal.

Degos syndrome (Erythrokeratoderma en cocardes): This again consists of two types of lesions, fixed scaly plaques, and round plaques with concentric erythema, this pattern is variable. There is no keratoderma, but palms and soles may show scaling as in summer erythrokeratolysis.

Symmetrical Progressive Erythrokeratoderma (Gottron's Syndrome)

This is an autosomal dominant disorder. The condition starts in childhood, shoulder girdle, cheeks and buttocks are mostly affected. The affected areas show large fixed erythematous and scaly plaques. Etretinate and acitretin are effective.

Parapsoriasis

The term parapsoriasis was first introduced by Brocq in 1902. Brocq referred to parapsoriasis as a group of maculopapular scaly disorders, of slow evolution, chronic in nature, resistant to treatment and absence of symptoms. The lesions look like psoriasis or lichen planus, but do not have any features of the disease. A unifying feature of parapsoriasis is that all of them appear to be cutaneous T cell lymphoproliferative disorders.

Parapsoriasis appears to comprehend the pathogenesis of both chronic dermatitis and mycosis fungoides. The T cells present in parapsoriasis belong to the skin-associated lymphoid tissue (SALT); mycosis fungoides is known to be a neoplasm of SALT T cells.

Parapsoriasis was initially grouped into four disorders: pityriasis lichenoides et varioliformis acuta, pityriasis lichenoides chronica, small and large plaque parapsoriasis. Pityriasis lichenoides acuta and chronica are now considered a form of immune complex vasculitis. (The disease is discussed in chapter 15).

Small and large plaque parapsoriasis will be discussed in this section.

Histopathology

Small plaque parapsoriasis shows parakeratosis, hyperkeratosis, mild to moderate acanthosis, some degree of spongiosis. T lymphocytes may be diffuse, and it may be perivascular. There is no epidermotropism.

In large plaque parapsoriasis, the histology is similar to small plaque parapsoriasis, epidermal oedema is less prominent and epidermal atrophy is frequent. The appearance of atypical lymphocytes (mycosis fungoides cell) in the dermis and epidermis is evidence of a change towards mycosis fungoides.

Small Plaque Parapsoriasis

This is an asymptomatic chronic eruption on the trunk and proximal extremities. The lesions are well-circumscribed plaques red or brown in colour, less commonly yellowish and nonindurated. The plaques are usually less than 5 cm in diameter. Initially a few lesions are present, usually on the trunk, later they become widespread. A distinctive variant, which is yellowish or fawn in colour with finger-like lesions is known as digitate dermatosis, it often follows the lines of cleavage of the skin. Small plaque shows a predominantly male preponderance of 3:1 ratio.

Large Plaque Parapsoriasis

Large plaque parapsoriasis is a disease of middle age and older people; with a peak incidence in the 5th decade. Large plaques 10 cm or more in diameter characterises the condition. The lesions are erythematous, may be irregular and show atrophy (cigarette-paper appearance). Large plaque parapsoriasis may undergo a malignant change towards a lymphoma. The lesions are found predominantly on the trunk and the flexures. Signs of malignant change in a plaque are:

- Induration
- Pruritus
- Poikiloderma
- Reddish hue in lesions that were formally of another colour
- Lymphadenopathy.

About 10–30% of large plaque psoriasis may progress to mycosis fungoides.

Retiform Parapsoriasis

Consists of a net-like or zebra striped distribution of red to brown, shiny flat topped papules. Poikilodermatous changes are characteristic. The lesions are present on the trunk and proximal extremities.

Treatment

Patients with small plaque parapsoriasis should be reassured; it is treated with emollients, topical tar or topical corticosteroids. They should be examined initially every 3–6 months and then every year to see that the disease is stable.

Large plaque parapsoriasis needs more aggressive therapy. It is treated by high potency topical corticosteroids, PUVA and narrowband UVB therapy. Nitrogen mustard may be used for the poikilodermic type of parapsoriasis. The patients should be examined every 3 months initially and then every 6 months subsequently to look for any progression towards mycosis fungicides. Topical steroids should be used with caution because of cutaneous atrophy.

Vitamin D_2 250,000 units daily has been used to treat parapsoriasis, intake of milk should be restricted in these patients to prevent hypercalcemia.

POROKERATOSIS

Porokeratosis are a group of disorders characterised histologically by the presence of cornoid lamella and specific varying degree of dysplasia, resulting in a keratotic lesion, which may progress to malignancy. The condition may be hereditary or acquired. It may be secondary to malignancy, renal transplantation and immunosuppression. Mibelli first described porokeratosis in 1893. Mibelli thought that the lesions had their origin in the orifice of the sweat glands, hence the name. It was in 1966 that the most common type of porokeratosis, the disseminated actinic porokeratosis was delineated by Chernosky.

Aetiology and Pathogenesis

The aetiology is unknown, multiple factors are probably involved. Involvement of several family members suggests expression of a genetic defect. Additional factors trigger the clinical manifestation. These factors include UVL, infectious/transmissible agents. High incidence of porokeratosis is found in transplant recipients, in imunosuppressed patients, HIV and patients with hepatitis C.

Histopathology

The border of the lesion should be biopsied, with a small spindle-shaped piece of tissue, with a long axis perpendicular to the prominent rim. The changes are only seen at the edge of the lesion. There is hyperkeratosis, parakeratosis and acanthosis. The cornoid lamella is a thickened column of keratin-containing parakeratotic nuclei extending outward from the acanthotic layer into the stratum corneum is characteristic of porokeratosis. The granular layer is absent beneath the cornoid lamella. Moderate lymphocytic infiltrate is present in the dermis.

Types of porokeratosis:

- Porokeratosis of Mibelli
- Disseminated superficial actinic porokeratosis
- Porokeratosis plantaris palmaris et disseminata

- Giant porokeratosis
- Linear porokeratosis (extremities)
- Punctate porokeratosis (palms and soles).

Porokeratosis of Mibelli

This is a chronic progressive disease, common in immunosuppressed patients. The disease is twice as common in males. It begins in childhood; it is characterised by the formation of atrophic patches surrounded by an elevated warty border. The sites of predilection are the hands and feet. It may also occur in the buccal mucosa, glans penis and on the scalp with resulting alopecia.

Porokeratosis begins as a small keratotic papule, which spreads peripherally and atrophies in the centre with the formation of well-defined keratotic wall or collar. The wall often has a groove or linear ridge running along its summit. If the nails are involved nail dystrophy occurs.

The pathognomonic features of porokeratosis of Mibelli are that it is unilateral, localised, the lesions are relatively large and have a prominent peripheral border exhibiting the diagnostic furrow.

Disseminated Superficial Actinic Porokeratosis

This condition is characterised by numerous annular keratotic reddish-brown papules found in the exposed areas of the body. The disease is common between of 20 years and 40 years of age. The condition is most often seen in women. The disease is of autosomal dominant inheritance. Exacerbation is seen in summer. Squamous cell carcinoma may occur in the lesions (Fig. 24).

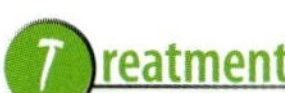

Treatment is disappointing in all forms of porokeratosis, recurrences can occur with any type of porokeratosis. Application of 5-FU solution under occlusion is commonly used for the treatment of porokeratosis. Cryotherapy, electrodesiccation, diclofenac gel can be used. Etretinate and isotretinoin are also effective.

Porokeratosis Plantaris Palmaris et Disseminata

The lesions first appear on the palms and soles and then extend over the entire body .

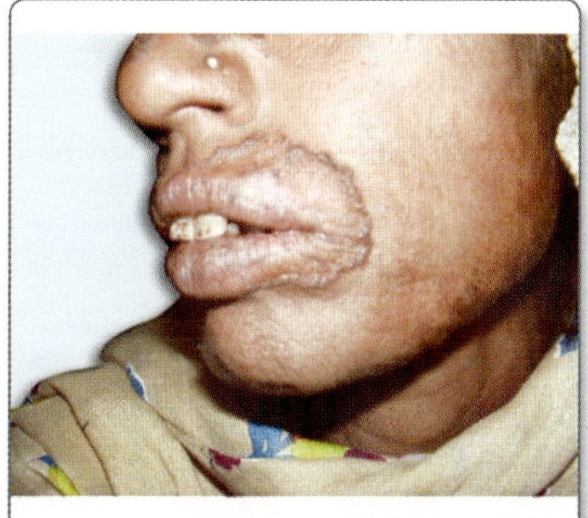

Fig. 24: Porokeratosis

Porokeratosis Striata

This is unilateral, onset is in infancy and childhood, and it should be differentiated from a verrucous epidermal nevus.

Giant Porokeratosis

The lesions are large10–20 cm in diameter; the surrounding wall may be raised to as much as 1 cm. The lesions are often found on the foot. Incidence of malignancy is high.

CONGENITAL DISORDERS OF KERATINISATION

Darier's Disease (Darier-White Disease)

Darier's disease is a dominantly inherited disorder of keratinisation, which affects the skin, nails and the mucous membranes. The cutaneous lesions comprise greasy papules on the upper trunk and scalp, palmar pits and nail dystrophy. The disease runs a chronic course.

Aetiology and Pathogenesis

Darier's disease is a genetic disorder determined by an autosomal dominant gene. The defect is in a calcium-channel regulating gene ATP-2A2 at 12q24.1. This results in a disturbance in calcium homeostasis, which leads to a defect in the synthesis or maturation of the tonofilament-desmosome complex.

Histopathology

The histological features of Darier's disease are distinctive; there is suprabasal acantholysis with premature and abnormal keratinisation resulting in the formation of corps ronds and grains. Corps ronds (cells with peculiar keratin inclusions) are cells that show premature partial keratinisation; these cells have a dark staining nucleus surrounded by a clear cytoplasm and a glistening ring simulating a membrane, present in the stratum malpighii. Grains (parakeratotic material) are cells formed from the corps ronds; they are small cells with a shrunken cytoplasm seen in the stratum corneum.

Clinical Features

The disease is not present at birth, but begins in the first or second decade. The disease is characterised by the appearance of yellowish-brown greasy crusted papules and plaques in the seborrhoeic distribution. The sites of predilection are scalp, forehead, ears, nasolabial folds and flexures especially axillae, groins and anogenital areas. The lesions of Darier's often become foul smelling due to secondary infection.

On the palms and soles, there are punctate keratoses or small pits. The pits are pathognomonic of Darier's disease. The nails show white and red longitudinal bands. There is often a V-shaped nick at the free end of the nail; this is typical of Darier's disease.

Mucous membrane lesions appear as white, centrally depressed papules on the mucosa of the cheek, hard and soft palate, known as "cobblestone lesions". Lesions are also seen on the rectal and genital mucosa.

The disease is exacerbated by use of steroids and exposure to sunlight. Patients with Darier's disease have an increased susceptibility to infection, perhaps due to a defect in the cell-mediated immunity (Fig. 25).

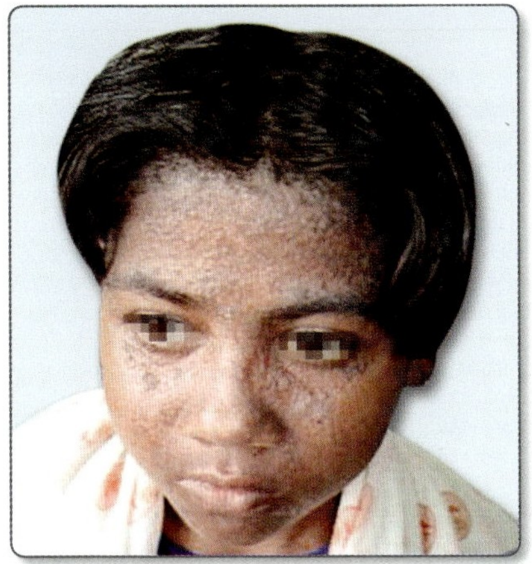

Fig. 25: Darier's disease

Differential Diagnosis

Mild forms of Darier's disease should be differentiated from acne and seborrhoeic dermatitis. The papules of Darier's disease are greasy, crusted and warty; there are no comedones, examination of the palms and nails help in differentiating the disease. Localised forms of Darier's disease must be differentiated from epidermal nevus.

Treatment

Sunscreens are essential in the management of Darier's disease. No treatment is required in mild cases apart from the use of emollients. In other cases tazarotene gel, adapalene and acitretin in severe cases is given in a dose of 0.5–1 mg/kg of body weight. However, in most cases, the disease relapses on stopping the drug. Appropriate antibiotics are required in secondary infection.

Pityriasis Rubra Pilaris

Pityriasis rubra pilaris (PRP) is a chronic disease characterised by follicular keratosis, palmoplantar keratoderma and erythroderma.

Aetiology

Genetic factors have been implicated in the aetiology, but it has not been proved with certainty. The cause of the disease is obscure. The age incidence curve is bimodal, the familial cases are seen in early childhood and the acquired type appears in the 5th and 6th decade. The essential defect is probably an overactive epidermis and an abnormality in vitamin A metabolism.

Histopathology

Hyperkeratosis is the most obvious feature of the disease. Parakeratosis is seen around the follicular orifices. Alternating vertical and horizontal parakeratosis in the interfollicular stratum corneum is characteristic of PRP. There is a mild mononuclear infiltrate in the dermis.

- Classic adult onset
- Classic juvenile onset
- Atypical adult onset
- Atypical juvenile onset
- Circumscript
- HIV associated PRP

Clinical Features

The disease is rare and affects both sexes equally. It can affect the adults (adult onset PRP) or children (juvenile onset PRP). The eruption starts on the face, neck and upper trunk and then spreads in a caudal direction. The affected areas are erythematous (reddish-orange) and scaly, with follicular papules, prominent on the dorsal aspect of proximal phalanges, elbows and wrists. The papules are the diagnostic features of the disease, being more or less acuminate, reddish-brown in colour, pinhead in size and topped by a central horny plug. In the horny centre, a hair is usually embedded. Pruritus is uncommon. Erythroderma may develop, but islands of normal skin (nappes claire) are characteristic. The palms and soles are hyperkeratotic and yellow (PRP sandal). The nails are grossly thickened and discolored, showing splinter haemorrhages. In majority of patients, spontaneous resolution occurs in 1–3 years. Recurrences are common. Teeth and hair are normal.

Lesions of the buccal mucosa include a diffuse whitish appearance, as well as lacy-white plaques and erosions.

In the atypical forms of the disease spontaneous healing does not occur. Circumscript PRP is localised; it is not associated with erythroderma and palmoplantar keratosis. Spontaneous healing does occur, but recurrences are common.

HIV-associated pityriasis rubra pilaris. Patients with HIV may have nodulocystic and pustular acneiform lesions. It is resistant to standard treatments, but they may respond to antiretroviral therapies.

Differential Diagnosis

Pityriasis rubra pilaris must be differentiated from follicular psoriasis and erythrokeratoderma. In psoriasis, the follicular papules are covered with the characteristic silvery-white scales. Erythroderma variabilis occurs shortly after birth, there are well-defined erythematous patches and hyperkeratotic generalised plaques, keratosis of the palms, soles may be present, nails, and mucous membranes are spared. There are no follicular papules.

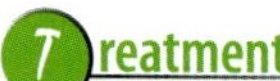

Treatment

The disease is difficult to treat. In mild cases, only emollients are required. Keratolytics, glucocorticoids and calcipotriol can be used topically. In erythrodermic phase, acitretin is given in a dose of 0.75 mg/kg of body weight. Oral steroids are ineffective, but methotrexate can be tried if retinoids fail. PUVA is not effective, but Re-PUVA has been effective in some cases. Cyclosporin is not effective in PRP.

Ichthyosis

Ichthyosis is a group of genetically determined disorders characterised by generalised, persistent scaling of skin surface that has been likened to the skin of the fish. There are different types of ichthyosis with different modes of inheritance. Ichthyosis is not one disease but a group of diseases in which the homeostatic mechanism of the epidermis cell replacement is accelerated or intercellular detachment is retarded, resulting in the clinical appearance of a scale.

A "brick and mortar" model of the epidermis helps in the understanding of ichthyosis. Mutation in the keratin of the epidermis is viewed as defective bricks; and defects in the intercellular cement is the defective mortar.

Ichthyosis Vulgaris

This is an autosomal dominant type of ichthyosis found in 1 in 300 persons. Reduction in filaggrin and delayed destruction of desmosomes, is seen in a number of cases, which results in decreased hydration of the stratum corneum. Histopathology reveals hyperkeratosis with a thickened stratum corneum and reduced or absent granular layer. Small white scales, involving the trunk and extensor aspect of the limbs, characterise the lesion. Flexures are spared. There is diffuse hyperkeratosis of palms and soles. Ichthyosis vulgaris is frequently

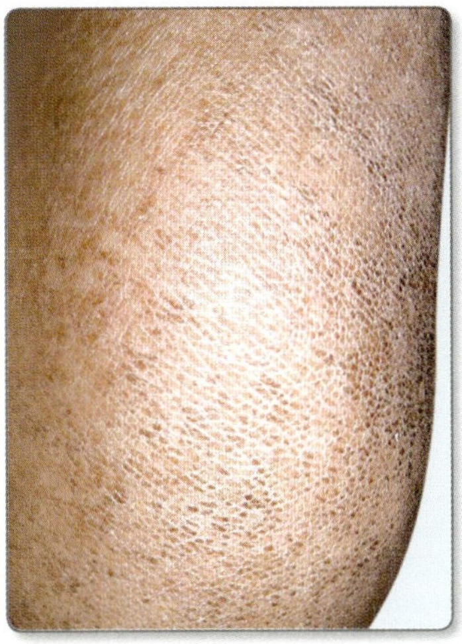

Fig. 26: Ichthyosis vulgaris—small thin scales

associated with keratosis pilaris and atopy. The disease runs a lifelong course with exacerbations in winter. It usually improves with age, but relapse is common in old age. Therapy produces a dramatic improvement, but the response is only temporary (Fig. 26).

X-linked Ichthyosis

This type of ichthyosis is common in males, although female carriers may show some features. It is found in 1 in 6,000 males. The disease is due to a deficiency of steroid sulphatase, due to which cholesterol sulphate cannot be broken down, and hyperkeratosis develops. Steroid sulphatase activity is also decreased in leukocytes and fibroblasts. Cholesterol sulphate levels are increased in the serum, epidermis and scale. There is an increased mobility of low-density lipoproteins on electrophoresis, a feature which can help in the diagnosis of X-linked ichthyosis.

Skin biopsy shows hyperkeratosis with a moderately increased stratum corneum and a granular layer present in contrast to ichthyosis vulgaris.

Large dark dirty scales are found on extremities, trunk, scalp, sides of neck and lower part of face. There is significant involvement of flexural surfaces. Palms and soles are often spared. X-linked ichthyosis is associated with corneal opacities, cryptorchidism and mental retardation (Fig. 27).

Pregnant women with this enzyme deficiency fail to metabolise steroid sulphate to oestrogen in the placenta. They have low oestrogen levels and a tendency to delayed onset of labour. The response to therapy is satisfactory.

Lamellar Ichthyosis (LI)

Lamellar ichthyosis is a rare ichthyosis (1 in 100,000 births) inherited by an autosomal recessive gene. Several genes are identified to cause LI, mutations in transglutaminase are the most common and several other loci are also known. A collodion baby is usually the initial presentation. Biochemically there is increase in sterols and fatty acids in scale.

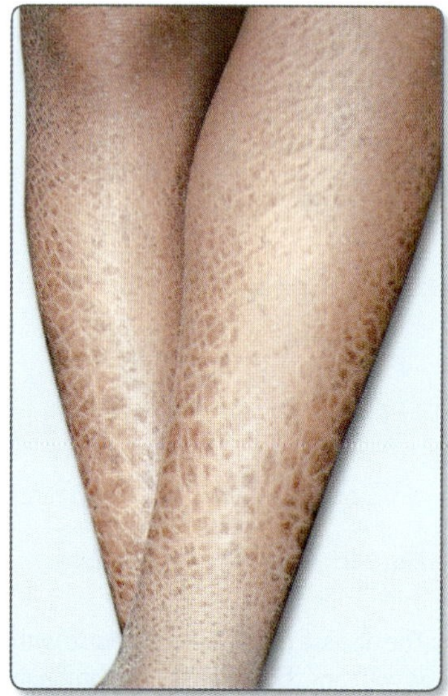

Fig. 27: X-linked ichthyosis—large thin dark scales

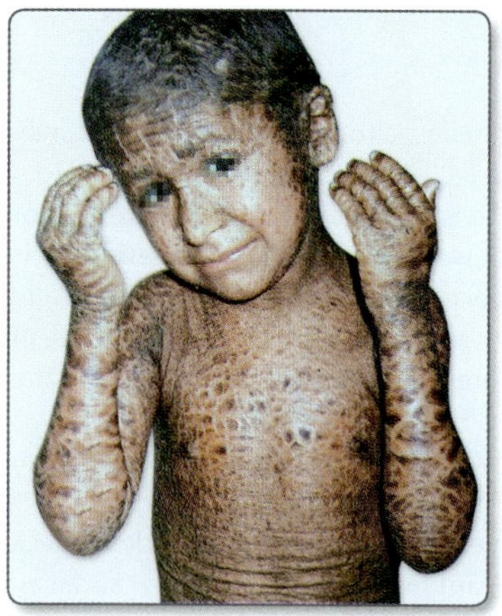

Fig. 28: Lamellar ichthyosis—large thick dark adherent scales

Skin biopsy shows hyperkeratosis, patchy parakeratosis, increased granular layer, acanthosis and papillomatosis.

Lamellar ichthyosis is characterised by generalised large adherent dark thick scaling, the scales are thicker than those of X-linked ichthyosis. The scales are said to be the largest on the lower extremities. The hyperkeratosis can result in obstructing the sweat ducts with resulting hypohidrosis. The scales tend to entrap hair, which together with tautness of the skin results in scarring alopecia. There is marked ectropion and crumpled ears. Palms and soles show diffuse hyperkeratosis (Fig. 28). The erythema is either mild or absent.

Lamellar ichthyosis is most refractory to treatment.

Non-bullous Ichthyosiform Erythroderma (Congenital Ichthyosiform Erythroderma)

This is a rare autosomal recessive disorder, associated with increased epidermal turnover. A collodion baby is the usual presentation. After shedding of the membrane, generalised erythema with fine scaling becomes evident. The erythema tends to decrease with age, but scaling is persistent and there may be hyperkeratosis around elbows, knees and ankles. Mild ectropion and crumpled ears may be present. Palms and soles are thickened. Dermatophyte infection of the skin and nails is common. It may be associated with immunological abnormalities, mental and physical retardation. Mutations in epidermal protein loricrin and other genetic loci have been found in congenital ichthyosiform erythroderma.

Bullous Ichthyosiform Erythroderma

Bullous ichthyosiform erythroderma [epidermolytic hyperkeratosis (EH)] is an autosomal dominant disorder characterised by generalised erythema, scaling and blistering. The condition is seen in 1 in 200,000–300,000 births.

Epidermolytic hyperkeratosis can be of two types: Brocq's and Siemens. In the Brocq type, there is mutation of keratin 1 and 10 and in the Siemens, type there is mutation of keratin 2e. Keratin 10 is the co-expressed partner of keratin 1, both of which are required to form intermediate filaments in the suprabasal layers of the epidermis. Six clinical types of EH are distinguished three with palmoplantar keratosis and three without palmoplantar keratosis.

Keratin 2e is a differentiation keratin of the suprabasal epidermis, but is expressed in the more superficial epidermal layers.

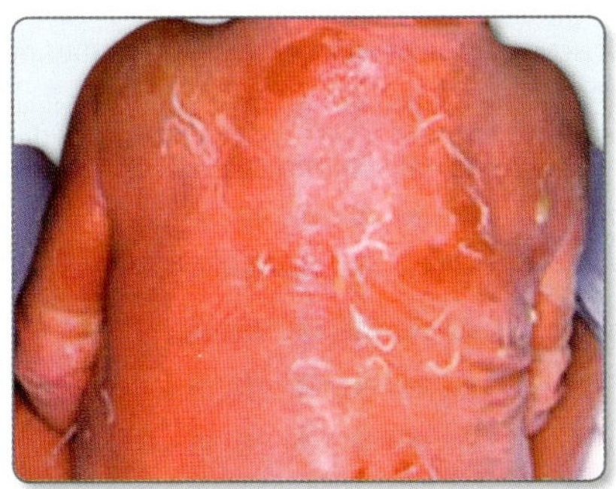

Fig. 29: Bullous ichthyosifrom erythroderma

Histopathology

Skin biopsy reveals hyperkeratosis and vacuolar degeneration (epidermolysis) of the upper epidermis, which leads to cell lysis. Electron microscopy shows clumping of the tonofilaments. The epidermal vacuolisation is confined to the granular layer in Siemens type of EH.

Clinical Features

The disease is present at birth with blisters, erythema and peeling. Erythema and blistering gradually decrease as the child grows older, but thick keratotic and verrucous lesions appear in late infancy, especially in the flexures, and persist throughout life. In severe cases, there is ectropion and crumpled ears. Palms and soles may be thickened. Secondary infection of the thick scales and bullae is common (Fig. 29).

Verrucous lesions develop later in the Siemens type of EH, it is not as severe as in the Brocq's type. Skin fragility is more superficial, resulting in the loss of stratum corneum, these results in a collarette like lesion, describes as moulting.

Acquired Ichthyosis

This type of ichthyosis is associated with vitamin and nutritional deficiencies, malignancies, blood dyscrasias, leprosy, hypothyroidism and the acquired immunodeficiency syndrome. It may follow ingestion of certain drugs like clofazimine, nicotinic acid and triparanol. Acquired ichthyosis is treated by removing the cause (Fig. 30).

Treatment of Ichthyosis

Lifelong treatment is required. The aim of treatment is to hydrate the skin and remove the scales. Ichthyotic skin has a decreased barrier function and increased transepidermal water loss. Pliability of the stratum corneum is because of its water content, hydration can soften the skin. Ichthyosis is nonsteroid responsive dermatosis. In children because of the high turnover of scales, nutritional requirements may be high. Fungal infections of the skin are common, these should be appropriately treated.

Treatment can be topical or systemic.

Topical therapy

- Emollients are a very important part of the therapy. Emollients should be applied after bath or shower when the skin is still moist. Salt-water baths may help in hydrating the horny layer
- Urea containing preparations act by virtue of water-binding properties of urea. It is used as 10–25% cream.
- Keratolytic agents. These are required if there is severe scaling. These include:
  - Salicylic acid (2–6% in suitable vehicle): Widespread use of salicylic acid may lead to salicylism
  - Alpha hydroxy acid (pyruvic acid, lactic acid and glycolic acid)
  - Topical retinoic acid.

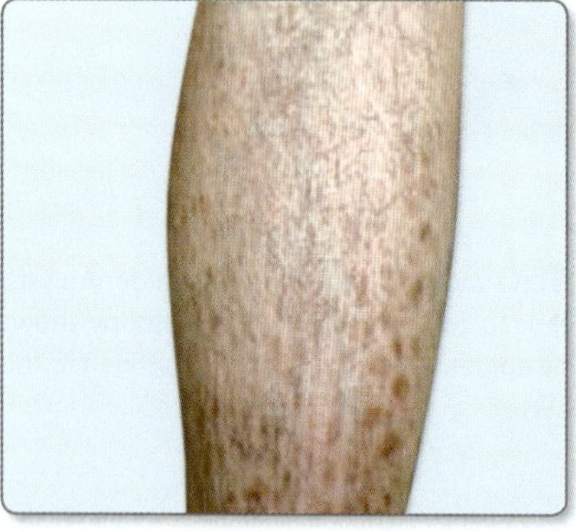

Fig. 30: Acquired ichthyosis

Table 3: Difference between ichthyosis vulgaris, X-linked ichthyosis, lamellar ichthyosis, & bullous ichthyosis erythroderma

Ichthyosis vulgaris	*X-linked ichthyosis*	*Lamellar ichthyosis*	*Bullous ichthyosis erythroderma*	*Non-bullous ichthyosiform erythroderma*
Mode of inheritance AD	X-linked recessive	AR	AD	AR
Aetiology Reduction of fillagrin and delayed destruction of desmosomes	Deficiency of steroid sulphatase	Mutations in epidermal transglutaminase	Mutations in keratin 1 and 10	Mutations in the cornified envelope protein loricrin.
Histopathology Hyperkeratosis, thickened stratum corneum, absence of granular layer	Hyperkeratosis, thickened stratum corneum, granular layer present	Hyperkeratosis, parakeratosis, increased granular layer, acanthosis and papillomatosis	Hyperkeratosis and vacuolar degeneration of the epidermis	Hyperkeratosis, acanthosis and parakeratosis
Scales Small and white	Large, dark and dirty looking	Larger, dark, thick adherent scales	Erythema, thick waxy scales and blistering	Erythema and fine scaling
Onset Disease apparent within the first year of life	Disease apparent at birth	Disease apparent at birth	Disease apparent at birth	Disease apparent at birth
Other features Flexures spared, diffuse hyperkeratosis of the palms and soles	Palms and soles spared, significant flexural involvement	Generalised scaling	Generalised scaling in 3 phenotypes, palms and soles spared in 3 phenotypes	Generalised scaling
Atopy and keratosis pilaris Frequently associated	Absent	Absent	Absent	Absent
Cholesterol sulphate levels Normal	Increased	Normal	Normal	Normal
Association with corneal opacities, mental retardation and cryptorchidism Not associated	Associated	Not associated	Not associated	Not associated
Association with prolonged labor and low estrogen levels in mothers urine No association	Associated with prolonged labor	No association	No association	No association
Associated with ectropion and crumpled ears No association	No association	Marked ectropion and crumpled ears	Only in severe cases ectropion and crumpled ears	Mild ectropion and crumpled ears present
Presents as collodion baby at birth No	No	Yes	No	Yes

Abbreviations: AD—Autosomal dominant; AR—Autosomal recessive

Systemic therapy: Acitretin is indicated in lamellar ichthyosis, non-bullous ichthyosiform erythroderma and bullous ichthyosiform erythroderma. The retinoids decrease the scaling, but erythema and blistering are unchanged. The retinoids should be considered only in those patients with severe and refractory disease not responding to conventional treatment. These should be combined with hydration and emollients.

Difference between ichthyosis vulgaris, X-linked ichthyosis, lamellar ichthyosis, and bullous ichthyosis erythroderma is given in Table 3.

Rare Ichthyosiform Disorders

Collodion Baby

Infants are sometimes born with a tough, inelastic, collodion-like membrane covering the body. The membrane in course of time fissures and peels off. Collodion babies are often seen with congenital ichthyosiform erythroderma or lamella ichthyosis, some patients may even have normal skin. Affected babies are often dehydrated and in danger of hypothermia. Mortality is high (Fig. 31).

Harlequin Foetus (Ichthyosis Congenita Gravis)

This disorder is of autosomal reccessive inheritance; the skin is covered with thick heavy armour-like plates covering the skin. The ears are rudimentary or absent, eclabium is present. The infant is often premature and of low-birth-weight, it may be stillborn, or may die soon after. There is no effective treatment. Some cases of recovery by etretinate have been reported (Fig. 32).

Refsum's Syndrome

This is a rare autosomal recessive disorder, resulting from a failure of breakdown of dietary phytanic acid and resulting in its accumulation in the tissues. Fine white scales resembling ichthyosis vulgaris are seen at adolescence. The

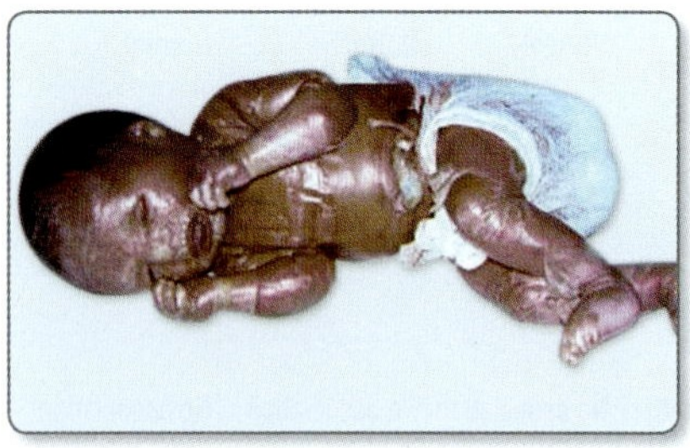

Fig. 31: Collodion baby

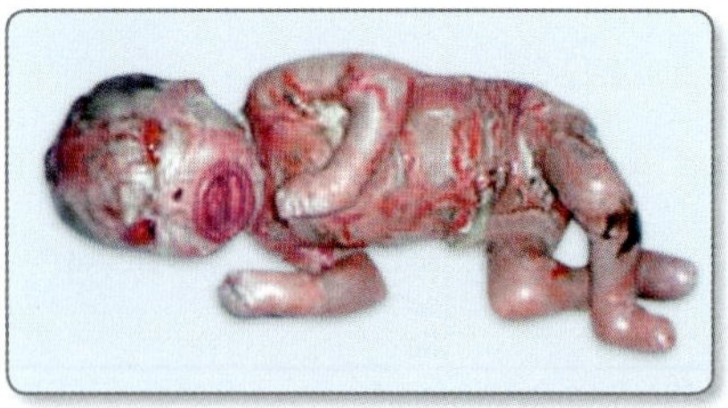

Fig. 32: Harlequin foetus

syndrome consists of polyneuritis both motor and sensory, nerve deafness, atypical retinitis pigmentosa and ichthyosis. Clinical improvement follows reduction of phytanic acid in the diet.

Sjögren-Larsson Syndrome

It is an autosomal recessive disorder; it presents as mild lamellar ichthyosis at birth. Later in childhood spastic paralysis, mental retardation, epilepsy and macular degeneration of the retina develop.

Rud's Syndrome

It is a poorly characterised disorder possibly of autosomal recessive inheritance, consisting of lamellar ichthyosis. Some patients with this syndrome have steroid sulphatase deficiency of the X-linked variety. The syndrome includes macrocytic anaemia, hypogonadism, epilepsy and dwarfism.

Conradi's Syndrome

This is a rare X-linked dominant disorder, lethal in males, presents as a mosaic pattern in females. It is a rare complex of skin, ocular and bone abnormalities. Skin at birth shows generalised erythroderma, more prominent on the face, and scaling of the skin in a whorl-like fashion. As the child grows follicular atrophoderma and pseudopelade develop. Usually the ichthyosis clears in the first year of life leaving behind a temporary pigmentation. The disease is associated with shortening of the humerus and femur, nasal hypoplasia, scoliosis, opacities of the lens, high arched palate and an apparent stippling of the epiphyses.

Ichthyosis Linearis Circumflexa (Netherton's Syndrome)

This is an autosomal recessive disorder that is present at birth or develops shortly after. Diffuse erythema and scaling are associated with polycyclic eruption with thickened migratory and hyperkeratotic margins. Many patients have hair shaft defects, such as trichorrhexis invaginata; there is generalised sparseness of the hair. Atopic manifestations are frequent, flexural accentuation dominates the picture. Other reported manifestations include mental retardation and aminoaciduria.

Keratitis, Ichthyosis and Deafness Syndrome

Keratitis, Ichthyosis and Deafness (KID) syndrome is an ectodermal dysplasia with an autosomal dominant (common) and recessive (rare) inheritance. The disease is characterised by erythematous discrete scaly plaques or mild generalised hyperkeratosis. The plaques have a discrete border, and a verrucous appearance. There is prominent follicular hyperkeratosis, which may result in scarring alopecia. The nails may be dystrophic and the teeth small. Affected individuals have an increased susceptibility to bacterial, fungal and viral infections. Deafness and keratitis are noticed in infancy. Connexin proteins 26, 30 and 31 are expressed in the stratified epithelium of the cochlea and epidermis, and abnormalities of these proteins are responsible for the sensorineural deafness and skin abnormalities.

Ichthyosis Hystrix

This is a severe disorder of keratinisation characterised by massive hyperkeratosis, with autosomal dominant inheritance. The term (hystrix means porcupine) is used to describe the various rare disorders of excessive keratinisation.

Types:

- Porcupine men of Lambert. Patients in this disorder have gross hyperkeratosis with quill-like projections
- Localised and linear warty epidermal naevus with histological features of epidermolytic hyperkeratosis
- Ichthyosis hystrix of Curth and Macklin. The condition is similar to that of localised linear warty epidermal nevus, but differs from it histologically. It shows continuous perinuclear tonofilament shell in the spinous and granular layer
- Ichthyosis hystrix gravoir Typpus Rhedt These patients develop ichthyosiform erythroderma, alopecia, nail and hair abnormalities and severe sensorineural deafness.

Drugs that alter lipids such as nicotinic acid and triparanol are potentially capable of causing ichthyosis
Think of ichthyosis vulgaris when a patient presents with extensive keratosis pilaris
Corticosteroids should not be used to treat ichthyosis.

FURTHER READING

1. Berneburg M, Rocken M, Benedix F. Phototherapy and Narrowband UVB. Acata Derm Venereol. 2005;85:1-11.
2. Block MM, Wilson-Jones E. The role of epidermis in the histopathogenesis of lichen planus. Arch Dermatol. 1972;105:81-6.
3. Bovenschen HJ, Seyger MM, Kerkhof VD. Plaque Psoriasis vs atopic dermatitis and lichen planus: A comparison for lesional T-cell subsets, epidermal proliferation and differentiation. Br J Dermatol. 2005;153:72-8.
4. Castio-Soccio L, Van Voorrhees AS. Long-term efficacy of biologics in dermatology. Dermatological therapy. 2009;22:22-33.
5. Crowly J. Scalp Psoriasis: an overview of the disease and available therapies. J Drugs Dermatol. 2010;9(8):915-9.
6. Dalton SR, Filman EP, Altman CE, et al. Atypical junctional melanocytic proliferation in benign lichenoid keratosis. Human Pathol. 2003;31:706-9.
7. Ibbotson SH, Speight EL, McLeod RJ, et al. The relevance and effect of amalgam replacement in subjects with oral lichenoid reactions. Br J Dermatol. 1996;134:420-3.
8. Klein A, Landthaler M, Karrer S. Pityriasis Rubra Pilaris: a review of diagnosis and treatment. Am J Clin Dermatol. 2010;11(3):157-70.
9. Marji SK, Marcus R, Moennich J, et al. Use of biological agents in pediatric psoriasis. J Drugs Dermatol. 2010;9(8):975-84.
10. Mirmirani P, Karnik P. Lichen planopilaris treated with a peroxisome proliferator-activated receptor- y agonist. Arch Dermatol. 2009;145(2):1363-6.
11. Menter A, Papp KA, Jan A, et al. Efficacy of tofacitinib an oral janus kinase inhibitor on clinical signs of moderate-to-severe plaque psoriasis in different body regions. J Drug Dermatol. 2014;13(3):352-6.
12. Mortel RM, Emer J. Prospective new biological therapies for psoriasis and psoriatic arthritis. J Drugs Dermatol. 2010;9(8):951-62.
13. Okulicz FJ, Schwartz AR. Hereditary and acquired ichthyosis. Int J of Dermatol. 2003;42:95-8.
14. Patterson JW. The spectrum of lichenoid dermatitis. J Cutan Pathol. 199;18:676-74.
15. Smith MC, AnsteyVA, Barker JN, et al. British Association of Dermatologists guideline for psoriasis 2009. Br J Dermatol. 2009;161:987-1019.
16. Warren BR, Lavery DB, Ashcroft MD, et al. Biological therapies for psoriasis: practical experience in a UK tertiary referral centre. Br J Dermatol. 2000;168:163-9.

Chapter 11

Connective Tissue Disorders

INTRODUCTION

Connective tissue disorders are a complex group of disorders without a unifying pathogenesis. Most of these disorders are associated with arthritis/arthralgia and have prominent skin lesions. Lupus erythematosus, scleroderma and dermatomyositis are frequently referred to as autoimmune connective tissue disorders. They are all associated with a high incidence of circulating autoantibodies and with widespread fibrinoid degeneration of collagen fibres.

LUPUS ERYTHEMATOSUS

Lupus erythematosus (LE) is a disease of autoimmune origin, its clinical spectrum ranges from benign cutaneous to a severe life-threatening systemic involvement. Numerous diverse types of autoantibodies are formed that produce the clinical signs, symptoms and laboratory abnormalities.

Pathogenesis

Lupus erythematosus is a multifactorial disease with genetic, environmental and immunopathological abnormalities. The release of nuclear antigens is a key factor in the production of LE. Defective immune regulatory mechanisms such as the clearance of apoptotic cells and immune complexes are important contributors of the disease. Ultraviolet radiations, medications, complement defects, genetic predisposition such as HLA B8, HLA DR2, HLA DR3, endogenous sex hormones such as estrogens, cytokines such as IL-10 are associated with LE. Transplacental transfer of maternal autoantibodies can result in neonatal LE.

Histopathology

The diagnostic features of all types of cutaneous lupus erythematosus involve changes in the epidermis, dermis and the pilosebaceous follicles. These changes are qualitatively similar but vary quantitatively in different types of LE.

The epidermal changes are damage to the basal layer, which is spotty and restricted, atrophy of the malpighian layer, hypergranulosis, hyperkeratosis and follicular plugging.

In the dermis the earliest follicular change is sebaceous atrophy, this usually takes weeks to develop and is therefore more marked in chronic cases, as is the conical keratotic plug, this also develops gradually. Damage to the follicular sheath is seen particularly on the scalp. The most prominent sign in the dermis is the lymphocytic infiltrate, this is more marked in the mid-dermis, it is arranged around the small vessels and near the hair follicles. The infiltrate practically approaches the epidermis in a few places and it is associated with basal cell degeneration. The infiltrate is heavy in chronic discoid lupus erythematosus (CDLE). Oedema in the dermis is usually associated with telangiectasis which is more marked in acute systemic lupus erythematosus (SLE) and subacute lupus erythematosus (SCLE).

Melanophages are present in the dermis, this is due to damage to the basal cells, which releases melanin granules. Spotty absence of elastic fibres is of considerable diagnostic value in chronic cases of lupus erythematosus.

Summary

Changes in the epidermis are characterised by hyperkeratosis and hypergranulosis, atrophy of the malpighian layer and focal liquefaction necrosis of the basal layer. The changes in the pilosebaceous follicles are characterised by sebaceous atrophy, follicular atrophy and there are conical keratin plugs in the opening of the pilosebaceous ducts. In the dermis there is lymphocytic infiltration, oedema, telangiectasia, subepidermal melanophagocytosis and focal destruction of the hair follicles in chronic lupus erythematosus.

Clinical Classification

- Chronic discoid lupus erythematosus
- Subacute lupus erythematosus
- Systemic lupus erythematosus

CHRONIC DISCOID LUPUS ERYTHEMATOSUS

This can present in many ways, the following are the more common presentations:

- Acral CDLE
- Generalised CDLE
- Chilblain CDLE
- Lupus profundus
- Lupus tumidus

Acral Chronic Discoid Lupus Erythematosus

This is a purely cutaneous disease occurring mainly on the exposed areas of the body; it is more common in middle-aged females. Ultraviolet light mainly UVB is the main exacerbating factor. The face is most commonly involved, lesions are asymmetrical, asymptomatic well-defined erythematous plaques with telangiectasia and fine adherent scales. The lesions heal from the centre, there is a red and pigmented advancing edge, the centre becomes atrophic and thin, and it is usually hypopigmented. Depressed scars may be found. Hyperkeratotic scales extending into the follicular infundibulum create keratotic spikes, when viewed from the undersurface scales resemble a carpet tack. This is a useful clinical sign in diagnosing CDLE. Atrophy and scarring are the hallmark of the disease (Fig. 1).

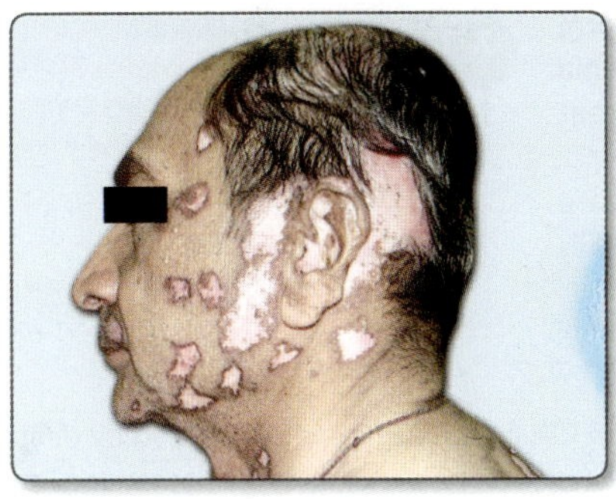

Fig. 1: Chronic discoid lupus erythematosus

Involvement of the scalp occurs in about 60% of cases often resulting in scarring alopecia. CDLE also affects the outer aspect of the external auditory canal, and vermillion border of the lips.

Laboratory Investigations

Most of the patients have no abnormality in their serum, a few have raised erythrocyte sedimentation rate (ESR), anemia, leukopenia, and antinuclear factor (ANF) (diffuse pattern) may be positive. Anti-DNA antibodies are not elevated.

Skin biopsy matches the clinical findings such as epidermal atrophy, telangiectasia, follicular plugging and lymphocytic infiltrate in the dermis.

Treatment

Sun block with high sun protection factor (SPF) against both UVB and UVA should be used.

Moderately potent topical fluorinated corticosteroids will reduce inflammation and scarring.

Systemic antimalarials like chloroquine (250 mg/day) or hydroxychloroquine (200 mg/day) for 4–6 months can be helpful. Antimalarial drugs give rise to corneal opacity and retinopathy, a monthly examination of the eyes is therefore required for patients on antimalarials.

Intralesional steroids, cryotherapy, topical tacrolimus and pimecrolimus can also be tried in resistant cases.

Dapsone 50–100 mg daily and thalidomide 50–200 mg daily have also helped a number of patients.

Systemic corticosteroids should be avoided, but if the disease is recalcitrant then prednisolone 40 mg daily can be used.

Generalised CDLE

Clinically it is similar to the acral variety, the lesions spread to the covered parts of the body and systemic symptoms of arthralgia and Raynaud's phenomenon may be present. Palms and soles may be the site of painful erosive lesions. Nail involvement is represented by nailfold erythema, telangiectasia, red lunulae, clubbing, paronychia, pitting, leukonychia and onycholysis.

This variety should be differentiated from the SLE. It is treated by low dose systemic steroids or antimalarial drugs.

Chilblain CDLE

This is a rare variety of CDLE; the patients are young women with a history of poor circulation. The fingers, toes, heels, calves, ears and nose are commonly affected. The lesions are raised and purple, scaling and fissuring may be present.

The lesions persist into the warm weather. Occasionally an erythema multiforme like rash may be present (Rowell's syndrome).

Laboratory investigations are similar to CDLE; however, the ANF is of the speckled pattern.

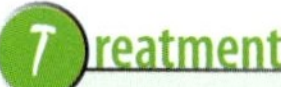

Treatment

As the lesions are due to cold injury to the microvasculature, the usual treatment of CDLE is ineffective. Systemic steroids and antimalarial drugs help a few patients. Warmth is the most important factor.

Lupus Profundus

This may be associated with both CDLE and SLE. It is characterised by deep dermal or subcutaneous nodules, firm in consistency, they are not tender. The lesions are most commonly seen on the face, head and the upper arm. The lesions heal with scarring and atrophy of the dermis (Fig. 2).

Histopathology

Shows lymphocytic panniculitis, hyaline degeneration of the fat, sharply circumscribed lymphocytic nodules in the lower dermis. The overlying epidermis may show basal liquefaction and follicular plugging.

Treatment

Antimalarials are as a rule dramatically successful. An initial dose of hydroxychloroquine 200 mg twice a day is reduced as soon as possible. Intralesional triamcinolone acetonide is also effective.

Lupus Tumidus

Erythematous papules, nodules or urticarial plaque are present on the face and upper trunk, lesions are very light sensitive. Histology shows abundant

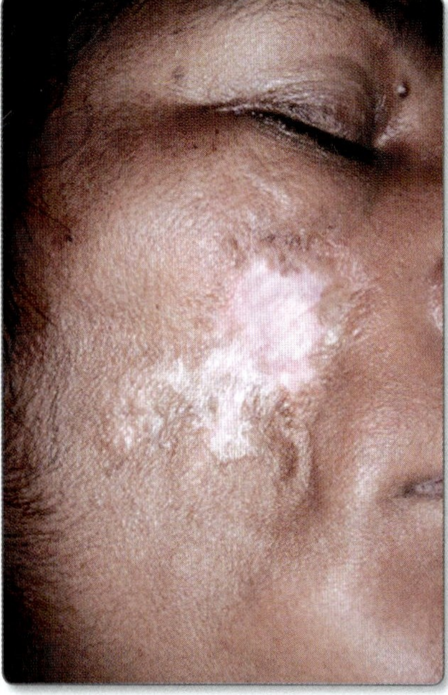

Fig. 2: Lupus profundus-scarring
Source: Dr S Janjua: Global Skin Atlas

mucin deposition, and superficial perivascular and periadnexal inflammation. Epidermal changes are minimal. Unlike CDLE, lesions resolve completely, without scarring or atrophy.

The condition is treated by antimalarials and intralesional corticosteroids. *Risk Factors in CDLE For Development Into SLE.* These are:

- Generalised CDLE,
- Diffuse scarring alopecia
- Periungual telangiectasia
- Unexplained anaemia
- Leukopenia
- ESR more than 50
- Non-lesional lupus band test positive
- High titres of ANA

SUBACUTE LUPUS ERYTHEMATOSUS

This encompasses the clinical spectrum of cutaneous lupus erythematosus between CDLE and acute SLE. Lesions of SCLE may last for months, but heal without scarring. Females are more commonly affected. Two varieties of clinical lesions occur; the papulosquamous and annular polycyclic, these are mainly found on the chest and back. On healing hypopigmentation and telangiectasia become more evident, both the lesions resolve after several months. Some patients of SCLE may share some of the features of acute SLE.

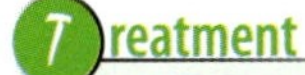

Similar to CDLE with sunscreens, topical steroids and antimalarials control SCLE in most patients. Patients not responding to antimalarial may require oral corticosteroids, acitretin or isotretinoin. nonsteroidal anti-inflammatory drugs (NSAIDs) for arthritis.

Course and Prognosis

The disease generally runs a mild course; renal, central nervous system and vascular complications are rare.

SYSTEMIC LUPUS ERYTHEMATOSUS

Systemic lupus erythematosus is a multisystem disease, characterised by a tendency to pancytopenia and immunological abnormalities, especially antibodies to nuclear antigens. It usually presents in females between the ages of 20 and 50.

Aetiology

Systemic lupus erythematosus is a multifactorial disease with genetic and immunological abnormalities. The presence of antinuclear antibodies is a key factor in diagnosis. The disease is predominant in females. Multiple abnormal immune responses are present that are responsible for the widespread manifestations of the disease.

HLA-B8, HLA -DR2, HLA-DR3, HLA-DQwl are some of the histocompatibility antigens associated with LE. The possible linkage to a virus, ultraviolet light both UVA and UVB, drugs such as hydralazine, sulphonamides, penicillins, procainamide, tetracyclines, anticonvulsants and TNFα blockers have precipitated or unmasked SLE. Drug-induced SLE is mild, renal and central nervous symptoms being unusual, anti-dsDNA antibodies are absent but antihistone antibodies are present in >95% patients.

Immunological abnormalities are due to the overproduction of antibodies by the B-lymphocytes against endogenous antigens; T suppresser cells are also reduced. There is evidence for externalisation of cellular antigens such as Ro/SSA in response to sunlight. This may lead to cell injury by the way of antibody-dependent cellular toxicity. A range of antibodies are produced, some are more specific such as anti-dsDNA, anti-Sm antibody and some are more commonly found such as ANA and anti-Ro. Genetic factors may play a role in the development of SLE.

Clinical Features

Middle-aged women are predominantly affected with a wide range of signs and symptoms. These may be either somatic such as profound weakness, fatigability or fever of undetermined origin, or on the other extreme fulminating toxaemia, widespread erythema, purpura and high fever. Skin involvement is seen in 80% cases of SLE.

Cutaneous Manifestations

This consists of a mid-facial erythematous rash (butterfly rash) Fig 3. Fine scales are present, but atrophy does not occur. Photosensitivity is present in 40–60% of cases; discoid rash is less commonly seen. Diffuse erythema may be present in the sun-exposed areas. Palmar and plantar erythema is also common. Bullae may occur due to damage to the basement membrane. Nailfold telangiectasia similar to those of systemic sclerosis and dermatomyositis are common.

Alopecia is scarring and non-scarring, lupus hair consists of fine short lustreless hair, prominent on the frontal area of the scalp. Alopecia sometimes precedes other manifestations of the disease, or it occurs with exacerbation of SLE. Scarring alopecia is a classic sign of CDLE.

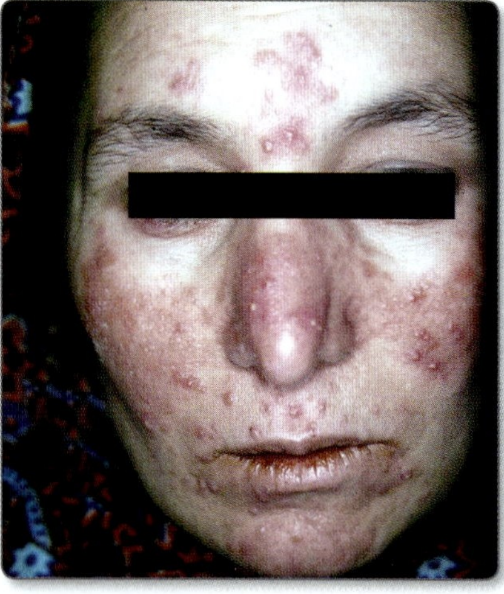

Fig. 3: Lupus erythematosus

Vasculitis presents as microinfarcts in the form of ulceration on the tips of the fingers, purpura, erosions and telangiectasia on the palms and soles. Dilated tortuous capillary loops are commonly reported on the nailfolds (Fig. 4). Raynaud's phenomenon occurs in 20% of SLE patients. Digital ischemia and gangrene may follow urticarial vasculitis in 7–28% of cases; the urticaria is painful and persistent.

Leg ulcers are deeply punched out, indolent with little inflammation, these are present on the pretibial and malleolar areas. Livedo reticularis and gangrene of the toes may occur. Other manifestations of vasculitis are nodular vasculitis and livedo reticularis.

Mucosal lesions vary from cheilitis to deep painful ulcerations involving the lips, buccal mucosa and the palate. Conjunctivitis is common.

Systemic Manifestations

Lassitude, malaise and fever are common; arthritis and arthralgia are frequent presenting symptoms. Myalgia with severe pain and myositis are common. It is often said that 'the bark of SLE is worse than the bite', i.e. the pain is very severe, but little structural damage occurs. 50% of the patients have renal involvement. This ranges from mild hematuria and proteinuria to nephrotic syndrome, nephritis, hypertension or renal failure.

Pleurisy is common, chest X-ray shows basal atelectasis or raised diaphragms (shrinking lungs).

Central nervous system (CNS) manifestations may be mild to life-threatening. These include headaches, nerve palsies, aseptic meningitis, fits and stroke. Psychiatric disturbances range from mild depression to psychosis.

Pericarditis, myocarditis and Libman-Sack's endocarditis may occur. Raynaud's phenomenon is a frequent symptom.

Gastrointestinal involvement is rare, ascites may be present, hepatitis is induced by drugs such as salicylic acid used for arthritis.

(Medical textbook should be consulted for details of systemic manifestations)

According to the American Rheumatism Association 1982, the following 11 criteria are enlisted for the diagnosis of SLE. These are:

I. Malar rash
II. Discoid rash
III. Photosensitivity

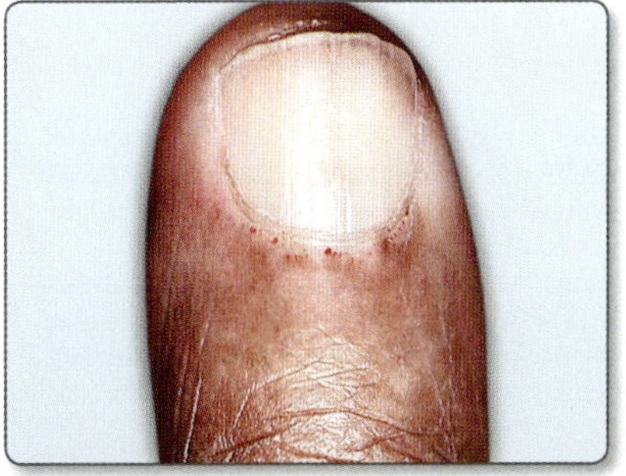

Fig. 4: Periungal telangiectasia

IV. Mucosal ulcers (oral)
V. Arthritis
VI. Serositis
VII. Renal disorders (proteinuria more than 0.5 gm/24 hours, RBC, casts)
VIII. Neurological disorders
IX. Anaemia, leukopenia, thrombocytopenia
X. Anti-dsDNA, anti-Sm antibodies in the serum, false positive tests for syphilis for 6 months, positive antiphospholipid antibodies
XI. ANA in the serum

If any 4 or more of the 11 criteria are present, serially or simultaneously, the patient is diagnosed as SLE.

Laboratory Diagnosis

Urine examination shows albumin, RBC and casts. Blood examination shows anaemia, leukopenia and thrombocytopenia. The ESR is raised. Coomb's test may be positive. Rheumatoid factor may be present. Albumin globulin ratio is usually reversed.

Immunological examination is characterised by the presence of a large number of antibodies such as ANA, anti-dsDNA (indicates a high-risk of renal damage), anti-La, anti-Ro, anti-Sm, anti-RNA and anti-snRNP antibodies. Serum complement levels are low.

Lupus erythematosus cells are polymorph leukocytes, which have ingested basophilic staining homogenous nuclear material from degenerative white cells in the presence of LE cell factor; this is an antibody to deoxyriboprotein present in the gammaglobulin fraction of the serum.

The LE cell test is also seen CDLE, systemic sclerosis, rheumatoid arthritis and in some drug reactions. The test is now superseded by the anti-DNA antibodies.

Immunofluorescence shows granular deposits of immunoglobulins and complements along the dermo-epidermal junction, the lupus band test. This is positive in the normal and lesional skin of SLE patients. In CDLE the deposits are found only in the lesional skin.

Differential Diagnosis

Systemic lupus erythematosus is also known as a great imitator of diseases, probably exceeded in this respect by syphilis and drug eruptions, because of its multisystem involvement. The rash on the face should be differentiated from rosacea, pemphigus erythematosus, dermatomyositis, seborrhoeic dermatitis, pellagra, and polymorphic light eruption. The disease should also be differentiated from rheumatoid arthritis, erythema multiforme, haemolytic anaemia, purpura, myasthenia gravis and nephritis.

SLE can be differentiated by many factors such as increased ESR, anaemia, leukopenia and thrombocytopenia, ANA and anti DNA antibodies in the serum, lupus band test and by a skin biopsy.

A number of drugs induce signs closely resembling LE (drug-induced LE). The common drugs are antihypertensives such as hydralazine, methyldopa, drugs used against arrhythmias such as procainamide and quinidine, biologics such as IFN-γ, anti-TNFα antibodies, minocycline, isoniazid and chlorpromazine are also responsible for LE like symptoms. The disease resolves when the drugs are stopped. Most of the patients who are affected are slow acetylators who metabolize drugs slowly. The disease produced is less severe, arthritis is common. History of drug intake is important in excluding these cases.

Treatment

The aim of treatment is to maintain optimal function with minimum of therapy. In acute cases bed rest is required, undue exposure to sun should be avoided. Mental and physical stress, secondary infection should be prevented.

The treatment of cutaneous lesions is similar to that of CDLE.

Mild systemic disease can be controlled by NSAIDs and antimalarial drugs.

Treatment with corticosteroids depends upon the severity of the illness; this can be judged by the severity of the symptoms, serum C3 complement levels and anti-DNA titres. Prednisolone 60 mg daily, once the disease is under control, the dose is gradually reduced to 10–15 mg daily.

Immunosuppressive drugs such as azathioprine (100–150 mg daily), methotrexate (7.5–20 mg weekly), cyclosporin (5 mg/kg daily), cyclophosphamide (1–3 mg/kg daily), and mycophenolate mofetil (2 g daily) are used for patients not responding to corticosteroids.

Dapsone, isotretinoin, thalidomide, sulphasalazine have also been used for the treatment of resistant cases of SLE.

Plasmapheresis may be helpful in small number of cases. Intravenous gammaglobulins can be used for severe thrombocytopenia. Biologics like anti-CD 20, anti-CD 40 and TNF–α inhibitors, rituximab and belimumab have also been used in recalcitrant cases.

Course and Prognosis

The disease is characterised by relapse and long periods of remission. Many patients survive for decades. Death is usually due to fulminating renal or central nervous system disease.

ANTIPHOSPHOLIPID SYNDROME (LUPUS ANTICOAGULANT SYNDROME)

The syndrome is characterised by livedo reticularis, thromboembolic complications, severe headaches and abortion. The syndrome is seen mostly in young women, secondary to SLE, chronic infections, lymphoma and drugs.

Antiphospholipid antibodies recognise phospholipid-binding proteins, they target β_2-glycoproteins; it then triggers activation of T cells, thrombocytes, and endothelial cells.

Lupus anticoagulant antibody which is present in about 10% of LE patients may be found in antiphospholipid syndrome. Although this antibody inhibits conversion of prothrombin to thrombin, it is associated with prolonged activated partial thromboplastin time, bleeding rarely occurs. It increases the risk to thromboembolism.

Clinical Features

Arterial emboli and venous thrombosis occur in about 30% of patients. Cutaneous signs include livedo reticularis, Raynaud's phenomenon, acral ulcerations and gangrene. Sneddon's syndrome is a combination of livedo reticularis and CNS thrombosis. Pregnancy often leads to abortion or intrauterine death due to placental insufficiency.

Diagnosis

Presence of antiphospholipid antibodies, and lupus anticoagulant antibodies if the condition is secondary to LE.

Treatment

Treat underlying disease. Anticoagulation therapy should be initiated. After thrombosis, lifelong anticoagulation with coumarin is required. Aspirin is used for prophylaxis.

NEONATAL LUPUS ERYTHEMATOSUS

Lupus erythematosus can be transmitted to the child if the mother has anti-Ro/SS-A and anti-La/SS-B antibodies. These antibodies cross react with fetal cardiac conduction system antigens.

The mothers may be normal, they may have SCLE or Sjögren's syndrome. The infant has mild features of SCLE, the lesions are usually annular, transient and heal without scarring. The major problem is congenital heart block, which is present in 70% of cases.

The cutaneous lesions should be differentiated from urticaria, erythema multiforme and annular erythemas. These are uncommon in childhood. Check the mother for anti-Ro/SS-A and anti-La/SSB antibodies.

Treatment

Skin lesions do not require any therapy. The heart block can be treated with a pace maker after birth. If the condition is diagnosed during pregnancy then plasmapheresis and dexamethasone (crosses the placenta) can be used.

Lupus erythematosus was first recognised as a cutaneous disorder, and for many years the systemic form of the disorder was unknown. Kaposi in 871 was the first to recognise the systemic component of the disease.

DERMATOMYOSITIS

Dermatomyositis (DM) is a rare inflammatory disease of the skin and the muscles. It is characterised by a specific rash and muscle weakness. Females outnumber males by the ratio of 2:1. Two age groups are affected, the children and the adults. Adult DM may be associated with malignancy especially those of the gastrointestinal tract, prostate, ovaries and the blood.

Aetiology and Pathogenesis

Dermatomyositis is a genetically determined disease with autoimmune response associated with the presence of circulating autoantibodies; these are muscle specific and overlapping. Important predisposing factors are environmental; the most important environmental factor is UVL, about 50% of patients experience photosensitivity. Other environmental stimuli include viruses, such as Human T-lymphotropic virus, Coxsackie, Parvovirus and Toxoplasma gondii infection.

The disease can be exacerbated with emotional and physical stress.

Histopathology

The histological features are similar to those of SLE. In the skin liquefaction, degeneration of the basal layer is present; the overlying epidermis is thin and atrophic. In the dermis, mucin deposits and sclerosis of collagen and blood vessels may be seen. Large number of melanin granules, are present in the dermis, due to pigmentary incontinence. Free RBC's are also seen due to capillary leakage.

Muscle involvement is variable; the affected muscle fibres show loss of transverse striations, hyalinisation of the sarcoplasm and an increase in sarcolemmal nuclei. Later the muscle fibres show granular and vacuolar degeneration. There is infiltration of the muscle fibres with lymphocytes, plasma cells and macrophages. The trapezius, deltoid and quadriceps seem to be always affected.

The immunopathology of cutaneous DM includes a deposition of IgG and complement at the dermal-epidermal junction and within the dermal vasculature. The predominant infiltrating cells are the macrophages and activated CD 4 T cells.

Dermal mucin is a predominant finding in DM; this could be due to the production of glycosaminoglycans by dermal fibroblasts as a result of immunological stimulation.

Clinical Features

Onset may be sudden or gradual; skin changes may accompany or follow the muscle changes.

The characteristic skin changes are erythema of the face and on the V area of the neck. The facial skin may have a violaceous hue; the eyelids are involved first (Fig. 5). They become swollen, are pinkish violet (heliotrope) in colour, tender to touch due to the involvement of the orbicularis oculi muscle. There is erythema on the dorsum of the hands and linear erythema on the dorsum of the fingers. Smooth violaceous flat-topped papules over the knuckles (Gottron's papules) (Fig. 6) are thought to be pathognomonic of dermatomyositis. Gottrons sign refers to the symmetrical confluent violet erythema, with or without oedema over the dorsal aspect of the interphalangeal joints, metacarpophalangeal joints, olecranon process, patella and medial malleoli.

Prominent ragged cuticles and dilated capillaries are present in the proximal nailfold.

Hand lesions of DM are non-pruritic hyperkeratotic eruptions, accompanied with scaling, fissuring and hyperpigmentation, giving a false appearance of a callosity. These changes are seen along the ulnar aspect of the thumb and radial aspect of the fingers, with occasional extension onto the palms.

There is erythema over the knees and elbows in some patients, calcified nodules on the elbows, knees and acral parts may occur. Shawl sign: erythema over upper back.

Dermatomyositis can be associated with poikiloderma vasculare atrophicans and calcinosis cutis. 10-20% of cases have oral ulcers.

Muscle involvement is variable. In some cases, there is little evidence of muscle disease, in others there is profound muscle weakness. Typically, there is pain followed by symmetrical weakness and wasting of the girdle muscles. Early weakness of these muscles is noted on climbing the stairs or raising the arms above the shoulders. Pharyngeal and oesophageal muscles may be involved leading to dysphagia. Cardiac involvement with cardiac failure may be the terminal phase of the disease. Strabismus is due to the weakness of ocular muscles.

Asymptomatic ECG changes are common; occasionally myocarditis and cardiac myopathy can occur.

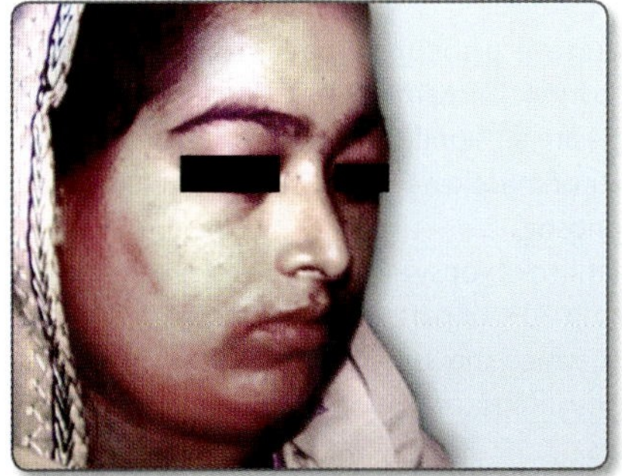

Fig. 5: Dermatomyositis—note the swollen heliotrope eyelids

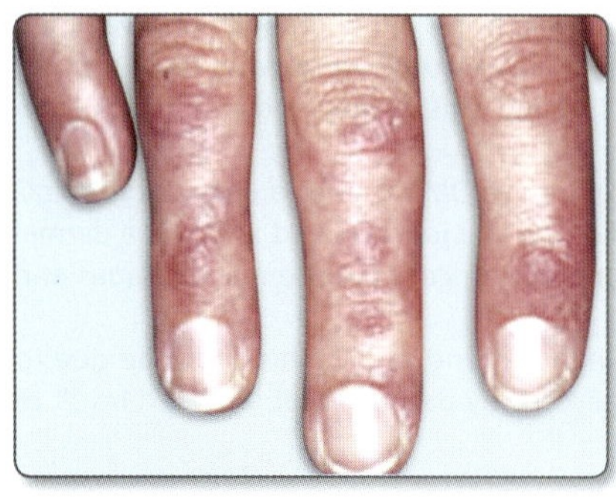

Fig. 6: Gottron's papule

Childhood Dermatomyositis

Several features differ from the adult form. The more common Brunsting type has a slow course, progressive weakness, calcinosis cutis is present and the disease is steroid responsive. Calcinosis may be subcutaneous, in the acral parts as in adults, or it may involve the intermuscular facial planes. The second type; Bankers variety is rapid in onset, characterised by vasculitis of the muscles and the gastrointestinal tract. There is severe weakness; the disease does not respond to steroids, death occurs early. This type is uncommon. Internal malignancy is seldom seen with either form.

Paraneoplastic Dermatomyositis

This is of late onset; it is associated with tumours, commonly of the breast, gastrointestinal tract, blood and head and neck. Pathogenesis of paraneoplastic dermatomysitis is unclear.

CORRELATION BETWEEN CUTANEOUS AND SYSTEMIC/MUSCLE MANIFESTATIONS

There is little correlation between skin and muscle disease. Patients who have both skin and muscle disease, which gets controlled by drugs, can have a return of cutaneous signs without any evident of muscle disease after discontinuation of medication.

Laboratory Investigations

Muscles enzymes [serum creatine phosphokinase, aldolase, lactic dehydrogenase, serum glutamic pyruvic transaminase (SGPT), serum glutamic oxaloacetic transaminase (SGOT)] are all significantly raised. Serum creatine phosphokinase is the best marker of muscle damage. 24-hour urine creatine level greater than 200 mg is diagnostic.

Electromyography (EMG) and muscle biopsy are other diagnostic aids. EMG shows the characteristic changes in 70% of patients. Muscle biopsy is one of the most reliable diagnostic tests, which shows necrosis and varying degrees of regeneration, with inflammatory infiltrates.

- ESR is elevated in 50% of cases.
- MRI scan shows inflamed muscles.

A large number of autoantibodies are present such as myositis-specific antibody (MSA), anti-Jo-I (antisynthetase), anti-SRP (signal reaction protein), and anti-Mi2 (helicase).

Others are rheumatoid factor, and ANA. Anti-dsDNA antibodies are not found. Routine medical check up should be done to exclude malignancy. Ovarian cancer is common; a pelvic examination should be done.

Treatment

Strict bed rest is essential during the acute phase of the disease. Antimalarials help in cutaneous lesions, as do topical corticosteroids. Sunscreens are essential, as UVL is an important environmental trigger of the disease.

Acetylsalicylic acid is given regularly (2 tablets given 4 times daily). Oral corticosteroids: prednisolone 40–60 mg/day gives symptomatic relief. The dose of prednisolone is reduced in line with the clinical response. SGOT and creatine phosphokinase assume normal levels as remission occurs.

Methotrexate when given early will produce remission in most cases. It is given in a dose of 5–15 mg weekly for 4–6 weeks.

Other immunosuppressive drugs such as azathioprine, mycophenolate mofetil and cyclosporin are also helpful.

Intravenous immunoglobulin (IVIG) 2 g/kg daily for 2 days, repeated every 4 weeks for 6–12 months, can be used in resistant cases.

For paraneoplastic dermatomyositis, appropriate treatment of the underlying malignancy is indicated.

Physiotherapy should be initiated once the disease is under control to avoid loss of function in the affected muscles.

Course and Prognosis

Prognosis is said to be better in dermatomyositis than in polymyositis. Patients without muscular involvement have a better prognosis. Calcinosis is a good prognostic sign. Removal of an underlying carcinoma in adults can lead to regression of dermatomyositis.

Only biopsy those muscles, that are shown to be affected by EMG or MRI.
The biopsy specimen should be kept in a special solution provided by the pathologist.
Keep the biopsy specimen under tension by a muscle clamp, otherwise the procedure is worthless.

SCLERODERMA

Scleroderma is a multiorgan disease characterised by hardening of the skin. It occurs in two forms; localised (morphea) and systemic.

Aetiology

The exact aetiology is unknown, but damage to the endothelial cells of the blood vessels is the initial target of the disease. Damage to the endothelial cells initiates the fibrotic process, either through the effects of ischaemia or via the growth modulating mediators, released from the platelets or from the inflamed cells.

The damage to blood vessels may be due to autoimmunity as seen by the presence of antibodies against the blood vessels, circulating immune complexes, anticentromere and anti-ScL-70 antibodies. There may be a genetic factor associated with the disease, chemicals, viruses, etc. are also said to be the causative factors.

The tick borne *spirochaete Borrelia* burgdorferi is said to play a part in the pathogenesis of morphea. Polymerase chain reaction has shown the presence of borrelial infection in cases of morphea reported from Europe but not in cases from USA.

Morphea (Circumscript Scleroderma)

This is the pure cutaneous form of the disease, the most striking feature is hardening of the skin. The disease is more common in females, it can occur in any age. The lesions are usually solitary of about 5–20 cm. The disease begins spontaneously, initially the affected area of the skin has a violaceous hue, but gradually these areas become thickened and ivory white in colour. The surface is smooth and shiny, as the pathological process destroys the hair follicles and the sweat glands, the plaque is devoid of hair and does not sweat. Eventually after many months, the sclerosis resolves leaving atrophic hypopigmented areas.

Clinical variants are: linear lesions on the limbs, circumscribed plaques on the trunk, guttate lesions present as multiple small plaques. Fronto-parietal lesion (en coup de sabre) involves the scalp, forehead and face with or without facial hemiatrophy (Fig. 7), and nodular variety resembling a keloid. Generalised morphea involving the whole body is mutilating, leading to crippled deformity of the limbs.

Histopathology

There is first oedema of the collagen tissue and a non-specific dermal infiltrate. Later the collagen becomes dense, the elastic tissue and the appendages eventually disappear. This is followed by fibrosis; the stage shows a marked deposition of collagen in the dermis and subcutaneous tissue. The epidermis becomes thin and atrophic.

Diagnosis

The clinical presentation is characteristic. A skin biopsy can confirm the diagnosis, but does not differentiate between morphoea and systemic sclerosis. ANA and anti-ss-DNA may be found in generalised disease. In widespread disease an evaluation of the joints and oesophagus should be done.

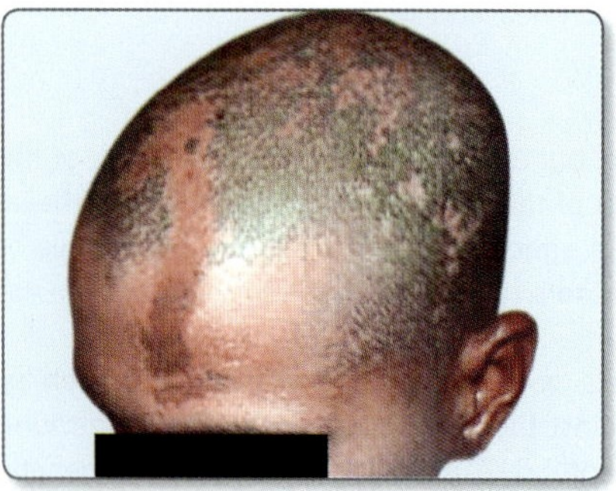

Fig. 7: Morphoea

Treatment

There is no effective treatment of morphoea. Intralesional steroids may help to resolve the induration. Topical steroids under occlusion also help. Hydroxychloroquine 400 mg/day may be considered when multiple inflammatory lesions are present. Pencillamine is said to be helpful in a few cases particularly in the linear morphea of childhood. En coup de sabre may be helped by plastic surgery. For widespread morphea treatment is similar to systemic sclerosis.

UVA-1 has shown good response in some cases.

Sometimes large plaques respond to penicillin. Repeated course of IM or IV penicillin are recommended.

Phenytoin sodium may also be used for the treatment of linear morphea.

Course and Prognosis

Plaque morphea usually resolves over a period of several years leaving atrophy or hyperpigmentation. En coup de sabre usually does not resolve. Some cases of generalised morphea progress inexorably until the patient is very disabled.

DIFFUSE SYSTEMIC SCLEROSIS

Systemic sclerosis is a multisystem disorder characterised by association of vascular abnormalities, connective tissue sclerosis, atrophy and autoimmune changes. Scleroderma may commence from childhood, but is most commonly seen between 30 and 60 years of age. Women outnumber males in the ratio of 4:1. Systemic sclerosis may have extensive skin lesions or the skin lesions may be limited.

Clinical Features

The following are clinical forms of scleroderma:

- Acrosclerosis
- CREST syndrome
- Acute diffuse scleroderma

Acrosclerosis

Acral systemic sclerosis Type 1 is the common variety, it involves only the hands and forearms. It begins with swelling of the fingers and Raynaud's phenomenon, which causes blanching of the fingers. Hardening and tapering of the distal digits (sclerodactyly) follow these changes. Progressive ischemia leads to ulceration of the tip of the fingers, followed by scarring to resorption and gangrene of the digit. The nailfolds show dilated capillaries and nailfold infarcts. Nails show changes of ischaemia, discolouration, brittleness and longitudinal ridging. The nails may also shed. Calcinosis cutis is seen in the skin of the hands and feet. Raynaud's phenomenon is often the presenting sign.

The hardening of the hands eventually spreads to the forearms.

Acral systemic sclerosis type 11 starts on the hand then spreads to the arms and trunk.

CREST Syndrome

This is an acronym for **C**alcinosis, **R**aynaud's phenomenon, **E**sophageal dysmotility, **S**clerodactyly and **T**elangiectasia. Immunologically anti-centromere antibody, appears to be highly specific for CREST syndrome.

It is positive in 50–90% of cases. This variant of systemic sclerosis has the most favorable prognosis, owing to the limited systemic involvement.

Diffuse Scleroderma

This is the most serious form of disease and affects both the sexes. The disease begins on the trunk or the face. The lesions are yellowish or ivory coloured hardened plaques that spread peripherally. Telangiectasia and pigmentary changes are often found. The telangiectasia in scleroderma, have a unique morphology; they occur as flat (macular) rectangular collection of uniform, tiny vessels so called the telangiectatic mat. These are most common on the face, lips, palms, back of the hand. The telangiectasia may also be present on the tongue and mucous membrane. On the face there is microstomia and tightening of the frenulum. Old patients may have difficulty in inserting and removal of dentures. There is reduced facial expression. Confetti-like hypopigmentation is common in dark skin people. There is widening of the periodontal membrane (Fig. 8).

The course of acute diffuse scleroderma progresses rapidly both externally and internally. Fibrosis, loss of smooth muscles of the internal organs and progressive loss of visceral function characterise this disorder. The gastrointestinal tract is frequently involved, followed by the lungs and then the cardiovascular and renal system. The central nervous system and musculo-skeletal system are less frequently involved.

Esophageal involvement is seen in 90% of cases, the distal two thirds is commonly affected, leading to dysphagia and reflux oesophagitis. Small intestinal atonia may lead to constipation, malabsorption and diarrhoea.

Pulmonary involvement includes pulmonary fibrosis with arterial hypoxia, dyspnea and cough. There may be bronchiectasis and cyst formation.

Cardiac involvement produces dyspnea and symptoms of congestive cardiac failure. Sclerosis of the myocardium produces conduction changes. Death is often due to cardiac or renal failure.

Kidney involvement leads to hypertension and progressive renal failure.

Skeletal manifestations are first noted by pain, swelling and inflammation of the bones. There is limitation of movement due to skin tautness followed by ankylosis. The hand joints are most frequently involved. Bones may show acro-osteolysis. Muscle involvement leads to myosclerosis and calcium deposits in the muscle.

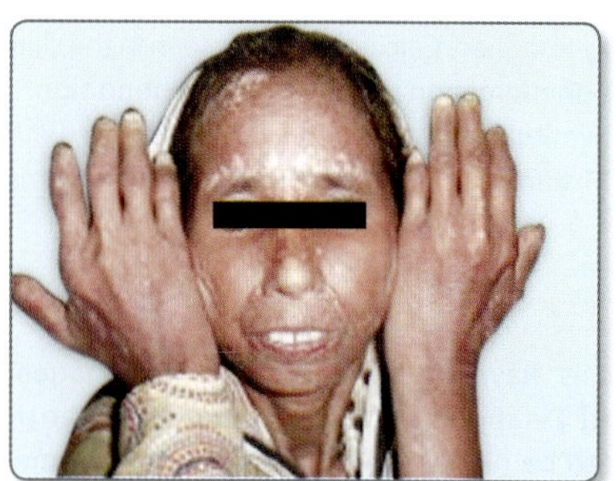

Fig. 8: Scleroderma

The Criteria of Diagnosis

Major Criteria

- Scleroderma of the digits, face, limbs neck or the trunk

Other Criteria

- Digital pitted scarring
- Bilateral basal pulmonary fibrosis
- Raynauds phenomenon
- Telangiectasia
- Abnormal pigmentation
- Distal oesophageal dysphagia and dysmotility
- Serological changes.

Laboratory Investigations

Anaemia, hypergammaglobinemia, increased ESR, positive rheumatoid factor, ANA antibodies (speckled), anti-Scl-70 and anti-centromere antibodies are found in a high proportion of patients. X-ray of the jaw shows widening of the periodontal membrane. A barium swallow shows loss of oesophageal peristalsis.

Differential Diagnosis

Scleroderma should be differentiated from scleredema a type of cutaneous mucinosis. Scleredema is a self-limiting, non-pitting oedema of the neck and upper trunk, seen in children and adults, after infections such as streptococci, measles, influenza, systemic disorders such as diabetes, rheumatoid arthritis, multiple myeloma and HIV. It is also associated with diabetes mellitus. The fingers and toes are not involved, Raynaud's phenomenon is absent, and there is no telangiectasia or ulceration. The disease is limited to the skin.

Sclerodermoid changes are seen in porphyria, carcinoid syndrome, Werner's syndrome, phenylketonuria, lichen myxoedematosus, Sjögren's syndrome, in these cases the cutaneous signs of the corresponding diseases are present.

Eosinophilic fasciitis is preceded by trauma, or unusual physical exertion, it usually involves the extremities. The skin is indurated and tightly bound to the underlying structures. There is no Raynaud's phenomenon or internal manifestations. The frequent laboratory finding is severe eosinophilia.

In graft-versus-host reaction, sclerodermoid changes occur in the late stages of transplantation.

A large number of chemicals produce scleroderma like lesions such as vinyl chloride workers, minerals like silica, ingestion of adulterated oil, and certain medicines such as bleomycin, pentazocine, cocaine, paraffin and silicone implants. In these conditions Raynaud's phenomenon is present, fingers may show pseudo-clubbing, osteolysis is frequent. Laboratory findings are usually negative; some patients may reveal ANA of a different pattern.

Other conditions to be differentiated are scleromyxedema, stiff skin syndrome and premature aging syndromes.

Treatment

There is no specific treatment but symptomatic treatment and management are important. Well-planned general exercises, regular massage and warmth, protection from trauma, exposure to cold should be avoided and smoking should be prohibited. Physiotherapy helps by increasing the circulation and avoiding strictures, thereby increasing mobility of the body.

Drugs used in scleroderma are the immune modulators, vasoactive drugs and the anti- fibrotics.

Prednisolone 10–15 mg daily; is said to reduce inflammation and skin thickness. Corticosteroids do not offer any lasting benefit, but the patient feels better and the joint symptoms may be ameliorated.

Contd...

Contd...

Methotrexate 20–30 mg weekly, cyclosporin 3–5 mg/kg daily, or cyclophosphamide 2 mg/kg daily or as pulse therapy 500–800 mg once monthly can be tried, if response to corticosteroid is unsatisfactory. Azathioprine, acitretin, colchicine and etanercept may also be used to reduce the inflammatory changes of scleroderma.

Nifedipine 5 mg thrice daily improves the peripheral circulation and reduces vasospasm. If postural hypotension is a problem then diltiazem 60–120 mg daily or verapamil 240-360 mg daily can be used. If the frequency of Raynaud's phenomenon is high and there is extreme vasospasm then prostaglandin analogues such as iloprost can be given by IV route daily over 6–8 hours. Topical nitroglycerine paste may help to avoid digital necrosis.

Captopril 150 mg daily and 2.5 mg/kg of prostacyclin infused IV in 24 hours can also be used.

In some cases D-penicillamine in doses of 150–300 mg daily may be used, it inhibits the synthesis of collagen crosslinks. Other antifibrotic agents are cyclofenil and colchicine. Griseofulvin in a dose of 750 mg daily, inhibits the proliferation of fibroblasts.

Recently phototherapy with ultraviolet A-1 (340–400 nm), has shown some promising results.

The involvement of the internal organs need appropriate treatment, e.g. angiotensin-converting enzyme inhibitors for renal hypertension, proton pump inhibitors help to treat oesophageal disease. A physician should be consulted in these situations.

Physiotherapy is required to treat and avoid muscle contractures and to retain function. Infrared light may help by increasing circulation and raising body temperature.

Course and Prognosis

The prognosis is very variable; life expectancy can be a few months to over 30 years. 50% of the patients usually die within 5 years. Death results from renal failure, cardiac dysrhythmias and intestinal perforation. The morbidity from Raynaud's phenomenon is considerable.

Maurice Raynaud (1834-1881)

Raynaud was to address the great Medical congress held in London and chaired by Sir James Paget in 1881. Lister, Kock, Pasteur and Osler were all there to hear Raynaud's paper, but his paper was read by someone else, Raynaud having died of coronary infarction, a month before. He was very religious and this probably prevented his achieving high professional status. His description of local asphyxia and gangrene was published in 1862.

MIXED CONNECTIVE TISSUE DISEASE

Mixed connective tissue disease (MCTD) also known as the Sharp syndrome is regarded by some as an entity characterised by clinical overlapping of LE, polymyositis, scleroderma and occasionally rheumatoid arthritis. The most striking finding is the presence of high tires of an antibody against U1-ribonucleoprotein (U1-RNP), which gives ANA a speckled pattern. The other antibodies to extractable nuclear antigens are usually absent.

The clinical picture usually consists of polyarthralgia, Raynaud's phenomenon, swollen hands, sclerodactyly, oesophageal dysmotility, pulmonary disease and inflammatory myositis. Anti-dsDNA antibodies may be present usually at low titres, serum complements may be depressed. Other features of LE such as serositis, leukopenia, anaemia and skin rashes. Other associations of anti-U1-RNP are myocarditis and trigeminal neuropathy. Severe kidney and CNS disease are infrequent in MCTD.

Improvement can be achieved by prednisolone in a dose of 1 mg/kg of body weight. Generally, the prognosis is good with long remissions. LE features of MCTD are most likely to improve and sclerodermal features least likely. Mild cases may respond to antimalarials.

SJÖGREN'S SYNDROME (Sicca syndrome)

Sjögren's syndrome (Sicca syndrome) is an autoimmune disease which has a predilection for epithelial tissues and exocrine glands. The syndrome may be primary, or secondary when associated with rheumatoid arthritis. It then comprises a triad of keratoconjunctivitis sicca, xerostomia and rheumatoid arthritis. Rheumatoid arthritis may be replaced by other connective tissue disorders such as scleroderma, MCTD, polyarteritis nodosa or SLE.

Aetiology

The pathogenesis is largely unknown. It may be immunogenetic. Anti-Ro and anti-La antibodies are present in some patients. The disease is associated with HLA-B8, HLA-DR3, HLA-DQw2 and HLA-DR w52.

Clinical Signs

The syndrome primarily affects the eyes and the mouth, resulting in dry eyes and mouth.

Oral Lesions

Include dry mouth, which is due to the destruction of major and minor salivary glands. The salivary glands may be enlarged due to blockage by mucoid salivary secretions. The oral lesions give rise to burning or pain and difficulty in swallowing. Dental caries are common.

Ocular lesions include dryness of the eyes, which may lead to corneal ulcerations due to rubbing. Conjunctivitis may be present. The lacrimal glands are enlarged due to blockage of its duct. Advanced cases show a decrease in the aqueous secretion of the eyes.

Vaginal dryness leads to dyspareunia. Bacterial and yeast infections are common.

Cutaneous manifestations include dry skin, and vasculitic changes such as palpable purpura, ulcers, urticaria, and erythema multiforme.

The patients are prone to lymphoreticular malignancies.

Histologically leukocytoclastic vasculitis or mononuclear vasculitis is found.

Diagnosis

Labial salivary gland biopsy is said to be the most definite diagnostic test for Sjögren's syndrome. There is a dense lymphocytic infiltrate with many plasma cells and few lymphocytes. Biopsy is taken from the lower lips.

Lacrimal secretion can be measured by the Schirmer's test.

Treatment

This is directed against the vascular manifestations of connective tissue disease. Artificial lubricants should be used for oral, nasal and vaginal dryness. Artificial tears for dryness of the eyes. Treat oral candisiasis when present.

Rheumatoid arthritis is described in Chapter 31.

MISCELLANEOUS DISORDERS OF COLLAGEN TISSUE

Keloids

Keloid is an excessive connective tissue response to cutaneous injury; it extends beyond the site of tissue damage.

Aetiology

Both local and constitutional factors are involved in the production of a keloid. It may follow surgical incisions, burns, infections, etc. Tension on the wound or the presence of a foreign body, exogenous or endogenous predisposes to keloid formation. Spontaneous keloids may occur from minor trauma such as acne lesions. A family history is found in some cases of keloids. Both autosomal dominant and autosomal recessive patterns of inheritance have been reported. There is a genetic association with other fibromatosis such as Dupuytren's contracture. Keloids are also reported in association with Ehlers-Danlos syndrome and pachydermoperiostosis.

In a keloid, collagen production is increased; collagen degradation appears to be normal. Keloid fibroblasts produce exorbitant collagen and glycosaminoglycans.

Histopathology

In a normal scar the collagen bundles run parallel to the skin surface. In a keloid, the collagen bundles produce curvilinear tracts and bundles, several of which form a whorl, the blood vessels are seen at the periphery. The collagen is also abnormal; Luxol blue stains normal collagen blue, keloid collagen is reddish in colour. The collagen filaments are half the diameter than those the normal skin. The interstitial tissue retains large amounts of mucopolysaccharides. Mast cells are also numerous. The overlying epidermis is flattened or normal. Neuropeptide containing nerves are present in a keloid, which contribute to its discomfort and itching.

In a keloid of recent onset, endothelial proliferation is surrounded by a number of fibroblasts. Mucinous deposition is present in keloids, but not in a hypertrophic scar.

Clinical Features

Keloids are firm, irregular, thickened, pink or red fibrous growths. Early growths are red and have a rubber like consistency, often surrounded by an erythematous halo, it may be telangiectatic. In course of time, the keloids become brown. Hyperesthesia may sometimes be present. It may be tender, painful and pruritic. The tendency to send out claw like projections is typical of a keloid. Keloids may become inflamed and drain purulent material.

Sites of predilection are chest, shoulders, upper back, pubis and lower legs. Keloids are common between the ages of 10 and 30 years; women are more commonly affected than men (Fig. 9).

Differential Diagnosis

Keloids should be differentiated from a hypertrophic scar, sclerotic basal cell carcinoma, malignancy in a scar and dermatofibroma. Blastomycosis and lobomycosis also cause keloidal reactions.

Differentiating points from hypertrophic scar are:

- Keloids extend beyond the site of trauma; hypertrophic scar is restricted to the site of injury
- Hypertrophic scar tends to flatten and become hypopigmented after 6-24 months; keloids remain active for years
- Keloids continue to enlarge in the absence of continued injury; hypertrophic scars grow with tissue injury only
- Keloids may be pruritic, tender, or painful. Purulent discharge and foul odour occasionally develops in a keloid. Hypertrophic scars are symptomless.

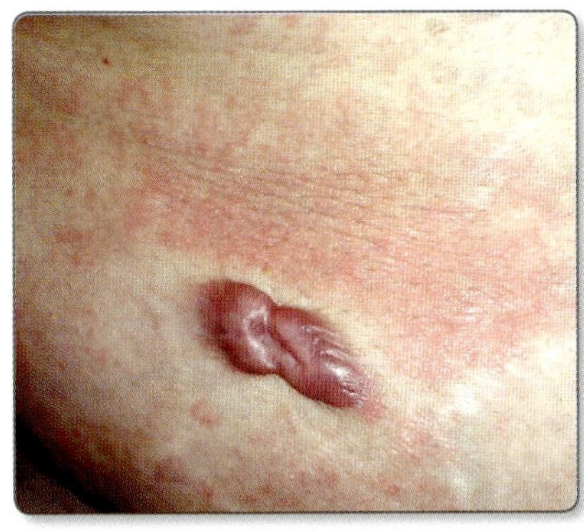

Fig. 9: Keloid

Prophylaxis

Nonessential surgery should be avoided at the sites where there is a tendency for keloids to occur. If surgery is essential then simple excision with sutures without tension should be applied. Pre and postoperative steroid injections should be given. Preoperative radiotherapy is also used in some cases. Precautions should be taken to avoid secondary infection. Electrocoagulation and caustic chemicals should be avoided at such sites.

Treatment

Intralesional injections of corticosteroids are used for early keloids. 40 mg/ml of triamcinolone is injected in the keloid; the treatment is repeated every 6-8 weeks. Several injections may be required. Prior freezing with liquid nitrogen before the injection, causes oedema, softens the keloid and helps the injection to penetrate in the keloid. Dermojet is used for keloid injection.

Pressure dressings with pressure greater than 24 mm Hg are useful for fresh wounds, especially for burn scars and for prophylaxis against keloid formation.

If surgical removal is required then pre- and postoperative injection of triamcinolone should be given in a dose of 10 mg/ml. Surgical excision and control with methotrexate has given good results. Methotrexate is given orally 15–20 mg in a single dose and repeated every 4 days, starting a week before surgery and for about 4 months after surgery.

Colchicine, which prevents fibrous tissue formation, has also been used in the treatment of keloids.

A cream containing 20% of silicon acid applied under occlusion has also been used for the treatment of keloids. Topical retinoic acid applied daily may be helpful in some cases. Systemic retinoids enhance keloid formation.

Intralesional IFN α-2b decreases production of collagen and glycosaminoglycans, it is not effective in mature keloids.

Knuckle Pads

Knuckle pads or holoderma are well-defined fibrous thickenings on the extensor surface of the proximal interphalangeal joints of the fingers. The toes are seldom involved. It is said to have an autosomal dominant inheritance. The age of onset is variable, commonly seen after the fourth decade. The growth is rapid initially; it grows to a diameter of 10-15 mm and then persists permanently. Knuckle pads are skin coloured or slightly brownish in colour, freely movable over the underlying structures (Fig. 10). It is often associated with Dupuytren's contracture and other fibromatous lesions.

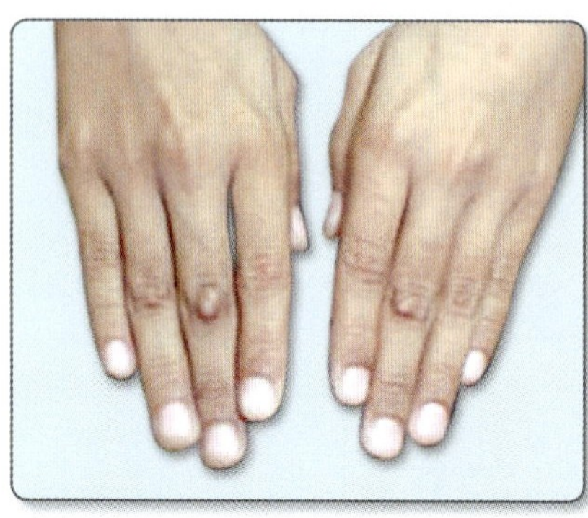

Fig. 10: Knuckle pads

Histologically there is hyperkeratosis and acanthosis. The collagen fibres are thickened, the lesion resemble palmar fibromatosis.

Treatment is unsatisfactory. Excision is often followed by keloid formation. Intralesional steroids may be beneficial.

Fibrous Papule of the Nose

This is usually a single dome-shaped sessile papule, skin coloured or slightly red in colour, asymptomatic, present on or near the side of the nose. It occurs in middle age. The lesion is said to be an angiofibroma. The connective tissue is oriented vertically towards the surface, the capillaries are prominent, dilated elastic fibres are also seen. On electron microscope, most of the cells are seen to consist of fibroblasts.

Fibrous papule of the nose should be differentiated from a fibrocytic nevus and a fibroma; it does not contain S-100 protein, which is characteristic of nevus cells.

On excision, recurrence is rare.

Striae distensae are described in chapters 33, 34 and 42.

HEREDITARY DISORDERS OF COLLAGEN AND ELASTIC TISSUE

Pseudoxanthoma Elasticum

Pseudoxanthoma elasticum (Systemised elastorrhexis) is an inherited disorder of connective tissue, characterised by elastorrhexis of the dermis, blood vessels and the Bruch's membrane of the eyes. Calcium accumulates in the abnormal elastic tissue. The disease may develop in early childhood and usually does so before the age of 30.

Pseudoxanthoma elasticum is also associated with sickle cell anaemia, thalassemia, amyloid elastosis and chronic renal failure. Penicillamine can cause cutaneous pseudoxanthoma elasticum, but not systemic involvement

Histopathology

The characteristic changes are seen in the mid-dermis, which consists of degenerated elastic fibres, on which calcium deposits readily. The abnormality is also found in the elastic tissue of the Bruch's membrane of the eyes, blood vessels and the heart.

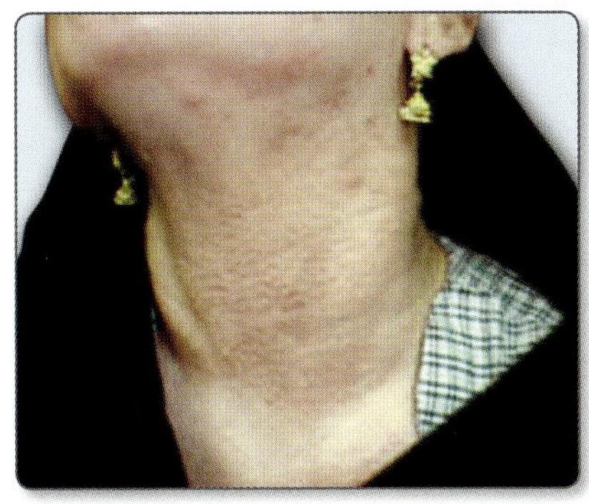

Fig. 11: Pseudoxanthoma elasticum

Clinical Features

The cutaneous manifestations consist of small yellowish papules in a linear or reticulate pattern, seen commonly on the flexural skin such as the neck, axillae and groins (Fig. 11). Thighs and abdomen are affected as the disease progresses. The skin is soft, lax and slightly wrinkled. The lesions on the neck give rise to a 'plucked chicken' appearance. Similar changes are also seen in the oral mucosa, mucous membrane of the stomach, rectum and the vagina. In the mouth, the lesions resemble Fordyce spots.

Systemic Manifestations

The arteries throughout the body are affected, resulting in intermittent claudication, decreased peripheral pulses, cardiac myopathy and hypertension. Abnormal blood vessels of the gastrointestinal tract result in haemorrhage. Striae occur in all pregnancies (Fig. 12).

Angioid streaks of the retina are caused by rupture of the elastic tissue in Bruch's membrane. They are seen as greyish streaks radiating from an incomplete greyish ring surrounding the optic nerve head.

Treatment

No definite therapy is available. Important aspect of the treatment is to prevent the complications of vascular involvement. Laser photocoagulation may be helpful in retinal hemorrhage. Cosmetic appearance of the skin can be improved by plastic surgery. Restriction of calcium and phosphate in the diet is helpful in a few cases.

Cutis Laxa

Cutis laxa (generalised elastorrhexis) is a rare condition characterised clinically by lax pendulous skin and histologically by loss of elastic tissue in the dermis. It may be inherited or acquired.

The inherited dominant form has only cutaneous manifestations; the recessive variety has both cutaneous and systemic manifestations. X-linked recessive forms are also seen. The patients often die young.

The acquired variety may appear at any age from early childhood to late fifties. It is secondary to urticaria, angioedema, systemic lupus erythematosus, syphilis, multiple myeloma, etc. D-Penicillamine can also induce cutis laxa.

Clinical Features

In all forms of cutis laxa, the skin appears too large for the body; the skin is inelastic and hangs in folds. The face and the neck are often affected; the skin has the effect of premature aging. The abdomen is frequently the site of large pendulous folds.

Besides the skin the cardiovascular system, gastrointestinal tract and the respiratory system may be affected. Pulmonary manifestations are emphysema, fibrosis of the lungs, tracheobronchomegaly. Cardiac involvement results in cor-pulmanale and aortic dilatation. Involvement of the gastrointestinal tract results in oesophageal dilation, dysphagia, gastric ulcers, rectocele, etc. There is a tendency to form multiple hernias and diverticula.

Differential Diagnosis

In psuedoxanthoma elasticum the face is usually not involved, it is distinguished histologically by the presence of calcification. In severe actinic damage, there is marked skin laxity but other signs of actinic damage are also present.

Treatment

Plastic surgery may reduce the cosmetic disability. Systemic complications need a physicians supervision. Regular evaluation of internal organ involvement is important in the management and prevention of major complications.

EHLERS-DANLOS SYNDROME

Ehlers-Danlos syndrome (cutis hyperelastica) is a group of generalised disorder of connective tissue; it is characterised by increased fragility of the skin and blood vessels, hyperextensibility of the skin and joint hypermobility. There is increased tendency towards scar formation and calcification of the skin to produce psuedotumors.

Clinical Features

There are eleven types of Ehlers-Danlos syndrome, classified on the basis of clinical and genetic grounds. The broad subtypes are:

- The classical type
- The hypermobile type
- The vascular type
- The kyphoscoliosis type
- The arthrochalasia type (Associated with multiple joint dislocations)
- The dermatosparaxis type (Associated with marked skin fragility)
- Associated with tenascin deficiency (Intermediate in severity between the classical and hypermobile forms).

Classical Manifestations

The skin may stretch out like rubber and snaps back with equal resiliency. This rubbery skin is most pronounced on the elbows, neck, and sides of the abdomen. Minor trauma may produce a gaping wound with large haematoma underneath. Trauma produces cigarette paper like thin scars. Approximately 50% of the people can touch the tip of the nose with their tongue (Gorlin's sign).

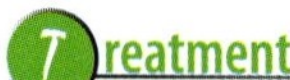

Is highly unsatisfactory, some cases may respond to ascorbic acid (those with ocular involvement). Patients should be told to avoid trauma and pregnancy for the fear of uterine rupture. Bleeding should be controlled conservatively as the fragility of the blood vessels makes surgical procedures dangerous and difficult. Tension in sutures should be avoided.

Internal manifestations include diverticulae in the gastrointestinal tract, intestinal perforation and haemorrhage. Aortic aneurysm, diaphragmatic hernia, intraocular haemorrhage and a tendency to the formation of keratoconus.

MARFRAN'S SYNDROME

This is an autosomal dominant disorder, with defect in fibrillin 1 (component of elastic fibers), with skeletal, cardiac, ocular and cutaneous abnormalities. Premature death is often due to cardiac abnormalities such as aortic rupture or aortic dissection.

Clinical Features

Skeletal Abnormalities

The patients are tall, with characteristic elongated facies and long narrow extremities. Shortening of the trunk is due to kyphoscoliosis. There is skeletal disproportion, the most obvious being the low ratio of the upper segment to the lower segment. There is depression of the sternum, and an asymmetry of the chest. The other skeletal abnormalities are pectus excavatum and pes vulgus.

The arm span (fingertip to fingertip) is often greater than height.

Ocular Changes

The most common finding is myopia, due to the long anterior-posterior axis of the orbit, and flattening of the cornea. Other changes are ectopia lentis, heterochromic irises, and retinal detachment.

Cardiac Abnormalities

These are the most severe. These include aortic root dilatation and mitral valve prolapse. Dilatation of the proximal aorta is progressive; it may lead to aortic rupture or aortic dissection. Regular cardiac monitoring is necessary for patients with Marfran's syndrome.

Cutaneous lesions include striae and elastosis perforans serpiginosa. Incisional and inguinal hernias are common.

Other features include high-arched palate, crowding of the anterior teeth, emphysema and pneumothorax

JUVENILE HYALINE FIBROMATOSIS

This is a rare hereditary disease of autosomal recessive inheritance, characterised by cutaneous tumours, gingival hyperplasia and joint contractures. Other associated features are stunted growth, osteolytic changes and muscle weakness. The mental development is normal. The disease is due to increased synthesis of glycosaminoglycans by the fibroblasts.

The disease is mainly described in the Asian skin. It usually manifests between 2 months and 4 years of age. The cutaneous changes consist of papules, nodules and subcutaneous swellings. The papules are prominent on the neck, ears and perianal area (Figs 12 and 13). The large subcutaneous swellings are seen on the ankles, spine and the scalp. Osteolytic changes are seen in the skull, long bones and the phalanges. Joint contractures are disabling. Gingival hyperplasia is seen early in life and often leads to falling of the teeth.

Treatment

There is no definite treatment, cardiac and ocular changes should be monitored and treated accordingly.

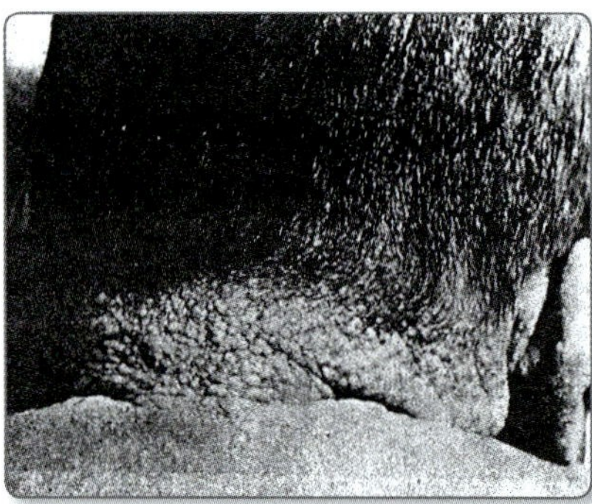

Fig. 12: Juvenile hyaline fibromatosis: papules on the neck

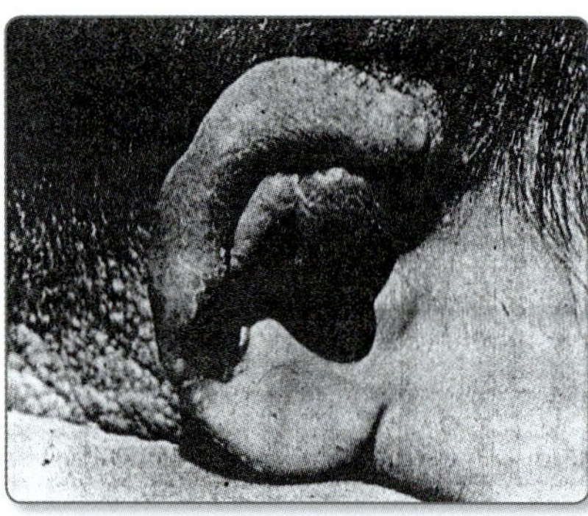

Fig. 13: Juvenile hyaline fibromatosis: papules and nodules on the ear

The disease should be differentiated from Winchester syndrome which is an extremely rare, autosomal recessive connective tissue disorder characterised by short stature, with multiple prominent and painful subcutaneous nodules, massive osteolysis in the hands and feet, and generalised osteoporosis. Coarse face, hirsutism, and abnormalities in the eyes and teeth are other features.

Treatment is unsatisfactory; steroids and cytotoxic drugs have been used. Capsulotomy gives temporary results.

FURTHER READING

1. Chung L, Liu J, Parsons L, et al. Characterization of connective tissue disease- associated pulmonary hypertension from REVEAL:identifying systemic sclerosis as a unique prototype. Chest. 2010;138(6):1383-94.
2. Dalakas MC, Hohlfeld R. Polymyositis and Dermatomyositis. Lancet. 2005; 362(9388):971-82.
3. Fusade T, Belanji P, Joly P, et al. Subcutaneous changes in Dermatomyositis. Br J Dermatol. 1993;128(4):541-3.
4. George C, Tsokos MD. Systemic lupus erythematosus. (Review article). N Engl J Med. 2011;365(22):2110-21.
5. Gill JM, Quisel AM, Rocca PV, et al. Diagnosis of systemic lupus erythematosus. Am Fam Physician. 2003;68(11):2179-87.
6. Goyal S, Nousari HC. Treatment of resistant discoid lupus erythematosus of the palms and soles with mycophenolate mofetil. J Am Acad Dermatol. 2001;45(1):142-4.

7. Hill CL, Zhang Y, Sigurgeirsson B, et al. Frequency of specific cancer types in Dermatomyositis and Polymyositis: a population based survey. Lancet. 2001;357(9250):96-100.
8. Holbrook KA, Byers PA. Skin is a window on hereditary disorders of connective tissue. Am J Med Genet. 1989;34(1):105-21.
9. Holbrook KA, Byers PA. Ultrastructural characteristics of the skin in a form of Ehlers-Danlos syndrome. Lab Inves. 1981;44(4):342-9.
10. Housman TS, Jonzzo JL, McCarty MA, et al. Low dose thalidomide therapy for refractory cutaneous lesions of Lupus Erythematosus. Arch Dermatol. 2003;139(1):50-4.
11. Jeffry P, Callen MD. Statins might benefit digital ulceration and Raynaud's Phenomenon. J Rheumatol. 2008;35(9):1801.
12. Haroon TS, Zaidi Z. Juvenile hyaline fibromatosis J Pak Med Assoc. 1990;40(8):194-6.
13. Kaufman LD, Gruber BL, Marchese MJ, et al. Anti-IgE autoantibodies in Systemic Sclerosis. Ann Rheum Dis. 1989;48(3):201-5.
14. Lapiere CM, Nusgene BV. Ehlers-Danlos type V111 has a reduced production of typr 111 collagen. J Invest Dermatol. 1981;76:422
15. Lebhwohl M, Phleps RG, Yannuzzi L, et al. Classification of Pseudoxanthoma Elasticum in patients with characteristic skin changes. N Engl J Med. 1987;317:347-50.
16. Lee JH, Wang LC, Lin YT, et al. Inverse correlation between CD4 and regulatory T cell population and autoantibody levels in paediatric patients with Systemic Lupus Erythematosus. Immunol. 2006;117:280-6.
17. Marvi U, Chung L. Digital Ischaemic loss in Systemic Sclerosis. Int J Dermatol. 2010;2010:1307-17.
18. Niewold TB, Wie SC, Smith M, et al. Familial aggregation of autoimmune disease in Juvenile Dermatomysitis. Pediatrics. 2011;127:1239-46.
19. Panjwani S. Early diagnosis and treatment of Discoid Lupus Erythematosus. J Am Fam Med. 2009;22(2):206-13.
20. Vilgoen DL, Bealty S, Beighton P. The obstetric and gynaecological implications of Pseudoxanthoma Elasticum. Br J Obstet Gynaecol. 1987;94:884-8.

Chapter

12

Bullous Disorders

Vesicles and bullae are physical signs that occur in a number of cutaneous disorders; these range from simple infections such as impetigo to immunopathological disorders such as pemphigus. Mechanism of blister formation differs in different diseases.

THE PATHOGENIC MECHANISM OF BLISTER FORMATION

Spongiosis: This is separation of keratinocytes from one another by the accumulation of fluid in the intercellular space, as seen in eczema.

Epidermal cell necrosis: When the keratinocytes are invaded by a foreign organism such as a virus, the cells become swollen and vacuolated to produce an appearance called "balloon degeneration", as seen in herpes simplex and varicella.

Acantholysis: In pemphigus vulgaris, antibodies are directed against the desmosomes. This causes the keratinocytes to loosen their cohesion and drift apart, a process called acantholysis (prickle cells are also called acanthocytes).

Basal cell damage: In epidermolysis bullosa simplex, there is disruption of the basal cells following mild trauma. Degeneration of the basal cells also occurs in other disorders such as lupus erythematosus (LE) and lichen planus.

Damage to the dermo-epidermal junction: Damage can occur in different layers of the dermo-epidermal junction. In bullous pemphigoid, the split is seen at the level of hemidesmosomes, presumably as a result of IgG antibody binding with the bullous pemphigoid antigen at this site. In recessive dystrophic epidermolysis bullosa, the split occurs just below the basal lamina in the anchoring fibrils.

Dermal damage: In dermatitis herpetiformis, there are granular deposits of immunoglobulin A (IgA) at the tips of the papillary dermis. In porphyria cutanea tarda, the blisters develop in the dermis and there is considerable edema of dermal papillae. Immunoglobulins and complement deposits are found around the blood vessels, presumably as a result of damage caused by solar irradiation due to excess of porphyrins in the blood.

From the above-mentioned mechanisms of bullae formation, we can appreciate that the site of bullae may be in the epidermis, dermo-epidermal junction or in the dermis. The intraepidermal bullae can be distinguished clinically from the subepidermal bullae. The epidermal blisters have a thin roof and thus can rupture easily, whereas the thicker roof of the subepidermal blister allows the formation of a tense shiny dome-shaped bulla. Blisters taken for biopsy must be a fresh bulla, because subepidermal blisters begin to re-epithelise within 24 hours and then can be mistaken for intraepidermal blisters.

Some causes of intraepidermal bullae are eczema, impetigo, fungal infections (zoophilic), superficial burns, viral infections and pemphigus. Some causes of subepidermal blisters are erythema multiforme, dermatitis herpetiformis, pemphigoid, vasculitis and porphyria.

PEMPHIGUS

The word pemphigus is derived from a Greek word "pemphix" meaning blister or a bubble. Pemphigus comprises a group of autoimmune blistering disorders, in which intraepidermal blisters occur due to acantholysis (separation of acanthocytes or prickle cells) and autoantibodies are directed against the desmosomes. It is a disease of middle age; it affects all races and both sexes. Acantholysis can occur in the deeper layers of prickle cells (pemphigus vulgaris and subtypes), or its superficial layers (pemphigus foliaceus and subtypes).

Classification

- Pemphigus vulgaris with subtypes:
  - Classic pemphigus vulgaris
  - Pemphigus vegetans
    - ➢ Neumann type
    - ➢ Hallopeau type
- Pemphigus foliaceus with subtypes:
  - Classic pemphigus foliaceus
  - Pemphigus erythematosus (Senear-Usher syndrome)
  - Pemphigus herpetiformis
  - Fogo salvagem (endemic)
- Others
  - Paraneoplastic pemphigus
  - Drug induced
  - Intercellular IgA pemphigus

Aetiology

Pemphigus is an autoimmune disease in which intercellular autoantibodies are found in the epidermis and oral mucous membrane while circulating autoantibodies are present in the serum. Autoantibodies attack normal proteins within desmosomal structures that cause cell-to-cell adhesion. Pemphigus may be a genetically determined disease as shown by the presence of various HLA antigens. Most patients are of the genotype HLA- DR4 or HLA-DRw6. Pemphigus vulgaris tends to be more common in people of Middle Eastern or Jewish descent, though it can affect people of all races.

Drugs such as penicillamine, rifampicin and captopril may cause pemphigus. Ultraviolet light (UVL) may aggravate the disease. Pemphigus may also be found in association with thymoma, myasthenia gravis, lupus erythematosus and lymphoproliferative diseases.

Pathogenesis

The basic pathological change in pemphigus is acantholysis (the separation of keratinocytes from one another) which leads to blister formation in the epidermis. Autoantibodies inhibit the function of desmosomes, resulting in acantholysis.

The probable mechanism of bulla formation is the binding of the circulating autoantibody to a cell surface glycoprotein; this results in activation of plasmin. The plasminogen-plasmin system may be involved in acantholysis. Keratinocytes in the lesional epidermis may express plasminogen activator. Plasmin causes destruction of the intercellular cement and desmosome, thus separating the keratinocytes.

Desmoglein 3 is the target antigen in pemphigus vulgaris; this is a desmosomal cadherin that causes intercellular adherence of the epidermis. The serum of pemphigus vulgaris patients also shows antibodies to desmoglein 3. Complement is not necessary in producing acantholysis but complement enhances the pathogenicity.

In pemphigus foliaceus, the antibodies target desmoglein 1. Patients with mucosal pemphigus are negative for antidesmoglein 1 antibodies but are positive for antidesmoglein 3. Desmoglein 2 is expressed in all desmosome possessing tissue. Desmoglein 1 and 3 are restricted to stratified squamous epithelium.

Drugs containing a sulfhydryl groups such as penicillamine and captopril are more likely to cause pemphigus foliaceus. While drugs without a sulfhydryl group such as β blockers, cephalosporins, penicillins and rifampicin are more likely to cause pemphigus vulgaris. But drugs from either group can cause pemphigus vulgaris or pemphigus foliaceus.

Histopathology

Histology shows intraepidermal suprabasal blister formation in pemphigus vularis and variants, subcorneal blister formation in pemphigus foliaceus and subtypes, with acantholytic cells. These are degenerating large prickle cell, which assume a rounded appearance. It has a large basophilic nucleus containing 2–3 nucleoli, with a rim of mildly eosinophilic cytoplasm and a densely staining basophilic cell outline. The blisters are suprabasal in pemphigus and variants, and subcorneal in pemphigus foliaceus and its subtypes. The dermis shows mild perivascular infiltration.

Clinical Features

Pemphigus Vulgaris

This is the most common and severe type of pemphigus. It accounts for 70% of all cases of pemphigus. The disease is characterized by appearance of bullae, on normal skin or on an erythematous base. The bullae are intraepidermal and they thus rupture easily, producing painful erosions (Fig. 1). The lesions may occur in any part of the body, with a predilection for the face, scalp, axillae, groins and pressure points. In some patients, only a few lesions are seen, while in others large areas of the skin may be involved. Nikolsky's sign is positive.

Contd...

Contd...

Pemphigus vulgaris may present in many ways. In most cases, the lesions first appear in the mouth, the oral cavity is affected in 50–70% of cases, the mucosae including the conjunctiva, pharynx, larynx, oesophagus, urethra, vulva and the cervix may be involved (Fig. 2). The oral lesions may precede the cutaneous lesions by months, in some cases the disease may be confined to the oral cavity for years, making the diagnosis difficult. The lesions present as painful erosions on a red base. Initially, the lesions are sparse, later they become generalised. These may vary from a few millimetres to large areas with a total loss of the upper epithelial surface.

Pemphigus Vegetans

This is a rare variety of pemphigus vulgaris, it is characterized by vegetating erosions primarily in the flexures (Fig. 3). There are two types of pemphigus vegetans: Neumann and Hallopeau. Hallopeau variety is the severe form of disease, pustules and not bullae are the primary lesions but on immunofluorescence the findings are similar to pemphigus vulgaris.

Pemphigus Foliaceus

In pemphigus foliaceus the autoimmune reaction is high-up in the epidermis, bullae are seldom seen, erosions are both painful and offensive, eventually the patient may become erythrodermic, with crusted oozing, red skin (Fig. 4). The lesions are generally well demarcated and do not extend into large eroded areas as in pemphigus vulgaris. Pemphigus foliaceus may remain localized for years. Oral lesions are uncommon.

Pemphigus Erythematosus (Senear-Usher syndrome): The patients have antibodies to both systemic lupus erythematosus and pemphigus antigens. Scaly lesions are formed over the nose and the cheeks, similar to lupus erythematosus, sunlight may exacerbate the disease and oral lesions rarely occur (Fig. 5).

Pemphigus Herpetiformis: Pemphigus herpetiformis combines the clinical features of dermatitis herpetiformis and histological features of pemphigus foliaceus. It presents with pruritic vesicles or papules often in a herpetiform pattern. Most cases have circulating antibodies to desmoglein 1.

Fogo Salvagem (Endemic or Brazilian pemphigus): This type of pemphigus is found in some rural areas of Brazil. Patients affected are usually children and young adults. A black fly is thought to be the vector of the disease.

The disease is similar to pemphigus foliaceus, the oral mucosa is not involved. The cutaneous lesions present as burning in denuded areas and erythroderma is frequent. The treatment is similar to pemphigus foliaceus.

The clinical features of pemphigus vulgaris, pemphigus vegetans, pemphigus foliaceus and pemphigus erythematosus are given in brief in Table 1.

Paraneoplastic Pemphigus

This is associated with overt or occult neoplasm. Neoplasms such as hepatocellular carcinoma, lung cancer, B cell lymphoma, thymoma, Hodgkin's disease, and malignant acanthosis nigricans. Paraneoplastic pemphigus is characterized by the presence of serum antibodies to a number of antigens. Presumably there is a cross reaction between tumour antigens and desmosomal antigens which includes all the plakins, and desmoglein and even bullous pemphigoid antigens.

Severe mucosal erosions are the most constant feature of paraneoplastic pemphigus. The lesions are present in the oral mucosa, pharynx and oesophagus. Lesions on the conjunctiva can result in blindness. Some patients develop bronchiolitis obliterans which can be fatal. Antibodies are found against epithelial proteins that are present in the desmosomes and hemidesmosomes in the epidermis and respiratory tract. Progressive respiratory failure is frequently the cause of death. Death may also be due to sepsis and multiple organ failure.

Biopsy shows necrosis of keratinocytes in addition to suprabasal clefting and acantholysis**.** Biopsy is similar too that of pemphigus and erythema multiforme. Direct immunofluorescence shows immunoglobulin or complement at the basement membrane zone as well on the surface of the keratinocytes.

IgG antibodies against desmogleins and plakins confirm the diagnosis. The underlying tumour should be investigated and diagnosed.

The disease is generally refractory to all treatment. Treat the underlying tumour. Some success has been reported with rituximab, an anti-CD20 antibody.

Drug-Induced Pemphigus

This is caused by drugs containing a sulphydryl (thiol) group such as penicillamine and captopril. Pemphigus can also be produced by nonthiol group of drugs such as angiotensin converting enzyme inhibitors. Pemphigus induced by the thiol group of drugs is mild and show spontaneous recovery, once the drug is withdrawn. The other drugs that can cause pemphigus are nifedipine, cephalosporin, penicillin and rifampicin. Pemphigus can also follow burns and radiotherapy.

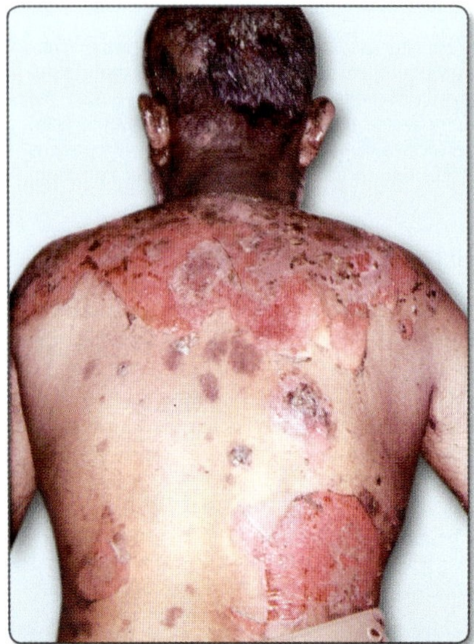

Fig. 1: Pemphigus vulgaris

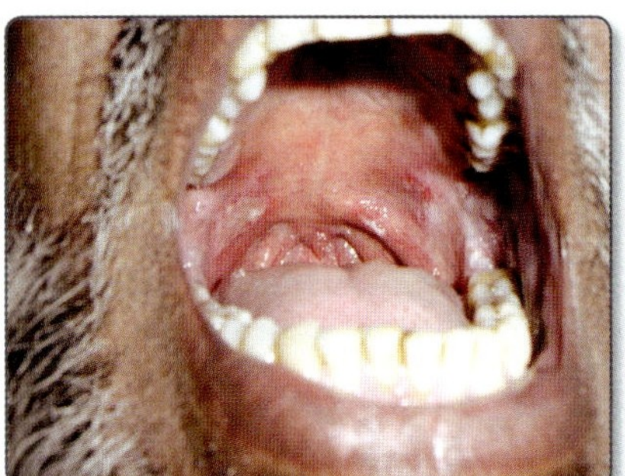

Fig. 2: Pemphigus vulgaris—oral ulcers

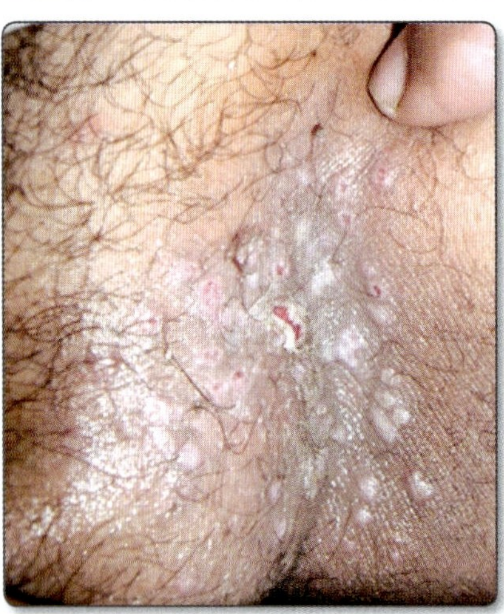

Fig. 3: Pemphigus vegetans
Source: Dr S Janjua: Global Skin Atlas

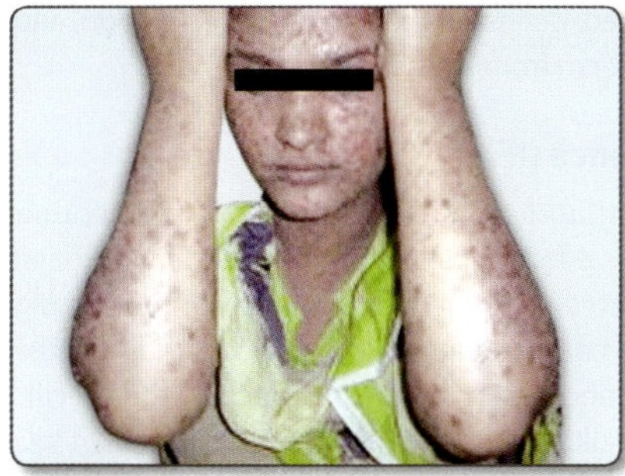

Fig. 4: Pemphigus foliaceus

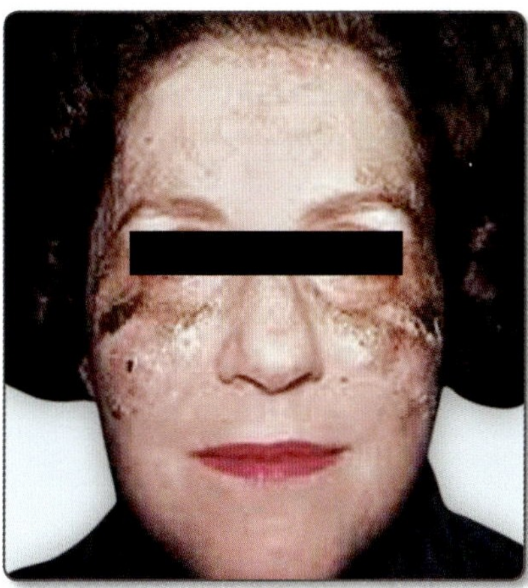

Fig. 5: Pemphigus erythematosus

Diagnosis

Nikolsky's Sign

Due to absence of cohesion in the epidermis, the upper layers of the epidermis can be separated easily by a slight twisting pressure or rubbing with the fingertips, thus leaving a moist surface.

Bullae Spreading Sign

A slight pressure on an intact bulla forces the blister fluid to wander under the skin from the present site to the surrounding skin, thus enlarging the bulla.

Tzanck's Test

The roof of a fresh bulla is removed, the base of the bulla is gently scraped, the contents examined for acantholytic cells under a microscope.

Direct Immunofluorescence (DIF)

Direct Immunofluorescence (DIF) shows the deposits of IgG in the intercellular space. IgG is found in both the normal and involved skin, but C3 is found only in acantholytic areas. Direct immunofluorescence should not be performed on a blister, as immunoreactants are often lost from the roof of the blister.

Two biopsy specimens are required: one from the edge of a fresh lesion, and the other best performed about 2 cm from a lesion.

Indirect Immunofluorescence (IF)

Indirect IF shows circulating antibodies against intercellular cementing substance, cadherins. These are a family of calcium-dependent cell-cell adhesion molecule. The substrates used are from monkey or guinea pig oesophagus. Thin sections of animal epithelium are first incubated with the patient's serum. Skin reacting antibodies in the serum attach to the specific components of the animal epithelium. Fluorescein-labeled anti-human IgG is then added for specific identification of the circulating antibody. They also help in assessing the prognosis of the disease.

Enzyme-linked Immunosorbent Assay (ELISA)

Enzyme-linked Immunosorbent Assay (ELISA) is used to detect antibodies against desmoglein 1 and desmoglein 3, this distinguishes between pemphigus vulgaris and pemphigus foliaceus.

Diagnostic Features

The following points help in diagnosing pemphigus vulgaris:

- Bullae appear in middle-aged persons
- Bullae appear on normal skin or on an erythematous base
- Bulla is flaccid and ruptures easily
- There is no sign of self -healing of these bullae
- Nikolsky's sign is positive
- Bulla spreading sign is positive
- Oral mucosa is usually involved
- Disease should be confirmed by a Tzancks test and by immunofluorescence.

Differential Diagnosis

Eczema may present as widespread scaly patches but the patient complains of pruritus and irritation. Pemphigoid occurs at a later age, the blisters are tense, and they do not rupture easily. Dermatitis herpetiformis is very pruritic, lesions appear on the elbows, knees and buttocks. In erythema multiforme, the lesions are symmetrical and target lesions are diagnostic. Occasionally, bullous impetigo and dyskeratotic acantholytic disorders such as Hailey-Hailey disease, Darier's disease and Grover's disease can cause diagnostic problems.

The difficulty arises when only oral lesions are present, the disease should then be differentiated from other causes of oral ulceration such as aphthous stomatitis, oral lichen planus, oral ulcers due to dentures, erosive candidiasis and herpetic gingivostomatitis. A proper history, oral and cutaneous examination with investigations can help in differentiating these disorders.

Treatment

Corticosteroids have greatly reduced the mortality and morbidity of pemphigus. All precautions should be taken to prevent secondary infection, by potassium permanganate baths and topical antiseptic applications. Good oral hygiene is important. Fluid and electrolyte balance should be maintained when patients have extensive blisters and erosions.

Contd...

Contd...

All forms of pemphigus are treated with corticosteroids. It works quickly and it is relatively safe when used appropriately. Some clinicians use corticosteroids with steroid-sparing drugs, to reduce the side effects of corticosteroids.

Pemphigus vulgaris and pemphigus vegetans require a high dose of prednisolone 1.5–2 mg/kg per day. The goal is to suppress blister formation within a week. If there is no effect in suppressing the disease and new blisters are forming, then double the dose of prednisolone. Once the blister formation has stopped and the old lesions have started to heal, the dose of prednisolone is decreased. Dosage may be tapered primarily by 1/3 total dosage, then 5 mg every 3 days to reach the daily dosage of 30 mg then tapered by 2.5 mg every week to reach daily dosage of 20 mg/day, then tapered by 1.25 mg every 2 weeks to reach daily dosage of 10 mg, then tapered by 1.25 mg monthly to reach daily dosage of 7.5 mg and continue this dosage for 6 months, then taper to 5 mg/day.

An immunosuppressive drug is added if there is no response to prednisolone, if side effects to prednisolone occur, or if the lesions flare up. The most common drug used is azathioprine 3–4 mg/kg given as a single dose daily. Other drugs that can be used are cyclophosphamide 2.5 mg/kg daily, mycophenolate mofetil 2 gm/daily, and cyclosporin 5 mg/kg daily.

Opportunistic infections are frequently the cause of death in immunosuppressed patients. Azathioprine induced immunosuppression can be predicted by detecting levels of thiopurine methyltransferase (TPMT). Azathioprine is best avoided in patients with very low TPMT levels.

High doses of intravenous immunoglobulin (IVIG), 2 gm/kg, infused in divided doses over 2–5 days monthly, will suppress the formation of autoantibodies, block the Fc receptors, and it has a modulatory effect on cytokine release and cellular response. IVIGs are effective in difficult cases of pemphigus. IVIG is most effective when used in conjunction with other drugs.

Plasmapheresis is the only method by which autoantibodies are rapidly removed. It is used in very extensive and active pemphigus. It involves a total of six high volume removals (3–3.5 liters), three times weekly for 2 consecutive weeks. Plasmapheresis is used in conjunction with other drugs, otherwise a rebound flare of pemphigus will occur.

Biologics like rituximab, have been used in recalcitrant cases, more controlled trials are needed for evidence. Rituximab is a chimeric monoclonal antibody against the protein CD20.

Intravenous pulse treatment with methylprednisolone. 250–1,000 mg of methylyprednisolone given over 3 hours in 24 hours for 4–5 consecutive days can result in long-term remission. This method can be used when the standard treatment with corticosteroids is not effective.

Pemphigus foliaceus and pemphigus erythematosus may respond to topical steroids, if control is inadequate then prednisolone in a dose of 20–40 mg per day may be required.

Meticulous protection against UVL is required for the treatment of pemphigus erythematosus. Antimalarials should be added.

Nicotinamide 1.5 gm/day with tetracycline 500 mg qid or minocycline 100 mg/day have also been used for the treatment of pemphigus foliaceus. Some studies have shown response of pemphigus vulgaris to tetracycline and nicotinamide.

Course and Prognosis

Before the advent of corticosteroids pemphigus was invariably fatal, the mortality is now below 25% and death is often due to the complications of steroids and immunosuppression. In a number of patients, the disease may go into remission and treatment can be stopped, in others, a small maintenance dose may be required.

American Academy of Rheumatology recommends the following daily doses for anyone taking oral corticosteroids for more than 3 months:
1,000 to 1,200 milligrams (mg) of calcium supplements
400 to 1,000 international units (IU) of vitamin D supplements

Table 1: Differentiation of pemphigus vulgaris, pemphigus vegetans, pemphigus foliaceus and pemphigus erythematosus

Pemphigus vulgaris	*Pemphigus vegetans*	*Pemphigus foliaceus*	*Pemphigus erythematosus*
Immunopathology IgG autoantibodies against the cell surface of keratinocytes throughout the epidermis	IgG autoantibodies against the cell surface of keratinocytes throughout the epidermis	IgG autoantibodies against the cell surface of keratinocytes throughout the epidermis	IgG autoantibodies against the cell surface of keratinocytes throughout the epidermis and IgG and C3 at the basement membrane zone
Pemphigus antigens Desmoglein 3	Desmoglein 3	Desmoglein 1	Desmoglein 1
Pathophysiology Bullae suprabasilar	Bullae suprabasilar	Bullae subcorneal	Overlap syndrome with features of pemphigus foliaceus and lupus erythematosus
Acantholytic cells present Basal cells may appear like a row of tombstones.	Acantholytic cells present Papillomatosis of dermal papillae, intraepidermal abscess with eosinophils	Acantholytic cells present Subcorneal pustules, may be present	Acantholytic cells present Acantholysis with basal cell alteration similar to lupus erythematosus
Lesions Skin and mucous membrane	Skin and mucous membrane	Mucosal lesions rare	Mucosal lesions rare
Anywhere on the skin	Usually localized to flexures	Anywhere on the skin	Localized to malar areas of the face and other seborrhoeic areas
Bullae flaccid	Bullae flaccid	Bullae flaccid, more easily ruptured	Bullae flaccid, more easily ruptured
Large erosions form once blisters rupture	Vegetating lesions, the reactive pattern of disease	Lesions scaly and crusted	Lesions scaly and crusted
Treatment High doses of steroids	High doses of steroids	Topical or low dose of steroids	Topical or low dose of steroids

OTHER ACANTHOLYTIC BULLOUS DISORDERS

Acantholysis may be primary (pemphigus, Darier's disease) or secondary (impetigo, viral diseases, solar keratosis, squamous cell carcinoma). The other causes of primary bullous acantholysis are:

- Transient acantholytic dermatosis
- Chronic benign familial pemphigus (Hailey-Hailey disease)
- Intercellular IgA pemphigus

Transient Acantholytic Dermatosis

The disease commonly occurs in men over the age of 50 years. The disease is of limited extent and duration. Clinically, the lesions consist of fragile vesicles that rapidly become eroded and crusted. The condition is confined to the chest, shoulder girdle and the upper abdomen. The disorder is often asymptomatic.

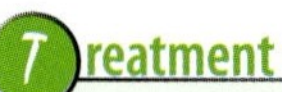

Potent topical steroids are the treatment of choice. Cases that do not respond can be treated with dapsone.

If the condition persists for more than 3 years, it is called persistent acantholytic dermatosis. It should then be differentiated from other acantholytic disorders such as pemphigus, benign familial pemphigus, Darier's disease and even simple spongiosis.

Familial Benign Chronic Pemphigus (Hailey-Hailey Disease)

This is a rare autosomal dominant disorder, unrelated to pemphigus.

Aetiology

The disease may be due to a genetic defect in the synthesis and maturation of tonofilament desmosome complex, or in the synthesis of intercellular cement.

Histopathology

The disease has the features of both pemphigus and Darier's disease. Acantholytic cells are viable unlike the degenerated cells of pemphigus. Acantholysis occurs at the suprabasal level. Dyskeratotic cells resembling corps ronds of Darier's disease are seen high-up in the epidermis. Antibodies are absent and the mmunofluorescence is negative.

Clinical Features

The onset is usually seen in the late teens or the early twenties. In the sun exposed areas the lesions appear as pruritic vesicles on an erythematous or nonerythematous base. These are grouped in an annular or serpiginous pattern. In the intertriginous areas the bullae rupture as soon as they are formed. The lesions present as moist red fissured areas, or as warty papules and plaques. These do not extend beyond the opposing skin surface.

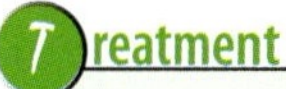

The treatment is difficult especially in obese women. Antibacterial agents (both local and systemic) are effective in controlling the exacerbation. Topical steroids and antibacterial creams are also helpful. Intralesional steroids given at weekly intervals have shown good results.

In chronic persistent cases, complete excision and replacement of the axilla by split skin grafts has been reported to be successful.

Intercellular IgA Pemphigus

IgA pemphigus is characterized by tissue-bound and circulating IgA antibodies targeting desmosomal or nondesmosomal cell surface components in the epidermis. Histologically, infiltrating polymorphonuclear cells (mainly neutrophils) are observed in the epidermis with formation of pustules and bullae at various levels. Clinically the lesions present as subcorneal flaccid pustules mainly on the abdomen (Sneddon Wilkinson disease), or as pruritic vesiculopustular eruption simulating dermatitis herpetiformis. Most cases are responsive to dapsone. Prednisolone and immunosuppressive drugs can be used as alternatives.

PEMPHIGOID

Pemphigoid is a disease of the elderly, in the classical form there are widespread large tense bullae, which develop on areas of pruritus, dermatitis or urticarial lesions. The autoantibodies are directed against the specific antigen in the hemidesmosomes (BP 230) and extracellular proteins of the basement membrane (BP 180).

Classification

- Bullous pemphigoid
- Cicatricial pemphigoid
- Pemphigoid gestationis

Aetiology and Pathogenesis

About 90% of patients have circulatory autoantibodies against BP antigens: BP 180 and BP 230. The binding of autoantibodies to antigens results in the activation of the complement, attraction of eosinophils, the release of proteases and separation of the dermoepidermal junction.

Drugs (furosemide, penicillins, sulphasalazine and benzodiazepine), ionizing radiation and sunlight, can also cause bullous pemphigoid. Diseases such as diabetes mellitus, rheumatoid arthritis, ulcerative colitis, multiple sclerosis and malignancy (gastric carcinoma being the most common) are other causes of pemphigoid like eruptions.

Histopathology

The bullae are subepidermal with a viable epidermis that forms the roof of the blister. The blister may contain numerous eosinophils and neutrophils, so does the dermal infiltrate. Blood eosinophilia may be present. Old blisters may demonstrate re-epithelialisation along the basement membrane giving rise to an artifactual intraepidermal blister. A fresh bulla should therefore be taken for biopsy; otherwise, a false result may occur.

Clinical Features

Pemphigoid frequently begins on the limbs; the trunk is invariably affected after a few days. In majority of the patients, the disease is widespread and symmetrical but occasionally the disease is localized to a small area, such as the lower legs (Fig. 6). The face and the scalp are usually not affected nor are the mucous membranes.

Prior to the blister formation, the disease presents as an urticarial or eczematous rash. When the lesions are urticarial, the prodrome lasts for 1–3 weeks, when eczematous the blisters may not develop for several months. The blisters are large and tense, which do not rupture easily, they may attain diameter up to 7 cm. Milia may be profuse during the healing phase.

Variants of Pemphigoid

Pemphigoid Nodularis

Patients present with intensely itching nodules, blisters are rarely reported. The nodules may be generalized or localized to the limbs. The disease should be differentiated from prurigo nodularis.

Localized Disease

Bullous pemphigoid may be localized on the lower extremities, it responds well to treatment. The disease can also be localized on the vulva of young girls, or on the gingiva.

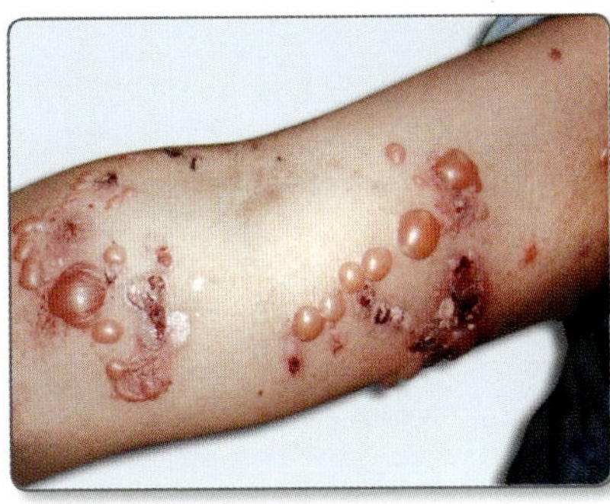

Fig. 6: Pemphigoid

Pemphigoid Vegetans

The clinical features are circumscribed hypertrophic lesions, with crusts, erosions, vesicles and pustules at the periphery. It usually affects the intertriginous areas.

Lichen Planus Pemphigoides

Bullous pemphigoid can occur with lichen planus. Blisters arise on the lesions of lichen planus as well as on the normal skin. They respond rapidly to treatment and the condition is short lived.

Herpetiform Pemphigoid

This clinically resembles dermatitis herpetiformis.

Dishidrotic BP

Occasionally BP can start as acute vesicular eruptions on the palms and soles.

Diagnosis of Pemphigoid

Peripheral blood eosinophilia is seen in 50% of patients, and an elevated IgE in 85% of cases. Remissions of BP parallel those of IgE.

The skin biopsy shows a subepidermal blister.

Direct Immunofluorescence (DIF)

This should not be performed on a blister, as immunoreactants are often lost from the roof of the blister. It should be best performed on peri-lesional skin, where it shows the presence of IgG and C3, or C3 alone in the basement membrane zone. The immune deposits are deposited in the hemidesmosomes or lamina lucida. The antibodies interfere with the cell-matrix adhesion, in contrast to the pemphigus antibodies which interfere with the cell-cell adhesion.

Indirect Immunofluorescence (Indirect IF)

In general, there is only a little correlation between the autoantibody titres and disease severity.

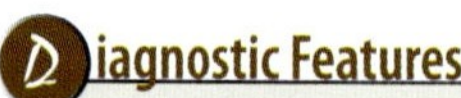

Diagnostic Features

The following features are characteristic of pemphigoid:

- Bullae appear in elderly persons
- Bullae appear on an erythematous or urticarial base
- Bullae are tense
- Bullae heal with time without treatment
- Oral mucous membrane is occasionally involved

Differential Diagnosis

Pemphigoid blisters should be differentiated from those of pemphigus, drug eruptions and erythema multiforme. In pemphigus, blisters usually arise on normal skin, they are flaccid and rupture easily, oral mucosa is usually involved, without treatment the blisters spread and there is no sign of healing, the blisters are epidermal with acantholytic cells which can be seen on Tzanck's smear. In erythema multiforme the lesions are usually seen on the distal parts of the extremities, they are polymorphic, target lesions are pathognomonic.

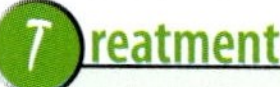

Treatment

The patients of bullous pemphigoid are elderly and usually on numerous drugs, they are susceptible to adverse drug reactions and side effects. Topical steroids are the mainstay of treatment. Oral prednisolone in a dose of 20–40 mg per day usually controls the disease; the drug is then gradually withdrawn. Measures to prevent osteoporosis should be implemented from the start of oral steroid treatment.

Successful treatment is also reported with tetracycline and nicotinamide. Tetracyclines suppress the inflammatory response at the basement membrane zone, inhibit neutrophil chemotaxis and increase cohesion at the dermoepidermal junction. The effect is enhanced by the synergetic effect of nicotinamide.

When the disease is widespread immunosuppressive drugs such as azathioprine, methotrexate and mycophenolate mofetil are effective.

For severe and refractory cases cyclophosphamide, plasmapheresis and high dose intravenous immunoglobulins have shown efficacy.

Localized variants usually respond to topical or intralesional steroids.

Course and Prognosis

Bullous pemphigoid is a relatively benign disease, usually self-limiting over a period of 5–6 years. With adequate treatment, most patients have a lasting remission; 10–15% may relapse once the therapy is stopped.

Exclude pemphigoid when an elderly patient complains of persistent urticaria

Cicatricial Pemphigoid (Benign Mucosal Pemphigoid)

This is a rare blistering disease of the mucosa and the skin. Oral mucous membrane and conjunctiva are usually involved along with the skin adjacent to it. The disease results in permanent scarring of the affected area. It is a disease of middle age mostly affecting women.

Pathogenesis

Cicatricial pemphigoid is an autoimmune disorder similar to that of pemphigoid, with IgG and C3 deposited at the basement membrane. The autoantibodies are directed against BP 180, BP 230, laminin 5 and integrins. Laminin is found in the lamina densa, a site slightly lower than that seen in Classical BP. Circulating antibodies are absent.

Clinical Features

The disease is characterised by the formation of bullae in the conjunctiva and mouth. Bullae also occur in the oesophagus, pharynx, genital mucosa and anus. The lesions are symptomless, they heal with scarring. Scarring leads to complications such as strictures and adhesions. On the conjunctiva and cornea scarring may lead to corneal opacity and impairment of vision and even blindness. Long standing cases may give rise to malignancy especially of the oral mucosa.

Cutaneous lesions are usually seen on the skin adjacent to the mucosa or they may be generalized.

In the localized variety (Brunsting-Perry pemphigoid), there are no mucosal lesions but there are one or several erythematous plaques on which recurrent crops of blisters appear. They heal with scarring.

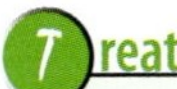

Treatment

Treatment is unsatisfactory, topical steroids are used without much improvement. In more aggressive cases such as those with ocular complications, dapsone alone or in combination with steroids may be tried. Other immunosuppressive drugs like azathioprine and cyclophosphamide have been used without much help. Lesions of the oral cavity respond better than the ocular lesions.

Although called benign, the disease causes blindness in 25% of patients.

Pemphigoid Gestationis (Herpes Gestationis)

Pemphigoid gestationis (PG) has many features similar to pemphigoid, it resembles it clinically, histologically and the immunofluorescence findings are similar. The disease is often called herpes gestationis. It has no relationship with the herpes virus infection. The term pemphigoid gestationis is preferable.

Aetiology

Pemphigoid gestationis is an autoimmune disorder, similar to pemphigoid. It is considered that an HLA mismatch between the mother and the foetus triggers an immune response that cross-reacts with the maternal skin. There is a clinical evidence of placental insufficiency; mothers have high titres of antibodies to HLA class 1 antigens. The autoantibodies are directed against the same hemidesmosomes target antigens such as bullous pemphigoid antigen BP 180, less often BP 230. The autoantibodies can also react with the basement membrane of the placenta, resulting in placental insufficiency. Pemphigoid gestations can be associated with premature delivery and low birth weight.

The disease occurs in the presence of paternal tissue such as the foetus, hydatidiform mole and choriocarcinoma. Once the disease is manifested, its course can be modulated by the changes of estrogen and progesterone levels. Exacerbations can occur with oral contraceptives and menstruation.

Clinical Features

Onset is usually in the second trimester. Urticarial papules and plaques develop around the umbilicus, the lesions then spread to the abdomen, chest, trunk and the extremities. Face, scalp and the oral mucosa are generally spared. Within these papules, vesicles and bullae erupt often in an annular or polycyclic configuration. Pruritus is severe. The disease usually flares up at postpartum and remits within 3 months. It recurs in subsequent pregnancies, in women taking oral contraceptives and during menstruation. Maternal health is usually not affected but adverse fetal deformities may occur.

The disease is more severe in successive pregnancies. Pemphigoid gestationis may also be associated with other autoimmune disorders such as Grave's disease, vitiligo and alopecia areata.

Differential Diagnosis

The disease should be differentiated from pruritic urticarial papules and plaques of pregnancy (PUPP). PUPP arise on the striae of pregnancy, it has no bullae and is not immunologically mediated.

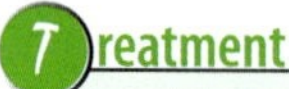

Topical steroids are helpful in most cases. In cases that do not respond, oral prednisolone 40 mg per day will be effective. Plasmapheresis and intravenous immunoglobulins can be used for severe cases. Most of the alternative drugs which can be used for pemphigoid are contraindicated during pregnancy and when the child is in breastfeeding.

Patients should avoid oral contraceptives while the disease is still active

DERMATITIS HERPETIFORMIS

Dermatitis herpetiformis (DH) or Duhring-Brocq disease is a rare intensely pruritic chronic papulovesicular disorder, occurring in all ages. Common sites of occurrence are the elbows, knees, extensor surfaces of the forearms, over the scapula and the shins. The vesicles occur in a group hence the name herpetiformis. There is an underlying associated gluten sensitive enteropathy that may be asymptomatic.

Aetiology

The disease occurs in all ages. The age incidence varies in different countries. In Italy it is seen in childhood, while in Sweden it occurs in old age; it is uncommon in the far East. There is a family history of DH in 10–15% of cases, an association with HLA B8 and DR3 and DQw2 is found in these cases.

All patients have an underlying gluten sensitive enteropathy similar to that of coeliac disease. This enteropathy may be asymptomatic. There is an association with exposure to infection with adenovirus as seen in coeliac disease.

It is possible that there is some underlying immunological abnormality, as patients with DH have deposits of IgA in the dermal papillae; they also have antithyroid antibodies, antireticulin antibodies and antinuclear antibodies.

There is an increased incidence of small bowel lymphoma in patients with DH.

Pathogenesis

Dermatitis herpetiformis and gluten sensitivity are closely related. Gluten is the main adhesive substance of many grains. DH is due to an abnormal immune response to the proteins present in gluten. The main sensitising protein in gluten is gliadin, which is a substrate for tissue transglutaminase. Autoantibodies against tissue transglutaminase of the gut also cross react with similar cutaneous transglutaminase in DH. The exact mechanism by which cutaneous transglutaminase is affected is not known; perhaps the cutaneous transglutaminase binds to the tissue transglutaminase of the gut, which circulates as an immune complex to be deposited in the skin.

The characteristic finding in DH is deposition of IgA in the dermal papillae. The IgA deposits are gluten sensitive. The true pathogenetic relationship between cutaneous IgA deposits, cutaneous manifestations of DH, and the associated GSE remains unknown. There may be a slight decrease in IgA deposits after a gluten free diet.

Immunoglobulin A bound to the skin stimulates the complement via the alternate pathway. The activated complement is chemotactic for the neutrophils. The surrounding collagen is degraded resulting in the separation of the dermis from the epidermis and the formation of subepidermal bullae.

Enteropathy is found in all patients of DH but clinical symptoms are found in only 10–20% of cases. In the early stages, there is infiltration of lymphocytes and later there is atrophy of the villi, giving a flat appearance to the jejunum. This is associated with increased antiendomysial antibodies. The other abnormalities found in coeliac disease are also found in DH such as anemia, Howell-Jolly bodies in blood film indicating splenic atrophy and antireticulin antibodies.

There is a strong HLA association, most of the patients are HLA-DQ2 positive, some are also HLA DQ8.

Patients of DH have an increased risk of developing B cell lymphoma.

Histopathology

Changes are best seen in the perilesional skin or in the lesional skin that has not been blistered.

Neutrophils and eosinophils are seen in the dermal papillae that form microabscesses. The surrounding collagen is degraded resulting in the separation of the epidermis from the dermis and formation of a bulla.

Clinical Features

The average age of onset is between the ages of 20–55 years. The manifestations differ widely according to the type of lesion. The lesions are mainly present on the knees, elbows, extensor surface of the forearms, buttocks and scapulae (Fig. 7). Involvement of the face and scalp is rare. The characteristic lesion is a small blister on an urticarial base, as the lesions are often grouped, they are called herpetiform. The lesions are extremely pruritic and are often excoriated due to scratching. Pruritic papules are a common feature of most eruptions. Mild eruption resembles prurigo or urticaria. Vesicles and bullae when present are thick walled and they occur in groups. In later stages of the disease, only pigmentation and grouped scars are present. Pigmented spots at the lumbosacral region should alert the suspicion of DH.

Mucous membrane involvement is rare; it is present only when bullae are numerous. Dryness of the oral mucosa and recurrent oral mucosal ulceration are the most common reported findings. Coeliac like dental enamel defects are seen in 50% of DH patients. This suggests that patients were already suffering from subclinical gluten induced enteropathy in early childhood, when the crowns of permanent teeth develop.

All patients with dermatitis herpetiformis have gluten sensitive enteropathy, but the clinical evidence is seen in only 10-20% of cases. The enteropathy resembles coeliac disease. There is an increased incidence of gut lymphomas in patients of dermatitis herpetiformis. The primary pathology seems to be in the bowel.

Patients of DH are not able to tolerate iodine, and flare up of the disease occurs after eating seafood. Iodine challenge is an old method of diagnosing DH.

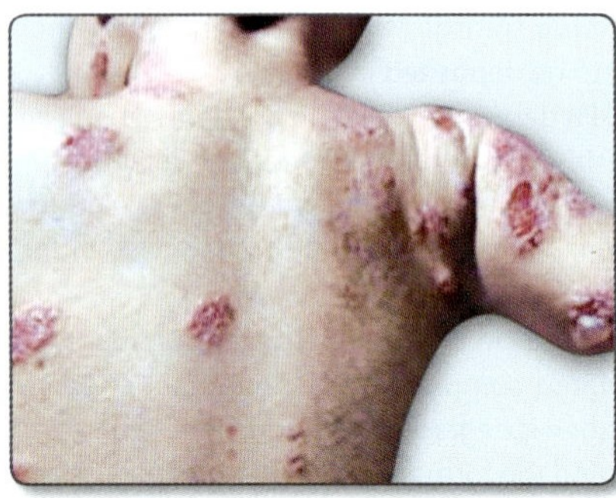

Fig. 7: Dermatitis herpetiformis

Diagnosis

Direct immunofluorescence (IF) shows the deposition of IgA in the dermal papillae. Indirect IF is negative for dermal antibodies.

A gluten sensitive enteropathy with patchy areas of villous atrophy and mild intestinal wall inflammation is found in majority of patients with dermatitis herpetiformis. A significant correlation is found between IgA endomysial antibodies (IgA-EmA) and DH severity of gluten induced jejunum damage. Serum IgA-EmA antibodies disappear after 1 year of gluten-free diet with regrowth of jejunum villi. These antibodies are a useful marker of enteropathy present in DH without symptoms of the disease.

Diagnosis can be confirmed by a skin biopsy (from a new red papular lesion that has not blistered.), direct IF test and biopsy of the jejunal mucosa.

- IgA deposits are found in the dermal papillae. A biopsy shows subepidermal blister and microabscesses in the dermal papillae, which is pathognomonic for DH. Because of the focal nature of deposits, multiple specimens may be needed for diagnosis. Antibodies to epidermal transglutaminase are present in DH but not in coeliac disease.
- Tissue transglutaminase (an enzyme that metabolizes gliadin), has been identified as the target antigen of antiendomysial antibodies (IgA-eMA)
- Haematology may show iron and folic acid deficiency due to gluten sensitive enteropathy.
- ELISA identifies IgA antibodies against tissue transglutaminase in at least 80% of patient.

Previously the disease was diagnosed by exacerbating the disease with iodides, given either by mouth or by the patch tests. It is now outmoded as a severe reaction may result. Skin cleansers containing iodine preparations should be avoided in DH.

Diagnostic Features

The following are some of the diagnostic features:

- ❑ Very itchy papulovesicular eruption arranged in groups
- ❑ Common sites are the elbows, knees, scapulae and the buttocks (Fig. 8)
- ❑ Vesicles and bullae are tense
- ❑ Age group is between 20 years and 55 years
- ❑ All patients are associated with a gluten sensitive enteropathy. Symptoms may be present in only 20% of cases.

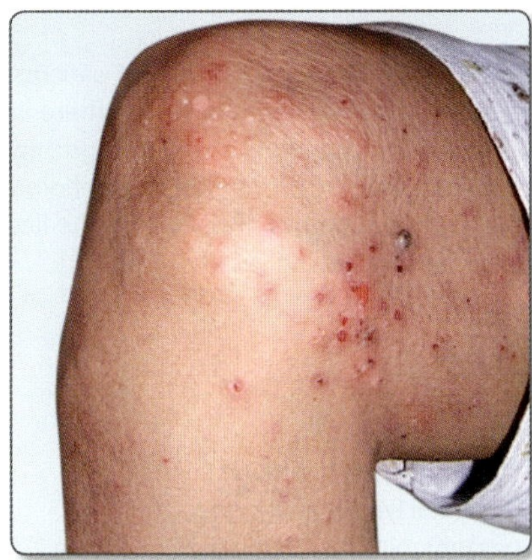

Fig. 8: Dermatitis herpetiformis: knee
Source: Dr S Janjua: Global Skin Atlas

Differential Diagnosis

The disease should be differentiated from the other blistering and pruritic disorders. It should be differentiated from bullous pemphigoid, pemphigus, and erythema multiforme. Papular urticaria is very pruritic and persistent if the source of the insects is not removed. Papular urticaria is usually found in the exposed areas of the body. Scabies is also a very pruritic condition, other members of the family are affected, itching is more at night and the characteristic burrow may be found. Nummular eczema is often very irritating but it is localized to the distal extremities.

Treatment

A gluten-free diet is essential for treatment and dapsone is highly effective for the rash. The pruritus disappears within 24-48 hours and the rash within a week.

The dose of dapsone varies from one person to another, it may be as high as 300 mg per day, or as little as 50 mg twice a week. The drug is started at 50 mg a day and then increased up to 100–200 mg daily. The clinical response is so specific that it may be used as a therapeutic test for DH. Dapsone is not without side effects, the most serious of which is hemolytic anemia, and it produces methaemoglobinaemia. The co-administration of cimetidine is reported to reduce dapsone dependent methaemoglobinaemia in DH.

Other drugs that may control the disease are sulphapyridine, in a dose of 0.5 gm three times a day initially. The dose is then increased to 1.5 gm three times a day.

The effects of a gluten-free diet may not be apparent for many months, the average time of stopping dapsone after adhering to gluten-free diet is about 2–3 years. Reintroduction of gluten in the diet brings about relapse of the disease. Gluten-free diet protects the patient from lymphoma.

Adherence to a gluten-free diet (avoid wheat, rye and barley) is monitored by measuring the titres of antiendomysial antibody, which should fall if gluten-free diet is strictly followed. With a gluten-free diet the bowel changes revert to normal.

The effects of dapsone are quick, and the effect of gluten-free diet is slow. Combine at the start of treatment; then slowly decrease the dose of dapsone.

Successful treatment is also reported with tetracycline (500 mg 1–3 times daily) or minocycline (100 mg bid) and niacinamide (500 mg bid). Colchicine, systemic steroids and cyclosporin have been reported to be useful in some studies.

Course and Prognosis

Dermatitis herpetiformis is a chronic disorder and less than 10% of patients have a spontaneous remission. Even in those patients in whom there is a remission, the disease may reappear. Lymphoma is a well-recognized complication of DH, role of a gluten-free diet for the prevention of lymphoma has recently been established. A gluten-free diet may also increase the life expectancy due to a decrease in the ischaemic heart disease.

Advantages of a Gluten-Free Diet

- It reduces the requirement for dapsone
- It improves associated gluten enteropathy
- It enhances nutrition and bone density
- It may reduce the risk of developing other autoimmune conditions
- It probably reduces the risk of intestinal lymphoma.

Differences between pemphigus, pemphigoid and DH are shown in Table 2.

OTHER SUBEPIDERMAL BULLOUS DISORDERS

Linear IgA Disease

The disease is a subepidermal blistering disorder characterized by the presence of linear IgA deposits in the basement membrane. It can occur in childhood (chronic bullous disease of childhood) and adults (linear IgA disease). There is a strong association between linear IgA disease and the extended autoimmune haplotype HLA- B8, CW7 and DR3, possession of these haplotypes is associated with early disease onset.

Multiple target antigens have been identified, some attach to lamina lucida, others attach to type V11 collagen in lamina densa.

Linear IgA disease is commonly seen after the age of 60 years. The eruptions are intermediate in size and characteristic to bullous pemphigoid and DH. The trunk is almost always involved, followed by the flexures. The skin lesions consist of papulovesicles or blisters which may have an arcuate or annular pattern. Mucosal involvement is common, involving the eyes, nose, pharynx, larynx and the genitals. There is no coexisting enteropathy. It can be produced by drugs such as vancomycin, lithium and diclofenac acid. There is an increase of lymphoproliferative disorders in adults with linear IgA disease. A number of precipitating factors have been observed such as infections and antibiotics like penicillin.

Diagnosis

Histology reveals subepidermal bullae. Within the papillary dermis and the blister cavity, there are numerous neutrophils with admixed eosinophils. Well-formed papillary microabscesses are not found. Direct immunofluorescence shows deposition of IgA in the lamina lucida or below the lamina densa.

Treatment

Patients usually respond to dapsone or sulphapyridine. Refractory cases may be given prednisolone in combination with dapsone or sulphapyridine. The other drugs that can be used are tetracycline and niacinamide, colchicine, mycophenolate mofetil, azathioprine and cyclosporin.

Table 2: Differentiation of pemphigus, pemphigoid and dermatitis herpetiformis

Pemphigus vulgaris	*Bullous pemphigoid*	*Dermatitis herpetiformis*
Bullae Flaccid, rupture within 24 hours	Tense, do not rupture easily	Tense, occur in groups
Distribution Generalized	Face and scalp usually spared	Elbows, knees, scapulae, buttocks commonly affected
Oral mucosa Affected in 80% of cases	Affected in 10-35% of cases	Not affected
Prodromal phase None	Eczematous or urticarial phase may be present	None
Age of onset Middle age	Elderly	20-55 years
Antigens In the desmosomes, desmoglein 1 and 3	In the hemidesmosomes, BP 180 and BP 230	In epidermal transglutaminase (TG)
Autoantibodies IgG	IgG	IgA
Circulating autoantibodies Used to assess the prognosis of disease	Not used for assessing prognosis	Not significant for prognosis
Pruritus Absent or mild	Moderate	Severe
Pain Painful erosions	Pain absent	Pain absent
Acantholytic cells Present	Absent	Absent
Gluten sensitive enteropathy Absent	Absent	Present
Resolution No sign of resolution without treatment	Remits in 5–6 years	Healing in course of time
Nikolsky's sign Present	Absent	Absent
Bullae spreading sign Present	Absent	Absent
Treatment High dose of steroids	Low dose of steroids	Dapsone and gluten-free diet

Epidermolysis Bullosa Acquisita

The disorder is characterized by skin fragility and blister formation following trauma to the skin in an elderly person. Sites commonly involved are those prone to trauma such as knees, elbows, back of the hands, toes and sacral areas. The lesions on the back of hand mimic those of porphyria cutanea tarda. Mucous membranes may or may not be involved. Healing occurs with scarring and milia formation.

A number of conditions are associated with epidermolysis bullosa acquisita (EBA) namely amyloidosis, inflammatory bowel disease, carcinoma of the lung, diabetes mellitus, multiple myeloma, lymphoma and systemic lupus erythematosus.

Rare Presentations

An inflammatory form similar to cicatricial bullous pemphigoid or DH is seen in some cases, the lesions heal with scarring. If the scalp is involved scarring alopecia occurs. Mucosal involvement is seen in 50% of cases.

Treatment

The treatment is very unsatisfactory; corticosteroids are the mainstay of treatment. Prednisolone in a dose of 40–60 mg is usually required. The dose is gradually withdrawn; maintenance therapy is usually not required. A combination of prednisolone with dapsone 100–200 mg daily, or azathioprine 1–2 mg/kg daily is often used.

Cyclosporin and colchicine are also reported to be helpful. Photopheresis and intravenous immunoglobulins have been helpful in resistant cases.

Histology

The blister is subepidermal. Direct immunofluorescence (IF) depicts deposition of IgG and C3 below the lamina densa, in the anchoring fibrils-type V11 collagen. Immunofluorescence on salt-split technique is on the dermal side of lamina lucida, whereas in bullous pemphigoid it is on the epidermal side of lamina lucida.

BULLOUS DISORDERS OF CHILDREN

The cause of bullae formation in children is the same as that of adults. The specific dermatoses of children are:

- Chronic bullous disease of childhood
- Epidermolysis bullosa
- Shabbir syndrome
- Bullous ichthyosiform erythroderma
- Acrodermatitis enteropathica

Chronic Bullous Disease of Chidhood (Childhood Linear IgA Disease)

This is a rare self-limiting bullous disorder of children, average age of onset is about 5 years, and it remits by the age of 13 years. A linear band of IgA is present at the basement membrane. It is HLA B8 positive.

Clinical Features

Three distinct clinical lesions characterize this disease: large tense bullae as seen in bullous pemphigoid, grouped vesicles as in DH or lesions similar to those seen in erythema multiforme. One lesion type may predominate or a combination of the three may be found. Bullae arise on normal skin, they are often arranged in a rosette; new bullae may cluster around the older lesions, forming a "cluster of jewels" arrangement. Healing is rapid with hyperpigmentation but without scarring.

Common sites involved are the inner thighs, the groin and pelvic areas, and the central facial area around the mouth. Mucous membrane is involved in about 90% of cases. Hoarseness indicates laryngeal involvement, there may be nasal bleeding, soreness of the eyes and conjunctivitis. Pruritus is mild or may be absent.

Differential Diagnosis

The disease should be differentiated from the other bullous disorders of childhood such as epidermolysis bullosa, in which bullae arise at the site of trauma. In incontinentia pigmentosa, bullae arise within the first few weeks of life; they later become warty and pigmented. In bulbous ichthyosiform erythroderma, bullae are generalized and the skin is covered with scales. Bullous impetigo may occur anywhere in the body, head and neck are the frequent sites affected. The disease should also be differentiated from juvenile pemphigus, juvenile pemphigoid and juvenile DH. Direct immunofluorescence studies differentiate these disorders.

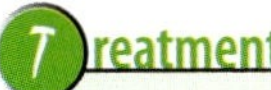

Treatment

Dapsone in a dose of 20–125 mg daily or sulphapyridine 250 mg-3gm daily usually controls the condition. In those, who do not respond, corticosteroids may be added. Conservative approach should be followed, as the disease is a self -limiting disorder.

Erythromycin has shown favourable results in some studies, suggests that this drug could be used as an alternative.

Histopathology

The histological features are not specific. The subepidermal vesicle may contain numerous eosinophils as in pemphigoid, or neutrophils as seen in dermatitis herpetiformis.

EPIDERMOLYSIS BULLOSA

These are a group of genetic disorders that results in the formation of blisters on minor injury. This is due to some defect of structural proteins in basal keratinocytes, dermo-epidermal junction and upper papillary dermis, that split easily and give rise to bulla formation.

Classification

- Epidermolysis bullosa simplex
- Junctional epidermolysis bullosa
- Epidermolysis bullosa dystrophica

Epidermolysis Bullosa Simplex (EBS)

The disease is usually inherited as autosomal dominant; the pathological change is seen in the basal cells. Mutations are seen in keratin 5 and 14. Blisters can be present at birth, or they may appear when the child begins to crawl, or walk, the blisters heal without scarring (Fig. 9). The hair nails and teeth are generally unaffected; the mucous membranes are occasionally involved. There is a little tendency to remission in the later life.

Types of EBS:

- Localized (Weber-Cockayne)
- Generalized (Koebner) 20% of these may be associated with nail dystrophy
- Herpetiform (Dowling-Meara) it may be associated with palmoplantar keratoderma, this is the most severe type, and the blistering is often generalized
- Abnormal plectin in EBS is associated with muscular dystrophy; localized blistering is seen in this disorder. Plectin abnormalities are also found in an endemic form of EBS, seen in Scandinavia and Germany (Ogna type).

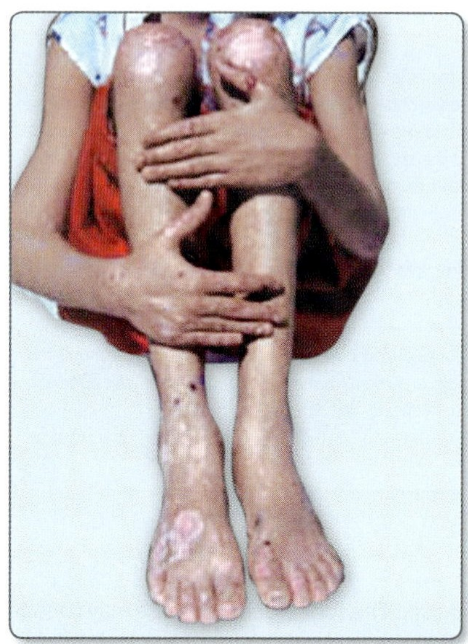

Fig. 9: Epidermolysis bullosa simplex

- Mutations in keratin 5 in EBS is associated with mottled hyperpigmentation. The disease is generalized, corneal dystrophy and mental retardation. Lesions heal with hypopigmentation
- Some rare types of EBS have an autosomal recessive inheritance, which involve other proteins of the dermo-epidermal junction, the lesions heal with scar formation.

Junctional Epidermolysis Bullosa

Junctional epidermolysis bullosa (JEB) is inherited as an autosomal recessive disorder and the abnormality lies in the lamina lucida; hemidesmosomes may be reduced in number. It is associated with abnormal laminin in the lamina lucida. The disease is present at birth or manifests soon after. Bullae appear at the site of trauma and there is little tendency to healing, raw denuded areas are seen which get secondarily infected. Healing occurs without scarring and milia formation. Mucous membranes are affected, drinking becomes difficult, and hoarseness develops due to laryngeal involvement. Nails are malformed and shed prematurely. Lesions heal with atrophy of the skin. Most of the children die due to secondary infection and failure to thrive. Laryngeal lesions lead to death in 50% of cases. Gene therapy and laminin 5 replacement are being tried in the treatment of JEB.

Types of JEB:

- Herlitz (lethal), laryngeal involvement leads to 50% mortality within the first 2 years of life, pyloric atresia is also common. Survivors have severe growth retardation and anaemia.
- Non-Herlitz (mitis), affected persons have normal growth and life span.
- Generalized atrophic JEB (Hinter-Wolff type). Defects are found in laminin 5, integrin β4 and bullous pemphigoid antigen 180 (BP 180). The onset is at birth, with generalized blistering, nail loss, scarring alopecia and moderate mucosal involvement.

Dystrophic Epidermolysis Bullosa

The inheritance may be autosomal dominant or autosomal recessive. The recessive variety is severe and is present at birth. The split is present at the level of the anchoring fibrils, which are rudimentary and reduced in number. Production of collagen VII is reduced or absent, or there is increased production of collagenase. Lesions of dystrophic epidermolysis bullosa (DEB) heal with atrophy and scarring (Fig. 10).

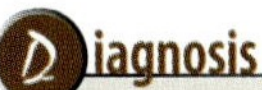

Diagnosis

Transmission electron microscopy is the gold standard investigation, alternative to it are fluorescent antigen mapping and monoclonal antibody studies.

The dominant variety occurs in late infancy or early childhood. Bullae heal with scarring and milia formation. However, the teeth and nails develop normally, mucous membranes are rarely involved.

Dominant epidermolysis bullosa dystrophica may be associated with hypertrophic lesions (Cockayne-Touraine) or atrophic lesions (Pasini).

Treatment

All efforts should be made to reduce the chances of getting trauma, e.g. drinking bottles should have soft nipples with slightly larger holes to make sucking easy, food should be soft. Elastic diapers should be avoided, knees and elbows should be padded to avoid trauma, and footwear should be soft and well ventilated.

Jobs should be suitable; those prone to trauma should be avoided. Farming, mechanical work, typing, sports should be prohibited especially in the dystrophic type of epidermolysis bullosa.

Once blistering has occurred, blisters should be drained followed by the application of topical antibiotics. In severe junctional type of epidermolysis bullosa fluid and electrolyte balance should be maintained, treatment of sepsis is most important in this type of disease, as septicaemia is the most important cause of death.

In severe recessive forms of epidermolysis bullosa, phenytoin is rapidly becoming the mainstay of treatment. Phenytoin works by inhibiting the synthesis and secretion of collagenase from the dermal fibroblasts. It is started in a dose of 2–3 mg/kg body weight in two divided doses and then gradually increased until the blood levels exceed 8 mg/l. Steps must be taken to keep the blood levels under 20 mg/l, as lethargy, dizziness and nystagmus are common at higher levels.

Prevention of infection is an important part of treatment. Antibiotics are routinely used, these should be rotated frequently to avoid development of resistance to infection. An active nutritional support should be given to patients with lesions in the oral cavity

Surgical treatment of syndactyly may be required to restore the function of the hands with fused digits. Because of the high incidence of carcinoma of the oesophagus, annual examinations beginning in early adolescence has been recommended in recessive dystrophic epidermolysis bullosa.

Hopes for the future include gene therapy. Adding the normal gene to the epidermal stem cells and then laying these onto the denuded skin.

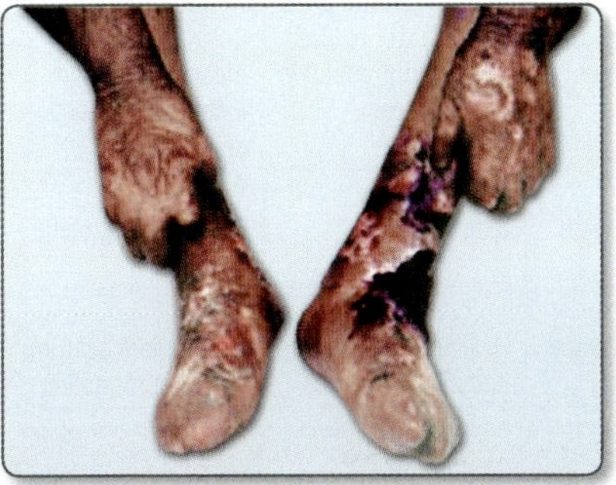

Fig. 10: Epidermolysis bullosa dystrophica (recessive type)

In the recessive variety the disease is present at birth, mucosa, teeth and nails are affected. The bullae heal with scarring and milia formation. The fingers and toes may fuse together to form a useless club like fist. Feeding becomes difficult because of oral ulceration; strictures may develop in the oesophagus leading to dysphagia. Corneal erosions with scarring affect visual acuity. Epidermal neoplasia can occur.

Types of Recessive DEB: Hallopeau-Siemens type is the severe type in which systemic involvement is maximum; there is severe involvement of mucous membranes and severe nail dystrophy. In the mitis type, the systemic involvement is minimal.

Diagnosis

Transmission electron microscopy is the gold standard investigation, alternative to it are fluorescent antigen mapping and monoclonal antibody studies.

Lesions of DEB can develop into squamous cell carcinoma of the skin and mucosa. Scarring of the hands and feet leads to mitten and sock deformity, due to fusion of digits secondary to scarring. Patients with epidermolysis bullosa should have a genetic counselling as prenatal diagnosis is now possible.

Differences between epidermolysis bullosa simplex, junctional epidermolysis bullosa and dystrophic epidermolysis bullosa are seen in Table 3.

Table 3: Differentiation of epidermolysis bullosa simplex, junctional epidermolysis bullosa and dystrophic epidermolysis bullosa dystrophica

Epidermolysis bullosa simplex	*Junctional epidermolysis bullosa*	*Dystrophic epidermolysis bullosa*	
Inheritance AD	AR	AD	AR
Age of onset Usually after birth, when child begins to crawl	At birth	Usually after birth	At birth
Aetiology Abnormality in basal cells, mutations in keratin 5 and 14	Abnormality in lamina lucida (Abnormal laminin), hemidesmosomes may be reduced	Anchoring fibrils reduced or absent. Collagen V11 reduced. Increased production of collagenase	Anchoring fibrils reduced or absent. Collagen V11 reduced. Increased production of collagenase
Sites affected Skin	Skin, mucosa, teeth and nails	Skin	Skin, mucosa, teeth and nails
Healing Without scarring	Little or no tendency to healing	Healing with scarring and milia formation	Healing with scarring and milia formation

Contd...

Contd...

Epidermolysis bullosa simplex	*Junctional epidermolysis bullosa*	*Dystrophic epidermolysis bullosa*	
Complications None, atrophy of skin can occur	Infection of eroded areas, septicaemia common Laryngeal involvement common, shedding of nails, Failure to thrive	Scarring and milia formation	Digits fuse to form a useless club like fist. Dysphagia, corneal ulcerations

SHABBIR SYNDROME

Shabbir syndrome (laryngo-onycho-cutaneous syndrome) is a rare epithelial disorder confined to the Punjabi Muslim population. It is an autosomal recessive disorder. The condition is similar to JEB, some authors consider it to be a type of JEB. The disease starts in infancy and affects both sexes. Ulcers appear at sites of trauma, the face is mainly affected; trunks, limbs and genitalia are seldom involved. The nails and teeth are affected, and so is the larynx resulting in hoarseness. The hemidesmosomes show ultrastructural and immunohistochemical abnormalities.

BULLOUS ICHTHYOSIFORM ERYTHRODERMA (EPIDERMOLYTIC HYPERKERATOSIS)

This is inherited as an autosomal dominant disorder with mutations in keratin 1 and 10. The disease manifests soon after birth and is characterized by generalized erythema, scaling and blister formation. The blisters may occur at any site but tend to be common at sites of trauma during infancy. The erythema and blistering gradually decrease as the child grows older, blistering is not a problem by 7–8 years of age, the erythema becomes scarcely noticeable at middle age. The palms and soles may be thickened, but hair, nails and mucosa are normal. Pyogenic infections are common causing a distinctive odour in these patients. Gradually the skin changes to a more diffuse hyprkeratotic almost verrucous appearance.

Treatment is symptomatic with emollients and keratolytics. Topical retinoids such as tretinoin and tazarotene, or calcipotriol can be used in resistant cases. In severe cases, oral retinoids may be required. Patients with epidermolytic hyperkeratosis should start with a low dose of retinoids, increasing the dose gradually to avoid exacerbation of blistering. Children on oral retinoids should be monitored for skeletal toxicity and growth. There is a risk of premature epiphyseal closure in children.

Topical and systemic antibiotics are used to treat pyogenic infection; sodium bicarbonate baths are effective in controlling the odour of these patients.

Acrodermatitis Enteropathica

Acrodermatitis enteropathica (AE) is a rare autosomal recessive disorder. It results from mutation in the gene which encodes the transport of zinc in the intestine. It has a number of findings similar to epidermolysis bullosa (EB);

the bullous nature of the disorder and the acral distribution, led many early investigators to classify AE with EB of the dystrophic type. Males and females are equally affected. Only a few hundred cases are reported in world literature.

The basic lesion in AE is a bulla, occurring typically on the hands, feet, and around the body orifices. The skin is often eroded, crusted and sharply marginated. A psoriasiform diaper eruption is present. The other characteristics are alopecia, nail dystrophy, gastrointestinal disturbances such as diarrhoea with exacerbations and remissions, and a peculiar apathy during periods of exacerbations.

The disease can be hereditary or acquired. Acquired form is seen in chronic wasting diseases, chronic infection, nutritional deficiencies and chronic alcoholism.

Aetiology

The disease is due to the failure of the gastrointestinal tract (duodenum and jejunum) to absorb zinc. Lesions usually manifest after weaning from breast milk, as human milk contains a factor that helps in the absorption of zinc. Paneth cells located at the bottom of the crypts of Lieberkuhn are rich in zinc; these may be involved in some phase of zinc absorption. The mucosa of the duodenal villi is flattened and there is loss of villous architecture.

Clinical Features

Lesions begin as a bulla usually on an erythematous base. These bullae quickly rupture, leaving oozing eroded plaques, which often become secondarily infected with candida. The distribution is acral, around the body orifices, on the occiput, elbows and knees. Lesions of the napkin area are often mistaken for candidiasis (Figs 11 and 12). Perlèche is an early clinical sign of AE. Paronychial bullae formation results in dystrophy of the nails. Scalp involvement is common resulting in alopecia. Glossitis and stomatitis are characteristics of AE; the lesions become secondarily infected with candida. Photophobia develops gradually. This is due to malfunction of zinc-dependent retinol-binding protein.

The children are often lethargic and irritable. Diarrhoea is a cardinal feature of AE; the stools are frothy and foul smelling.

Diagnosis

Serum zinc levels are below 50 μg/100 ml. Decreased zinc levels are found in the RBC, hair and urine. Serum alkaline phosphatase level is also in the low-normal range, which becomes normal after zinc therapy. Histologically intraepidermal clefts with acantholytic cells can be seen, making the histological picture similar to that of pemphigus.

Normal serum zinc level is 80–120 μg/100 ml.

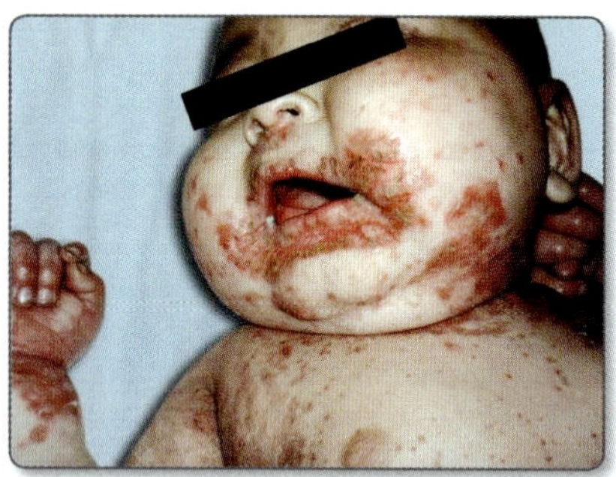

Fig. 11: Acrodermatitis enteropathica

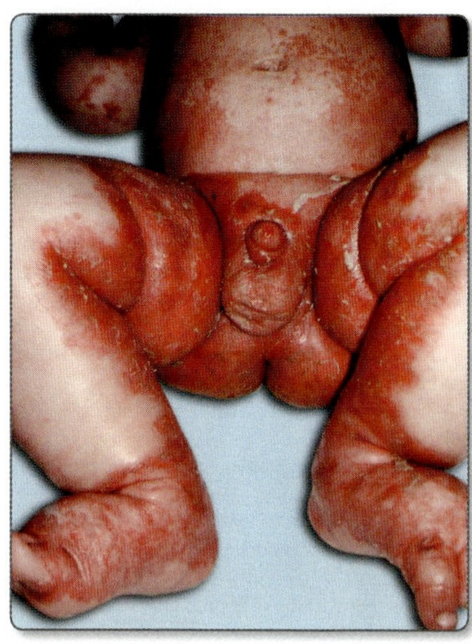

Fig. 12: Acrodermatitis enteropathica

Treatment

Oral zinc gluconate or sulphate in a dose of 5 mg/kg in two to three divided doses brings about complete remissions, symptoms respond in 1–2 weeks before zinc reaches normal levels.

Foods containing phytates should be avoided, phytates are known chelators of zinc.

Diiodohydroxyquin was used until recently to treat AE. It is said to contain zinc, but due to the complication of optic neuritis, it is now no longer used.

The body normally stores 4 gm of zinc, the average daily requirement is 10–15 mg.
Zinc is an important trace element, required for growth, reproduction, immune functions and it has anti-oxidant activities.
The classical triad of AE are acral dermatitis, alopecia and diarrhea.
The hallmark of zinc deficiency is acral dermatitis.

Weary-Kindler Syndrome

This is an autosomal recessive disorder. The disease starts at the age of 1–3 months, it has manifestations of both epidermolysis bullosa and congenital poikiloderma. Vesicopustules occur on the hands and feet often following trauma, which resolve in childhood. Photosensitivity develops early in life, gradual appearance of poikiloderma, which persists until adult life. Keratotic papules develop on the hands, feet, knees, and elbows that persist indefinitely. Early exfoliation of deciduous teeth, severe periodontal disease, and fragile bleeding gingiva are key features of the syndrome. The defect lies in kindlin-1, a protein found in basal keratinocytes.

FURTHER READING

1. Colllier P, Wojnarowske F, Welsh K, et al. Adult Linear IgA Disease and Chronic Bullous Disease of Childhood: The association with human leukocyte antigens Cw7, HLA DR3 and human necrosis factor, influences disease expression. Br J Dermatol. 1999;141(5):867-75.

2. Fry R. Dermatitis Herpetiformis: problems, progress and prospects. Eur J Dermatol. 2002;12(6):523-31.
3. Hale EK, Bystryn JC. Laryngeal and nasal involvement in Pemphigus Vulgaris. J Am Acad Dermatol. 2001;44(4):609-11.
4. Hardy K, Perry H, Pingru G, et al. Benign Mucous Membrane Pemphigoid. Arch Dermatol. 1971;104(5):467-75.
5. Kaneko K, Kakuta M, Ohtomo Y, et al. Renal amyloidosis in Recessive Dystrophic Epidermolysis Bullosa Dystrophica. Dermatology. 2000;200(3):209-12.
6. Kirtschig G, Murrell D, Wojnarowska F, et al. Interventions for Mucous Membrane Pemphigoid/Cicatricial Pemphigoid, and Epidermolysis Bullosa Acquisita: a systematic review of literature. Arch Dermatol. 2002;138(3):380-4.
7. Kitajima Y, Inoues S, Yaoita H. Abnormal organization of keratin intermediate filaments in cultured keratinocytes of epidermolysis bullosa simplex. Arch Dermatol Res. 1989;281(1): 5-10.
8. Luke MC, Darling TN, Hsu R, et al. Mucosal morbidity in patients with Epidermolysis Bullosa Acquisita. Arch Dermatol. 1999;135(8):954-9.
9. Matuo K, Komani A, Ishii K, et al. Pemphigus foliaceus with prominent neutrophilic pustules. Br J Dermatol. 2001;145(1):132-6.
10. Mellerio JE, Mcmillan JR, McGrath JA, et al. Recessive eidermolysis Bullosa Simplex associated with plectin mutation; infantile respiratory complication in two unrelated cases. Br J Dermatol. 1997;137(6):898-906.
11. Mustakallio KK, Blomqviss K, Laiho K. Papillary deposition of fibrin, a characteristic initial lesion of Dermatitis Herpetiformis. Ann Clin Res.1970;2(1):13-8.
12. Orange AP, van Joost T. Pemphigoid in children. Pediatr Dermatol. 1998;6(4):267-74.
13. Powell J, Kirtschig G, Allen J, et al. Mixed immunobullous disease of children. A good response to antimicrobials. Br J Dermatol. 2001;144(4):769-74.
14. Sacher C, Konig C, Scharffelter Kochanek K, et al. Bullous Pemphigoid in a patient treated with UVA 1 Phototherapy for Disseminated Morphea. Dermatology. 2001;202(1):54-7.
15. Sapadin AN, Anhalt GJ. Paraneoplastic Pemphigus with a Pemphigus Vegetans like plaque as the only cutaneous manifestation. J Am Acad Dermatol. 1998;39(5):867-71.
16. Schmidt E, Obe K, Brocker EB, et al. Serum levels of autoantibodies to BP 180, correlate with disease activity in patients with bullous pemphigoid. Arch Dermatol. 2000;136(2):174-8.
17. Wong SN, Chua SH. Spectrum of subepidermal immunobullous disorders seen at the National Skin Centre, Singapore: a 2 year review. Br J Dermatol. 2002;147(3):476-80.

Chapter

13 Sarcoidosis

SARCOIDOSIS (BOECK'S DISEASE)

Sarcoidosis is a multisystem granulomatous disorder of unknown aetiology. It most commonly affects young adults, and presents most frequently with bilateral hilar lymphadenopathy, pulmonary infiltrates, skin and eye lesions. The course and prognosis depends upon the mode of onset. An acute onset heralds a self-limiting course and spontaneous resolution, whereas an insidious onset may be followed by relentless progressive fibrosis. The common cutaneous manifestation is erythema nodosum. Sarcoidosis can also occur on old scars and tattoos, with papules and nodules.

Sarcoidosis is mainly a disease of colder climate. Its incidence, especially the cutaneous manifestations, in tropical countries is extremely low. Young female adults between the ages of 20–40 years are commonly affected. Male to female ratio is 1:5.

AETIOLOGY

The cause of sarcoidosis is unknown, many hypotheses have been put forward. It may be associated with an imbalance between the subsets of T lymphocytes and other disturbances of cell-mediated immunity. B lymphocytes are also present at the site of activity. Activated macrophages and helper T cells are increased in sarcoid granulomas. The increased T lymphocytes could be recruited from the blood, which explains the leukopaenia in sarcoid patients. The T cells are also responsible for the activation of B lymphocytes and immunoglobin synthesis at the site of activity. Circulatory immune complexes are also present in the serum.

Tuberculosis has drawn attention as a major cause of sarcoidosis, because of a similar histopathology and increased incidence of tuberculosis in some cases of sarcoidosis. In some patients, the tuberculosis preceded the development of sarcoidosis. It is also seen that in areas where tuberculosis is widespread, sarcoidosis is rarely seen, but as tuberculosis is brought under control, sarcoidosis becomes more frequent. It has been demonstrated that DNA from *Mycobacterium tuberculosis* can be found in tissue sections of sarcoid lesions. Some authors predict the role of atypical mycobacteria, as a cause for sarcoidosis. There is a relative anergy to tuberculin in sarcoid patients. The disease resembles tuberculosis histologically but tubercle bacillus and caseation are not found.

Chronic beryllium poisoning produces a disease similar to sarcoidosis but exposure to beryllium is very rare. The occasional occurrence of familial sarcoidosis suggests genetic influences.

The decrease of T cells in the peripheral blood is responsible for the anergy to tuberculosis, mumps, candida and trichophyton antigens; the anergy is relative, not absolute.

HISTOPATHOLOGY

The central histological feature of sarcoidosis is the presence of non-caseating epithelioid cell granulomas in all tissues affected. The sarcoid granuloma consists of tightly packed collection of modified macrophages, abundance of epithelioid cells, few or no Langhans giant cells and closely admixed lymphocytes. Cellular inclusions such as asteroid bodies and Schaumann bodies are frequent, these increase in number as the disease progresses. Caseation is absent, there is no peripheral lymphocytic infiltration surrounding the granuloma. Sarcoid granuloma is often called the "naked tubercle".

> **Clinical Features**
>
> Sarcoid is rare in childhood, young female adults are commonly affected. All races are susceptible; it is rare in Asians. It is a multi-system disorder.

Cutaneous Manifestations

Cutaneous manifestations of sarcoidosis may be specific or non-specific.

Specific Lesions

Several morphological lesions have been described. The lesions are multiple, firm and elastic when palpated. It may extend deeply to involve the entire dermis; the overlying epidermis is usually thin. The colour varies according to the stage of development from dull tint of red to purple, brown or yellow. The lesions are asymptomatic, some may itch. Constitutional symptoms are usually present at the onset with fever and arthralgia.

Papular lesions: These present as crops of small papules, most commonly seen on the face and extensor surface of the limbs. On the face, these are mostly present around the eyelids, nasal alae, nasolabial folds and cheeks. These papules are purplish red or yellowish color, without scarring. They are associated with good prognosis (Fig. 1A).

Nodular lesions: These are found on the face, trunk and proximal portion of the limbs. They may be superficial or deep, yellowish or purple in color (Fig. 1B).

Plaques: Occur on the shoulders, buttocks and thighs. These are usually associated with chronic disease and the prognosis is poor. The plaques of sarcoidosis are always violaceous and often transparent. Telangiectatic vessels may be seen on the surface.

Annular sarcoid: Confined to the head and neck, the lesions have a peripheral scaly edge and central hypopigmented scarred area. These are associated with chronic disease and have a poor prognosis.

Scar sarcoid: Old scars become infiltrated with sarcoid granulomas, these scars become purplish in color resembling keloids. They occur in acute disease.

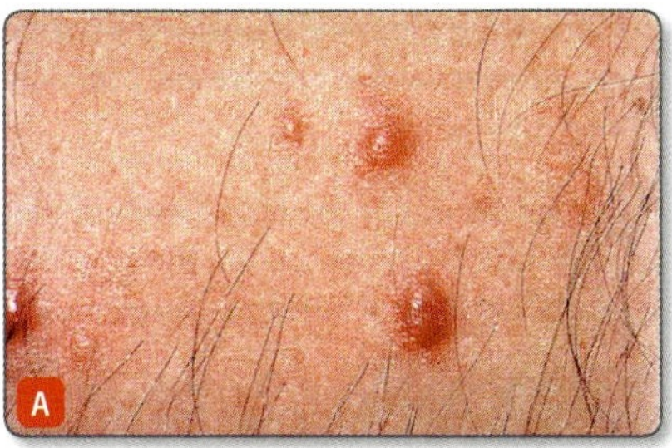

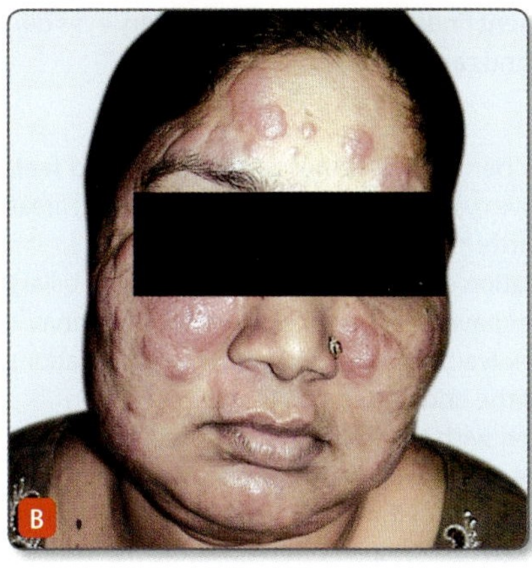

Figs 1A and B: Sarcoidosis: (A) Papular lesions; (B) Nodular lesions

Lupus pernio: This affects the poorly perfused areas, i.e. the nose, ear lobes and fingers. Once involved these areas become swollen and indurated, which have a deep purplish red color. The phalangeal bones may contain cysts of sarcoid granulomas. Nasal bones may erode. Lupus pernio is a sign of bad prognosis.

Non-specific Lesions

These may present as erythema nodosum, which is frequently one of the earliest manifestations of sarcoidosis. Other lesions are subcutaneous calcium deposition; erythema multiforme scarring and non-scarring alopecia.

Lofgren syndrome consists of erythema nodosum, hilar lymphadenopathy and arthritis.

Sarcoidosis can also occur in children and infants; they tend to have more joint involvement and rashes, less pulmonary and eye problems. The skin lesions are eczematous and papular. Erythema nodosum can involve multiple sites, such as the soles and limbs. The joints show multiple boggy synovitis without much pain or limitation of movements.

Systemic Manifestations

Many cases of sarcoidosis are asymptomatic. The disease is often diagnosed on a routine X-ray examination of the chest. In some cases, there is an acute onset with erythema nodosum, bilateral hilar lymphadenopathy, peripheral arthropathy and occasional fever. In chronic cases, the disease manifests by cough, breathlessness and with extra-pulmonary manifestations, weight loss and malaise. Any system of the body may be involved, the lungs and eyes involvement is more common.

Pulmonary Changes

The most frequent manifestation is involvement of the hilar lymph nodes, these are asymptomatic. Pulmonary infiltration is more serious; this may lead to pulmonary fibrosis. Bronchial stenosis and obstruction may also occur.

Ocular Changes

The eyes are involved in 25–30% of cases. Granulomatous anterior and posterior uveitis is the most frequent finding. Conjunctivitis and dry eyes due to involvement of the lacrimal glands are also common.

Bony Involvement

This is often present with lupus pernio. The bones of the hands and feet, especially the distal phalanges have cystic changes seen as punched out areas on X-rays. Arthralgias and acute arthritis can also occur.

Enlargement of the liver, elevation of serum alkaline phosphatase, biliary cirrhosis and portal hypertension have been reported. The central nervous system and the heart are rarely involved, but when affected the complications are serious. Almost any system of the body can be involved.

Sarcoidosis may be associated with Sjogren's, Mikulicz and Heerfordt's syndromes. Heerfordt's syndrome consists of uveitis, swollen parotid glands, fever and facial nerve palsy. Involvement of the lacrimal glands and associated changes in the salivary glands and cervical lymph nodes constitute the Mikulicz syndromes. Common features of Sjogren syndrome consist of dryness and atrophy of the conjunctiva and cornea, dry mouth and rheumatoid arthritis.

Differential Diagnosis

The disease should be differentiated according to the type of clinical presentation:

- Lupus pernio, from perniosis and lupus vulgaris.
- Maculopapular form from generalized lichen planus, secondary syphilis, generalized granuloma annulare.
- Nodular form from lymphocytoma cutis, cutaneous amyloidosis, and also from foreign body granulomas, such as beryllium, zinc, silica and zirconium.

Diagnosis

In most cases, the skin sensitivity to tuberculin is depressed or absent. The Mantoux test is, therefore, a useful screening test. A positive reaction to tuberculin test virtually excludes sarcoidosis.

Blood examination shows lymphocytopaenia, mild eosinophilia, increased ESR and elevated levels of serum angiotensin-converting enzyme (ACE). The source of ACE in most cases is the granulomas. The serum levels do not correlate with disease activity. It is an additional test to support the diagnosis of sarcoidosis.

Biopsy of the skin or lymph nodes shows the typical sarcoid granuloma. Kveim's test is a useful diagnostic procedure. The antigen (0.1 ml) is injected intradermally, when the test is positive, a small nodule develops at the site in about 4 weeks. Biopsy of the nodule shows the typical sarcoid follicles.

X-ray of the chest will show bilateral hilar lymphadenopathy, and typical punched out lesions of the distal phalanx. Gallium-67 scan (Panda and Lambda sign), gadolinium enhancement on nuclear magnetic imaging (MRI) and by fluorodeoxyglucose positron emission tomography (PET) scanning may also be helpful in diagnosis.

Treatment

Eighty to ninety percent cases of acute sarcoidosis show spontaneous resolution, so therapy is seldom indicated. Most patients require only symptomatic therapy like NSAIDs.

For small or localized cutaneous lesions topical or intralesional potent corticosteroids are required. Tetracyclines have shown promise for the treatment of cutaneous sarcoidosis. If the lesions are diffuse the treatment is similar to that of systemic sarcoidosis.

For systemic sarcoidosis corticosteroids are required in acute sarcoidosis, when accompanied by lesions of the eyes, the central nervous system and cardiovascular system, patients with pulmonary diseases and functional disability. Prednisolone is given in a dose of 1 mg/kg/day which is tapered to every other day when improvement occurs. Long-term therapy is needed over several weeks. Most patients who require long-term steroids can be treated using 10–15 mg of prednisolone every other day.

In chronic sarcoidosis, the treatment with oral steroids has to be continued for several years.

Chloroquine and hydroxychloroquine are antimalarial drugs with immunomodulating properties, have been used for treatment of cutaneous lesions, hypercalcaemia, neurological sarcoidosis, and bone lesions. Chloroquine has also been shown to be efficacious for the treatment and maintenance of chronic pulmonary sarcoidosis

Methotrexate, azathioprine, and thalidomide have also shown promising results.

Allopurinol has been successful in some cases of sarcoidosis. It can be combined with pentoxifylline. Infliximab has been reported recently to be effective in treating patients with sarcoidosis. A few studies have shown fumaric acid esters effective in recalcitrant cutaneous sarcoidosis.

Lung transplantation remains the only hope for patients with advanced sarcoid-induced pulmonary fibrosis.

COURSE AND PROGNOSIS

Acute sarcoidosis resolves in a few months, the chronic disease extends over many years. Mortality is 5%. Death usually follows pulmonary and cardiac diseases.

FURTHER READING

1. Georgi T. Cutaneous Sarcoidosis. The great imitator: morphology, differential diagnosis and clinical management. Am J Clin Dermatol. 2006;7(6):375-82.
2. Katta R. Cutaneous Sarcoidosis: a dermatologic masquerade. Am Fam Physician. 2002;65(8):1581-5.
3. Nowack U, Gambichler T, Hanefeld C, et al. Successful treatment of recalcitrant sarcoidosis with fumaric acid esters. BMC Dermatol. 2002;5:15.
4. Sharma OP. Cutaneous sarcoidosis: clinical features and management. Chest. 1972;61(4):320-5.
5. Wilson NJ, King CM. Cutaneous sarcoidosis (Research article). Postgrad Med J. 1998;74(877):649-52.

Chapter

14 Amyloidosis

Amyloid is a proteinaceous substance that can be deposited in many organs, or it is restricted to a single site. Deposition can be primary or secondary; its deposition is associated with considerable tissue dysfunction. Amyloidosis is associated with Alzheimer's disease, plasma cell dyscrasias, multiple myeloma and many chronic infections. Skin deposits are present in all varieties except in secondary systemic amyloidosis.

AETIOLOGY

The exact aetiology of the deposition remains unknown. It is said that amyloid fibrils are of intermediate type (100 Å diameter), similar to that of the keratinocytes. They also respond to anti-human keratin antibody indicating an epidermal origin of the fibrils. This type of amyloid is known as amyloid K, for keratin.

The amyloid fibrils in primary systemic amyloidosis are derived from immunoglobulins (amyloid IO), for immunoglobulin origin. This type is also found in the nodular form of cutaneous amyloidosis, which may progress to systemic disease.

The amyloid fibrils in secondary systemic amyloidosis are unrelated to immunoglobulins, it is designated as amyloid A. Its precursor is serum amyloid A protein, which is an acute phase protein reactant, increased in various inflammatory states.

Electron microscope reveals that the amyloid fibrils are non-branching, anastamosing often irregularly like the tonofilaments of the epidermis. A second minor component of amyloid appears doughnut-shaped, outer diameter of 9 nm and inner diameter of 4 nm, this resembles the glycoprotein.

Genetic factor may be associated, as some cases are familial.

HISTOPATHOLOGY

In the macular and papular forms of amyloidosis amyloid deposits are found in the papillary dermis, the overlying epidermis shows irregular acanthosis and hyperkeratosis. Near the amyloid deposits, there are sparse lymphohistiocytic perivascular infiltrates.

In the nodular form of primary cutaneous amyloidosis, the amyloid deposits are found diffusely in the dermis, subcutaneous tissue and in the blood vessel walls. In addition, there may be a perivascular infiltration of plasma cells, which is similar to that of systemic amyloidosis.

Amyloid is weakly periodic acid-Schiff (PAS) positive and diastase resistant. In hematocrit and eosin stains amyloid looks like eosinophilic collagen. Stain specific for amyloid is Congo red. It can also be stained with crystal violet and thioflavin T.

Clinical Features

Primary Cutaneous Amyloidosis

The disorder commonly affects middle-aged people of either sex. The deposits may be macular, papular or nodular.

Macular Amyloidosis

Macular amyloidosis is uncommon; it is the most subtle of cutaneous amyloidosis. It appears as brown rippled macules, characteristically located in the interscapular region; it is also found on the shins, thighs, arms, breast and buttocks (Figs 1A and B). The disease is common in Orientals.

Lichen Amyloidosis

Lichen amyloidosis is the most common form of amyloidosis, it is common in Asians. The lesions present as itchy papules typically on the shins. The papules are small, brown, discrete and slightly scaly (Fig. 2). These may coalesce to form plaques. The thighs, forearms and upper arms may also be affected. Recently a type of cutaneous amyloidosis has been recognized that appears as grouped papules on the concha.

Nodular Amyloidosis

Nodular amyloidosis is a rare variant of cutaneous amyloidosis. Most of the patients are females. Single or multiple nodules or plaques are seen on the scalp, trunk, limbs and on the vulva. The overlying skin is often atrophic showing the underlying yellowish fat. There may be petechial haemorrhages in the nodules. Although nodular amyloidosis is seen without systemic involvement, in some cases progress may occur to involve the internal organs. A long-term follow up is necessary for this form of amyloidosis.

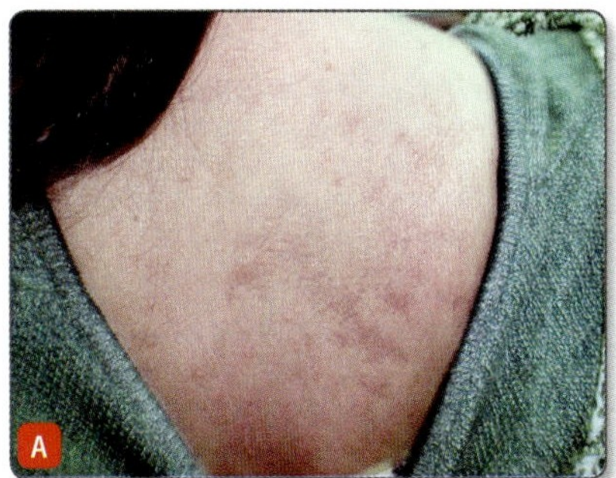

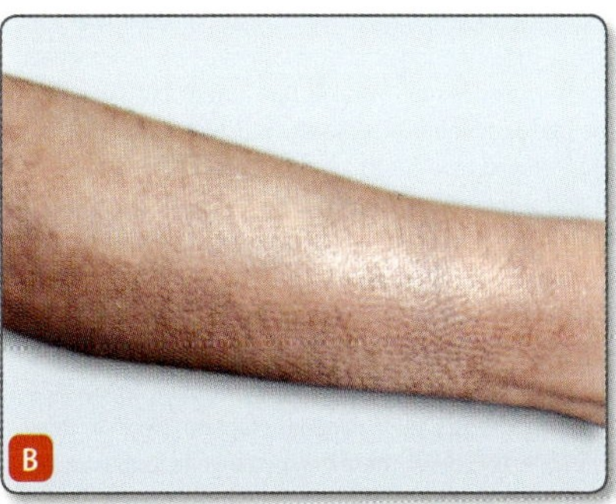

Figs 1A and B: Macular amyloidosis: (A) Common site; (B) Rippled appearance

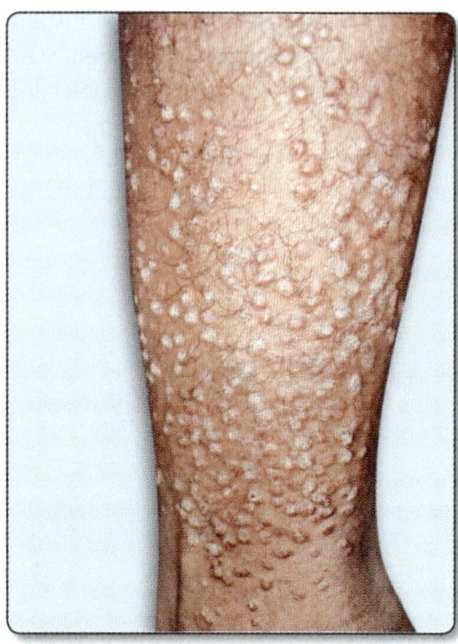

Fig. 2: Lichen amyloidosis

Familial Syndromes Associated with Amyloidosis

These include familial Mediterranean fever and Muckle-Well syndrome. Microscopically amyloid appears in the shape of cylinders, flakes or rods, except in the nodular form in which plasma cells and calcification are often present.

Secondary Cutaneous Amyloidosis

Secondary deposits are often found on histology as incidental findings. Amyloid can be deposited secondary to certain cutaneous disorders such as psoriasis, hidradenitis suppurativa, certain intradermal melanocytic naevus, seborrhoeic warts, dystrophic epidermolysis bullosa, stasis ulcers, porokeratosis of Mibelli, some skin tumours such as basal cell carcinoma, trichoepithelioma, sweat gland tumours, etc. Amyloid is also deposited following long-term photochemotherapy.

Systemic Amyloidosis

Amyloid is deposited in the skin in primary systemic amyloidosis, amyloid deposition does not occur in secondary systemic amyloidosis. Secondary systemic amyloidosis is also called the wear- and- tear amyloidosis, in which amyloid deposits are seen secondary to inflammatory diseases, such as tuberculosis, rheumatoid arthritis, inflammatory bowel disease, etc.

Primary Systemic Amyloidosis

(Immunoglobulin derived amyloidosis). Immunoglobulin deposit of amyloid is associated with diseases such as multiple myeloma, plasma cell dysplasia. The immunoglobulin deposits are seen in numerous sites. Signs and symptoms are very variable. The most common initial feature is nephrotic syndrome, with a protein loss of more than 20 g per day. Cardiac abnormalities present with biventricular cardiac failure. Neurological features include carpal tunnel syndrome due to compression of the median nerve by amyloid deposits, peripheral neuropathy and autonomic neuropathy.

Amyloidosis is also associated with familial Mediterranean fever, (intermittent fever, erysipelas like lesions on the lower leg and urticaria), Muckle-Well syndrome (urticaria, fever, limb pains, progressive perceptive nerve deafness and renal amyloidosis). About a quarter of patients with primary systemic amyloidosis, develop skin lesions. Glossitis and macroglossia is seen in 20% of cases. The tongue is painful, enlarged and furrows develop. The mucous membranes of the lips and cheeks have a similar hypertrophic appearance.

Cutaneous lesions in primary systemic amyloidosis: The cutaneous eruptions begin as shiny smooth, firm, flat topped or spherical papules of waxy colour. These may coalesce to form nodules and plaques of various sizes. The regions around the mouth, nose, eyes as well as the mucocutaneous junctions are commonly involved. Lesions on the vulva should be differentiated from condylomata lata.

Diffuse amyloid infiltrations in the skin resembles a scleroderma like appearance of the face, hands and feet. Amyloid deposits on the scalp may resemble cutis verticis gyrata, or amyloid deposits may result in alopecia. Bullae may occur due to shearing forces within dermal amyloid deposits.

Common manifestations of systemic amyloidosis are petechiae, purpura and ecchymosis occurring spontaneously or after minor trauma (pinch purpura). These are the result of amyloid deposits in the blood vessel walls. Purpura and ecchymosis are common; it is seen chiefly on the eyelids, limbs and in the mouth. Bullae are rare, alopecia occurs if the lesions occur on the scalp. Nodular lesions are also present along with the blood vessels. Purpura of the eyelids on pinching and perianal purpura (post-proctoscopic purpura) is seen on proctoscopic examination, Valsalva's manouvre or vomiting also produces periorbital haemorrhage. Periorbital purpura is diagnostic of immunoglobulin amyloid deposits.

Nails are brittle and may produce longitudinal striation, partial or complete anonychia may be a presenting sign.

Amyloid elastosis is a cutaneous systemic pattern of amyloidosis. Eruptions of yellowish brown rubbery, discrete papules and nodules occur, sparing only the head, hands, feet and the mucosa.

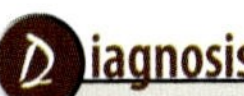

Diagnosis

Cutaneous Amyloidosis

The diagnosis of cutaneous amyloidosis depends on skin biopsy, which shows deposits of amyloid in the cutaneous lesions. Special stains such as Congo red are used for detecting amyloid deposits. When the sample is examined in polarized light, amyloid is doubly refractive and apple green in color. With thioflavin T, a yellow fluorescence is seen and with acridine orange a red fluorescence appears.

Biopsy of even normal forearm skin has been reported to be positive in about 50% of cases. Plasma cell dyscrasia can be diagnosed by the detection of Bence-Jones proteins in the urine.

The most useful sites for biopsy of primary systemic amyloidosis are rectal mucosa (85%) and transverse carpal ligament (100%).

A few studies have shown some characteristic dermatoscopic features in primary cutaneous amyloidosis. Dermatoscopic findings show a central hub which is white or brown, surrounded by various configurations of hyperpigmentation.

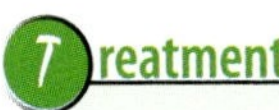

Treatment

Cutaneous Amyloidosis

Treatment is difficult because amyloid deposits are insoluble. Mild cases can be helped with a potent topical steroid or intralesional injections of corticosteroids. Topical application of 10% dimethylsulphoxide (DMSO) has been used in the treatment of amyloidosis in Equador where amyloidosis is very common. Tacrolimus 0.1% used twice a day is also used to treat cutaneous amyloidosis.

Acitretin appears to be helpful in relieving the troublesome pruritus of lichen amyloidosis. PUVA, UVB, helpful in some cases. The nodular forms should be surgically excised. Dermabrasion, pulse-dye and carbon dioxide lasers, cryotherapy, electrocautery have been used to treat cutaneous amyloid deposits. Recurrences are common.

Capsaicin used topically once daily may reduce pruritus.

Systemic amyloidosis should be managed in a multidisciplinary fashion. Systemic amyloidosis can be treated with melphalan, colchicine, thymosin, various chemotherapy regimens and autologous peripheral blood stem-cell transplantation. A marked improvement is seen with the long-term use of DMSO, this therapy often results in bad odour. Renal transplantation may be of benefit in renal failure.

Course and Prognosis

Primary cutaneous amyloidosis persists indefinitely; there are no systemic complications. In systemic amyloidosis, death usually occurs within 2 years.

It is often due to heart failure due to the involvement of the cardiac muscle. Myelomatosis often develops and may be responsible for death.

If a patient presents with bilateral carpal tunnel syndrome, think of amyloidosis.
Amyloid IO and amyloid A do not itch.
In pure cutaneous amyloidosis with Amyloid K, there are no perivascular deposits of amyloid.
Think of systemic amyloidosis in cases of spontaneous purpura, such as pinch purpura.
A cardiac evaluation should be done in all cases of systemic amyloidosis, as congestive cardiac failure is the most common cause of death.

FURTHER READING

1. Brownstein MH, Helwig EB. The Cutaneous Amyloidosis: localized forms. Arch Dermatol. 1970;102(1):8-19.
2. Chuang YY, Lee DD, Lin CS, et al. Characteristic dermatoscopic features of primary cutaneous amyloidosis. A study of 35 cases. Br J Dermatol. 2012;167(3):548-54.
3. Gorgoi DJ. Treatment of Primary localized cutaneous amyloidosis with cyclophosphamide. Ind J Dermatol Venereal Leprosy. 2003;69(2):163-4.
4. Hashimoto K, King LE. Secondary localized cutaneous amyloidosis associated with actinic keratosis. J Invest Dermatol. 1973;61(5):293-9.
5. Sakuma TH, Hans-Filho G, Aarita K, et al. Familial primary localized cutaneous amyloidosis in Brazil. Arch Dermatol. 2008;145(6):695-9.

Chapter

15

Diseases of Blood Vessels and Lymphatic System

The skin has an abundant blood supply that is finely regulated by the sympathetic nervous system. The blood vessels of the skin have dual functions to perform: to maintain the normal body temperature and to supply nutrition to the skin. The blood vessels are involved in many diseases. These can be broadly classified as:

- Vasculitis
- Erythemas
- Telangiectasia
- Tumours and naevi

VASCULITIS

Vasculitis is a term applied to inflammation and necrosis of the blood vessels. The vessels affected may be the arteries, arterioles, capillaries, venules or the veins. The small blood vessels with a slow rate of flow are usually affected. The stagnant circulation in the capillaries and venules of the legs makes the site a predilection for vasculitis. Vasculitis may be primary or secondary.

The clinical signs depend upon the severity of inflammation. The degree of damage ranges from increased permeability of the blood vessels; causing oedema resulting in urticaria, leakage of red blood cells causing purpura, to occlusion of the blood vessels resulting in ischaemia and necrosis.

Many agents have been postulated to cause vasculitis. Allergic factors such as food, drugs, and pollens, systemic autoimmune diseases such as systemic lupus erythematosus (SLE), infections, infestations, or malignancies. Vasculitis may be primary or it may be associated with systemic disease.

Classification of vasculitis continues to be difficult. It may be classified according to the size of the blood vessels involved: large, medium or the small blood vessels, or according to the type of infiltrate present: neutrophilic, lymphocytic or granulomatous. Vasculitis may be cutaneous or systemic.

CLASSIFICATION

ACCORDING TO THE INFILTRATE

- **Neutrophilic Vasculitis**
  - Leucocytoclastic vasculitis
  - Polyarteritis nodosa
  - Erythema elevatum diutinum

- **Lymphocytic Vasculitis**
  - Cutaneous pityriasis lichenoides
  - Collagen tissue disease vasculitis
- **Granulomatous Vasculitis**
  - Granuloma faciale
  - Wegener's granulomatosis (WG)
  - Temporal arteritis

ACCORDING TO THE SIZE OF VESSEL INVOLVED

- **Large Vessel Involvement**
  - Takayasu disease
  - Temporal arteritis
- **Medium Vessel Involvement**
  - Wegener's granulomatosis
  - Churg-Strauss syndrome
  - Polyarteritis nodosa
  - Kawasaki disease
- **Small Vessel Involvement (Arterioles, capillaries and venules)**
  - Anti-Neutrophilic Cytoplasmic Antibody-associated (ANCA-associated)
  - Non-ANCA-associated
    - Leukocytoclastic vasculitis
    - Henoch-Schonlein purpura
    - Urticarial vasculitis
    - Inflammatory bowel disease vasculitis

CUTANEOUS AND SYSTEMIC VASCULITIS

- **Cutaneous Vasculitis**
  - Leucocytoclastic vasculitis
  - Urticarial vasculitis
  - Erythema elevatum diutinum
  - Granuloma faciale
- **Systemic Vasculitis**
  - Wegener granulomatosis
  - Churg-Strauss syndrome
  - Polyarteritis nodosa
  - Temporal arteritis
  - Takayasu disease

NEUTROPHILIC VASCULITIS

Cutaneous Leucocytoclastic Vasculitis (Allergic Vasculitis, Palpable Purpura)

This is an inflammation of the small vessels (often venules) with marked perivascular infiltration of fragmented polymorphs and variable number of eosinophils. Allergy to drugs or microorganisms is often blamed for the disease.

Many clinical patterns have been recognized, in many cases the lesions are confined to the skin, in others systemic involvement occurs.

Aetiology

There can be many possible triggers; leucocytoclastic vasculitis is due to the deposition of immune complexes in the venules. This leads to complement activation and production of polymorph chemotactic factors. Polymorphs attracted to the area release lysosomal enzymes that damage the vessel wall. Drugs, bacterial and viral infections may act as antigenic triggers, but often the initiating factor is not identified. This type of vasculitis may also be associated with infections, malignancy, rheumatoid arthritis, SLE, Sjogren's syndrome and drugs. The disease is common in children and young adults. In older patients it is often due to drug reaction or is a manifestation of systemic disease.

Histopathology

There is fibrinoid necrosis of the small blood vessels and a perivascular infiltrate composed mainly of neutrophils, extravasated red blood cells and fragments of polymorph nuclei (nuclear dust). A biopsy is essential for the diagnosis.

Clinical Features

Cutaneous manifestations: The classical sites are the lower legs and the feet, but the arms, hands, lower trunk, ears and even the mucosa may be involved in severe cases. The hallmark of leucocytoclastic vasculitis is purpura, which is present in about 90% of cases. Vasculitis commences as palpable purpura and often progresses to haemorrhagic bullae, necrosis and ulceration. There may be ulcerated nodules; ulcerated lesions are very slow to heal when situated on the lower leg (Fig. 1). Urticarial lesions and oedema of the ankles may occur. Urticarial lesions are less evanescent than the ordinary hives and subside after a few days, leaving residual hyperpigmentation. Pain, burning and stinging sensation may be present.

Systemic manifestations: In the more severe forms of allergic vasculitis, in addition to the skin other organs are also involved. Henoch-Schonlein purpura is a type of leucocytoclastic vasculitis that occurs predominantly in children. The syndrome comprises an urticarial or purpuric rash, flitting arthralgia, gastrointestinal symptoms (pain, vomiting and bloody diarrhoea) and a focal proliferative glomerulonephritis. The prognosis depends upon the degree of renal damage.

Gastrointestinal involvement causes ulceration, haemorrhage and perforation. The lungs may be affected with haemoptysis, oedema, infiltration and infarction. Peripheral nerves and the central nervous system are involved in severe cases.

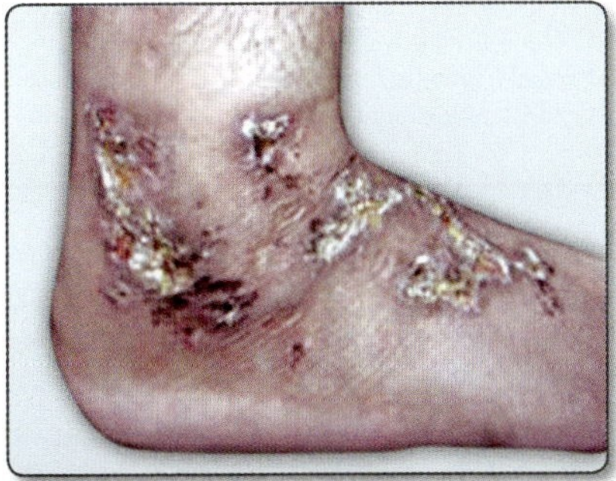

Fig. 1: Leucocytoclastic vasculitis

Treatment

Treatment of leucocytoclastic vasculitis should in general be non-aggressive since the majority of the cases are acute and self-limiting. Rest and elevation of the legs are likely to be helpful. Analgesics for pain, avoidance of trauma and cold are prudent general measures.

An identified drug or antigen should be eliminated and any identifying infection, collagen or neoplastic disease treated.

Aggressive treatment depends upon the severity of systemic involvement. Most cases are treated by moderate to high doses of prednisolone (60–80 mg daily), often with a cytotoxic drug. In cases that do not respond dapsone 100–150 mg daily may be given. Colchicine is also effective.

Course and Prognosis

The cutaneous form may be an episode of a few weeks, but in some cases, it is very persistent. The systemic form may have a similar time course, but it may be fatal in the acute stage.

Polyarteritis Nodosa (Kussmaul-Maier Disease)

This is a disease characterised by widespread vasculitis of the small to medium sized arteries with predictably lethal consequences without treatment. The involvement is segmental, and is found in areas where branching of the vessels occur. Small aneurysms frequently develop, thrombosis leads to tissue infarcts. Polyarteritis nodosa may be associated with hepatitis B and human immunodeficiency virus.

The disease may involve any organ, but it has a strong predilection for renal and visceral vasculature. There is no pulmonary involvement in polyarteritis nodosa. The systemic illness is associated with fever, malaise, tachycardia, leucocytosis (a count as high as 40,000 may occur, mainly of polymorphs) and a high erythrocyte sedimentation rate (ESR).

Clinical Features

The skin changes are seen mainly on the lower limbs, but may occur anywhere else on the body (Fig. 2). The lesions appear as palpable subcutaneous nodules along the course of the superficial arteries. Other cutaneous findings are livedo reticularis, purple necrotic plaques, and haemorrhagicbullae or deep punched out ulcers with an irregular margin. The lesions may remain localised in the skin for long periods of time.

Postprandial abdominal pain is a sign of gastrointestinal involvement. Serious complications include ischaemic bowel perforation, mesenteric artery thrombosis or rupture.

Vascular neuropathy occurs in a number of patients, it involves the larger peripheral nerves with sensory and motor symptoms. Kidneys are involved in almost all cases; it is usually subclinical, except for hypertension. Myocardial infarction, congestive cardiac failure and there is a risk of strokes due to involvement of the central nervous system.

Diagnosis

Segmental involvement makes it hard to find the site for biopsy. Initial inflammatory infiltrate is neutrophilic, later replaced by mononuclear cells with intimal proliferation. Granuloma and fibrosis is seen in the late stage.

Angiography reveals microaneurysms, in the gastrointestinal or renal arteries.

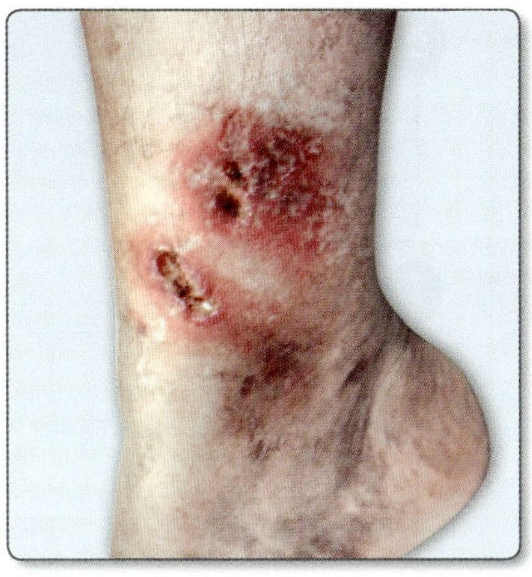

Fig. 2: Polyarteritis nodosa

Treatment

Bed rest is essential in early stages.

Corticosteroids have increased the survival rate to over 90% (without treatment survival rate was only 13%). The steroids are given as prednisolone in a dose of 1 mg/kg/day or a pulse dose of methylprednisolone 1 g daily for 3 days. If unresponsive, cyclophosphamide and other immunosuppressive agents can be used.

For the cutaneous variety of polyarteritis nodosa, local treatment with bland topical application with supportive therapy will be more successful than oral steroids. Fibrinolytic therapy with stanozolol or nicotinic acid may be helpful in some cases. Infection is treated with antibiotics; special care is taken to avoid drugs to which the patient is sensitive.

There is no pulmonary involvement in polyarteritis nodosa

Erythema Elevatum Diutinum

Erythema elevatum diutinum is a chronic vasculitis; a streptococcal infection may exacerbate the disease. The disease is frequent in adults, but may be present at any age, it is usually, distributed symmetrically over the extensor surfaces of the extremities especially the hands and knees. The condition is usually painful, but the patient can be asymptomatic.

Histopathology

There is dense perivascular infiltrate consisting mainly of neutrophils. Some neutrophils show leucocytoclasis. In the late stages, fibrosis replaces the cellular components. The association of neutrophils and fibrosis is often said to be pathognomonic for erythema elevatum diutinum. Occasional cholesterol deposits can also be seen.

Clinical Features

This is a rare disease characterised by persistent painful elevated erythematous papules which progress to plaques and nodules. These lesions are usually found over the joints, especially those of the fingers, wrists, elbows, knees, ankles and toes (Fig. 3). The forearms and the legs may also be involved. The plaques may become annular. Bulla formation and haemorrhagic crusting may occur. Old plaques may also become fibrotic. The trunk and mucous membranes are usually spared. Condition may last for many years and then involutes without scarring.

Erythema elavatum diutinum can be associated with rheumatoid arthritis, Crohn's disease, or chronic upper respiratory tract infection.

Diagnosis

Most patients have an increased ESR. There is often a positive reaction to intradermally injected streptokinase-streptodornase products of streptococci. Histology shows features of leucocytoclastic vasculitis.

Treatment

For limited disease intralesional corticosteroids are effective.

Dapsone is the drug of choice for widespread lesions; it produces dramatic response in 48 hours after the start of therapy. 50 mg is given daily for 3–4 days; the dose is then doubled. Systemic steroids are of limited value. Nicotinamide and tetracyclines may help.

LYMPHOCYTIC VASCULITIS

Cutaneous Pityriasis Lichenoides

Pityriasis lichenoides exists in acute and chronic forms with occasional transformation from acute to the chronic form. The acute condition is called pityriasis lichenoides et varioliformis acuta (PLEVA) and the chronic form is called pityriasis lichenoides chronica. Mucous membranes may be involved in the acute form. The rash is asymmetrical.

PLEVA

Most patients are children and young adults. The cause is unknown, viral infection may be a preceding factor. Fever and constitutional symptoms may precede the eruption. The initial lesion is a small, red papule, this becomes vesicular and haemorrhagic. Some lesions undergo necrosis and ulceration. The lesions heal with the formation of pitted scars. The eruption is polymorphous; all stages of the lesions are present. New crops may cease to develop after a few weeks, many cases clear within 6 months. The acute form should be differentiated from chickenpox.

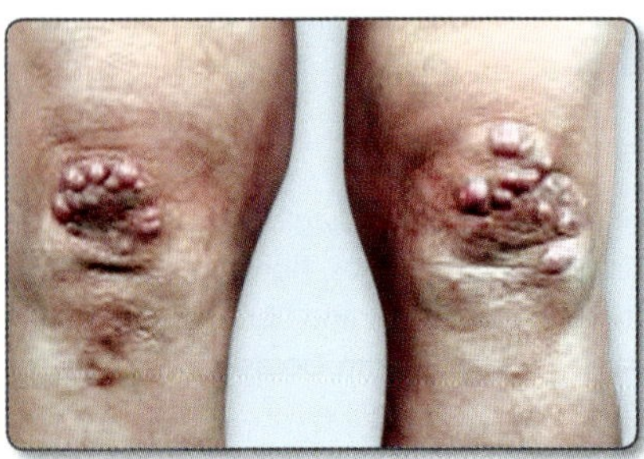

Fig. 3: Erythema elevatum diutinum

Pityriasis Lichenoid Chronica

There is no constitutional upset, small red papules are the earliest lesion, these may become purpuric, brownish in colour and are covered by a characteristic "mica scale". This is a shiny scale attached centrally to the papule; it can be scraped off to leave a slightly brown surface. The papule resolves slowly leaving hyperpigmentation, which may be a presenting sign. Lesions may develop from time to time over the years. The chronic form should be differentiated from secondary syphilis and guttate psoriasis.

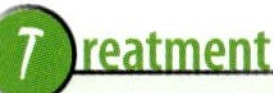

A short course of systemic steroids may curtail the acute attack. Tetracycline in a dose of 1–2 g daily for 3–4 weeks may also be used for both the acute and the chronic forms. Ultraviolet light and PUVA are sometimes successful in healing the chronic lesions.

Course and Prognosis

The acute form may present as a single attack lasting for a few weeks or there may be recurrent attacks. A few cases undergo transition to the chronic forms. The chronic form is often persistent for many years.

GRANULOMATOUS VASCULITIS

Cutaneous Granuloma Faciale

Granuloma faciale is a chronic form of leucocytoclastic vasculitis, characterised by the formation of reddish brown, soft, facial plaques or nodules, these are usually solitary. It is not a granuloma as the name suggests. The lesions are confined to the cheeks, forehead, chin, and ears. In some cases there may be multiple plaques and these are widespread. The plaques are soft, poorly circumscribed and are asymptomatic. In some patients annular lesions may form. The lesions are slowly progressive, occasionally they involute.

Extracutaneous involvement is rare; few cases have been reported in the oral mucosa and upper respiratory tract.

The disease is diagnosed by a biopsy, which shows the features of leucocytoclastic vasculitis. A characteristic clear Grentz zone is seen between the infiltrate and the epidermis. The perivascular infiltrate consists of lymphocytes, neutrophils and eosinophils. Extravasated red blood cells, melanin and hemosiderin contribute to the brown colour.

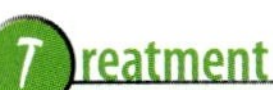

The disease is difficult to treat; an intralesional injection of steroid or dapsone 0.5–2.0 mg/daily sometimes produces prompt remissions. Destruction by pulse dye laser and cryotherapy has also been used to treat granuloma faciale.

Wegener's Granulomatosis with Polyangiitis

Wegener granuloma is a systemic vasculitis, with aseptic granuloma formations. WG primarily affects the upper and lower respiratory tract. Changes in the other organs also occur with less frequency. Changes are seen in the kidneys, joints, eyes, ears, skin, nerves and heart. The cause is unknown, infections have been suspected in a number of cases. **A**nti-**N**eutrophilic **C**ytoplasmic **A**ntibody (c-ANCA) is present in a number of patients.

Histology

A triad of necrotizing leucocytoclastic vasculitis, necrosis and granuloma formation are seen in WG. The granulomas are in the vessel wall or adjacent to it, these can be palisading and may be rich in giant cells. The necrosis is irregular, often described as geographic.

Clinical Features

In the initial stage there is fever, malaise and signs of upper respiratory tract infection such as rhinitis and sinusitis. Later the lower respiratory tract is involved, with dyspnoea, haemoptysis and pleuritis. In the later stage of disease there is generalised involvement including the skin.

The cutaneous lesions are similar to those of leucocytoclastic vasculitis, urticarial vasculitis, pyoderma gangrenosum and panniculitis.

Diagnosis

A tissue biopsy reveals the characteristic granulomas. Estimation of cytoplasmic pattern of c-ANCA with anti-PR3 specificity in the patient's serum, is other diagnostic criteria.

Treatment

The treatment requires two immunosuppressive drugs. Prednisolone 1 mg/kg daily with cyclophosphamide 2 mg/kg daily is the treatment of choice. As recovery occurs, prednisolone is tapered; cyclophosphamide is continued for another year before being slowly tapered down. Other immunosuppressive regimens such as methotrexate have also been used to treat WG.

Some authors have suggested the use of trimethoprim-sulphamethoxazole as an adjuvant therapy given three times a week to prevent *Pneumocystis carinii* infection. Local nasal and sinus care is of utmost importance care. An otolaryngologist should be involved in the treatment of WG.

Localised disease and recurrences can be treated with co-trimoxazole; the mechanism of action is unclear.

Temporal and Takayasu's Arteritis

These are progressive granulomatous arteritis affecting the large and medium sized arteries, particularly the aorta and vessels of the skull. Temporal arteritis can cause blindness if not recognized and treated early.

Clinical Features

Temporal arteritis is seen mainly in the elderly people over the age of 70 years. Classical a temporal arteritis presents as severe headache, which may be unilateral or bilateral. Tender red nodules are seen on the scalp in the temporal area. The skin over the scalp is red inflamed and tender. Thinning and loss of hair may occur in the affected area. There may be difficulty in opening the mouth and pain on eating due to ischaemia of the muscles of mastication. Loss of vision usually monocular occurs abruptly due to involvement of the ophthalmic artery or central retinal artery.

Takayasu's disease (pulseless disease) is a chronic inflammatory disease affecting the aorta and its main branches. It is seen in relatively younger patients predominantly females in the reproductive age. The disease is associated with stenosis and aneurysms. It is often associated with erythema nodosum. The characteristic features of the disease reflect the ischaemia produced by the stenosis of the aorta and its main branches, such as hypertension due to renal ischaemia, arm claudication due to the involvement of the subclavian artery. Stroke is common often related to hypertension. Severe central hypertension due to renal disease may not be recognized due to coexistent arm artery stenosis. Blood pressure should therefore be checked in all four extremities, and monitored on a frequent basis.

Other features of large vessel involvement are fever, general malaise; the patient usually has a very high sedimentation rate. There may also be involvement of the coronary, mesenteric and coeliac arteries. Dysphagia and peripheral neuritis may occur. Glossitis occurs in 10% of patients, senile purpura and gangrene of the legs may be the other occasional features.

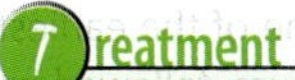

Corticosteroids should be given in large doses (40–60 mg daily). Once remission has occurred, the dose is gradually tapered. The ESR is a guide to progress; the patient may require a maintenance dose of 2.5–20 mg for at least 24 months.

VASCULITIS-MISCELLANEOUS

Anti-Neutrophilic Cytoplasmic Antibody Positive Vasculitis

Anti-neutrophilic cytoplasmic antibody (ANCA) are specific antibodies for antigens in cytoplasmic granules of neutrophils and monocyte lysosomes, first reported in 1982. These antibodies can be detected with indirect immunofluorescence microscopy. Two major patterns of staining are present: cytoplasmic ANCA (c–ANCA) and peri-nuclear ANCA (p–ANCA).

Anti-neutrophilic cytoplasmic antibodies positive vasculitis can be c-ANCA or p-ANCA. In c-ANCA antibodies are directed against proteinase 3 as seen in Wegener's granulomatosis. In p-ANCA the antibodies are directed against myeloperoxidase, this is most common in microscopic polyangitis.

Vasculitis associated with ANCA:

- Microscopic polyangiitis
- Wegener's granulomatosis
- Churg-Strauss syndrome.

Microscopic Polyangiitis

This is a necrotising vasculitis, involving the smallest blood vessels, with a predilection for the blood vessels of the lungs and the kidneys. The condition is characterised by fever, malaise and weight loss. The kidneys manifest necrotising glomerulonephritis, and the vasculitis of the lungs is manifested by haemoptysis and alveolar haemorrhage.

The disease is diagnosed by the changes seen the lungs and the kidneys. The blood is positive for p-ACNA in 60% of cases.

Treatment is by prednisolone and cyclophosphamide.

Kawasaki's Disease (Mucocutaneous Lymph Node Syndrome)

Kawasaki's disease is an acute multisystem vasculitis of unknown aetiology. The disease is common in children. The age range is from 7 weeks to 12 years. The disease is rare in adults. Kawasaki's disease is associated with marked activation of T cells and monocytes/macrophages. The coronary arteries are often involved. Kawasaki's disease is the most common acquired heart disease of children in the United States of America.

Clinical Signs

Three clinical stages are recognized:

1. Acute febrile phase: This phase lasts from 7–14 days. One of the earliest sign is an erythematous eruption, prominent in the perineum, followed by desquamation. Desquamation in the perineum is earlier than that of the palms and soles. There is associated inflammation of the conjunctiva, oral cavity and lips. The lips are cherry red, and the tongue strawberry like. The lymphadenopathy is non-suppurative and often limited to the cervical glands.

2. Subacute stage: This phase covers the period of about 25 days. In this phase there is desquamation of the fingers and toes. There is associated arthralgia, arthritis, aseptic meningitis, abdominal pain, jaundice, cardiac arrhythmias, coronary aneurysm and heart block.

Aneurysm may also be found in the axillary, common iliac, coeliac and mesenteric arteries.

3. Convalescent stage: This phase begins when clinical signs disappear and continues until the ESR becomes normal, usually 6–8 weeks after the onset of symptoms.

Diagnostic Criteria: Fever, conjunctivitis (spares the area around the limbus), inflammation of the oral mucous membrane, changes in the extremity—oedema, pain and desquamation of the fingers and toes, Beau's lines on the nails, rash which may be maculopapular or urticarial, dermatitis in the diaper area. Perineal desquamation starts before that of the finger tips and toes, cervical lymphadenitis.

Laboratory Evaluation

Leucocytosis, thrombocytopaenia, anaemia, T cell and monocyte/macrophage activation, raised ESR, transaminase elevation, an ECG should be done as soon as the diagnosis is suspected.

After the acute stage repeat ECG, ESR at 2–3 weeks interval till normal figures occur. Repeat again at 6–8 weeks.

Treatment

Intravenous gammaglobulin 2 g/kg/day given over 10–12 hours. If gammaglobulin is not administered at an early stage about 25% of patients may develop coronary artery aneurysm.

Aspirin 80–100 mg kg/day every 6 hours (blood salicylate levels should be 20–25 mg/dl). The dose of aspirin should be reduced to 3–5 mg/kg/day as a single dose when the fever has resolved. Aspirin is discontinued after 6–8 weeks if the ECG shows no evidence of coronary artery disease. If abnormalities are detected then aspirin should be continued indefinitely.

A cardiologist should be consulted if the patient has cardiac involvement.

Kawasaki's disease is the most common cause of acquired cardiac disease in children in US. The vasculitis involves the coronary arteries.

Churg–Strauss Syndrome (Eosinophilic Granulomatosis with Polyangiitis)

Churg-Strauss syndrome (CSS) also affects the small and medium-sized vessels. It is associated with a triad of asthma, granulomatous vasculitis of the lungs and the skin, with eosinophilia of the blood and tissues. CSS may also involve the gastrointestinal tract, kidneys, peripheral nerves, and the kidneys. Cardiac disease can be severe, leading to death.

Cutaneous manifestations: Purpura is the most common cutaneous sign. Urticaria and polymorphous skin eruption including cutaneous nodules may occur on the scalp, and extensor surface of the arms.

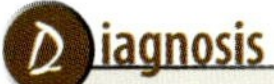

Biopsy of the lungs or skin shows striking palisading granulomas with necrosis, marked eosinophilia, nuclear dust and giant cells. Blood examination shows marked eosinophilia, increased ESR and elevated IgE.

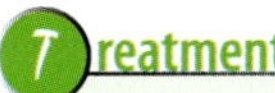

Churg-Strauss syndrome responds to treatment with glucocorticoids. Patients with severe systemic involvement need combined treatment with cyclophosphamide, methotrexate or azathioprine. IFN-α and intravenous immunoglobulins have also shown positive response.

ERYTHEMAS OF THE SKIN

Erythema is redness of the skin, due to the increase in blood flow within the small vessels of the skin. Erythema is often the first sign of a cutaneous disorder. Erythema can be localised or generalised.

Generalised erythema may be due to heat, fever, exercise, diseases such as viral exanthems, erythroderma, drug reactions etc. Localised erythema may be due to insect bites, burns, infections such as fungal, bacterial or viral, eczema, etc. The precise shade of the erythema, pink, purple, yellowish, red etc. are due to a number of factors. These are thickness of the cornified layer, amount of epidermal pigment present, degree of involvement of dermal vasculature, presence of dermal oedema, macrophages, or extravasation of red blood cell and inflammatory or non-inflammatory infiltrates.

Localised Erythema

Flushing

Flushing is a transient vasodilatation of the face that may occur in normal persons due to heat, exercise or emotion (blushing). Flushing is also produced by ingestion of alcohol, or after hot drinks. The hot beverages increase the temperature of the blood draining the oral cavity. The heat exchange between the internal jugular vein and the internal carotid artery may result in slight increase in temperature in the hypothalamus, which responds by providing heat-dissipating reaction such as sweating and flushing.

Alcohol induced flushing is uncertain. It is probably related to acetaldehyde levels. Flushing is also seen in alcoholics after taking chlorpropamide and disulfiram. It is thought that endogenous opioids such as enkephalins may play a role in chlorpropamide-induced flushing.

Flushing is a feature of rosacea, carcinoid syndrome, menopause; systemic diseases associated with flushing are dumping syndrome and various forms of malignancy. It is probably due to release of prostaglandins. Pheochromocytoma may also induce flushing.

Flushing may also occur after taking monosodium glutamate; this is often called "Chinese restaurant syndrome". Drugs producing flushing include calcium channel blockers and vasodilators such as amyl nitrate, fumaric acid esters used in the treatment of psoriasis, IL-2 and mast cell degranulators.

Diagnosis and treatment of flushing will depend upon the cause of flushing. A detailed history of the patient, pattern of flushing, drug intake, systemic disease etc., will help in the diagnosis of flushing. Investigations will be required depending upon the cause, such as levels of 5-hydroxyindole acetic acid (5-HIAA) in the urine for carcinoid syndrome. Treat the patient accordingly.

Erythema Palmare

This is usually most marked on the hypothenar eminences. It is associated with carcinoma of the pancreas, cirrhosis of the liver, pregnancy, thyrotoxicosis, graft-versus-host reactions, chemotherapy and SLE. Erythema palmare may be hereditary in some cases.

Generalised Erythema

Many generalised erythemas may resemble the rash produced by scarlet fever and measles. These are named scarlatiniform and morbilliform rash. It may be due to heat, exercise, drugs, viral infections, erythroderma or may develop during the course of a systemic illness.

Scarlatiniform Erythema

The rash consists of two elements; a diffuse erythema on which are superimposed punctate areas of increased redness, but either of these two elements may be absent (Fig. 4). The punctate lesions are about the size of goose pimples. In some cases the punctate rashes are larger, and the erythematous element indistinct.

Morbilliform Erythema

This is a generalised maculopapular eruption with a characteristic blotchy appearance, resembling the rash of measles (Fig. 5).

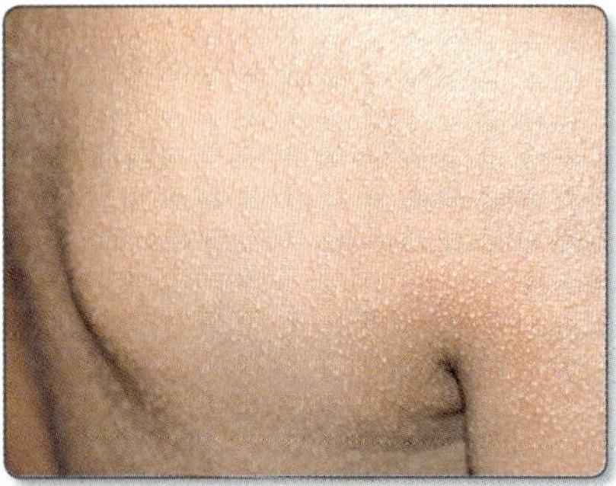

Fig. 4: Scarlatiniform rash

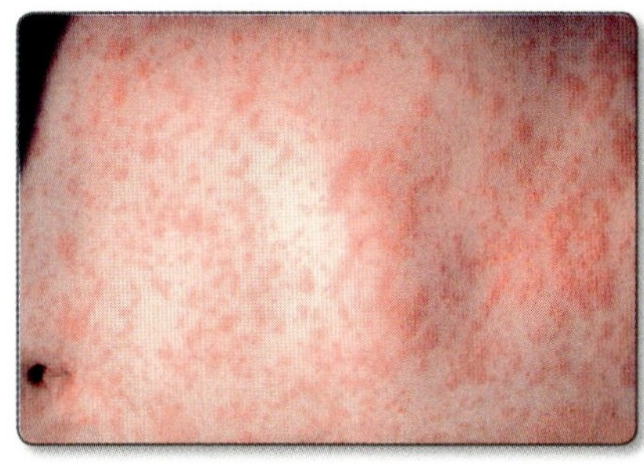

Fig. 5: Morbilliform rash

Annular Erythemas

Annular erythemas arise as a consequence of both peripheral spread and central recession within individual lesions or may result from an aggregate circular configuration of many individual lesions. Annular erythemas may be a manifestation of cutaneous disease such as tinea corporis, boderline tuberculoid leprosy, nummular eczema, annular psoriasis etc. It may appear as a hypersensitive reaction to various etiological factors, or it may evolve during a disease process, e.g. malignancy.

Erythema Annulare Centrifugum

Erythema annulare centrifugum (EAC) is considered as the paradigm of annular erythemas, it is a recurrent hypersensitivity reaction pattern to a diverse group of underlying conditions such as malignancy, drug ingestion, bacterial, fungal and viral infections etc. In most cases the underlying condition is unknown.

Erythema annulare centrifugum most often involves the trunk and extremities. The lesions begin as papules that enlarge peripherally and clear centrally resulting in gyrate, serpiginous or polycyclic configurations. There is a thin fine scaly line towards the edge of the lesion.

The center is often yellowish covered by a fine scale, the margins are pink or reddish in colour, slightly raised, with a firm rubber like induration and covered with fine scales. The lesions grow for several weeks, break up and disappear. These are replaced by new elements that follow a similar course.

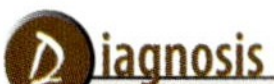

Diagnosis

Since there are numerous causes of EAC, laboratory investigations should be directed towards the most probable cause based on the history and examination of the patient. In most cases the epidermis is normal; there is an infiltration of lymphocytes and histiocytes around the blood vessels. In other cases the histopathology findings depend upon the cause. Erythema marginatum is the most transient of all annular erythemas. Investigations are similar in pattern to those of chronic urticaria.

The course of EAC generally parallels the underlying disease. Treatment is directed towards the aetiology of EAC. Oral corticosteroids have a dramatic effect in clearing the disease; recurrence follows on discontinuation of the drug.

Erythema Chronicum Migrans (Lyme Disease)

Erythema chronicum migrans (ECM) is due to a spirochaete, Borrelia burgdorferi that is introduced into the human body by the bite of a tick: Ixodes dammini. It may also occur following bite by a mosquito or thorn prick.

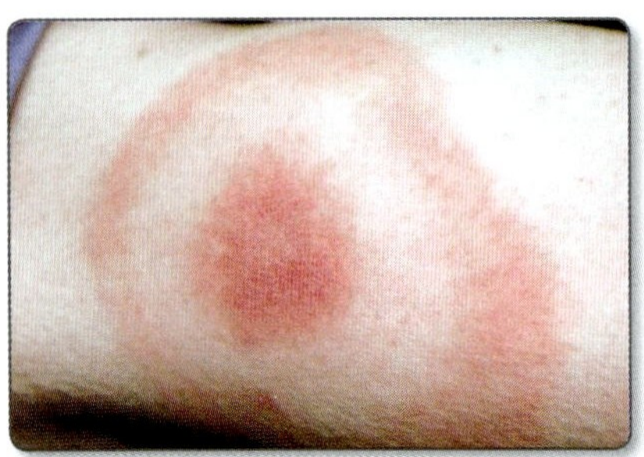

Fig. 6: Erythema chronicum migrans

Clinical Features

The lesion is usually single most often present on the trunk or proximal extremities. The lesion begins as a small papule, then expands peripherally and clears in the centre. A central punctum is sometimes seen. Most lesions are several centimetres in diameter. Lesions are bluish red, non-scaly with raised borders (Fig. 6). Patients usually have constitutional symptoms such as fever, malaise, arthralgias, myalgias etc. 10% of patients may also have myocarditis, pericarditis, meningitis and Lyme's arthritis; this is an acute sterile large joint monoarthritis. Lyme's arthritis was first described in Lyme County, Connecticut, but since then it has been reported in other forest areas of North America and in other continents.

Biopsy of the centre of the lesion demonstrates the characteristic tick bite findings, while that of the periphery shows superficial and deep perivascular lymphohistiocytic infiltrate. Spirochaetes when present in the lesion are diagnostic.

Erythema Gyratum Repens

This is a rare migratory erythema often associated with internal malignancy. Lesions are multiple, mainly involve the trunk and proximal extremities, rapidly spreading, usually enlarging in waves within a matter of hours. Regular waves of erythema spread over the body, to produce a pattern resembling grains of wood. The erythematous bands may be flat or indurated, with fine marginal desquamation.

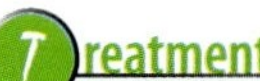

Treatment

Lymes disease

Doxycycline is the drug of choice, amoxicillin can be used as an alternative. Removal of the ticks in the first 24 hours is important.

The disease is described in detail in chapter 4.

Treatment

Necrolytic Migratory Erythema

Treatment consists in treatment of the underlying malignancy. Removal of the malignancy results in complete resolution of the lesion.

Necrolytic Migratory Erythema

Patients with glucagon secreting pancreatic tumours may experience a rare striking superficial migratory eruption. Lesions of necrolytic migratory erythema (NME) are generally confined to the periorificial areas and frictionally irritated intertriginous areas such as the groin, buttocks and thigh. Less common sites of occurrence are the shins, ankles, feet and fingertips (Fig. 7). NME can also occur in hepatic disease, gluten sensitive enteropathy, pancreatic insufficiency and in malabsorption or malnutrition.

There is a cyclic pattern in the course of the eruption. First to develop is a macule with central bulla. In about 7–14 days, the central part heals leaving

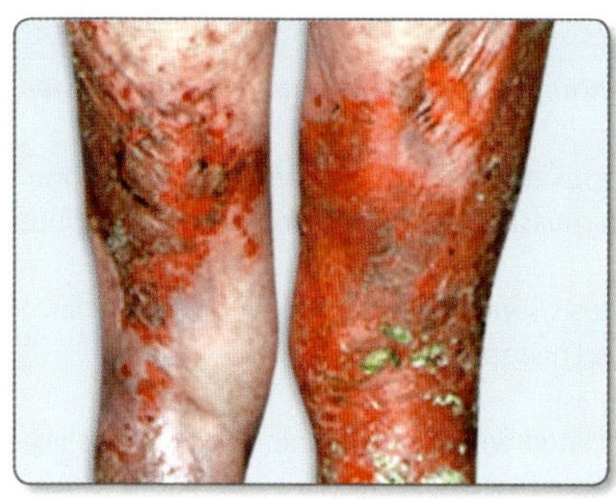

Fig. 7: Necrolytic migratory erythema

postinflammatory pigmentation while the erythematous periphery becomes crusted. There is centrifugal extension of the annular lesion. Lesions coalesce to form serpiginous patterns. Burning and itching accompany the lesion. Associated abnormalities include diabetes, glossitis, stomatitis, dystrophic nails, and weight loss.

Histology shows necrolysis of the outer cells of the stratum malpighii. In the dermis, there is mild perivascular lymphocytic infiltration.

Diagnosis rests on finding an elevated glucagon levels and demonstration of the pancreatic tumour. Removal of the tumour results in clearance of the skin rash within 48 hours. NME in the absence of glucagonoma should focus towards the correction of nutritional deficiencies such as essential fatty acids, amino acids and zinc deficiency.

Erythema Marginatum Rheumaticum

Erythema marginatum rheumaticum (EMR) is seen in about 18% of patients with acute rheumatic fever. It is one of the five major Jones Criteria for the diagnosis of acute rheumatic fever. Lesions are multiple; these involve the trunk, axillae and proximal extremities. Beginning as small patches or papules, they assume polycyclic or festooned configurations. The lesions are mildly pruritic, rapidly migratory and transitory, not lasting for more than 7 hours. It usually follows the onset of arthritis, and is frequently associated with rheumatic carditis. EMR seldom lasts for more than several weeks.

The five major Jones Criteria are: (1) polyarthritis, (2) carditis, (3) chorea, (4) subcutaneous nodules and (5) erythema marginatum.
The minor criteria are: arthralgia, fever, elevated acute phase reactants, prolonged PR interval on electrocardiogram

OTHER ERYTHEMAS

Erythema Multiforme (EM)

This is an acute cell-mediated immune reaction due to a variety of provoking factors. The hallmark of the disease is the target lesion. It is a relatively common condition, seen in patients of all ages, but is predominant in adolescence and young adults. The term multiforme implies there are a variety of other lesions ranging from red macules to large bullae.

Aetiology

Erythema multiforme (EM) is a symptom complex of many infective processes. These may be:

- Viral: as many as 1/3 of the cases of EM are due to herpes simplex virus. Other viral infections include measles, mumps, poliomyelitis, infectious mononucleosis etc.
- Bacterial: Diphtheria, tuberculosis, leprosy, typhoid fever, mycoplasma
- Fungal: coccidioidomycosis and histoplasmosis
- Protozoal: filariasis, trichomoniasis
- Collagen disorder: EM is associated with both chronic discoid lupus erythematosus (CDLE) and SLE
- Drugs: a number of drugs cause EM such as sulphonamides, tetracyclines, trimethoprim sulphamethoxazole, phenytoin, phenobarbitone, antipyretics and digoxin
- Vaccines: BCG, DPT, Hepatitis B, MMR, poliomyelitis
- Internal malignancies: Hodgkin's disease, lymphoma, myeloma and leukaemia
- Miscellaneous: hormonal changes such as pregnancy, menstruation, radiotherapy
- Sometimes ingestion of food as, e.g. shellfish or meat can cause may cause EM.

Pathogenesis

In EM, the epidermal damage appears to be the primary process. Foreign antigens are sequestrated in the epidermis, cytotoxic cell-mediated immune responses lead to epidermal cell damage. Circulating immune complexes have been documented. Vascular deposits of IgM and C3 are seen under direct immunofluorescence. Vasculitis does not appear to be a primary process.

Histopathology

The characteristic epidermal change is necrosis. In mild cases, foci of epidermal necrosis is seen. In severe cases, the whole epidermis appears to have a homogenous eosinophilic appearance. There is vacuolar degeneration of the basal layer and perivascular lymphocytic infiltrate is present in the upper part of the dermis. The papillary dermis is oedematous.

Clinical Features

The disease can occur at any age. The eruption develops over a few days and resolves in 2–3 weeks. Recurrences are common. The disease may be mild to severe. The lesions may be macular, papular, nodular, vesicular or bullous. The typical lesion is the target lesion, which has 3 zones: a central area of purpura or dusky red erythema, the middle area is pale, and the outer zone is well-defined erythema (Fig. 8). The central area bears the brunt of the disease. Atypical target lesions have two out of the three zones. The central area can be bullous or urticarial. A central bulla with a peripheral ring of vesicles is called the 'Herpes iris of Bateman'. Lesions first appear on the acral parts of the body, which then spreads centripetally.

EM Minor (maculopapular form)

The sites of predilection are the acral parts of the body, upper parts of the face, neck, forearms, legs, hands and feet (Fig. 9). The lesions are small red maculopapular that may increase in size in 48 hours. The target lesions are

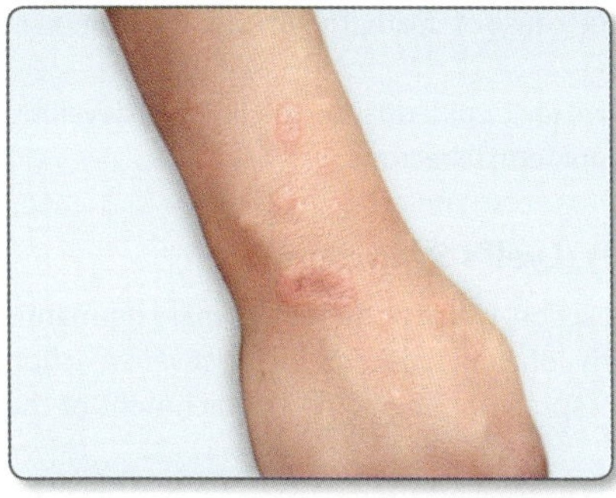

Fig. 8: Erythema multiforme

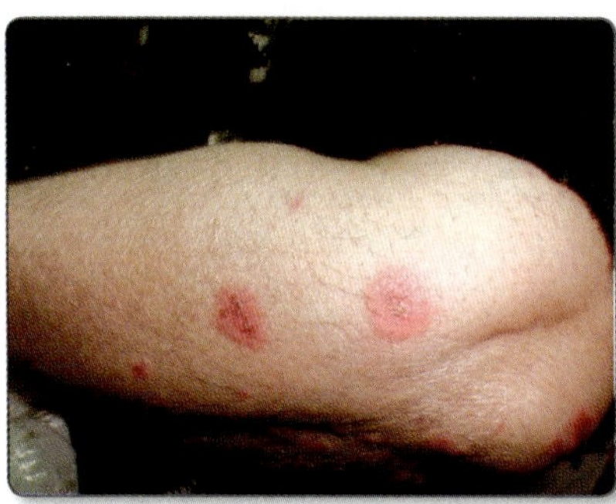

Fig. 9: Erythema multiforme

especially prominent on the palms. Mucous membrane is not involved.

Localised EM

This is an intermediate form of EM. The skin lesions present as erythematous macules or papules. The mucous membranes may be involved, distribution is acral.

Severe EM (Stevens-Johnson Syndrome)

The onset is sudden, manifested by fever, malaise, headache and sore throat. Joint pains and stomatitis are early and conspicuous symptoms. Vesicles and ulcers are present in the oral cavity, eating and drinking become difficult. Keratitis with corneal ulcers, conjunctivitis, rhinitis, epistaxis, vulvovagintis, and balanitis may also occur.

Systemic symptoms such as pneumonia, gastrointestinal disturbances develop. In severe cases central nervous system is involved, cardiac arrhythmias and pericarditis

Treatment

In mild cases treatment is symptomatic. The underlying factor causing EM should be removed. Local measures should be used to treat the burning and itching. Antibiotics should be avoided unless there is secondary infection. Acyclovir is used when EM is due to herpes simplex. In recurrent attacks suppressive therapy with acyclovir is useful.

In severe cases (Stevens-Johnson syndrome), good nursing care is of primary importance. Patient should be treated as for burns in an intensive care unit. Intake-output chart should be maintained, electrolyte levels corrected. The use of corticosteroids is hotly debated. 30–60 mg of prednisolone may be given in severe cases and tapered over a period of 1–4 weeks. Ocular involvement requires the consultation of an ophthalmologist.

may occur. Septicaemia is often the cause of death. The disease is common in children and young men.

If lesions become more extensive toxic epidermal necrolysis (TEN) develops, often-called acute disseminated epidermal necrosis.

Toxic Epidermal Necrolysis (Lyell's Syndrome)

This is a severe mucocutaneous reaction, which occurs as a primary dermatitis or as a complication of EM (Stevens-Johnson syndrome). It is a severe reaction of the skin characterised by widespread erythema and detachment of the epidermis.

Aetiology

Toxic epidermal necrolysis is a cytotoxic immune reaction to a number of aetiological factors. Most frequently drugs are responsible; these include long acting sulphonamides, anticonvulsants, antibiotics such as aminopenicillins, quinolones, cephalosporins, nonsteroidal anti-inflammatory drugs (NSAIDs), phenobarbitone, valproic acid and allopurinol. TEN may also be associated with malignancy, graft-versus-host reaction. Some cases are idiopathic.

Histopathology

Full thickness epidermal necrosis is prominent, at first it is patchy, and then it gradually spreads to involve larger areas of the skin. Signs of inflammation are scanty. Dermal vessels show endothelial swelling but no necrosis or vasculitis. In contrast in staphylococcal scalded skin syndrome (SSSS), the stratum corneum is only lost.

Clinical Features

The initial prodromal phase of fever, malaise and headache depends upon the underlying cause of TEN. The cutaneous onset is acute in some cases a prodromal phase of burning sensation of the conjunctiva, fever, malaise and arthralgia may occur. A morbilliform rash then appears predominantly on the face and extremities; it then spreads to other parts of the body. Vesiculation within the macular lesion occurs, these coalesce to form bullas, and they rupture easily resulting in large areas of denuded skin. Denuded skin is tender and painful. Nikolsky's sign is positive in the erythematous areas. In more severe cases there is loss of fingernails, toenails, loss of eyelashes and eyebrows.

Mucous membranes are also severely involved, which show erythema, vesiculation and erosions. Mucous membranes of the oral cavity is involved in all patients, bulbar conjunctiva and anogenital mucosa are involved in about 40% of cases. Healing is slow, scarring may therefore result.

Systemic signs include high fever, leucocytosis, albuminuria, and salt and water imbalance. These may lead to pulmonary oedema and renal failure. There is severe involvement of the respiratory tract and gastrointestinal tract, leading to bronchopneumonia and haemorrhages from the gastrointestinal tract. Toxicity, dehydration and electrolyte imbalance leads to haemodynamic shock. Mortality rate is from 30% to 50%.

Scarring is a serious complication of mucosal involvement. The most serious effect is on the eye leading to ectropion, synechiae, trichiasis, corneal opacities due to scarring and blindness. Oral lesions often heal without scarring, but strictures develop in the esophagus, bronchi, vagina, urethra and anus.

Differential Diagnosis

Toxic epidermal necrolysis should be differentiated from severe erythema multiforme and SSSS.

Treatment

There is no specific treatment; all cases of TEN should be treated as second degree burns in a burns ward. There should be good nursing care, fluid and electrolyte balance should be maintained. Secondary sepsis should be avoided with topical antibacterial agents. Eyelids and conjunctiva should be lubricated with paraffin to avoid adhesions. Ophthalmic monitoring is essential to prevent blindness. Necrotic areas should be removed, and the eroded areas treated with biological dressings.

Infection is the most important threat to a patient of TEN. Local and systemic infection should be promptly treated. Bacterial and fungal cultures should be done twice a week. Skin sepsis avoided by the use of local antiseptics. The use of prophylactic antibiotics is controversial. Some authors do not use it for the fear of precipitating TEN. Others are of the opinion that antibiotics are uncommon in causing TEN, start the treatment with a course of penicillin, and then adjust according to the culture report.

Intravenous immunoglobulins have been used with success; they should be used in severe cases.

Cyclosporin and cyclophosphamide have been used successfully.

The role of corticosteroids is controversial. There is a general agreement that should not be used if TEN has involved more than 20% of the body surface. Corticosteroids increase the risk of infection and delays healing.

Erythema Dyschromicum Perstans (Ashy Dermatosis)

The condition is poorly understood, the dermatosis consists of an inflammatory phase followed by postinflammatory dermal melanosis. Some authors consider it to be a variant of lichen planus; others consider it to be an idiopathic dermatosis. The condition is prevalent in Latin America and in other dark-skinned people.

Histology

In acute phases, the histology resembles that of basal cell damage and band like lymphocytic infiltration of the dermis. In the chronic stage, histology resembles that of post-inflammatory hyperpigmentation, with deposits of melanin in macrophages.

Clinical Features

In the inflammatory phase the lesions consist of erythematous patches, mainly on the trunk, with a fine erythematous, non-infiltrated or slightly infiltrated margin. Growth by centrifugal extension leads to bizarre polycyclic patterns. The lesions slowly turn into bluish-grey (ashy) patches with indistinct borders (Fig. 10). Sometimes extensive areas of the body may be involved.

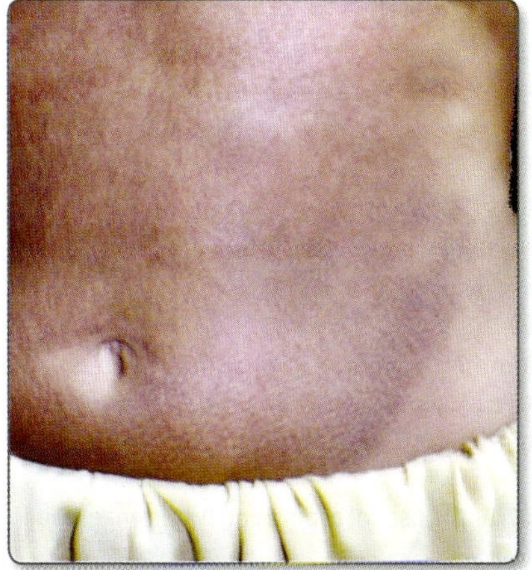

Fig. 10: Ashy dermatosis

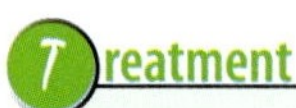

Treatment

The response to treatment is poor. Chloroquine and PUVA have shown some positive results.

HYPERSENSITIVITY SYNDROMES (TOXIC ERYTHEMAS)

These syndromes are caused by 'superantigens'. Superantigens are those antigens that act directly on the T cells without being processed by the Langerhans cells. These antigens directly activate the T cells and cause the release of inflammatory mediators such as cytokines. The cytokines especially the tumour necrosis factor-α, interleukin-1 and interleukin-2 are mainly responsible for the inflammatory reaction. The common hypersensitivity syndromes are:

- Group-A β-hemolytic streptococci, produce an erythrogenic toxin, this is responsible for scarlet fever
- Staphylococcal scarlatiniform eruption and staphylococcal scaled skin syndrome (SSSS) are due to toxins produced by phage 11 *Staphylococcus aureus*
- In toxic shock syndrome, several staphylococcal toxins are isolated, but the one of most commonly implicated is an exoprotein designated toxic shock syndrome toxin-1. This toxin is different from that of SSSS. Streptococcal toxins are also responsible for producing toxic shock syndrome
- The pathogenesis of Kawasaki's disease is unclear. An infectious origin is probably responsible; toxin-producing bacteria have been isolated in a few cases. The use of gammaglobulin in the treatment helps in neutralizing the toxin.

Clinical Features

The clinical features of these erythemas are characteristic; the skin is generally red, the erythema is accentuated in the skin folds, it feels like sandpaper. Erythema of the hand, feet, palms and soles is characteristic, followed by peeling and desquamation. Mucous membrane involvement is common, except in SSSS. The eyes, oral cavity, and lips are bright red in colour. The skin is desquamated, once the inflammation is over. Most of the cases occur in childhood except toxic shock syndrome.

Treatment

All of the toxic erythemas are treated with appropriate antibiotics except Kawasaki's disease.

Kawasaki's Disease

It has all the features described above, the differentiating points are:

- Fever is more prolonged more than 5 days
- Cervical lymph nodes are enlarged
- Diaper dermatitis is common
- Acquired heart disease is common in children, when not treated early. It is the most common cause of acquired cardiac disease in America. Cardiac disease is manifested by coronary aneurysm, arrhythmias and cardiomegaly
- The disease is treated early with high doses of aspirin and IV gammaglobulin, to prevent heart disease.

Toxic Shock Syndrome

The differentiating points are:

- It occurs in adults (tampons were a common cause)
- It is due to the toxins of *Staphylococcus* or *Streptococcus*. Streptococcal toxic shock syndrome often has bacteraemia, but the focus of skin disease is usually not found in staphylococcal disease
- High fever (above 38.9°C) and hypotension (systolic pressure of less than 90 mm) are characteristic
- Loss of hair and nail may be seen after about 2 months of infection.

Staphylococcal Scalded Skin Syndrome (Ritter's Disease)

There are two hypotheses for this syndrome; it may be caused by an antigen-antibody reaction to the toxin, or the staphylococcal toxin acts as a superantigen. Nikolsky sign is positive. The points in favour of the toxin being a superantigen are:

- The disease occurs in children
- Erythema of the skin followed by desquamation. Erythema accentuated in the flexures

Points against the favour of superantigen:

- Mucous membranes not affected
- Superficial blisters form after the generalised scarlatiniform erythema
- Prodromal symptoms absent or mild.

  Scarlet fever is described in chapter 6.

  Staphylococcal scalded skin syndrome is described in chapter 4.

TELANGIECTASIA

Telangiectases are permanently dilated capillaries and post-capillary venules, usually arising from the subpapillary plexus. They appear as small dull red, linear stellate or punctate markings. Telangiectasia may be primary or secondary.

PRIMARY TELANGIECTASIA

- Angioma serpiginosum
- Hereditary haemorrhagic telangiectasia
- Ataxia telangiectasia
- Generalised essential telangiectasia.

SECONDARY TELANGIECTASIA

These may be present secondary to a number of disorders such as collagen disease, varicose veins, rosacea, AIDS, occupational (mat like telangiectasia are present on the upper back of men working in aluminum plants), Bloom's syndrome, basal cell carcinoma, poikiloderma, etc.

Angioma Serpiginosum

The disease occurs predominantly in females, usually in children. The eruption is mainly present on the lower extremities, but may be present on any part of the body, except the palms, soles and mucocutaneous junctions (Fig. 11). The disease is characterised by minute erythematous puncta, which has a tendency to become papular. The puncta are arranged peripherally, and those at the center fade. Frequently there is a background of diffuse erythema.

The puncta, are due to a single large ectatic capillary, lined by normal endothelial cells. The background erythema is due to dilatation of subpapillary venous plexus. The condition should be differentiated from Schamberg's disease. Treatment if necessary is done with lasers and diathermy.

Hereditary Haemorrhagic Telangiectasia (Osler-Rendu-Weber Disease)

The disease has autosomal dominant inheritance, with defects in transforming growth factor-beta receptors. It affects both the skin and internal organs, with a tendency to bleeding. Symptoms such as epistaxis appear in childhood or infancy. Cutaneous lesions are usually seen at puberty. The basic defect is probably in the vessel wall.

The cutaneous lesions are numerous, these may be present anywhere on the body, but are most prominent on the upper half of the body. They appear as punctate or linear telangiectases. In some case, stellate telangiectasia appear but these do not pulsate. The lesions are symptomless and do not bleed.

Most important presenting feature is nasal bleed in childhood. At puberty, telangiectases appear in the oral and nasal mucosa. Systemic lesions include the involvement of the gastrointestinal tract, respiratory tract and genitourinary tract. Lesions in the eye and central nervous system are uncommon. Aneurysms of vessels such as the aorta and splenic artery have occurred. Haemorrhages from the gastrointestinal and urinary tract, will lead to anaemia. Lesions may form in the spinal cord or brain leading to apoplectic syndromes. Repeated haemorrhages result in iron deficiency anaemia.

Cutaneous lesions usually do not require treatment; these may be destroyed by laser or diathermy.

Ataxia Telangiectasia (Louis-Bar Syndrome)

The syndrome consists of cerebellar ataxia, oculocutaneous telangiectases, and sinopulmonary infections. The disease is autosomal recessive. The carriers have an increased risk of internal malignancy, usually lymphoreticular. There is marked IgA and IgE deficiency with decreased lymphocytes, absent or small thymus. The combined immune deficiency is responsible for multiple infections. The disease is associated with a defect in the repair of DNA damage.

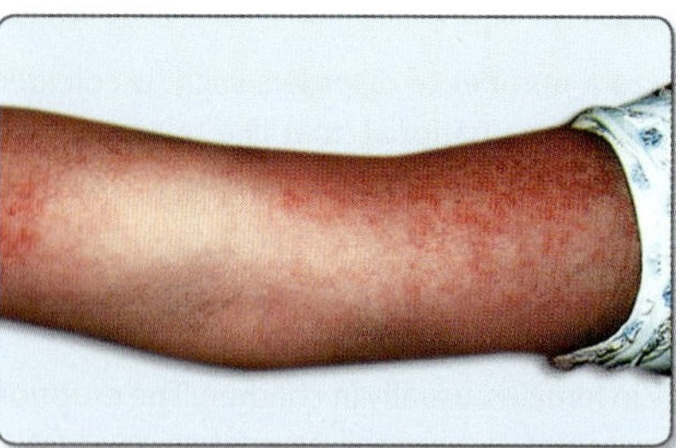

Fig. 11: Angioma serpiginosum

The affected children are apparently normal until the second year, when they are noticed to have difficulty in walking; they have a swaying gait and are unable to walk by about 2 years of age. The telangiectasia appears when the child is between the ages of 3–6 years. The telangiectasia first appears on the conjunctiva, later on the face, and then they become widespread.

The cutaneous lesions include telangiectases on the butterfly area of the face, inside the helix of the ear, behind the ears, on the V of the neck, back of the elbows and knees, and on the dorsum of the hands and feet. Other cutaneous stigmata include café-au-lait patches, hypopigmented macules, seborrhoeic dermatitis, premature graying of the hair and progeroid facies. The skin later becomes dry coarse, inelastic as in scleroderma. Non-infectious granulomas are common.

The major problem is progressive cerebellar ataxia; the children are usually bedridden early in life. Pseudopalsy of the eyes and nystagmus are common manifestations.

Treatment aims at controlling the secondary infection. Use of gammaglobulin has been reported to be helpful. Bone marrow transplantation at an early age is advised.

Prognosis is poor; patients often die due to infection or lymphoreticular malignancies by late childhood or early adolescence.

Generalised Essential Telangiectases

The condition is characterised by dilatation of the veins and capillaries over a wide area of the body, or it may be localised to an area of the legs, arms or trunk. It is not associated with systemic illness.

The disease is usually seen in women after the age of 40 years. It is differentiated from telangiectasia of systemic disease, as the telangiectatic vessels do not have alkaline phosphate activity. The telangiectasia are usually linear, but small angiomas may be present.

Spider Telangiectases (Naevus Araneus)

The condition is known as spider naevi, as the lesions are suggestive of a spider like appearance. The central arteriole represents the body, and the fine radiating vessels are suggestive of the multiple legs of the spider.

The sites of predilection are on the back of the hands, toes and the face. It is present in 15% of normal persons. They are common in children, pregnant women, and in patients with liver disorders. In pregnant women, palmar erythema is usually present with spider naevi. It is due to increased estrogen levels.

Treatment

When required the central arteriole can be destroyed with a cautery or diathermy. Pulsed dye laser is also effective.

Cutis Marmorata Telangiectatica Congenita

The condition is also known as Van Lohuizen syndrome. Cutis marmorata telangiectatica congenita (CMTC) is present at birth, the dilated vessels giving rise to a striking marbled appearance of the skin, which may be localised or generalised. Segmental lesions are often found on the extremities. The telangiectasia becomes more prominent when the patient cries, during exercise or in cold temperature. Midline naevus flammeus is often present. Other abnormalities include mental retardation, glaucoma, craniofacial abnormalities. Cutaneous abnormalities include hypertrophy or atrophy.

Histopathology reveals dilatation of the capillaries and veins, associated with vascular fibrosis.

There is no known treatment.

The other hereditary telangiectasias such as Bloom's syndrome and Cockayne's syndrome are described in chapter 20. Urticarial vasculitis is discussed in chapter 16. Tumours and naevi of blood vessels discussed in chapters 27 and 28.

DISORDERS OF THE LYMPHATIC SYSTEM

The lymphatic system is an accessory route by which interstitial fluid can be returned to the blood. Under normal conditions slightly more fluid is filtered out of the capillaries into the interstitial fluid, less is reabsorbed back into the plasma. This extra fluid of about 3 litres is picked up by the lymphatic system.

Small blind-ended terminal lymph vessels (initial lymphatics) permeate almost every tissue of the body. Once interstitial fluid enters the lymphatic vessel it is called lymph. Initial lymph vessels converge to form large lymph vessels, which eventually empty into the venous system (at the junction of the internal jugular and subclavian veins), through the right and left (thoracic duct) lymphatic ducts. Lymph vessels resemble veins but have thinner walls and more valves. At intervals along the lymphatic vessels, are the lymph nodes. In the skin the lymphatic vessels, lie in the subcutaneous tissue; and generally follow the veins.

Functions of the lymphatic system:

- Return of excessive interstitial fluid
- Transporting dietary lipids
- Defence against disease, through the immune response
- Return of filtered protein.

The primary lymphatic organs of the body are the red bone marrow (in flat bones and epiphyses of long bones) and the thymus. These are termed primary lymphatic organs because they produce T and B cells, the lymphocytes that carry the immune responses. The major secondary lymphatic organs are the lymph nodes and the spleen. Thymus is the organ where the T cells are processed and matured. Bone marrow is the site for the processing and maturation of B lymphocytes. Lymphatic nodules are collection of lymphocytes that stand guard in all mucous membranes.

LYMPHOEDEMA

Lymphoedema is oedema, due to inadequate lymphatic drainage. It may be primary or secondary.

Primary lymphoedema may be congenital, or appears at puberty (praecox) or after the age of 35 year (tarda). Primary lymphoedema is associated with defective or absent lymphatics, leading to swelling of the limbs. Milroy's disease is familial of autosomal dominant inheritance. Lymphoedema is present at birth or infancy; it usually involves both legs, associated with pleural effusion and ascites. Familial lymphoedema praecox (Meige syndrome), has the onset at puberty, it is unilateral and not associated with other findings. Lymphoedema tarda occurs in patients over the age of 35 years, it usually affects one or both the legs. There is a family history of similar swelling. The disease can be diagnosed by lymphoscintigraphy.

Yellow nail syndrome, is a triad of primary lymphoedema, yellow nails, and chylous pleural effusion or ascites.

Secondary lymphoedema is often seen in the lower limbs due to infections, such as cellulitis and filariasis. Silica dust damages the lymphatic vessels; a condition found in developing countries where people often walk barefoot. It may be seen secondary to inflammation as in rosacea or acne. Lymphoedema may follow lymphatic blockage by tumours, and destruction of lymphatics by surgery.

Lymphangioma is described in chapter 28. Lymphangitis is discussed in chapter 4. Filariasis is discussed in chapter 7.

Clinical Features

Lymphoedema develops gradually, and the patient often does not notice the swelling till it becomes prominent. In the initial stages the swelling is soft and pitting; later the swelling becomes non-pitting and indurated. The overlying skin becomes thick and hyperkeratotic. The process is known as elephantiasis. Cellulitis is a common complication.

The defect in the lymphatic system can be detected by lymphangiography or radiolabelled lymphoscintigraphy.

Complications

Swelling and infection are common complications of lymphoedema. The swelling may restrict movement; this can be especially troublesome if there is associated scarring and fibrosis. Malignancy and some rare disorders such as necrotising fasciitis, and TEN can also occur.

Diagnosis

The diagnosis is obvious on clinical examination. Invasive tests are unnecessary in most cases. Blood, urine examination, ultrasound of the pelvis should be done in females suspected of a pelvic pathology. Males should be examined for prostate cancer. Patients from endemic areas should be tested for filariasis.

Treatment

Treatment should aim to minimise oedema and prevent subcutaneous fibrosis. Patients with lymphoedematous limbs should be taught meticulous skin care, to prevent secondary infection. Good antiseptics following abrasions and minor trauma are important measures to be taken. Tight bandaging, massage, bed rest and elevation of the affected limb, may help to control lymphoedema.

Prompt diagnosis and treatment of bacterial erysipelas and cellulitis is important in preventing further lymphatic drainage and worsening of the existing elephantiasis.

Drug therapy is generally disappointing. Diuretics alone have little benefit in lymphoedema, because their mode of action is to limit capillary filtration, by reducing the blood volume. Improvement by diuretics suggests that the predominant cause of oedema was not lymphatic. The benzopyrone group of drugs have been advocated to treat lymphoedema, but their clinical effects seem to be small.

Surgery may be of value in a few patients, in whom the size and weight of the limb inhibit its use and mobility. Relief may be obtained by removal of excessive tissue, but recurrences are common, unless new lymphatic drainage is established. Lifelong non-surgical measures such as hosiery must be continued post-operatively.

FURTHER READING

1. Callen JP. A clinical approach to the vasculitis patient in dermatologic office. Clin Dermatol. 1999;17(5):549-53.
2. Daroczy J. Pathology of lymphoedema. Clin Dermatol. 1995;13(5):433-44.
3. Graham-Smith DG. The Carcinoid syndrome. Am J Cardiol. 1968;21(3):376-87.
4. Guillevin L, Lhote F, Gherardi R. Polyarteritis Nodosa, Microscopic polyangiitis, and Churg-Strauss syndrome: clinical aspects, neurological manifestations and treatment. Neurol Clin. 1997;15(4):865-86.
5. Hazen PG, Michael B. Management of necrotizing vasculitis with colchicine: improvement in patients with cutaneous lesions and Behcet's syndrome. Arch Dermatol. 1979;115(11):1303-5.
6. Ioannidou DJ, Krasagakis Sotsiou F, Tosca AD. Cutaneous small cell vasculitis: an entity with frequent renal involvement. Dermatology. 2002;138(3):413-4.
7. Kohler JK, Lorincz AL. Erythema elevatum diutinum treated with niacinamide and tetracycline. Arch Dermatol. 1980;116(6):693-5.
8. Lotti T, Ghersctich I, Comacchi C, et al. Cutaneous small vessel vasculitis. J Am Acad Dermatol. 1998;39(5 Pt 1):667-87.
9. Mortimer PS. Managing lymphoedema. Clin Exp Dermatol. 1995;20(2):98-106.
10. Nordborg E, Nordborg C. Giant Cell Arteritis: epidemiological clues to its pathogenesis and an update on its treatment. Rheumatology (Oxford). 2003;42(3):413-21.
11. Scott DG, Watts RA. Systemic vasculitis: epidemiology, classification and environmental factors. Ann Rheum. 2000;59(3):161-3.
12. Sias G, Vidaller A, Jucgla A, et al. Prognostic factors in Leukocytoclastic vasculitis: a clinicopathological study of 160 patients. Arch Dermatol. 1998;134(3):309-15.
13. Stone JH, Calabrese LH, Hoffman GS, et al. Vasculitis: a collection of pearls and myths. Rheum Dis Clin North Am. 2001;27(4):677-728, v.
14. Weinberg J, Kristal L, Chooback L, et al. The clonal nature of Pityriasis Lichenoides. Arch Dermatol. 2002;138(8):1063-7.
15. Wilkin JK, Rountree CB. Blockade of carcinoid flush with cimetidine and clonidine. Arch Dermatol. 1982;118(2):109-11.
16. Wilkin JK. Flushing reactions, consequences and mechanism. Ann Intern Med. 1981;95(4):468-76.

Chapter 16

Urticaria

Urticaria is common acute or chronic relapsing dermatosis, caused by temporary increase in capillary permeability leading to exudation of fluid in the dermis, this results in an oedematous blotchy eruption often with a central pallor, the wheal is pathognomonic. The rash fades within 24 hours leaving no trace, but new patches develop at other sites. Urticaria may be acute with only a single or a few attacks lasting for a few days. It may be chronic when the lesions persist for more than 6 weeks. The lesions of urticaria are very pruritic.

Angioedema may occur alone or in combination with urticaria. Angioedema is less pruritic, of a longer duration and the pathology lies in the subcutaneous tissue. Angioedema of the submucosa of upper respiratory tract may lead to laryngeal oedema and respiratory obstruction. Angioedema particularly affects the loose subcutaneous tissue around the eyelids, mouth and male genitalia.

AETIOLOGY

Urticaria may be produced by the degranulation of mast cells directly or indirectly after IgE or IgE receptor dependent reactions, in association with abnormalities of the complement system and other plasma effector systems that release histamine and other mediators. Urticaria can also be due to vasculitis, or by activation of cellular arachidonic acid metabolic pathways. The common causes of urticaria are:

- *Food and food additives:* Common foods responsible for urtcaria are sea foods, eggs, nuts, strawberries, tomatoes, mushrooms and dairy products. Possible food allergens are: food dyes such as tartrazine group of dyes found in yellow and orange colored drinks, benzoates used as preservatives, antioxidants such as tocopherol, butyl hydroxyanisole, taste enhancers such as monosodium glutamate, fragrance, etc.
- *Drugs:* Salicylates such as aspirin, penicillin, codeine, morphine, polymyxin B, and vaccines. Traces of penicillin in the food may also cause chronic urticaria.
- *Parasitic infestation:* Intestinal parasites such as round worm, tapeworm, biting and stinging arthropods, fleas, lice and caterpillars.
- Physical agents such as friction, pressure, heat and cold.
- Inhalants such as house dust, pollen, perfume, insecticides.
- General medical problems such as infections of the urinary tract, upper respiratory tract, systemic lupus erythematosus, lymphomas, etc.
- Neoplasms and endocrinal causes.
- Psychogenic
- Autoimmunity

PATHOGENESIS

Urticaria can be produced by a variety of physical, chemical and immunological stimuli. It may be reproduced experimentally by the intradermal injection of histamine. Histamine produced by degranulation of mast cells is the most frequent cause of urticaria. Histamine produces the triple response of Lewis (erythema, oedema and the surrounding flare). Other vasoactive mediators such as kinins, neuropeptides and prostaglandins may also be involved in producing urticaria. Neutrophils and platelets are also released by the activation of mast cells. The release of histamine may be by the direct stimulation of mast cells, by IgE related mechanism or by the components of the complement cascade.

Urticaria can also be produced by immunological reactions as seen in vasculitis. In vasculitis, there is inflammation of the endothelial cells of the blood vessels, resulting in the escape of red blood cells and plasma into the dermis, so that both urticaria and purpura are produced. In severe vasculitis, there is complete thrombosis of the vessels with fibrinoid necrosis of its walls.

Trauma such as stroking may produce urticaria; this is known as dermographism.

Urticaria may also be produced on exposure to cold, water, exercise etc.; these are known as physical urticarias.

About one third of patients with chronic urticaria have circulating functional histamine releasing IgG autoantibody that binds to high affinity IgE receptor, or less commonly with IgE that resides on the surface of the mast cells and basophils. Most cases of chronic urticaria may ultimately be associated with an autoimmune disease rather than an allergic reaction.

CLASSIFICATION

- IgE mediated such as atopic diathesis, specific antigen sensitivity due to food, aeroallergens, animal dander and autoimmune urticaria
- Complement mediated such as hereditary angioedema, acquired angio-edema, urticarial vasculitis, serum sickness, infections
- Direct mast cell degranulation by opiates, polymyxin B and radiocontrast media
- Abnormalities of arachidonic acid metabolism by aspirin, NSAIDs, pressure urticaria
- Idiopathic such as cyclic episodic urticaria.

Physical Urticaria

Dermographism (Skin Writing)

This is an exaggerated triple response of Lewis seen on stroking the skin firmly. It appears soon after applying pressure and disappears within 30 minutes of releasing the pressure. Delayed dermographism develops 3–6 hours after stimulation, with or without an immediate reaction. It lasts for 24–48 hours. It appears as red nodules. It may be associated with delayed pressure urticaria.

Clinical Features

Urticaria may occur at any age, but most commonly presents between the ages of 10–40 years. There is a slight female preponderance. The lesions of urticaria can occur anywhere on the body, but commonly affects the limbs and the trunk. The lesions vary in size from a few millimeters to several centimeters; they are transient and last for minutes or hours, but resolve within 24 hours. Urticaria presents as raised wheals that may be white or red with surrounding erythema (Fig. 1). Urticarial lesions are very itchy.

Urticaria may be acute or chronic. Urticaria that lasts more than 6 weeks is termed as chronic. Acute urticaria is short lived, often caused by food, drugs, infections and infestations. No routine testing is required and antihistamines are the mainstay of therapy.

- The subsets of chronic urticaria are:
  - Chronic idiopathic urticaria
  - Autoimmune urticaria
  - Physical urticaria
  - Urticarial vasculitis
- There are several varieties of physical urticaria such as:
  - Dermographism
  - Cholinergic urticaria
  - Delayed pressure urticaria
  - Solar urticaria
  - Aquagenic urticaria
  - Cold urticaria
  - Vibratory urticaria

A dermographometer can be used to measure the amount of pressure applied on the skin. The dermal mast cells are within normal limits. Histamine is released at the site of pressure, and antihistamines are the mainstay of treatment. Loose fitting clothing is advocated.

Cholinergic Urticaria

This occurs in about 20% of individuals and is often unnoticed in its milder forms. This usually occurs secondary to exercise, warm temperature, ingestion of hot spicy food or emotional stress. The disease presents as small wheals, surrounded by large erythematous flare. The rash of cholinergic urticaria is intimately associated with eccrine sweating, but is not dependent on it, for cholinergic urticaria can occur in anhidrotic individuals. It can be diagnosed by provocation by hot baths or exercise. Cholinergic urticaria responds better to hydroxyzine.

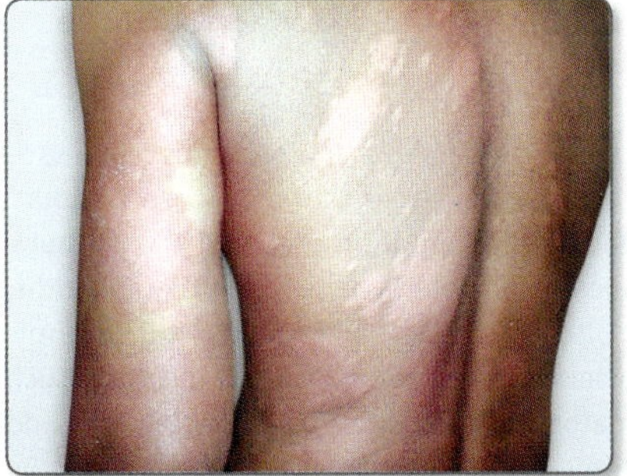

Fig. 1: Urticaria

Delayed Pressure Urticaria

Whealing occurs 2–6 hours after application of pressure. Wheals usually last for more than 24 hours. Delayed pressure urticaria is often accompanied by symptoms such as fatigue, arthralgia and myalgia. It is generally unresponsive to antihistamines, but the lesions improve with NSAIDs because it is due to abnormalities of arachidonic acid metabolism.

Solar Urticaria

Wheals occur within 5 minutes of exposure to the sun. Lesions usually fade within 15 minutes if the patient covers the affected skin. The lesion is often misdiagnosed as polymorphic light eruption. It responds poorly to antihistamines. Tolerance following repeated exposure to ultraviolet light may be used as a mode of treatment. Chloroquine, beta carotene, and PUVA have been used successfully in a few cases.

Aquagenic Urticaria

This urticaria develops in areas which are in contact with water. The pruritic follicular cholinergic-like wheals, appear within 2–3 minutes of the contact. It is the most difficult chronic urticaria to treat. Coating the skin with inert oil may be effective. 10 mg propranolol given half an hour before a bath has been helpful in some cases.

Cold Urticaria

This can be primary or familial and acquired or secondary. In both varieties contact of the skin with cold surfaces and fluids cause immediate local whealing and itching. It may be associated with acute systemic symptoms such as flushing, headache, faintness or even collapse. Fatalities have been reported of acute anaphylaxis following sea-bathing. The cardinal objective is to prevent anaphylaxis during aquatic and other cold exposures. Antihistamine administered 30–60 minutes before cold exposures are effective in aborting urticarial episodes. Cyproheptadine has antihistamine, antiserotonin and anticholinergic properties. Desensitisation has been shown to be beneficial.

Vibratory Urticaria

Urticaria develops within minutes of massage or other vibratory movements. There is no known effective treatment.

Urticarial Vasculitis

This is an immune complex vasculitis. Classically urticarial vasculitis presents as wheals often tender on palpation, persistent, lasting for more than 24 hours, with inconsistent itch, often leaving pigmentation secondary to purpura. Urticarial vasculitis may be normocomplementemic which is usually idiopathic or hypocomplementemic. It is often associated with underlying systemic lupus erythematosus or other autoimmune connective tissue disorders such as Sjogren's syndrome, inflammatory bowel disease, cryoglobinaemia and hepatitis B or C. Systemic symptoms include arthralgia and malaise. Treat the underlying disorder, antihistamines, corticosteroids, colchicine, and other immunosuppressant drugs have been used to treat these disorders.

Autoimmune Urticaria

Some cases of chronic urticaria have recently been classed as autoimmune. IgG class antibodies against IgE and receptors for IgE have been demonstrated in the serum of patients of chronic urticaria. Many autoimmune diseases are also associated with autoimmune urticaria such as autoimmune thyroiditis, coeliac disease, insulin dependent diabetes mellitus and ulcerative colitis. The auto-antibodies to IgE can be detected in the patients serum, by the autologous serum skin test (ASST). Peripheral blood basophils are reduced or absent in patients with autoimmune chronic urticaria. The clinical course of autoimmune urticaria does not differ much from that of non-immune urticaria. It does tend to be more prolonged and less responsive to antihistamines. Severely affected patients may respond to immunotherapy such as cyclosporin, intravenous immunoglobulins or plasmapheresis.

DIFFERENTIAL DIAGNOSIS

Urticaria is easy to diagnose, but sometimes other diseases such as early lesions of bullous pemphigoid, multiple arthropod bites, and drug reactions such as serum sickness should be differentiated.

Approach in the Management of Chronic Urticaria

There are different schools of thought to the management of chronic urticaria. One school of thought is that the treatment of urticaria is the same regardless of the cause, and routine investigations would rarely be able to detect a cause. The second school of thought recommends a major effort to determine a cause for chronic urticaria including numerous diagnostic tests. If these fail then elimination regimens are advised to remove the offending agent. Therapeutic trials are conducted to treat occult infections.

A midline approach probably seems to be more appropriate. A thorough history and physical examination is required in every case of chronic urticaria. There are compelling reasons for pursuing the cause of chronic urticaria. First a systemic disease if present is removed, and if the tests are negative, the patient is reassured that there is no systemic problem.

A routine blood test, urinalysis, stool examination, serum creatinine, liver function test, and X-ray chest is done to reassure if any systemic disease is present or not. In some patients serum complement and immunoglobulin estimations may be required to exclude serum sickness. It is worth including thyroid function tests because urticaria can be associated with hyperthyroidism. Exclude the possibility of vasculitis if urticarial wheals are persistent, painful, and associated with systemic symptoms.

Avoidance where possible should be the mainstay of therapy for allergens. Challenge with relevant foods, food additives, drugs or physical stimuli may be done to remove the possible cause of urticaria. Ice cube test is done for cold urticaria, phototesting for solar urticaria, and exercise challenge for cholinergic

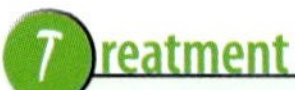

Treatment

Acute urticaria is easily treated by H_1 antihistamines and eliminating the cause of urticaria such as food, drug, infection, etc.

Problem arises in case of chronic urticaria when a cause cannot be found. In treating chronic urticaria H_1 histamines are again the treatment of choice. It should initially be administered at a low dose and then increased to tolerance. If the initial drug is ineffective then another antihistamine from another group should be used. A combination of two antihistamines from two different groups is effective in some patients. If this fails then a combination of H_1 and H_2 antihistamines can be tried.

The tricyclic antidepressant doxepin has activity against both H_1 and H_2 receptors; it can be used in some cases of chronic urticaria. Other drugs used for the treatment of chronic idiopathic urticaria are terbutaline (β-adrenergic agonist), zafirlukast and montelukast (leukotriene receptor antagonists), sulphasalazine, methotrexate, and cyclosporin.

Penicillinase has been successfully used in the treatment of patients with chronic urticaria who have a history of penicillin allergy.

Some studies have shown that vitamin D deficiency can be a cause of chronic urticaria in adults. Administration of high doses of vitamin D (50,000 units weekly), improves chronic urticaria in patients who have low level of serum 25-hydroxy-vitamin D. Omalizumab has also shown promising results in chronic idiopathic urticaria.

urticaria. Food sensitivity can be tested, by eliminating a certain food from the diet for a period and then seeing whether urticaria develops or not. Keeping a food diary is often helpful.

Course and Prognosis

The natural history is very variable, acute allergic urticaria usually resolves within days or weeks. Very occasionally respiratory tract involvement may be fatal. Chronic urticaria persists for many years but its activity varies. Although it causes discomfort to the patient, it rarely causes severe problems.

ANGIOEDEMA (QUINCKE'S OEDEMA)

Angioedema is a reaction characterized by swelling of the subcutaneous tissue of the skin and mucous membrane due to increased vascular permeability. It may be an antigen associated IgE dependent reaction, or mediated via the complement such as seen in systemic lupus erythematosus and necrotizing vasculitis. In a few cases it may be hereditary.

Angioedema can occur at any site, but particularly affects the periorbital region, lips, ears, hands, feet and the male genitalia. Involvement of the tongue or the respiratory tract can lead to airway obstruction. The incidence of anaphylaxis is high in angioedema, as compared to urticaria. Urticaria is rarely seen in hereditary and acquired angioedema. Pruritus is uncommon, patients complain of a burning sensation. The subcutaneous swellings of angioedema are skin coloured but may be erythematous. Patients with underlying bronchial asthma, ischaemic heart disease or cardiac failure are more likely to suffer from anaphylactic reactions.

Hereditary Angioedema

Hereditary angioedema (HAE) is an autosomal dominant disorder, caused by the lack of a specific C1-esterase inhibitor, which normally keeps the complement cascade in check. Most patients have ancestors who died suddenly from asphyxia. Any stimuli that activate the complement will initiate a chain of reactions, resulting in a massive liberation of kinins.

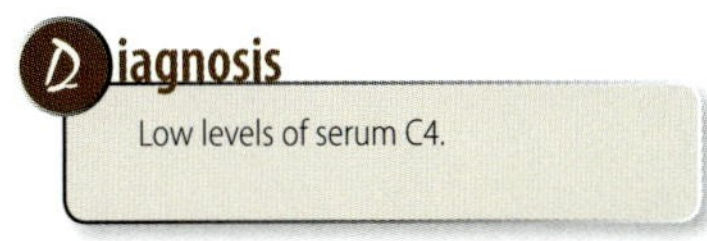

The disease may start in early childhood or the symptoms may begin in the second decade or even later. The disease becomes worse at puberty, later the attacks decrease in severity and after the age of 50 years may even disappear.

Hereditary angioedema affects the skin and the internal organs. Clinically the subcutaneous lesions of HAE are characterized by recurrent non-pruritic, non-pitting, circumscribed oedema. Cutaneous angioedema develops over several hours over a particular site, often preceded by a faint erythema. Patients may have a prodromal feeling of twitching or tingling in the area. Swelling in the face and lips may involve the respiratory tract. Patients do not have urticarial lesions. All patients of HAE have some involvement of the gastrointestinal tract. Laryngeal oedema can be life-threatening.

Prophylaxis

Anabolic steroids such as danazol 200–600 mg daily, stanozolol 2 mg/day have a very beneficial effect in preventing the attacks. It acts by stimulating the synthesis of deficient protein in the liver. The drug should not be given to pregnant women and prepubertal children. It should be given 4–5 days before triggering factors such as tooth extraction, intubation, etc.

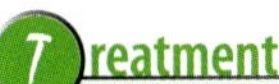

Acute attack: C1 esterase inhibitor concentrate should be administered immediately; if this is not available then an infusion of fresh plasma 500–2000 mL, supplies the necessary C1 esterase inhibitor.

MASTOCYTOSIS

Mastocytosis may be localized to the skin or it may be systemic. The condition is characterized by accumulation of mast cells in the skin or the internal organs.

Cutaneous Mastocytosis

This present as:

- Urticaria pigmentosa
- Diffuse cutaneous mastocytosis
- Telangiectasia macularis eruptiva perstans
- Solitary mastocytoma

Urticaria Pigmentosa

It usually develops in childhood, but the onset may be delayed until adulthood. The abnormal skin is recognized as yellowish brown macules or papules, which urticate and itch when they are rubbed (Darier's sign) (Fig. 2). Palms and soles are spared. Sometimes the release of chemical mediators is severe enough to cause systemic signs and symptoms such as hypotension, tachycardia, headache and dizziness. Most cases improve by adolescence, mast cell

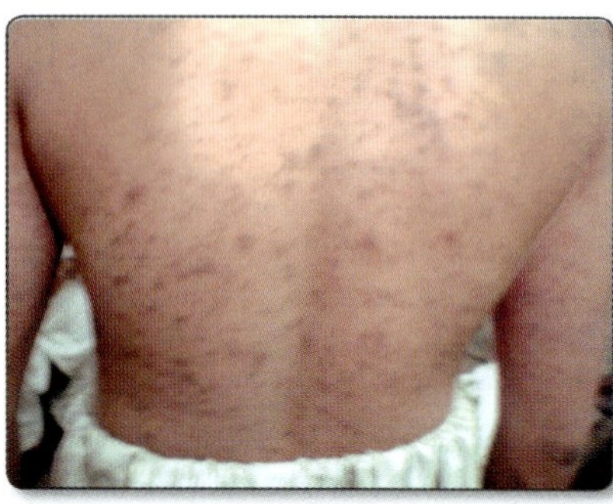

Fig. 2: Urticaria pigmentosa

leukaemia can occur in 25% of cases. If the condition persists in adults there is risk of systemic disease.

Diffuse Cutaneous Mastocytosis

This may present as an erythroderma or as a diffuse infiltration of the skin; the skin is thickened, reddish brown in colour, oedematous with an orange peel like texture. Dermographism with hemorrhagic blister formation is common. The disease begins in childhood and spontaneously resolves by the age of 15 months to 5 years.

Telangiectasia Macularis Eruptiva Perstans

Telangiectasia macularis eruptiva perstans (TMEP) is the rarest form of cutaneous mastocytosis. It is limited to adults. The lesions consist of widespread telangiectasia which resembles freckles. The disease is due to sparse but widespread distribution of mast cells in the skin.

Solitary Mastocytosma

This is the most common form of cutaneous mastocytosis. The lesion is often single, but may be multiple. Darier's sign is positive. The lesion is present in infancy as a localized plaque or nodule; which urticates or blisters spontaneously; it usually involutes spontaneously in 2–3 years.

Systemic Mastocytosis

This may occur at any age, but generally seen in older children and adults. Cutaneous lesions range from 50% to 100%. Mast cells are found in many organs often with cutaneous involvement. Bone is the most common organ involved, presenting with pain and osteoporosis, with

Diagnosis

- Lesions show a positive Darier's sign (urticaria produced on rubbing or scratching the skin).
- Skin biopsy shows increase in mast cells, in which more than 25% of the cells have an abnormal morphology. The most useful stain for mast cells is tryptase, although other metachromatic stains can also be used.
- Analysis for the chemical markers of mast cells, urinary and serum tryptase levels should be assessed. Patients should not consume histamine rich foods 24 hours before urine collection.
- Bone marrow biopsy and total serum tryptase levels more than 20 ng/ml may be required in the diagnosis of systemic mastocytosis.
- Elevated plasma histamine levels in diffuse cutaneous mastocytosis.

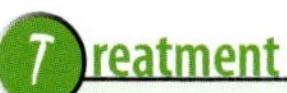

Treatment is symptomatic, most cases resolve spontaneously. Antihistamines are the mainstay of treatment. Photochemotherapy (PUVA) and mast cells stabilizers such as disodium cromoglycate may be helpful, vascular lasers (pulse dye and Nd:YAG 532 nm) have also been used. Alcohol and other mast cell degranulating agents should be avoided such as insect bite, drugs (morphine, codeine, polymyxin B, vancomycin, aspirin, NSAIDs, muscle relaxants, sympathomimetic drugs), change of temperature and bacterial infections.

proliferation of mast cells and other blood cells. Involvement of the gastrointestinal tract results in nausea, vomiting and diarrhoea. Involvement of the liver, spleen and lymph nodes leads to hepatosplenomegaly, lymphadenopathy. Mast cell leukaemia may occur in 2% of cases.

PAPULAR URTICARIA

Papular urticaria is due to hypersensitivity to bites of arthropods such as mosquitoes, mites, bedbugs, fleas, gnats, etc. Mites are important cause of urticaria in people who keep pets such as birds and animals.

The distribution of lesions depends upon the insect. Bites by bedbugs are found on the covered parts of the body, and mosquito bites are on the exposed parts. The lesions pass through two stages: an urticarial wheal that fades in 1–2 days, it is replaced by a firm papule. The pruritic papules often have a central punctum. These papules are excoriated, secondarily infected and lichenified, due to rubbing and itching. Sometimes impetiginous crusts or ecthymatous ulcers develop.

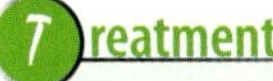

Elimination of the insect that is responsible for the urticaria is necessary. The house should be disinfected and treated with insecticide sprays twice weekly. Infected pets should also be treated. Anti-pruritic lotions are used topically. Antihistamines help to reduce itching.

The lesions recur in crops, usually at night. Each lesion may persist for 2–12 days. The attacks may persist for months or years. The attacks may be seasonal. There are no palpable lymph nodes and no constitutional symptoms. Residual pigmentation is common.

FURTHER READING

1. Delong KL, Culler DS, Saini SS, et al. Annual direct and indirect care costs of chronic idiopathic urticaria. A cost analysis of 50 nonimmunosuppressed patients. Arch Dermatol. 2008;144(1):33-9.
2. Greaves MW. Pathophysiology of chronic urticaria. Int Arch Allergy Immunol. 2002;127(1):3-9.
3. Heymann WR, Canden MD. Chronic Urticaria and angioedema associated with thyroid autoimmunity. J Am Acad Dermatol. 1999;40(2 Pt 1):229-32.
4. Sabroe RA, Grattan CEH, Francis DM, et al. The Autologous Skin Test: a screening test for autoantibodies in chronic idiopathic urticaria. Br J Dermatol. 1999;140(3):446-52.
5. Sicherer SH. Clinical implications of cross-reactive food allergies. J Allergy Clin Immunol. 2001;108(6):881-90.
6. Thorpe WA, Goldner W, Meza J, et al. Reduced vitamin D levels in adult subjects with chronic urticaria. J Allergy Clin Immunol. 2010;126(2):413-4.
7. Tong LJ, Balakrishnan G, Kochan JP, et al. Assessment of autoimmunity in patients with urticaria. J Allergy Clin Immunol. 1997;99(4):461-7.

Chapter

17 Purpura

Purpura is a red or purplish discolouration of the skin caused by the extravasation of blood into the skin or the mucous membrane. Small lesions less than 5 mm are called petechiae; larger ones usually subcutaneous are called ecchymosis. Linear purpuric lesions are called vibices. Bleeding occurs when the platelet count falls below 50,000 per mm^3. The risk of serious haemorrhage is increased at levels below 10,000/mm^3 and grave complications such as intracranial haemorrhage occur at counts below 2,000 per mm^3.

As the purpuric lesions grow older the colour changes from red to purple, bluish green and finally to yellow. These colour changes are due to chemical changes in the haemoglobin of red blood cells (RBCs). Purpuric lesions do not blanch on pressure as opposed to those of erythema caused by the dilatation of the blood vessels. In inflammations such as vasculitis, the purpuric lesions are raised and palpable.

AETIOLOGY

Spontaneous bleeding or excessive bleeding following trauma may be due to:

- Increased fragility of blood vessels
- Platelet deficiency or dysfunction
- Derangement in clotting mechanism.

Increased Fragility of Blood Vessels

The increased fragility of blood vessels; may be due to severe infections, vitamin C deficiency, infective endocarditis, rickettsial disease, typhoid fever, vasculitis, collagen disorders, etc. Vascular fragility is manifested by:

- Spontaneous appearance of petechiae and ecchymosis in the skin and mucous membrane
- Positive tourniquet test
- Normal platelet count and clotting time.

Decrease in Platelet Number and Function

Deficiency of platelets may occur due to a variety of clinical settings including bone marrow suppression from any cause, disseminated intravascular coagulation (DIC); these result in consumption of both clotting factors and platelets, platelet function can be deranged in spite of normal platelet count such as uraemia or from idiopathic thrombocytopaenic purpura.

Decrease in platelet number and function is manifested by:
- Petechiae and ecchymosis
- Excessive bleeding from minor trauma
- Tourniquet test is positive
- Platelet count is low
- Clotting time is normal
- Bleeding time is prolonged.

Derangement in Clotting Mechanism

Derangement in clotting mechanism differs in many respects from those due to defects of the vessel wall and platelet dysfunction, e.g. haemophilia. It is characterized by:
- Prolonged clotting time
- Bleeding time is normal
- Petechiae and ecchymosis are usually absent
- Massive haemorrhage follows trauma
- Haemorrhage is present in areas of body subject to trauma, such as joints of the lower extremities.

INVESTIGATIONS

The following are some of the investigations, which should be done in cases of purpura when the cause is unknown.

A simple diascopic examination helps to distinguish purpura from erythema and telangiectasia. Palpable purpura is usually inflammatory.

Platelet Count

The normal count is 150–400 $\times$ 10^9/l. It varies from person to person and in the same person, it differs at different times. Apart from the variation in number, variation in function can also be observed *in vitro* tests.

A full blood count will reveal the degree of blood loss, and levels of blood cells.

Capillary Resistance

If there is an increased pressure between the tissues and the capillaries, leakage of blood cells occurs. Capillary fragility can be measured by the Hess test. Inflating the sphygmomanometer cuff around the upper arm to a constant pressure of 80 mm Hg for about 5 minutes, petechiae will develop in the presence of abnormalities of the vascular wall. The number of petechiae is counted, a count of up to 5 in a measured area of 5 cm below the antecubital fossa is considered normal.

Bleeding Time

This is the time taken for the bleeding to stop after making a tiny incision on the skin. The bleeding normally stops due to the formation of a platelet thrombus at the site of incision. Normal bleeding time is 4–10 minutes. It is prolonged in platelet disorders.

Coagulation Screen

A clotting screen can exclude major defects of coagulation. These include prothrombin time, clotting time, fibrinogen levels and individual clotting factors.

Capillary Microscope

Direct microscopic examination of the capillaries is disappointing in bleeding disorders. Purpura may be seen in the nailfold capillaries, it may also be possible to see the exact point in the capillary at which extravasation of blood occurred.

SYSTEMIC CAUSES OF PURPURA

Disseminated Intravascular Coagulation

Disseminated intravascular coagulation is an acute, subacute or chronic disorder, characterized by intravascular fibrin deposition, principally within the arterioles and capillaries with resulting bleeding diathesis from depletion of clotting factors and platelets.

About 50% cases of DIC are obstetric patients following complications of pregnancy. Another 33% of patients have cancer; the remaining disorders are varied. These may be due to tissue damage such as burns, trauma, transplant rejection, haemolysis from mismatched blood, autoimmune disorders. DIC may be due to miscellaneous causes such as severe infections, e.g. meningococcaemia, malignant hypertension. Children with cavernous haemangioma are at risk from this consumptive coagulopathy (Kasabach-Merritt syndrome).

Clinical Features

The clinical picture is an apparent paradox, with a bleeding tendency in the face of widespread coagulation. Typically, the abnormal clotting occurs only in the microcirculation, only occasionally are the large vessels involved. The manifestations may be minimal or there may be oliguria, with acute renal failure, dyspnoea, cyanosis, convulsions and coma. Hypertension is characteristic when the haemolysis is brisk: fever, back pain and jaundice may occur (Fig. 1).

Prolonged bleeding may occur from venous puncture, or there may be petechiae and ecchymoses in the skin, purpura fulminans may supervene.

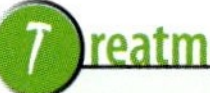

Treatment

Control of the underlying disease is of paramount importance, together with correction of haemostatic abnormalities with heparin. The dose is adjusted to keep the clotting time two to three times the normal.

Laboratory Findings

These show decreased platelets, decreased fibrinogen, elevated prothrombin and partial thromboplastin time (PT and PTT) and fibrin degradation products (d-dimers).

Prognosis

Prognosis of DIC is highly variable depending upon the underlying disorder as well as the degree of intravascular clotting, activity of the reticuloendothelial system and fibrinolysis. In some cases, it is self-limiting, in others it responds to prompt treatment with heparin, often it runs a fulminant course leading to death within a few days.

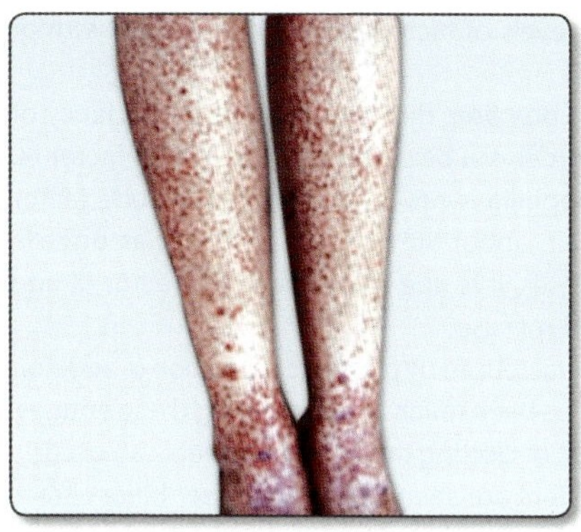

Fig. 1: Purpura

Thrombocytopaenia

Platelet deficiencies may be primary or secondary to some disorder. In either case, thrombocytopaenia is characterised by a prolonged bleeding time with a normal coagulation time. Petechiae are often present and showers of them suddenly develop, distal to the cuff as the blood pressure is taken (positive tourniquet test), platelet counts are diminished.

Secondary thrombocytopaenia may be a component of myelophthisic pancytopaenia; hypersplenism or it may be due to drugs and toxins. Thrombotic thrombocytopaenia is characterised by intravascular aggregation of thrombocytes; it may be related to DIC.

Treatment

Corticosteroids, immunosuppressive drugs, blood transfusion and splenectomy. Prednisolone in a dose of 60 mg daily is usually effective in bringing about a remission.

Colchicine 0.6 mg, two to four times daily is also effective. Other drugs used for treatment are danazol, vincristine and vinblastine. Platelet transfusions may be life-saving. They do not increase the platelet count and are only useful in emergencies.

Idiopathic thrombocytopaenia (ITP) is a mysterious disorder probably of autoimmune origin. Often it is the first manifestation of SLE. In most cases it appears as an isolated disorder. Patients are usually children or young adults; females are slightly more affected than males.

Haemorrhages are seen dispersed throughout the body, particularly in the serosal and mucosal linings, petechiae and ecchymosis are seen in the skin, haemorrhagic bullae in the mouth may be a presenting sign of the disease, gingival bleeding may occur. Malena, haematemesis and menorrhagia may occur in young women.

An antiplatelet IgG has been identified in the serum of patients with ITP; spleen is the site of destruction of platelets, presumably coated with IgG. Spleen may be involved in the production of antiplatelet IgG. The bone marrow is nondiagnostic; it may have increased number of megakaryocytes.

Coagulation Disorders

These can be hereditary or acquired. There are a number of hereditary disorders of coagulation, most important of these are a heterogenous group of inherited disorders characterized by low levels of factors VIII or IX (or both), with or without platelet dysfunction.

The term haemophilia was at one time defined simply as a deficiency of factor VIII; a clinically similar disorder can be seen with low level of factor IX, as well as factor XI. Thus, haemophilia is now considered to include factor VIII deficiency (Haemophilia A) in about 80% of cases. Christmas disease (Haemophilia B) in 10–15% of cases, it is due to deficiency of factor IX and deficiency of factor XI in about 5% of cases.

Von Willebrand's disease is characterized by platelet dysfunction in addition to low levels of factor VIII. There has been much overlap among these entities, any combination of derangement of clotting factor and platelets can occur.

Acquired coagulation disorders are seen in liver disease, biliary tract obstruction, malabsorption, drug ingestion, etc. Haemorrhagic manifestations are severe similar to the hereditary forms. Ecchymosis and subcutaneous hematomas are common especially on the legs. Severe haemorrhage may follow trauma, haemarthrosis is common. Other haemorrhagic manifestations include haemorrhages in the gastrointestinal tract and in severe case haemorrhages in the central nervous system.

Dysproteinemic Purpura

Purpura may be a presenting symptom of disturbances of plasma proteins. It may occur with cryoproteinaemia, hyperglobinaemia, sarcoidosis, myeloma, etc. The mechanism is unknown. It may be due to immune complex vasculitis. Hyperviscosity leading to stasis and endothelial damage may play a part. Lesions appear in crops as small erythematous papules mainly on the legs and then progress to form punctate purpuric lesions.

Henoch-Schonlein Purpura (Anaphylactoid Purpura)

This is seen in leucocytoclastic vasculitis, due to deposition of immune complex in the walls of the arterioles and venules, which subsequently are damaged. It is associated with abdominal pain, and acute arthritis affecting one or more joints for a few days at a time. The disease frequently follows an upper respiratory tract infection. Intussusception, rectal bleeding and renal involvement are features of severe disease.

PURPURA OF DERMATOLOGICAL INTEREST

Drug Eruption

The drugs may either cause thrombocytopaenia or damage the vessel walls. Those causing capillary damage are barbiturates, carbromal, chlorpromazine, isoniazid, quinine, quinidine and sulphonamides. Carbromal causes a distinctive type of purpura. The widespread areas of capillary leakage combined with erythema produce a picture similar to Schamberg's disease.

Drugs causing bone marrow suppression include chloramphenicol, some cytotoxic drugs such as nitrogen mustard, heparin, sulphonamides, thiazides, indomethocin, rifampicin, quinidine, penicillin and furosemide.

Contact Purpura

Certain substances cause contact purpura with little or no eczematous reaction. This distribution of purpura corresponds to the area of contact. Khaki clothing, azo dyes, optical whiteners, various rubber additives and benzoyl peroxide cause contact purpura.

Infection

Purpura is associated with severe infections, such as thrombocytopaenia due to DIC. The infections include bacterial endocarditis, viral haemorrhagic fevers and rickettsial infections.

Systemic Disease

These include renal disease, diabetes mellitus, collagen disorders, liver diseases, hemochromatosis, carcinomatosis, amyloidosis and malnutrition. It may also occur with ovarian and endocrine disease such as Cushing's syndrome.

Senile Purpura

This is a harmless condition caused by changes in the collagen that supports the dermal blood vessels. It is seen in the elderly due to the cumulative effect of sunlight on the exposed areas, especially the forearms. The lesions are triggered by minute trauma, large ecchymosis may occur.

Scurvy

The condition begins with perifollicular haemorrhages, usually on the thighs and later on the buttocks, abdomen and arms. Hypertrophic gingivitis, haemorrhages and other signs of scurvy are present. It is treated by ascorbic acid 200 mg daily. Rapid response is seen in a few days, a diet containing green leafy vegetables and citrus fruits should be taken regularly with adequate proteins.

Pigmented Purpuric Dermatosis (Capillaritis of Unknown Origin)

Pigmented purpuric dermatosis (PPD) is a purely local inflammatory process characterised by petechiae, pigmentation and occasionally telangiectasia. The Aetiology is unknown. Gravity and increased venous pressure are important localising factors. Exercise is a provoking factor. Most cases are chronic, the legs are the common site of involvement. The condition is occasionally due to drugs, mycosis fungoides and rheumatoid arthritis. There are a variety of PPD, which have different morphological features, but all have a similar histology. The superficial vessels show narrowing of the lumen, swelling of the endothelial cells and a perivascular lymphocytic infiltrate. There is extravasation of RBC, hemosiderin deposits are present in the dermis.

Schamberg's Disease (Progressive Pigmented Purpuric Dermatosis)

The eruption is more common in males found most frequently on the lower shin and ankles, but it may occur in any part of the body. It may occur at any age from childhood onwards. Gravity and increased venous pressure are important localizing factors in the pathogenesis of Schamberg's disease (Fig. 2). Exercise may be a provoking factor.

Histopathology

The lesion is characterized by narrowing of the lumen, endothelial swelling of the superficial blood vessels, accompanied by perivascular infiltrate of T lymphocytes, extravasation of erythrocytes and haemosiderin deposits in macrophages.

Clinical features

The lesions appear as irregular patches or plaques of orange or brown pigmentation due to haemosiderin, with pinhead-sized reddish puncta, resembling the grains of red pepper. The lesions develop insidiously on one or both legs. It is usually symptomless or is associated with slight itching. The condition is usually persistent; there may be occasional clearing in some cases.

Eczematoid-Like Purpura (Purpura of Doucas and Kapetanakis)

It is seen frequently in adult men, purpuric lesions commence around the ankles and spread to involve the whole leg. The lesions are more pronounced at the site of friction and clothing. Spongiosis may be seen in the epidermis. The lesions consist of erythematous and purpuric macules, which may become confluent; the eruption has a characteristic orange colour. Spontaneous improvement may occur after a few months, but recurrences occur. It may respond to topical steroids.

Pigmented Purpuric Lichenoid Dermatosis of Gourgerot and Blum

The eruption occurs in men between the ages of 40–60 years. The lesions are seen on the legs, but may be present elsewhere. Minute rust coloured lichenoid papules appear that tend to form plaques, purpuric lesion are also seen. The term lichenoid describes the similarity of the papules to lichen planus in appearance but not on histology.

Lichen Aureus

This condition is seen more often in the younger age group; in the second or third decade. The lesions appear as gold-brown flat papules, which form plaques, linear pattern may sometimes occur. The condition is common on the

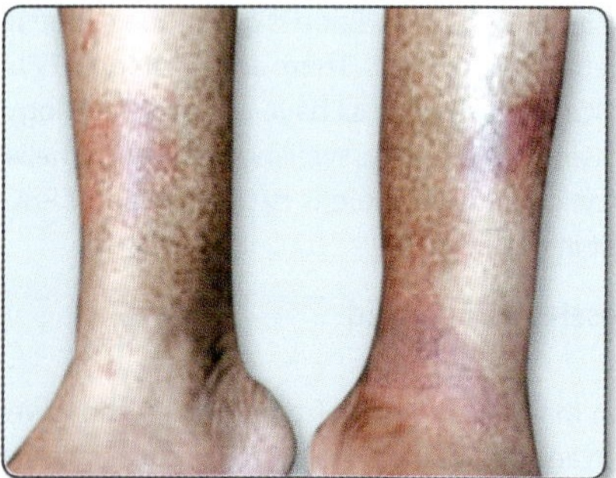

Fig. 2: Schamberg's disease

lower limbs, usually over or near a perforating vein. In some cases the lesions can be seen on the upper limbs. The condition is asymptomatic. The condition resembles lichen planus in appearance and histology.

Purpura Annularis Telangiectodes (Majocchi's Disease)

The eruption occurs in adolescents and young adults of either sex. The lesion consists of small plaques often annular from the onset. These are purple, yellow or brown in colour; they often contain "cayenne pepper" spots and telangiectasia. The centre is hypopigmented with slight atrophy.

Gravitational Purpura

This is a common dermatosis, although associated with venous insufficiency; other factors may also be involved. It is more frequent in men, the lesions occur on the lower leg, but may extend to the feet and toes. They appear as minute purpuric macules that coalesce to form irregular plaques one to several centimetres across. Oedema, ulceration and other signs of venous insufficiency may be present. The disease is characteristically chronic. Treatment is unsatisfactory.

Treatment of PPD

The condition is resistant to any form of therapy. The disorder may persist for years. Simple supportive hosiery is the most appropriate approach. Topical steroids may help especially for itchy lesions; prolonged use should be avoided. PUVA, cyclosporin, and griseofulvin have also been used.

Some trials have shown the disappearance of the lesions with oral rutoside 50 mg bid and ascorbic acid 500 mg bid.

MISCELLANEOUS PURPURIC DISORDERS

Easy Bruising Syndrome (Purpura Simplex)

This is seen in young women who bruise easily but have normal coagulation profile and normal platelet count. There may be an increase in megakaryocytes; some patients may have antibodies to platelets.

Painful Bruising Syndrome (Autoerythrocyte Sensitisation)

The condition occurs in young and middle aged women, who usually have emotional and personality problem. Painful tender ecchymosis is seen most commonly on the extremities. The lesion evolves in a few hours, it resolves in 5–8 days. New lesion may occur in crops. Many patients have premonitory signs before the eruption of lesions.

Some authors have reported that intracutaneous injection of erythrocytes evoked a similar lesion. Similar reactions have occurred with autologous whole blood and packed RBC transfusion. Many believe that the lesions are artifactual, other feel that they are spontaneous. Similar lesions have been reported with DNA sensitivity.

Devil's Pinches

These are transitory painful sensations on the upper leg of postmenopausal women, who subsequently develop ecchymoses at the site of pain.

Achenbach's Syndrome

In this syndrome, there are recurrent episodes of burning sensation in the palm and fingers followed by bruising. This is mostly seen in the elderly.

FURTHER READING

1. Berndt MC, Andrew's RK. Thrombotic thrombocytopenic purpura: reducing the risk? J Inves Clin Dermatol. 2011;121(2):522-4.
2. Detrana C, Hurwitz RM. Painful purpura: an adverse effect to a thrombolysin. Arch Dermatol. 1990;126(5):690-1.
3. George JN, Shetti SJ. The clinical importance of acquired abnormalities of platelet function. N Eng J Med. 1991;324(1):27-39.
4. Nishioka K, Kataya I, Masuzawa M, et al. Drug-induced pigmented purpura. J Dermatol. 1989;16(3):220-2.
5. O'Leary ST, Glanz JM, McClure DL, et al. The risk of immune thrombocytopenic purpura after vaccination in children and adolescence. J Pediatr. 2012; 129(2):248-55.

Chapter 18

Leg Ulcers

The lower legs are the common site of both arterial and venous ulcers. The most common ulcer is the venous ulcer; other causes include trauma, ischaemia, vasculitis, chronic infections, malignancies, and some haematological and metabolic disorders. Acute ulcers show signs of healing in less than 4 weeks, these include traumatic ulcers and post-operative wounds. Chronic ulcers are those that persist longer than 4 weeks.

CLASSIFICATION OF LEG ULCERS

Venous ulcers	Varicose veins Post-thrombotic ulcers
Infection	Tropical phagedaenic ulcer Tuberculosis Swimming pool granuloma Leprosy Deep fungal infections
Parasitic	Leishmaniasis
Metabolic	Gout Diabetes mellitus
Vasculitis and autoimmune disorders	Leucocytoclastic vasculitis Pyoderma gangrenosum Rheumatoid arthritis Systemic lupus erythematosus
Arterial	Atherosclerosis Hypertension
Blood disorders	Sickle cell anaemia Thallassaemia
Neuropathic	Diabetes mellitus Leprosy Tabes dorsalis Syringomyelia
Bullous disorders	Pemphigoid
Malignancy	Squamous cell carcinoma, melanoma Kaposi's sarcoma
Traumatic	Burns Footballers, ulcer Artefacts

VENOUS ULCERS

Venous ulcers are the most common ulcers of the lower leg. These arise because of increased venous hydrostatic pressure in the venules, particularly

Clinical Features

All venous ulcers have the following characteristics:

- Varicose ulcers are shallow, have irregularly shaped shelving edges, that are often characterised by a thin blue line of growing epithelium. The base of the ulcer is formed of pink granulation, pale granulation tissue or slough. Often one or more feeding veins can be seen proceeding from the edge of the ulcer (flare sign). When the surrounding skin is scarred, the feeding veins are no longer visible, but is palpated.
- The site of the venous ulcer is remarkably constant; it is situated on the medial side of the leg, above or behind the medial malleolus. Most venous ulcers are painless.
- *Lipodermatosclerosis:* Chronic accumulation of tissue fluid may eventually lead to induration and fibrosis of the tissue around the ankle. This further limits the action of the calf muscles. When lipodermatosclerosis is circumferential, the tissue above the ankle is enlarged, giving the leg a classical inverted champagne bottle appearance.
- *Eczema:* Redness, irritation and swelling are common. The condition may be severe, and secondary spread to other parts of the body may occur.
- *Pigmentation:* There may be postinflammatory hypermelanosis, in addition to haemosiderin deposits derived from the extravasated RBCs.
- *Atrophie blanche:* This is a white plaque of sclerosis, stippled with telangiectasia, and often surrounded by hyperpigmentation.

on standing. This causes leakage of plasma through the endothelial pores of the capillaries. It then forms a layer of pericapillary fibrin; this interferes with the transfer of blood gases and metabolites. The leakage of plasma causes local oedema. Oedematous tissue is more vulnerable to trauma than the healthy skin, and is less able to combat infection. The ulcers can attain a large size.

Venous ulcers coexist with incompetent superficial veins, incompetent perforating veins that pierce the deep fascia and link the superficial and deep veins. A small number of venous ulcers also arise due to deep venous thrombosis. The former two are called varicose ulcers. There is an adequate functioning lower limb arterial function with ankle brachial index of greater than 0.80 (Fig. 1).

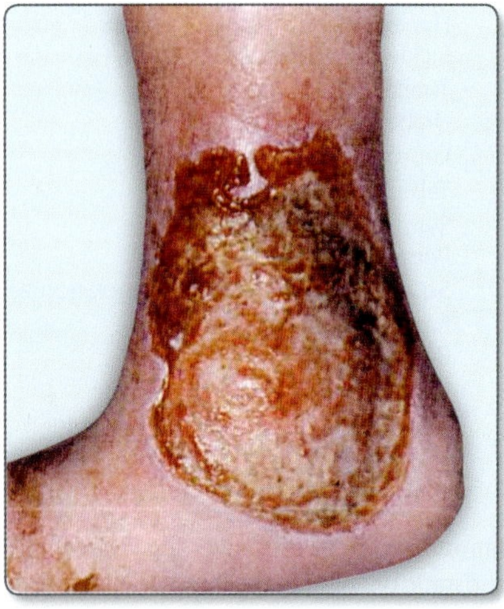

Fig. 1: Venous ulcer

Post-thrombotic Ulcer

In contrast to varicose ulcer, this ulcer is painful. The site and morphological characters are similar to varicose ulcers. Often there is a clear-cut history of venous thrombosis following childbirth, an abdominal operation or an accident to the leg. Bursting pain may be complained if the deep veins are blocked, varicose veins are lacking. The skin is firm and seems to be tethered to the underlying structures.

Complications of Venous Ulcer

Infection: Pathogenic organisms are often found in leg ulcers of all types. Culture and sensitivity should be done to initiate therapy.

Eczema: This may be due to contact sensitivity to medicaments, or it may be infective due to the bacteria present in the ulcer. The eczema should be carefully treated. Potent topical steroids on leg ulcers may inhibit healing for several weeks, by producing an indolent arterial type ulcer, with deep adherent slough called a steroid ulcer.

Haemorrhage: Spontaneous haemorrhage often occurs from large ulcers. This can lead to death if severe and not treated immediately.

Lymphoedema: The distortion and obliteration of lymphatics in long standing ulcers give rise to lymphoedema.

Lipodermatosclerosis: Chronic venous hypertension in the legs causes tightening and thickening of the subcutaneous tissue leading to fibrosis (Fig. 2).

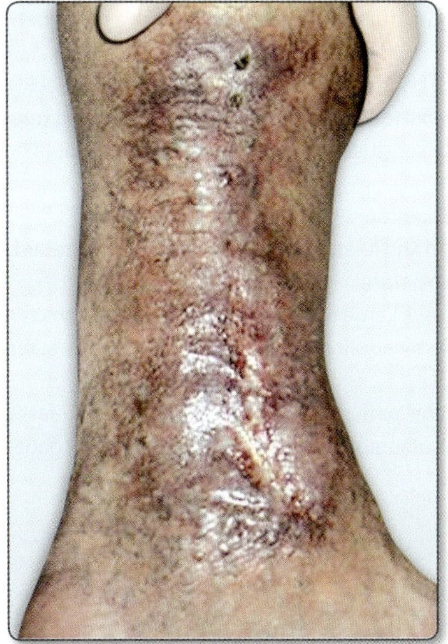

Fig. 2: Lipodermatosclerosis

Bone changes: Periostitis is common; fibrosis and ankylosis of the ankle joint are seen in neglected cases. X-ray of the lower leg should be done in long standing venous ulcers.

Zinc depletion: Low zinc levels are often found in patients with venous ulceration, improvement is reported with zinc sulphate therapy.

Malignant change (Marjolin's ulcer): Malignant change is rare, but carries a bad prognosis. The edge of the ulcer becomes heaped up and cauliflower like, induration is marked in squamous cell carcinoma. Basal cell carcinoma may remain flat and undetected. The ulcer may become painful. Lymph nodes should be examined. These ulcers should be biopsied and treated accordingly.

Treatment of Venous Ulcers

Venous ulcers take a long time to heal; many patients never achieve complete wound healing. About 30–60% of healing is seen in 24 weeks and about 70–80% may take a year or longer.

The primary aim is to treat venous hypertension by compression bandages, so that natural healing occurs. Bandages support the leg, and reduce swelling. Different types of bandages can be used. A paste bandage covered by elastic adhesive is usually the most satisfactory. It is important to exclude arterial insufficiency by measuring the arterial pressure, and by feeling the pulses such as dorsalis pedis. The arterial pressure is measured with a Doppler probe. If the resting ankle/brachial pressure index is greater than 0.8, then there is no arterial disease.

Patient should be encouraged to walk (not stand) with the bandage on. This will increase the arterial blood flow, improve the muscle pump, this prevents deep venous thrombosis and contractures that readily develop in a recumbent patient.

In a clear granulating ulcer, the bandages are changed once or twice weekly. A bland antiseptic is used to clean the ulcer. Systemic antibiotics should treat secondary infection; possibility of sensitisation to topical antibiotics should be kept in mind.

For obese patients weight reduction is required.

Deficiency of iron, ascorbic acid and folate may occur. Zinc deficiency retards healing, oral zinc therapy may be helpful.

Firm sloughs should be removed. Large ulcers which have granulations can be re-epithelialised more quickly by application of multiple skin grafts taken from the thigh.

Once the ulcer has healed, the patient should continue to wear elastic stocking, and should protect the vulnerable skin from further damage by gauze pads.

Other Measures

These include hyperbaric oxygen, but this requires a system for pressurised administration, precautions should also be used against fire.

The role of surgery for the removal of varicose veins is a matter of dispute. A recurrence rate of 30–50 % has been reported within 5 years.

Stripping, ligation and sclerotherapy are the procedures frequently undertaken. The newer procedures of deep vein bypass, valvuloplasty and brachial vein transplant are still under assessment by different centers concerned with the treatment of leg ulcers.

Skin grafting is helpful in reducing the time taken for the ulcer to heal.

ARTERIAL ULCER

This is rare as compared to a venous ulcer and is extremely painful. Varicose veins are usually absent but their presence does not exclude the diagnosis. Both sexes are affected after the age of 60 years.

The ulcer appears on the area most susceptible to trauma, usually the shin, lateral malleolus or the toes. The ulcers are sharply defined, punched out and are deep. The ulcer may penetrate the deep fascia; at times even the tendons are exposed at the base.

The pedal pulsations are absent, and the foot is cold. Intermittent claudication is usual; sometimes discolouration of the toes is present, indicating the onset of gangrene.

Treatment

- Treat the cause such as diabetes, vasculitis and atherosclerosis.
- Increase the blood flow by peripheral vasodilators, such as nifedipine, pentoxifylline.
- Leg should be placed in a dependent position, this helps to reduce the pain and increase the arterial flow.
- If it is not possible to improve the vascular supply, the patient should be referred to a vascular surgeon.
- Treat the ulcer itself, remove the slough and clean the ulcer. Once the ulcer is clean, it should be covered with a nonadherent dressing. The dressing is covered with a light bandage. A tight bandage will further impede the blood supply.

Arterial ulcers may occur in advanced age due to atherosclerosis, vasculitis, diabetes, following radiation, increased blood viscosity and platelet adhesiveness (Fig. 3).

The difference between arterial and venous ulcer is shown in Table 1.

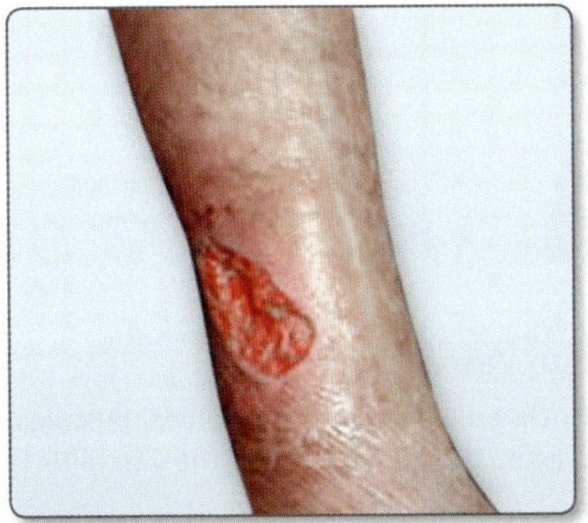

Fig. 3: Arterial ulcer

Table 1: Table showing the difference between arterial and venous ulcer

Arterial ulcer	*Venous ulcer*
Site Shin, lateral malleoli, toes	Medial side of the leg above and behind the medial malleolus
Clinical features Deep sharply defined, surrounding skin normal	Shallow, irregular edges, surrounding skin pigmented and oedematous
Painful	Not painful
Eczematisation absent	Eczematisation present
Foot cold, pedal pulsations absent	Foot warm, pedal pulsations present
Intermittent claudication present	Intermittent claudication absent

MISCELLANEOUS CAUSES

Hypertensive Ischaemic Ulcer (Martorell's Ulcer)

It is caused by thrombosis of the cutaneous arterioles. The painful ulcers are shallow; edge is reddish or yellowish, with livedo pattern at the peripheries. The ulcers are usually bilateral, seen mostly on the mid and lower parts of the leg. Varicosities are usually absent. The peripheral pulses are present (Fig. 4).

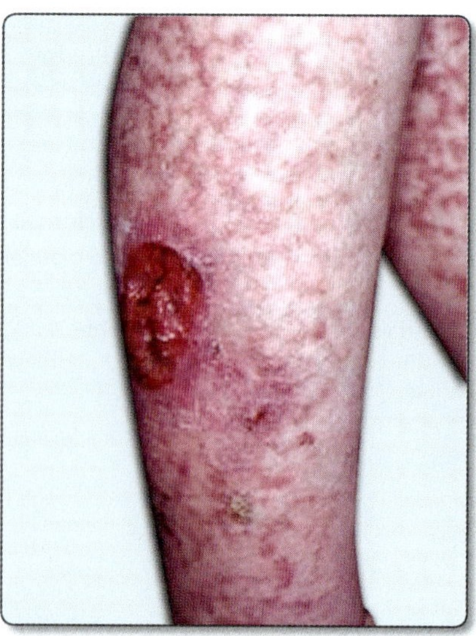

Fig. 4: Hypertensive ischaemic ulcer—note the livedo pattern at the periphery

Leg Ulcers due to Cutaneous Vasculitis

Leucocytoclastic ulcers are associated with purpura, papules, pustules, nodules, urticaria and livedo racemosa. The hallmark of the vasculitis is palpable purpura.

Leg Ulcers due to Blood Diseases

Ulcers of the leg are common in sickle cell anaemia, thalassaemia, hereditary spherocytosis, Felty's syndrome and other hemolytic anaemias. The spleen should be examined when the cause is not clear.

Factitious Ulcer (Dermatitis Artefacta)

A self-induced ulcer is sometimes encountered in a highly neurotic individual. The mode of production varies. The ulcer is present in an accessible part, often on the anterior or lateral part of the leg. The ulcer is unusual in shape.

When such an ulcer is placed in a plaster cast so that it is not tampered, healing readily occurs. A psychiatrist should treat the neurosis.

Leg Ulcers in the Tropics

There are three ulcers specific to the tropical and subtropical region. These are yaws, tropical phagedaenic ulcer and the diphtheritic desert sore.

Yaws

The primary sore of yaws is sometimes found on the leg, foot or the buttocks in children before walking. It appears as an infected abrasion in which *Treponema pallidum pertenue* can be found. It heals within a few weeks. In the tertiary stage, multiple deep ulcers are seen which also contain the spirochetes. The ulcers are painless; on healing they form tissue paper like scars.

Tropical Ulcer (Chronic Phagedaenic Ulcer)

The ulcer occurs in the monsoon ridden humid zones, where it is endemic, but breaks out as seasonal epidemics. The infection develops in a breach of continuity of the skin due to trauma or by an insect bite; the onset of ulceration is then rapid. It occurs exclusively on the lower leg, seen in people who walk barefoot. The bacterial picture is nonspecific; *Bacillus fusiformis* and *Borrelia vincenti* are almost always present. Malnutrition appears to be a predisposing factor.

The lesion commences as a papule which soon becomes a pustule, within hours it is surrounded by a zone of inflammation and induration. There is accompanying tender lymphadenitis. In 2–3 days, the pustule bursts, and an ulcer forms that spreads rapidly, the edges are undermined. There is a copious foul smelling serosanguineous discharge with pain.

If untreated the ulcer remains of the same size for months, or even a year or two. Sometimes it assumes phagedaenic characteristics and attains large dimensions. On healing, a scar is left which is characteristically circular, parchment like, and faintly pigmented. Occasionally squamous cell carcinoma develops (Fig. 5).

Treatment

Depends upon the culture and sensitivity results. Ciprofloxacin and metronidazole is usually effective. Topically wet compresses and antibiotic ointments are helpful. The chronic ulcer requires occlusive dressings with adhesive tape or light plaster cast. Reconstructive surgery may be necessary.

The ulcer should be differentiated from venous ulcers and mycobacterium ulceration.

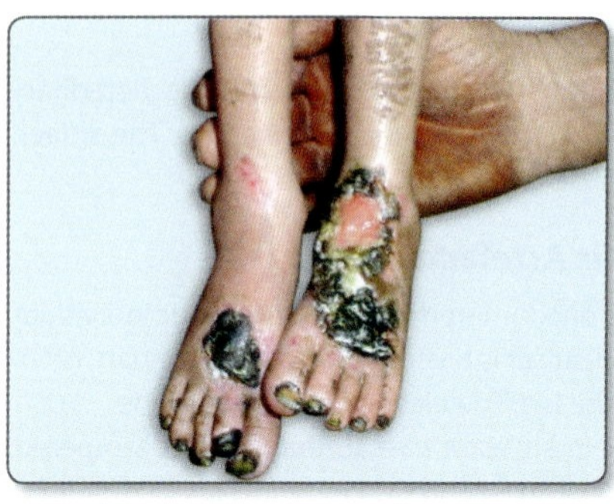

Fig. 5: Tropical ulcer

Diphtheritic Desert Sore (Veldt Sore, Barcoo Rot)

As the name implies the ulcer is found in the hot parched deserts of the world. It is caused by *Corynebacterium diphtheriae*; other pathogens such as staphylococci and streptococci are often present. The lesion presents as grouped papulo-pustules or vesicles, within a few days the papules become necrotic, and ulcer forms. The ulcer slowly enlarges, until it attains a diameter of 1–2 cm. Usually a diphtheritic membrane covers the floor of the ulcer, this is removed with difficulty. The ulcer runs a chronic course. The ulcer has a hard rolled elevated edge, with a pale blue tinge. Rarely there are signs of peripheral neuritis, due to toxic products by the diphtheria bacillus.

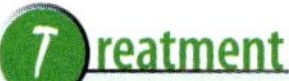

The desert sore is treated with diphtheric antitoxin. Systemic and topical antibiotics are also given for other pathogenic organisms.

Pyoderma gangrenosum is described in chapter 38.

Exclude malignancy in long standing ulcers.
X-ray chronic ulcers to exclude osteitis.
Topical antibacterial creams should be avoided to prevent sensitisation.

FURTHER READING

1. Burnard K, Clemenson S, Morland M, et al. Venous lipodermatosclerosis: treatment by fibrinolytic enhancement and compression. BMJ. 1980;280(6206):7-11.
2. Charles H. Compression healing of ulcers. J Dist Nurs. 1991;4:6-7.
3. Gambichler T, Avermaetic A, Wilment M et al. Generalized essential telangiectasia successfully treated with High Energy Long Pulse frequency doubled Nd; YAG Laser. Dermatol Surg. 2001;27(4):355-7.
4. Goslen JB. Autoimmune ulceration of the leg. Clin Dermatol. 1990;8(3-4):92-117.
5. Greaves MW, Ive FA. Double blind trial of zinc sulphate in the treatment of chronic venous ulceration. Br J Dermatol. 1972;87(6):632-4.
6. Koelemay MJW, Den Hartog D, Prime MH, et al. Diagnosis of arterial disease of the lower extremities with duplex ultrasonography. Br J Surg. 1996;83(3):404-9.
7. Leu IJ. Hypertensive ischaemic leg ulcer (Martorell's ulcer): a specific disease entity? Int Angiol. 1992;11(2):132-6.
8. Long CC. Treatment of angioma serpiginosum by Pulsed Tunable Dye Laser. Br J Dermatol. 1997;136(4):631-2.
9. Nelzen O, Bergquist D, Lindhogen A. Venous and non-venous leg ulcers: clinical history and appearance in a population study. Br J Surg. 1994;81(2):181-7.

Chapter 19

Diseases of Pigmentation

INTRODUCTION

The colour of the skin is important to us; any change in colour from the normal can lead to psychological problems. The colour of the skin depends on melanin, degree of vascularity (oxidized and reduced haemoglobin), presence of carotene, and thickness of the horny layer. The pigment of the human skin is contained in the keratinocytes, the pigment is manufactured by melanocytes, it is then transferred in packages called melanosomes. The racial difference in colour is not due to the number of melanocytes, which is constant in human beings, but due to the production, degradation and distribution of the melanosomes.

Melanin production is influenced by genetic factors, amount and type of ultraviolet light received, melanocyte-stimulating hormone and by the effect of melanocyte-stimulating chemicals, such as psoralens.

There are three types of melanin pigment present in human beings: (1) eumelanin, (2) pheomelanin and (3) neuromelanin. Eumelanin and pheomelanin are formed in the epidermis from melanocytes. Eumelanin is found in ellipsoidal melanosomes, it imparts brown-black colour to the skin, eyes and hair. Pheomelanin is found in spherical melanosomes, it gives yellow-red hair. A small amount of pheomelanin is present in most melanocytes. Red-haired people may only contain pheomelanin. Neuromelanin is black pigment formed in nerve cells, such as substantia nigra.

On light microscopy melanin appears brown, but when seen through the intact skin it may look black and when melanin accumulates in the deeper layers of the dermis it is blue due to the scattering effect of light by the overlying tissues.

There are important genetic differences in the individual's ability to respond to ultraviolet radiation, called the skin type. The following are the different types of skin (Fitzpatrick skin types):

- Type I — Burns easily, tans very poorly
- Type II — Burns easily, tans poorly
- Type III — Burns moderately, tans gradually and uniformly
- Type IV — Burns minimally, tans easily
- Type V — Rarely burns, tans easily; genetically brown skin of Mongoloids and Indians
- Type VI — Rarely burns, tans easily, genetically black skin of Afro-Caribbeans.

Disorders of melanin production are common; these may be in the form of hypermelanosis, hypomelanosis, and depigmentation due to loss of previously existing melanin. Wood's lamp is used in the diagnosis of epidermal pigmentary disorders. Hypomelanosis appears whiter in epidermal lesions, epidermal hyperpigmentation becomes accentuated. Dermal melanosis is not enhanced, it may become less apparent.

PHYSIOLOGY OF PIGMENTATION

Hyperpigmentation can be epidermal or dermal. Most cases are epidermal due to increased production of melanin in the epidermis; it is generally brown in colour. Increased production of melanin from the existing melanocytes is called melanotic hyperpigmentation. Increased production from active proliferation of melanocytes is called melanocytotic hyperpigmentation.

Dermal hyperpigmentation or ceruloderma is due to the presence of melanin in the dermis. Due to Tyndall effect dermal pigment is perceived as blue, grayish-blue or grayish-brown. Dermal hyperpigmentation may be postinflammatory, due to drugs or failure of migration of melanocytes to the epidermis, e.g. Mongolian spot and dermal naevi.

Hyperpigmentation can be generalised or patchy.

Generalised Hyperpigmentation

It may be due to the following causes:

Genetic: There is a considerable variation in skin colour even in the same race, e.g. light colour may occur in Afro-Caribbeans.

Radiation: Ultraviolet radiation of the sun is the best-known cause of tanning.

Hormonal: Hypoadrenalism such as Addison disease causes diffuse pigmentation more marked in the sun exposed areas, and in areas already hyperpigmented, such as the axillae and oral mucosa. A similar change may occur in Cushing's syndrome that is more marked after adrenalectomy. Chronic renal failure causes hypermelanosis due to the increase in circulating β-melanocyte stimulating hormone, the hormone is normally degraded by the kidney.

Estrogens also stimulate melanogenesis, pregnancy causes a generalised increase in skin pigmentation, especially of the nipples and lower abdomen, such as linea nigra. There may be a patchy pigmentation on the cheeks (chloasma) by oral contraceptives, especially those containing a high content of estrogens.

Metabolic: Any severe wasting disease, such as tuberculosis or malnutrition may cause diffuse hyperpigmentation.

Malabsorption and biliary cirrhosis: These are also important causes of hyperpigmentation; the latter causes pruritus in addition. In hemochromatosis (bronze diabetes), a characteristic skin colour is seen, which is due to a combination of melanin and haemosiderin.

Drugs: Arsenic was used extensively in the past for the treatment of nerve, blood, and skin diseases; it caused a characteristic diffuse hyperpigmentation with multiple small spots of pale normal skin. Busulfan used for the treatment of leukaemia also causes hypermelanosis similar to that caused by Addison's disease. Chlorpromazine occasionally causes slate gray discolouration due to a metabolite that binds to the melanin.

Hereditary Diffuse Pigmentation

Fanconi's Syndrome

This is an autosomal recessive disorder with a high frequency of chromosomal abnormalities, characterised by pancytopenia, developmental defects, and high incidence of neoplasm. Around 80% of the patients have cutaneous disorders.

There is diffuse pigmentation of the skin often interspersed with hypopigmented raindrop-like macules. Generalised dusky brown pigmentation is most intense on the lower trunk, flexures and on the neck. The other developmental defects include absence of the thumbs, aplasia of the radius, testicular hypoplasia, strabismus and generalised hyper-reflexia. The condition is associated with anaemia, neutropenia and thrombocytopenia. The syndrome is associated with increased risk of myelomonocytic leukaemia, squamous cell carcinoma and hepatic tumours.

The course is progressive; death usually results from infection, haemorrhage or neoplasms.

Localised Hyperpigmentation

This can be hereditary or acquired:

Hereditary Patchy Pigmentations

Freckles: Ephelides are probably of autosomal dominant inheritance. They appear at about the age of 5 years as small brown macules on the sun-exposed skin. It is more common in persons of fair complexion or in red-haired individuals. In freckles, the number of melanocytes is normal, but the melanosomes are abnormally large and are more active than those of the surrounding skin. The freckles therefore tend to darken on exposure to sunlight; people with freckles tend to sunburn easily (Fig. 1).

Differential Diagnosis

Freckles should be differentiated from lentigines, which are prominent and are present anywhere on the skin. Junctional naevi are larger, fewer and darker in colour. Xeroderma pigmentosum is associated with photosensitivity, photophobia and skin neoplasms.

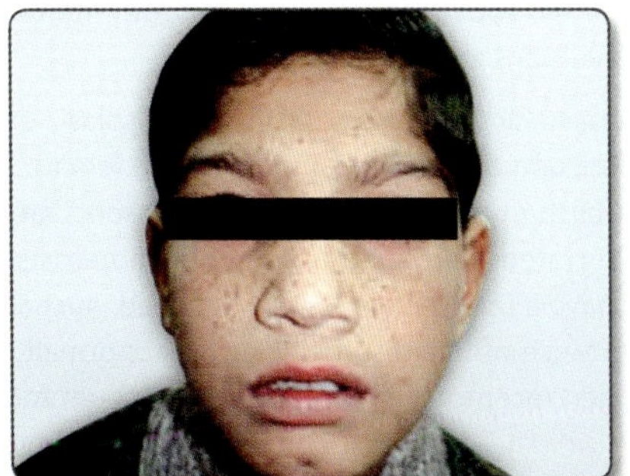

Fig. 1: Freckles

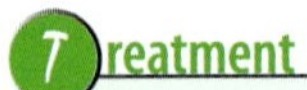

Treatment may be required for cosmetic reasons. Topical sunscreens during summer are helpful. The freckles may be peeled off with a brief application of solid carbon dioxide or phenol. Lasers are also helpful.

Periorificial lentigines (Peutz-Jeghers disease): This rare autosomal dominant disease is characterised by multiple small deep brown macules around the mouth with multiple polyps throughout the intestinal tract. These tend to cause recurrent intussusception.

Incontinentia Pigmenti (Bloch-Sulzberger syndrome): This is a neurocutaneous hereditary disorder often apparent at birth. It has an X-linked dominant inheritance, usually lethal in males.

Cutaneous lesions comprise of three stages: Vesiculobullous stage is seen at birth or within the first 2 weeks. The verrucous stage may begin from the 2–6 weeks and pigmentary stage from 12–26 weeks of age. The lesions are present on the trunk and extremities; they do not correspond to any dermatome. The lesions are scattered irregularly that may coalesce to form irregular patterns. The hyperpigmentation is in the form of whorls, streaks or bands. The pigmentation gradually fades and continues to do so throughout adolescence and adulthood.

Other cutaneous lesions include patchy alopecia of the vertex of the scalp. Atrophic changes similar to acrodermatitis chronica atrophicans are present on the hands, onychodystrophy, subungual tumours and palmoplantar hyperhidrosis are characteristic.

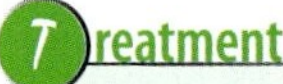

No treatment is required; pigmentation usually fades in early adulthood. As with the other genetically determined disorders, genetic counselling should be offered.

Eye changes include cataract, strabismus, optic atrophy, blue sclera and exudative chorioretinitis.

Skeletal abnormalities include syndactyly, skull deformities, spina bifida, clubfoot and shortening of the legs and arms.

Teeth may show delayed dentition, pegged or conical crowns, malformed and missing teeth.

Abnormalities of the central nervous system (CNS) include mental retardation, spastic paralysis, convulsions and microcephaly.

Albright's syndrome: This syndrome includes polyostotic fibrous dysplasia of the long bones, endocrine dysfunction and precocious puberty in females. café au lait spots are present at birth or appear soon after. These spots are larger, darker and have more serrated margins than neurofibromatosis, they tend to be unilateral. They have a predilection for the forehead, nuchal area, sacrum and buttocks. The cause of this disorder may be abnormally functioning ovarian cysts. Estrogen receptors in the bone may account for the bony lesions.

Acquired Patchy Pigmentations

Lentigines: These are brown macules due to localised increase in epidermal melanocytes. They appear in childhood and increase until adult life. They may be flat or slightly raised; they do not darken on exposure to sunlight. Elderly people often develop large lentigines on light exposed areas. Lentigines also develop in patients receiving photochemotherapy (PUVA therapy); cellular atypia may be seen in these lentigines. Several systemic and genetic disorders are associated with localised or generalised lentigines.

Postinflammatory pigmentation: In some inflammatory diseases, such as eczema and lichen planus hypermelanosis occurs, especially in pigmented races. This is probably due to the release of proteolytic enzymes, which activates tyrosinase. The patch of pigmentation that follows fixed drug eruption also belongs in this category. Persistent rubbing or scratching also provokes patchy pigmentation.

Melasma (Chloasma): This is a common disorder of the facial skin, pigmentation occurring mainly in women. The highest incidence is during the reproductive years, often precipitated by pregnancy and taking of oral contraceptives with a high oestrogen content. It may be associated with ovarian disorders. There are reports of melasma occurring after use of cosmetics. Chloasma is uncommon in men, but when present it is more difficult to treat. Drugs, such as hydantoin sodium can cause chloasma in both men and women. Acquired immunodeficiency syndrome (AIDS) may also give rise to similar pigmentation. The cause of melasma is unknown, sunlight and genetic factors are important.

The lesions are pale or dark brown patches of pigmentation with irregular borders, sites of predilection are the cheeks, nose, upper lip and forehead. Three patterns are seen; centrofacial, malar and mandibular. The pigmentation is frequently bilateral. The pigmentation may be predominantly epidermal (brown), dermal (bluish) or epidermal/dermal (brownish-blue) (Fig. 2).

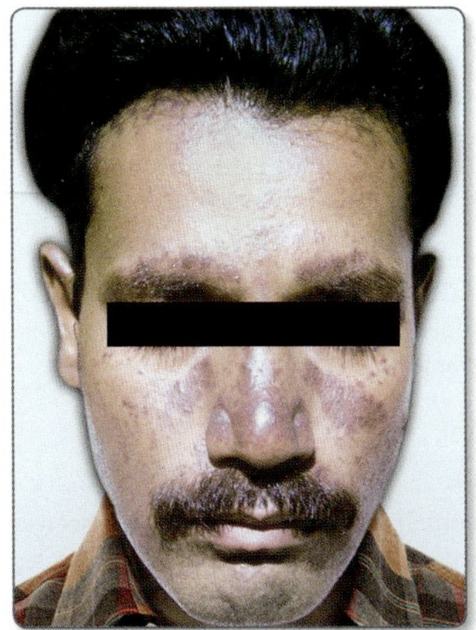

Fig. 2: Melasma

Histologically, there are three forms of melasma depending upon the distribution of the pigment: epidermal, dermal or both epidermal and dermal. The "epidermal type" is the most common in which the pigmentation appears more intense under Wood's lamp examination. Epidermal melasma is most responsive to therapy.

Differential Diagnosis

Hyperpigmentation on the face after using photosensitising agents in soaps and cosmetics must be considered. Some drugs may cause photosensitivity and subsequent pigmentation, such as chlorpromazine, nalidixic acid and tetracyclines.

In peribuccal pigmentation of Brocq there is diffuse pigmentation around the mouth. In poikiloderma of Civatte reticular pigmentation, atrophy and telangiectasia are found on the sides of the cheek and neck. Postinflammatory pigmentation on the face may be confused with melasma. In Addison's disease diffuse hyperpigmentation also occurs at other sites.

Periorbital Hyperpigmentation

The pigmentation may be genetic with an autosomal dominant inheritance. The genetic factors are more frequent in people with dark skin. The pigmentation may extend to the eyebrows and the cheeks. The pigment is melanin. There is an increase in basal melanocytes with upper and mid dermal melanophages.

Treatment

Topical hydroquinone is the most commonly used depigmenting agent. It is more effective when used in combination with tretinoin and dexamethasone, exposure to sunlight should be avoided, and a sunblock should be used daily. Hydroquinone may cause allergic sensitization and exogenous ochronosis. Recent evidence has shown that it can be carcinogenic when taken orally. The study has been done on animals.

Topical azelaic acid, kojic acid alone or in combination with glycolic acid or hydroquinone, has produced good results.

0.1% Adapalene gel used for 3–4 months has shown a similar response as 0.05% tretinoin cream.

Arbutin cream is also used for the treatment of hyperpigmentation, it is a derivative of hydroquinone. It inhibits the action of tyrosinase, and does not have the side effects of hydroquinone. It is natural extract found in bearberry plant.

Other creams that have been used are: liquirtin cream (a flavonoid derived from liquorice) used twice daily for 4 weeks has shown good results in some patients.

A few studies have shown some response to a phenolic thioether (N-acetyl-4-S-cysteaminyl-phenol), applied daily for 4 weeks. The cream is less irritating than hydroquinone and is specific for melanocytes.

Chemical peels may induce temporary bleaching; the area treated first turns red and then black. The black eschar peels off usually within a week. Lasers have also been used for melasma, it is not suitable for dark skin. Lasers (Q-switched ruby, erbium:YAG, fractional), intense pulsed light have also been used.

Periorbital pigmentation may be due to cosmetics or it may be a part of generalised pigmentation, such as Addison's disease. It may be due to chronic diseases such as chronic renal and liver failure (Fig. 3).

Reticular Hyperpigmentation

Localised Reticular Pigmentation

Acroreticular pigmentation of Kitamura: This rare disorder is primarily seen in Japan. The disease is associated with depressed reticular pigmented macules on the hands and feet, associated with palmoplantar pits and interrupted dermatoglyphics. The disease is autosomal dominant.

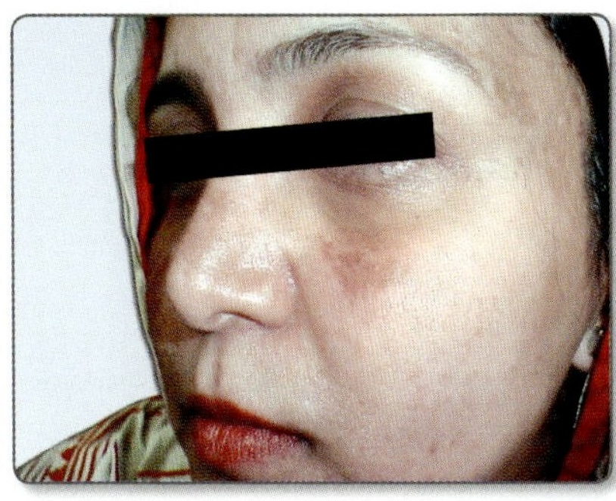

Fig. 3: Periorbital pigmentation

Reticulated pigmented anomaly of the flexures (Dowling-Degos disease): The disease is similar to Kitamura disease, but this involves the flexures. It also has an autosomal dominant inheritance.

Galli-Galli disease: The condition is similar to Dowling-Degos disease, but histology shows acantholysis.

Erythema ab igne: This follows local application of heat-like sitting in front of a heater or fire to keep warm in winter. The erythema later becomes pigmented when melanin is deposited in the dermis.

Generalised Reticular Pigmentation

Dermatopathia pigmentosa reticularis: There is a generalised reticular pigmentation of the trunk and extremities. Non-scarring alopecia, nail dystrophy, occasional hypohidrois and absence of fingerprints are other associated features. This is a rare dermatosis with autosomal dominant inheritance (Figs 4 and 5).

Naegeli-Franceschetti-Jadassohn syndrome: This is a rare genodermatosis with autosomal dominant inheritance. Generalised reticular hyperpigmentation, marked in the groins, axillae and the neck. It is associated with palmoplantar hyperkeratosis, adermatoglyphia, hypohidrosis and dental anomalies. The hair is normal.

Confluent and reticulated papillomatosis of Gougerot and Carteaud: This is a distinctive acquired dermatosis associated with dark scaly papules and plaques in reticulated pattern on the central trunk: interscapular and intermammary region. The lesion bears a clinical resemblance to pityriasis versicolor. Clinical response to minocycline suggests that the condition could be due to an abnormal response to infection. Topical keratolytics and systemic antibiotics or retinoid are the treatment of choice.

Dyskeratosis congenita (Zinsser-Cole-Engman syndrome): Dyskeratosis congenita (DC) is an inherited bone marrow failure syndrome, primarily caused by defects in the maintenance of chromosome telomeres. It is characterised clinically by the triad of abnormal nails, reticular skin pigmentation, and oral leucoplakia. Early mortality is often associated with bone marrow failure, infections, fatal pulmonary complications, or malignancy.

It is an X-linked recessive disorder, although occasional cases of autosomal recessive inheritance have been documented.

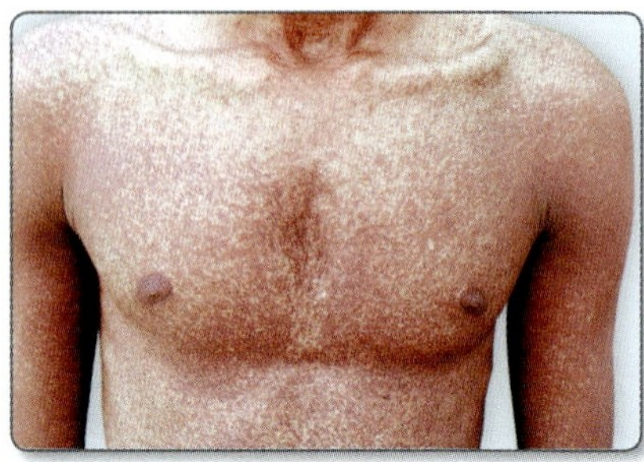

Fig. 4: Dermatopathia pigmentosa reticularis

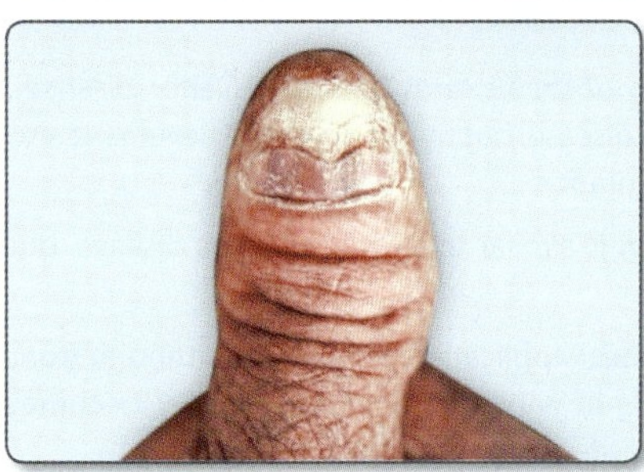

Fig. 5: Dermatopathia pigmentosa reticularis—nail dystrophy

Nail dystrophy is the first sign of disease, which manifests below the age of 5 years, the nails are lost by the time the child is 10 years. Poikiloderma is present on the neck and thighs. Oral leucoplakia has the risk of developing into squamous cell carcinoma. Pancytopenia is usually the cause of death.

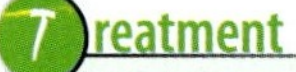

The oral lesions should be monitored for malignant change. Pancytopenia may benefit from bone marrow transplantation.

Dyschromatosis

Symmetrical hereditary dyschromatosis of Dohi: This keratosis (hypo- and hyperpigmentation) is also seen primarily in Japan, it has an autosomal dominant inheritance. The dorsal aspect of the extremities is mostly affected; the trunk is involved in some cases.

Dyschromatosis symmetrica universalis hereditaria: The condition is similar to that of Dohi, but with generalised involvement.

GENERALISED HYPOPIGMENTATION

Hypopigmentation can be melanocytopenic, such as due to failure of migration of melanoblasts to the skin, e.g. piebaldism, or due to the failure of mitosis of melanocytes, or due to destruction of melanocytes, e.g. vitiligo.

Hypopigmentation can be melanopenic, due to failure of synthesis of tyrosine as seen in albinism, due to defects in the transfer/defects of melanasomes, e.g. Chediak-Higashi syndrome, or defects in the transfer of melanasomes to keratinocytes, e.g. pityriasis alba and postinflammatory hypopigmentation.

Hypopigmentation can be generalised or localised.

Generalised Hypomelanosis

Albinism is transmitted as a simple recessive trait with consanguinity playing a prominent role; it is due to a congenital inability to form melanin. The number of melanocytes is normal. The reduced melanin synthesis in melanocytes of the skin, hair, and eyes is termed as oculocutaneous albinism.

Classification

- Tyrosinase negative albinism
- Tyrosinase positive albinism

Tyrosinase Negative Albinism

This is due to mutation in tyrosinase gene, melanosomes contain no melanin. Patients with absence of tyrosinase have white hair, white skin and blue eyes. The pupils are red in colour; patient have poor vision with photophobia and nystagmus. These patients do not tans on exposure to light.

Hair bulbs are negative for tyrosinase.

The patients should strictly avoid sunlight; eyes should be protected by glasses that block UVL. A regular dermatological and ophthalmic examination should be done at frequent intervals.

Tyrosinase Positive Albinism

This is the common form of albinism. There is a reduction in the synthesis of eumelanin primarily, less effect on pheomelanin. There are many phenotypes; skin colour varies from creamy white to yellow, freckles and some pigmentation may develop with age. The patient slightly tans on exposure to light. There is some pigment present in the eyes; eye defects are less severe than those of tyrosinase negative albinism.

Hair bulb test is positive for tyrosinase.

Hair bulb test for tyrosinase: Incubating the plucked hair bulbs *in vitro* with tyrosinase or DOPA can differentiate the two varieties. The hair bulb shows pigment deposition in tyrosinase positive patients, there will be no pigment formation in tyrosinase negative patients (Fig. 6).

Treatment

No treatment is available; prevention of sun damage is essential with a sun protection factor of 30 or more. Eyes should be shielded by glasses that block UVL. Regular clinical check-up is essential for early diagnosis of skin tumours. Ocular problems require ophthalmological supervision.

Patients have a high risk of developing multiple skin cancers because of the poor protection against ultraviolet light.

Table 1: Difference between tyrosinase positive and tyrosinase negative albinism

ALBINISM (Tyrosinase positive)	*ALBINISM (Tyrosinase negative)*
Inheritance Autosomal recessive	Autosomal recessive

Contd...

Contd...

ALBINISM (Tyrosinase positive)	*ALBINISM (Tyrosinase negative)*
Hair bulb darkens when incubated with tyrosine	Hair bulb does not darken when exposed to tyrosine
Skin colour Pale yellow to yellowish brown	White to pale pink
Hair colour Pale yellow to yellowish brown	White
Skin and hair darken over the years	Colour remains the same
Eye Error of refraction + Nystagmus + Iris- bluish gray or lightly pigmented Photophobia + Visual acuity improves with age	Error of refraction ++ Nystagmus ++ Iris- translucent, pink, Photophobia ++ Visual acuity does not improve
Melanosomes develop up to stage 3	Melanosomes develop up to stage 2
Pigmented naevi, lentigenes and freckles often develop over the years	No pigmented lesions develop

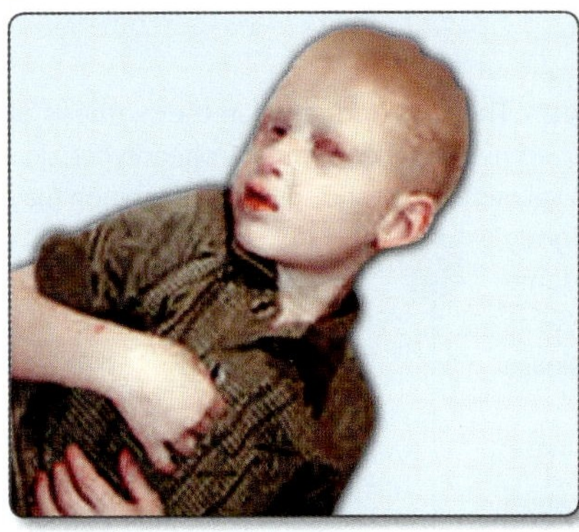

Fig. 6: Albinism

Hermansky-Pudlak syndrome: In this syndrome oculocutaneous albinism is associated with bleeding diathesis, and a lipofuscin like lysosomal storage in a number of tissues. It is autosomal recessive in inheritance. The disease affects the melanocytes, platelets and other tissues, such as the lungs, kidneys and intestines, causing intestinal and pulmonary fibrosis and renal insufficiency. Patients have blond hair, blue eyes, freckling, and multiple melanocytic naevi. The disease is rare, found more frequently in Caribbean Island. It is caused by a mutation of seven different genes.

Sun protection and regular monitoring is required.

Aspirin is contraindicated in Hermansky –Pudlak syndrome.

Chediak-Higashi syndrome: This is an autosomal recessive disorder characterised by severe immunological defects, hypopigmentaion and bleeding tendency. The skin is pale with silvery hair, bluish-white or light brown irises.

The immunological defect is due to the presence of large peroxidase-positive lysosomes in the peripheral blood granulocytes. Like Hermansky-Pudlak syndrome, this syndrome affects many tissues. The hypopigmentation is due to the defect in the granules of the melanocytes. The hypopigmentation is not prominent, it is noted when the patient is compared with other family members.

The infections should be promptly treated. Bone marrow transplantation is helpful.

Phenylketonuria: Is due to congenital deficiency of phenylalanine hydroxylase, with subsequent accumulation of phenylketones that are toxic to the cerebral neurones. Phenylalanine is a competitive inhibitor of tyrosinase and the patients are therefore of light complexion, who look like angels, but behaving like devils, because of their mental deficiency and aggression. It is important to detect this disease at birth in order to restrict dietary phenylalanine.

Hypopituitarism: It causes the skin to become pale because of adrenocorticotropic hormone (ACTH) and melanocyte-stimulating hormone (MSH) deficiency. Pallor with axillary hair loss suggests the diagnosis. The possibility may be considered in any woman whose periods fail to recur after the birth of a child.

Localised Hypopigmentation

This may be due to vitiligo, pityriasis versicolor, pityriasis alba, postinflammatory hypopigmentation, leprosy, pinta, etc. Most of these diseases have been discussed in their respective chapters. Vitiligo and idiopathic guttate hypomelanosis will be discussed here.

VITILIGO

It is a common disorder, manifested by depigmented white patches, surrounded by a normal or a hyperpigmented border. Vitiligo affects about 3% of the population, and shows no racial, sexual, or regional differences. The condition is asymptomatic, but in dark skin individuals, the colour contrast causes considerable social embarrassment. It often misinterpreted as leprosy by the common man.

Vitiligo begins before the age of 20 years, men and women are equally affected. There is a family history in about one third of the cases. Vitiligo is often associated with other autoimmune disorders, such as pernicious anaemia, Addison's disease, diabetes mellitus, thyroid disorders and alopecia areata. About 40% of vitiligo patients have some subclinical pigmentary abnormalities of the retina.

Pathophysiology

The following mechanisms for vitiligo have been proposed:

- Autoimmune - patients with vitiligo also have increased organ specific antibodies, including antibody against thyroid, adrenal and pancreas
- Neurogenic - some neurotoxic agent is liberated near the melanocytes, causing depigmentation
- Self-destructive - melanin production makes a toxin that destroys melanocytes
- Exogenous chemicals - thiols, phenols, catechols, mercaptoamines and several quinones produce depigmentation by inhibition of tyrosinase; some may also have a direct action on the melanocytes.

Clinical Features

Depigmented patches (chalky white) are first noticed in the sun-exposed areas of the body, such as the face and hands, these are liable to sunburn. Other sites of vitiligo are those subject to trauma, such as the knees, elbows and ankles, or those areas, which are normally hyperpigmented, such as axillae, groins, genitals and areolae. It also commonly affects the periorbital, perioral and anogenital areas. The distribution of the lesions is usually symmetrical but, sometimes it may be unilateral and may have a dermatomal arrangement. Rarely vitiligo may be generalised. The hair in patches of early stage of vitiligo remain normally pigmented, but later the hair may also turn white.

Spontaneous re-pigmentation is seen in 10–20% of patients, most frequently in the sun-exposed areas. The pigmentation is first perifollicular. Premature graying of the hair, uveitis, abnormalities of the fundus, and deafness may occur in some cases.

Segmental vitiligo may or may not follow a dermatome. The segmental variety is seen at an earlier age, it is not associated with autoimmune diseases, and spontaneous re-pigmentation occurs more often in this type of vitiligo.

A typical macule of vitiligo is chalky white in colour; it is round or oval with an irregular border, surrounded by normal skin. A patch of vitiligo may be a few millimetres to several centimetres. In trichome vitiligo there is a narrow or broad uniform tan interface between the patch of vitiligo and the normal skin. This tan colour usually evolves into a normal white vitiligo macule. A quadrichrome vitiligo includes the perifollicular pigmentation with trichome vitiligo. Blue vitiligo occurs in regions of postinflammatory hyperpigmentation (Figs 7 to 9).

Mucosal involvement is frequent, vitiligo involving the lips, nipples, genitalia and the gingival mucosa. Other cutaneous abnormalities associated with vitiligo are alopecia areata, halo naevi, premature gray hair and leucotrichia. Poliosis is associated with about 9–45% vitiligo patients.

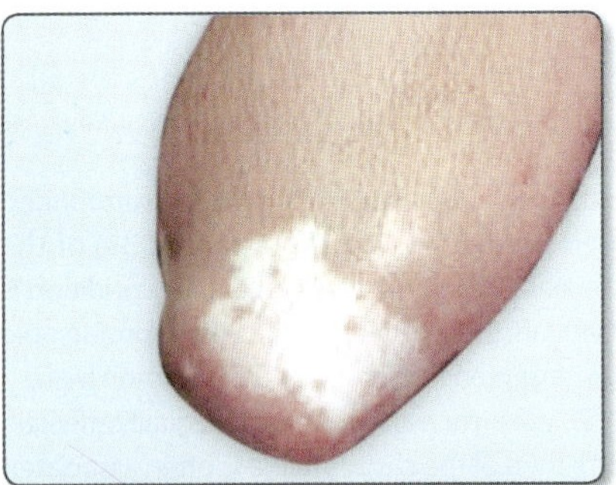

Fig. 7: Vitiligo

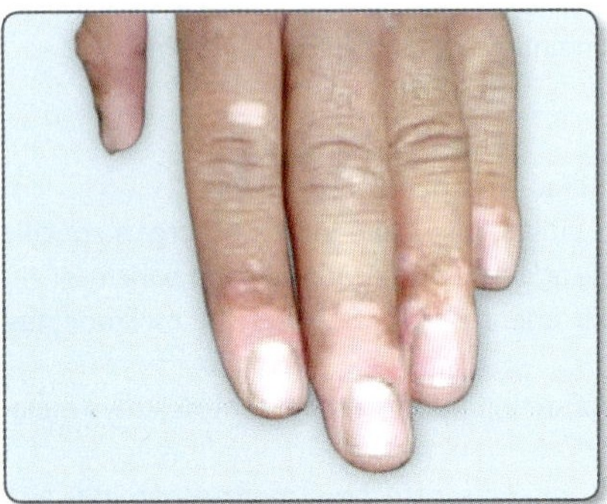

Fig. 8: Vitiligo (fingertip—bad prognosis due to absence of hair follicles

Differential Diagnosis

Pityriasis versicolor is confined to the upper parts of the body, the patches are hypopigmented and scaly, they are not chalky white as in vitiligo. Scraping of the lesion will show the fungus.

In postinflammatory hypopigmentation, there is a previous history of inflammation, the texture of the skin is not normal as in vitiligo, but may manifest irregularity and roughness. Pityriasis alba is seen in children as hypopigmented scaly patches usually on the face. Albinism is present at birth it is generalised and not progressive.

Hypopigmented patches of leprosy have no hair, sweating is absent and the lesion is anaesthetic. A smear examination and a biopsy can confirm the diagnosis.

Lichen sclerosus et atrophicus and morphea have hypopigmented areas but have abnormal skin texture.

Treatment

The treatment is unsatisfactory in most cases; an effective cosmetic camouflage for lesions on the exposed skin is required. Cosmetic cover up with Vitadye and Dy-o-Derm stains are used. These cosmetics are mixed to match the skin hues to mask the white skin. In sunny climates, sunscreens are necessary.

A small percentage may respond to topical steroid therapy. Topical steroids may be used with careful monitoring. These are especially effective on the face of dark skinned people.

Narrowband UVB therapy (311 nm), 2–3 times weekly is used as firstline therapy, both in adults and children, as it is free of psoralen side effects.

Psoralens and ultraviolet light. The best results are obtained with oral psoralens. The treatment is time consuming and may have to be continued for up to 2 years. Asians and Afro-Caribbeans respond better to treatment than Caucasoids. If follicular pigmentation has not occurred in 3 months, it should be considered as a therapeutic failure and treatment should be stopped.

Psoralens can be applied topically or taken orally. Topical treatment is usually meant for localised lesions. The local psoralen should be diluted before application or else the skin will show marked irritation. Oral psoralens (tri-psoralen or 8-methoxy psoralen), are given in a dose of 0.6 mg/kg of body weight, 2 hours before exposure to sunlight. Starting with a 15 minutes exposure and then increasing to 5 minutes per exposure until a faint persistent erythema is obtained. About 30–100 treatments may be required to elicit repigmentation. A sunscreen should be used in the non-vitiliginous area to avoid sun tanning and thereby increasing the colour contrast. Spectacles that protect against UVL should be worn, and the patient should avoid sunlight for the rest of the day.

Tacrolimus and narrow band UVB therapy are also effective in the treatment of vitiligo, but the two should not be given at the same time.

Topical calcipotriol has been used in combination with topical corticosteroids, narrowband UVB and PUVA for the treatment of vitiligo with some success.

Khellin is a furanochromone; it is being tried for the treatment of vitiligo. Furanochromone is a photosensitiser in combination with ultraviolet light. It does not produce phototoxic erythema.

Patients with vitiligo involving more than two-thirds of the body may prefer to have the normal skin bleached with hydroquinone preparation. Twenty percent monobenzyl ether of hydroquinone cream or 20% hydroxyquinone cream is applied to the skin in qd or bid dose. Depigmentation of the normal skin takes 2–3 months to show initial lightening and may take 1–3 years to complete. Bleaching is permanent.

Minigrafting: Grafts of pigmented skin are transplanted to non-pigmented areas. Melanocyte and stem cell transplants, in which single cell suspensions are made from unaffected skin and applied to the dermabraded affected skin is also used to treat vitiligo.

Micropigmentation (tattooing) involves injecting coloured pigments, mostly iron oxide into the dermis. This may be most useful in the lip area, particularly those with dark skin. Unfortunately, many patients experience significant pigment loss within the first several weeks after the procedure. It is difficult to obtain a perfect match of the colour of the surrounding skin.

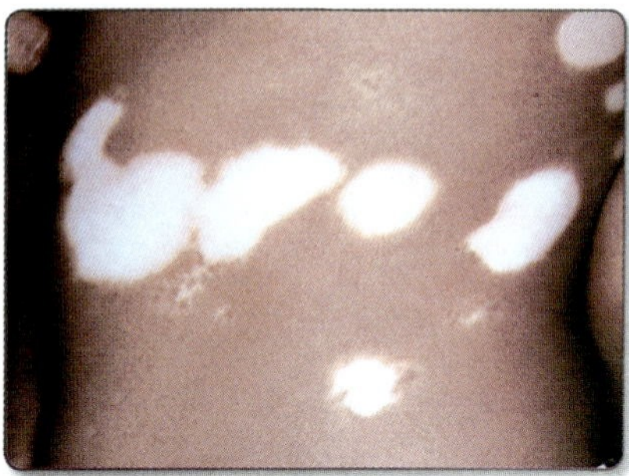

Fig. 9: Segmental vitiligo

Histopathology

There is a decrease and eventually disappearance of melanocytes, which may be partially or completely replaced by Langerhans cells.

Course and Prognosis

The course of vitiligo is unpredictable; lesions may stay stable for years or progress rapidly. About 10–20% of the patients may have some degree of spontaneous regression.

Piebaldism: Piebaldism is an autosomal dominant disorder. It is characterised by a white forelock (poliosis), often with white medial eyebrows, usually present at birth. Permanent and non-progressive amelanotic macules involving forehead, upper chest and back are present in 20% of cases. Hyperpigmented macules within the amelanotic macule and on normally pigmented skin are characteristic of piebaldism.

Piebaldism should be differentiated from vitiligo. Piebaldism is present at birth and is not progressive.

Treatment is by autologous minigrafts.

Waardenburg's syndrome: This is a rare autosomal dominant disorder associated with piebaldism. It is characterised by lateral displacement of the inner canthi, broad nasal bridge, heterochromia, congenital deafness, white forelock and hypomelanotic macules.

Alezzandrini's syndrome: This is also associated with poliosis. The syndrome is characterised by unilateral facial vitiligo, poliosis, deafness and retinal degeneration on the same side as the vitiligo. The cause is unknown, a viral and autoimmune hypothesis have been postulated. The skin lesions are treated on the same pattern as vitiligo.

Vogt-Koyanagi-Harada syndrome (VKHS): The syndrome is characterised by vitiligo, poliosis, uveitis, dysacousia and alopecia. The syndrome appears in three stages:

The first stage is that of meningoencephalitis with fever, headache, nausea and vomiting. The degree of cerebral involvement is variable.

The second stage appears rapidly and lasts for 10 or more years. It is associated with decreased visual acuity, photophobia, uveitis and retinal detachment. Dysacousia is usually bilateral; it is present in 50% of cases.

The convalescent phase starts as uveitis begins to abate; this stage is characterised by alopecia, poliosis and vitiligo.

Hypomelanosis of Ito (Incontinentia pigmenti achromians): The condition is characterised by bizarre pattern of hypopigmentation in a whorled, streak and marble-cake like configuration. The lesions correspond to the lines of Blaschko. Any part of the body can be involved. The lesions are present at birth. It is often associated with other abnormalities, such as mental or motor retardation, microcephaly, ataxia, deafness, strabismus, nystagmus, symblepharon, myopia, and skeletal defects.

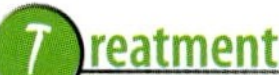

Systemic corticosteroids are indicated for eye involvement. Skin lesions are treated as for vitiligo.

Histology shows rounded melanocytes, with reduced or absent dendrites, and reduced epidermal-melanin pigmentation.

Naevus depigmentosus: Three clinical forms are described: isolated, which can be circular or rectangular, a dermatomal pattern, or in the form of streaks or whorls. The lesions remain stable throughout life. Its aetiology is debated, whether it a distinct entity or a manifestation of cutaneous mosaicism.

IDIOPATHIC GUTTATE HYPOMELANOSIS

This is a common disorder first described by Matsumoto in 1923. The lesion occurs chiefly on the shins and forearms. The lesions are chalky-white, round about 2–6 mm in diameter; they are usually less than a dozen or two in number. They are not found on the trunk or face. The lesions are commonly seen in women after the age of 40 years. The borders are sharply defined, often angular and irregular. It is probably due to somatic mutation of melanocytes (Fig. 10).

Tyndall effect reflects the change that light undergoes as it passes through the skin. Colours of longer wavelength, such as red, orange and yellow continue travelling forward, while those of shorter wavelength, such as blue, indigo and violet are scattered. This scattered light is seen by the viewer. Tyndall effect thus explains why subcutaneous lesions have a bluish tinge.
John Tyndall was a 19th century physicist.
Melanocytes originate in the neural crest; they then migrate to the skin, retina, uvea, cochlea and labyrinth. Any disorder that affects the migration of melanocytes in the skin, can also affect the eyes, ear and the central nervous system.

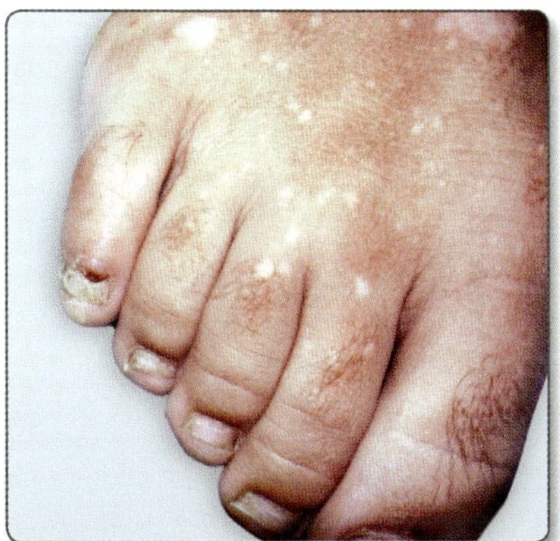

Fig. 10: Idiopathic guttate hypomelanosis

FURTHER READING

1. Dermatopathia Pigmentosa Reticularis. A Case report. Z Zaidi, N Jafri, S Ebeidat, H Thawerani. JPMA. 1995;11(1):73-7.
2. Falabella R, Eseobar C, Giraldo N, et al. On the pathogenesis of idiopathic guttate hypomelanosis. J Am Acad Dermatol. 1987;16(1):35-44.
3. Full CS. Primary disorders of hypopigmentation. J Am Acad Dermatol. 1984;10(1):1-16.
4. Gordon B, Sparano BM, Iatropoulos MJ. Hyperpigmentation in the skin associated with minocycline therapy. Arch Dermatol. 1985;121(5):618-23.
5. Parsad D, Kanwar JA, Kumar B. Psoralen Ultraviolet A vs Narrowband Ultraviolet B phototherapy in the treatment of vitilgo. J Eur Acad Dermatol Venereol. 2006;20(2):175-7.
6. Pinto FJ, Bolognia JL. Disorders of hypopigmentation in children. Pediatr Clin N Am. 1991;38(4):991-1017.
7. Slominski A, Tobin DJ, Shibahara S, Wortsman J. Melanin pigmentation in mamamlian skin and its hormonal regulation. Physiol Rev. 2004;84(4):1155-228.
8. Smith AG, Shusyer S, Thoday AJ, Peberdy M. Chloasma, oral contraceptives and plasma immunoreactive-melanocytic stimulating hormone. J Ivest Dermatol. 1977; 68(4):169-70.
9. Uhle P, Norvell SS. Generalised lentiginosis. J Am Acad Dermatol. 1988;18(2):444-7.
10. Witkop CJJ. Inherited disorders of pigmentation. Clin Dermatol. 1985;3(1):70-134.
11. Zaynoun ST, Aftimos BG, Tenekjian KK, et al. Extensive pityriasis alba: a histological, histochemical and ultrastructural study. Br J Dermatol. 1983;108(1):83-90.
12. Zaidi Z, Jafri N, Ebeidat S, et al. Dermatopathia pigmentosa reticularis. A case report. J Pak Med Assoc. 1995;11(1):73-7.

Chapter

20 Skin and Ultraviolet Radiation

INTRODUCTION

Skin is the only organ, which is exposed to the direct hazards of external environment. Our survival is offered by protective mechanisms provided by the skin. Sunlight exposure, which is moderate for a short duration of 10–15 minutes daily, is healthy. Moderate sunlight exposure has a useful effect on the human body; it helps in the production of vitamin D, and has a positive influence on psyche. Ultraviolet radiation (UVR) is used for the treatment of cutaneous disorders, such as vitiligo, psoriasis, atopic dermatitis and pruritus. But exposure to strong sunlight even for a short duration is harmful. It leads to photoageing, immunosuppression and malignancy.

Spending vacations in sunny climate, tanning with artificial light should be discouraged, because ultraviolet light (UVL) is a potent carcinogen. It is responsible for extrinsic ageing, demonstrated by stochastic theory of ageing. This theory states that cumulative environmental damage to genes and proteins; ultimately produces ageing and homeostatic failure.

Radiation passes through various layers of the skin, from the stratum corneum to the viable layers of the epidermis, to the dermal connective and the cells of the dermis. The absorption of UVL by the skin is dependent on the wavelength. Radiation of shorter wavelength, such as ultraviolet B (UVB) is reflected or absorbed by the epidermis. By contrast radiation of longer wavelength, such as ultraviolet A (UVA), penetrates deeply into the dermis. Small amounts of radiation reaching the basal cells, is likely to cause important biological reactions.

The sun emits a continuous spectrum of electromagnetic energy, from the short cosmic rays to the long radio waves. This includes the UVL (200–400 nm), visible light (400–700 nm), infrared rays (>760–10^5 nm), and radio waves and microwaves >10^5 nm (Fig. 1). The atmosphere absorbs most of the short wavelengths and none shorter than 280 nm reaches the ground level. UVR spectrum consists of 3 wavebands — ultraviolet C (UVC) (200–290 nm), UVB (290–320 nm), narrow band UVB is at 311 nm, and UVA (320–400 nm) (Fig. 2). UVA is further subdivided in to UVA 11 (320–340 nm) and UVA 1 (340–400 nm). Solar UVR on the earth's surface is approximately 95–98% UVA and 2–5% UVB.

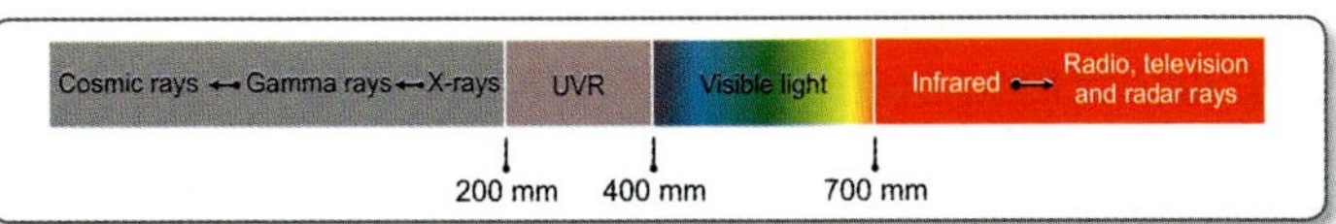

Fig. 1: Spectrum of sunlight

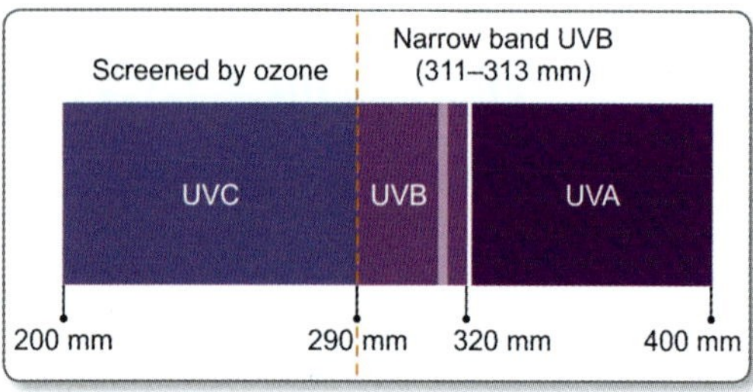

Fig. 2: Spectrum of ultraviolet radiation (UVR)

Sunburn in the human skin, is produced by a narrow band of radiation that extends from (290–320 nm) UVB. Shorter wavelengths UVC (200–290 nm) are more effective in producing sunburn, because these do not reach the sea level and are blocked by the ozone layer of the atmosphere. With the break in the ozone layer, the chances of sunburn and malignancy to the skin are high. The radiations of longer wavelength UVA have relatively little effect on the normal skin, it is invisible to man; this wavelength is sometimes called the "black light". UVA causes certain substances to emit fluorescence; it is important in some diseases, such as porphyria and drugs, such as psoralens that sensitize the normal skin to UVA. Most window glass absorbs the wavelengths less than 315 nm and thus prevents sunburn. Infrared rays (700–5000 nm) generally do not cause biological damage, unless they are of sufficient intensity to generate heat. These are generally used for diathermy. Gamma rays, X-rays are of very short wavelength (smaller than 200 nm) penetrate the skin deeply into the tissues where it can cause extensive damage.

SITES OF PHOTOSENSITIVE ERUPTION

The areas exposed to sunlight are the forehead, nose, cheeks, rim of the ears, sides and back of the neck, V area of the chest, extensor surface of the forearms, dorsum of the hands, shins and feet when exposed.

Sparing of the shielded areas is characteristic of photosensitive eruption; these include the retro-auricular folds, sub-mental region, upper eyelids protected by the supraorbital ridge, nasolabial folds and flexor aspect of the forearms.

STANDARD ERYTHEMA DOSE

Standard erythema dose (SED) is equivalent to an erythematous effective exposure of 100 J/m^2; it is independent of individual sensitivity to UVR and specific UVR spectrum. An exposure of 2–4 SED would be expected to produce mild sunburn on previously unexposed skin.

ULTRAVIOLET RADIATION AND ITS INTERACTION WITH THE SKIN

About 5% of the UVR falling on the skin is diffusely reflected back, the remainder is transmitted, scattered, absorbed or passed out of the medium.

Radiation below 300 nm is largely removed through the epidermis by urocanic acid, deoxyribonucleic acid (DNA), ribonucleic acid (RNA), tryptophan, tyrosine and melanin. Any remnants passing through are presumably absorbed by the dermal DNA, RNA and amino acids in elastin and collagen. Radiation above 300 nm passes mostly into the dermis after variable melanin absorption followed by reflection back from the dermal collagen bundles to the environment. In addition, minor absorption also occurs through the intravascular haemoglobin, tissue bilirubin and β carotene in the fat.

EFFECTS OF ULTRAVIOLET RADIATION ON THE SKIN AT MOLECULAR LEVEL

Skin cells respond to UVR by release of inflammatory mediators, transient growth arrest, followed by hyperplasia and special adaptive changes, such as increased melanin production. In the absence of further radiation, the cells return to baseline status. But with increased exposure to radiation the adaptive mechanisms get exhausted, it is followed by cellular atrophy, loss of function, or by mutation.

Epidermal Changes

Keratinocytes

In the epidermis, there are areas of hyperplasia and atrophy of keratinocytes. The atrophy represents depletion of competent cells from the germinative epithelium; while hyperplasia represents compensatory hypertrophy of UVR damaged cells. Loss of germinative cells is due to direct effect of the cells by UVR. This results in the generation of reactive oxygen species, which damages the cell membrane as well as cellular proteins. The natural scavengers for reactive molecular oxygen include enzymes, such as superoxide dismutase, glutathione peroxidases and catalase. These enzymes are decreased by UVR.

Epidermal cytoskeleton proteins are also affected by UVR. The protein reticular network is broken down with the formation of a microfilament ring at the periphery of the cell.

Melanocytes

The irregular pigmentation is characteristic of photodamaged skin. The hyperpigmentation is due to hyperplasia of melanocytes leading to the formation of freckles, lentigines and hyperpigmented macules. These are interspaced by areas of hypopigmentation due to depletion of melanocytes, or severely damaged melanocytes, which cannot transfer melanin to the surrounding keratinocytes.

After UV exposure leukotriene C4 and D4 increase, which are mitogenic to melanocytes. Topical application of arachidonic acid, such as prostaglandin E2 is said to increase the number of dopa-positive melanocytes. Other melanocyte stimulants are fibroblast growth factor and transforming growth factor alpha (TGF-α). Direct effect of UVR on melanocyte membrane also contributes to irregular pigmentation in photoaged skin.

Photocarcinogenesis

Ultraviolet radiation is the most important factor responsible for cutaneous malignancy. UVR produces DNA mutations along with suppression of cutaneous immune response. Tumours develop in a stepwise process, which include molecular alteration in cellular DNA. This involves activation of growth promoting genes (proto-oncogenes), or inactivation of tumour suppression genes. Proto-oncogene proteins, such as c-Fos proteins and H-Ras proteins are increased by UVR leading to their mutation, which predispose to malignancy.

Dermal Changes

Ultraviolet A penetrates deeper in the skin than UVB. Most of the changes in the dermis are produced by UVA, but UVB also plays an important role. Fibroblasts are main cells of the dermis responsible or the production of elastin, collagen and ground substance. Normally fibroblasts proliferate at a slow rate and synthesize low levels of proteolytic enzymes. Under UVR the fibroblast are activated by IL-1 and TNF-α, similar to changes that occur in the epidermis. The usual fibrillar structure of the dermis is replaced by connective tissue, which is arranged in irregular clumps and strands. The immediate sub-epidermal zone (Grenz zone), is free of elastotic change, the reason for this is unclear.

Changes in Elastin

The histologic hallmark of dermal photoageing is elastosis. Under UVR fibroblasts are stimulated to produce increased amounts of elastin, which is abnormal. When elastin is deposited on the microfibrils, it becomes abnormally wide and susceptible to enzymatic degradation. Elastin fibres are digested by elastase or chymotrypsin like enzymes.

Changes in Collagen

Normally about 85% of collagen in the dermis is collagen 1, and 10% is collagen 111. Under UVB sun exposed areas show a decrease in collagen 1 and increase of collagen 111. The collagen fibre is also photodamaged. It displays abnormal basophilic degeneration and homogenisation. Sometimes the increased deposition of abnormal homogenised collagen in the dermal papillae appears on the surface as colloid milium. This is often seen after a very heavy sun exposure. Since UVR produces cross-links between collagen molecules, which render it more susceptible to enzymatic degeneration. The increase of collagenase is due to release of IL–6, which is released by fibroblasts. Collagenase is also produced by mast cells and keratinocytes. The other enzymes that produce homogenisation of collagen are cathepsin and chymotrypsin like enzymes.

Changes in the Ground Substance

The biochemical changes in the ground substance are increased production of glycosaminoglycan/proteoglycan complexes. The increased proteoglycans are mainly hyaluronate and dermatan sulphate. These are due to metabolic changes in the fibroblasts.

EFFECTS OF SOLAR RADIATION ON THE SKIN

These can be studied under the following headings:

- Acute reactions
- Chronic reactions.

Acute Reactions

Sunburn is due to UVB, it is manifested by painful erythema and oedema that develops in 2–3 hours after exposure to the sun. It reaches its maximum in 24 hours and is then followed by peeling of skin in a few days. Use of sunscreens can prevent sunburn. It is treated by the use of soothing lotions, such as calamine; liberal application of talcum powder and in some cases a topical steroid lotion or spray. Systemic steroids are indicated in severe cases. Prostaglandins are produced in the skin in sunburn; indomethacin, which inhibits the enzyme prostaglandin synthetase, can decrease the sunburn due to UVB.

Tanning

Both UVA and UVB stimulate the formation of melanin for some days following exposure to the sun. UVA produces immediate and UVB produces late tanning. The new melanin forms a 'cap' over the keratinocyte nuclei to protect DNA from further damage.

Epidermal Thickening

The epidermis may double its thickness following radiation, it is important in providing protection against further damage by UVL.

Vitamin D Production

Vitamin D_3 (calciferol) is formed in skin from dehydrocholesterol with the help of UVR. Exposure to sunlight is thus helpful in preventing rickets and osteomalacia in individuals who have a deficient intake of this vitamin.

Immunological Effects

It is now well established that PUVA therapy causes a temporary suppression of type 4 or delayed hypersensitivity reactions in the skin. This is associated with a depletion of epidermal Langerhans cells. The success of PUVA therapy in treating T cell lymphomas suggests that this irradiation also affects the lymphocytes. Recent work suggests that ordinary sunburn can also produce immunosuppression. In medieval age, patients with tuberculosis were advised to avoid sunbathing as it was supposed to exacerbate the infection; the reason being immunosuppression.

Chronic Reactions

Many of the changes associated with ageing of skin, such as wrinkling, solar keratosis, lentigines, dryness, inelasticity and thinning of the skin are due to chronic exposure of skin to UVR of the sun. There is some evidence that UVA can potentiate the damaging effects of UVB. Chronic exposure of the sun is precancerous and can lead to malignancy. The following are the changes due to prolonged exposure to the sun.

Actinic Keratosis

These are premalignant scaly lesions, which develop on skin exposed to UVB; common sites are the back of the hands, forehead and ears. Clinically they appear as scaly hyperpigmented plaques. The histology shows dysplastic changes with loss of normal keratinocyte maturation, and areas of parakeratosis. There is usually a period of several years between the development of solar keratosis and its transformation to squamous cell carcinoma.

Actinic Elastosis

Small yellowish papules and plaques develop on the face or back of the hands. The skin assumes a dull yellowish colour with deep furrows and wrinkles. Histologically there is an increase of elastic tissue staining in the dermis; it is due to deposition of abnormal elastic tissue in the dermis produced by fibroblasts.

Annular Elastolytic Granuloma

Annular elastolytic granuloma (actinic granuloma), is seen on the forearms, upper back and over the head and neck. Pink translucent papules develop, which enlarge into annular lesions 1–3 cm in diameter. Histological examination shows a granuloma, with evidence of destruction of elastic tissue.

Nodular Elastoidosis (Favre-Racouchot Syndrome)

This is seen mainly around the eyes and extends on the cheeks seen in elderly especially in men. The lesions consist of comedones, follicular cysts and large folds of furrowed and yellowish skin. Treatment consists of removal of the comedones and cysts. Retinoic acid cream is often helpful.

Pseudo Colloid Milium

This is another uncommon lesion due to severe elastosis. Translucent papules and plaques are seen on the back of the hands and face.

Cutis Rhomboidalis Nuchae

The skin over the back of the neck becomes thickened, rough, and leathery, the normal skin markings become exaggerated. The condition is often seen in farmers, sailors or people who are exposed to excessive sunlight.

Actinic Cheilitis

This occurs on the lower lips, excessive sunlight produces dryness, scaling, atrophy and telangiectasia. Fissures, keratosis, leucoplakia and carcinoma may develop. It responds well to cryotherapy and 5% fluorouracil.

Triradiate Scars

Irregularly shaped scars are found on the back of hands and forearms in individuals who are chronically exposed to UVR. The scars are linear, triradiate, angulate or stellate; they are usually 1–2 cm in length. The scars occur spontaneously or in response to minor trauma. The scars are perhaps due to an abnormality in tissue repair.

Telangiectasia and Purpura

Telangiectasia and purpura are due to the lack of support to the cutaneous blood vessels. The telangiectasias are prominent on the cheeks; while the purpura is common on the forearms and back of arms. The extravasated blood takes longer to disappear due to depressed macrophage activity.

Senile Comedones and Other Pilosebaceous Abnormalities

Dilated follicular orifices with comedonal plugging are found on the back and face of the elderly. On the face they are found around the eyes and upper cheeks. These are probably due to elastotic degenerative changes.

Sebaceous gland hyperplasia is very common in the elderly. Small yellowish papules are found with a cental puncta over the cheeks and nose.

Poikilodermic Changes

This is characterised by telangiectasia, hyperpigmentation, hypopigmentation and atrophy are often seen on the sides of neck, and V of the chest.

Skin Cancer

Squamous cell carcinoma basal cell carcinoma and, malignant melanoma are enhanced by the total hours of exposure to UVB and perhaps UVA. These are more common in fair skinned people. The more sensitive skin types (skin type 1–3) should take care to avoid excessive exposure to the sun and should use sunscreens.

DISORDERS OF THE SKIN CAUSED BY ULTRAVIOLET LIGHT

The disorders can be studied under the following headings:

- Acquired idiopathic photodermatoses
- Exogenous photosensitisation:
  - Phototoxic reaction
  - Photoallergic reaction
- Endogenous photosensitisation by chemicals, e.g. porphyrias
- DNA repair disorders e.g. Xeroderma pigmentosum
- Dermatoses exacerbated by UVL.

Acquired Idiopathic Photodermatoses

These idiopathic dermatoses are characterised by an abnormal reaction of the skin to UVL. These include the following:

- Polymorphous light eruption
- Actinic prurigo
- Hydroa vacciniforme
- Solar urticaria
- Chronic actinic dermatitis.

Polymorphous Light Eruption

Polymorphous light eruption (PLE) is the most common photosensitisation due to intermittent exposure of sunlight. The eruptions are polymorphous they consist of itchy, erythematous papules or plaques, vesicles on the sun exposed areas of the skin. The eruptions may be uniform or polymorphous in any one patient. The eruptions can also be haemorrhagic or purpuric. It occurs within hours or days after exposure to the sun. The eruptions last for several days, and then resolve spontaneously without scarring. PLE is a type IV hypersensitivity reaction. It is severe in spring and summer and is common in young women.

Actinic Prurigo

The condition is common in both North and South America. Some cases are associated with atopy, conjunctivitis, cheilitis and pterygium formation. Onset is usually in childhood; the lesions consist of itchy papules or nodules these are often excoriated. Facial lesions often heal leaving minute linear or pitted scars.

Hydroa Vacciniforme (Prurigo of Hutchinson)

This is a rare intermittent bullous scarring eruption, the onset is in childhood and resolution often occurs by adolescence or early adult life. On exposure to the sun, erythema develops on the face and less commonly on the hands, blisters soon develop, which are often haemorrhagic. The lesions heal with scarring. Systemic symptoms, such as malaise, fever and headaches often accompany the attack. The condition is difficult to manage. Psoralen ultraviolet A (PUVA) therapy is helpful. Anti-malarials have also been used, but these need careful supervision due to ocular toxicity.

Solar Urticaria

Urticarial reactions are rare. Patients develop stinging and pruritic hives on areas exposed to the sun. Systemic reactions, such as chills, fever, fatigue, syncope and abdominal cramps may also occur. The symptoms subside in several hours. Solar urticaria may occur at any age and in either sex.

Chronic Actinic Dermatitis

Chronic actinic dermatitis (CAD) is an uncommon persisting and often disabling photoallergic dermatitis due to a wide range of light spectrum, it can be UVB, UVA and possibly visible light. The patients are also often sensitive to artificial light, such as fluorescent light.

The histology shows acanthosis, dermal fibrosis and lymphocytic infiltrate. Progression to lymphoma is uncommon.

Chronic actinic dermatitis is seen in elderly men; it may appear on a previously normal skin or follows endogenous eczema. CAD can affect any skin type. The lesions begin as photosensitive eczema; this leads to thick, erythematous lichenoid skin often with indurated plaques. Some patients of CAD are so light sensitive that they are unable to go out during the day; they are unable to tolerate light even in the room. These patients are often depressed and even prone to suicide.

The disease is diagnosed by a phototest. The back is exposed to different wavelengths of light: UVA, UVB and visible light. The test will reveal, to which wavelength the patients is sensitive to. It may be one or more wavelengths.

Photopatch testing is done to remove any other allergen to which the patient may be sensitive.

The disease is treated as any other eczema, paying special attention to photosensitivity. Systemic steroids are used in acute erythroderma secondary to CAD. Azathioprine and cyclosporin also produce remission. Desensitisation by PUVA or UVB is helpful in some cases. Many cases persist for life.

Actinic reticuloid is the term used when histology shows atypical lymphocytes.

Exogenous Photosensitisation

Exogenous photosensitisers are widely distributed in nature; they are present in plants, plant extracts, cosmetics, industrial products, drugs, etc. The photosensitive reactions are:

- Phototoxic reactions
- Photoallergic reactions.

Phototoxic Reactions

These reactions are elicited in any individual provided there is enough light energy of appropriate wavelength and adequate concentration of the phototoxic agent. The immune system does not take part in the reaction. The reaction may begin within a few minutes to a few hours of irradiation. The eruption may be painful, burning and pruritic, in some cases vesicles and blisters are produced, similar to that of sunburn. The phototoxic reactions are common; these may be due to plants, dyes, oils, cosmetics or drugs.

The common drugs that give rise to phototoxic reactions are tricyclic antidepressants, such as imipramine; chloroquine, ciprofloxacin, furosemide, doxycycline and retinoids. Griseofulvin, nalidixic acid, phenothiazine and sulphonamides can cause both phototoxic and photoallergic reaction. Crude coal tar is produced by the destructive distillation of coal. It a mixture of over 10,000 products, these include many phototoxic hydrocarbons. Dyes, such as Rose Bengal used in ophthalmic examination, eosin used in lipsticks are phototoxic.

A number of plants cause phototoxicity. The most important are those containing furocoumarins. Furocoumarins are found in a number of plants, such as compositae species, Umbelliferae, Rutacae and Leguminosae family. These include fruits and vegetables like lime, lemon, fig, celery, parsley, parsnip, and psoralens. In the past patients with vitiligo would rub the juice of these plants and then expose themselves to the sun. This is similar to the principle of phototherapy used today.

Photoallergic Reactions

In photoallergic reactions, the absorbed light energy promotes a photochemical reaction between the chemical and skin proteins, resulting in the formation of a photoallergen. There is photosensitisation to this photoallergen and on subsequent exposure to the allergen, an eczematous response is elicited. An incubation period of 1–3 weeks follows the second or the subsequent exposure to the allergen. The eruption is eczematous and may show flares at a distant from the previously exposed site. Photoallergy is mainly caused by UVA irradiation. It is a type IV hypersensitivity reaction. The eruption is eczematous, in contrast to a burn like reaction in phototoxicity.

Most common photoallergens are sunscreens; the photoallergens are benzophenone and dibenzoylmethane. Fragrances are the second most common cause of photosensitivity. Methylcoumarin, sandalwood and musk ambrette frequently cause photosensitivity. Other photosensitizers include soaps containing halogenated salicylanilides. Skin cleansers, such as chlorhexidine, bithionol, triclosan and dichlorophen are photoallergic.

A number of drugs can cause photosensitivity, some of these are quinine, griseofulvin, quinolone, sulphonamides, non-steroidal anti-inflammatory drugs (NSAIDs), such as ketoprofen and piroxicam.

Photo-onycholysis: It is an unusual form of exogenous photosensitisation that affects the finger nails. There is pain in the fingertips followed by onycholysis; nails may separate from the nail bed. It is usually caused by tetracycline and PUVA therapy. The reaction occurs several weeks after commencing the therapy.

Persistent light reactors: These are rare individuals with photocontact allergy in whom the eruptions persist for months or years in spite of avoidance of the causative sensitiser. These persons are totally intolerant to sunlight.

Diagnosis of photoallergic eruptions: This is done by the photopatch test. The photosensitizers are applied in duplicate on the back of the patient, after 24 hours one set of the applied substance is exposed to UVA irradiation and then covered again. Both tests are observed after 48 hours of application. A positive response in the irradiated site is diagnostic of photoallergic dermatitis.

Evaluation of a Patient with Phototoxicity and Photoallergy

A detailed history is of paramount importance. Development of lesions after the first exposure points towards phototoxicity, and a reaction, which develops after a lapse period is indicative of photoallergy. Try and assess the causative agent by history and examination. Widespread eruption is suggestive of systemic photosensitisers. Vesicular and bullous lesions, like that of a burn suggest phototoxicity. Eczematous like lesions suggest photoallergy.

A skin biopsy, which shows necrotic keratinocytes, suggests phototoxicity; while a spongiotic epidermis is indicative of photoallergy. Finally a photopatch test will differentiate the two conditions.

Unless diagnosis is certain, exclude dermatoses exacerbated by UVR.

Endogenous Photosensitisation

Endogenous photosensitisation due to metabolic disorders.

Porphyria

The porphyrias are a group of metabolic photosensitive disorders in which there is an overproduction of porphyrins (endogenous photochemical), due to the deficiency of enzymes required in the production of haem. Haem is an important cellular constituent, required for the transport and binding of oxygen (e.g. haemoglobin), electron transport (e.g. cytochrome), and for fixed function oxidases (e.g. cytochrome P450). The amount of haem normally produced is sufficient for the metabolic requirements of the human body. The major part of haem synthesis takes place in the bone marrow (about 85%); the rest is produced in the liver. Haem synthesis is regulated by a number of factors, and it is directly dependent upon its concentration in the cell and upon its requirement.

The biochemical defect in the synthesis of haem is either in the bone marrow or the liver depending upon the site of porphyrin production. Porphyrias can therefore be erythropoietic, hepatic or erythrohepatic. Porphyrins when exposed to light react with molecular oxygen to form oxygen radicals, these injure the cells. Most of these disorders are inherited as autosomal dominant, except congenital erythropoietic porphyria (CEP), which is autosomal recessive.

All specimens for porphyria should be taken in the dark at room temperature, as porphyrinogens are spontaneously oxidised to porphyrins outside the body in sunlight. The samples should be analysed within 48 hours of collection.

A number of drugs can precipitate acute hepatic porphyrias, such as aminopyrine, amphetamine, barbiturates, dapsone, chloroquine, dramamine, ethyl alcohol, griseofulvin, hydralazine, methyldopa, pyrazinamide, rifampicin, sulphonamides, and theophylline.

Pathogenesis: Photons of UVL with a wavelength of 408 nm (Soret band), transform porphyrin molecules into excited singlet state. The singlet oxygen destroys tissue both directly and indirectly. Indirectly by complement activation, mast cell degranulation and matrix metalloproteinase activity.

The ability to synthesize haem is dependent upon a series of eight intracellular enzymes, as shown in Figure 3.

CLASSIFICATION

- Based on the enzymatic defect and organ involved:
  - Erythropoietic porphyria
  - Hepatic porphyria
  - Hepatoerythropoietic porphyria.
- Based on the clinical features:
  - Acute porphyrias. Acute intermittent prophyria, variegate porphyria (VP), hereditary coproporphyria,
  - Non-acute porphyrias. Congenital erythropoietic porphyria, erythropoietic protoporphyria (EPP), hepatoerythropoietic porphyria and porphyria cutanea tarda.

Erythropoietic Porphyrias

Congenital erythropoietic porphyria (CEP) Gunther's disease: This manifests soon after birth; the inheritance is autosomal recessive. It is due to the deficiency of uroporphyrinogen III synthase, this results in the accumulation of hydroxymethylbilane that converts spontaneously to urogen 1.

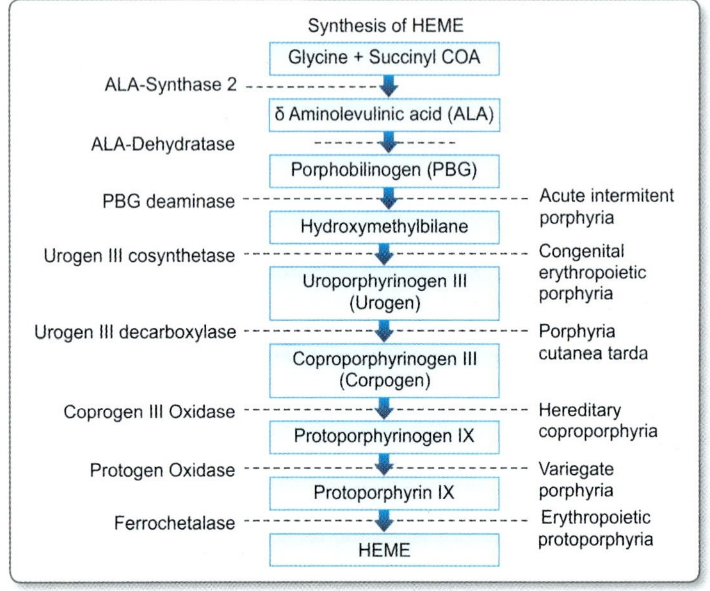

Fig. 3: Synthesis of heme

There is extreme photosensitivity with erythema and blister formation on exposure to sunlight associated with pinkish-red urine. Scarring is severe with sclerosis, hyperpigmentation and hypopigmentation. Hypertrichosis is always present in CEP, hairs are present on the cheeks and eyebrows are profuse. Eyelashes are long; this associated with hypertrichosis has prompted the term 'monkey face' or 'werewolf' for these patients. The nose, ears and fingertips become obliterated. Eyes are affected by photosensitivity, blindness may occur. There is hemolytic anemia and splenomegaly. Porphyrins in the bone and the teeth cause fluorescence and fragility.

Erythropoietic protoporphyria (EPP): The disease is autosomal dominant, it is due to deficiency of the enzyme ferrochelatase in the red blood cells (RBCs), this leads to an increased level of protoporphyrin levels in the RBCs and/or in the faeces, which shows transient fluorescence. In addition there may be increased protoporphyrin in plasma and coproporphyrin in faeces.

In EPP the photosensitivity is seen at 3–5 years of age, photosensitivity is not so severe. There is no hemolysis of RBC on exposure to the sun, urticarial plaques and eczematous lesions appear, several hours after exposure to the sun. There is immediate pain on exposure to light. The skin over the knuckles and fingers appear thickened, wrinkled and waxy, scarring is also seen on the bridge of the nose. Symptoms often improve spontaneously after the age of 10–12 years, but the porphyrin abnormality persists throughout life. There is no hypertrichosis, milia and sclerodermoid change. Gallbladder stones are common and these are composed of protoporphyrins.

Hepatic Porphyrias

These appear at a later age, it is usually seen at puberty or later, except in hereditary hepatic coproporphyria. Most of these porphyrias have acute abdominal and nervous symptoms except porphyria cutanea tarda; this has cutaneous lesions only. The hepatic porphyrias are:

- Porphyria cutanea tarda
- Acute intermittent porphyria
- Variegate porphyria
- Hereditary coproporphyria.

Porphyria cutanea tarda: This is the most common porphyria; it is congenital (autosomal dominant) or acquired. Congenital porphyria cutanea tarda (PCT) is due to the deficiency of uroporphyrinogen decarboxylase. There is an elevated level of iron stores in all forms of PCT, manifested by increased levels of serum iron, ferritin, and/or hepatocellular iron. The exact relationship between iron overload and PCT is not clearly understood. It has been suggested that there is an increased absorption of iron. Increased levels of porphyrins are found in the urine, and increased secretion of isocoproporphyrin in the faeces.

The acquired form of PCT is due to liver damage caused by alcohol, drugs, viral hepatitis and hemochromotosis.

Porphyria cutanea tarda is characterised by photosensitivity, especially on the face and back of hands, resulting in bullae and erosions that heal with scarring, milia and hypo or hyperpigmentation. There is increased fragility of the skin, especially on the dorsum of hands. Hypertrichosis of the face especially over the cheeks and temples is common. There may be purplish-red suffusion of the central part of the face. Sclerodermatous thickening and calcification may develop. Although the signs are due to photosensitivity, patients hardly complain of sun sensitivity, although they give the history of symptoms increasing in summer months.

Acute intermittent porphyria: Acute intermittent porphyria (AIP) is due to deficiency of porphobilinogen deaminase, with increased amounts of porphobilinogen, aminolevulinic acid, uroporphyrin and coproporphyrin in the urine. The disease is autosomal dominant.

Acute intermittent porphyria is characterised by acute attacks of abdominal pain, gastrointestinal disturbances, paralysis, psychiatric disorders, tachycardia and hypertension. It has no cutaneous symptoms. The symptoms are similar to lead poisoning; increased blood levels for lead should be done to exclude this if required.

Variegate porphyria: Variegate porphyria (VP) is an autosomal dominant disorder, due to defect in protoporphyrinogen oxidase. Increased levels of uroporphyrin and coproporphyrin are found in the urine, and protoporphyrin and coproporphyrin in faeces.

Variegate porphyria is characterised by a combination of cutaneous lesions, abdominal crisis and neurological manifestations. The cutaneous lesions may or may not be associated with the acute symptoms. The cutaneous lesions are similar to PCT. Hypertrichosis is seen in the temporal area, hyperpigmentation of the sun-exposed area is similar to that of pellagra. Gastrointestinal and neurological manifestations are similar to that of AIP. The abdominal symptoms comprise acute attacks of lower abdominal pain, usually colicky that may last from a few hours to a few days. There is no abdominal rigidity of an acute abdomen. Urine should be examined for porphyrins in an emergency to avoid unnecessary surgery. Other symptoms include nausea, vomiting, constipation and back pain. The peripheral neuropathy may be a major feature of the disease. Psychiatric symptoms result in depression, anxiety, fits, delirium and coma.

Hereditary coproporphyria: Hereditary coproporphyria (HCP) is an autosomal dominant disorder, due to defect in hepatic coproporphyrinogen oxidase. Increased levels of coproporphyrin are present in the urine and faeces.

Hereditary coproporphyria has both the cutaneous symptoms and the acute attacks similar to that of AIP. The cutaneous symptoms are less severe than porphyria variegata; haemolytic anaemia is seen in childhood.

Hepatoerythropoietic Porphyria

Hepatoerythropoietic porphyria (HEP) is an extremely rare disorder that has the clinical features of CEP and the biochemical profile is like that of PCT. Excess of porphyrins is produced both in the liver and the bone marrow. Dark urine is passed from birth; extreme photosensitivity is present since the 1st year of life. Blisters heal with scarring, mutilation, hypertrichosis and sclerodermatous changes. Haemolytic anaemia and splenomegaly are present. Liver may show mild lymphocytic infiltration (Table 1).

TREATMENT OF PORPHYRIA

The management in general is based on preventing violet light of wavelength 408 nm (Soret band) from entering the epidermis. Most of the sunscreens do not protect the skin against violet light of 408 nm. Sunscreens containing the reflective particles like zinc oxide and titanium dioxide, can to some extent protect against violet light, but it is not very effective. Dundee sunscreen is available commercially, which can provide protection up to 430 nm. Management in general is based on sun avoidance, sun protective clothing and sun protection. Elimination of drugs causing acute hepatic porphyrias is essential.

Protection from sunlight is important in all forms of porphyrias. β carotene 150 mg/day is an active oxygen radical quencher and can be used in most cases of porphyrias. Low dose of chloroquine 125 mg twice a week is helpful in a number of cases. How chloroquine works is not fully understood, it seems to form a complex with porphyrins deposited in the liver to form water-soluble compounds that are excreted in the urine. Chloroquine must be given with care as higher doses may exacerbate the symptoms, or produce ocular changes and hepatic toxicity.

Phlebotomy: In PCT there is increased iron overload, 500 mL of blood is removed weekly till the haemoglobin level falls to 10 g/dL, and serum iron falls to 50–60 µg/dL. Iron chelation therapy with desferrioxamine, plasmapheresis have been used to decrease the iron levels.

Table 1: The difference between erythropoietic, hepatitic and hepatoerythropoietic porphyria

Erythropoietic porphyrias		*Hepatic porphyrias*				*Hepatoerythropoietic porphyria*
Congenital erythropoietic Porphyria	Erythropoietic protoporphyria	Porphyria cutanea tarda	Acute intermittent porphyria	Variegate porphyria	Hereditary coproporphyria	
Inheritance AR	AD	Acquired (80%) and AD (20%)	AD	AD	AD	AR
Enzyme defect Urogen 111 synthase	Ferrochelatase	Urogen decarboxylase	Porphobilinogen deaminase	Protogen oxidase	Coprogen oxidase	Urogen decarboxylase
Incidence Very rare	Second most common	Most common	Rare-incidence higher in Scandinavia	Rare-incidence high in white South African population	Very rare	Extremely rare
Onset Early infancy	3–5 years	Middle age	Adult, after puberty	2nd-3rd decade	Adults	Early childhood
Photosensitivity +++	++	+	Nil	+	+	++
Clinical signs Blistering and skin fragility positive Scarring, most mutilating skin lesions Urine colour Burgundy red	No blisters or skin fragility Immediate pain on exposure to sun, burning and itching Normal	Blisters and skin fragility positive Scarring, milia, hypertrichosis, sclerodermoid plaques Normal	No cutaneous lesions Normal	Blisters and skin fragility positive Scarring, milia, hypertrichosis, sclerodermoid plaques Normal	Blisters and skin fragility positive Scarring, milia, hypertrichosis, sclerodermoid plaques Normal	Blistering and fragility Scarring, milia, hypertrichosis, sclerodermoid plaques Dark urine

Contd...

Contd...

Erythropoietic porphyrias		*Hepatic porphyrias*				*Hepatoerythropoietic porphyria*
Congenital erythropoietic Porphyria	Erythropoietic protoporphyria	Porphyria cutanea tarda	Acute intermittent porphyria	Variegate porphyria	Hereditary coproporphyria	
Other signs Erythrodontia + Haemolytic anaemia Common Fluorescence of RBC +, stable Splenomegaly Present No gall-stones Iron stores normal No acute attacks Fluorescence at 622 nm	Erythrodontia absent Present Fluorescence transient, 5–30% cases Present Gall stones present Iron stores normal No acute attacks Negative	Absent Absent Absent Absent Absent Increased iron load No acute attacks Negative	Absent Absent Absent Absent Absent Iron stores normal Acute attacks-GIT and neurological Negative	Absent Absent Absent Absent Absent Iron stores normal Acute attacks-GIT and neurological Positive	Absent Absent Absent Absent Absent Iron stores normal Acute attacks-GIT and neurological Negative	Absent Present Present Present Absent Iron stores normal No acute attacks Negative
Treatment Preventive and symptomatic Splenectomy	Preventive and symptomatic β-carotene	Preventive and symptomatic Phlebectomy Antimalarials Remove precipitating factors-alcohol, drugs	Preventive and symptomatic - Remove precipitating factors-alcohol, drugs Glucose loading Haem arginate	Preventive and symptomatic - Remove precipitating factors-alcohol, drugs Glucose loading Haem arginate	Preventive and symptomatic - Remove precipitating factors-alcohol, drugs Glucose loading Haem arginate	Preventive and symptomatic

Glucose loading decreases levels of aminolevulinic acid (ALA) synthase. Alkalization of the urine also increases porphyrin excretion.

Patients with acute porphyrias can be treated by glucose loading and I/V infusion of haem arginate (3 mg/kg body weight once daily for 4 days). Haem arginate can repress the synthesis of ALA synthase; it can normalize the excessive urinary excretion of porphobilinogen and aminolevulinic acid (ALA). Acute symptoms usually disappear during the infusion of haem arginate; the correction of neuropathy takes about 2 months.

The first known reported case of porphyria was by Schultz. He described a patient with cutaneous photosensitivity and splenomegaly, which he called 'Pemphigus Leprosus'. Studies by Gunther led to the first classification of porphyrias.

PHOTOSENSITISATION DUE TO ABNORMALITIES IN DNA REPAIR

Xeroderma Pigmentosum

This is an autosomal recessive disorder occurring in childhood, characterised by photosensitivity, dryness of skin, and abnormalities of pigmentation, premature skin ageing and malignancy. It is due to an abnormal DNA repair. Some patients have neurological abnormalities. The patient is sensitive to light with wavelength of 280–340 nm.

Etiology

In xeroderma pigmentosum the sunlight damaged DNA strands in the skin cells cannot be repaired due deficiency of DNA endonuclease. This enzyme paves the way for DNA polymerase to repair the damaged DNA. This causes cumulative defects in the epidermal DNA that predisposes to malignancy.

There are different types of xeroderma pigmentosum (A-I plus variant); each type has a separate defect to repair the damaged DNA. Group A, C and D variants comprise over 90% of all cases of xeroderma pigmentosum. Variant or 'pigmented xerodermoid' has a later onset; it has a defect in the post-replication DNA repair.

This is an autosomal recessive disorder characterised by photosensitivity, facial telangiectases, short stature and high frequency of malignancy. It is common in Ashkenazi Jews. There is a high incidence of chromosomal breakage, re-arrangement and sister chromatid exchanges.

Clinical Features

The skin is normal at birth; the symptoms are noted between the 6th months to the 3rd year in about 75% of cases. Freckling and increased dryness of the skin on the light exposed areas are the earliest manifestations of disease, hence the name xeroderma pigmentosum. These changes usually follow an acute sunburn. The freckles initially become lighter in winter but later they become permanent. In between these freckles, telangiectasia and senile angiomas appear. Angiomas also occur in the buccal mucous membrane. Small atrophic spots appear on the face; these may be secondary to photosensitivity or may occur independently. Superficial ulcers heal with scarring and contractures. Actinic keratosis are frequent, these may undergo malignant change. Basal cell carcinoma is the most

Contd...

Contd...

common tumour to occur. Other tumours that can occur are malignant melanoma, squamous cell carcinoma, angiosarcoma and fibrosarcoma.

The disease is often fatal before the age of 10 years. Multiple metastases from squamous cell carcinoma or malignant melanoma is the common cause of death. Patients may also die from secondary infection or neurological complications. Internal malignancies are also increased by 10–20 folds. These include oral squamous cell carcinoma, CNS tumours and other organ involvement.

Ocular abnormalities are common. Clinical abnormalities are confined to the eyelids, cornea and conjunctiva. Photophobia and lacrimation are common, conjunctivitis, keratitis, corneal opacities and tumours of the lid may cause loss of vision.

Neurological abnormalities are seen in about 30% of cases. These include low intelligence, areflexia, impaired hearing and abnormal speech. De Sanctis-Cacchione syndrome comprises of xeroderma, microcephaly, mental deficiency, dwarfism and gonadal hypoplasia.

Pigmented xerodermoid is a variant of xeroderma pigmentosum. It has a later onset with defective post-replication DNA repair.

Bloom Syndrome

Facial erythema and telangiectases resembling lupus erythematosus are present in the first few weeks after birth. Sun exposure accentuates these abnormalities. Other cutaneous changes are *café-au-lait* spots, ichthyosis and acanthosis nigricans.

The other abnormalities include irregular dentition, hypoplastic malar areas and a receding chin. There are abnormalities of immune system and frequent gastrointestinal and respiratory infections occur. Although the risk of cutaneous malignancy is low, leukaemia, lymphoma, adenocarcinoma of the sigmoid colon, oral and oesophageal carcinoma occur.

Treatment

Avoid exposure to sunlight. Actinic keratosis should be thoroughly treated before malignant change takes place. 5-Flourouracil has been especially helpful, oral retinoids help in reducing skin cancers, a trial of prophylactic therapy should be considered.

Topical bacterial endonuclease has shown improvement in some cases.

Cockayne Syndrome

Cockayne syndrome is an autosomal recessive degenerative disease with cutaneous, ocular, neurological and somatic abnormalities. There is progressive neurological degeneration. It is not associated with increased incidence of malignancy. There is a delayed recovery of chromosomal damage after UV light exposure.

The disease is characterised by dwarfism, deafness, and pigmentary retinal degeneration. The skin exhibits photosensitivity, telangiectases, atrophy, scarring and hypopigmentation. There is marked loss of subcutaneous fat resulting in typical bird like facies. Ocular findings include cataract and optic atrophy, the ears are large and protruding suggestive of a 'mickey mouse appearance'. The hands and feet are cold and cyanotic. Neurological abnormalities include deafness, peripheral neuropathy, hydrocephalus and microcephaly.

Fibroblasts in patients with Cockayne syndrome show decrease in DNA and RNA synthesis after UVA irradiation, which is the basis for prenatal diagnosis.

Rothmund-Thomson Syndrome (Poikiloderma Congenitale)

This autosomal recessive disorder occurs predominantly in girls. Many patients have a defect in DNA helicase. The lesions begin between 3–6 months of age. Photosensitivity, poikiloderma, alopecia, cataracts, short stature, hypogonadism and premature canities characterise the syndrome. Poikiloderma begins at the age of 6 months. Pink oedematous patches appear on the cheek, hands, feet and buttocks; this is followed by reticulate or punctate atrophy and pigmentation.

Short stature, absence of eyebrows, eyelashes, alopecia of the scalp and congenital bone defects are frequently observed. Sensitivity to sunlight is manifested by the development of bullae and erythema on exposure to the sun. Defects are seen in nails, teeth and hair, there is a high risk of osteosarcoma. Squamous and basal cell carcinoma may occasionally occur.

SKIN DISEASES AGGRAVATED BY ULTRAVIOLET RADIATION

Some skin diseases are aggravated by sunlight, such as herpes simplex, lupus erythematosus, rosacea, pellagra, carcinoid syndrome, actinic lichen planus, disseminated actinic porokeratosis, congenital photosensitizing disorders. Diseases helped by sunlight are psoriasis, vitiligo, and some cases of acne. PUVA is an important method of treating cutaneous disorders, such as vitiligo and psoriasis. Venous leg ulcers appear to be helped by UVR, it is said to decrease secondary infection and promote healing. Acne vulgaris and eczema usually benefit from UVR, but some cases deteriorate. Sunlight has been used for thousands of years as a therapeutic modality, but its precise mode of action is unknown.

PROTECTION AND TREATMENT OF SKIN AGAINST UVR

Clothing: Protective clothing should be worn, such as long sleeve shirts, broad brim hats. Dark coloured clothes tend to absorb light and heat and these should therefore be avoided.

Time of the day: UVB reaching the earth's surface is most intense between 11.30 am–4 pm, avoid sun exposure at this time. Window glass prevents UVB but it does not prevent UVA. Clouds absorb 70% of the sunrays and so it is quite possible to sunburn on a cloudy day. Snow reflects 85% of the rays of sun, sand 17–25% and water vapour up to 5%. People easily burn on a snowy day.

Sunscreen: These are of two types, those that absorb the UVR and those that reflect the UVR. Para aminobenzoic acid (PABA), absorbs the UVR, they are cosmetically acceptable. Some also permit tanning, this is especially useful for the skin types I and II. The others are the opaque sunscreens, such as zinc oxide and titanium dioxide, these are very effective, they reflect the UVR, but are cosmetically less acceptable.

Sunscreens containing cinnamates and benzophenones are also efficient and cosmetically acceptable, sensitisation may occur rarely.

Sun protecting factor (SPF), is the ratio of the dose of UVL to produce minimal erythema dose (MED) of the skin, to which a sunscreen has been applied, to the dose of UVL to produce minimal erythema of the skin without the use of a sunscreen. SPF of 10 means that a person would remain out of doors 10 times longer than if the sunscreen was not applied to the skin to achieve the same effect.

$$SPF = \frac{\text{MED sunscreen protected}}{\text{MED unprotected}}$$

Sun protecting factor is a measure against UVB. It is difficult to measure and express protection against UVA. In general the protection against UVA provided by sunscreens is often expressed as a ratio of protection against UVB to that of UVA in the 'star system', in which four stars express the best ratio.

There are two methods employed to measure the SPF. One is pigment darkening method, in which the time taken to produce a transient darkening of the skin is measured. The other is *in vitro* method by a spectroscope.

Chemical photo-protective agents: Antimalarial drugs, such as chloroquine 250 mg/day helps to protect the skin against UVL. They probably absorb the UVL and have anti-inflammatory properties. β carotene absorbs the visible light and psoralens are used to increase the pigment production and thereby help in tanning.

Ultraviolet protective adhesive films are used in car and home windows to stop UVL coming through. This is especially useful in patients with chronic actinic dermatitis.

Photosensitivity in infants, exclude neonatal lupus erythematosus and erythropoietic porphyria.
A widespread blistering sunburn is comparable to a second degree burn, it should be treated accordingly.

Pellagra is described in chapter 29.
Hartnup's disease is described in chapter 31.

FURTHER READING

1. Dabski C, Beutner EH. Studies of laminin and type 1V collagen in blisters of porphyria cutanea tarda and drug induced pseudoporphyria. J Am Acad Dermatol. 1991;25(1):28-32.
2. Dawl RS, Crombe IK, Ferguson J. The natural history of chronic actinic dermatitis. Arch Dermatol. 2000;136(10):1215-2029.
3. Michael J, Kowertz MD. The therapeutic effect of chloroquine: hepatic recovery in porphyria cutanea tarda, JAMA. 1973;223(5):515-9.
4. Poh-Fitzpatrick MB. The porphyrias. Dermatol Clin. 1985;15:55-61.
5. Rocchi E, Gibertini P, Cassenelli M et al. Iron removal therapy in porphyria cutanea tarda: phlebotomy versus slow subcutaneous desferrioxamine infusion. Br J Dermatol. 1986;114(5):621-9.

Chapter 21

Cutaneous Reactions to Cold

Normal body temperature has traditionally been considered to be 98.6°F. However, a recent study indicates that normal temperature varies throughout the day, ranging from 96°F in the morning to 99.9°F in the evening. Furthermore, there is no fixed body temperature; temperature varies from organ to organ. From a thermoregulatory point of view, the body may be regarded as having a central core, surrounded by an outer shell. The temperature within the inner core consists of the central nervous system and skeletal muscles; these are subject to precise regulation to maintain homeostatic constancy. The core tissues function best at a constant temperature of 100°F. The skin and the subcutaneous tissue constitute of the outer shell. In contrast to the constant high temperature of the inner core, the temperature within the outer shell is generally cooler and may vary substantially. Skin temperature may fluctuate between 68°F and 104°F without damage. The skin temperature is deliberately varied as a control measure to help maintain the core thermal constancy.

The skin vessels constrict up to a temperature of 15°C (59°F); at this point, they reach the maximum degree of vasoconstriction. The vessels then begin to dilate. This dilatation is caused by direct local effect of cold on the vessels. Extreme cold causes paralysis of the contractile mechanism of the vessel walls. This vasodilatation in severe cold plays a purposeful role in preventing freezing of the exposed parts of the body, particularly hands and ears. This is known as the 'Hunting reaction of Lewis'.

The ability of the hypothalamus to regulate temperature is impaired when the body temperature falls to 94°F. This ability is completely lost when the temperature falls below 85°F. The rate of heat production in each cell is depressed almost two-fold for each 10°F decrease in body temperature.

On exposure to cold, the body reacts by vasoconstriction; this prevents heat loss. Shivering is very effective in increasing heat production. Contraction of the arrector pilorum muscles of the skin lifts the hair follicles and traps a layer of poorly conductive air between the skin surface and the environment, thus increasing the insulating barrier between the core and the cold air, and thereby reducing heat loss.

Newborn babies have a special type of adipose tissue known as the brown fat, which is capable of converting chemical energy to heat.

All the metabolic processes of the body are slowed down because of decreasing temperature. Higher cerebral functions are first affected by cooling of the body, leading to a loss of judgement, apathy, disorientation, and tiredness. As the body temperature continues to fall, depression of the respiratory centre occurs, breathing becomes slow and weak. Activity of the cardiovascular system is also reduced. The heat rate falls and cardiac output decreases. Ventricular fibrillation leads to death.

Most of the body tissues can sufficiently withstand cooling. The cooled tissues require less nourishment than at normal body temperature. This pronounced reduction in metabolic activity and lowered oxygen requirement of the cooled tissue accounts for the occasional survival of drowning victims.

On exposure to extreme cold, the blood viscosity increases, platelet adhesiveness is increased, and there is slowing of dissociation of oxyhaemoglobin to haemoglobin. The concentration of electrolytes in the cell increases because of water withdrawal during ice crystal formation. Ice crystals are formed both inside and outside the cell, leading to denaturing of proteins. All enzymatic and vital activities of the cell are depressed. Vascular stasis and constriction results in necrosis of the tissues.

Melanocytes are very susceptible to cold injury, damage occurs at −4 to −7°C (19.4°F). This explains the hypopigmentation that follows cryosurgery. Nerve axons are easily damaged by cold, leading to axonal degeneration of myelinated fibres. Autonomic fibres are also affected; this results in abnormal sweating often seen after cold injury. Severe cold can lead to desolidification of lipids in adipose tissue, damage the endothelial lining of the blood vessels and lymphatics, with disturbances in the permeability and flow of blood. Nerve sheaths, cartilage, and bone are quite resistant to cold.

Three stages are seen after extreme cold injury:

- Stage 1: There is massive vasoconstriction and blanching, with fall in temperature. This serves to maintain the central core temperature. This is followed by the "Hunting reaction of Lewis", with painful erythema. This is a protective mechanism against skin necrosis.
- Stage 2: Cold injury becomes more extensive, with oedema and blister formation.
- Stage 3: If cold exposure continues then tissue damage occurs, with vascular injury and necrosis.

The above changes are similar to the pathological changes seen after thermal burns.

REACTION OF SKIN TO COLD- PHYSIOLOGY

Asteatosis (Chapping)

This is the most common skin problem in winter. Cold as well as dryness lowers the extensibility of the stratum corneum. The outer layers of the skin exchange water in the air in terms of relative humidity. In winter, the dry air contains less moisture, which leads to dryness and winter itch (pruritus hiemalis). This may become severe enough to produce visible fissures through the stratum corneum. This is described as "eczema craquele". The dry skin requires water and oil to retain moisture.

Cutis Marmorata

This is a physiological, mottled, cyanotic reaction to cold, seen in about 50% of normal children and in some adults. The mottling is diffuse, mild, and usually symptomless. Chilblain, acrocyanosis, and erythrocyanosis may be associated.

Cold induces a reticulate pattern of purple, dilated blood vessels overlying the fat of legs and arms. The fat insulates the skin and peripheral vasoconstriction causes stagnation of blood in dilated capillaries, giving rise to livedo reticularis. This physiological livedo reticularis should be differentiated from livedoid vasculitis, which occurs irrespective of weather. In livedoid vasculitis painful ulcers may develop; poor perfusion of the skin leads to atrophie blanche. Fibrinolysis may be defective. No therapy is required in physiological livedo reticularis.

Chilblains (Perniosis)

It is the mildest form of cold injury. It is common in cold countries during winter, especially seen in people working outdoors or in poorly heated houses.

Aetiology

Cold induced vasoconstriction causes stagnation of blood in small blood vessels, which damages the vessel wall. Skin biopsy shows vasculitis.

Chilblains occurs on cold, poorly diffused areas usually the fingers, toes, ears, and nose. In obese persons areas insulated from the warm core by fat are involved, such as the calves and thighs.

Clinical Features

The first sign of chilblain is erythema accompanied by burning and itching. The lesions become purple, papular, may blister and ulcerate (Fig. 1). The affected extremities are often cold, cyanotic, and hyperhidrotic.

Chilblains occur throughout winter and cease as the warm weather approaches. Chilblain like lesions may also occur in chronic discoid lupus erythematosus (CDLE) and systemic lupus erythematosus (SLE).

Treatment

There is no specific treatment. Prevention is by warmth. The whole body as well as the peripheries should be kept warm. Smoking should be avoided as it causes vasoconstriction. Nicotinamide or nifedipine may be used to increase the circulation. Systemic steroids are used to treat chilblains due to CDLE and SLE.

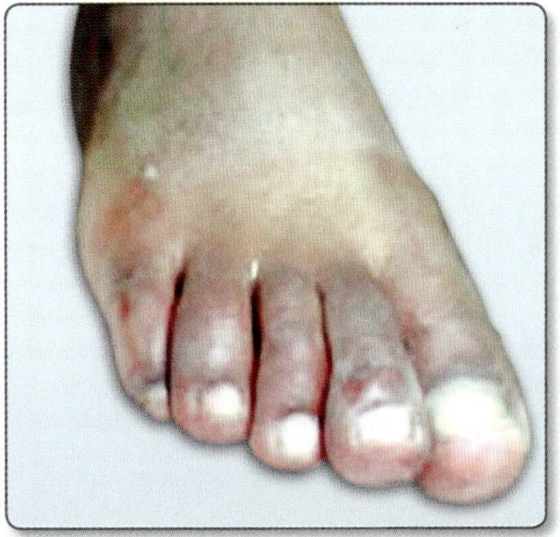

Fig. 1: Chilblain

Acrocyanosis

This is persistent mottled cyanosis with coldness and hyperhidrosis of the fingers, hands, and face, sometimes of the feet and toes, accentuated by cold. The peripheral pulses are normal. It occurs chiefly in girls and young women. There is often a family history indicating a genetic basis for acrocyanosis. The aetiology is unknown.

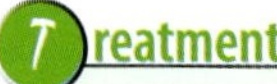

There is no medical cure. Peripheral vasodilatation is not very effective. Topically applied minoxidil may help. Smoking should be avoided.

Erythrocyanosis

It is a persistent dusky erythema, deep cyanosis occurring over the areas of thick layers of subcutaneous fat such as the thighs and buttocks. It is exacerbated in winter. It is often associated with diseases which involve areas of slow circulation, e.g. tuberculosis of the leg, sarcoidosis, SLE. The affected limbs are cold to touch. There may be a history of cramps in the legs at night. On palpation, small tender nodules may be found as a result of fat necrosis in the deep dermis. Spontaneous improvement occurs after a few years.

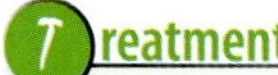

Warm clothing, exercise, weight reduction and elastic support are helpful. Vasodilatation has no effect.

Frostbite

This is due to acute freezing of the tissues on exposure to extreme degrees of cold; the temperature is at freezing point.

Clinical Features

The ears, nose, cheeks, fingers, and toes are most affected. The clinical signs can be grouped in three stages depending upon the tissues affected. These are:

- Stage 1 (Frostnip): The skin is only affected. There is a sensation of cold followed by numbness. Erythema is present on the ears, nose, toes, and fingers.
- Stage 2 (Superficial frostbite): This affects the skin and subcutaneous tissue. There is numbness of the acral parts of the body. Later there may be pain and a feeling of warmth. The skin has a waxy appearance. Small blebs form after thawing.
- Stage 3 (Deep frostbite): The damage extends deeper to the subcutaneous tissue. The skin becomes white, with varying degrees of anaesthesia. The discomfort of feeling cold disappears. Muscles, nerves, blood vessels and even the bone may be damaged. Large blisters form on thawing. Gangrene may follow.

The extent and severity of tissue damage becomes apparent on rewarming. Erythema and soreness is seen in mild cases; blistering and destruction of the dermis occurs in more severe cases. In extreme cases, there is necrosis and gangrene.

Treatment

Rapid rewarming by immersion in water at 40–42°C (104–107.6°F) for 20 minutes is now recommended. Slow thawing results in tissue damage. Analgesics should be given as pain is experienced with rapid thawing. When the skin flushes and becomes pliable, thawing is complete. After thawing, the patient should be kept in bed with legs slightly elevated. Penetration by a heat cradle may be desirable. Surgical removal of the gangrenous tissue should be delayed for weeks or months to allow for tissue regeneration after maximum vasodilatation therapy.

Supportive therapy with bed rest, wound care, avoidance of trauma is imperative. Antibiotics should be given as a prophylactic against infection. Use of anticoagulants to prevent thrombosis or gangrene has been advocated. Nicotinic acid may be given to reduce vasospasm. Recovery may take several months. Topical nifedipine may also help.

Trench Foot (Immersion Foot)

Previously immersion foot was used to describe the signs and symptoms produced by immersing the feet in cold water for 48 hours or more, the temperature being above 0°C (32°F). Today trench and immersion foot are regarded as identical processes. Trench foot results from prolonged exposure to cold without actual freezing. This word is derived from "trench warfare" in World War I, when soldiers sometimes stood for hours in trenches with a few inches of cold water in them. The changes result from chronic dependency and cold-induced ischaemia. Smoking and vascular disease are said to aggravate the lesions. The lack of circulation produces paraesthesias and oedema. The limb feels cold. Gangrene can occur in severe cases.

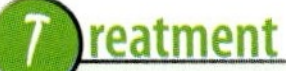

Removal from the environment, analgesics, antibiotics, and restoration of circulation are required.

DERMATOSES ASSOCIATED WITH COLD SENSITIVITY

These include Raynaud's phenomenon, cold urticaria, cold panniculitis, cryoglobulinaemia, cryofibrinogenaemia, cold haemolysis, and cold erythema. The diseases of neonates due to cold injury include sclerema neonatorum and subcutaneous fat necrosis.

Raynaud's Phenomenon

'Asphyxia of the fingers,' so it was described by Maurice Raynaud in 1862 who had first set down the clinical phenomenon associated with spastic closure of the digital blood vessels; pallor, cyanosis, and rubor provoked by cold exposure or emotional stress (Fig. 2). The digits have varying but symmetrical pallor, cyanosis, and rubor. The phenomenon is more frequently observed in cold winter. The digits are affected in paroxysms by attacks of ischaemia, which causes them to become pale, cold to touch and numb. In due course of time, the digits fail to regain their normal circulation between the attacks and become persistently cyanotic and painful. Gangrene may even occur.

Raynaud's phenomenon can be primary often called Raynaud's disease or it may be secondary due to a number of underlying causes. Raynaud's

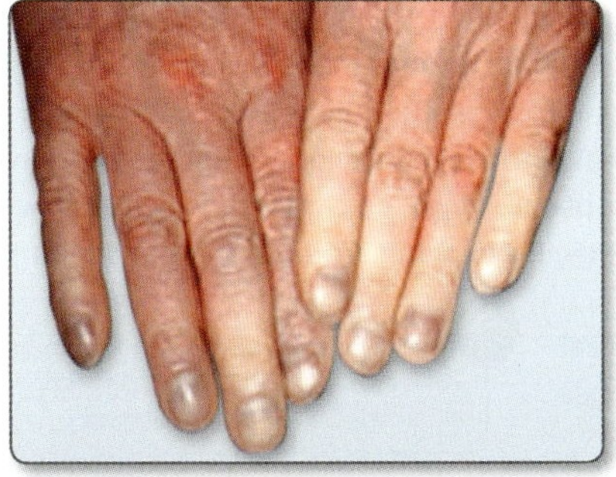

Fig. 2: Raynaud's phenomenon

phenomenon can occur secondary to collagen disorders, occlusive arterial diseases such as thromboangiitis obliterans. It may be secondary to drugs such as ergot alkaloids, adrenergic antagonist and bleomycin. A number of neurological disorders such as poliomyelitis, syringomyelia, carpal tunnel syndrome, and intervertebral disc compression can also cause Raynaud's phenomenon. It may be due to blood dyscrasias such as cryoglobulinemia. A number of neoplastic disorders such as multiple myeloma, leukaemia, phaeochromocytoma and occupations such as vinyl chloride manufacture, sequel of blunt trauma such as pneumatic hammer disease may cause Raynaud's phenomenon. Some miscellaneous disorders such as mitral valve prolapse, myxoedema, heavy metals such as lead and arsenic, and pulmonary hypertension lead to Raynaud's phenomenon.

Treatment

Primary Raynaud's phenomenon (Raynaud's disease) is generally benign and the patient can be managed without vasodilators. The patient should avoid cold exposure, wear woollen gloves, and protect the hands from mechanical trauma. Smoking should be stopped.

Secondary Raynaud's phenomenon: The primary disease should be treated. Vasodilators counteract the cause of digital spasm, dilating specifically those vessels supplying the ischemic zone should be given. Generalised vasodilators may produce the 'steal' phenomenon diverting blood flow from the ischaemic area. Nifedipine 10–20 mg tds has benefitted about 60% of patients. Diltiazem may be effective when combined with oral sympatholytic drugs.

Other drugs include losartan, iloprost (prostaglandin analogue), phosphodiesterase inhibitors (sildenafil), bosentan (endothelin receptor antagonist), botulinum toxin.

Pentoxifylline improves the membrane flexibility of the RBC, reduces blood viscosity, and retards platelet aggregation.

Local application of 2% nitroglycerine in ointment base, rubbed well into the skin several times gives relief in some patients. In severe cases, symphathectomy has been advocated.

Prognosis is good in Raynaud's disease. Prognosis of secondary Raynaud's phenomenon depends upon the underlying disease.

Cryoglobulinaemia

Cryoglobulins are single (Type I cryoglobulin) or mixed immunoglobulins (Type II and III cryoglobulins) that undergo reversible precipitation at low temperatures. The clinical manifestations vary by cryoglobulin type. Type I cryoglobulins are usually associated with lymphoproliferative diseases such as multiple myeloma and B cell lymphoma. Mixed globulins are usually associated with diseases such as hepatitis B, leprosy, subacute bacterial endocarditis and autoimmune disorders. Symptoms are usually due to intra-vascular precipitation of cryoglobulins. These include purpura of the exposed parts on cooling, cold urticaria, Raynaud's phenomenon, patchy livedo reticularis and atypical ulceration of the legs. Systemic symptoms are those of the underlying disease.

The unifying cutaneous clinical features include acral skin changes in response to cold.

Diagnosis

The blood is cooled to temperature below 4°C and the proteins are then analysed.

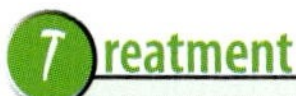

Avoid exposure to cold, treat the underlying disease. If associated with hepatitis C, interferon and ribavirin are indicated. For progressive disease, cyclophosphamide and systemic steroids are indicated; these can be combined with plasma exchange. Anticoagulants and corticosteroids have provided symptomatic relief. The treatment is unsatisfactory when the cause cannot be found.

Cryofibrinogenaemia

In cryofibrinogenaemia, fibrinogens aggregate at low temperatures. It can be primary or secondary. Secondary cryofibrinogenaemia may occur in patients with collagen tissue disease, infections or malignancy. The clinical signs and symptoms depend upon thrombosis and coagulation defects. Skin findings include Raynaud's phenomenon, acrocyanosis, urticaria and purpura.

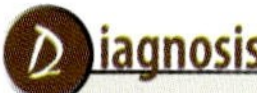

The abnormal fibrinogen can be detected on cooling the blood.

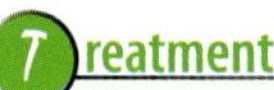

Streptokinase or urokinase is indicated for acute thrombosis. Plasma exchange prevents complications.

Paroxysmal Cold Haemoglobinuria (Cold Haemolysis)

In 1903, Landsteiner described the presence of cold agglutinins in the blood, which were capable of agglutinating red blood cells, but the association of red-to-brown urine with exposure to cold was established in 1872. Cold agglutinins are IgM antibodies.

Transient acute haemolysis may occur secondary to certain infectious diseases such as *Mycoplasma pneumoniae* and infectious mononucleosis. Other viral infections, such as influenza, HIV, cytomegalovirus, rubella, varicella, and mumps, have been reported to be associated with haemolytic anaemia due to cold agglutinins. Other associated illnesses include subacute bacterial endocarditis, syphilis, and malaria.

Clinical Features

Acrocyanosis follows exposure to cold, accompanied by paraesthesias, and at times necrosis. The condition may be associated with cold urticaria and livedo reticularis. In severe cases, there is hepatosplenomegaly.

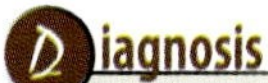

Erythrocyte sedimentation rate is raised, measure cold agglutinins.

Treatment

Avoid exposure to cold. Treat any predisposing cause such as syphilis, HIV, or any other infection. Steroids are commonly employed, but these agents have not shown to shorten the clinical course of paroxysmal cold haemoglobinuria. In severe cases, immunosuppression with chlorambucil or cyclophosphamide is combined with plasmapheresis.

Cold Panniculitis

Following exposure to cold, well-demarcated erythematous warm plaques develop, particularly on the cheeks of young children. The lesions usually develop 2 days after exposure to cold, the lesions involute spontaneously in 2–4 weeks.

The condition is believed to be due to excessive amounts of saturated fatty acids in the immature subcutaneous fat. Patient usually outgrows this susceptibility. No treatment is indicated.

Sclerema neonatorum and subcutaneous fat necrosis are discussed in chapter 33, "Ages of Man and their Dermatoses."

FURTHER READING

1. Dowd PM, Rustin MH, Lanigan S. Nifedipine in the treatment of chilblains. BMJ. 1986;293(6552):923-4.
2. Fritz RL, Perrin DH. Cold exposure injuries: prevention and treatment. Clin Sports Med. 1989;8(1):111-28.
3. Gage AA. What temperature is lethal to cells? J Dermatol Surg Oncol. 1979;5(6):459-60.
4. Goette DK. Chilblains (perniosis). J Am Acad Dermatol. 1990;23(2):257-62.
5. Kellem RE, Ray TC, Brown GR. Sclerema neonatorum. Report of a case and analysis of subcutaneous and epidermal-dermal lipids by chromographic methods. Arch Dermatol. 1968;97(4):372-80.
6. Mehta RC, Wilson MA. Frostbite injury: prediction of tissue viability with triple phase bone scanning. Radiology. 1989;170(2):511-4.
7. Page EH, Shear NH. Temperature dependent skin disorders. J Am Acad Dermatol. 1988;18(5):1003-19.
8. Walls LM, Smith NP. Perniosis: a histopathological review. Clin Exp Dermatol. 1981;6(3):263-71.

Chapter

22

Pruritus

Pruritus or itching is the sensation that produces the desire to scratch the skin. Pruritus is the most common presentation of cutaneous disorders; the cause can be systemic or cutaneous.

ITCH RECEPTORS

Both itch and pain sensations are the result of activation of a network of free-nerve endings situated at the dermo-epidermal junction. Mechanical, thermal, or electrical stimuli produce itching when applied in a pin-point fashion to "itch point" in the skin. Using methylene blue staining of nerve endings, itch points coincided with an increased density of unspecialised free-nerve endings. These nerve endings are equipped with specialised receptors vital to the cycle of induction and continuation of pruritus. It is however surprising that face and wrist, which have low threshold for itching, have no microscopic differences in the nerve ending density and distribution as compared with the less sensitive areas.

CENTRAL ITCH

Central itch is itching that actually originates in the central nervous system due to dysfunctional processing of sensory information in the central pathways. Itch is due to the combination of peripheral excitation and central disinhibition. Opioid peptides could play a role in producing central itch. Morphine administered spinally causes intense itching of the face; this is relieved by naloxone.

TYPES OF ITCH

Itch can be:

- Pruritoceptive or cutaneous. Caused by cutaneous disorders
- Neuropathic. This is due to lesions of afferent pathways of the nervous system, e.g. peripheral neuritis
- Neurogenic. Due to centrally acting mediators such as opioids
- Psychogenic. Due to stress, anxiety or depression.

Response of the Skin to Itch Stimuli

There are two distinct responses on application of a stimulus that causes itching. An itch that is well localised to the site of stimulus, and persists only briefly after the stimulus has been removed, is called spontaneous itching. The other type of itch is diffuse, poorly localised, and does not itch spontaneously on application of the stimulus, but responds with intense itching when subjected to light touch or minor stimulus. The phenomenon of itching skin is seen in urticaria, chronic lichenified eczema and chronic pruriginous disorders.

NEURAL PATHWAYS OF ITCHING

Both pain and itch are transmitted through the same pathways, although these two sensations are perceived as quite distinct entities. Itch produces scratching while pain evokes withdrawal. Opioids relieve pain while they make itch worse. There could be separate receptors for itch and pain. Itch receptors are also sensitive to temperature.

The sensation from the itch receptors by the free-nerve endings at the dermo-epidermal junction is relayed to the dorsal horn root of the spinal cord. Crossing of fibres is complete in the segment above the segment of entrance; fibres from the dorsal roots are added progressively above the cord. The fibres from the dorsal horn are passed to the contralateral thalamus via the lateral spinothalamic tract. From the thalamus, the thalamocortical tracts relay itch fibres to the cortex. The phenomenon of referred itch is probably due to the spread of excitation from the thalamus.

There seems to be a pattern of central sensitisation to itch, especially in patients with atopic dermatitis. When a painful stimulus is applied to the skin of such patients due to the chronic itch stimuli, a central sensitisation occurs over time resulting in elicitation of itch instead of expected result of such stimulus, i.e. pain.

Gate Control Theory of Melzack and Wall

The theory states that that non-noxious stimulation of large Aβ fibres, inhibits the response to painful stimuli with wide dynamic range. The spinal processing of pain and itch can be modulated, resulting in a hypersensitivity or hyposensitivity to pain or itch. Itch sensation can be reduced by painful scratching. The inhibition of itch by painful stimuli has also been shown experimentally by use of noxious thermal, mechanical, and chemical stimuli

The dorsal horn of the spinal cord receives afferent impulses from the peripheral nervous system; it is also subjected to control by the descending fibres from the central nervous system. The histamine-induced discharge of the dorsal horn in pruritus is suppressed by the stimulation of the fibres from the midbrain. This suppression is decreased at night, which explains the reason why itching is more severe at night.

PERIPHERAL AND CENTRAL PHARMACOLOGIC MEDIATORS OF ITCH

Mediators, both peripheral and central, are an essential link between the itch-producing stimulus applied to the skin and the production of itch. However, chemical, mechanical and thermal stimulus can produce pruritus directly upon application to the itch spots.

The chemical mediators of itch are as follows:

Histamine

Application of low concentration of histamine at the level of dermo-epidermal junction causes itching; deeper intracutaneous injection causes pain. Histamine receptors, H1–H4 are located in keratinocytes and in the sensory nerve endings throughout the skin. H1 receptors are most commonly associated with pruritus but recent studies suggest that H3 and H4 receptors are also involved in mediation of itch. Antihistamines including disodium cromoglycate, which prevents the release of histamine from the mast cells, reduce itching produced by histamine. More recent studies have suggested a lower level of histamine in the skin of chronic atopic dermatitis patients suggesting a down-regulation of histamine receptors, which explains inefficacy of antihistamines in controlling itch in these patients.

Neuropeptides

It has been observed that insertion of cowage (*Mucuna pruriens*) into the skin causes intense local itching. Cowage contains proteinase as the active principle. Subsequent studies revealed that endopeptidase produces itching. On a molecular basis peptidases are more potent than histamine in producing itching. No potent itch producing peptide has been isolated from the human skin. Bradykinin present in the blister fluid causes considerable pain, but little or no itch.

Opioid Peptides

Morphine has long been known to provoke itching, similar to morphine-like analgesics. Two types of peptide receptors, μ and δ are found in sensory-nerve endings. The opioid peptides are β-endorphin, leucine, enkephalin and methionine. Enkephalins are extensively distributed in the peripheral and central nervous system. Opioid peptide antagonists inhibit the release of inflammatory neuropeptides that cause itch; this is the mechanism by which naloxone, a μ-receptor opioid antagonist, can relieve itching.

Substance P

Substance P is an undecapeptide and a tachykinin. When injected in human skin, it causes itch in some subjects. Very likely the results are indirect, probably due to the ability of substance P to induce local histamine release, as well as its activation of neurokinin receptor.

Other Neuropeptides

Several other neuropeptides including neuropeptide Y (NPY), vasoactive intestinal peptide (VIP) and somatostatin are also known to play a role in induction and mediation of itch most likely due to an imbalance of these neuropeptides in relation to others.

Cytokines

Cytokines play a role in mediation of pruritus by activating release of neuropeptides from sensory nerve endings. Some interleukins including IL-2 and IL-8 are thought to play an indirect role by activating other mediators of pruritus.

Platelet Activating Factor (PAF)

This is an ether phospholipid with pro-inflammatory properties. Platelet activating factor (PAF) is a powerful itch-producing agent that is released by mast cells, neutrophils, eosinophils, and basophils. PAF causes increased vascular permeability and liberates histamine from the mast cells.

Prostaglandins and other Eicosanoids

These are metabolites of arachidonic acid. They are found in a wide range of inflammatory skin diseases. Prostaglandin E1 does not cause itching, but it lowers the threshold of human skin to histamine-produced itching. Prostaglandins and related compounds also induce itching due to a specific sensitising effect on the free nerve-ending receptors.

PATTERNS OF ITCHING

There are great variations in the pattern of itching. It varies from person to person and even in the same person. There may be different patterns at different times. Emotional trauma, absence of distraction, anxiety or fear, all enhance itching. Itching is often more severe at night. Variations are also found in different regions of the body. Ear canal, eyelids, nostrils, perianal and genital areas are easily susceptible to pruritus. Pruritus is temperature dependent; heat aggravates pruritus.

Pruritus may be mild, moderate, severe, recurrent, or paroxysmal. Paroxysmal itching is characteristic of lichen simplex chronicus, atopic dermatitis, nummular eczema, dermatitis herpetiformis, neurotic excoriations, and prurigo nodularis. Itching may be so intense that it may produce bleeding in the skin leaving hyperpigmentation, scarring or both. Urticaria leaves scratch marks, scabies produces only short excoriations. Patients with lichen planus often rub their skin to relieve itching.

INFLUENCE OF SKIN TEMPERATURE ON ITCHING

The relationship between temperature and itching is well recognised. Itching is aggravated when the skin is warm as in thyrotoxicosis. Itching is more distressing later in the day as the temperature rises in the afternoon. Measures to lower skin temperature help to relieve itching.

CAUSES OF PRURITUS

- Cutaneous
- Systemic
- Psychosomatic.

Cutaneous

Any skin lesion may itch. The major dermatoses that itch are scabies, dermatitis herpetiformis, eczema, especially atopic dermatitis, lichen planus, urticaria, drug eruptions, arthropod bites, prurigo, ichthyosis, phototoxic reaction, viral exanthems, and dryness of the skin.

The rapidly increasing incidence of AIDS has introduced a new spectrum of pruritic dermatological disorders. Two conditions deserve particular attention; these are seborrhoeic dermatitis with severe pruritus covering large areas of the face, scalp, and chest. The other condition is eosinophilic folliculitis, which produces extremely pruritic erythematous follicular papules on the chest. These two conditions are highly suggestive of AIDS.

Notalgia paraesthetica is localised persistent pruritus, often seen in the midscapula areas. The patients complain of persistent burning pruritus, in the midscapula area, often spreading to a widespread distribution. On examination there is hyperpigmentation, lichenification, with or without evidence of macular amyloidosis. The exact cause of it is unknown; it may be due to amyloidosis, increased cutaneous innervation or perhaps nerve root entrapment. Capsaicin cream offers relief in some patients.

Systemic

These cases are more difficult to evaluate. Itching can be due to many systemic diseases. Hepatic disease such as obstructive jaundice may present with intense itch. Pruritus is a hallmark of chronic renal failure and patients undergoing dialysis. Many endocrine disorders are associated with pruritus, including diabetes mellitus, hyperthyroidism especially thyrotoxicosis, and hyperparathyroidism. Many neoplastic disorders present with pruritus such as lymphomas, especially Hodgkin's disease.

Psychosomatic

Psychosomatic connection is not more prominent in any other area than in skin conditions. Stress and psychological illness can manifest as pruritus. There is a clear correlation of relapse and worsening of pruritis in skin conditions like urticaria, atopic dermatitis, psoriasis, etc. Psychogenic pruritus or prurigo nodularis is a condition where psychological factors trigger, aggravate or play a central part in the persistence of pruritus. Patients suffering from factitious dermatitis have multiple dugout superficial or deep ulcers of the skin, which generally do not meet the diagnostic criteria of any dermatological disorder. The patients complain of severe intractable pruritus. In delusions of parasitosis, the patient complains of parasites crawling under the skin, leading to intense itch and scratch cycle. These patients need a careful empathic team approach including dermatologic and psychiatric treatment.

CLASSIFICATION

Itching can be:

- Localised
- Generalised.

Localised Pruritus

Localised causes are often dermatological such as eczema, prurigo nodularis, lichen planus, fungal infections, insect bites, etc. Localised itching can also be due to systemic disease, but this is rare. It may be psychosomatic, or as a manifestation of internal malignancy, e.g. pruritus of the nose may be due to malignancy of the central nervous system.

Pruritus Ani

The anal area is a frequent cause of itching; it may be due to threadworm infestation, ringworm, candidiasis, anal psoriasis, seborrhoeic dermatitis, contact dermatitis, erythrasma, etc. Rectal diseases, haemorrhoids and anal fissures also cause pruritus. Anal neurodermatitis is characterised by paroxysmal attacks of violent itching; manifestations are identical to lichen simplex chronicus.

Pruritus Vulvae

The common causes of pruritus vulvae are candidiasis, *Trichomonas vaginalis*, contact dermatitis, lichen simplex chronicus and ringworm infection. Urinary incontinence and diabetes should be kept in mind. Leucoplakia and lichen sclerosus also cause pruritus vulvae; these conditions should be carefully followed up, as they are premalignant. Neurodermatitis should also be kept in mind.

Pruritus of the Scalp

This is especially common in the elderly. Common causes of itching scalp are pediculosis, seborrhoeic dermatitis, psoriasis and neurodermatitis. In the elderly, cause is often unknown.

Notalgia Paraesthetica

This is localised persistent pruritus, often seen in the midscapula region. The cause is unknown; it may be due to increased cutaneous innervation, nerve root entrapment or cutaneous amyloidosis. Treatment is unsatisfactory; capsaicin cream is effective in some patients.

Brachioradialis Pruritus

A rare entity brachioradialis pruritus (BRP) is localised to the skin of the lateral aspects of the arms, and is more commonly seen in areas with high level of sun exposure. Although main cause of BRP is thought to be due to high UVL exposure, cervical root impingement is also considered as a possible cause.

Generalised Pruritus

The cause may be cutaneous or systemic. The dermatological causes of generalised pruritus are scabies, dermatitis herpetiformis, xerosis, urticaria, generalised neurodermatitis, viral exanthems, drug eruptions, etc. As these conditions are visible, they can easily be diagnosed and treated. In some cases, the cutaneous lesions are not easily detectable such as clean scabies, fibreglass dermatitis, a thorough history taking is essential in such cases.

Generalised pruritus without skin lesions may be anything from dry skin to occult carcinoma. A detailed history and investigations are required in these cases.

Liver Disorders

Chronic liver disease with obstructive jaundice causes severe generalised pruritus. Conjugated bile acids do not cause pruritus, but unconjugated bile acids and bile salts on the skin surface are effective pruritogens. Cholestyramine is an effective anti-pruritic in obstructive jaundice.

Certain metabolites of cholesterol have also been proposed as a cause of itching in liver disease. Itching is common in infective hepatitis, but does not occur in jaundice of haemolytic anaemia.

Pruritus of pregnancy is due to cholestasis. Itching may be a presenting complaint of carcinomas causing extra-hepatic biliary obstruction.

Renal Disorders

Chronic and acute renal failure is a common cause of pruritus. It is also seen after dialysis. The pruritus may be persistent and extensive or transitory and localised. The exact cause of pruritus in renal disease is not known. It may be due to increased density of mast cells in the skin, raised levels of serum parathyroid hormone, abnormal sprouting of enolase myelinated nerve fibres, elevated plasma met-enkephalin levels and dryness of the skin.

Uraemic patients can be treated by phototherapy, ultraviolet light B (UVB) is frequently effective. Parathyroidectomy in patients with raised parathyroid hormones is helpful. Emollients relieve the itching of dry skin. Topical capsaicin has been effective in localised pruritus. Patients who are on hemodialysis are reported to respond to cholestyramine, low protein diet, ultraviolet phototherapy, lowering of magnesium content of the dialysate, IV heparin, IV lignocaine, oral charcoal and antihistamines. Itching does not occur in patients after successful renal transplants.

Haematological Disorders

Pruritus is a presenting symptom of polycythaemia rubra vera. Iron deficiency anemia has been implicated as a cause of severe pruritus. Correction of the iron deficiency leads to an improvement in pruritus.

Internal Malignancy

In Hodgkin's disease, itching is usually continuous and at times accompanied with severe burning. The pruritus of leukaemia is more generalised and less severe than Hodgkin's disease. Other malignant conditions can also present with pruritus as a prominent symptom, e.g. cutaneous T-cell lymphoma and multiple endocrine neoplasia type 2A (MEN 2A).

Thyroid Disorders

Intractable itching may be a presenting complaint of thyrotoxicosis. This is perhaps due to vasodilatation, which leads to an increase of skin surface temperature; this in turn lowers the itch threshold. Myxoedema may cause itching due to dryness of the skin.

Diabetes Mellitus

Although often reported that diabetes is a cause of pruritus, itching due to diabetes is rare. Pruritus vulvae in diabetes is due to candidiasis.

Carcinoid Syndrome

This is associated with itching, perhaps due to decrease in itch threshold, caused by the vasodilatory effect of serotonin.

Postmenopausal Pruritus

This may give rise to persistent or episodic widespread itching. It is frequently associated with other menopausal symptoms such as flushing. It responds to hormone-replacement therapy.

Psychogenic Pruritus

Itching can be either local or generalised. Diagnosis of psychological itch should be done after excluding cutaneous and systemic causes of itching. Psychogenic pruritus may be so extensive that it can result in disfiguring excoriations and even self-mutilation. Patients with severe itching may become secondarily depressed, this further lowers the threshold of itch and thus a vicious cycle is set up.

Drugs

Many commonly used medications can cause pruritus. Some of these are opiates and its derivatives, anti-hypertensive drugs including beta-adrenergic blockers, ACE inhibitors, angiotensin II antagonists, calcium-channel blockers, clonidine and methyldopa. Diabetic medications include metformin and gliclazide. Statins include lovastatin and simvastatin. Analgesics include aspirin and nonsteroidal anti-inflammatory drugs. Chemotherapeutic medications include chlorambucil, tamoxifen, gemcitabine, and paclitaxel. Exogenous sex hormones include estrogens, progestins, testosterone. Many psychotropic medications include selective serotonin reuptake inhibitors (SSRIs), tricyclic anti-depressants, and phenothiazines and other neuroleptics. Many antibiotics such as penicillins, macrolides, cephalosporins, quinolones, carbapenems, and glycopeptide are all known to cause generalised itching. Vancomycin can cause 'red man syndrome' which is characterised by intense flushing of upper body along with pruritus.

Unusual Causes of Pruritus

These include the 'Dumping syndrome', Sjögren's syndrome, multiple sclerosis; sometimes even coffee intoxication can produce severe itching.

Pruritus of Undetermined Origin

Pruritus of undetermined origin is defined as continuous or daily itching of more than 2 weeks duration, the cause of which remains undiagnosed after 2 weeks of initial investigation and management. Pruritus of undetermined origin (PUO) should be taken as seriously as fever of unknown origin. Every possible investigation should be done to exclude the possible cause of itching.

DIAGNOSIS AND EVALUATION OF THE ITCHING PATIENT

A detailed history is the single most important step toward diagnosing the cause of itching. This includes a detail of drug intake, personal or family history of any systemic illness, history of exposure to any physical or chemical irritant, and history of travel, etc. History of the onset and course of pruritus should be noted such as specific time (nocturnal/day), whether gradual or sudden, continuous or paroxysmal. Paroxysmal itching that awakens the patient from sleep may be of organic origin.

A history of animal pets should always be taken in PUO; fleas and mites of pets are often a cause of itching in household individuals. Unusual environmental causes such as beetle-infested carpets, fowl mites from air conditioner, where birds choose to build their nests, may be a cause of unusual itching.

A thorough physical examination, along with obtaining pertinent laboratory and other diagnostic studies are of utmost importance in diagnosing the aetiology of pruritus. Specific dermatological disorders with pathognomonic signs can be excluded by a thorough physical examination of the skin such as scabies and other conditions. Scratch marks and excoriations indicate the degree of itching. Scratch marks of scabies are quite short; those of pediculosis corporis are often several centimetres long. Deep gouged-out excoriations may be present in delusional parasitosis and neurotic excoriations; subtle signs of persistent rubbing include the barnished nail sign.

Signs of dermatological disease require no further investigations. More generalised itching without any cutaneous sign points to a systemic illness. Itching after a hot bath may point to polycythemia rubra vera or aquagenic pruritus. Failure to obtain relief from symptomatic measures indicates severity. Itching from wool often points to atopy.

For practical purpose, itching may fall into one of the following four groups:

1. Itching due to recognisable dermatological disease, e.g. atopic dermatitis, lichen planus, etc.
2. Itching in which excoriations may in fact be the primary lesion such as fibreglass dermatitis.
3. Itching due to a primary dermatological disorder in which the primary lesions are camouflaged by secondary lesion such as eczema, infection.
4. Itching with no detectable primary or secondary lesion.

Preliminary working diagnosis is required in the last two groups. They usually require a complete blood examination, tests for thyroid, hepatic and renal function and a chest X-ray examination.

Patients with PUO should be considered to have an internal disorder unless proved otherwise. Additional tests such as stool for occult blood, Papanicolaou smear and further radiological examinations may be necessary. Radiocontrast studies and CT scans are usually not indicated as a part of evaluation in every case, but in some cases it may lead to the diagnosis of a disorder that can be treated.

Treatment

Symptomatic treatment falls into the following categories:

- Patient education and reduction of provocative factors
- Topical preparations
- Oral medications
- Physical modalities

Patient education and reduction of provocative factors

If the underlying cause of pruritus is known, treatment is straightforward. When the cause cannot be determined, symptomatic treatment is required. Symptomatic treatment is also required when investigations are underway.

Stimulants such as tea, coffee may aggravate itching; patients should be protected from external irritants such as wool, and certain synthetic fibres should be avoided. Soaps and detergents should not be used with dry skin. Baths containing small amounts of oil is helpful for dry skin. Nails should be kept short and clean. As pruritus is elevated by an increase of temperature, wearing light clothes, cool environment, and taking a shower before sleep is helpful. Dryness of the skin produces itching, simple emollients such as white soft paraffin, cold creams; moisturisers help to reduce the itch.

The patient should also be taught to break the itch-scratch cycle. When the urge to scratch comes, a cool washcloth, pressure or will power may be helpful.

Fabrics that have been contaminated in the laundry, e.g. by fibreglass curtains, may have to be discarded. Drugs known to cause pruritus should be avoided.

Topical preparations

Calamine lotion is one of the commonly used topical anti-pruritic agents. One percent menthol in aqueous cream relieves itching; it has a cooling sensation on the skin. The local anaesthetics as benzocaine, xylocaine are good anti-pruritics, but they cause contact dermatitis and therefore cannot be used. Liquor picis carbonis 2–10% in alcohol, thymol, and tincture of benzoin are other topical anti-pruritics.

Phenol, menthol, and camphor may be added to a variety of vehicles such as calamine lotion. Camphor is used in a concentration of 1–5%, menthol in 0.5–2% and phenol in 0.5–2%. Phenol should not be prescribed to infants and pregnant women. Doxepin cream may be helpful in some cases, but it can only be used in localised areas. Capsaicin is effective in treating pruritus of various types especially in cases of disorders with severe itching like nostalgia paraesthetica.

The following are some of the baths recommended for itching:

- ***Oatmeal baths:*** One cup of starch is added to a tubful of water, for generalised pruritus.
- ***Bath oils:*** 5–25 millilitres of olive oil are added to a tub of warm water, for dry and sensitive skin.
- ***Tar baths:*** 100 millilitres of coal tar solution is added to a tubful of water for pruritus due to psoriasis.

Oral medications

There are no effective antipruritic drugs. Antihistamines relieve itching by inhibiting the release of histamine and by sedation. Promethazine, diphenhydramine, cyproheptadine and hydroxyzine are commonly used. Benzodiazepines like diazepam may provide useful sedation in an agitated or disturbed person. Use of opioid receptor antagonist, including naloxone, is helpful in the management of intractable pruritus.

Cholestyramine may be effective in relieving the pruritus of renal and hepatic origin. It is also useful in relieving the itching of polycythaemia rubra vera. It acts by removing the pruritogenic substances in the gut.

Activated charcoal is useful for the treatment of pruritus in patients undergoing renal dialysis.

Use of opioid receptor antagonist, including naloxone, is shown to be helpful in the management of intractable pruritus. Naloxone was used to treat pruritus of primary biliary cirrhosis. Enkephalin and endorphin blockage by naloxone is not used routinely for the treatment of pruritus, but holds considerable promise. Because of the close relationship between pain and itch, aspirin is used for the treatment of itching in some patients. It is used in the treatment of polycythaemia rubra vera. It blocks the release of prostaglandins and serotonin.

Thalidomide can be used in the treatment of recalcitrant prurigo nodularis.

Contd...

Contd...

Other modalities

Other suggested methods for the treatment of pruritus are transcutaneous nerve stimulation, phototherapy, and acupuncture. Narrowband ultraviolet light B (UVB) therapy is especially useful in pruritus of renal failure and after dialysis. UVB radiation is administered 2–3 times a week starting with an initial dose of 75% of minimal erythema dose. Improvement is seen in 2–3 weeks, remission of several weeks or months may be obtained. Narrowband UVB and Psoralen plus ultraviolet A (PUVA) are helpful in the treatment of atopic dermatitis. Ultraviolet light A (UVA) alone has not been used in the treatment of pruritus as UVA itself may cause itching.

Stress can make anything worse, itching is no exception. Every effort should be made to reduce stress. A team approach with having expertise of dermatologists, psychiatrists, and social workers working in conjunction of each other along with having the input from patient and family members will help to relieve itching due to stress.

FURTHER READING

1. Bauer A, Geier J, Elsner P. Allergic contact dermatitis in a patient with anogenital complaints. J Reprod Med. 2000;45(8):649-54.
2. Bernstein JE, Swift R. Relief of intractable pruritus with naloxone. Arch Dermatol. 1979;115(11):1366-7.
3. Davies MG, Greaves MW. Sensory responses of human skin to synthetic histamines analogues and histamine. Br J Clin Pharmacol. 1980;9(5):461-5.
4. Fruhstorfer H, Hermanns M, Latzke L. The effects of thermal stimulation on clinical and experimental itch. Pain. 1986;214(2):259-69.
5. Grudmann S, Strander S. Chronic pruritus: clinics and treatment. Ann Dermatol. 2011;23(1):1-11.
6. Hagermark O, Wahlgren CF. Some methods for evaluating clinical itch and their application for studying pathological mechanisms. J Dermatol Sci. 1992;4(2):55-62.
7. Harrington CI, Lewis FM, McDonagh AJ, et al. Dermatological causes of pruritus ani. BMJ. 1992;305(6859):955.
8. Khigman AM, Greaves MV, Steinman H. Water induced itching without cutaneous signs in aquagenic pruritus. Arch Dermatol. 1986;122(2):183-6.
9. Krause L, Shuster S. Mechanism of action of antipruritic drugs. BMJ.1983;287:1119-2000.
10. Lowman MA, Benyon RC, Church MK. Substance P causes selective histamine release from human skin. Br J Pharmacol. 1988;95(1):121-30.
11. Lynn B. Capsaicin: action on C fibre afferents that may be involved in itch. Skin Pharmacol. 1992;5(1)8:9-13.
12. Szepietowski JC, Schwarz RA. Uraemic Pruritus. Int J Dermatol. 1998;37(4):247-53.
13. Zylicz Z, Smits C, Chem D, Krajnic M, et al. Paroxetine for pruritus in advanced cancer. J Pain Symptom Manage. 1998;16(2):121-4.

Chapter

23

Disorders of the Sebaceous, Sweat and Apocrine Glands

ACNE VULGARIS

Acne vulgaris is a common chronic inflammatory disorder of the pilosebaceous unit. The disease occurs primarily in adolescents, both sexes are equally affected. The lesions are pleomorphic, comprising comedones, papules, pustules, cysts and nodules, and pitted or hypertrophic scars as sequelae. The usual sites affected are the face, shoulders, chest and upper back.

Aetiology

A number of factors are involved in causing acne vulgaris. There is often a family history, indicating a genetic factor. The hormonal role is evident, as the disease has its onset at puberty; androgens play an important role in the pathogenesis of acne. Climate also affects acne. Slight exposure to the sun is beneficial but extreme heat and humidity often aggravates acne. Acne is less common and milder in Mongoloids and Negroids than the Caucasoids.

The other factors that affect acne are stress, menstruation, sweating, dust, cosmetics and oil. Some individuals claim that eating fatty foods and sugar products aggravate acne, a fact yet to be proven.

Factors Regulating Sebum Production

Factors regulating sebum production are predominantly androgens. The most powerful androgens are testosterone and dihydrotestosterone (DHT). Although androgens correlate to the severity of acne, yet acne can occur in people with normal androgen levels. It is not known if these hormones are taken from the serum by the sebaceous glands or if they are locally produced in the sebaceous glands, or there is an increased sensitivity of these hormones by the glands. The reaction of these hormones on molecular and cellular level is still not clear. Androgen receptors are found in the basal layer of the sebaceous glands and outer root sheath of the hair follicle. The increased hypersensitivity to androgens locally in the sebaceous glands may be due to increased number of androgen receptors or abnormal binding response. A number of enzymes are present in sebaceous glands which act on androgens at tissue level.

The weak adrenal androgen, dehydroepiandrosterone sulphate (DHEAS) might play a significant role in acne production by its peripheral conversion to testosterone and DHT. Levels of DHEAS are high in newborns, fall in childhood, and rise again when sebum production increases at puberty. Steroid sulphatase is widely distributed in human tissues; it is also present in the lesional skin of acne patients but not in the unaffected skin. The enzyme converts DHEAS to dehydroepiandrosterone (DHEA).

The enzymes required to convert DHEA into the potent androgens testosterone and DHT are present in the sebaceous glands. These include type 1 3β-hydroxysteroid dehydrogenase (13β-HSD) which acts on DHEA to convert it to androstenedione. Type 2 17β-hydroxysteroid dehydrogenase (17β-HSD) plays a protective role in skin by metabolizing testosterone back into the less potent androgen androstenedione. Type 1 5α-reductase, this enzyme converts testosterone to the more potent androgen, DHT.

The levels of type 2 17β-HSD are greater in nonacne prone areas as compared to acne areas, as it converts the potent androgens into the less active androgens. Whereas the enzymes type 1 5α-reductase and type 1 3β-HSD are higher in acne prone areas.

Isotretinoin is the most potent inhibitor of sebum. Reduction in sebum secretion can be seen within 2 weeks after its use. It inhibits sebum production by decreasing sebaceous gland size and down-regulates androgen receptors in the skin.

The other hormones that effect sebum production are growth hormone, insulin like growth factor (IGF), keratinocyte growth factor, epithelial growth factor and prolactin. Acne is prevalent at a time when growth hormone is maximally secreted and serum levels of IGF are high. Oestrogens on the other hand inhibit sebum production. The dose of oestrogens required to suppress sebum production is higher than the dose required suppressing ovulation. The major oestrogen, estradiol is produced from testosterone by the enzyme aromatase. Aromatase activity is also present in the skin, but the expression of oestrogen receptors in the sebaceous glands is not understood clearly.

Pathogenesis

Four major factors are involved in the pathogenesis of acne, these are:

1. Increased production of sebum
2. Cornification of the pilosebaceous ducts
3. An abnormality of the microbial flora
4. Production of inflammation

Acne results from an overactivity of the sebaceous glands which leads to the blockage of its duct. The gland is under the control of androgens, which is activated at puberty. It produces sebum, mixture of lipids that may be comedogenic; this results in follicular hypercornification and development of a microcomedone. The microcomedone prevents the passage of sebum to the skin surface. Follicular occlusion with the formation of white and black comedones, results in the proliferation of *Propionibacterium acnes*, which generates a T cell response resulting in inflammation.

It is important to target the microcomedone while treating acne, because the whole cascade of follicular obstruction is arrested by its removal.

Sebum Secretion

Sebum secretion is increased in acne, the secretion is greater in severe acne. However, acne is not a particular feature of certain greasy states such as acromegaly and Parkinson's disease. Acne usually remits in the early twenties and yet sebum secretion does not fall precipitously at that time.

The composition of sebum is altered in acne such as reduced linoleic acid. The hypercornification may be due to the altered sebum.

Cornification of Pilosebaceous Ducts

The primary change in the sebaceous follicle is the alteration in keratinisation of the pilosebaceous duct, and the formation of a microcomedone. Initial changes are seen in the lower end of the follicular infundibulum. The exact cause for these changes are still not known, several hypotheses are put forward.

The excess of sebum is acted upon by lipases of *P. acnes* that converts triglycerides of sebum to fatty acids. These acids are said to be comedogenic, it produces an alteration of keratinisation in the follicles, so that the keratinous squames are not shed correctly. Instead, the keratinous squames adhere to one another and along with bacteria and sebum block the gland. This results in the formation of comedones, at first white comedones (closed comedones) are formed, later as the keratin sheds, oxidation of keratin occurs, and the black comedones are formed (open comedones).

Acne may thus be said to be due to the cohesive hyperkeratinisation of the hair follicle. Cytoplasmic organelles called membrane-coating granules are necessary for the normal desquamation of the keratin. These granules are said to be sparse in comedones, produced experimentally by the application of fatty acids. Contents of the comedones are both chemotactic and cytotoxic.

Several other factors are implicated in the induction of hypercornification; these include the sebaceous lipids, local cytokine production and bacteria. Linoleic acid is significantly reduced in epidermal and comedogenic lipids, this returns to normal with the resolution of acne. Other lipids involved in the production of comedones are squalene and free fatty acids. Cytokine production by ductal keratinocytes is also important in the production of acne. Interleukin-1α (IL-1α) is present in many comedones and may be responsible for formation of comedones.

Androgens may play a part in follicular keratinisation. Androgens regulate the production of sebum, and androgen receptors are present in the outer root sheath of the infundibular region of the pilosebaceous duct.

The microcomedone is the first lesion produced by hypercornification of the follicular epithelium. It prevents the passage of sebum on to the skin surface. As the microcomedone enlarges, it forms the white (closed) and black (open) comedones. These occlude the follicular opening which results in the proliferation of anaerobic *P. acnes*.

Abnormality of Microbial Flora

Three major organisms are isolated from the surface and pilosebaceous ducts in patients with acne. These are *P. acnes*, *Staphylococcus epidermidis* and *Malassezia furfur*. Subgroups of propionibacterium are *P. acnes*, *P. granulosum* and *P. avidum*. Their growth is dependent on oxygen tension, pH and nutrient supply. With the blockage of the ducts by comedones, oxygen tension decreases in the follicle, this is important for the growth of *P. acnes*, this grows well in low oxygen. Activation of *P. acnes* results in a T cell response, which results in inflammation, this leads to the development of papules and pustules.

Production of Inflammation

P. acnes generates components that produce inflammation such as lipase, protease, hyaluronidase and chemotactic factors. Lipase act on the triglycerides to produce free fatty acids and glycerol. Free fatty acids are comedogenic and irritant. Chemotactic factors attract neutrophils which besides producing inflammation (papules and pustules), also weakens the wall of the pilosebaceous follicle by the enzyme hydrolase. The thin wall of the follicle becomes inflamed and ruptures, releasing the contents of the comedone into the dermis.

P. acnes also produce proinflammatory cytokines such as tumour necrosis factor-α, IL-1α and IL-8. Inflammation triggered through toll-like receptors (TLR) is also important in the production of acne. *P. acnes* induces monocyte cytokine production (IL-2, and IL-8) through a TLR2-dependent pathway. The inflammation in acne represents a classical type IV immunological reaction. Immune response may be involved with complement fixation in the late stages when the reaction becomes granulomatous.

Acne improves after about 25 years of age. This may be due to the change in host response of the follicle; it no longer produces cohesive hyperkeratinisation. There may be a change in the host response to various inflammatory stimuli; or there may be changes in the duct function.

Clinical Features

Acne often begins at adolescence when the sebaceous glands first become active. Its severity peaks at about 14–18 years and thereafter the disease gradually subsides; in some cases, it may go until middle age. Acne vulgaris tends to wax and wane, various precipitating factors have been incriminated such as premenstrual flare, stress, some patients blame food although scientific evidence is lacking.

The acne lesions are polymorphic, these may comprise of comedones, papules, pustules, nodules, cysts and scars. The lesions are present on the face, less commonly on the chest and back. The hallmark of a preclinical lesion is the microcomedone. This lesion may evolve into noninflammatory or inflammatory lesion of acne.

The microcomedone represents a distension of pilosebaceous follicles with accumulation of a large number of corneocytes which appear to be shed in layers that are tightly compact. The microcomedone initiates follicular obstruction, which leads to the development of white and black comedones (Fig. 1).

Comedones (noninflammatory lesions) are important diagnostic aid in acne. Closed comedones are a large mass of sebaceous material behind a very small follicular orifice. They are as white or yellow in colour; they occur as small papules, which are slightly elevated. Sometimes these are difficult to visualise; stretching the skin helps in visualising them. As the follicular orifice dilates, and the superficial keratin sheds, open comedones are formed. These are black in colour; the black colour is perhaps due to the oxidation of keratin, or due to the presence of melanin. The white comedones that are difficult to treat are the precursors for cysts and nodules.

Papules and pustules (inflammatory lesions) are relatively superficial lesions, these develop on an erythematous base; these may be itchy or painful (Fig. 2). They resolve over the course of a few days. New lesions may arise at the same place in a number of cases (Fig. 3).

Nodules and cysts are deep-seated lesions; they are less common than the papules and pustules (Fig. 4). They often heal by scarring; the scars can be atrophic or hypertrophic. Hypertrophic scars, such as keloids, are common on the trunk. The characteristic scar of acne is the "ice pick" scar found on the face.

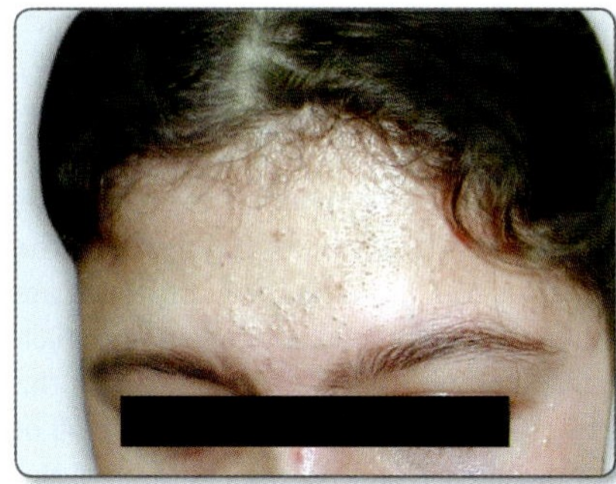

Fig. 1: Acne vulgaris (black and white comedones)

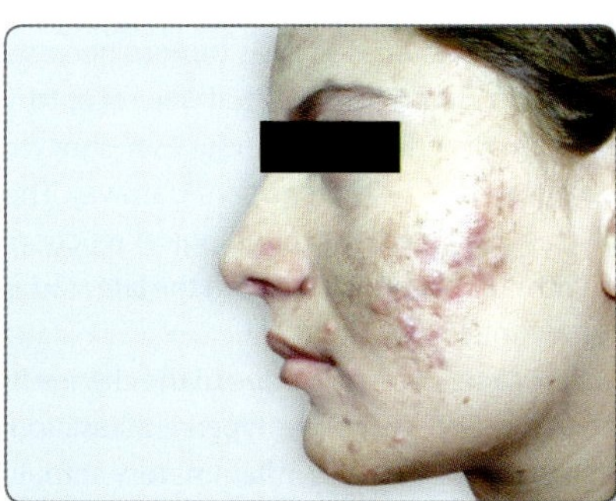

Fig. 2: Acne vulgaris (papules and pustules)

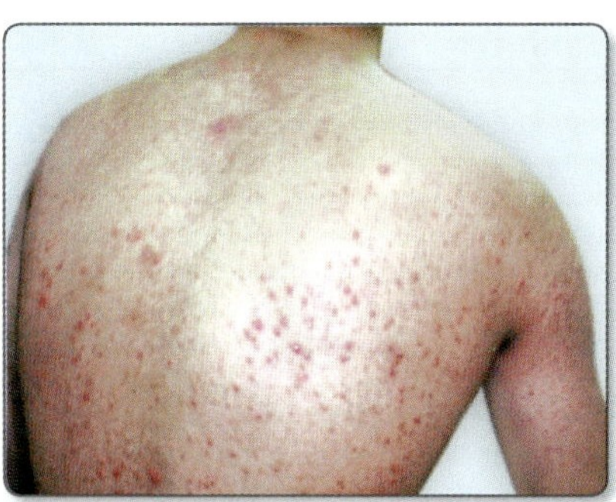

Fig. 3: Acne vulgaris (lesions on the back)

Clinical Variants of Acne

Adolescent Acne

This is the most common form of acne, it begins when the sebaceous glands become active at puberty, severity peaks are seen at 14–18 years of age, the disease then gradually declines. Although in some unfortunate youngsters, the disease may continue until middle age. Severe acne with hirsutism in a female should suggest the possibility of virilism.

Postadolescent Acne

This is common in women in their thirties who invariably state that they did not have acne in adolescence. The condition usually clears by middle or late thirties,

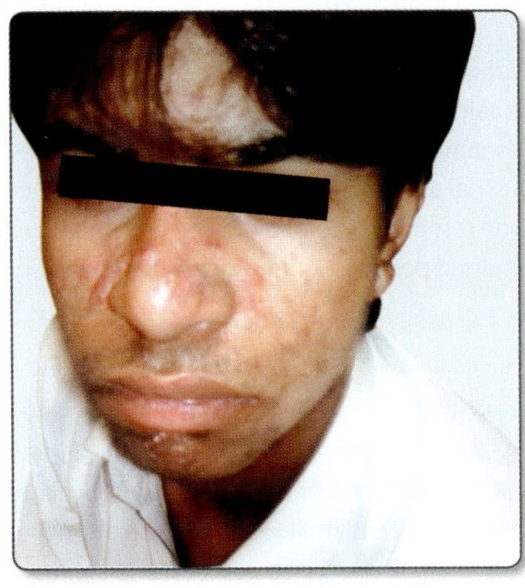

Fig. 4: Acne vulgaris (nodules and cysts)

but not always. It has a characteristic predilection for the muzzle area of the chin and jaw, painful and deep nodules appear, especially premenstrually. Most patients have low levels of sex hormone binding globulin, and the subsequent rise in free circulating testosterone levels is responsible for acne. Some patients have the polycystic ovary syndrome. The more progesterone containing pills (levonorgestrel and ethynodiol) probably aggravate the acne; the minimally androgenic progestogens combined with ethinyloestradiol may be beneficial. Post-adolescent acne may be due to stress; this leads to increased secretion of androgens and acne formation.

Infantile Acne (Milk Spots)

This commonly occurs in early infancy, it may be due to transplacental stimulation of sebaceous glands by maternal adrenal androgens. Rarely, it is the presenting feature of congenital adrenal hyperplasia or a virilising tumour.

Acne Excoriee

This is a facial disorder secondary to an obsessional and neurotic tendency to excoriate and interfere with the skin lesion. The diagnostic features are unhappy women, in whom excoriations, postinflammatory hyperpigmentation and scars are seen.

Drug Induced Acne

Halogens produce acne when used therapeutically or diagnostically. Iodides in cough mixtures, in radiological contrast media and in the drugs used in the treatment of thyroid disease may cause acne. Iodine in seaweed if eaten in large amounts may be responsible for acne. Bromides are rarely given nowadays also cause acne. Phenobarbitone, troxidone, isoniazid, androgens and lithium precipitate may aggravate acne.

Steroids both oral and topical produce acneiform lesions. They are said to induce cornification of the upper part of the pilosebaceous duct. Steroid acne is more monomorphic than acne vulgaris.

Occupational Acne

Exposure to halogenated hydrocarbons such as chloronaphthalene can cause severe and persistent type of acne called "chloracne". Chloracne can also occur after accidental environmental poisoning. One hundred and ninety-three cases of chloracne resulted from an industrial accident in Seveso, Italy in 1976. Other causes of occupational acne include tars and mineral oils. Acne developing in an unusual distribution in a middle-aged person should suggest the possibility of occupational acne.

Occlusive Acne

Acne may be produced by changes in the microenvironment of the skin. Tight-fitting clothes may occlude the pilosebaceous ducts, so that acne may develop on the buttocks and thigh. Sitting on high-backed chairs for a long time, particularly if they are made of materials such as plastics cause follicular occlusion and acne.

Tropical Acne

People working in hot humid conditions develop acne probably due to the hydration of pores of the pilosebaceous ducts, this block the ducts and precipitate acne. This condition is commonly seen in housewives and cooks of tropical countries.

Severe Forms and Complications of Acne

Acne Conglobata

If the cysts and nodules predominate, acne is called the nodulocystic acne or acne conglobata. This is seen particularly in males, the lesions are common on the trunk, face and limbs, and they fuse to form draining sinuses. Multiple fused comedones and extensive scarring are characteristic features. Therapy is difficult, oral isotretinoin is the treatment of choice.

Acne Fulminans

This is a severe form of nodulocystic acne with systemic signs and symptoms. It is an acute febrile illness with arthritis, anorexia, malaise and leucocytosis. Splenomegaly and erythema nodosum have been reported. Bone involvement is common resulting in osteomyelitis.

Oral prednisolone therapy 1 mg/kg/day is the treatment of choice, the steroids are tapered over a period of 6 weeks. Few patients develop severe vasculitis and pyoderma gangrenosum like lesions. This can be treated by isotretinoin.

Synovitis, Acne, Pustulosis, Hyperostosis, and Osteitis (SAPHO Syndrome)

This is a reactive infectious osteitis, genetic, immunological and bacterial mechanisms are implicated. Patients often have acne and arthritis, or acne and anterior wall osteitis. It is associated with pustular skin disease and arthritis, seen also in association with hidradenitis suppurativa, dissecting cellulites of the scalp and pustular psoriasis. The disease is chronic and self-remitting, nonsteroidal anti-inflammatory drugs (NSAIDs) and isotretinoin are helpful.

Pyoderma Faciale

In this condition, the acne suddenly develops purulent nodulocystic lesions; there are no systemic symptoms. It is often seen in females associated with stress. The prognosis is good. It is treated with oral steroids along with the treatment of acne. Isotretinoin is the treatment of choice.

Gram-Negative Folliculitis

This is seen when the patient has been on treatment with antibiotics for a long time for acne. Sudden eruption of small follicular pustules occurs, some patients have nodulocystic lesions. Gram-negative organisms such as Klebsiella, *E. coli*, Proteus or Pseudomonas are responsible for the condition. For treatment, the prescribed antibiotics have to be replaced by ampicillin 250 mg given four times daily. Isotretinoin is again the treatment of choice.

Scars

These can be hypertrophic and keloidal, or the scars can be associated with the loss of collagen such as the "ice pick" scars.

Calcification in the scarred area is an unusual complication of acne, it needs no treatment.

Pyogenic Granuloma

This is a rare complication of healing nodular lesions, it occurs more frequently with isotretinoin therapy.

Solid Facial Oedema

This may be symmetrical or asymmetrical; it is due to abnormal lymphatics. The condition is slowly progressive and it should be treated aggressively.

Granuloma Formation

Extensive localised acne can become granulomatous; its response to therapy is poor. Antibiotics and isotretinoin are of limited benefit. Oral steroids may help, but relapse is frequent.

Associations of Acne

1. Hidradenitis suppurativa
2. Dissecting cellulitis of the scalp
3. Pilonidal sinus
4. Apert's syndrome: This is an androgen mediated early epiphysial closure. The patients have a flat face, fused digits and extensive acne.

Acne with 1 and 2 is called the follicular occlusion triad, and acne with 1, 2 and 3 is called follicular occlusion tetrad.

Systemic Therapy

Indications:

- Extensive lesions
- Painful, deep papules or nodules
- Active acne causing postinflammatory hyperpigmentation and scarring
- Acne excoriee

Differential Diagnosis

Acne vulgaris is easy to diagnose; it has a mixture of findings, comedones, papules, pustules, with nodules and cysts in some cases. The sites are also characteristic. But at times, it can be confused with rosacea, which starts at a later age, papules and pustules, absence of comedones, and the presence of telangiectasia are differentiating features.

Acne should also be differentiated from acne agminata (lupus miliaris disseminatus faciei). These appear as multiple monomorphic, symmetrical, reddish-brown papules on the chin, cheeks and eyelids. Diascopy reveals apple jelly nodules indicating their granulomatous appearance. The lesions are self-limiting and often heal with scarring. It is most unlikely to be tuberculous, it is a distinct entity. Response to tetracycline is variable, so is the response to isotretinoin. Dapsone may be effective, so is low dose prednisolone.

Treatment

Mild acne may be acceptable to a teenager if his or her peers are similarly affected, but moderate acne may be more difficult to cope, it can sometimes significantly interfere with the patient's life. The treatment of acne depends upon its severity, duration and the previous medications used.

Sebum is produced by a holocrine process; cells at the periphery of the gland break down and are completely converted into lipid secretion as they move to the gland centre, from where they are secreted through the sebaceous duct into the hair follicle. The sebaceous gland takes about a month to reach maturity; this explains why therapy takes this length of time to act. The patients should be told of the slow response to treatment at the initiation of therapy.

The treatment can be topical or systemic. Physical modalities such as comedone extraction, intralesional injection are often used in association with topical and systemic treatment.

Topical Treatment

This is satisfactory for mild adolescent acne vulgaris; these are mainly antibacterial or keratolytic drugs.

Keratolytic drugs: Topical retinoids result in the modification of several acne pathogenic factors; they are comedolytic and they normalize the altered pattern of follicular keratinisation. Topical retinoids act on the noninflamed lesions of acne. It may cause irritation that may be unacceptable to some patients. The commonly used retinoids are tretinoin (0.025% and 0.01%), isotretinoin (0.05%) and adapalene (0.1%). Start with the lowest concentration of tretinoin, every night or every other night, and then gradually increase the strength of tretinoin over 6 weeks.

Side effects include burning, dryness and stinging. Adapalene is less irritant than other topical retinoids. Use of sunscreen and avoidance of sunlight is recommended after the use of retinoids. Topical retinoids should not be used in pregnancy.

A combination of topical retinoids with antibacterial is also available.

Benzoyl peroxide is an effective antibacterial, and it is also comedolytic. Benzoyl peroxide acts as an antibacterial against ***P. acnes*** by releasing oxygen in the anaerobic follicular microenvironment. It is sometimes combined with sulphur or antibiotics such as erythromycin and clindamycin. It is available in strengths of 2.5%, 5% and 10%. As it causes irritation, it should be applied initially on alternate nights.

Sulphur, resorcinol and salicylic acid also act as keratolytics.

Topical antibiotics: The commonly used topical antibiotics include 1% clindamycin, and 2% erythromycin. Neomycin and chloramphenicol are available as such, or in combination with preparations containing sulphur and a weak steroid.

Other topical preparations: Azelaic acid (20%) reduces comedones; it normalises the disturbed terminal differentiation of keratinocytes in the follicle infundibulum. Azelaic acid is not sebosuppressive; it reduces the number of ***P. acnes***. It is less likely to cause dryness and irritation caused by retinoids and benzoyl peroxide, but it is less effective therapeutically.

Topical nicotinamide (4%) is anti-inflammatory; it also causes dryness and irritation of the skin.

Topical antiandrogens such as topical cyproterone have been tried but without much success.

Dapsone gel 5% has been approved by US Food and Drug Administration (FDA) for the treatment of acne, for adults and children over the age of 12 years. It is applied twice daily. It is antibacterial and anti-inflammatory. Application of dapsone gel followed by benzoyl peroxide causes a temporary local yellow or orange discolouration of the skin and facial hair; this reaction resolves in 1–8 weeks.

Systemic antibiotics: Tetracycline, erythromycin, azithromycin, cotrimoxazole, flucloxacillin are affective, as they concentrate in the pilosebaceous apparatus. They decrease the free fatty acid concentrations in sebum by modifying the action of bacterial lipases. They also reduce the inflammation of acne by inhibiting neutrophil chemotaxis.

Before initiation of therapy, the patient should be warned not to expect quick therapeutic response. It is usual to start with tetracyclines such as oxytetracycline 500 mg twice a day, half an hour before meals; it must not be taken with milk products, which reduce its absorption. Doxycycline 100 mg daily and lymecycline 400 mg daily are alternatives to oxytetracycline. Doxycycline is photosensitive, patients should be told to avoid exposure to sunlight after its use. Minocycline 50 mg or 100 mg twice daily is effective. It is highly fat soluble, giving it good tissue penetration and it can be taken with meals. Although minocycline has greater antimicrobial activity, it is associated with increased risk of systemic lupus erythematosus like syndrome, and it causes irreversible pigmentation. Lymecycline is a relatively cheap tetracycline with a long half-life, its absorption is not affected by food in the stomach, and it does not have the side effects of minocycline such as systemic lupus erythematosus.

Erythromycin 500 mg twice daily, azithromycin 250 mg 3 times a week, trimethoprim 300 mg twice daily, are alternatives when tetracycline has failed to produce a therapeutic response, and in pregnancy.

Hormonal therapy: Cyclic oestrogen therapy: Oral contraceptives containing 50 μg of ethinylestradiol are of some benefit in mature women with a pronounced premenstrual flare of acne.

Oral steroids in a dose of 5 mg prednisolone in the morning and 2.5 mg in the evening are effective in some cases of severe acne.

Combined antiandrogen oestrogen therapy: The antiandrogen, cyproterone acetate limits the conversion of testosterone to the highly potent androgen, dihydrotestosterone. A combination of 2 mg cyproterone acetate with 35 microgram of ethinyl estradiol reduces sebum production. In severe cases, an extra 50 mg or 100 mg of cyproterone acetate may be added from day 5 to day 15 of the cycle. This approach is ideal for a female already taking an oral contraceptive, as this drug will feminise a male.

Spironolactone in a dose of 200 mg/day, suppresses sebum production by 75%, it can also reduce lesion counts by 75% over a period of 4 months. In low doses 50–100 mg/day, it is used as an adjunct with other therapies. Side effects are menstrual irregularities, breast tenderness, decreased libido, mild hyperkalemia, headache, giddiness, nausea, vomiting and diarrhoea.

Systemic retinoid therapy: 13-cis-retinoic acid/isotretinoin (Roaccutane) is a potent synthetic derivative of vitamin A, which influences all the major features of the pathogenesis of acne.

- It reduces sebum excretion by 90% within a month. The sebaceous glands are reduced to their prepubertal state by the drug's influence on epidermal proliferation and differentiation.

- It reduces the microorganism's activity in acne, particularly *P. acnes*, both at the surface and within the pilosebaceous duct.
- It decreases the hyperkeratinisation in the duct.
- It reduces inflammation and chemotaxis.

It is the treatment of choice in nodulocystic acne, for acne unresponsive to adequate conventional therapy, and for acne causing scarring. It is given in a dose of 1 mg/kg, orally for 4 months. Improvement occurs within 6 weeks. The side effects are dryness of the skin especially of the lips; occasionally, nose bleeds, arthralgias, myalgias, headaches and benign intracranial hypertension. Retinoids should not be given with tetracycline to reduce the risk of intracranial hypertension. Diffuse interstitial hyperostosis, a temporary hyperlipidemia (liver function tests and lipid levels should be done before and during therapy) and most importantly, the drug is teratogenic, pregnancy should be avoided during and 4 weeks after cessation of treatment.

In older patients isotretinoin can be given in a dose of 0.25 mg/kg or 0.5 mg/kg for 1 week, every month for 6 months.

Isotretinoin may be started early in patients who have a propensity for scar formation. Patients vary in their tendency for scar formation. Some demonstrate little scarring even after a significant inflammation; others scar after developing small papules or pustules.

Other modalities

Manual removal of comedones: The orifice of the closed comedone is enlarged before applying pressure. Following the angle of the follicle, the scalpel point is inserted with the sharp edge up, approximately 1 mm into the orifice. After the head of the comedone is nicked, the contents can be evacuated with a comedone extractor.

Mild cautery or cryotherapy is helpful to treat resistant white comedones.

Intralesional triamcinolone: Large inflamed cysts may be injected with less than 0.1 mL of 2.5mg/ml triamcinolone after evacuating any material within the cyst. Atrophy will result if the steroid is injected too deeply.

Persistent non-inflamed cysts may be excised.

Evidence based reviews on lasers, light sources and photodynamic therapy in treatment of acne have concluded that optical treatment only possess the potential for improving inflammatory acne on a short-term basis. The best outcome was with photodynamic therapy. These are not the first line interventions.

Acne scars can be treated by punch excision, punch elevation, subcutaneous incision (subcision), scar excision, laser skin resurfacing or dermabrasion. It is always advisable to refer cases of scarring to plastic surgeons or laser therapists.

The importance of diet in acne is also gaining popularity, but it is not yet scientifically proved to be effective. It is said that a high carbohydrate diet, sets off a series of hormonal changes, which results in the secretion of insulin, this affects the secretion of other hormones. Low glycaemic diet of fruits and vegetables might offer a new treatment option for the treatment of acne. Two westernised populations of New Guinea and Ache hunter gatherers of Paraguay do not have acne. They eat fruit, fish and tubers. They do not eat cereals nor use sugar in their diet.

Future medications would focus on enzymes in the skin that produce androgens locally. Therapies that could block the action of these enzymes may be useful in the treatment of acne.

ROSACEA

Rosacea is a chronic inflammatory disease of unknown aetiology. It is characterised by flushing, erythema, papules, pustules and telangiectasia occurring on the muzzle area of the face. It is associated with hyperplasia of the sebaceous glands. The disease is common in the fair skinned people, especially seen the Celtics of North Europe, hence the disease is also called the "Curse of the Celtics".

Aetiology

The cause of rosacea is unknown; many hypotheses have been proposed and discarded. The disease is common in women between the ages of 30 years and 50 years; this suggests an endocrine factor, since vasomotor instability is also pronounced in menopause. Migraine is also associated with vasomotor instability, it is common in patients of rosacea. Hot drinks such as hot tea and coffee may be responsible for causing rosacea; it is the heat and not caffeine that causes flushing. Flushing is said to be linked to a heat regulating reflex involving countercurrent thermal exchange between the internal jugular vein and the common carotid artery. The heat is responsible for flushing.

In the dermis, there is a damage to the collagen and elastic tissue; and degenerative changes in the perivascular tissue are suggestive of a climatic damage. These changes lead to telangiectasia and erythema. Probably sunlight plays an important part in the pathogenesis of rosacea. Repeated vascular dilation or damage by ultraviolet (UV) light releases inflammatory mediators that trigger off an inflammatory reaction.

Demodex folliculorum is frequently found in the inflamed follicular pustules, the mite could play a part in the inflammatory reaction seen in rosacea. There is an increased prevalence of *Helicobacter pylori* with rosacea. It has been suggested that *H. pylori* synthesises gastrin, which may stimulate flushing.

Histopathology

Most of the changes found are those caused by UV light. In the early stages, there is a moderate hyperplasia and damage of elastic tissue. These fibers are curled and thickened. Elastosis is more marked in the second stage of the disease. In the third stage of the disease, there is hyperplasia of the sebaceous glands with diffuse expansion of connective tissue. The elastic tissue is degenerated, it appears as amorphous masses. *Demodex folliculorum* is found in all forms of disease.

Variants

Ocular Rosacea

About one-third of the patients with rosacea suffer from inflammation of the eyes. Conjunctivitis is common but blepharitis, scleritis and even keratitis may occur. This may give rise to corneal ulceration and even blindness.

Clinical Features

Rosacea is a disorder that affects the face. It usually begins as flushing attacks and then persistent erythema develops. Subsequently telangiectasia, papules and finally pustules appear against a background of erythema. The skin looks shiny and greasy, but seborrhoea is not a feature of rosacea. The shiny appearance is due to lymphoedema, which may occasionally be marked with considerable swelling of the forehead and periorbital areas (Fig. 5). The following are the four stages of rosacea:

Stage 1: Flushing of the face occurs, which is triggered by hot drinks such as tea and coffee. In the early stage the erythema is temporary, later it becomes persistent. There are no comedones or pustules.

Stage 2: Papules and pustules develop the erythema is persistent.

Stage 3: A small number of patients develop large inflammatory nodules, and tissue hyperplasia. The facial contours become coarse, thick and irregular. Finally, the skin becomes inflamed, and oedematous, having a peau d'orange appearance. Sebaceous hyperplasia is represented by yellowish umbilicated papules on the cheeks, nose, forehead and temples.

Rhinophyma finally develops, probably mediated by tumour necrosis factor-β (TNF-β). Rhinophyma is a florid hypertrophy of the lower third of the nose with marked erythema, telangiectasia and dilated follicular orifices. The sebaceous glands are markedly increased in size. Rhinophyma is a disorder generally seen in men. Apart from the nose, there may be enlargement of the chin (gnathophyma), forehead (metophyma), eye (blepharophyma), and ear (otophyma).

Stage 4 (Ocular rosacea): This is characterised by watery or bloodshot appearance of the eyes, foreign body sensation, burning or stinging, dryness, itching, blurring, light sensitivity, telangiectasia of the conjunctiva and lid margin, blepharitis and conjunctivitis.

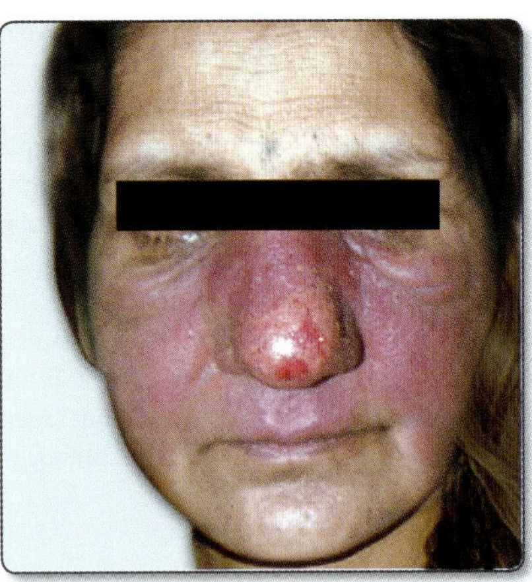

Fig. 5: Rosacea

Lupoid or Granulomatous Rosacea

Tiny reddish-brown papules are found around the periorbital area. Histological examination reveals perifollicular and perivascular, noncaseating epithelioid granulomas. The disease is chronic and prognosis poor. The condition is also called rosacea-like tuberculid of Lewandowsky. The disease should be differentiated from lupus miliaris disseminatus faciei.

Steroid Rosacea

When rosacea is treated with topical steroids, for a long time, telangiectasia, thinning of the skin appears. Later papules, pustules and nodules and even comedones develop.

Rosacea Fulminans

This is a severe inflammatory reaction, similar to acne fulminans. Conglobate nodular lesions develop suddenly, mainly on the chin, cheeks and forehead. The prognosis is good, once the disease is brought under control, it usually does not recur.

Rosacea Conglobata

This also resembles acne conglobata with nodules, cysts, and plaques. The course is chronic and progressive.

Differential Diagnosis

Rosacea should be differentiated from acne, it does not have comedones and acne appears in younger people. Systemic lupus erythematosus (SLE) does not have pustules; it is characterised by follicular plugging, scaling and other systemic signs. Long-term use of potent corticosteroids results in erythema and telangiectasia of the face and pustules tend to develop when steroids are stopped. A careful history and attacks of flushing should differentiate the two conditions.

Gram-Negative Rosacea

This is a complication of long-term treatment with oral antibiotics. The common organisms found are Klebsiella, *E. coli*, pseudomonas and proteus.

Treatment

Hot drinks, spices, alcohol and exposure to sunlight should be avoided. Sunscreens are an important part of treatment, these should be broad spectrum acting against both UVB and UVA. All sources of local irritation should be avoided such as soaps, detergents, peeling agents, etc.

Stage 1: Topical erythromycin and clindamycin are effective on topical application. Tetracyclines are not effective topically.

Topical metronidazole (0.75–1%), 1–2% sulfur ointment, 20% azelaic acid, are effective. Most topical agents are applied twice a day on the affected areas. Patients require 3 months of therapy for optimal diminution in erythema, papules and pustules.

Topical imidazoles are also helpful in treating rosacea. Best results are with ketoconazole cream applied once or twice daily.

Erythema of rosacea is thought to result from abnormal cutaneous vasomotor activity. Brimonidine tartrate (BT) is a highly selective α2-adrenergic receptor agonist with vasoconstrictive activity. It has helped to reduce the erythema of rosacea.

Topical corticosteroids are contraindicated.

Stage 2: Systemic tetracyclines are the most effective form of treatment. The dose is 250 mg twice daily, until the condition is cleared; this usually takes 2–3 months. The dose should then be reduced to 250 mg daily for a further period of 6 weeks. If there is no recurrence the tetracycline should be stopped. Tetracycline also improves the eye lesions, but have no effect on rhinophyma.

The effectiveness of tetracyclines is due to their nonantibiotic effects, such as inhibition of angiogenesis, inhibition of neutrophil chemotaxis, and inhibition of proinflammatory cytokines.

A low dose doxycyline (oracea) is the first oral medication approved by FDA for rosacea in USA. It is a 40 mg capsule of doxycycline monohydrate, containing 30 mg immediate-release, and 10 mg delayed-release doxycycline beads. The capsule is given once daily, it is a promising drug therapy for papulopustular rosacea.

If the tetracyclines are ineffective or if the patient is pregnant, erythromycin, azithromycin or clarithromycin can be used.

Metronidazole 200 mg twice daily is also effective. The duration of treatment is the same as that for tetracyclines.

Isotretinoin should be reserved for patients with severe involvement. The dose is 0.5–2.0 mg/kg per day for 16–20 weeks.

For rosacea fulminans a short course of systemic corticosteroids and isotretinoin are recommended.

Stage 3: Surgical intervention is usually required for the treatment of rhinophyma. Lasers are also helpful.

Flushing and telangiectasia do not respond to the above treatment. Oral clonidine 50 μg twice a day may be effective in reducing flushing. β-blockers such as propranolol twice daily may also be effective. Pulsed dye laser, KTP laser, diode laser and Nd:YAG laser are useful for erythema and CO_2 and Er:YAG lasers for rhinophyma.

Tetracyclines improve the eye lesions, but it has no effect on rhinophyma. Mild ocular lesions respond to oral tetracyclines and steroid eye drops, but keratitis needs the care of an ophthalmologist.

PERIORAL DERMATITIS

Perioral dermatitis has become more common since the introduction of potent corticosteroids. It tends to affect young women; erythema, papules and pustules occur around the mouth and the nasolabial folds. It is probably a variant of rosacea and responds to the same treatment if topical steroids are avoided.

Aetiology

Perioral dermatitis occurs predominantly in young females. Topical steroid therapy on the face is said to be the causative factor in producing perioral dermatitis. Application of potent topical steroids on the face over a time leads to burning sensation, papules and pustules in the muzzle area of the face. The more potent the steroid, the more likely is the severity of perioral dermatitis.

In a small percentage of cases perioral dermatitis occurs in patients who have never used topical steroids. This could probably be due to the overuse of moisturisers, leading to follicular occlusion. The condition is worse in people with atopic dermatitis.

Infection by candida, demodex, falliculorum, fusiform bacteria and cosmetics are also said to be probable aetiological agents causing perioral dermatitis.

Clinical Features

The eruption begins at the nasolabial folds, spreading rapidly to the perioral zone sparing the lip margin. The lesions comprise of papules, pustules along a background of erythema and scaling. Facial flushing and telangiectasia seen in rosacea are absent. The lesions can also be periorbital (Fig. 6).

Treatment

The condition can be eradicated if patients stop applying potent topical steroids on their face.

Topical tetracyclines or 1% metronidazole cream with a short course of oral tetracycline or erythromycin for 6 weeks is the treatment of choice.

Differential Diagnosis

The condition should be differentiated from seborrhoeic dermatitis, contact dermatitis, and late onset acne vulgaris. Although often said to be a variant of rosacea, perioral dermatitis does not have telangiectasia and facial flushing. Seborrhoeic dermatitis affects other sites such as scalp, ears, eyebrows and the trunk. Contact dermatitis does not spare the vermillion border of the lips. Acne vulgaris shows evidence of comedones, papules, and cysts.

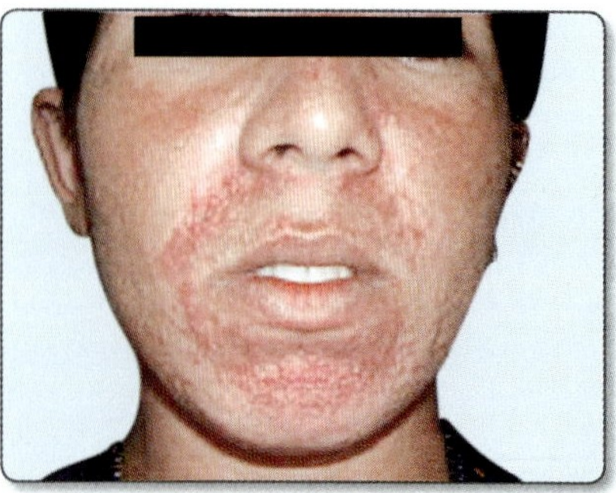

Fig. 6: Perioral dermatitis

The topical steroid that the patient was using should not be stopped suddenly; otherwise, there will be a rebound and worsening of the reaction. The strength of steroid should be gradually reduced.

Course and Prognosis

With appropriate treatment perioral dermatitis has a good prognosis. Only weak topical steroids should be used on the face for any subsequent dermatoses.

TUMOURS OF THE SEBACEOUS GLANDS

Sebaceous Adenoma

These are yellowish or flesh coloured benign tumors present on the face or the scalp. The tumour may form plaques that often become ulcerated. Treatment is by excision.

Sebaceous Carcinoma

This is an uncommon tumour seen in men over the age of 40 years. It is firm, yellowish in colour, situated over the face or the scalp. The tumours are slow growing, except those that arise from the meibomian glands. Treatment is by excision.

Steatocystoma

These are nevoid sebaceous cysts that show a mixture of keratinizing epithelium and sebaceous lobules attached to the skin by a thin epidermal strand. When these cysts are multiple they are inherited as autosomal dominant. Steatocystoma can be of the following types:

- Steatocystoma simplex: This is a single flaccid cyst resembling an epidermoid cyst.
- Steatocystoma multiplex: These are multiple cysts, smooth, yellowish, in colour present on the trunk and proximal aspect of the limbs. There is no punctum but a number of comedones may be present. An oily fluid can be expressed from the cysts. Both sexes are equally affected. Age of onset is adolescence or early adult life.

  Steatocystoma multiplex may be hereditary, with an autosomal dominant inheritance, many cases are nonhereditary. Histologically, the cyst wall consists of several layers of epithelial cells. The sebaceous lobules lie in or close to the wall of the cyst. In some cases hair follicles may also be seen, these are labelled as dermoid cysts.

  In some patients, steatocystoma multiplex is associated with pachyonychia congenita type 11, in which natal teeth are present.
- Oldfield's syndrome: In rare cases steatocystoma may be associated with familial polyposis of the colon; relationship is controversial.

Treatment is by excision: This is often difficult because of the multiple cysts (Naevus sebaceous is discussed in chapter 28).

DISEASES OF THE SWEAT GLANDS

There are two kinds of sweat glands: (1) the eccrine and (2) the apocrine sweat glands. The eccrine sweat glands are concerned with thermoregulation and are present over the entire body surface. The apocrine glands are found chiefly in the axillae and the groins, they have no apparent function but are said to contribute to body odour.

DISEASES OF THE ECCRINE GLANDS

Most diseases of the sweat gland result in either excessive production of sweat (hyperhidrosis) or decreased production of sweat (hypohidrosis). Hyperhidrosis may lead to disorders such as bacterial infections, fungal infections, intertrigo and pitted keratolysis.

HYPERHIDROSIS

Different centers in the nervous system control the production of sweat. Sweating may be generalised or localised depending on which centre is stimulated.

Generalized Hyperhidrosis

This may result from fever, exercise, heat, alcoholic intoxication, metabolic disturbances such as gout, hypoglycsemia, phaeochromocytoma, hyperthyroidism or malignancy. When no cause is found for excessive sweating, it is called essential hyperhidrosis. Generalised hyperhidrosis is due to stimulation of the heat-regulating center of the hypothalamus.

Localised Hyperhidrosis

Hyperhidrosis of the Hands and Feet

Mental or cortical sweating occurs due to stress or emotion; it is usually localised to the palms and soles. Most cases of sweating seen by the dermatologist are of this type. Due to excessive sweating of the hand, the patients find it difficult to work such as typing, stitching, and writing. When these workers work in factories handling metals, rusting of the metal occurs, for this reason these patients are called "rusters". The hands may be cold and show a tendency to acrocyanosis. Hyperhidrosis may lead to contact dermatitis, bacterial and fungal infections. Hyperhidrosis may persist for some years; there is a tendency to spontaneous improvement after the age of 25 years.

Hyperhidrosis of the Axillae

These patients often have a bad odour similar to bromhidrosis. About 25% of cases have associated hyperhidrosis of the hands and feet. But unlike palmar and plantar sweating, axillary hyperhidrosis is relatively easy to control.

Gustatory Sweating

Certain individuals experience reflex sweating after eating hot and spicy food, chocolates, coffee, tea or hot soups. This type of sweating is localised to the forehead, upper lip, nose and perioral region, it occurs within a minute or two after eating. It can be associated with encephalitis, syringomyelia or invasion of the sympathetic trunk by a tumour.

Frey's Syndrome

Gustatory sweating may be localised to the region of distribution of the auriculotemporal nerve following injury often surgical such as operations on the parotid glands.

Olfactory hyperhidrosis has been described in which amitriptyline was effective.

Asymmetrical Hyperhidrosis

This is due to a lesion in the central nervous system, spinal cord or peripheral nerves. Localised hyperhidrosis can be due to cutaneous disease such as blue rubber bleb naevus, POEMS syndrome (*P*olyneuropathy, *O*rganomegaly, *E*ndocrinopathy *M*-protein and *S*kin changes). The skin lesions include hyperpigmentation, hyperhidrosis, apparent skin thickening, white nails, digital clubbing, peripheral oedema, verrucous angiomata and telangiectasia.

Asymmetrical hyperhidrosis is also seen in painful pretibial myxoedema, pachydermoperiostosis, and Goplan's disease (burning feet syndrome).

Asymmetrical sweating may also occur reflexly from visceral disturbances, or due to an axon reflex stimulation. Compensatory hyperhidrosis occurs in normal sweat glands when those elsewhere are not functioning because of some abnormality of their nerve supply. Asymmetrical hyperhidrosis may also be due to psychological disturbances.

Treatment

The treatment is not satisfactory. Topical drugs are generally used to treat hyperhidrosis. For emotional sweating affecting the axillae, 20% aluminium chloride in absolute ethanol is applied at night, initially daily and then at weekly intervals. It should be applied after washing and then drying the axillae with or without a polythene occlusion. Mild irritation of the skin occurs, which can be treated with topical steroids.

For the palms and soles aluminium chloride is not very successful, 1% formalin solution or 10% glutaraldehyde in a buffered solution of pH 7.5 swabbed into the feet three times weekly has helped some persons.

Iontophoresis is another method of treating hyperhidrosis of the hands and feet, using either tap water or anticholinergic drugs. A direct current of low voltage can be used to introduce ionised drugs into the skin. The electric current selectively damages and blocks the sweat duct.

Botulinum toxin inhibits the release of acetylcholine; it is used to treat in severe cases of hyperhidrosis. It is more popular in the treatment of hyperhidrosis of the axillae and feet. On the hand, there is the disadvantage of paralysing the intrinsic muscles of the hand. Subdermal injections are given, one area in a single session. Sweating is abolished after 2–3 days. Repeat injections (after 6–8 months) are necessary as the toxin gets absorbed.

Systemic drugs such as propantheline in a dose of 15 mg three times a day may be used; the dose is increased gradually to 150 mg daily if tolerated. However, the side effects of the drug such as dryness of the mouth, glaucoma, hyperthermia and convulsions limit its use.

Surgical Treatment

Axillary hyperhidrosis can also be cured by excision and undercutting of the affected skin. The area of the densest sweat glands is the first identified by staining with iodine and starch, which is then removed.

Cervical and lumbar sympathectomy will reduce hyperhidrosis of the hands, feet and axillae, but the operation is not free from risks; some patients may develop compensatory hyperhidrosis of the trunk.

INTERTRIGO

This is a superficial, inflammatory dermatosis occurring when two skin surfaces are in apposition, such as axillae, groins, intergluteal folds, beneath the pendulous breasts and between the toes. The folds are red, tender and itchy, fissures may develop (Fig. 7). Maceration leads to secondary infection with pyogenic bacteria and candida; infective eczema may result.

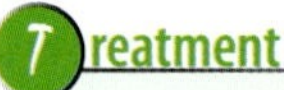

Treatment

This is similar to that of superficial dermatitis. Appropriate antibiotics or fungicides are applied locally. The apposing skin surfaces may be separated with gauze or appropriate dressings. Castellani's paint and liberal use of dusting powder is helpful.

PITTED KERATOLYSIS

This is a bacterial infection of the skin, often seen in men with sweaty feet, during the hot and humid climate; palmar infection is rare. No marked discomfort is produced although the lesions are malodourous (Fig. 8).

The disease is bacterial in origin; several bacteria have been implicated, most likely caused by *Micrococcus sedentarius* and in some cases by *Corynebacterium* species or *Dermatophilus congolensis*. These bacteria produce and excrete exoenzymes (keratinase) that are able to degrade keratin and produce pitting in the stratum corneum, when the skin is hydrated and the pH rises above neutrality.

Clinically numerous tender superficial erosions are found, mainly on the weight bearing areas of the sole, coalescing to form polycyclic patterns. The course is chronic and recurrent. The clinical presentation is so characteristic that laboratory confirmation is usually not necessary.

Treatment

Excessive sweating is reduced by 1% formalin or 10% buffered glutaraldehyde or 10–20% aluminium chloride. Topical antibiotics such as erythromycin or clindamycin are curative. Whitfield's ointment, miconazole or clotrimazole cream, 5% benzoyl peroxide gel preparations are all helpful.

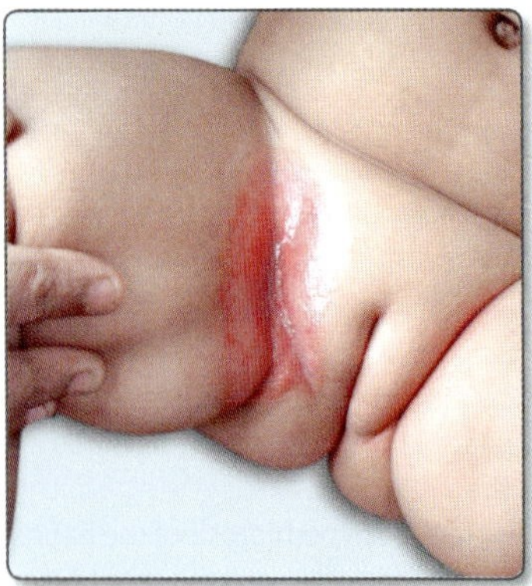

Fig. 7: Intertrigo

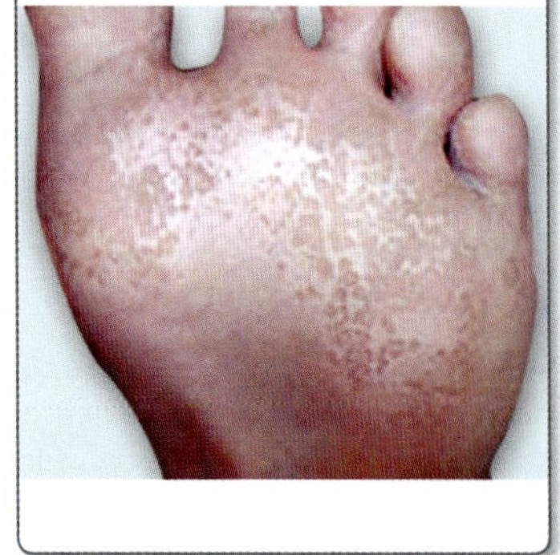

Fig. 8: Pitted keratolysis

ANHIDROSIS

Anhidrosis may be due to lesions of the central nervous system, peripheral nerves or of the sweat glands themselves. The most common cause of anhidrosis in tropical countries is miliaria. Other causes are congenital ectodermal dysplasia, diabetic neuropathy, ichthyosis, Sjögren's syndrome, atopic dermatitis, leprosy, poliomyelitis, multiple sclerosis, etc. Many premature babies do not sweat even when pyrexial.

Miliaria

Miliaria is very common in newborns in the first week of life, when the infant is adjusting to the new environment. In later life, it is seen in countries where the climate is hot and humid. Miliaria is due to the blockage of the sweat ducts caused by overhydration of keratin in hot and humid climates. It produces a distinct papulovesicular eruption. The disease is common in children; men are more affected than women.

The excessive production of sweat in the tropics leads to maceration of the orifice of the sweat duct, resulting in a keratin plug. With further increase of sweating, the obstructed duct breaks and the sweat leaks into the surrounding epidermis, producing vesicles and irritation. The sweat retention can occur at different levels, which causes three different clinical types: (1) miliaria crystallina (stratum corneum), (2) miliaria rubra (living layers of epidermis and upper dermis) and (3) miliaria profunda (dermis).

Clinical Features

Miliaria crystallina: This is characterised by very small clear vesicles without an inflammatory reaction. The trunk, axillae and the groins are the common sites affected. The lesions are often seen in bed-ridden patients, whose fever produces excessive perspiration. In miliaria crystallina, the rupture of the duct is superficial in the stratum corneum (Fig. 9).

Miliaria rubra (prickly heat): The lesions appear as itchy vesicles or papules on an erythematous base. Common sites are the flexures: the antecubital and popliteal fossae, inframammary areas, inguinal region and the trunk. Pruritus and pricking sensations are severe; scratching may lead to secondary infection. The course is variable depending upon temperature, amount of exertion and sweating. Recurrences in the same part of the body are common. In miliaria rubra the rupture is at the level of the prickle cell layer (Fig. 10).

Miliaria profunda: It is manifested by skin coloured elevations resulting from deep vesicles. This gives the skin a goose flesh appearance, there is no redness or itching, the trunk is mainly affected. The lesions develop following persistent or recurrent miliaria rubra.

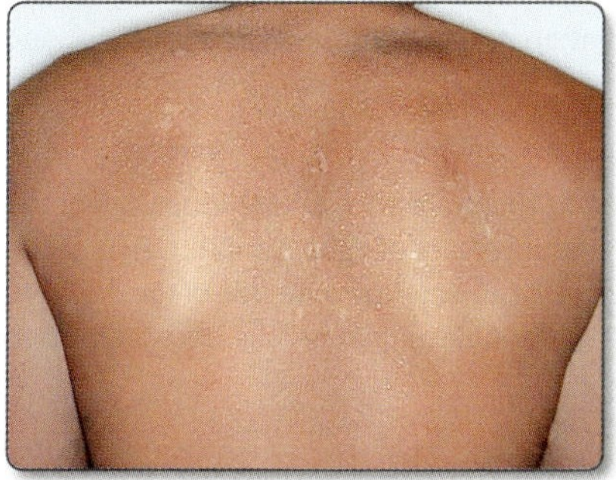

Fig.9: Miliaria crystallina

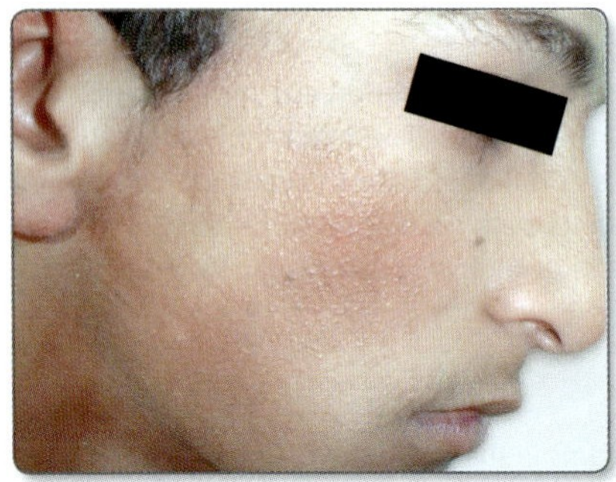

Fig. 10: Miliaria rubra

Complications

In children, miliaria rubra may result in the development of sweat gland abscess. Tropical anhidrotic asthenia is relatively common in the tropics, it often follows several attacks of miliaria rubra or is seen after prolong exposure to heat. The patient has low-grade fever, tachycardia, fatigue, dyspnoea, vertigo, headache and exhaustion. The skin may later develop miliaria profunda.

Treatment

It is essential to cool the patient. This can be achieved by cooling lotions such as calamine, baths, liberal application of dusting powders, the use of electric fans or if possible air conditioning. Removal of the keratin plugs can be attempted by salicylic acid lotion. Vitamin C 1 g daily may be helpful. Topical and systemic antibiotics should be used to control secondary bacterial infections.

TUMOURS OF THE SWEAT GLANDS

There are a number of tumours of eccrine sweat glands; syringomas are the most common. Syringomas and cylindromas are of uncertain histogenesis. The dermal cylindromas are said to be of eccrine origin, although histochemical reactions show an apocrine derivation.

Syringomas

Syringomas are benign skin tumours, more common in females than males. They usually appear at adolescence, subsequent lesions appear later in life. The lesions are small papules, 2–3 mm in diameter, usually skin coloured, sometimes they may have a cystic appearance. The lesions are multiple, symmetrical and the common sites of involvement are the face, around the eyes, neck and upper chest (Fig. 11).

Histopathology

Collections of convoluted and cystic ducts are seen in the upper half of the dermis. The ducts are lined by a double layer of cells, similar to that of the eccrine glands. A tail like strand of cells projects from one side of the duct into the dermis; giving resemblance to a tadpole or comma. The duct is enclosed in a fibrous stroma.

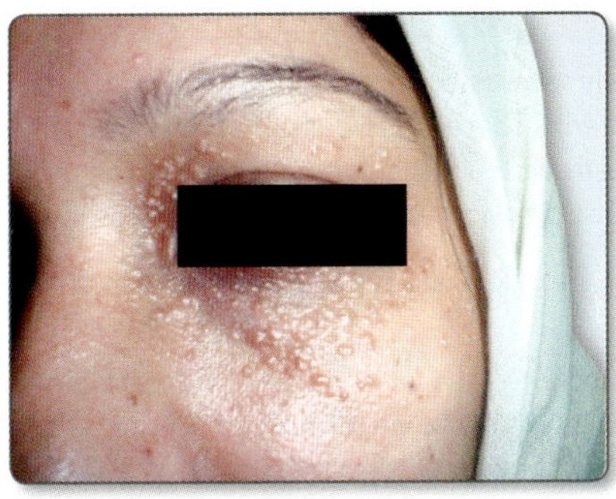

Fig. 11: Syringomas

Differential Diagnosis

The tumour should be differentiated from trichoepithelioma, these appear on the nose or sides of the nose, these are larger than syringomas, and often have a family history. The lesions on the eyelids should be differentiated from xanthelasma but syringomas lack the orange colour. The eruptions on the chest may be mistaken for disseminated granuloma annulare.

Treatment

This may be required for cosmetic reasons. Electrocautery, laser ablation or cryotherapy are used to treat syringomas, care should be taken to avoid scarring.

Cylindromas (Turban Tumour)

This is a skin tumour of uncertain origin, either eccrine or apocrine. It may be hereditary or acquired. Women are chiefly affected in early adult life.

The dominantly inherited form manifests as numerous round masses, pink to red in colour, on the scalp soon after puberty. The lesions resemble bunches of grapes or small tomatoes. Sometimes, they cover the entire scalp like a turban (Fig. 12).

The solitary or the nonhereditary variety occurs predominantly on the scalp and the face, it is firm, rubber-like nodule, blue or pink in colour, ranging from a few millimetres to several centimetres in size.

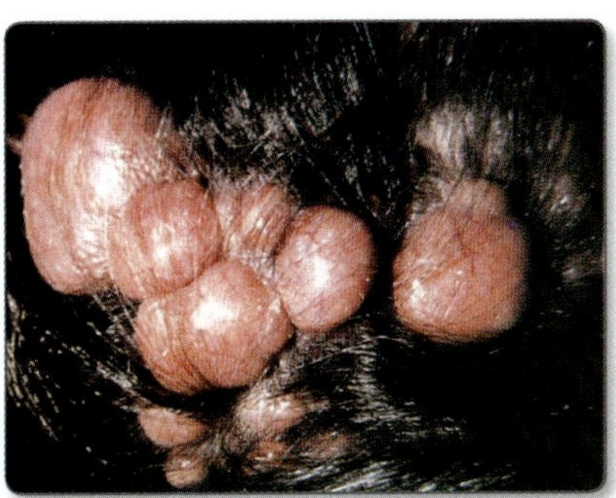

Fig. 12: Cylindromas

Histopathology

The tumour is composed of closely set masses or columns of cells, surrounded by a narrow mass of hyaline material. There are two types of cells: one large with a large amount of cytoplasm with a vesicular nucleus, and the other small with little cytoplasm and a compact nucleus. The small cells tend to be peripheral.

Treatment

Surgery is the treatment of choice. Extensive involvement of the scalp may require wide excision and replacement of the area by a graft. It can also be treated by removal of a few tumours at a time.

Eccrine Poroma

The tumour occurs at middle age, it is derived from the intraepidermal and/or upper dermal component of the eccrine duct. The tumours are asymptomatic, smooth, dome-shaped pink to red papules or nodules, situated on the soles, palms or the scalp (Fig. 13). They can be verrucous and bleed easily. Ulceration is uncommon. Malignant changes in long standing cases have been recorded; these lesions present with pain, sudden increase in size, bleeding or itching.

Eccrine poromas should be differentiated from pyogenic granuloma, verruca vulgaris and intradermal naevus.

Treatment is by excision.

Eccrine Spiradenoma

Eccrine spiradenoma occurs in late adolescence. They present as painful skin coloured or reddish blue papules or nodules, on any part of the body, usually less than 1 cm in diameter. The pain is either spontaneous or secondary to pressure, touch or injury. Ulceration is uncommon.

The tumour should be differentiated from other painful tumours such as blue rubber bleb naevus, angiolipoma, neuroma, glomus tumour and leiomyoma.

Treatment is by excision.

(Painful skin tumours can be studied by the acronym *BANGLES*: **B**lue rubber bleb naevus, **A**ngiolipoma, **N**euroma, **G**lioma, **L**eiomyoma and **E**ccrine **S**piradenoma)

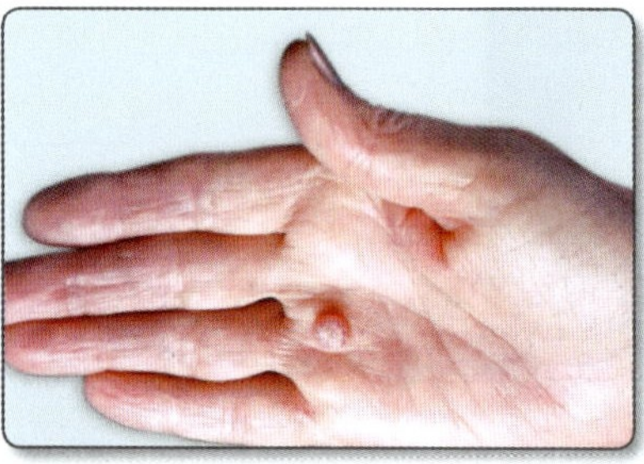

Fig. 13: Eccrine poroma
Source: Global Skin Atlas (Dr Ian McColl)

CONGENITAL DISORDERS OF THE SWEAT GLANDS

Anhidrotic Ectodermal Dysplasia

The classical triad of this disorder consists of hypotrichosis, anodontia and anhidrosis. The inheritance is X-linked recessive, males are commonly affected. Histology shows reduction, absent or poor development of the sweat glands and hair follicles. The number of sebaceous glands is variable. The epidermis is thin and flattened, dermal connective tissue appears normal. In some cases, collagen and elastic tissue may be fragmented.

These patients have a typical facies suggestive of congenital syphilis. The nasal bridge is depressed forming a saddle shaped nose. The supraorbital ridge is prominent, cheekbones are high and wide, the eyebrows are scanty, there are radiating furrows at the buccal commissures, and lips are thickened (Fig. 14). There is partial or complete anodontia. The incisors and/or canines if present are conical and pointed (Fig. 15). Nails may be thin and brittle. Hypotrichosis is generalised. The alopecia is not complete, the hairs are thin, sparse and dry. Mental retardation is present in some cases.

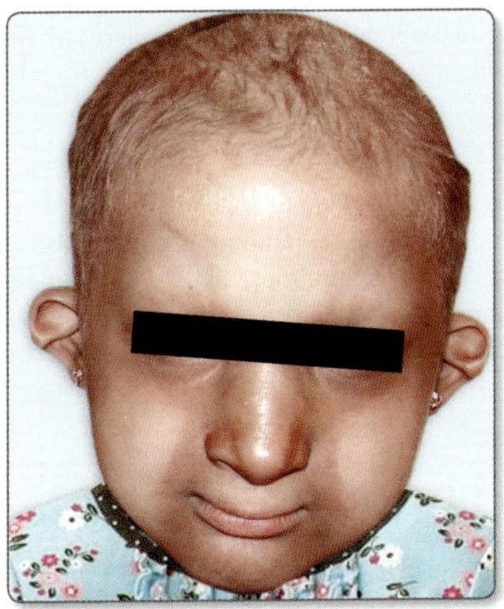

Fig. 14: Anhidrotic ectodermal dysplasia

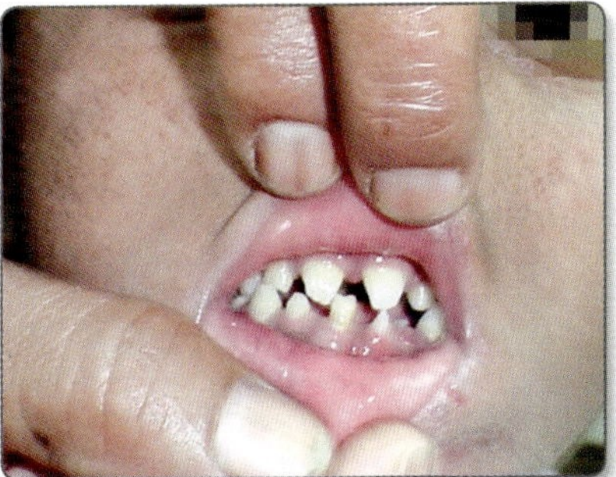

Fig. 15: Anhidrotic ectodermal dysplasia (note the conical incisors)

The patients are unable to tolerate heat, fever-induced sweating is absent or slight. Seizures may occur.

Differential Diagnosis

The condition should be differentiated from hypohidrotic ectodermal dysplasia in which the clinical findings are similar to anhidrotic ectodermal dysplasia. The disease has an autosomal recessive inheritance, hypohidrosis is less severe, and sweat glands are reduced in number but not absent.

In hidrotic ectodermal dysplasia, there is no abnormality of the sweat glands. The disease is characterised by nail dystrophy, hair defects and palmo-plantar keratosis.

Congenital syphilis has other stigmata, VDRL is positive.

Treatment

The patients should be advised against physical exertion, choice of a suitable occupation, avoidance of warm climate. Regular dental supervision is essential. Genetic counselling should be advised, the condition could be diagnosed on prenatal examination.

DISEASES OF THE APOCRINE GLANDS

The diseases of the apocrine glands are generally localised in the areas such as the axillae, around the nipple and the anogenital region, or in places where ectopic apocrine glands are found.

HIDRADENITIS SUPPURATIVA (ACNE INVERSA)

This is a chronic suppurative, recurrent, debilitating, painful disease of the apocrine glands, the earliest change is follicular occlusion. It begins at puberty and gradually fades in middle life; women are more affected than men. Exacerbations are common during menstruation and hot weather. Excessive perspiration appears to macerate and plug the apocrine sweat duct. Obesity and cigarette smoking are often associated with hidradenitis suppurativa.

Clinical Features

Deep-seated, tender, red nodules resembling furuncles develop in the axillae, anogenital region or around the nipples (Fig. 16). These nodules rupture with the formation of sinus tracts. Recurrent lesions result in the formation of fistulas. The lesions heal with irregular hypertrophic scars. In advanced lesions, bands of scar tissue and fibrosis develop that may limit mobility of the tissue.

The three clinical stages of hidradenitis suppurativa described by Hurley are:

Stage 1: Solitary or multiple nodules, isolated abscesses; without scarring and sinus tracts.

Stage 2: Recurrent abscesses, single or multiple, widely separated lesions with sinus tracts and scarring.

Stage 3: Diffuse or almost diffuse involvement of the axillae or groins or multiple interconnected tracts with scarring.

A total of 75% of cases stay in stage 1, 24% may progress to stage 2, and 1% of cases progress to stage 3.

Complications

Sinus tract formation and scarring can result in strictures. Urethral and vaginal strictures can develop with perineal involvement. Mild arthritis of the axial or peripheral type may develop in acute phases of the disease. Squamous cell carcinoma may develop in long standing cases; it behaves aggressively and has high mortality. Other complications include amyloidosis, interstitial keratitis and anaemia.

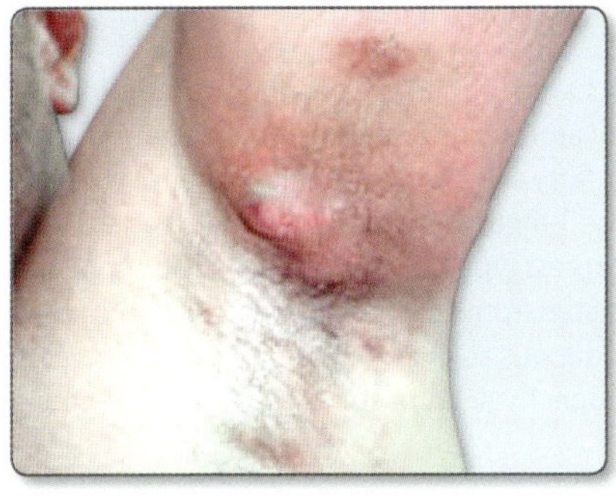

Fig. 16: Hidradenitis suppurativa

Histopathology

Follicular plugging and portal occlusion are prominent features. Folliculitis and perifollicular inflammation are seen in about two-thirds of cases. Active inflammation around the apocrine glands is less common. Varying degrees of inflammation and fibrosis are present according to the stage of disease. The inflammatory cells are neutrophils, lymphocytes, plasma cells and occasional eosinophils. Areas of frank dermal abscess are seen.

Differential Diagnosis

Single deep-seated tender nodule may resemble a furuncle or infected epidermoid cyst. Multiple lesions in the axilla should be differentiated from scrofuloderma, deep mycosis, and actinomycosis (Table 1). Groin and genital lesions should be differentiated from lymphogranuloma venereum.

Treatment

Despite numerous forms of treatment, possibilities for a permanent cure are elusive. In the early stages, hot compresses are useful. Topical clindamycin may prevent new lesions from developing. Long-term systemic antibiotic usually tetracycline is given for 4–6 months. Systemic antiandrogens help some women. Abscess which is pointing and painful may be incised and drained. In these lesions, intralesional corticosteroid injections should be given at the same time. If inflammation is severe, a short course of systemic corticosteroids is often needed. The other antibiotics effective in hidradenitis suppurativa are clindamycin, rifampicin, trimethoprim/sulphamethoxazole and dapsone.

When associated with acne, it can be treated by isotretinoin given in a dose of 1 mg/kg/day for 3 months.

In resistant cases, wide surgical excision and skin graft is indicated . Biologics, CO_2 laser and Nd:YAG (1064 nm) laser, radiotherapy have also been used..

Table 1: The differentiating features of hidradenitis suppurativa and scrofuloderma

Hidradenitis suppurativa	*Scrofuloderma*
Bilateral or unilateral	Unilateral
Nodules and sinuses	Nodules and sinuses
Etiology—blockage of the follicular unit	Infection with *Mycobacterium tuberculosis*
Age of onset: after puberty	No relationship to puberty, can occur at any age
Comedones present	Comedones absent
May be associated with acne conglobata, dissecting cellulitis of the scalp and pilonidal sinus	May be associated with tuberculous foci in other parts of the body

APOCRINE BROMHIDROSIS

The disease affects young adults after puberty. Apocrine bromhidrosis is commonly encountered in the axillae; it is due to the bacterial decomposition of the apocrine sweat, producing fatty acids with distinctive offensive odour. The main component appears to be 3-methyl-2-hexenoic acid. Androgens may also play a part; apocrine glands express type 1 5α- reductase activity. Apocrine bromhidrosis should be differentiated from eccrine bromhidrosis, which may be keratogenic, metabolic or exogenous such as due to garlic or amino acid disorders. Co-factors include improper hygiene, bacterial and fungal infections and nonabsorbent clothing.

Treatment

Axillary bromhidrosis can be controlled by reducing the bacterial flora by using antibacterial soaps; many commercial deodourants are quite effective in controlling the odour, because they contain antibacterial components. Frequent bathing and changing of underclothes are helpful. Reduction of eccrine sweating by using aluminium chloride may help reduce local bacterial flora. Aluminium chloride (20%) in anhydrous ethanol applied at bedtime, with or without occlusion, may be used on two consecutive nights, then every three to seven nights thereafter.

- Treatment of secondary bacterial or fungal infection is essential. Ultrasonic surgical aspiration of the axillary apocrine glands, or open surgical removal of axillary skin and subcutaneous tissue have been used to treat apocrine bromhidrosis. The use of double frequency Q switched Nd-YAG by lasers has been reported to be effective.

APOCRINE CHROMHIDROSIS

Apocrine chromhidrosis refers to coloured secretion by the apocrine glands. It is a localised disease affecting the axillae or the face (due to ectopic apocrine glands). Lipofuscins are the responsible pigment. The condition is seen after puberty when apocrine gland function is activated. Slow regression of the disease is seen with advanced age, which parallels the regression of apocrine glands.

Apocrine chromhidrosis is rarely a clinical problem; as the quantity of apocrine secretion at the follicular orifice is relatively small (0.001 mL or less). The most common colour in axillary chromhidrosis is yellow, while on the face it is dark blue or black. When dried the secretion is adherent at the follicular orifice, the skin of the affected region is otherwise normal.

Differential Diagnosis

Patients with ochronosis may have brown coloured sweat; sweat can also be contaminated by corynebacteria, piedra, drugs such as clofazimine, or from dye of clothes. The presence of lipofuscin granules in apocrine cells and the characteristic fluorescence confirm the diagnosis.

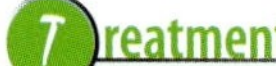

Treatment

There is no satisfactory treatment for apocrine chromhidrosis. Capsaicin cream depletes the neurons of substance P, an important transmitter in apocrine sweat production, has been successively used in the treatment of apocrine chromhidrosis. The disease is chronic and slowly fades with age.

FOX-FORDYCE DISEASE

This disorder of the apocrine glands can be compared to the prickly heat (miliaria) of the eccrine glands. The disease is common in women during adolescence or soon afterwards. The disease is due to the keratinous obstruction of the distal part of the apocrine duct. Retention of apocrine secretion results in dilatation of the duct and its rupture. A genetic predisposition could be a factor; the condition is seen in families and monozygotic twins.

Clinical Features

It is characterised by conical, flesh or greyish coloured discrete pruritic papules in the areas of apocrine distribution. The hair in these areas is likely to be scanty.

The disease may be regulated by endocrine factors but the primary cause of apocrine duct occlusion by a keratinous plug is not known. The disease runs a prolonged course and may persist until menopause. Some remission may occur in pregnancy. The disease is worse in summer, and it is usually pruritic. It improves with the use of oral contraceptives.

Treatment

Response to treatment is unsatisfactory. Topical clindamycin used twice a day may reduce itching and burning. Topical corticosteroids, UV radiation, topical retinoic acid and oral contraceptives may be helpful. Severe cases may require surgical excision of the affected area.

John Fordyce (1858–1925)

"Fordyce was a professor of dermatology and syphilology in the Columbia University College of Physicians and Surgeons. Fordyce described multiple cystic epitheliomas, pseudocolloid of the lips (Fordyce spots), and Fox Fordyce disease along with GH Fox."

APOCRINE HIDROCYSTOMA

Apocrine hidrocystomas are solitary cystic tumours usually periorbital, usually at the lateral canthus or in a pretemporal location. They are blue-black to purple dome-shaped cystic nodules. On the eyelids, they arise from the glands of Moll.

The tumour should be differentiated from a cavernous or thrombosed haemangioma, blue naevus and pigmented basal cell carcinoma.

Treatment is by excision.

FURTHER READING

1. Alikhan Ali, Lynch JP, Essen BD. Hidradenitis suppurativa: a comprehensive review. J Amer Acad Dermatol. 2009;60(4):539-61.
2. Chen W, Thiboutot D, ZC Zouboulis, et al. Cutaneous androgen metabolism.: basic research and clinical perspectives. The Journal of Invest Dematol. 2002;1198(5):9923-10073.
3. Ebling FJG. Apocrine glands in health and disease. Int J Dermatol. 1989;28:501-11.
4. Foster KG, Hey EN, Katz G. Eccrine sweat glands functions in the newborn baby. J Physiol. 1968;198:36-7.
5. Giacobetti R, Caro WA, Roenigk WH. Foxfordyce disease. Arch Dermatol. 1979;115:1365-6.
6. Haedersdal M, Togsverd-Bo K, and Wulf HC. Evidence-based review of lasers, light sources and photodynamic therapy in the treatment of acne vulgaris. J Eur Acad Dermatol VenereolJEADV. 2008;22:267-78
7. Holzle E, Kligman AM. The pathogenesis of miliaria rubra. Br J Dermatol. 1978; 99:117-37.
8. Korting HC, Schollmann C and Korting HC. Current topical and systemic approaches to treatment of rosacea. J Eur Acad Dermatol VenereolJEADV. 2009;23:876-82.
9. McDonald A, Fewel F. Perioral dermatitis: aetiology and treatment with tetracyclines. Br J Dermatol. 1972;87:315-9.

10. Melnik CB, and Schmitz G. Role of insulin-like growth factor-1, hyperglycaemic food and milk consumption in the pathogenesis of acne vulgaris. Experimental Dermatology. 2009; 18:833-41.
11. Moon SE, Lee YS, Youn JI. Eruptive vellus cysts and steatocystoma multiple in a patient with pachyonychia congenita. J Am Acad Dermatol. 1994;30:275-6.
12. Moore A, Kempers S, Murakawa G, et al. Topical Brimondine Tartarte Gel 0.5% for the treatment of moderate to severe facial erythema of rosacea. Results of a one year open trial. J Drugs Dermatol. 2014;13(1):56-61.
13. Parks WR, Parks GT. Pathogenesis, clinical features and management of hidradenitis suppurativa. Ann R Coll Surg Engl. 1997;79:83-9.
14. Porter AMW. Why do we have apocrine and sebaceous glands?. J R Soc Med. 2001;94(5): 236-7.
15. Shuster S. Direct disruption; a new explanation of miliaria. Acta Derm Venereol (Stockh). 1997;77:111-3.
16. Sigmore RJ. A pilot study of 5% permethrin cream versus 0.75% metronidazole gel in acne rosacea. Cutis. 1995;56:177-9.
17. Strauss JS, Ebling FJG. Control and functions of skin glands in mammals. Mem Soc Endocirnol. 1970;18:341-71.
18. Thiboutot D, Chen W. Update and future of hormonal therapy in Acne. Dermatology. 2003; 206:57-67.
19. Thiboutot D, Weiss J, Bucko A, et al. Adapalene-benzoyl peroxide, a free-dosed combination for the treatment of acne vulgaris. Results of a multicentre, randomized double-blind control study. J Am Acad Dermatol. 2007;57(5):791-9.

Chapter

24 Hair Disorders

INTRODUCTION

Although hair has no vital function in human beings, it plays an important part in the psychological build-up of man. It is very distressing to have excessive hair or loss of hair. Eyebrows and eyelashes provide protection to the eyes. Pubic and axillary hair enhance dissemination of odour from the apocrine glands, vellus hair of the body partly plays a role in protection against cold by piloerection. Hair such as nasal cilia play a part in preventing foreign antigens entering the body. Scalp hair and beard have cosmetic importance to man. Scalp hair protects the scalp from ultraviolet radiation; bald men are more prone to skin cancer.

Hair disorders can be studied under the following headings:

- Hypertrichosis, hirsutism and alopecia
- Pigmentary abnormalities
- Structural defects of the hair
- Hair cosmetics.

APPROACH TO A PATIENT WITH HAIR DISORDERS

A proper history with a complete scalp, cutaneous and systemic examination will in most cases help in coming to a diagnosis, or differentials of hair disorders. A history of drug intake, any systemic illness, pregnancy, family history in cases of hirsutism, and androgenetic alopecia (AGA) is important. Contact with animals should be taken for dermatophyte infections. A dietary history, especially of iron, zinc and proteins, is essential for generalised hair loss. Assess the hair loss, especially the type (cicatricial, noncicatricial), pattern (patchy, regular or irregular, diffuse, universal), and duration of hair loss. Always compare the distribution of scalp hair and body hair before coming to any conclusion of hair loss.

Investigations are sometimes required to confirm the diagnosis. These include a scraping, and Wood's light examination for fungal infections. Hormonal assessment, such as free testosterone, dehydroepiandrosterone sulfate (DHEAS), androstenedione, prolactin, follicle-stimulating hormone and luteinising hormone (LH) levels, is required for hirsutism. Complete blood picture, urinalysis, and anti-nuclear antibody (ANA) for lupus erythematosus are helpful in alopecia.

Hair-Pull Test

A bundle of hair, about 50–60 hair, are pulled in the direction of the hair shaft; the pull should be firm, but not forceful. The test should be done 5 days after shampooing. On the day of shampooing, all the telogen hair are removed by washing. The test is positive if more than six hairs are pulled out, indicating increased hair shedding. If less than six hairs are pulled, it is normal physiological hair shedding. The test is not standardised and is not much used nowadays. Under normal conditions about 100 hairs are lost daily.

Dermatoscopy

It is a useful tool before a skin biopsy; it also helps to determine the site of biopsy. It is especially helpful in detecting hair-shaft defects, exclamation mark hairs, tapered hair and pediculosis. Dermatoscopy is also helpful in scalp disorders such as psoriasis, lichen planus, scarring alopecia, etc. The normal scalp shows simple fine red loops that represent capillaries in the dermal papilla. In psoriasis, typical scaly plaques are seen under high magnification. In alopecia areata (AA), yellowish dots are very characteristic. The dots represent follicular opening filled with keratin debris and sebum. AGA is characterised by diversity in hair diameter due to miniaturisation of the hair follicle. Variability in hair shaft diameter of more than 20% is diagnostic of androgenetic alopecia. In lichen planus, dermatoscopy reveals the absence of follicular openings and presence of perifollicular scales at the periphery of the lesion. Scalp atrophy is represented by diffuse white colour of the scalp.

Microscopic Examination

Simple microscopic examination of the hair is a useful diagnostic tool in the detection of hair disorders in children. Diseases such as Menkes disease, Netherton's syndrome, trichothiodystrophy, Chédiak-Higashi syndrome, loose anagen syndrome, and other structural defects can be seen under a microscopic examination.

The hairs are cut close to the scalp; they are embedded in a standard medium, and covered with a coverslip, then examine under a microscope.

Trichogram

It is useful to find out the degree of alopecia, to study the hair cycle and its anomalies; it is also used as follow-up for prognostic purpose. It should be done in a standard way and by an experienced person. The study is carried out 5 days after the last washing. About 40–60 hair are plucked from two sites; either frontal and occipital, or one from the affected area and one from the unaffected area. The sites should be selected by a dermatologist. The hair are held by a needle holder with rubber tipped ends, then pulled briskly in the direction of the hair shafts. The hair are then put on a glass slide with a mounting solution and cover slip applied. Then examine the hair under a microscope.

Trichoscan

It is used for the measurement of hair density, hair diameter, growth rate, and anagen/telogen ratio. It is also used to study the effects of drugs and lasers on hirsutism and hypertrichosis. A small area of the scalp is shaved about 2 cm behind the anterior hairline. This site can be covered by most patients. After 3 days, the area is dyed with a special dye. A digital image is then taken. A software then analyses the picture measuring the hair density, anagen/telogen ratio, and the growth rate.

Scalp Biopsy

A scalp biopsy is done to confirm the cause of scalp disorders such as cicatricial alopecia. Early diagnosis with proper treatment prevents cicatricial alopecia from spreading. It is also useful in diagnosing the type of hair loss. In these cases, both transverse and longitudinal sections are required. A transverse section indicates the density of hair follicles, and a longitudinal study shows the ratio of vellus hair to the terminal hair. In female pattern hair loss (FPHL), the ratio of terminal (T) to vellus hair (V) is T:V < 4:1. In telogen effluvium, the ratio is T:V > 8:1.

HYPERTRICHOSIS

Hair can be vellus, lanugo or androgen-dependent. Increased growth of vellus hair is known as hypertrichosis. Lanugo hair is normally present in intrauterine life and is shed before birth. Increased growth of such hair when found after birth is termed as hypertrichosis lanuginosa. It may be congenital or acquired.

Congenital Hypertrichosis Lanuginosa

This is usually present at birth; the entire body is affected except the palms and soles. The hair is long; it may be 10 cm or more. Long eyelashes and eyebrows are conspicuous. In some cases, the scalp may have normal androgenic hair and the face may be spared. The condition may be associated with other abnormalities such as dental and gingival fibromatosis, hypodontia or adontia. Physical and mental development is normal. These children are often referred to as "dog facies" or "human werewolf".

Acquired Hypertrichosis Lanuginosa

This is often secondary to malignancies of gastrointestinal tract, bronchus, breast, urinary bladder, and other organs. In milder forms, only the face may be affected. In other cases, the change from vellus to lanugo hair may affect the whole body. Usually androgen-stimulated hair are not affected. The hair growth is rapid usually about 2.5 cm per week.

Hypertrichosis of the Vellus Hair

This may be localised or generalised. Localised hypertrichosis may be seen in some melanocytic nevi, Becker's nevus, and spina bifida. Hypertrichosis of the exposed skin is seen in porphyria. In Cornelia-de-Lange syndrome, increased growth of hair is seen on the face. In hyperthyroidism, hypertrichosis is seen over the tibia in pretibial myxoedema.

Generalised hypertrichosis is seen in Hurler's syndrome, Winchester syndrome, hypothyroidism, hyperthyroidism, pituitary disorders, malnutrition, and anorexia nervosa.

A number of drugs cause hypertrichosis. These include corticosteroids, diphenylhydantoin, penicillamine, psoralens, minoxidil, benoxaprofen, cyclosporin and streptomycin. Hypertrichosis may also be produced by local stimulation such as application of plaster over inflamed joints, after recurrent thrombophlebitis and epidermolysis bullosa.

HIRSUTISM

Hirsutism is defined as the terminal hair growth in a woman, the face or body in a male pattern. It is due to the action of androgen on the hair follicles. Skin is the target tissue for these hormones.

Not all hair follicles are androgen-dependent; those of the eyebrows, eyelashes, corona of the scalp, forearms and lower legs are androgen-independent; those of the upper lip, beard, nasal tip, ears, pubis, upper legs, thorax, axillae, and frontal and temporal scalp are androgen-dependent. Hirsutism is defined as vellus-to-terminal hair transformation of androgen-dependent hair follicles in a female (Fig. 1).

Normal and Abnormal Action of Androgens

The following are the determinants of androgen action:

- Androgen production
- Biological availability of androgen to the target tissues
- End-organ sensitivity to circulatory androgens
- Utilisation of androgens by the target tissue

There are several steroids present in the plasma that have androgenic activity. For practical purposes, testosterone (T) is the important androgen present extracellularly, and dehydrotestosterone (DHT) present intracellularly. The other major androgens present in the circulation are the 17-ketosteroids, androstenedione (A), dehydroepiandrosterone (DHEA) and dehydroepiandrosterone sulphate (DHEAS). These steroids are androgenic via their eventual conversion to T and DHT. These hormones are considered as prehormones.

The potent androgen, testosterone and androgen precursor androstenedione (A) are secreted by the ovaries. The adrenals contribute to prehormones: DHEA, DHEAS and A. These require peripheral conversion in the skin and liver to testosterone.

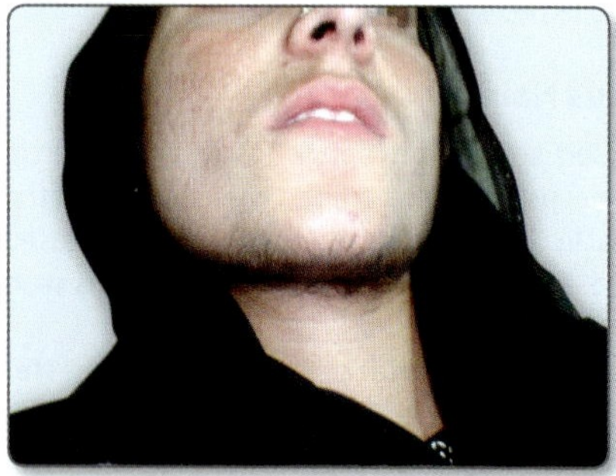

Fig. 1: Hirsutism

Androgen Production

The ovaries and adrenals, each secrete 25% of the circulating T; the remaining 50% is derived from extra-glandular metabolic conversion of other androgens, mainly A. This arises equally from direct ovarian and adrenal glandular secretion. Eighty percent of DHEA is secreted by the adrenals and 20% by the ovaries. DHEAS is secreted entirely by the adrenals.

Under normal circumstances, the fate of the ovarian androgens is to produce oestrogen, and the fate of adrenal androgens to produce adrenal cortisol and aldosterone. Ovarian androgen production is under control of pituitary gonadotrophin LH.

Adrenal androgen production is under control of adrenocorticotrophic hormone (ACTH). Hence, the feedback of both ovarian and adrenal androgens is via oestradiol and cortisol respectively.

In pathological conditions, androgen production can be increased by increased glandular secretion of T, or increased production of prehormones A, DHEA and DHEAS. These can be due to abnormalities in the ovaries, adrenals, or due to increased trophic hormone stimulation, i.e. LH or ACTH.

Biological Availability of Androgen to the Target Tissues

Most of the androgens (80%) are bound to proteins: sex hormone-binding globulin (SHBG), rest to the albumin; only a small amount is found as free testosterone. It is the level of free testosterone that reflects clinical evidence of androgen excess rather than total testosterone. Free-androgen index (FAI) is a ratio of total testosterone and SHBG. Furthermore, compounds that have a higher affinity for SHBG than endogenous steroids will displace them, thus increasing their bioavailability.

Utilisation of Androgens by the Target Tissue

In androgen target tissues, such as the hair follicle, biologically active T enters from the circulation by diffusion. This intracellular T is metabolised further by 5-α-reductase to the more potent androgen DHT; this then binds to the androgen receptor in the cell.

Testosterone may also bind to the androgen receptors in the cell without conversion to DHT, e.g. in the muscle cells.

In the hair follicles, intracellular DHT is further metabolised to 3-diol-androstanediol. The 3-diol-androstanediol is converted irreversibly at a variety of sites to 3-α-diol glucuronamide. Both blood and urinary levels of 3-α-diol glucuronamide correlate closely with the measurements of 5-α-reductase activity in androgenic target tissues.

Target tissue androgen requires the presence of intracellular androgens receptors. Abnormalities of such receptors are seen in testicular feminisation.

Hirsute women have increased 5-α-reductase activity; peripheral levels of 3-α-diol glucuronamide reflect this abnormality.

Androgens are a major cause of acne, seborrhoea, hirsutism, and hidradenitis suppurativa. Each individual is endowed with a fixed number of hair follicles at birth.

Factors Governing the Action of Androgen

Race

Iranian women have more hair as compared with oriental women. In the Mediterranean region, the incidence of hirsutism is high; it is rare in Japanese women. Jewish and Irish women have more hair as compared with Danish women.

Age

Facial hirsutism tends to increase until old age. It is said that 40% of old women have slight hirsutism.

Hair Colour

Brunettes are more hairy than blonde women.

Hereditary

This plays an important part in hirsutism; it tends to run in families. Ninety percent hirsute women were found to have an increased incidence of hirsutism in their female relatives.

Obesity

Although many hirsute women are obese, the role of adipose tissue is undefined. Weight loss by obese hirsute women with menstrual irregularities may result in regulation of menses and reduction in body hair growth.

Assessment of Hirsutism

It can be done by assessing the androgen levels. Normal levels of androgens in males and females are shown in the Table 1.

Table 1: Testosterone levels in male and females

Testosterone measurement	*Females*	*Males*
Free Testosterone level ng/dL	0.3–1.9	9–30
Testosterone glucuronamide excretion µg/24 hours	4–10	40–200
Testosterone production rate mg/24 hours	1–3	4–12

Ferriman-Gallwey Scoring System

The system determines the severity of hair growth from 0-4 in nine body areas. The scorecard of every body location under survey begins from 0 (no excessive terminal hair growth) to 4 (extensive terminal hair growth) and the numbers are added up to a maximum count of 36. Total score 0-36. A score of ≥ 8 is labeled as hirsutism.

The nine areas are: upper lip, chin, chest, upper abdomen, lower abdomen, upper back, lower back, arms and thighs.

Aetiology of Hirsutism

- Idiopathic
- Ovarian causes
  - Polycystic ovaries
  - Leutomas of pregnancy

  - Virilising tumours
    - ➢ Hilar cell tumours
    - ➢ Arrhenoblastoma
    - ➢ Theca cell tumours
    - ➢ Leydig cell tumours
- Adrenal causes
  - Congenital adrenal hyperplasia
  - Virilising adrenal tumour
  - Cushing's syndrome
- Causes in the pituitary
  - Acromegaly
  - Prolactin-secreting adenomas
- Drugs
  - Androgens
  - Testosterones
  - Anabolic steroids such as danazol, levonorgestrel containing oral contraceptives
- Miscellaneous
  - Achard-Thiers syndrome
  - Turner's syndrome
  - Leprechaunism
  - Cornelia de Lange syndrome

Ovarian Causes

These include the polycystic ovaries and a variety of ovarian tumours, both benign and malignant. The polycystic ovary syndrome (Stein-Leventhal syndrome) is characterised by hirsutism (50%), acne (20%) and signs such as amenorrhoea, anovulation, obesity, and small breasts. The ovaries are frequently palpable on physical examination. Pelvis ultrasound is also helpful. Serum-free testosterone and LH are elevated, but FSH is normal or decreased.

Hirsutism caused by ovarian tumours, especially malignant, is usually rapid, often associated with virilism. Free testosterone level is high (generally greater than 2 ng/dL).

Adrenal Causes

These include adrenal hyperplasia, adrenal tumours, the adrenogenital syndrome, or congenital adrenal hyperplasia. Adrenogenital syndrome is an autosomal dominant disorder which results from the deficiency of enzymes, 21-hydroxylase (most common), 11-hydroxylase and 3-β-hydroxysteroid dehydrogenase. Onset is generally in childhood with large genitalia, precocious growth and virilism. However, adult onset with partial enzyme deficiencies is seen as a familial trait.

Pituitary Causes

Causes include Cushing's disease due to increase in ACTH, acromegaly, and prolactin-secreting adenomas. Prolactin-secreting tumours have a 20% incidence of hirsutism and acne. Other conditions in which prolactin levels are increased include hypothyroidism, phenothiazine intake and hepatorenal failure.

Idiopathic Hirsutism

This usually starts at puberty and may slowly become more extensive over the next three decades. The testosterone and other androgen levels are normal. In some women, hirsutism first develops at pregnancy and then tends to recur at each pregnancy. Hirsutism confined to the face is common after menopause. Hirsutism may follow severe emotional stress.

Other Causes

These include exogenous intake of androgens and high progesterone birth-control pills. End-organ hypersensitivity may be a mechanism in patients with normal levels of testosterone.

Evaluation of Hirsutism

A detail history and physical examination are essential in all cases of hirsutism. The history should focus on the age and acuteness of onset, progression, virilisation, menstrual history, family, and racial background.

Physical examination may reveal signs of Cushing's disease, acromegaly, and other endocrinal disorders. Other signs to be evaluated are distribution of muscle mass, body fat, size of clitoris, voice depth, and galactorrhoea.

Laboratory evaluation should include a free testosterone level, DHEAS level, a 17-hydroxyprogesterone level and a prolactin level. Free testosterone level above 2 ng/dL, suggests ovarian tumour.

Elevation of 17-hydroxyprogesterone levels should suggest congenital adrenal hyperplasia. Prolactin levels above 200 ng/mL suggests a pituitary gland tumour, the patient should be referred for further evaluations.

Twenty-four-hour urinary specimen for increased levels of 17-ketosteroids. Level of 30 mg in 24 hours also suggests adrenal pathology.

ACTH stimulation test and adrenal suppression tests may be done to distinguish between pituitary and adrenal disorders.

In other cases, the cause probably is idiopathic; a re-evaluation is required every 6–12 months.

History should rule out Cushing's disease, acromegaly and drug intake. Galactorrhea is present in prolactinoma, polysystic ovaries and acromegaly.

Diagnosis

A major elevation of DHEAS (above 9,000 ng/mL) suggests adrenal neoplasm, elevation of 17-hydroxyprogesterone levels should suggest congenital adrenal hyperplasia. Prolactin levels above 20 ng/mL should be referred for further evaluation.

Twenty-four-hour urinary specimen for increased levels of 17 ketosteroids (>30 mg in 24 hours) also suggests adrenal pathology.

ACTH stimulation test and adrenal suppression test may be done to distinguish between pituitary and adrenal disorders.

In other cases, the cause is probably idiopathic and proper treatment should be started. A re-evaluation is required every 6–12 months.

History should rule out Cushing's disease, acromegaly and drug intake. Galactorrhoea is present in prolactinoma, polycystic ovaries and acromegaly.

Patients with rapid onset of hirsutism who have elevated free testosterone levels, above 2 ng/mL, or presence of virilism, suggest underlying ovarian malignancy.

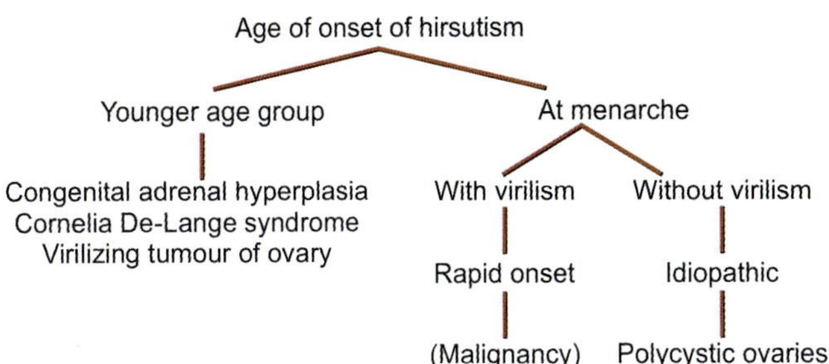

Treatment

This may be:

- Cosmetic
- Suppressive
- Anti-androgenic

Cosmetic: Cosmetic methods are the cheapest and easiest therapy for hirsutism. These include shaving, wax depilatories, chemical depilation, bleaching of the hair, and electrolysis. Chemical depilatories previously contained barium sulphide; these corrode the projecting hair shaft, and they have no action on the intrafollicular growing portion of the hair. It also irritates the skin and is therefore not used. Present depilatories contain sodium thioglycolate; this acts by reducing the disulphide bond of the hair follicles. These are non-irritating. Hair re-grows after these methods.

Hair removal by lasers and epilation is permanent. But the problem with permanent hair removal is that multiple treatments are required. Also permanent removal of stem cells will deprive the person of wound healing and regeneration of epidermis after deep burns and injuries.

Suppressive Therapy: These include oral contraceptives and glucocorticoids. These suppress hirsutism caused by ovaries and adrenals. Ovarian suppression can be achieved by a combination of ethinyl oestradiol 35 microgram and norethindrone 0.5 mg. Birth pills are helpful in 75% of hirsute women. These drugs should not be given to patients with thromboembolism, liver tumours, and hypertension. The therapy should be continued for 1 year. Serum T levels monitor oestrogen therapy.

Glucocorticoids are indicated in the treatment of congenital adrenal hyperplasia. DHEA levels monitor dexamethasone therapy. Dose of 0.25 mg of dexamethasone at bedtime can suppress adrenal androgens. Improvement in hirsutism can be seen in 6 months to 1 year of therapy.

Anti-Androgens: These include cyproterone acetate and chlormadinone acetate (primary anti-androgens), and spironolactone, cimetidine and ketoconazole (secondary anti-androgens). Cimetidine is a weak anti-androgen and is not used widely. Ketoconazole is hepatotoxic; it has not been well evaluated for the treatment of hirsutism.

Combination of cyproterone acetate and ethinyl oestradiol has been widely used to treat hirsutism. Cyproterone acetate, 100 mg a day, from 5–14 days of the menstrual cycle, and ethinyl oestradial from 5–25 days of the cycle. Strict contraception is indicated during its use.

Spironolactone is a stronger anti-androgen. It is used in a dose of 75–200 mg/day. A combination of spironolactone and oral contraceptives is also used to treat hirsutism. It limits menstrual irregularities and prevents contraception.

Eflornithine used topically is effective, but only as long as it is used; it shortens the anagen phase of the hair cycle.

Application of topically applied anti-androgens is not very effective, probably due to its poor penetration.

Other Drugs

5-α-Reductase Inhibitors

Finasteride, a 5-α-reductase inhibitor has been used with promising results in males; its effects are seen after 6 months of therapy. It may feminise a male fetus; it is therefore a drawback for women of childbearing potential.

Flutamide

This is an anti-androgen that binds to androgen receptors. It has no anti-gonadotrophic effects. It is given with oral contraceptives for 6 months to 1 year. It should be used with extreme caution as it can cause severe hepatic toxicity.

Gonadotrophic-Releasing Hormone Agonists (GnRH)

This inhibits LH production and thus reduces androgen production. It is presently under investigation.

Bromocriptine

This is a dopamine agonist used in the treatment of hyperprolactinaemia. It can also be used in the treatment of women with polycystic ovaries. It is given in a dose of 2.5 mg twice daily for 6 months to 1 year. It should be started with a smaller dose to prevent orthostatic hypotension.

Combined Drug Therapy

Additional therapeutic benefit can be obtained by combining oral contraceptives, glucocorticoids, and anti-androgens. Indications for such therapies are persistent hyperandrogenism and poor clinical response to a single agent. The risk of combined therapy is additive and not synergistic.

ALOPECIA

The world alopecia is derived from a Greek word, alopex, for fox. Fox are said to develop areas of baldness, when it rubs its skin to relieve itching. Alopecia may be scarring or non-scarring. It can be localised or diffuse.

Causes of Non-Cicatricial Alopecia

- Androgenetic alopecia (AGA)
- Alopecia areata (AA)
- Associated with systemic disease
  - Telogen effluvium
  - Deficiency disorders
  - Endocrine disorders
  - Syphilis
  - Drugs
- Traumatic
  - Trichotillomania
  - Traction alopecia
- Hereditary syndromes
  - Anhidrotic ectodermal dysplasia
  - Congenital alopecia universalis

  - Progeria, metageria and pangeria
  - Moynahan syndrome
  - Congenital triangular alopecia
  - Congenital poikiloderma
  - Cockayne's syndrome
  - Dyskeratosis congenita
  - Pachyonychia congenita
- Infection
  - Fungal infection, e.g. Tinea capitis (mild-moderate)
  - Bacterial infection, e.g. folliculitis (mild-moderate).

NON-CICATRICIAL ALOPECIA

Androgenetic Alopecia (Male-Pattern Baldness)

Androgenetic alopecia is believed to be inherited as an autosomal dominant pattern with incomplete penetrance. It is due to a conversion of terminal hair into vellus hair, which later becomes atrophic. Common male pattern baldness results from a combination of adequate androgen levels and appropriate genetic background. This hypothesis is difficult to reconcile as androgen results in terminal hair differentiation in other parts of the body. It is now felt that AGA probably results from local differences on the scalp in the amounts of enzymes that convert weak androgens such as DHEA into more potent androgens such as testosterone and dihydrotestosterone. Two of the enzymes required for conversions are 5-α-reductase and aromatase.

Androgenetic alopecia is a more appropriate term than androgenic alopecia as it is often called. This process can affect both men and women and affects people of all races.

The progression of terminal hair to vellus hair is gradual with successive follicular cycles producing hair of shorter length and decreased diameter. Males usually exhibit loss in the fronto-temporal and vertex area. In extreme cases, only a rim of hair is seen in the lateral and posterior aspect of the scalp. Females exhibit a more diffuse hair loss. The process may become apparent at any time after puberty in either sex.

Pathogenesis

Characteristics of AGA are:

- It has an autosomal dominant inheritance with variable penetrance
- Both sexes are affected
- Coexistence of greasy skin, hirsutism and acne in some cases

Hippocrates stated the fact that androgens are responsible for androgenetic alopecia in 400 BC, "Eunuch's are not subject to gout, nor do they become bald." Hippocrates was bald except for a small rim of hair covering the lower parietal and occipital scalp. If a person is castrated before puberty, he does not get bald. Following administration of testosterone, baldness appears in those people who are genetically predisposed. In women, maximum change of hair pattern occurs after menopause, when oestrogen level falls, and there is a more androgenic environment.

Sebaceous glands are under androgenic control. The pilosebaceous unit has the ability to metabolise a wide range of androgens. The enzyme 5-α- reductase has the ability to convert testosterone to dehydrotestosterone. Adult males with a genetic determined deficiency of 5-α-reductase have reduced levels of DHT, and lack the tendency to develop AGA.

There are two isoenzymes of 5-α-reductase, type 1 and 2. Type 1 is found in the dermal papillae, outer root sheath of the hair follicles, sebaceous glands, and basal layer of the epidermis. Type 2 is found predominantly in the prostate. Type 2 is more widespread in the skin of infants. This could play a conditioning role in programming the follicles to respond to post-pubertal androgens in a genetically determined manner.

Testosterone secreted by the testis is the principal circulating androgen in men. In women, the ovarian and adrenal steroids, androstenedione and DHEA are androgenic.

Human skin is an important site for the biotransformation and metabolism of androgens. The skin is also a major site for the peripheral conversion of T to DHT by 5-α-reductase. 5-α-reductase activity is especially higher in areas of higher sebaceous gland density. The pathogenesis is centred around the lengthening of the telogen phase and shortening of the anagen phase of hair growth. The shorter the anagen phase, the shorter is the length of hair.

Testosterone may be bound to the globulin or it may be free in the plasma. It is only the free testosterone that is biologically active testosterone to produce alopecia. Factors that increase plasma SHBG are estrogen therapy, pregnancy, hyperthyroidism, and liver cirrhosis. SHBG is decreased by increased androgen production, hyperinsulinemia, hyperprolactinaemia, corticosteroid therapy, hypothyroidism. and acromegaly.

Despite the wealth of knowledge regarding the mechanism of action of steroid hormones, the mechanism by which androgens regulate the hair follicles is still unclear. The paradox remains why androgens cause hirsutism on one hand and AGA do on the other hand. The basis of this functional mosaicism remains unclear.

In AGA, each anagen hair is a little shorter than the previous one and its Arao-Perkins body will be left behind a little distance above the first one. Eventually in scalps that form good elastic tissue, there will be a row of elastic clumps stacked within the remnants of the collapsed fibrous tissue sheath, like the rungs of a ladder. This picture is an absolute proof of male or female pattern alopecia.

Pattern of Hair Loss

Hamilton introduced the first grading scale for AGA, Norwood later modified this.

Hamilton's Classification

Type I	Normal pre-pubertal scalp pattern
Type II	Slight recession of the fronto-temporal region
Type III	Deeper recession of the fronto-temporal region
Type IV	Associated patch of baldness at the vertex

Type V Patch at the vertex enlarges

Type VI Joining of the fronto-temporal patch and that of the vertex by a narrow path

Type VII Widening of the joining patch, both fronto-temporal patch and that of the vertex appear as a single patch

Type VIII Only a narrow rim of hair remains at the occipital and parietal region

Diagnosis

Clinical diagnosis is obvious, investigations are not necessary. Hormone levels are normal; a family history is often present. A trichogram reveals reduced anagen/telogen ratio.

Clinical Features

AGA may begin at any age after puberty. The replacement of the terminal hair by vellus hair occurs in a particular manner. In men, hair is lost from the fronto-temporal region so that the hairline recedes on each side, and the forehead appears high (Fig. 2). The hair is then lost from the vertex. Eventually the entire top of the scalp becomes devoid of hair. The rate of hair loss varies amongst individuals. The parietal and occipital areas are often spared (Fig. 3).

In women, the pattern of hair loss is quite different. Women generally have diffuse hair loss throughout the scalp, sparing the frontal hairline. The changes that occur are same as that of male AGA, i.e. reduction of the anagen phase, reduced diameter and reduced growth of hair, followed by hair loss. Overlap form of male and female AGA is common in both the sexes.

Early in the process when the thinning is not apparent, creating a part in the frontal or vertex area and comparing it with an area on the posterior scalp may demonstrate subtle thinning. A hair-pull test should be performed by firmly grasping 50–60 hairs and then pulling them. The hair should be immediately examined. In a normal scalp, it should not yield more than five normal club hairs. Hair-pull test is normal in AGA. The hair examination should be carried out at a standard time, at least 5 days after the last washing of the hair. The areas should be carefully selected and specified.

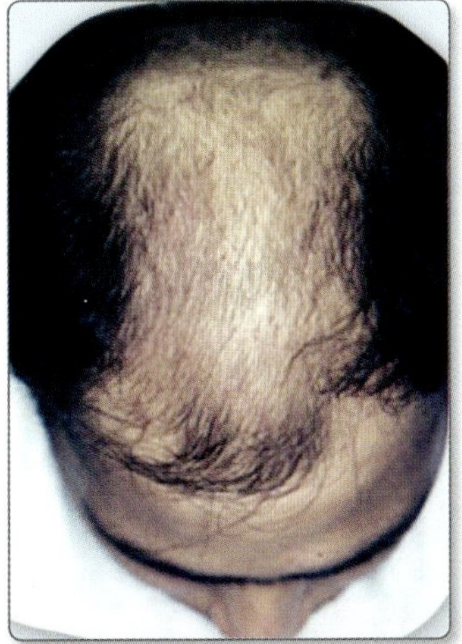

Fig. 2: Androgenetic alopecia—patient on minoxidil

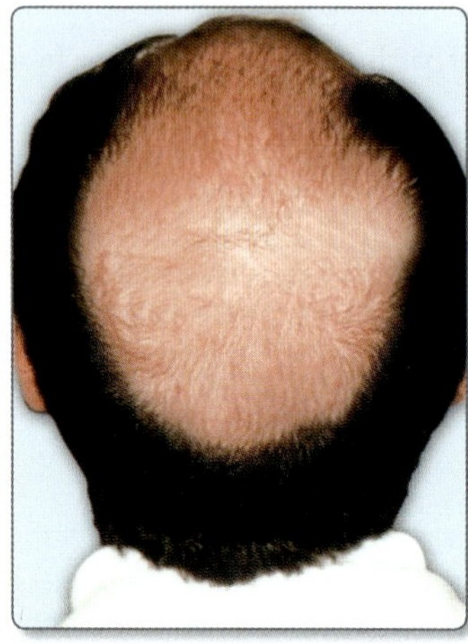

Fig. 3: Androgenetic alopecia—spared rim of hair

Treatment

Treatment of baldness dates back over 5000 years ago, record of its treatment is found in the Egyptian papyri. Hippocrates prescribed opium mixed with an essence of roses or lilies and oil of vinegar, olive oil or acacia juice.

Even today, treatment cannot be directed against genetic or time-dependent factors. Treatment should be mainly directed against DHT, reducing its production from T, preventing the binding of T to androgen receptors in the cell. No clinical effects can be expected in less than 3 months.

Most of the medical treatment is ineffective. Minoxidil, a potent peripheral arterial vasodilator, is used in the treatment of resistant hypertension; hypertrichosis is a frequent side effect. Ideal candidate for minoxidil are men younger than 30, who have hair loss less than 5 years.

Topical application of minoxidil is said to increase blood flow but how it produces hair, growth is not established. Perhaps by increasing the cutaneous perfusion by increase of skin temperature, the hair growth may increase. Systemic side effects are not recorded. Local tolerance is also good. Two-to-five percent solution of minoxidil is applied locally; clinical improvement is seen after 3–4 months of treatment. The medication should be applied on dry scalp, and the scalp should not be wet for 1 hour afterwards. Hair growth is evident in 8–12 months. This treatment has to be continued for life; for baldness reappears when minoxidil treatment is stopped.

More recently, 0.5% minoxidil has been studied in combination with topical tretinoin for AGA.

Topical 17-α-estradiol is used in some countries, but not a very effective treatment. It does not exert oestrogenic effect, but it inhibits 5-α-reductase activity.

Finasteride, an anti-androgen, is given in a dose of 1 mg/daily, is an effective therapy for men. Finasteride inhibits the conversion of testosterone to dihydrotestosterone. It slows further hair loss and improves hair growth. The effects are seen within 3 months of therapy. Side effects include decrease in libido and sexual potency. The drug is not effective in men after the age of 60, because 5-α-reductase activity may not be as high as in younger men. About 20–30% of men do not respond. Finasteride is not as effective in women; it should not be given to pregnant women. In both the sexes, there is a risk of development of breast cancer.

Surgical Treatment of AGA. AGA can be treated with full thickness hair bearing punch autografts obtained from AGA-resistant occipital hair. Many surgeons practice follicular unit transplant nowadays. In their new position, the transplanted follicles continue to produce hair of the same texture and colour, at the same rate as it did in the occipital area

Scalp reduction techniques can reduce the area requiring hair transplants.

In Women. The increased androgen production by the adrenals can be decreased by glucocorticoids, 2.5 mg prednisolone taken orally at bedtime, or 60 mg triamcinalone IM given once every month.

Contd...

Contd...

When both adrenals and ovaries are producing AGA, a combination of glucocorticoids and oestrogen may be effective. Oral anti-androgens and oestrogens are not effective; it may benefit acne and hirsutism, but is efficacy on AGA is not established.

Antiandrogens given in a cyclical form may be of benefit. It has increased the thickness of the hair.

Supplementary zinc therapy 60 mg/day has been used to inhibit 5-α-reductase activity, but the role of zinc in AGA remains hypothetical.

Topical minoxidil can also be used for AGA in women. Topical retinoids can be used with minoxidil; it increases the absorption of minoxidil through alterations in the stratum corneum.

Surgery is difficult, as the hair loss is diffuse. A wig or hairpiece is preferred; it can conceal such a hair loss better.

ALOPECIA AREATA

Alopecia areata (AA) is a common disorder in which sudden hair loss occurs. It is characterised by asymptomatic, non-inflammatory, clear-cut patches of baldness usually on the scalp or beard region. It may occur at any age, but is more common in children and young adults. Autoantibodies to anagen hair follicles are present in 90% of patients with AA. The trigger that initiates the process is unknown.

Aetiology

The aetiology of AA is still unknown. Much evidence points towards it being an autoimmune disease, modified by genetic factors and aggravated by emotional stress.

Alopecia areata has been associated with a number of autoimmune diseases such as Hashimoto's thyroiditis, pernicious anemia and vitiligo. Antibodies are present against the thyroid gland, parietal cells of the stomach and adrenal glands. Antibodies against the hair follicles have not been found. The disease remits with steroid therapy.

Genetic susceptibility appears to play a role in AA as suggested by the possible HLA associations. Nearly 25% of patients have a family history of AA. An autosomal dominant mode of inheritance with variable penetrance has been suggested.

Physical or emotional stress has often been cited as a precipitant of the disorder. Definite data in support of this is lacking.

Histopathology

The histopathology depends upon the stage of the disease. Anagen/telogen ratio varies with the stage of disease and its duration. In the early active phase of AA, the majority of the follicles are in telogen or late catagen phase. Peribulbar lymphocytic infiltration (mainly T cells) and Langerhans cells are seen around the follicles.

There is evidence of non-specific injury to the anagen hair. The hair passes prematurely into the telogen phase, here the hair is said to be safe from the damage. However, when the hair re-enters the anagen phase the attack is resumed. The cyclic phase goes on; this explains why the hair is not permanently destroyed.

In severe cases, the hair is damaged and weakened in the keratogenous zone. Such hair breaks within the keratogenous zone; this hair reaches the surface of the scalp and is later extruded as the "exclamation mark hair". These are short hair, which when plucked, can be seen to have a constriction just above the rounded hair bulb. These "exclamation mark hair" are found at the edge of a bald patch, these are pathognomonic for AA.

Cadaver hair are hair that are broken before they reach the skin surface; these hair also indicate signs of activity and progression of disease.

Ikeda's Classification of AA

Type I This accounts for 83% of patients. It occurs between the ages of 20 and 40 years. It runs a course of less than 3 years. Individual patches tend to re-grow in less than 6 months.

Type II The atopic type accounts for 10% of cases. The disease runs a lengthy course of 10 years or more. Individual patches tend to persist for about a year.

Type III The pre-hypertensive type accounts for 4% of cases. It is found in young adults, and runs a rapid course with alopecia totalis developing in 39% of cases.

Type IV This is the combined type, it accounts for 5% of cases of AA, seen in people over 40 years of age. It runs a prolonged course. Alopecia totalis develops in 10% of cases.

The re-growth of hair usually starts in the periphery of the patch and then spreads towards the centre. The new hair are at first non-pigmented and thin; they gradually become pigmented and the diameter of the hair increases. New patches may occur as the older ones are resolving, thus prolonging the total duration of the episode.

If alopecia extends along the parietal and occipital scalp margin, it is termed as ophiasis; it indicates poor prognosis. Alopecia areata tends to be more aggressive in young patients from families with a history of hypertension.

The hair of Marie Antoinette are said to have turned white overnight after hearing her death sentence. Middle-aged people often have a mixture of black and white hair. The diffuse form of AA preferentially affects the black hair, this fall out leaving the white hair intact.

Clinical Features

The disease is generally seen in children and young adults. One or more localised patches of alopecia occur, commonly on the scalp or beard. These patches are totally devoid of hair; there are no signs of inflammation (Figs 4 and 5). Exclamation mark hair may be present at the periphery of the lesion. These are better visualised by a dermatoscope. The disease occurs in three degrees of severity.

Common type of AA: This is the least severe form, single or multiple patches of well-demarcated hair loss are present. This is usually present on the scalp or beard.

Alopecia totalis: In this type of alopecia, there is total involvement of the scalp.

Alopecia universalis: This is the severest form of AA; there is generalised loss of body hair.

Other Anomalies in Alopecia Areata

In about 10% cases of AA, especially those of long duration, associated with alopecia totalis or alopecia universalis, the nails show uniform pits, with transverse or longitudinal striations.

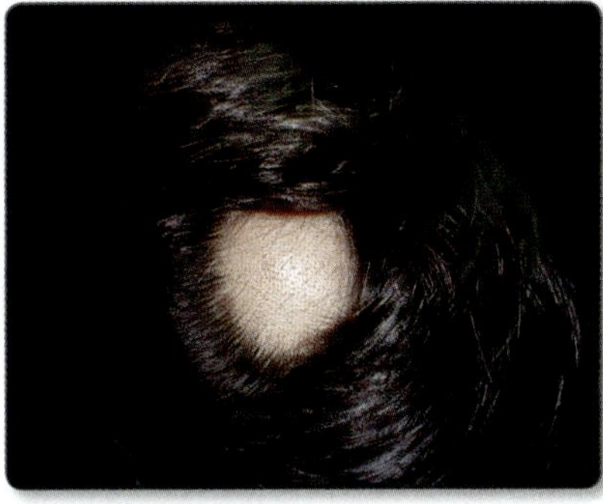

Fig. 4: Alopecia areata

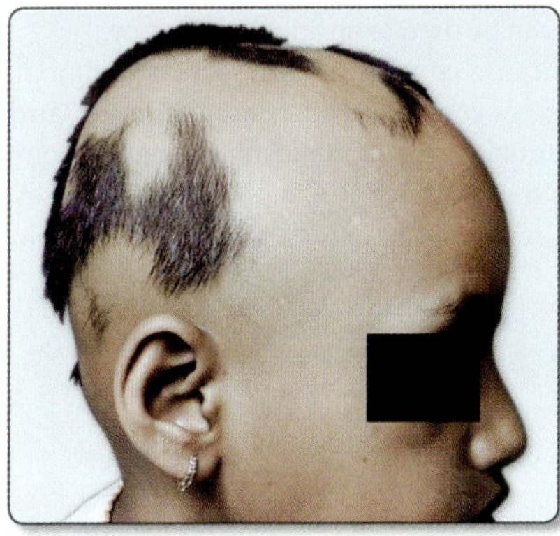

Fig. 5: Alopecia areata—extensive

Some cases of AA are associated with ocular and testicular abnormalities, atopy, Down's syndrome, thyroid disease, pernicious anaemia and Addison's disease.

Bad Prognostic Signs

- Alopecia totalis and alopecia universalis
- Ophiasis
- Cases associated with atopy or auto-immune diseases
- Prolonged history
- Multiple episodes
- Pitting of the nails
- Involvement of the eyelids and eyelashes

Treatment for Limited Scalp Involvement

When the lesions are small and few, no treatment may be necessary; spontaneous regrowth may often occur.

For others, intra-lesional steroids are usually given as first-line therapy. Triamcinolone injection is administered in a concentration of 5–10 mg/mL in the affected areas and the periphery of the patches. Less than 0.1 mL is injected

Differential Diagnosis

Alopecia areata should be differentiated from other causes of hair loss. In trichotillomania, the hair loss is irregular, hair of varying length are present in the alopecic patch, and exclamation mark hair is absent. In children, tinea capitis should be excluded, signs of inflammation are marked in the zoophilic species of dermatophytes, scaling and hair loss is obvious. Scraping should be done to confirm the diagnosis. In cicatricial alopecia, a previous history will give a clue to the cause of alopecia such as chronic discoid lupus erythematosus and severe infection. The skin markings are absent and the opening of the hair follicles is not seen.

per site, and the injections are spread out to cover the affected areas. Multiple injections at about 1 cm apart are given. Treatment is repeated every 3–6 weeks until resolution occurs. A concentration of 2.5 mg/mL should be used for the eyebrows and the beard.

Oral zinc aspartate 50 mg bid can be used as an adjuvant therapy.

Other topical applications include counterirritants such as dithranol, immunomodulators such as tacrolimus and pimecrolimus, and dinitrochlorobenzene (DNCB), squaric acid dibutylester, diphencyprone (DPCP). Minoxidil 5% applied bid may be helpful in unresponsive cases. DNCB has become less popular as a result of reports that it is mutagenic. Diphencyprone (DPCP). The patient is first sensitised to DPCP directly on the scalp with a 2% concentration on a small area (2 cm). The following week, a low concentration (0.0001%) is applied. The concentration is increased slowly every week as needed until a mild tolerable allergic contact dermatitis is elicited. Many concentrations are available that achieve this goal ranging from 0.001 to 0.1%. DPCP is more effective for extensive long-standing cases of AA.

Treatment

No curative treatment is available for AA; however, a number of modalities are available, which have resulted in hair growth. One useful way of deciding what modality is appropriate for the treatment is to see whether the patient has limited or extensive involvement.

The patient should be informed that initially vellus hair will replace the bald patch, which may be white; regrowth of terminal hair will occur later. The white hair will later pigment.

Treatment for Extensive Scalp Involvement

For severe cases of AA, such as alopecia totalis and alopecia universalis, a short course of systemic steroids is prescribed. A high dose 40–80 mg of prednisolone is used; even then many patients experience a loss of hair after the treatment. As an alternative dexamethasone, 4 mg daily on 2 consecutive days in a week can be tried, for a 6-month period with appropriate bone protection measures.

Minoxidil 5% applied bid may be helpful in unresponsive cases.

Immune modulators such as oral cyclosporin, is a powerful modulator of T cell function; it has produced regrowth of hair in alopecia totalis. Topical immune modulators such as tacrolimus, pimecrolimus can be used in difficult cases.

Phototherapy with 8-methoxypsoralen plus UVA has claimed success in some cases. UVB therapy is also helpful. A wig may help intractable cases of alopecia totalis.

> *My hair is gray, but not with years,*
> *Nor grew it white,*
> *In a single night.*
> *As men's have grown with sudden fear.*
> *(Byron)*

Telogen Effluvium

In telogen effluvium, there is an increased shedding of normal club hair; it follows a premature precipitation of anagen phase into telogen. Telogen effluvium is justified when the telogen count is over 25%.

Diffuse hair shedding is the only symptom. Normally about 100 scalp hair are lost every day. In telogen effluvium, about 120–400 hair are lost each day. When increased amount of hair loss occurs, AGA, which was previously unapparent may become obvious. Spontaneous regrowth occurs in about 6 months. In some cases such as severe infections, hair follicles may become destroyed, so that only partial recovery occurs. In postpartum effluvium, if successive pregnancies occur, regrowth may be incomplete.

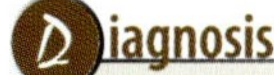

A trichogram shows more than 25% of hair in telogen phase. Complete blood screening should be done with liver and kidney functions, to exclude any systemic cause.

The patients complain of increased hair loss after combing and hair wash.

Treatment

There is no specific therapy for telogen effluvium. In most cases, the hair loss stops spontaneously within a few weeks, and then the hair regrows. If it becomes a cosmetic problem, a single injection of triamcinolone may help.

Any inflammatory scalp disease increases the shift to telogen phase; the infection should be treated promptly. Correct the predisposing factors such as thyroid disease, iron deficiency, stop the drugs causing telogen effluvium.

Causes of Telogen Effluvium

- Physiological effluvium of newborn
- Postpartum
- Postfebrile
- Severe systemic infections
- Chronic debilitating illness
- Postsurgical
- Hypothyroidism and other endocrinopathies
- Extensive dieting
- Drugs such as retinoids, anti-coagulants, anti-convulsants, anti-thyroid, heavy metals, lithium, indomethacin.

Anagen Effluvium

This usually follows the use of chemotherapeutic agents such as antimetabolites, alkylating agents, mitotic inhibitors, etc. With high doses, loss of anagen hair occurs immediately over a week or two of treatment. The hair becomes very thin and breaks when it reaches the surface of the scalp. With the cessation of therapy, the hair returns to normal. Mitotic inhibition stops the reproduction of matrix cells, but does not destroy the follicle. A pressure cuff applied to the scalp during chemotherapy can prevent such an arrest. Scalp hypothermia may also prevent anagen effluvium.

CICATRICIAL ALOPECIA

Scarring alopecia refers to permanent destruction of the hair follicles; these are replaced by fibrous tissue. There is a loss of follicular openings, which gives the scalp a smooth shiny appearance. The scalp may be soft or it may be indurated.

Classification of Cicatrical Alopecia

Developmental Defects and Hereditary Disorders

- Epidermal nevi
- Aplasia cutis
- Epidermolysis bullosa dystrophica
- Darier's disease
- Conradi's syndrome

Infection

- Severe bacterial infections
- Severe tinea capitis (kerion, favus)
- Viral (herpes zoster)
- Protozoal (leishmaniasis)

Neoplasia

- Basal cell carcinoma
- Squamous cell carcinoma
- Metastatic tumours
- Lymphomas
- Adnexal tumours

Physical and Chemical Agents

- Burns
- Radiation
- Mechanical trauma

Other Cutaneous Dermatoses

- Collagen diseases
- Sarcoidosis
- Lichen planus
- Pseudopelade of Brocq
- Folliculitis decalvans
- Dissecting folliculitis of the scalp
- Acne keloidalis
- Necrobiosis lipoidica diabeticorum

PSEUDOPELADE OF BROCQ

Pseudopelade is a term used for progressive cicatricial alopecia without any marked inflammation. It may be regarded as a clinical syndrome that may be the result of different pathological entities, known and unknown. Some known causes are lichen planus and systemic lupus erythematosus.

Clinical Features

The disease is commonly seen in women after the age of 40 years. The hairdresser or the patient herself notices a patch of cicatricial alopecia usually by chance. Initially a single patch is seen on the vertex, but it may occur anywhere; later other patches appear. The extension is usually gradual. The affected patches are smooth, round or oval, soft and slightly depressed. The patches are ivory white or slightly pink in colour. No sign of any inflammation is present. Large patches may form by coalescence of smaller patches.

Histopathology

Numerous lymphocytes are seen around the upper two-thirds of the follicles. Later the follicles are destroyed and the epidermis becomes thin and atrophic, the dermis is usually sclerotic.

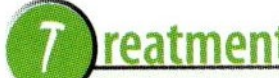

If the alopecia is secondary to a disease, such as lichen planus, it should be treated. However, baldness is irreversible. Skin grafts may be required.

FOLLICULITIS DECALVANS

This is an inflammatory reaction of the hair follicles that leads to cicatricial alopecia.

Etiology

The cause is unknown, it may be related to seborrhoeic dermatitis, *Staphylococcus aureus* may be found in some cases. Some patients have a defect in cell-mediated immunity. It seems probable that folliculitis declavans may be caused by local failure in the immune response or in leukocytic function. All patients should be investigated for these underlying defects.

Clinical Features

Initially small follicular pustules are seen, with erythema and crusting, later smooth shining depressed scars are apparent (Fig. 6). When the pustules have healed, the condition looks identical to psuedopelade of Brocq.

Treatment

If *Staphylococcus* aureus is present, appropriate antibiotic should be prescribed. In many cases, no pathogenic organisms are discovered. Chronic inflammatory reaction can be helped by topical and intralesional corticosteroids. Improvement has also been reported with a 10-week course of rifampicin.

Histopathology

Intra-follicular abscess and perifollicular lymphocytic infiltrate is present; these may contain plasma cells. In many cases, no pathogenic organisms are seen; in others coagulase positive *Staphylococcus aureus* are present.

DISSECTING CELLULITIS OF THE SCALP (PERIFOLLICULITIS CAPITIS ABSCEDENS ET SUFFODIENS)

This is a chronic progressive inflammatory disorder of the scalp, which affects predominantly the vertex and occipital scalp of males. The specific aetiology

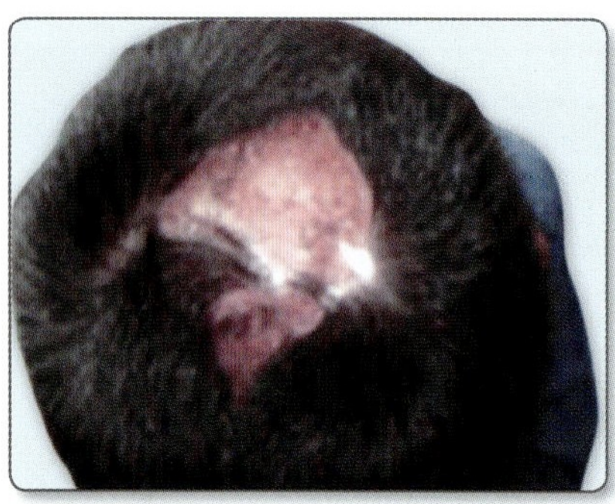

Fig. 6: Scarring alopecia. Note the absence of the opening of hair follicles

of this uncommon condition is unknown. The pathophysiology is believed to involve follicular blockage, it may occur in association with acne conglobata, and hidradenitis suppurativa (Follicular occlusion triad). The clinical signs include nodules and abscesses with intercommunicating sinuses. This is followed by patchy alopecia, extensive fibrosis and scarring. The treatment is similar to acne conglobata and hidradenitis suppurativa.

PIGMENTARY ABNORMALITIES OF THE HAIR

Hair derives its natural colour from melanin pigments, eumelanin in brown and black hair, and pheomelanin in red and blonde hair. These pigments are derived from the metabolism of tyrosine; pheomelanin also contains cysteine residues. Hair pigment is present in the cortex and medulla of the hair, pigment is generally not found in the cuticle or inner root sheath cells.

Hair colour is produced not only by variations in the amount of and type of melanin, but also by reflection and refraction of light at various interface of the mature hair shaft layers. It is not unusual to find heterochromia (hair of different colours) in the same person. A man can have different colours of the scalp and beard hair.

Canities (Graying of the Hair)

The normal greying of hair is related to physiological changes. This is due to the decrease in the amount of pigment present in the hair shaft. It occurs with aging process. Melanocytes are virtually absent in bulbs of white hair.

The age of onset of greying is different in different races and varies with the body site. Caucasians exhibit pigment loss earlier than blacks. Beard hair is the first to grey. Greying of the scalp hair begins in the temporal region, and then spreads towards the crown and occipit. Trunk and extremity hair grey later.

Premature Canities

This is greying of the hair before the aging process. It may be genetically determined, due to autoimmune diseases, or may be a part of the aging syndromes. Large doses of para-aminobenzoic acid, 300 mg/day, have been reported to darken grey hair in over 80% patients. Hair becomes grey again on discontinuation of treatment. Dyeing is the best method of treating grey hairs.

Poliosis

This is localised loss of hair pigment; often it is genetically based, such as the white forelock of piebaldism, and vitiligo. Early hair growth in AA is commonly white. Other causes of poliosis are Vogt-Koyanagi syndrome and tuberous sclerosis.

Other Causes of Greying of the Hair

Nutritional deficiencies such as kwashiorkor, iron, copper, and vitamin B12 deficiency may result in greying of the hair. Metabolic disorders such as phenylketonuria and homocystinuria also affect hair pigmentation. Drugs such as hydroquinone, triparanol (anti-hypercholesterolemic drug) and fluorobutyrophenone (an anti-psychotic) disturb keratinisation and pigmentation. Mephenesin carbamate (anti-spasmodic) causes lightening of hair colour on withdrawal of the drug. Chloroquine inhibits pheomelanin synthesis; it therefore affects red and blonde hair.

Other Causes of Hair Discolouration

Darkening of White Hair

This has followed treatment with carbidopa and bromocriptine therapy for parkinsonism. Accidental hair discolouration may be due to copper in swimming pools, the hair turns greenish in colour. Cobalt workers may get blue hair. Yellow hair colour is seen in heavy smokers. Yellow hair colour may also result from picric acid and dithronol. Trinitrotoluene (TNT) workers may have yellow shins and reddish-brown hair.

STRUCTURAL DEFECTS OF THE HAIR

Structural defects of the hair shafts may result in increased fragility of the hair; hair is susceptible to injury or minor trauma, and it may cause cosmetic disability (Figs 7A to K). These defects may be hereditary or acquired due to metabolic abnormalities.

Classification

Structured Defects with Increased Fragility

- Monilethrix
- Pseudomonilethrix
- Pili torti
- Bamboo hair
- Trichorrhexis nodosa

Structured Defects without Increased Fragility

- Pili annulati
- Woolly hair
- Uncombable hair syndrome

Other Abnormalities of the Hair Shaft

- Trichoptilosis

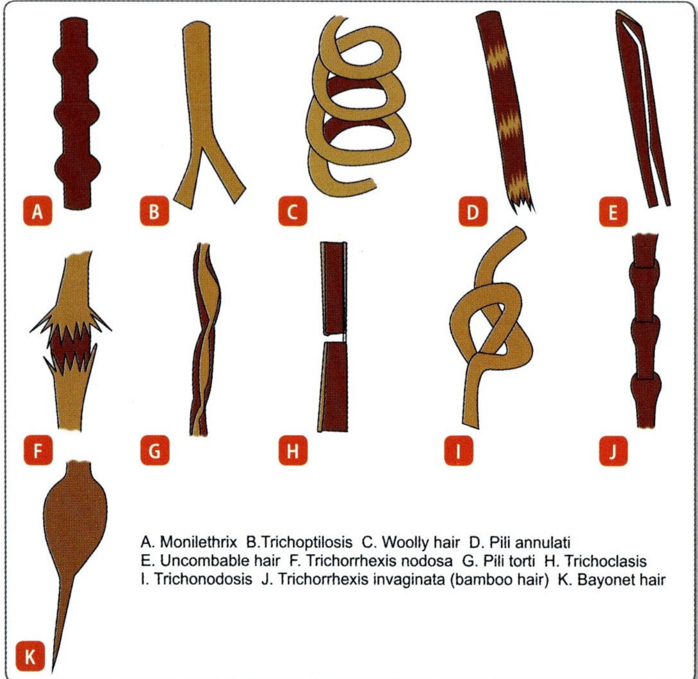

Figs 7A to K: Hair shaft disorders

- Pohl-Pinkus constriction
- Trichonodosis
- Trichostasis
- Weathering of the hair shaft

Monilethrix (Regular Beading of the Hair)

The defect is usually present at birth, but the onset may be delayed till adolescence. The hair shaft is beaded and breaks easily. Elliptical nodes at regular intervals are separated by narrow internodes. It is characterised by dryness, fragility and sparseness of the scalp hair. The hair tends to break at the delicate internodes. The disease is often associated with keratosis pilaris. Hair in regions other than the scalp may be affected. Leukonychia is occasionally seen; improvement may occur with age, pregnancy and in summer.

Pseudomonilethrix (Irregular Beading of Hair)

It usually presents from the age of 6 onwards. In this condition, two of the following three abnormalities should be present:

1. The nodes are placed at irregular intervals
2. Irregular twists of the hair, without flattening of the hair
3. Breaks or brush like ends in a hair shaft

Psuedomonilethrix is not associated with keratosis pilaris.

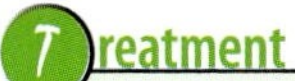

Patients with structural hair defects should refrain from hair styling procedures such as straightening of the hair; this causes more damage to the already fragile hair. Oral retinoids have induced some hair re-growth, but as it also causes alopecia, its use is limited. Systemic corticosteroids may be effective in some cases.

Pili Torti (Twisting of the Hair)

In this condition, the hair is flattened and twisted along its long axis. Scalp hair, eyebrows and eyelashes may be affected. The hair is brittle and breaks easily. Affected hairs have a spangled appearance in reflected light. In the classical type, unassociated with other disorders, pili torti may improve after puberty.

Pili torti may be associated with other syndromes such as Menkes syndrome, Bjornstad's syndrome, Bazex syndrome, hypohidrotic ectodermal dysplasia and pseudomonilethrix. Pili torti can also be associated with keratosis pilaris, nail abnormalities, dental abnormalities, corneal abnormalities, and mental retardation.

Bamboo Hair (Trichorrhexis Invaginata)

The hair defect is caused by intussusceptions of the hair shaft at the zone of keratinisation. It is due to softness of the cortex due to impaired keratinisation in the keratogenous zone. This allows the intussusceptions of fully keratinised and hard distal shaft into the soft proximal portion of the shaft. The bamboo hair has ball and socket deformities with the socket forming the proximal and the ball forming the distal portion of the node along the hair shaft.

These hair are associated with Netherton's syndrome or ichthyosis linearis circumflexa; atopic manifestations are usually present. The bamboo hair is not only present on the scalp, but is also seen in the eyebrows and eyelashes; rarely at other body sites. Hair scarcity is noted all over the body. Bamboo hair may become normal after a couple of years.

Trichorrhexis Nodosa

The condition may be genetically predetermined; it may be due to trauma such as hair styling procedures or associated with metabolic disorders such as arginosuccinic aciduria, Menkes kinky hair syndrome. It may also occur as a side effects of tretinoin therapy.

Trichorrhexis nodosa is a common defect seen due to trauma of hairstyling procedures. The cuticle is damaged and frayed, allowing cortical cells to protrude out; this leads to the formation of nodes. The nodes are found at irregular intervals along the hair shaft. Depending upon the extent of injury, fracture of the hair can occur at nodular swellings. The fractured hair is mainly found on the scalp, other sites are pubic, axillary and chest hair

Pili Annulati (Ringed Hair)

The hair has light and dark colours when seen in reflected light. The light bands are due to clusters of abnormal air filled cavities that scatter light. The hair growth is normal, and there are no associated abnormalities in the other organs. The mode of inheritance is autosomal dominant.

In pseudopili annulati, there are alternate dark and light bands in the hair, but the light colour is due to reflection and refraction of light by flattened and twisted surface of the hair. There are no abnormal air filled cavities.

Woolly Hair

These are tightly coiled hair, occurring over the entire surface of the scalp or in a local patch. It is often most severe in childhood, when it is impossible to brush the hair. The hair usually does not grow beyond a length of 12 cm.

Various subgroups have been identified: hereditary woolly hair with an autosomal dominant inheritance, familial woolly hair with an autosomal recessive inheritance, and woolly hair nevus with partial scalp involvement; the hair of the nevus has reduced diameter and is pale in colour. Woolly hair may also be associated with pigmented or epidermal nevus. Ocular defects may be present.

Microscopically, the hair is oval shape on cross section; pili torti like twisting may be present along the long axis. Trichorrhexis nodosa and pili annulati may be associated.

Uncombable Hair Syndrome (Spun Glass Hair)

The defect is only noticed in infancy as dry blonde shiny hair that stands straight from the scalp and cannot be combed.

On electron microscopy, longitudinal grooves are seen; it makes the hair stiff. Perhaps the internal root sheath keratinises before the hair shaft. There may be abnormal fibrous proteins in the hair. Oral biotin 0.3 mg three times daily has shown improvement in some cases.

Trichoptilosis

This is often referred to as a split end by the patient. There is longitudinal splitting of the hair by vigorous brushing, physical and chemical hair procedures applied to the hair. Trichorrhexis nodosa and trichoclasis are often present in the same patient. Further damage to the hair should be avoided.

Trichostasis Spinulosa

This is a common disorder of the hair follicles seen on the nose and forehead of elderly people. The lesions appear like blackheads. They are actually a tuft of several telogen hairs in the hair follicles, which are derived from a single matrix. These hair instead of falling off are present in the follicular infundibulum, due to a partial obstruction of the follicular orifice due to hyperkeratosis.

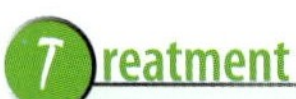

Keratolytic agents are effective, after using a wax depilatory; 0.5% tretinoin applied for 2–3 months is also effective.

Trichonodosis (Knotting of the Hair Shaft)

Knots are found in the hair shafts; the hair most commonly affected are the short curly hair with a flat diameter. The condition is common in Negroes, and in short, curly hair of Caucasoid. It is not found in the long straight hair. The trauma of brushing or combing may break the hair at the knot.

Pohl-Pinkus Constriction

This is analogous to the Beau's line of the nail. A zone of decreased shaft diameter appears in the hair shaft coinciding with illness, surgical operations, and intake of cytotoxic drugs. Hair in early anagen is most commonly affected.

Bayonet Hair

These are spindle shaped 2–3 mm hyperpigmented expansion of the hair cortex just proximal to the tapered tip of the hair. They are probably related to the hyperkeratinisation of the upper third of the follicle.

Hair Cast

Many scalp hair bear white keratinous plugs about 3–5 mm long that are found within 1–3 cm of the scalp. They look like nits, but can be slid along the hair shaft. These hairs show bluish-yellow fluorescence under Wood's lamp. The hair cast is formed by the retention and desquamation of segments of the root sheath.

The condition may occur as an isolated abnormality or may be associated with seborrhoeic dermatitis, psoriasis, lichen planus, or trichotillomania.

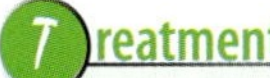

The causative scalp disease should be treated. Keratolytic shampoos may decrease the scaling but fail to remove the cast; 0.025% tretinoin may be effective.

MISCELLANEOUS CONDITIONS OF THE SCALP

Pityriasis Amiantacea

This is a disease characterised by thick asbestos (amiantaceous) like shiny scales on the scalp. This is usually localised to one or more areas of the scalp or it may be generalised. A tuft of hair is matted together by laminated crusts. The cause is unknown, in some cases it is thought to be secondary to psoriasis, seborrheic dermatitis, neurodermatitis, and perhaps bacterial infections, secondary to pediculosis.

Clinical Features

The condition is commonly seen in young girls and complicates recurrent infection of the scalp. The condition is often confined to small areas of the scalp, where the proximal part of the hair is matted together by laminated crusts (Fig. 8). The crusts are silvery white or dull gray. There is no structural damage to the hair, but in some patches where the crusting is thick, some purulent exudate is seen under the crusts and temporary alopecia is seen when the condition heals.

Histopathology

The asbestos-like scaling is due to diffuse hyperkeratosis, parakeratosis, and follicular hyperkeratosis, which surrounds each hair. The other findings are spongiosis and migration of lymphocytes in the epidermis with variable degree of acanthosis.

Treatment

The thick crust should be removed with appropriate keratolytics such as salicylic acid ointment. The underlying disease should be treated such as antibiotics for bacterial infections.

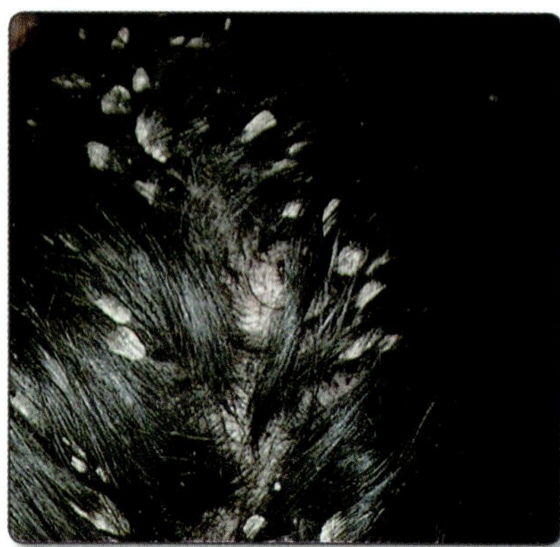

Fig. 8: Pityriasis amiantacea

Menkes Kinky Hair Syndrome

The light coloured hair of the syndrome is seen in a hereditary defect of intestinal copper transport. The inheritance is X-linked recessive, seen only in boys. The hair shaft defects such as pili torti, monilethrix, or trichorrhexis nodosa are often associated. Hair resembles steel wool. The characteristic ivory colour of the hair appears between 1 to 5 months of age. Drowsiness, lethargy, convulsions, and severe neurological deterioration occur. The skin is pale and the lips have an exaggerated cupid bow configuration.

Trichothiodystrophy (TTD)

The hairs in TTD are brittle with abnormally low sulphur content. The sulphur content is reduced to 50% of the normal value; various syndromes are associated with TTD. These are:

BIDS: Brittle hair, intellectual impairment, decreased fertility, and short stature.

IBIDS: Ichthyosis and BIDS.

PIBIDS: Photosensitivity with ichthyosis and BIDS.

The hair is brittle and breaks easily. It may form nodes as in trichorrhexis nodosa. The hair is flattened and can be twisted in various shapes. With polarised microscope, alternating dark and light zones are seen. There is decrease in the sulphur content of the hair shaft.

Pseudofolliculitis and Acne Keloidalis Nuchae

Pseudofolliculitis and acne keloidalis nuchae occur when a tightly curved hair re-enters the skin as it grows, causing intense perifollicular inflammation and scarring. This commonly occurs in black adolescents in the beard area (pseudofolliculitis) and along the posterior hairline (acne keloidalis nuchae) (Figs 9 and 10). Affected areas show localised pustules which develop into scars if left untreated. The scars continue to discharge purulent material. The problem is more severe at the neck, where the hair follicles are oriented at low angles to the skin, making penetration of the skin more likely.

Treatment

The treatment is difficult. intralesional steroids may be effective when treated early. The patient should let the hair grow for 4–6 weeks, then shave leaving about 1 mm of hair. This can be achieved by specially designed razors or electrical clippers. Avoid close shave with double or triple razor blades. Lifting of re-entered hair is helpful but tedious. Brushing with an abrasive brush is quicker but less effective. Plucking should be avoided. Definitive therapy is hair removal by lasers.

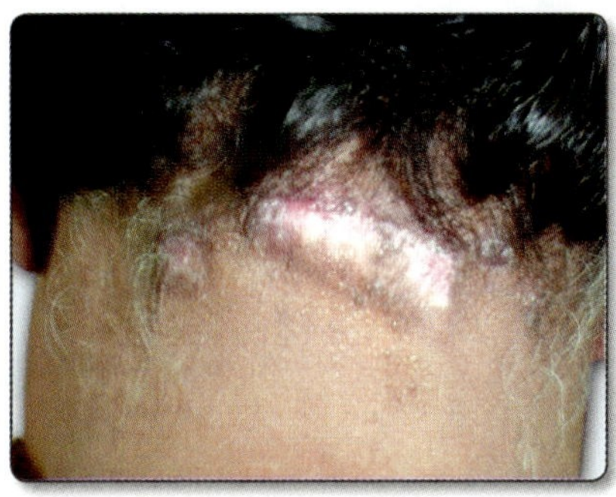

Fig. 9: Acne keloidalis

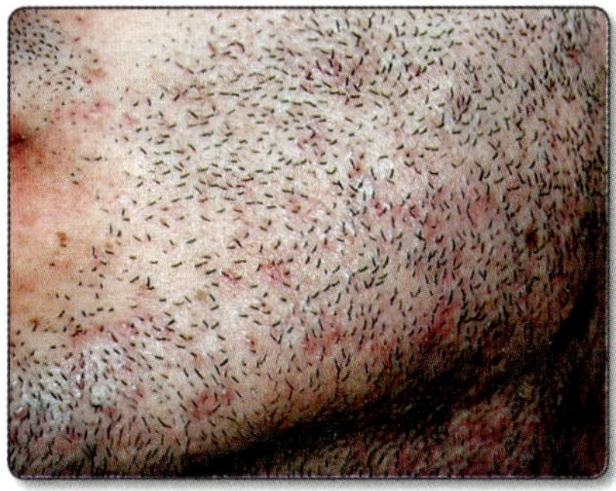

Fig. 10: Pseudofolliculitis barbae

TUMORUS OF THE HAIR FOLLICLE

Trichoepithelioma

These can be single or multiple.

Multiple Trichoepithelioma (Epithelioma Adenoides Cysticum)

Brooke first described this tumour in 1892. Multiple trichoepithelioma are hereditary; they have an autosomal dominant inheritance. The tumours appear as multiple, cystic and solid nodules, and papules on the face, especially about the upper lip, nasolabial folds, and eyelids. Other sites are the scalp, neck, and trunk.

Clinical Features

The lesions appear at puberty, it is more common in females, the tumours are multiple, small, rounded, smooth, shiny, translucent papules and nodules. These are skin coloured or pinkish, the centre may be depressed. The lesions are symmetrical on the face (Fig. 11). Generalised trichoepitheliomas are reported with alopecia and myasthenia. Continued growth, ulceration, induration and malignant changes have been reported in trichoepitheliomas.

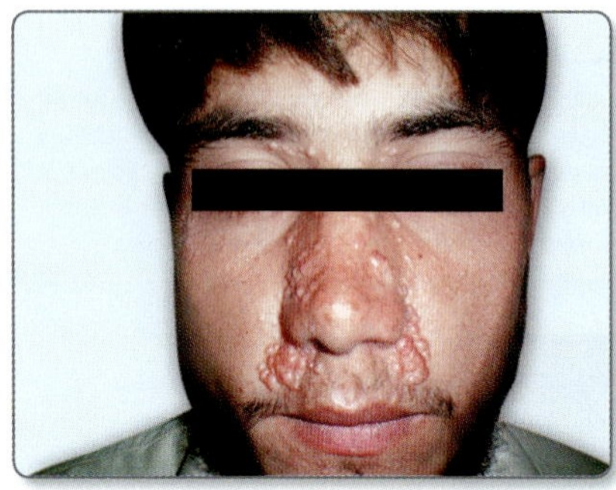

Fig. 11: Trichoepithelioma.

Histopathology

The lesions in trichoepithelioma are well-circumscribed; horny cysts are characteristic. These consist of fully keratinised inner shell, surrounded by an outer shell of flattened basophilic cells that appear similar to the cells of basal cell carcinoma. The keratinisation of the horny cysts is abrupt and complete as in the outer root sheath of the hair follicle. Occasionally the tumour attains a high degree of differentiation and shows primitive hair papillae and even hair shafts.

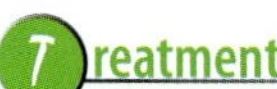

Treatment

Treatment is only required for cosmetic reasons, or if a change towards malignancy is suspected. Treatment is by surgical excision.

Solitary Trichoepithelioma

This appears as a solitary, smooth nodule, usually appearing on the nose, it closely resembles non-ulcerated basal cell carcinoma. Solitary giant trichoepithelioma presents as a large polypoid lesion on the lower trunk, frequently in the perianal area. The lesion causes discomfort because of its size and site.

Pilomatricoma

This is the most common tumour of the hair follicle. It is a benign tumour, which arises from the matrix cells. These often undergo calcification.

Histopathology

The tumour is found in the dermis, often extending into the subcutaneous tissue. It is well-circumscribed. Irregularly shaped islands are seen in the dermis that consists of two types of epithelial cells, basophilic cells, and shadow cells.

The basophilic cells have round and oval nuclei with scanty cytoplasm. These cells are arranged around the periphery of the tumour

Clinical Features

The tumour can occur at any age from infancy onwards. It is frequently seen in children. Females are more affected than males. The tumour is usually present on the face, neck or arms. It is a symptomless deep nodule, covered by normal skin, or the skin may be pinkish in color. It has a firm to stony hard consistency, which on stretching shows the "tent sign" with multiple facets and angles. The tent sign is due to calcification occurring in the lesion. It may be subject to periodic inflammation, and on occasion presents as a granulomatous swelling. Malignant change has been recorded.

island. The shadow cells are present in the centre of the island. The cytoplasm is acidophilic and there is gradual loss of nuclei. Due to the loss of nuclei, there is a central unstained area in the cell; it is a shadow of the lost nucleus. The cytoplasm contains keratin pigments.

Calcification occurs in most cases; it appears as dusting of basophilic substance in the shadow cells, or as solid purple amorphous masses. Ossification may also occur. Sebaceous glands and keratohyalin granules are present in the tumour mass.

HAIR COSMETICS

Both men and women are concerned with improving their appearance. Hair forms a very important part of the face. Well-groomed hair definitely has an impact on the personality of the person. Hair cosmetics includes:

- Hair dyeing
- Hair bleaching
- Temporary or permanent waving
- Hair straightening
- Hair removal.

Hair Dyeing

Women have used dyes since ancient times. Today even men are conscious of their looks. They use hair dyes along with other cosmetics. The penetration of the dye in the hair depends upon molecular size of the dye, aqueous swelling of the hair at the time of application, and basicity of the dye.

Classification of Dyes

- Vegetable dyes
- Metallic dyes
- Organic dyes

Vegetable Dyes

The most common vegetable dye is henna; this is obtained from the shrubs of *Lawsonia (L.) alba, L. spinosa and L. inermis*. The dye is produced from the dried leaves before the plant flowers. The active principle is an acid napthoquinone. The effect of henna lasts for about 10 weeks.

Other vegetable dyes are obtained from logwood and walnut shell. These can be used if the patient is sensitive to paraphenylenediamine.

Metallic Dyes

Men generally use these dyes as the colour change is less rapid, and the colour change is not immediately obvious. Inorganic salts are mainly used. These salts reduce keratin; this gives a dull metallic appearance to the hair. Commonly used metallic dyes are sodium thiosulphate (brown to black colour) and silver nitrate (shades of brown).

The metallic dyes damage the hair when used too often. Metallic dyes cannot be removed without hair damage; these should be left to grow out.

Synthetic Organic Dyes

These dyes are popular because of the range of natural colours that can be obtained from them. Most of these dyes penetrate the cuticle and some are potentially permanent dyes. These may be:

- Temporary
- Semi-permanent
- Permanent

Temporary organic dyes: These are deposited around the hair shaft, and can be washed out with one shampoo, often used by dramatists. These are azo, azine or thiazine derivatives that are available as organic sprays. The disadvantage is that they can flake off and discolour the clothing.

Semi-permanent organic dyes: These dyes are of low molecular weight, they penetrate the cuticle of the hair shaft, and do not undergo any reaction in the hair shaft, e.g. nitro-phenylenediamine, nitro-aminophenol.

Permanent organic dyes: These dyes contain colourless precursors that react with hydrogen peroxide inside the hair shaft to produce the permanent colour. The hydrogen peroxide produces smaller molecules of the dye, e.g. paraphenylenediamine (PPD), para-aminophenol. The disadvantage of these dyes is, that they damage the hair structure, they are potential irritants, can cause cross sensitisation with local anaesthetics and sulphonamides. They can be possible carcinogens; they can produce aplastic anaemia, carcinoma of the urinary bladder.

Bleaching of the Hair

Bleaching is used to lighten the colour of the hair. It is used by women with hypertrichosis and hirsutism, and to prepare the hair to take up darker dyes. Bleaching oxidises and bleaches melanin.

The disadvantage is that it may damage the hair, renders it dry, porous, and prone to tangle. Six percent hydrogen peroxide is often used for bleaching the hair. Ammonia is used to speed the reaction that alone would take about 12 hours.

Waving of the Hair

Women perhaps are not satisfied with what hair they have. Women with straight hair often want to have a perm, and those with curly hair want to have them straightened. The stages involved in hair waving are:

- Softening of the hair
- Reshaping of the hair
- Hardening the hair fibres to retain the re-shaped position.

Softening of the Hair

The hair is first softened with a perming lotion. The lotion breaks the disulphide bonds of the hair. Thioglycolates are potent reducers of disulphide bonds in the keratin molecule. The perm lotion gets through the cuticle of the hair to the cortex, making the hair soft.

Reshaping the Hair

The hair is then reshaped by rollers and curlers. The degree of curl or tightening of the permanent wave depends upon the diameter of the roller size, and size of the strand wound round the roller. The reshaping is a great test to the hair dressing skills and experience.

Hardening of the Hair

The process involves a reversal of the softening step. The reduced hydrogen and disulphide bonds have to be oxidised. Atmospheric oxygen may neutralise the waving process. This method is slow and may take several hours. Chemical oxidation by hydrogen peroxide is quicker. Hydrogen peroxide is a bleaching agent, so the hair is lighter after permanent waving. Other oxidizing agents are sodium percarbonate or sodium and potassium borate. These changes are only temporary.

Removal of the Hair

There are various methods for removal of excessive hair such as plucking, shaving, waxing, chemicals, electrolysis and laser.

- Shaving although unacceptable to most women as being too masculine is safe and causes no reaction. In some cases folliculitis may occur.
- Waxing is one of the oldest methods of hair removal. Warm wax is applied to the skin, the cooled hardened wax is then pulled off the skin, the hair is pulled out by its root. It then takes weeks for the new hair to appear on the skin surface.
- Cold waxing includes glucose and zinc oxide waxing; this has the advantage of the effect lasting for several weeks.
- Plucking is satisfactory for localised hair growth.
- Chemical depilatories: Chemicals are used to weaken the disulphide bond of the keratin in the hair follicle. Sulphides and stannites were previously used for hair removal; they cause irritation and have a strong odour. Mercaptans are slower in action. Thioglycolates in a concentration of 2–4% are applied for 5–15 minutes. It does not have a bad odour. Chemical depilatories attack the most recently formed part of the hair shaft, i.e. the part closest to the skin surface. The effect is like that of a very close shave. Chemical depilatories are marketed as foams, creams, liquids, and aerosol sprays.
- Electrolysis: It is destruction of tissue by an ionising electrical current. It is used to remove excessive hair; it can also be used to remove certain skin lesions such as dilated blood vessels on the skin surface. For removing the hair, an extremely fine platinum wire, serving as a negative electrode, is passed along a hair shaft down into the bottom of the hair follicle. Here it comes into contact with the hair papilla. The current is then gradually turned on and after 5–10 seconds, the papilla is destroyed. The hair is then pulled out. This is a method for permanent hair removal. Electrolysis can be used for both white and black hair.
- Lasers: Lasers target melanin granules in the hair, in an effort to destroy the hair follicles. The laser energy is absorbed by the melanin of the hair and transferred to the surrounding follicles, causing follicular damage. The

anagen follicle is the major target for laser energy and represents the most vulnerable phase of the hair cycle. The telogen and the catagen phase are more resistant at a given site. These hair follicles have to be targeted again, when they enter the anagen phase. A period of one to three months is required between the treatments. Lasers only target pigmented hair.

The most common alopecia is AGA, followed by alopecia areata and telogen effluvium. The scarring alopecias are uncommon. Always have a sympathetic approach towards a patient of alopecia.

Approach to a patient of alopecia

1. Careful history taking
   The following points should be noted:
   - ❑ Duration of hair loss
   - ❑ Amount of hair loss
   - ❑ Family history of hair loss
   - ❑ Any systemic illness
   - ❑ Contact with animals, source for fungal infections
   - ❑ Dietary habits
   - ❑ Psychosocial history, any stress, anxiety or depression
2. Examination (Local)
   - ❑ Pattern of hair loss
   - ❑ Degree of hair loss
   - ❑ Hair parting; normal or increase in width
   - ❑ Scarring or non-scarring
   - ❑ Any hair shaft defect
   - ❑ Scalp inflammation present or absent
   - ❑ Nails normal or pitted
2. Examination (Systemic)
   - ❑ Exclude systemic disease

FURTHER READING

1. Bath JH, Wojnarowska F, Dawber RP, et al. R. Acanthosis nigricans, insulin resistance and cutaneous hirsutism and virilism. Br J Dermatol. 1998;118:613-20.
2. Boyd AS, King LE. Thalidomide-induced remission in lichen planopilaris. J Am Acad Dermatol. 2002;47:967-8.
3. Brodin MB. Drug-related alopecia. Clin Dermatol. 1987;5:571-9.
4. Cotsarelis G, Sun TT, Lavker RM. Label-retaining cells reside in the bulge area of pilosebaceous unit: implication for follicular stem cells, hair cycle and skin carcinogenesis. Cell. 1990;61:1329-37.
5. Cunliffe WJ, Hall R, Stevenson CJ, et al. Alopecia areata, thyroid disease, and autoimmunity. Br J Dermatol. 1969;81:877-81.
6. de Beker D, Ferguson DJJP, Dawber RPR. Monilethrix: a clinicopathological demonstration of the defect. Br J Dermatol. 1993;128:327-9.
7. Demitsu M, Manaber M, Harima N, et al. Hypertrichosis induced by latanoprost. J Am Acad Dermatol. 2001;44:721-3.
8. Foulds IS. Lichen sclerosus et atrophicus of the scalp. Br J Dermatol. 1980;103:197-9200.
9. Gummer CL. Cosmetics and hair loss. Clin Exp Dermatol. 2002;27:418-21.
10. Hautmann G, Hercoqova J, Lott T. Trichotillomania. J Am Acad Dermatol. 2002;46:807-21.
11. Karaman GC, Sendur N, Basar H, et al. Localized monilethrix with improvement after treatment of iron deficient anaemia. J Eur Acad Dermatol Venereol. 2001;15:362-4.
12. Karniq P, Tekeste Z, McCormick ST, et al. Hair Follicle Stem cell defect-specific PPAR gamma Deletion causes scarring alopecia. J Invest Dermatol. 2009;129:1243-57.
13. Langtry JA, Ive FA. Pityriasis amiantacea; an unrecognized cause of scarring alopecia, described in 4 four patients. Acta Derm Venereol.19991;71:352-3.

14. Lord JM, Flight IHK, Normal RJ. Metformin in polycystic–ovary syndrome: systemic review and meta-analysis. BMJ. 2003;327:951-5.
15. Onayemi O, Soyinka F. Squamous cell carcinoma of the scalp following a chemical burn and chronic lupoid discoid lupus erythematosus. Br J Dermatol. 1996;135:342-3.
16. Powell JJ, Dawber RPR, Gatter K. Folliculitis decalvans and tufted folliculitis: clinical, histological and therapeutic findings. Br J Dermatol. 1999;140:328-33.
17. Rittmaster RS. Hirsutism. Lancet. 1997;349:191-5.
18. Sharma VK, Dawn G, Kumar B. Profile of alopecia areata in Northern India. Int J Dermatol. 1996;35:22-7.
19. Sharma VK. Pulsed administration of corticosteroids in the treatment of alopecia areata. Int J Dermatol. 1996;35:133-6.
20. Sinclair RD, Dawber RPR. Androgenetic alopecia in men and women. Clin Dermatol. 2001;19:167-78.
21. Vexiau P, Chaspoux C, Boudou P, Fiet J, Jouanique C, Hardy N and Reygagne, et al. Effects of minoxidil 2% versus vs. cyproterone acetate treatment on female androgenetic alopecia: a controlled, 12-month randomized trial. Br J Dermatol. 2002;146:992-9.
22. Whiting DA. Cicatricial alopecia. Clin Dermatol. 2001;19:211-25.

Chapter 25

Nail Disorders

INTRODUCTION

Nail disorders are common; these represent either a cutaneous or systemic disease, or the pathology can be in the nail itself. The most frequently encountered problems that affect nails are trauma, fungal infections, bacterial infections and dermatoses such as psoriasis, lichen planus and eczema. Vascular diseases and diabetes mellitus are often associated with nail changes. Exposure to certain cosmetics can also cause nail damage.

Nails take a long time to grow from proximal to the distal end. The fingernails take about 3–6 months to grow out completely from the base to the outer edge while toe nails take about 12–18 months. Fingernails grow at approximately 1 cm every 3 months and the toenails at one-third the rate of fingernails. While treating nails for any disease, this time-factor should be taken into consideration.

NAIL CHANGES IN SYSTEMIC DISEASE

Beau's Lines

These are transverse depressions on the nail plate due to temporary interference with nail formation. These lines are commonly seen during convalescence from severe diseases such as pneumonia, measles, mumps, coronary thrombosis, and other conditions causing prolonged fever. The line appears first at the cuticle and then moves forward with the nail growth. It is a self-limiting condition and requires no treatment.

Koilonychia

Koilonychia is the name for flat or spoon-shaped nails classically seen in iron-deficiency anaemia; correction of iron deficiency usually results in return to normal growth of the nails. Koilonychia can be familial or associated with conditions causing decreased peripheral circulation.

Clubbing

Clubbing is characterised by loss of angle between the nail and the posterior nail fold, later there is enlargement of longitudinal and transverse diameter of nail curvature and hypertrophy of the soft tissue components of distal phalynx.

There are three forms of geometric assessment that can be performed in clubbing. Lovibond's angle between the nail plate and the proximal nail fold is normally less than 160°; this angle in clubbing is 180° or more. Curth's angle at the distal interphalangeal joint is normally 180°; it is decreased to less than 160° in clubbing. Schamroth's window is seen when the dorsal aspect of the two fingers from the opposite hands is apposed at the distal interphalangeal joint. It reveals a window of light at the proximal nail fold. This window is obliterated in clubbing. Clubbing may be seen in following conditions:

- Lung
  - Bronchiectasis
  - Pulmonary tuberculosis
  - Bronchogenic carcinoma
- Heart
  - Congenital cyanotic heart disease
- Gastrointestinal tract
  - Crohn's disease
  - Ulcerative colitis
- Hyperthyroidism
- Biliary Cirrhosis
- Pachyonychia, pachydermoperiostosis

Hippocratic Nails

A swelling at the tip of the fingers causes a drumstick clubbing. It is seen in chronic pulmonary disease, hepatic, and thyroid disorders.

Half-and-Half Nails

In these nails, there is a proximal white zone and the distal part of the nail has a brownish colour. The histology shows an increase in the vessel wall thickness and melanin deposition in the nail bed. These nails are seen in patients with chronic renal failure and those on chemotherapy.

Terry's Nails

The distal 1–2 mm of the nail shows a normal pink colour; the proximal end is white. It is seen in patients with cirrhosis of the liver, chronic congestive heart failure, adult onset diabetes mellitus, and in the very elderly. Nail-bed biopsy shows hyperplasia of the nail bed.

Periungual Erythema

This is a valuable pointer to collagen vascular disease such as lupus erythematosus, dermatomyositis, and scleroderma. The dilated and tortuous capillaries can easily be seen with hand lens.

Muehrcke's Lines

Narrow white transverse bands occurring in pairs are present on the nails; it is a sign of hypoalbuminaemia. These are seen on the nail bed and not on the nail plate. Similar lines are also seen in patients receiving chemotherapy.

Mee's Lines

Single or multiple white lines on the nails that are seen in inorganic arsenic poisoning are also reported in thallium poisoning, dissecting aortic aneurysm, and acute and chronic renal failure.

NAIL CHANGES DUE TO CUTANEOUS DISORDERS

Psoriasis

In psoriasis, nail involvement can occur in 25–50% cases. The most common feature is the pitting of nails and this is due to psoriasis involving the nail matrix. Pitting is irregular, deep, large, and irregularly distributed (Fig. 1). Pitting is due to the detachment of parakeratotic cells in the superficial layers of the nail plate. Yellowish discolouration, thickening of nails, and onycholysis are due to involvement of the nail bed. The other abnormalities are subungual hyperkeratosis, splinter haemorrhages, and nail plate abnormalities such as splits, atrophy and fragility. Pustules on the nail bed are found in pustular psoriasis.

Nail psoriasis is difficult to treat. Methotrexate, cyclosporin, intralesional steroids, retinoids, and PUVA have all been tried; the results are not very satisfactory. Trauma should be avoided; it may trigger a Koebner response.

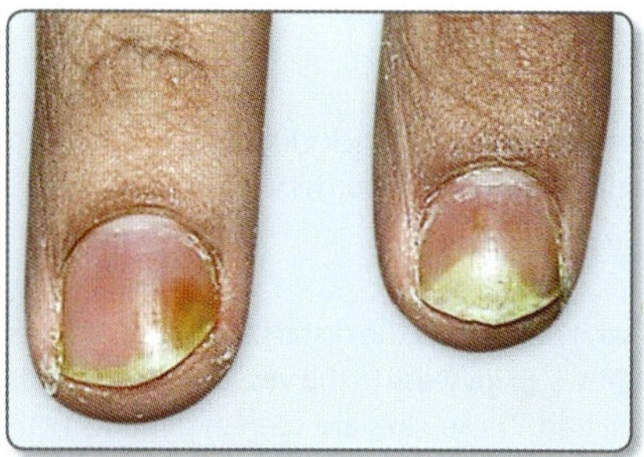

Fig. 1: Nail psoriasis

Lichen Planus

Nail changes are seen in about 10% cases of lichen planus. When the nail matrix is involved, diffuse nail scarring occurs. The most common changes include thinning, onychorrhexis, longitudinal ridging, brittleness of the nails and dorsal pterygium formation. This is a fibrotic band fusing the proximal nail fold with the nail bed (Fig. 2).

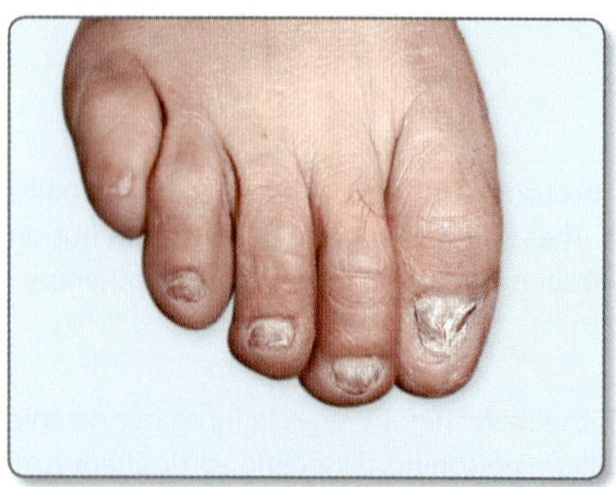

Fig. 2: Nail-lichen planus

Nail bed changes include subungual hyperkeratosis and onycholysis.

Treatment consists of intralesional injection of steroids or systemic triamcinolone 0.5–1 mg/kg IM every month. Acitretin is also effective.

Eczema

Nail changes depend upon the type of eczema, whether exogenous or endogenous. In atopic dermatitis, pitting of the nail is seen without any sign of inflammation. Nail matrix disturbances produce changes such as pitting, thickening, nail loss, transverse ridges, and furrows (Fig. 3). Nail bed pathology results in changes such as subungual hyperkeratosis and onycholysis. Nails may be smooth and shiny especially when itching is severe.

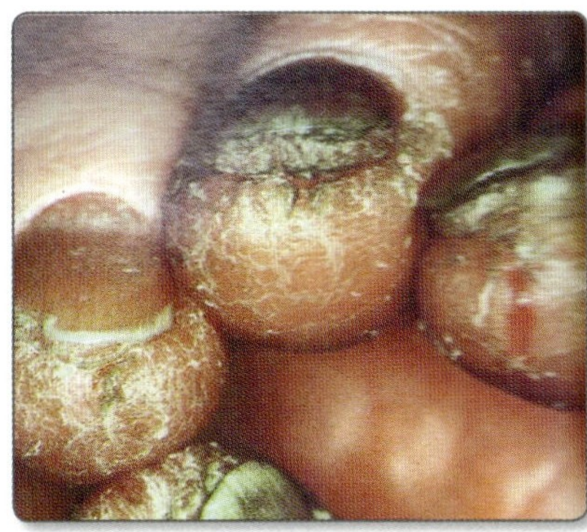

Fig. 3: Nail eczema

Darier's Disease

Nail changes are common in Darier's disease. The changes include red and/or white longitudinal streaks often terminating in a V-shaped nick. The streak may represent a zone of fragile or thin nail that is prone to fragmentation at the tip with the consequent nick. Subungual hyperkeratotic papules can be found in the hyponychium. Other occasional changes include ridging, leuconychia and roughness of the nail plate.

Alopecia Areata

Nail changes associated with alopecia areata are pitting, mottled erythema of the lunula and trachyonychia. Pits are small, superficial, and distributed in a geometrical pattern. Trachyonychia is characterised by nail roughness caused by excessive longitudinal striations.

Onychomycosis

Fungal infection of the nail is common in adults, usually affecting the toe nails. Dermatophytes are the most common cause of fungal infection. The

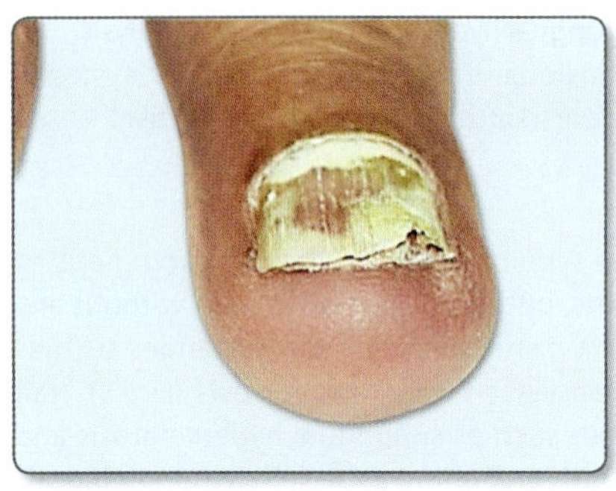

Fig. 4: Onychomycosis

most common finding is distal subungual onychomycosis. The fungus penetrates the hyponychium causing onycholysis and crumbling. There is subungual hyperkeratosis with yellowish discolouration (Fig. 4). Superficial white onychomycosis is infection of the nail plate, causing scaly white dots. Proximal onychomycosis occurs when the fungus penetrates the proximal nail fold, leading to severe nail dystrophy with diffuse involvement of the nail.

Recurrence is common after treatment of onychomycosis; remove the predisposing causes.

Haemorrhage

Subungual splinter haemorrhages may be seen in both local and systemic disorders of the nail. It may be due to trauma, systemic disease, e.g. subacute bacterial endocarditis, trichinosis, rheumatoid arthritis, hypertension, malignancy, systemic lupus erythematosus or skin diseases, e.g. psoriasis. Severe trauma may cause subungual haematoma which cause black discolouration of nails, onycholysis and sometimes nail loss.

Table 1: Showing the difference between nail psoriasis and onychomycosis

Nail psoriasis	*Onychomycosis*
Nails are thick, yellowish-white	Thick, yellowish-white
Subungual hyperkeratosis present	Subungual hyperkeratosis present
Pitting and onycholysis characteristic of psoriasis	Occasionally seen
Oil drop sign maybe present	Absent
Splinter hemorrhages may be present	Absent
Nails not friable	Nails friable
Psoriatic arthritis often present	Absent
Psoriatic lesions present at other sites: knees, elbows, scalp, lumbosacral areas	Absent
Fungal scrapings negative	Fungal scrapings positive

DISCOLOURATION (CHROMONYCHIA)

White Colouration (Leukonychia)

- White nails may occasionally be seen in healthy individuals, it may be hereditary. Leukonychia is generally due to systemic disease such as renal failure, cirrhosis of the liver, diabetes, systemic sclerosis, Raynaud's phenomenon and cryoglobulinaemia. It can also be due to extreme malnutrition (Fig. 5).
- White bands present as Mee's lines and Muehrcke's lines. White punctate spots are due to trauma or onychomycosis. An isolated longitudinal leukonychia may be due to an underlying nail bed tumour.

Yellow Colouration

- Dyes: turmeric, saffron, nail varnish.
- Drugs: tetracyclines, mepacrine
- Psoriasis
- AIDS
- Pulmonary diseases and malignancies

Black Discolouration

- Bands of pigmentation under the nail plate in Negroids are a common feature.
- Junctional nevus in the nail matrix also gives rise to a pigmented streak in the nail plate.
- Other causes of black pigmentation on nails include trauma, malignant melanoma, fungal infection, Addison's disease, drugs such as chloroquine, cytotoxic agents, and adriamycin.
- In Caucasians, the occurrence of pigmented streaks requires further investigations including a biopsy to rule out the possibility of malignant melanoma.

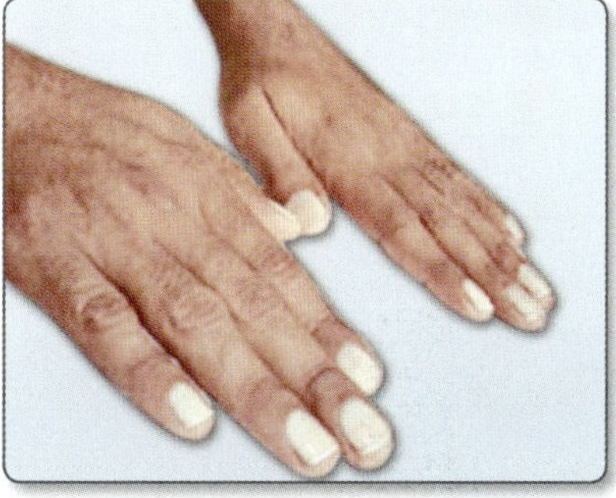

Fig. 5: Leuconychia

Blue Discolouration

- Cyanosis
- Drugs such as gold, mepacrine and chloroquine give a blue-black pigmentation. In fixed drug eruption, the pigmentation is dark blue. A blue lunula is seen in Wilson's disease.

DISEASES OF THE NAIL FOLD

Paronychia

Acute paronychia is usually due to Staphylococcal infection and is characterised clinically by painful swelling of posterior nail fold, sometimes with a purulent discharge (Fig. 6); there may be history of preceding trauma. The condition responds promptly to appropriate systemic antibiotics.

Chronic paronychia is a persistent condition and causes considerable therapeutic problem. It is common in housewives, nurses, cooks, hairdressers, and those who frequently immerse their hands in water. Diabetes mellitus is another predisposing factor. *Candida albicans* is the most important pathogenic agent. Acute exacerbations can be caused by secondary bacterial infection with *Staphylococcus aureus*, *Proteus*, *Pseudomonas* and *E. coli*. There is swelling at the base of the nail with loss of cuticle. The nail itself is affected later with discolouration, pitting, and ridging (Fig. 7).

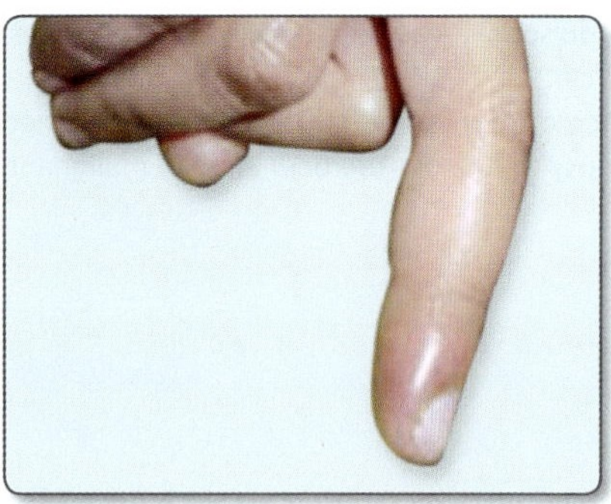

Fig. 6: Acute paronychia

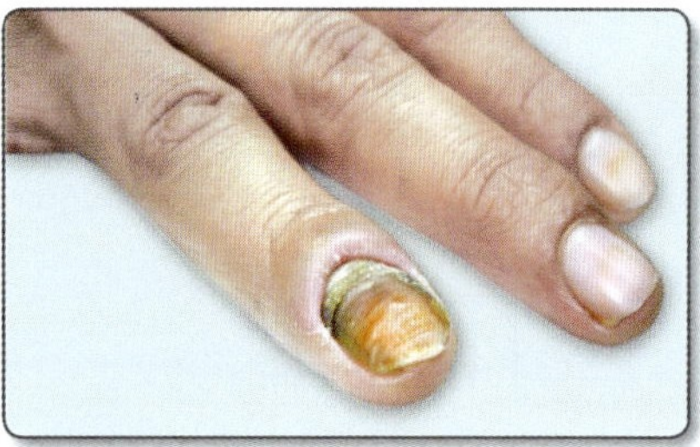

Fig. 7: Chronic paronychia

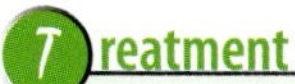

The importance of keeping the hands dry and the use of gloves when performing wet tasks should be emphasised. Topical anti-fungal agents like imidazole creams, nystatin ointment, and gentian violet paint are effective remedies. Oral antibiotics are required in acute exacerbations. Castellani's paint or sulphacetamide in alcohol are also effective agents.

Ingrown Toe Nails

This is due to ill-fitting shoes, improper or excessive trimming of the nail, or it may be traumatic. The toe nail is most frequently involved. The nail plate gets embedded in the lateral nailfold, which stimulates formation of granulation tissue, with subsequent pain and sepsis (Fig. 8).

In recent years, it may also be caused by successful therapy of fungal infections of the nail by oral anti-fungal drugs. A nail that has been infected for a long time is reduced in size and the nail-bed shrinks around it. When the infection is partly overcome, the nail plate is increased in size and the nail bed is no longer large enough to accommodate the whole new nail. The lateral nail fold may then be penetrated from each side.

Prevention

Cut the nails straight instead of in a semi-circle. The nail should be allowed to grow, until its edges are clear of the end of the toe, before it is cut. This prevents the formation of marginal spicules. Use of proper fitting shoes should be advised to prevent the compression of ill-fitting footwear.

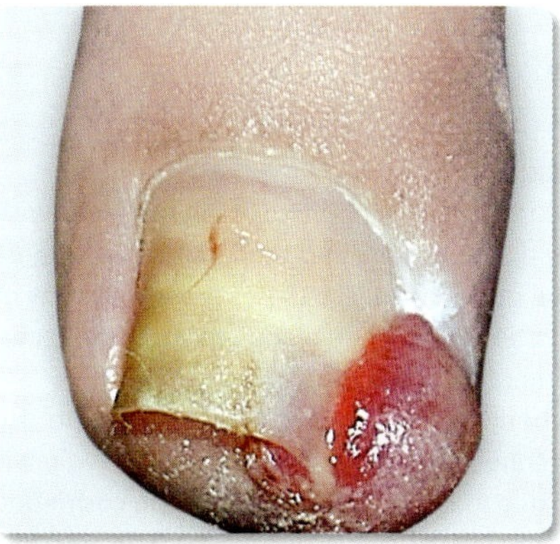

Fig. 8: Ingrown toe nail

Treatment

Ingrown toe nail without inflammation: Separate the toe nail gently from the nail fold with a wisp of absorbent cotton coated with collodion. Pain is relieved immediately. The collodion fixes the cotton in place and waterproofs the area. The cotton insert may need replacement after 3–4 weeks.

Ingrown toe nail with inflammation: Local antiseptics are used if infection is mild and systemic antibiotics if infection is severe. Remove the nail that is embedded in the nail fold under local anaesthesia. Granulation tissue is removed chemically by silver nitrate or surgically. The new nail is forced up and over the lateral nail fold by inserting cotton under the lateral nail margin and allowing it to remain in place or a few days or weeks.

Recurrent Ingrown nail: This may require permanent destruction of the lateral portion of the nail matrix by liquid phenol. In some cases, nail avulsion may be required.

Periungual Warts

Warts developing on the nail fold or beneath the nail plate may cause considerable therapeutic problems. The habit of nail biting or picking encourages the growth and spread of human papilloma virus. Recurrence rate is very high in periungual warts. Salicylic acid preparations are most useful for the treatment of periungual warts. If the wart extends beneath the nail, it should be trimmed to facilitate treatment. The duration of the treatment is 4–6 weeks. Salicylic acid 40% plaster can also be applied over the periungual warts. The plaster is cut to the shape and size of the wart and removed after 24 hours. The area is gently debrided and the plaster is re-applied until the lesions become soft and complete debridement is possible.

ABNORMALITIES OF THE NAIL PLATE

Onycholysis

Onycholysis is the separation of nail plate from the underlying nail bed. The detached portion of nail appears whitish. It can be seen in certain skin disease such as psoriasis and systemic disorders such as thyrotoxicosis. Certain drugs such as captopril and cytotoxic agents can also cause onycholysis. Tetracyclines cause photo-onycholysis that occurs on exposure to sun. Onycholysis of the great toe may result from trauma due to tennis and jogging. Long nails are also vulnerable to traumatic onycholysis. Nail cosmetics and use of nail file is a common cause of nail separation that is often overlooked. Excessive exposure to water, detergents and chemicals may also be responsible.

Pterygium

Pterygium can be dorsal or ventral.

Dorsal pterygium occurs due to progressive thinning of the nail plate, with fusion of the proximal nail fold to the nail matrix and then to the nail bed. As the disease advances, there is total loss of the nail with permanent atrophy of the nail. Dorsal pterygium is characteristic of lichen planus. It can also be seen in severe digital ischaemia, radiotherapy, or trauma.

Ventral pterygium occurs when the hyponychium is anchored to the undersurface of the nail; this obliterates the distal groove. Ventral pterygium is seen in scleroderma, trauma, and due to formaldehyde-containing cosmetics.

Median Nail Dystrophy

There is a longitudinal central split in the nail, with a fir tree-like appearance. Thumbs are most commonly involved; it is often bilateral. The thumbs show an enlarged lunula, probably from firm pressure at the base of the nail (Fig. 9). It is traumatic or occupational. There is no effective treatment.

Brittle Nails

This is a common complaint of many patients. The brittleness of nails is determined by its hydration. It is important to protect such nails from trauma,

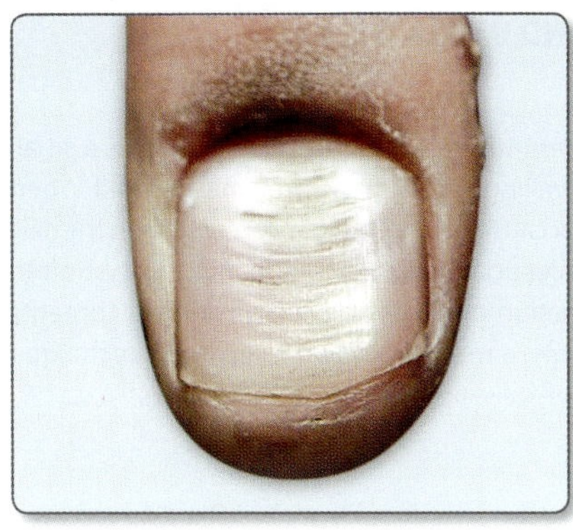

Fig. 9: Median nail dystrophy

water, detergents, and cleaning agents. Use of cotton gloves should be advised while doing household chores to avoid trauma to nails. This not only protects the nail from irritants but also reverses the undesirable nail changes. Nail polishes and nail solvent can sometimes cause this problem.

Onychogryphosis

This is a horn-like thickening of the nail. The nail is thickened, yellow and twisted; the big toe nail is most often affected (Fig. 10). The condition is commonly seen in the elderly. Injury and medical foot problems may precipitate changes earlier in life.

Onychogryphosis may be due to insufficient matrix as seen in old age, the nail bed contributing to the keratin of the nail. The nail increases in thickness, the elderly often fail to trim these nails due to neglect, as a result of which the nail increases in length; this later becomes curved. Nail infections such as onychomycosis may also be a contributing factor.

Treatment

Trimming is difficult; it may be facilitated by the use of 20% urea preparation. A chiropodist may trim thickened nails. When the condition occurs in young patients, the nail should be avulsed, so that a new nail grows.

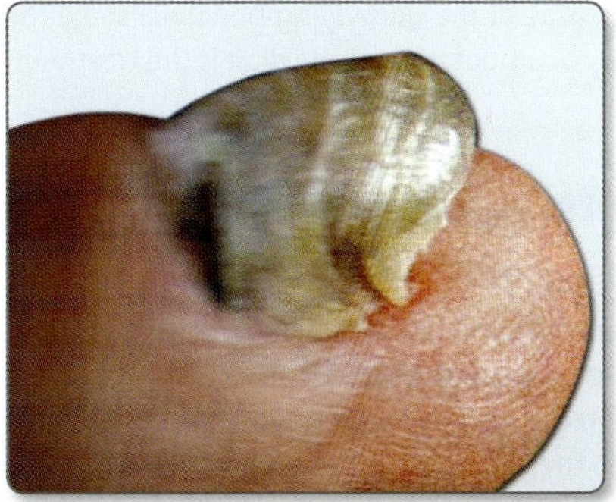

Fig. 10: Onychogryphosis

TUMOURS ADJACENT TO AND UNDER THE NAIL

Myxoid cyst

The most frequent tumour adjacent to the nail is mucoid cyst. This is a small translucent, non-inflammatory swelling, often on the proximal nail fold. When they persist, pressure on the matrix causes a longitudinal depression on the nail. Puncture elicits a viscous fluid. Injection of triamcinolone into the cyst often gives favourable results. Combination of squeezing the gelatinous contents and then freezing with cryotherapy, a method known as Epstein's technique is also quite successful.

Subungual Exostosis

This is a benign bony outgrowth of the distal part of the terminal phalanx; the nail plate is elevated but rarely damaged by the tumour. X-ray is used for the diagnosis. The condition is treated by the removal of the tumour.

Glomus Tumour

These are most characteristic of the vascular nail-bed tumours. The characteristic triad are pain, tenderness, and temperature sensitivity. Pain may be spontaneous or evoked by mild trauma. Nail-plate changes depend upon the site of the tumour. Tumours of the nail matrix cause splitting and distortion of the nail plate. Nail-bed tumours appear as reddish or blue lesions beneath the nail. MRI scan reveals the exact site of the tumour. Histology confirms the diagnosis. It is treated by excision.

Malignant Tumours

These may be squamous cell carcinoma or malignant melanoma. These present as chronic paronychia, ingrown nail, pyogenic granuloma, onycholysis, or as a nail dystrophy.

Malignant melanoma begins as pigmented streaks on the nail plate; the pigment then spreads to the periungual region, as macules and nodules (Hutchinson's sign). The lesion should be biopsied to rule out malignant melanoma. Dermatoscopy is a useful tool to distinguish between a nevus and melanoma.

Symptoms such as pain, itching, and throbbing may occur; metastasis is rare but local spread may occur. X-ray of the underlying bone will show the secondary changes. Mohs surgery or amputation of the digit is the treatment of choice.

CONGENITAL NAIL DISORDERS

The nail-patella syndrome

The nail-patella syndrome is an autosomal dominant disorder. It involves both the ectodermal and mesodermal structures; changes in the nails and bones are common. The nails are grossly defected; being about one-third or one-half of the normal size, they never reach the free edge of the finger. The nails of the thumb are most affected and the remaining nails, if involved, are progressively less damaged from index to little finger. The patella are smaller or rudimentary, knees are therefore unstable. Other abnormalities such as hyperextension of the joints, abnormalities of the iliac bones, scapulae and elbow are often seen. Skin laxity and renal abnormalities may be associated.

Pachyonychia Congenita

Pachyonychia congenita is generally an autosomal dominant disorder, although cases of autosomal recessive inheritance have been reported. The disease is characterised by hypertrophy of the nails; in some cases there is nail bed and hyponychial hyperkeratosis. Pachyonychia can be of the following types:

Type I (Jadassohn-Lewandowsky): The classical findings are hyperkeratosis of the palms and soles, follicular keratosis, and oral leucoplakia. Warty skin lesions are seen on the knees, elbows buttocks, legs, ankles, and popliteal region. Acral bullae, hyperhidrosis, and dyskeratosis of the cornea may occasionally occur.

Type II: Nail thickening is associated with mucocutaneous candidiasis, suggesting an immune deficiency.

Type III: This is similar to Type I, but is associated with epidermal cysts, lustreless kinky scalp hairs and eyebrows.

Type IV: Nail thickening and keratosis are associated with pigmentation, mainly flexural. Cutaneous amyloidosis may occur.

Yellow Nail Syndrome

This is an autosomal dominant disorder, with a triad of yellow nails, primary lymphoedema and bronchopulmonary disease. The nails are yellow due to thickening of the nail plate, lunula is obscured, and cuticle is lost. Occasionally there is chronic paronychia with onycholysis and transverse ridging. The nails grow at a reduced rate of 0.1–0.125 mm/week for the fingernails; all 20 nails may be involved. The syndrome is associated with lymphedema at one or more sites, with respiratory and nasal sinus disease. The condition may be associated with nephrotic syndrome, hypothyroidism, and AIDS.

FURTHER READING

1. Albom MJ. Avulsion of a nail plate. J Dermatol Surg Oncol. 1977;3:34-5.
2. Borgers Bongers EM, Gubler MC, Knoers NV. Nail-patella syndrome. Overview on clinical and molecular findings. Pediatr Nephrol. 2002;17:703-12.
3. Dawber RP, Sonnex T, Leonard J. Myxoid cysts of the finger: treatment by liquid nitrogen spray cryosurgery. Clin Exp Dermatol. 1983;8:153-7.
4. Haber RM, Rose TH. Autosomal recessive pachyonychia congenita. J Am Acad Dermatol. 1986;122:919-23.
5. Pechman KJ, Bergfield WF. Hyperhidrosis in Nail- patella syndrome. J Am Acad Dermatol. 1980;3:627-3032.
6. Ronger S, Touzet S, Lingeron C, et al. Dermoscopic examination of the nail pigment. Arch Dermatol. 2002;138:1327-33.
7. Samman DDPD. Idiopathic atrophy of the nails. Br J Dermatol. 1985, 1969;81:746-9.

8. Shelly WB, Shelly ED. Intralesional bleomycin sulphate sulfate therapy for warts.: A novel bifurcated needle puncture technique. Arch Dermatol. 1991;127:234-6.
9. Wegener EE. Glomus tumours of the nail unit: a plastic surgeon's approach. Dermatol Surg. 2001;27:240-1.
10. Zaias Zaiac MN, Weisse E. Mohs micrographic surgery of the nail unit and squamous cell carcinoma. 2001;27:246-51.
11. Zaias N, Ackerman AB. The nail in Darier-White disease. Arch Dermatol. 1973;107:193-9.
12. Zaias N. The nail in lichen planus. 1970;101:264-71.

Chapter 26

Diseases of the Subcutaneous Fat

INTRODUCTION

The subcutaneous tissue is an important metabolic organ; it functions as a thermal and mechanical insulator. It has three major components: lipocytes, fibrous septa and blood vessels. The fibrous septa contain the blood vessels, nerves and lymphatics. Small blood vessels branch from these septal vessels, traverse between the fat lobules and surround each lipocyte with its capillary network. Although the vessels of the septa supply the deep vascular plexus of the dermis, there are no connections between the deep plexus of the dermis and the capillary plexus of the subcutaneous lobules. There are no lymphatics and very little intervening connective tissue in the subcutaneous layer, and the vasculature is slow flowing; this renders the subcutaneous fat vulnerable to a variety of noxious insults, e.g. cold injury and enzymatic damage.

Brown fat is a special type of granular fat that differs from white fat in distribution, histology and function. It is multilobular, very active with many mitochondria so that it is capable of producing heat. It is most prominent in the neck and upper thorax of fetus. Brown fat is known to persist in adults and is said to prevent obesity. Warm patches develop in the skin 1 hour after taking ephedrine orally; these warm patches indicate the site of thermogenic fat.

Panniculitis represents an inflammatory reaction of adipose tissue involving the cutaneous or extra-cutaneous sites. The inflammation may affect fat lobules or the septa; this may overlap. Clinically, they present as erythematous or violet nodules, frequently in the legs which may or may not ulcerate. Diagnosis of panniculitis requires a deep skin biopsy to include an adequate amount of subcutaneous fat, a fully evolved lesion should be biopsied, not a new or a resolving one.

When fat cells are damaged, the liberated lipid undergoes hydrolysis to glycerol and fatty acids; this provokes a foreign body type of granulomatous reaction. Macrophages are attracted and foam cells are produced. After this phase of reaction, there is a period of reconstitution. The ease of repair depends upon the initial lipocyte damage and the efficacy of local circulation. Atrophy is a consequence of many types of inflammation in the fat lobules. In other cases there is extensive fibrosis with the formation of subcutaneous fibrotic nodule.

In certain types of panniculitis, a slow chain reaction is set up in the small focus of fat necrosis. This provokes a peripheral inflammatory reaction which leads to further necrosis thus allowing the lesion to spread centrifugally.

Panniculitis may be primary such as erythema nodosum, erythema induratum, and sclerema neonatorum. It may be secondary to diseases such as collagen disorders, pancreatic disease, steroid injections, or it may a part of other diseases such as benign cutaneous polyarteritis nodosa.

PANNICULITIS

Erythema Nodosum

Erythema nodosum is a hypersensitive reaction that occurs in response to a number of antigenic stimuli. This is a self-limiting panniculitis, with a sudden onset of reddish-brown macules and nodules on the shin. The condition often heals by itself in a few weeks. The eruption commonly affects the outer aspect of the legs, less commonly the thighs and forearms. Young women are mostly affected.

Aetiology

It is an immunological reaction to a variety of precipitating factors such as staphylococcal infection, streptococcal infection, tuberculosis, sarcoidosis, viral infections, such as hepatitis B and C, drugs (sulphonamides, oral contraceptives, penicillin), malignancy, deep fungal infections, such as coccidioidomycosis, and pregnancy. Circulating immune complexes have been found in some cases.

Clinical Features

There is a sudden eruption of bilateral tender nodules and plaques, 1–5 cm in diameter on the shins. The skin over the nodules is red, smooth and shiny, ulceration does not occur (Fig. 1). Lesion may occur in crops, individual lesion lasts for weeks and the eruption can last for months, but generally, the condition resolves without any sequelae. As resolution occurs the lesions become flat, and undergo colour changes like that of a bruise. The lesions later become purple and then greenish-yellow. The lesions heal without scarring or atrophy. Accompanying the outbreaks, fever, arthralgia and malaise may be present. In some cases, the lesions can also occur on the arms, thighs, face and neck.

Erythema nodosum migrans is a variant of erythema nodosum, instead of small bilateral nodules, one or more large unilateral nodules appear, these undergo central clearing, peripheral migratory satellite nodules develop, tenderness is absent; eruption lasts for years rather than months. Accompanying systemic signs and symptoms are less frequent than the acute form. Scarring and ulceration are absent.

Lofgren's syndrome comprises sarcoidosis, erythema nodosum, hilar lymphadenitis and arthritis.

Course and Prognosis

One attack usually lasts for a few weeks. The prognosis is good unless there is some serious underlying disease.

Differential Diagnosis

In nodular vasculitis, the nodules are smaller, harder and more persistent. They are often asymmetrical. In erythema nodosum leprosum, lesions are present in other parts of the body, signs of leprosy are present. Thrombophlebitic plaques affect the sides of the lower leg and hand; they are hard, irregular and fibrotic. Erythema induratum affects the back of the legs and are seen in people with erythrocyanotic circulation, and lesions break down to form ulcers.

Erythema Induratum

It is a panniculitis, associated with granulomatous vasculitis, involving the medium sized vessels. It was long

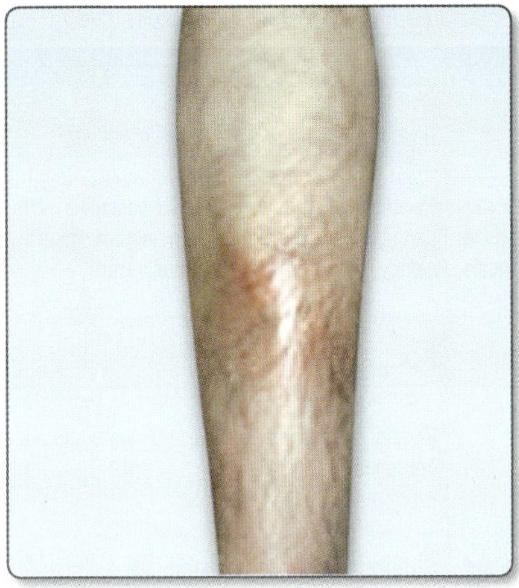

Fig. 1: Erythema nodosum

presumed to be a hypersensitivity to tuberculosis (Bazin disease), possibly immune complexes deposit on stagnant blood vessels. In most cases, relation to tuberculosis is not found, but venous insufficiency is present. The condition is found mainly in obese middle-aged women.

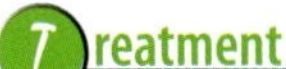

Treatment

In acute cases, bed rest and analgesics are required in the early stages. In the resolving stage when bed rest becomes impossible firm supportive bandages should be worn. Corticosteroids under occlusion speed resolution in the severe cases. Potassium iodide has recently been used again for the treatment of erythema nodosum.

Clinical Features

Ill-defined reddish-violet, bilateral nodules manifest the disease but the nodules are asymmetrical, usually situated on the posterior aspect of the lower limb (Fig. 2A). They often break down to form well-defined painful irregular ulcers that heal with depressed, hyperpigmented atrophic scars (Fig. 2B). Two types are recognised, one that affects middle-aged women with venous insufficiency, or it may be associated with tuberculosis, known as Bazin disease. Repeated infections acting on the vasculature already damaged may be important in the pathogenesis.

Associated signs of venous insufficiency such as cutis marmorata and erythrocyanosis are present.

Treatment

General measures as keeping the legs warm, reduction in weight are important. Treat the venous insufficiency or tuberculosis when present.

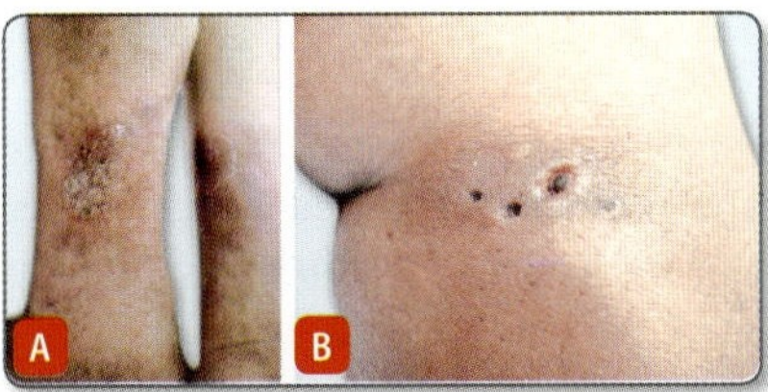

Figs 2A and B: Erythema induratum

Table 1: The difference between erythema nodosum and erythema induratum

Erythema nodosum	*Erythema induratum*
Site Anterior aspect of leg	Posterior aspect of leg
Aetiology Not associated with vasculitis. Reactive dermatosis in response to myriad of conditions: bacterial, fungal, viral, drugs, malignancies, sarcoidosis, etc.	Reactive inflammatory nodular vasculitis with panniculitis, associated with venous insufficiency (common) or tuberculosis (rare)
Onset Acute	Chronic
Clinical Features Tender-red nodules that do not ulcerate	Reddish-violet nodules, these ulcerate and are not tender
Association *Cutaneous* Not associated with changes of venous insufficiency *Systemic* Depends upon the cause	Erythrocyanosis, cutis marmorata, features of venous insufficiency present Systemic involvement absent when due to venous insufficiency Tuberculosis in Bazin disease
Resolves spontaneously Lesions heal without scarring	Treatment of venous insufficiency or tuberculosis Lesions heal with scarring

Course and Prognosis

Some cases respond spontaneously after a few months, others persist for years. There are no systemic complications.

Ernest Bazin (1807–1878)

"Ernest Bazin studied scabies thoroughly and revolutionised its treatment at the Hospital St. Louis. He used epilation in addition to parasiticides in the treatment of ringworm of the scalp and favus. He described acne keloidalis and erythema induratum."

WEBER-CHRISTIAN DISEASE

The disease occurs predominantly in men between 30 years and 60 years. It has been suggested that it results from an immunologically-mediated reaction to diverse antigenic stimuli. It may be secondary to jejunoileal bypass surgery, glomerulonephritis and α_1-antitrypsin deficiency. The disease has both systemic and cutaneous manifestations.

Histopathology

Weber-Christian disease is said to evolve through three stages; an acute inflammatory stage, in which lobules of fat are replaced by neutrophils, lymphocytes and histiocytes. An intermediate stage in which degenerated fat is ingested by the macrophages and results in the formation of foam cells. Finally the foam cells are replaced by fibroblasts, collagen tissue is laid down and fibrosis results. The epidermis and the dermis usually do not show any changes.

Clinical Manifestations

These may be systemic and cutaneous.

Systemic Manifestations

Systemic manifestations are due to the involvement the omentum, mesenteric and perivisceral fat. Inflammation at these sites, leads to nausea, vomiting, and abdominal pain. If the bone marrow is involved, anaemia and leucopenia may result.

Cutaneous Manifestations

Subcutaneous tender nodules appear on the trunk and extremities, chiefly on the thighs. The skin over the nodules may be erythematous, mottled or pigmented. The nodules regress spontaneously leaving localised depressed atrophic scars. Each attack is accompanied by fever. In time, the attacks become fewer and eventually they stop. Sometimes these nodules undergo liquefaction and discharge oily fluid.

Erythrocyte sedimentation rate (ESR) is useful in evaluating the disease; it rises steeply at the onset of the disease, and falls to normal at its conclusion.

Treatment

No effective therapy is recognised. Therapeutic response to sulphapyridine, dapsone, azathioprine, thalidomide, cyclophosphamide and tetracyclines is reported. The use of corticosteroids during the acute inflammatory phase is sometimes beneficial.

ROTHMAN-MAKAI SYNDROME

It is a disease of childhood, the patient developing large tender subcutaneous plaques and nodules over the trunk, legs and face. It has no systemic and visceral manifestations. The condition subsides spontaneously within a year. It is considered by some to be a variant of Weber-Christian panniculitis.

PANNICULITIS AND PANCREATIC DISEASE (NODULAR FAT NECROSIS)

This is an association of panniculitis with pancreatic disease. The pancreatic disease may have a number of underlying causes; it may be due to alcoholism, collagen disorders, carcinoma, and pancreatic pseudocyst.

Pathogenesis

Subcutaneous fat necrosis is primarily an enzymatic disorder; a damaged pancreas releases large amounts of lipolytic and proteolytic enzymes. These enzymes are relayed to distant sites by lymphatic and haematogenous spread. This results in lipolysis and saponification of fat with the deposition of calcium triglyceride complexes.

Histopathology

The histopathology is pathognomonic, the adipocytes become shrunken, the cell membrane thickens, and these are the ghost cells. Surrounding the cell membrane and in the adjacent connective tissue is a basophilic granular material which stains for calcium.

Systemic Manifestations

The patients are often extremely ill with fever, vomiting and abdominal distension, an associated large joint arthritis is present in about 60% of patients. The most common site is the ankle. Ascites, pleural and pericardial effusion indicates a poor prognosis.

Clinical Features

The patient is often a middle aged or elderly man, who has both systemic and cutaneous lesions.

Cutaneous Manifestations

The lesions usually begin in the leg as tender or non-tender subcutaneous nodules. The lesions may also occur on the trunk or buttocks, spontaneous liquefaction and drainage may occur.

Laboratory Finding

Serum amylase, lipase, and other proteolytic enzymes are elevated. Peripheral eosinophilia is especially seen in pancreatic carcinoma.

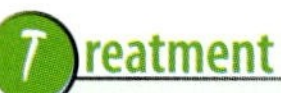

Treat the cause of the underlying pancreatic disease.

α_1-ANTITRYPSIN DEFICIENCY-ASSOCIATED PANNICULITIS

This is a rare panniculitis due to the deficiency in the serine proteinase inhibitor α_1-antitrypsin.

The cutaneous manifestations are characterised by ill-defined erythematous plaques, commonly seen on the lower extremities, face, arms and trunk. The lesions ulcerate with an oily fluid coming out of the lesion. The condition heals with atrophy and scarring. The disease commonly follows trauma. Other cutaneous manifestations are vasculitis, severe psoriasis and cutis laxa.

Systemic manifestations include hepatitis, emphysema and cirrhosis.

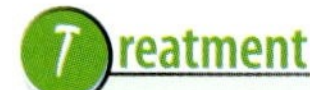

Therapies include dapsone, corticosteroids, doxycycline and intravenous infusion of exogenous α_1-protease inhibitor concentrate. The prognosis is poor.

SCLEROSING PANNICULITIS

This is a common panniculitis seen in obese middle-aged women. It is due to venous insufficiency of the lower extremities, often due to deep venous thrombosis and varicose veins. This is a lobular panniculitis without any vasculitis. Venous Doppler ultrasound studies indicate the venous insufficiency.

Clinical Features

The clinical features range from acute inflammatory disease to chronic fibrotic stage at the other end. In the acute phase of the disease symmetric erythematous plaques are seen on the lower extremities. Features of venous insufficiency such as oedema, hyperpigmentation and ulceration are also associated. As the disease progresses, there is extensive sclerosis and atrophy of the subcutaneous tissue, resulting in an inverted champagne bottle deformity.

Treatment

Treat the venous insufficiency with elastic compression bandages. Fibrinolytic agents such as stanozolol may help.

DERCUMS DISEASE (ADIPOSIS DOLOROSA)

The disease affects menopausal women, characterised by local overgrowth of fat with painful subcutaneous plaques and ecchymosis. Multiple areas of the body are affected; the painful areas feel like a bag of worms (subcutaneous lumps). Juxta-articular tissue is commonly involved, pain is spontaneous on palpation. Dercum's disease begins gradually, later makes the movements difficult and the patient can become immobilised. Classic triad: obesity, painful plaques and ecchymosis.

Treatment

Pain is unresponsive to analgesics, surgical excision is often required. Pain can be relieved by intravenous injection of local anaesthetics. Mexiletine 150–750 mg orally may be helpful.

LIPODYSTROPHY

Lipodystrophies are rare conditions in which there is atrophy of the subcutaneous fat. It can be generalized or partial, congenital or acquired.

Partial Lipodystrophy

The cause of partial lipodystrophy is unknown, 80% of the patients are females and the disease usually manifests before the age of 15 years. There is loss of fat usually from the face, it spreads downward and may stop at any level above or middle of the thigh. Most cases are of the cephalothoracic type. Buccal fat disappears leaving a relative prominence of the chin and zygomas. Because of the loss of periorbital fat, the eyes appear sunken. Many wrinkles are present on the face, and the patient appears prematurely aged. Because of the absence of subcutaneous fat, the muscles and veins appear prominent. The overlying skin is of normal colour, texture and elasticity. Some patients have glomerulonephritis and pancreatitis, eosinophilia has also been reported.

Barraquer-Simons Syndrome

There is loss of fat on the face, trunk, and arms, but there is a normal distribution on the buttocks, and lower extremities. In some cases, it is associated with renal failure.

Dunnigan Type of Lipodystrophy

This is a genetic disorder with autosomal dominant inheritance. There is loss of fat over the limbs and trunk, but an increased deposit of fat on the neck and labia. It is often associated with acanthosis nigricans, diabetes mellitus and hepatosplenomegaly. The diabetes is insulin resistant.

Kobberling Type of Lipodystrophy

This is associated with loss of adipose tissue on both upper and lower extremities, the face, neck and trunk are normal.

Laboratory Findings

Patients frequently have hypertriglyceridemia, and insulin resistant diabetes. The most common laboratory finding is decreased C3 levels. This is seen in 70% of cases.

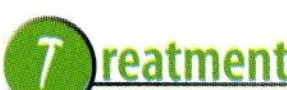

Effective therapy is not available. Injection of silicone can improve the appearance.

Generalised Lipodystrophy (Lawrence-Seip Syndrome)

The disease has an autosomal recessive inheritance. Girls are commonly affected.

Pathogenesis

Some investigators have postulated that adipose cells are defective; there is diversion of fat from the subcutaneous fat to other organs, which results in organomegaly, or it may be due to hypothalamic dysfunction. A urinary peptide that causes lipodystrophy is found in some patients.

Clinical Features

Patient lacks both the subcutaneous fat and extra-cutaneous adipose tissue. Acanthosis nigricans, hypertrichosis, generalised hyperpigmentation, thick curly scalp hair are often present. During infancy, linear growth is accelerated but adult height is normal. Patients have prominent teeth and small chin, liver is enlarged. Because of the absence of subcutaneous fat, muscles appear hypertrophic. The external genitalia are often enlarged. A fatty liver later leads to cirrhosis. Significant kidney disease, mental retardation, crippling schizophrenia can occur. Some patients have frank virilization with polycystic ovaries. Diabetes develops in the second or third decade which is usually fatal.

Laboratory Findings

There is decreased glucose tolerance. Diabetes is insulin resistant. Insulin resistance may be due a genetic defect in the insulin receptor or post-receptor pathway. Hyperlipoproteinemia is present; there is increase of total lipids, cholesterol and triglycerides. Bone changes comprise sclerosis and cystic changes.

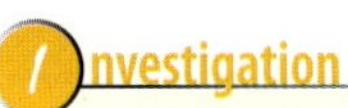

Blood glucose levels, lipids profile and liver functions should be done at regular intervals.

Leprechaunism

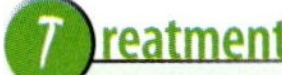

Pimozide has helped a few patients, probably by correcting the disturbed hypothalamic functions.

These patients have a generalised decrease or absence of subcutaneous fat as in congenital generalised lipodystrophy. The cutaneous features resemble those of other lipodystrophies, but there is no organomegaly or liver disease. The patients have muscular wasting, retarded bone age, retarded growth and early death.

Acquired Lipodystrophy

Acquired lipodystrophy can be due to drugs such as following injections of corticosteroids, truncal and nuchal lipodystrophy is sometimes seen after highly active antiretroviral therapy (HAART) of HIV infection. Buffalo hump and moon facies is seen in Cushing's syndrome and after steroid therapy. Linear depressed bands on the thighs of women following the use of tight pants.

CELLULITE

This is an altered topography of the skin that occurs mainly in women in the pelvic region. It is due to structural changes in the dermal microcirculation of lipocytes. The exact aetiology is not known, oestrogens is said to play a role in its production as the condition is predominant in females. It is found in young women who perform physical activity, or in inactive women who suddenly reduce weight. The surface of the skin looks dimpled. Fat deposits that push and distort the connective tissue, contribute to the lumpiness.

Cellulite is graded according to its clinical appearance and histology.

Grade I: No symptoms, no clinical changes, there is increased thickness of areola tissue and increase in capillary permeability.

Treatment

Weight reduction should be gradual, regular exercises improve the circulation, the use of non-hormonal contraceptives may help in preventing cellulite. The condition is difficult to treat; ultrasound, mesotherapy and thermotherapy may be helpful.

Grade II: No skin changes at rest, but on muscular contraction several clumps appear. There is local pallor, decrease in temperature and decrease in elasticity of the skin.

Grade III: The skin is orangish pink in appearance; pain may or may not be present. On histology, there is fatty tissue destruction.

Grade IV: Skin surface appears wavy; there are visible painful purple nodules. The lobular structure of adipose tissue has disappeared, and the nodules are encapsulated by dermal connective tissue.

Sclerema neonatorum, and subcutaneous fat necrosis are described in chapter 33, lupus profundus in chapter 11, and cold panniculitis in chapter 21.

FURTHER READING

1. Barnhill RL. Panniculitis and fasciitis. In: Barnhill RL (Ed). Textbook of Dermatopathology. New York: McGraw-Hill publication; 1998: pp. 233-56.
2. Garg A, Wilson R, Barnes R, et al. A gene for congenital lipid dystrophy maps to Chromosome 9q34. Journal of Endocrinology and Metabolism. 1999;16:4-8.
3. Horio T, Danno K, Okamoto H, et al. Potassium iodide in erythema nodosum and other erythematous disorders. J Am Acad Deramatol. 1983;9:77-81.
4. Houseman C, Johanson A, Varma M, and Blizzard RMet al. Congenital lipodystrophy: an endocrinal study in three siblings. J Pediatr. 1978;93:221-6.
5. Jafri NZ, Zaidi Z. Congenital generalized lipodystrophy. J Pak Med Assoc.JPMA. 1992;42: 72-76.
6. Psychos DN, Voulgaris PV, Skopouli FN, Drosso AA, Moutsopoulos HM et al. Erythema nodosum: the underlying conditions. Clin Rheumatol. 2000;19:212-6.

Chapter

27 Tumours of the Skin

INTRODUCTION

The tumours of the skin may be benign, premalignant or malignant. The incidences of tumours differ in different countries. Malignant tumours predisposed by sunlight are rare in dark-skinned population and present less serious problems than those of the fairer complexion. The racial and cultural diversity is another factor affecting the incidence of tumours and skin disease. Submucous fibrosis is a disease of the Indian subcontinent confined to people using areca nut and betel leaves; it is precancerous. Premalignant conditions in developing countries are commonly mucosal than cutaneous. In general, owing to limited medical facilities in the rural areas, especially of under developed countries, malignant tumours reach an advanced stage by the time they are seen by the physician.

MALIGNANT TUMOURS OF THE SKIN

Skin cancer in general is the most common form of malignant neoplasia. It has been estimated that almost half of all the people who have reached 65 years of age have had, or will have at least one skin cancer. Amongst the skin cancers, 30% are squamous cell carcinoma (SCC), 60% are basal cell carcinoma (BCC) and 2% are melanomas. The remaining 8% include Kaposi's sarcoma, lymphomas and other rare forms of skin malignancies.

Squamous cell carcinoma arises from the keratinising epithelium. BCC belongs to a group of organoid adnexal tumours. It appears to arise from the immature pluripotent cells, and they may also originate from the outer root sheath of the hair follicle. Malignant melanoma arises from the melanocytes.

All malignant tumours display some degree of anaplasia; anaplasia is one of the hallmarks of malignancy. Malignant tumours enlarge progressively and erratically. The malignant tumours are usually un-encapsulated, invasive and metastatic. The nucleus is extremely hyperchromatic and large. The nuclear cytoplasmic ratio may reach 1:1, instead of the usual 1:4 or 1:6. Giant cells may be present; these possess large nucleus or several nuclei. Anaplastic nuclei are variable and bizarre in shape. The chromatin is coarse and clumped, while nucleoli are large. Mitosis is numerous and atypical. Anaplastic cells grow in sheets or masses with total loss of structure. The changes are irreversible.

Predisposing Factors

Radiation

Ultraviolet irradiation is the most common cause of skin malignancy. They are mostly found on the sun-exposed areas. They are more common in individuals of lighter skin. The incidence increases with advancing age because of the cumulative damage of ultraviolet radiation (UVR). X-ray is also an increasing cause of skin cancer; radiation dermatitis is premalignant. Chronic infrared radiation causes erythema ab igne, which may also undergo malignant change.

Chemicals

People are continuously exposed exogenously to varying amounts of chemicals that have been shown to have carcinogenic or mutagenic properties, such as benzpyrene, chromates, coal tar, arsenic and mineral oil. These have caused skin cancer in industrial workers.

Scars and Chronic Inflammations

Malignancy may arise on old scars, burns, chronic ulcers and chronic inflammations, such as leprosy, lupus vulgaris, syphilis, epidermolysis bullosa, etc. Some human papilloma viruses are associated with SCC.

Immune Response

Some malignant cells are destroyed by the body's immune defence mechanisms. Immune deficiency predispose to skin cancer. Patients with multiple solar keratoses have a greater incidence of skin cancer after receiving immunosuppressive drugs.

Genetic Factors

Some congenital diseases predispose to malignancy such as xeroderma pigmentosum.

Basal Cell Carcinoma

This is the most common skin tumour; it outnumbers the SCC by the ratio of 4:1. It is a slow growing tumour, locally malignant that does not metastasise. If left untreated, the tumour invades the subcutaneous tissue, muscles or even the bones. Perineural invasion may result in pain, paraesthesias or even paralysis.

Histogenesis

Basal cell carcinoma is a fibroepithelioma consisting of an epithelial parenchyma interdependent with a mesodermal stroma. This intimal epidermal and mesodermal relationship is the outstanding feature that separates BCC from SCC or other adnexal tumours.

Epidermal portion: Epithelial cells are basaloid cells that resemble the basal cells of the epidermis and matrix cells of the appendages. The peripheral cells form a continuous layer of columnar cells resting on a basement membrane. Centrally situated cells may show no particular arrangement; they may be more or less fusiform. Basal cells usually do not have a well-developed system of tonofilaments; this may account for their softness. Desmosomes are present.

Mesodermal portion: The stroma is often less mature, more cellular and less fibrous. A periodic-acid-Schiff (PAS) positive basement membrane surrounds the epithelial portion. Another component of BCC is a cell-mediated inflammatory reaction that consists mainly of T lymphocytes and may include a few plasma cells and eosinophils.

Histopathology

The histopathological findings are diagnostic. Groups of small compact uniform cells with deeply staining nuclei grow downwards from the basal layer in irregular columns; these cells show a palisade arrangement at the periphery of their masses. Dermal stroma is an integral part of the BCC. The tumour does not terminate at the bottom of the epithelial nests, but actually extends into the newly formed matrix to constitute a fibroepithelial neoplasm. BCCs do not metastasise because they are highly dependent on the connective tissue stroma on which they lie. The interaction of the epidermis with the dermis produces the characteristic palisade of tumour cells and the well-organised stroma around it.

There is a great diversity in the patterns of BCC. Frequently melanocytic proliferation occurs in the tumour and the tumour appears pigmented. Mucin deposition commonly occurs in the tumour, particularly at the margins or may be encysted in it. Cystic cavities also form when the central cells undergo necrosis.

Clinical Features

This is the most common form of skin cancer and the lesion may present in a number of ways. Both the sexes are equally affected, mostly seen in the elderly people. The most common site is the face. There are many types of BCC, such as the nodular, ulcerative, pigmented, cystic, morphea-like, cicatricial and superficial basal cell carcinoma.

Ulcerated Type (Rodent Ulcer)

This is the most common presentation. The lesion has a raised pearly edge with a central ulcer. Telangiectases may be seen in the pearly edge of the lesion. The lesion usually ulcerates when it reaches a diameter of about 5 mm. This type of BCC may invade inwards forming a deep ulcer with destruction of the underlying tissues and spreads laterally over the surface of the skin (Fig. 1).

Nodulocystic BCC

The lesion commences as a small cystic papule; this gradually enlarges forming a lobulated cystic swelling (Fig. 2). The lesion does not ulcerate; it can be mistaken for a benign cyst, but it has telangiectasia on its surface and its pearly colour, are important differentiating features.

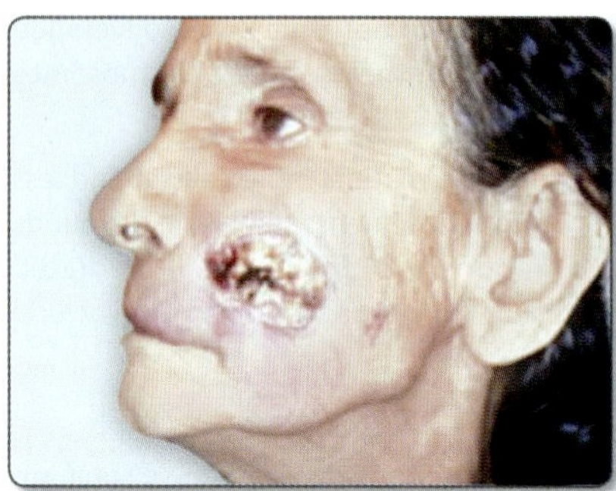

Fig. 1: Basal cell carcinoma—ulcerated.

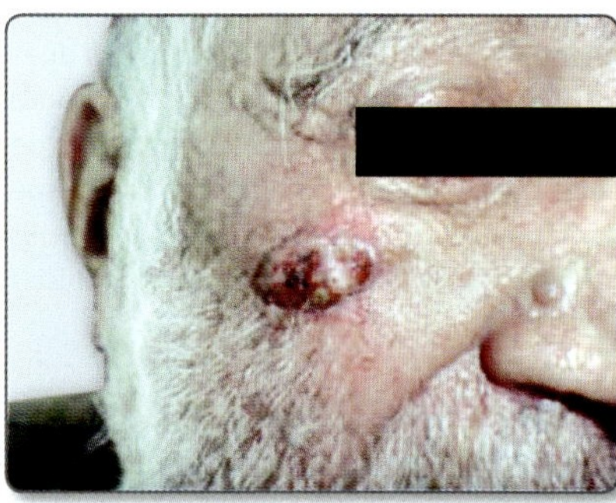

Fig. 2: Basal cell carcinoma—nodulocystic

Morphoeic BCC

This is so called because the lesions present as a firm red plaque resembling morphoea. The morphology is due to fibrosis; it is an attempt by the body at healing or containing the lesion. It can be mistaken for a scar; nests of tumour cells often infiltrate beyond the clinical margins of the plaque. Incomplete excision is therefore not unusual.

Superficial BCC

These are often seen in patients who have received arsenic early in life. It appears as red scaly plaques on the trunk or the limbs. It is often mistaken for psoriasis. On careful examination, a thin rolled border is seen. As its name implies, it spreads laterally and not inwardly.

Pigmented BCC

The ulcerated, cystic and superficial types may have varying amounts of pigment present (Fig. 3); this should be differentiated from a melanocytic nevus and seborrhoeic keratosis. Fragments can be removed by cytolysis for diagnosis.

The characteristic features of most BCCs are that they are found frequently on the face, they have a history of bleeding, telangiectasia are present on the surface, they appear translucent or pearly, and the edge of the lesion has a characteristic rolled border. It is one of the easiest tumours to recognise.

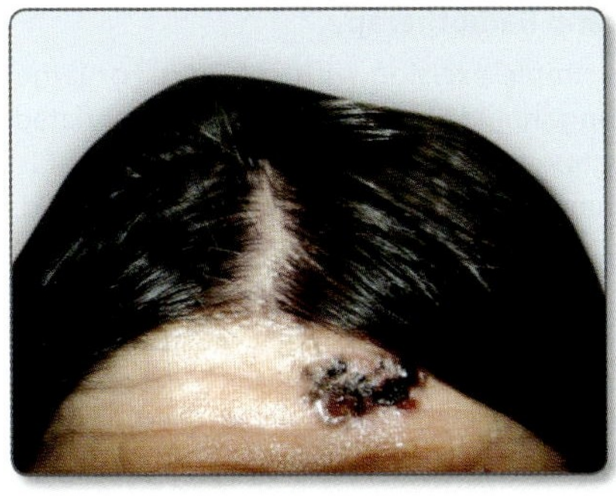

Fig. 3: Pigmented basal cell carcinoma. Note the rolled border

The typical BCC runs a slow progressive course of peripheral extension that produces a thread-like margin, a nodule with central depression or an expanding rodent ulcer. These tumours, if neglected, may cause mutilation of the face or scalp or the underlying structures.

Although ultraviolet light increases the incidence of BCC, it is not the only cause. It is unusual to find BCC on the back of the hands and forearms, sites exposed to sunlight. Inner canthus and the eyelids are areas shielded from sunlight, but these sites are commonly involved in BCC. BCC appears on the solar protected areas as the vulva.

Diagnostic Features

- Well-defined tumour
- Rolled pearly margins
- Site is usually the face (superficial BCC on the trunk)
- Telangiectasia is present
- History of bleeding and crusting.

Differential Diagnosis

The ulcerated type should be differentiated from SCC and keratoacanthoma. Telangiectasia is present in both keratoacanthoma and BCC. BCC is usually asymmetrical and the ulcer is less deep than a keratoacanthoma. Keratoacanthoma has a typical history of rapid growth, a quiescent phase and then a period of involution. On the pinna, BCC should be differentiated from chondrodermatitis helicis nodularis. The latter is usually painful. The superficial BCC should be differentiated from Bowen's disease, psoriasis or a patch of eczema. Cystic BCC should be differentiated from benign cysts of the skin. Pigmented BCC should be differentiated from the other pigmented lesions such as seborrhoeic warts and melanoma.

Diagnosis

- Biopsy
- Cytology: The lesion is scraped by a large scalpel blade; the cells which are removed are smeared on a slide and fixed as for cervical smears. Clumps of malignant basal cells are seen.

Treatment

Each tumour has to be evaluated individually for treatment. Age, sex, site and type of the tumour are important factors to be considered. The aim of the treatment is permanent cure and best cosmetic results. The BCC can be treated by surgical excision.

Local Destruction, Curettage and Radiotherapy

The ideal treatment for BCC is simple excision with suturing. For large tumours, excision with skin grafting should be done. The well-differentiated tumours are best suitable for surgery, whereas radiotherapy is more suitable for large, poorly-differentiated tumours. Some areas as dorsum of the hand, shin, ear and the skull are not suitable for radiotherapy due to necrosis of the bone and cartilage. Radiation should not be performed in the regions near the eyelids and angle of the mouth, as these present great problems to the reconstructive surgeon. Radiotherapy is the best suited for the elderly patient and those with extensive lesions. Radiotherapy should not be used for recurrences and for treating morphoeic lesions, as these are radio-resistant.

For recurrences and morphoeic type of tumours, Mohs surgery is preferable. This surgery is also suitable for tumours at the nasolabial fold, nasal alae, periorbital and periauricular region, and in certain scalp tumours. This technique ensures complete tumour clearance with minimal loss of normal tissue. The tumour is removed in thin slices and histopathological examination is carried out at the same time.

Local destruction by curettage, cryosurgery and topical cytotoxic therapy can be used for small nodular tumours, cystic lesions or superficial multicentric type, especially in the older population.

Oral retinoids, such as isotretinoin and acitretin, are reported to be useful in reducing the size of multiple carcinomas developing on the sun-exposed area of the skin. 5% imiquimod cream, photodynamic therapy and vismodegib (hedgehog pathway inhibitor) have also been used.

Course and Prognosis

As a rule, BCC has a good prognosis if treated correctly. The ulcerative lesions may invade deep tissues and eventually cause death. This will, however, take many years after the first appearance of the lesion. The good prognosis probably depends upon the fact that BCC does not metastasize like the other forms of cancer. The recurrence rate after treatment is less than 5% and further treatment usually results in cure.

Associations of BCC

- Naevoid BCC syndrome
- Basosquamous BCC
- Bazex syndrome
- BCC with arsenic keratosis (described earlier).

Naevoid BCC syndrome

This is a genetic autosomal dominant disorder associated with multiple BCCs, palmoplantar pits and defects in the other tissues, such as cysts of the jaw, abnormalities of the ribs, vertebrae and multiple other disorders. A characteristic facies is present with frontal bossing, hypoplastic maxilla, broad nasal root and hypertelorism.

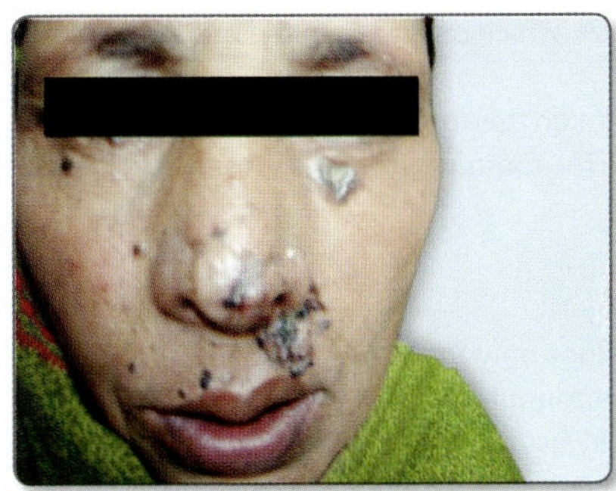

Fig. 4: Naevoid BCC syndrome showing multiple basal cell carcinomas

Clinical Features

Naevoid BCC syndrome appears between the ages of 13 and 17. The distribution is usually bilateral and symmetrical. Any area of the body may be affected; they have a tendency to be most marked on the central part of the face. Jaw cysts occur in 70% of cases. The patients may complain of pain, tenderness and difficulty in opening and closing the mouth (Fig. 4).

Pits of the hands and feet: An unusual pitting of the hands and feet is a distinguishing feature of the disease. They usually become apparent in the second decade of life.

Skeletal defects: Numerous skeletal defects are present, such as spina bifida, scoliosis, kyphosis, deformed ribs, etc. The shortened fourth and fifth metacarpals result in a dimple over the metacarpal joints (Albright's sign).

Disorders of the central nervous system: Calcification of falx cerebri, falx cerebelli, dura mater or the basal ganglia are common.

Other defects: Ophthalmic abnormalities, ovarian cysts, uterine fibroids, and renal calculi may occur.

Treatment: Mohs surgery for cutaneous tumours shows the best cure rates and cosmetic appearance. Genetic counselling is essential.

Bazex's Syndrome (Follicular Atrophoderma and BCC)

This is another disorder with multiple BCC; this has an autosomal dominant or X-linked recessive inheritance. Follicular atrophoderma is present at birth; it occurs as ice-pick marks. Facial eczema is present soon after birth. There may be hypotrichosis and anhidrosis of the face and hands. The BCC appear on the face in the second or third decades.

Basisquamous or Metatypical BCC

This tumour on histopathology shows the features of both BCC and SCC. It has a higher incidence of metastasis. Aggregates of cells embedded in fibrous tissue stroma are seen; these aggregates lack the palisading pattern of BCC. The cells are larger with a large pale nucleus and have eosinophilic cytoplasm.

Premalignant Epithelioma of Pinkus

This is a premalignant tumour composed of cells resembling BCC, arranged around a prominent papillary stroma. The tumour is composed of enlarged dermal papillae, which are more cellular and fibrotic. These papillae are surrounded by strands of dark cells, which extend from the underside of the epidermis.

Most of the tumours are present on the abdomen or loins. They are sessile, dome-shaped, and skin-coloured. The tumour is often diagnosed as a fibroma. Treatment is by surgical excision.

Squamous Cell Carcinoma

Squamous cell carcinomas arise not only from the skin, but also from the mucous membranes, such as the tongue, lips, oesophagus, cervix and the vagina. Most cases arise on the skin, usually on the exposed parts of the body. It is common after the age of 55, twice more frequent in men than women. In tropical countries, it mostly grows over chronic ulcers and granulomatous diseases. In Western countries, it is mostly secondary to UVR. The first clinical evidence of malignancy is induration or thickening of the skin.

Histopathology

Squamous cell carcinoma arises from the epidermis or from the adnexal epithelium. There is an invasion of the dermis by irregular nests of polygonal epidermal cells. The squamous cancer cells preserve their ability for keratinization to a greater or lesser degree, or lose it completely. The cells of SCC may be large, well-differentiated polygonal cells with prominent nucleoli and abundant cytoplasm. The cytoplasm contains tonofilaments and well-developed intercellular bridges. Towards the centre of the nodule, the cells undergo normal keratinisation; irregular horny pearls are produced. On the other hand, the tumour may be completely anaplastic with basophilic cytoplasm; it provides no cytological evidence of its origin. The tumour produces an inflammatory response in the dermis. Broder's histological grading is based on:

- Grade I: 75% or more differentiating cells
- Grade II: 50–75% differentiating cells
- Grade III: 25–50% differentiating cells
- Grade IV: > 25% differentiating cells.

Broder's Grade I includes well-differentiated tumours having keratin pearls. Broder's Grade IV has little keratinisation, marked anaplasia, tumour giant cell formation and numerous mitosis.

Many pathologists prefer to grade SCC as well-differentiated, poorly differentiated and undifferentiated tumours. No basal cells are seen, even the outermost cells are relatively large and pale staining and show little tendency to palisade.

Verrucous SCC

These are slow-growing exophytic growths with a variety of clinical patterns. Their malignant potential is low and often described as warty; they develop at sites of chronic irritation. Four subtypes are described as follows:

- Buschke-Lowenstein or giant condyloma: This is a large genital wart that occurs on the penis, scrotum, vulva, vagina, cervix or the anus.
- Ackerman's carcinoma or verrucous carcinoma is a unique clinico-pathological variant of SCC, occurring mainly in the oral cavity and larynx, buccal

Clinical Features

Squamous cell carcinoma usually arises on an abnormal skin or mucous membrane. The initial lesion may be a small nodule, plaque, or an ulcer with an indurated and thickened edge. The indurated plaque grows laterally and vertically; gradually it becomes fixed and nodular. Eventually the surface becomes ulcerated or crusted. The ulcers often have a purulent base. The margin is firm and more raised than a BCC; it is often everted and irregular in shape. It grows more rapidly than a BCC, but not as fast a keratoacanthoma. The nodule may later become papillomatous or cauliflower-like and invades the underlying tissue. Early enlargement of lymph glands is due to secondary infection of the ulcer; metastasis occurs late, the glands then become hard and fixed (Figs 5 and 6).

Squamous cell carcinoma is indurated, more likely to demonstrate an overlying scale; at times the scales may project above the skin surface producing a cutaneous horn. Verrucous carcinomas are a variant of SCCs; they look like warts and are often misdiagnosed.

On the lower lip, SCC develops over actinic cheilitis. From repeated sun exposure, the lower lip becomes dry, scaly, fissured and keratosis develops. Carcinoma usually arises on a fissure or keratosis. It begins as a small thickening; they later grow inwards with destructive ulceration. A history of smoking is an important predisposing factor. Use of sunscreen with a sun-protection factor of at least 30 for the first 18 years of life would reduce the lifetime incidence of nonmelanotic skin cancers by 78%.

Marjolin's ulcer is the name given to SCC that develops on a chronic ulcer, sinuses or burns.

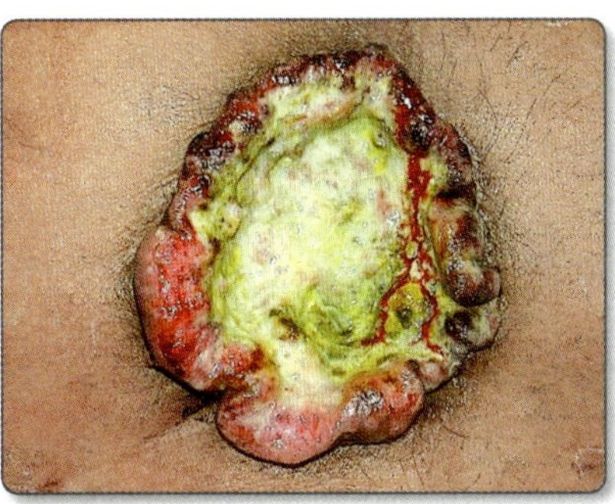

Fig. 5: Squamous cell carcinoma

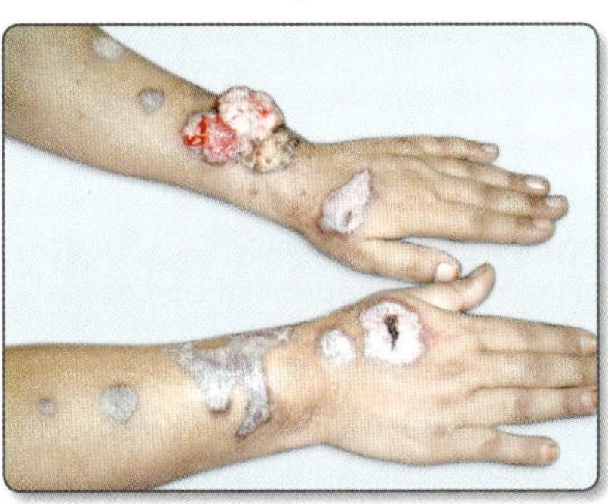

Fig. 6: Squamous cell carcinoma secondary to leishmaniasis

mucosa. It is commonly seen in elderly men who have a chronic history of tobacco chewing. This is often referred as oral florid papillomatosis.

- Epithelioma cuniculatum: This is a malodorous destructive plantar wart found in the feet of old men. This is often called "rabbit burrows", due to the invasive nature of the tumour.

- Papillomatosis cutis carcinoides: These are irregular nodules present over the shins, scalp and trunk. These are probably also related to the HPV.

Differential Diagnosis

Keratoacanthoma occurs at similar sites and has a similar morphology, but it grows more rapidly in the initial stages. Amelanotic melanoma, BCC and chronic granulomata that ulcerate may also give a similar appearance.

Diagnostic Features

- Usually solitary
- Opaque growth, not translucent like BCC
- Indurated nodule or plaque
- Surface may become crusted or ulcerated
- Margin of the ulcer is more raised than BCC, often everted and irregular in shape
- Solar sites are commonly involved, or superimposed on a chronic lesion.

Treatment

Because of the possibility of metastasis, treatment should be thorough. Ideally, surgical excision is imperative. If the lymph nodes are affected then their removal is also essential. Mohs surgery is indicated for recurrent disease, large lesions, those at special sites such as posterior auricular sulcus, in SCC arising in scarred or irradiated skin.

Radiation therapy is also effective. For metastatic or advanced lesions, cytotoxic drugs are preferred.

Factors Governing the Prognosis of SCC

- Preceding lesion: SCC arising on preexisting lesions such as Bowens disease, solar keratosis or tuberculosis is likely to metastasize earlier than those arising de novo.
- Site: Lesions on the ear, vermillion border of the lips, external genitalia, and on the mucosal surfaces metastasize early.
- Degrees of differentiation: Well-differentiated tumours have a better prognosis than poorly differentiated ones.
- Degree of invasion: The greater the invasion, the poorer the prognosis.

Treatment

Because of the possibility of metastasis, treatment should be thorough. Ideally surgical excision is imperative. If the lymph nodes are affected, these should be removed. Mohs surgery is essential for recurrence, and for SCC at special sites such as posterior auricular sulcus, and in squamous carcinoma arising in scarred or irradiated skin.

Radiation therapy is also effective. For metastatic and advanced lesions cytotoxic therapy is preferred.

Prevention

It is said that a sun protection factor of at least 30 for the first 18 years of life would reduce the lifetime incidence of nonmelanoma skin cancers.

Course and Prognosis

Squamous cell carcinoma has the potential to metastasize and thus if not treated will eventually kill the patient. However, many of the lesions are slow growing and do not metastasize early. The overall cure rate is 90% after treatment.

Percivall Pott (1714–1788)

Percivall Pott was a London surgeon who first gave the description for the fracture of the ankle, commonly known as Pott's fracture. Pott is said to have suffered this fracture himself, when crossing the London Bridge. He also described Pott's disease of the spine, due to tuberculosis. Pott was the first man to identify a cause of cancer. Chimney sweeps cancer of the scrotum resulted from repeated contamination with soot.

Malignant Melanoma

Melanoma is an uncommon highly invasive malignant tumour arising from the melanocytes. It is the most malignant skin tumour. It may appear at any time after puberty on normal skin or earlier on a pre-existing melanocytic nevus. It is extremely rare before puberty. Intense exposure to ultraviolet light is the major contributing factor for the development of a melanoma.

The incidence of malignancy has increased over the last 2 decades. This has been attributed to the increased exposure to the sun as a way of life. The damage to the ozone layer of the atmosphere by aircraft, and the use of aerosols, which allows more damaging ultraviolet (UVC) rays of the sun to reach the surface of the earth.

Once the malignant transformation has occurred, virtually all melanomas undergo a relatively long phase of radial growth during which the melanocytes spread centrifugally within the epidermis. This radial growth is now thought to be the earliest stage of malignant melanoma with a metastatic potential. Sooner or later the cells enter the vertical growth stage with extension in the dermis and subsequent metastasis. The exception to this is the nodular melanoma in which the radial growth phase is very short or absent; the vertical growth phase begins early or even before the radial growth phase.

Clinical Features

There are four main clinical varieties of malignant melanomas:

1. Superficial spreading melanoma accounts for 70% of all melanoma cases. The tumour is characterised by irregularly pigmented small arciform plaques with indented edges usually on the trunk or legs. It is most common on the legs in women and upper back in men. Absence of pigmentation within a tumour is a sign of regression (Fig. 7).
2. Nodular melanoma may arise at any site, rarely on a previously pigmented naevi. It accounts for 20% of melanomas. It presents as a reddish-brown, bluish or black nodule; ulceration and bleeding may occur. Satellite lesions are present. Lymphatic and haematogenous spread occurs early.
3. Lentigo maligna melanoma accounts for 5% of melanomas. It arises as a precursor lesion known as lentigo maligna, also known as the Hutchinson's melanotic freckle. Lentigo maligna is a form of melanoma *in situ* that occurs on sun-damaged skin. It is a slow-growing flat or brown macule occurring on the face of an elderly person. The nose and cheeks are the most common sites. Lentigo maligna is flat, but when palpable, it indicates a sign of invasion (Fig. 8).
4. Acral melanoma (Palmoplantar, subungual type): This tumour accounts for 2–10% of melanomas, found on the palms, soles and nail beds. This tumour is uncommon in the white population; it is the most common form of melanoma in darker pigmented races. It is a common variety in Mongoloids, Afro-Carribeans and in tropics. It begins as a pigmented macule, which develops to a papule, nodule and then ulcerates. Soles and heels are common sites; the big toe is commonly affected. Acral melanomas are also said to be more aggressive and with poorer prognosis (Fig. 9).

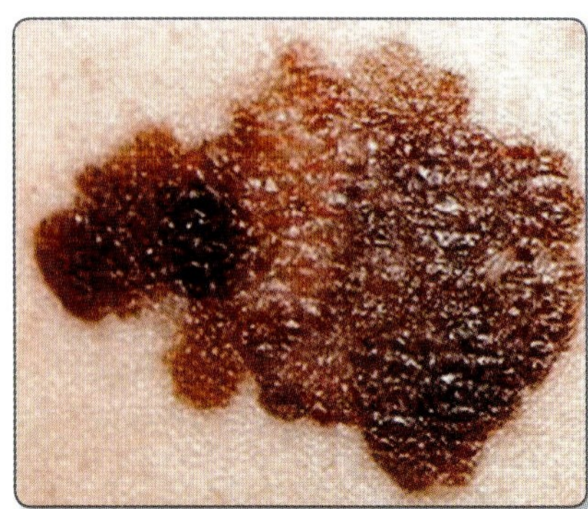

Fig. 7: Superficial spreading melanoma

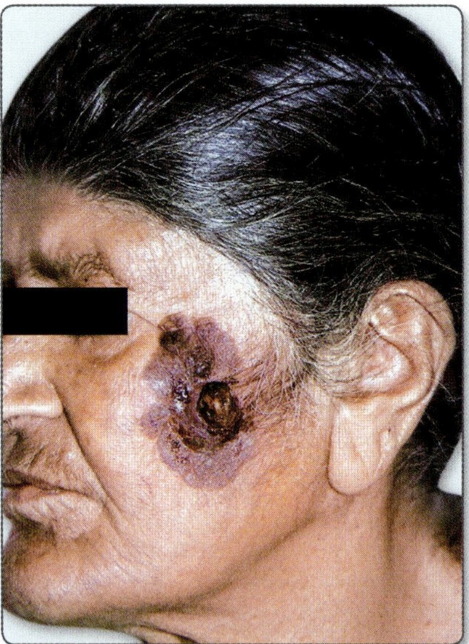

Fig. 8: Lentigo maligna melanoma

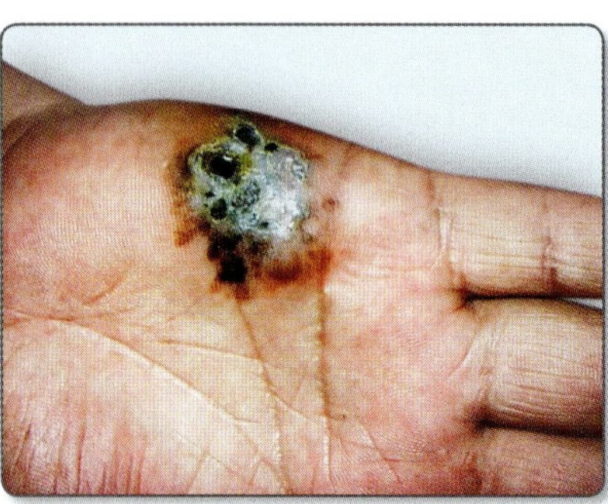

Fig. 9: Acral melanoma

Variants of Nodular Melanoma

- Polypoid melanoma: This is a pedunculated melanoma; it does not appear to descend for any appreciable distance into the dermis.
- Verrucous melanoma: These are hyperkeratotic uniformly pigmented, sharply demarcated tumours.
- Desmoplastic melanoma: This is a deeply infiltrating tumour, sometimes amelanotic, and often requiring S-100 stains for the diagnosis. The neurotropic melanoma may be a variant of this. It occurs most commonly on the hands and feet.
- Inflammatory melanoma: Inflammation near the site of the tumour indicates bad prognosis.
- Amelanotic melanoma: This does not differ from a melanoma except in lacking the melanin pigment. The lesion is pink, erythematous or skin-coloured. It can be mistaken for a pyogenic granuloma. Amelanotic melanoma is the typical variant seen in Albinos.
- Mucosal melanoma: Primary melanoma of the mucous membrane is rare. It may occur in the nasal mucosa with or without pigment; it is usually polypoid. On the lip, it appears as an indolent ulcer. In the mouth, the lesion is usually pigmented and ulcerated. The most common site is the palate. A tumour often pruritic, ulcerated with bleeding, manifests melanoma of the vulva.

Desmoplastic-neutrotropic Melanoma

These tumours are locally aggressive with a high rate of recurrence. These are mostly found in the head and neck of elderly people. These tumours have the tendency to invade the perineurium and endoneurium of the cutaneous nerves. Clinically the lesion presents as a pigmented macule or a nodule, without any surrounding pigmentation. The lesions may be firm, sclerotic or indurated.

Histopathology

Melanomas arise from the melanocytes of the epidermis and invade into the underlying dermis. The depth of invasion of the dermis is important for prognostic purpose. The criterion for diagnosis of a malignant melanoma is the presence of mitosis, inflammatory reaction composed of lymphocytes, dermoepidermal junctional activity and the absence of dermal stroma which is destroyed by the malignant melanoma.

The following features may help in differentiating a melanoma from dysplastic nevus:

- Atypical melanocytes present in the entire epidermis and dermis
- There are more single melanocytes than nests of melanocytes at the dermoepidermal junction, abnormal mitosis in all levels of the tumour
- There is lack of maturation of melanocytes at the deeper levels and variations in the size, shape and colour of infiltrate.

Diagnosis

Clinical (Naked eye examination): The ABCDE rule is applied to diagnose all types of melanoma. The early indication of a melanoma developing in a nevus is the change in size and colour. Always palpate the lesion to assess the infiltration. Infiltration, ulceration and bleeding indicate a more advanced primary melanoma. Infiltration indicates vertical spread of the tumour and chances of metastasis are therefore high. Changes of regression correspond to appearance of white, pink or red colour in a melanoma.

The development of a new pigmented lesion in a person above the age of 40 should be inspected closely to exclude the development of a melanoma. The appearance of halo naevi is also indicative of malignancy developing in a benign nevus. It is important to examine the entire skin. The use of magnifying lens and dermoscopy will help in examining the lesion in detail.

The other diagnostic procedures are listed below:

Dermoscopy (Epiluminescence microscopy)

This is a noninvasive examination technique to examine a pigmented lesion. This helps to differentiate benign from malignant lesions. The points to be noted are:

Pigmented network: This represents the pigmentation along the rete pegs. The clear holes represent the apex of the dermal papillae. Regular delicate pigmentation which gradually thins at the margin represents a benign lesion. Irregular pigmentation which ends abruptly at the margin indicates malignancy. Broad pigmented network is also a sign of melanoma; this indicates broad rete pegs and increased number of atypical melanocytes.

Black dots: These represent collection of aggregates of melanocytes in the stratum corneum; it is an indication of malignancy.

Brown globules: These represent pigmented nests in the papillary dermis and dermoepidermal junction. It is an indication of malignancy if irregular and nevus if regular.

Depigmentation: If this is in the centre and regular in an indication of a benign lesion. If the depigmentation is at the periphery and irregular, it suggests malignancy.

Blue-grey veil: This represents a wide papillary dermis, with fibrosis and melanophages in the papillary dermis. It also indicates a melanoma with signs of regression.

A maple leaf-like appearance on dermoscopy is suggestive of aggregates of basaloid cells, which represent a BCC, rather than a melanoma. While presence of horn-like aggregates and comedone-like openings are indicative of seborrhoeic keratosis.

Image Analysis

Computerised digital imaging is another noninvasive method of diagnosing melanomas. The images can be kept for comparison and analysed later. Digital dermoscopy uses a computer image analysis of the lesion.

Other Methods

Ultrasonography, magnetic resonance imaging (MRI) and confocal scanning, and laser microscope are also used to distinguish benign from malignant lesions.

Markers

There is yet no one specific marker for melanoma. S-100 has the highest sensitivity, but it is positive for other cells, such as Langerhans cells; it also identifies melanocytes of all types, both normal and abnormal. HMB-45 and Melan-A/Mart 1 are more specific for malignant melanoma. Proliferation markers such a Ki-67/MIB 1 are also useful.

Histological Diagnosis

Lesions showing a slight suspicion of melanoma should be immediately excised as a whole with 2 mm margin to exclude malignancy. If the lesion is large, such as lentigo maligna, then a biopsy is an acceptable alternative. This not only confirms the diagnosis, but also indicates the level of invasion, degree of anaplasia, helping in the staging of the melanoma for prognosis.

The differentiating points from a dysplastic nevus are that there are more single melanocytes than a nest of cells as seen in a naevus. The melanocytes are atypical; these are present in all the layers of the epidermis and dermis. Mitosis is abnormal at all levels of the tumour, while mitosis is normal in a naevus.

Bad Prognostic Signs

- Individuals with a fair complexion
- Individuals with numerous atypical appearing melanocytic naevi or large congenital melanocytic naevi
- Persons who have had a melanoma previously or have an immediate family member diagnosed with melanoma. Five percent of melanomas are familial
- Excessive exposure to UVR.

The following naevi should be suspected of becoming malignant:

- Asymmetry of any mole should be thoroughly evaluated
- Borders of a pigmented naevi are usually smooth, with clear demarcation between the naevi and the surrounding skin. Naevi that develop irregular or ill-defined borders or notching should be evaluated
- Bleeding from a mole needs observation.
- Colour of a mole is tan or brown, any variation from the normal should be suspected. Uneven distribution of shades and colours in a naevi should be suspected of malignant change.
- Diameter of a nevus is usually less than 6 mm: most melanomas are over 6 mm in diameter. Sometimes a small lesion may also become malignant.

The nevus should be considered as changing into a melanoma if it bleeds, crusts, itches, increases in size, becomes irregular or inflamed.

The acronym ABCDE is a useful reminder of some of the clinical features that should raise the suspicion of melanoma in a pigmented lesion: **A**symmetry of the lesion, **B**order irregularity, **C**olour variation, **D**iameter greater than 6 mm, and **E**levation of the lesion. The elevation indicates infiltration of the lesion. The asymmetry of the lesion is the least useful criterion, but the other three criteria seem to have diagnostic significance. Another worrisome feature is regression in a pigmented lesion, which appears as a new flat grey or white area in a previously completely pigmented lesion.

The "ugly duckling sign" is the appearance of pigmented lesion that is different from all the other pigmented lesions on the patient should arouse suspicion of a change to a melanoma.

Tumour Prognosis

Pathologists show an inverse relationship between the tumour thickness and survival so that the more superficial a lesion, the better the prognosis. *Breslow's thickness* is measured in millimeters from the granular layer of the epidermis to the deepest tumour cell in the dermis.

The following is the prognosis according to Breslow:

- Hundred percent survival in tumours less than 0.76 mm thickness (five-year survival)
- Fifty percent survival in tumours greater than 3.5 mm thickness.

Clark's prognostic criteria: This also relates to the depth of the tumour:

- Level I confined to the epidermis
- Level II confined up to the papillary dermis
- Level III confined up to the junction of the papillary and reticular dermis
- Level IV confined up to the reticular dermis
- Level V infiltration in the subcutaneous tissue.

Differential Diagnosis

The malignant melanoma should be differentiated from the other melanin-pigmented lesions and those that are pigmented due to haemorrhage. Those with melanin pigment include melanocytic naevi, seborrhoeic warts and pigmented BCC. The pigmented lesions due to haemorrhage include pyogenic granuloma, BCC, histiocytoma and subungual haematoma. The amelanotic melanoma should be distinguished from SCC and other granulomatous disease.

Treatment

- Early diagnosis and treatment, excision with a narrow margin of normal skin should be performed without delay. Margin of safety for tumours less than 1 mm thickness is 1 cm, and that for tumours exceeding 1 mm thickness is 2 cm excision.
- Radiolymphatic sentinel node mapping and biopsy is used for melanomas greater than 1 mm thickness and which do not have enlarged nodes on clinical examination. A radioactive dye is injected at the site of the melanoma. The first draining lymph node (sentinel lymph node) is identified by lymphoscintigraphy. This is examined for metastasis after biopsy. Regional lymph node dissection is performed if the sentinel lymph node was involved. This is followed by adjuvant immunotherapy.
- Patients with lymph node metastasis have a poorer prognosis than those who have no metastasis. If metastasis has occurred then chemotherapy with dimethyl triazeno imidazole alone or in combination with other chemotherapeutic agents is preferred.
- Immunotherapy is indicated for disseminated melanomas, with cytokines (interferons and interleukins), monoclonal antibodies, autologous lymphocytes and specific immunisation.
- For palliation of bone and brain metastasis, radiotherapy is used.
- For facial melanomas, Mohs surgery is preferred.
- In subungual melanomas, amputation of the affected digit is imperative. Involved lymph nodes should be removed.
- Lentigo maligna occurs in the elderly in areas of actinic damage and can leave unsatisfactory scars. Results with 5% imiquimod cream (aldara) have given satisfactory results.
- In all cases, follow-up is indicated, as recurrences are common. Once melanomas have spread beyond the skin, prospects for survival are very poor. Chemotherapy and radiation therapies are not very effective in the treatment of malignant melanomas.
- Melanoma vaccines: These vaccines were developed to stimulate the immune response to melanoma associated antigens. Tumour vaccines are developed using viruses (Newcastle vaccine), mechanical lysates and nonspecific adjuvants such as BCG vaccine. They are not of proven evidence up-to-date.
- Development of gene therapy to genetically alter melanoma cells, to produce cytokines which will destroy the tumour cells, is under study.
- A recent promising biologics injection ipilimumab has been approved by FDA to treat inoperable metastatic melanoma. It appears to be promising, although it is associated with severe adverse effects.

Tumour markers such as S-100, tyrosinase, and MIA may be done to see the response to therapy. Periodic follow-up of melanoma patients should be done at regular intervals to determine recurrences and to detect the development of a new tumour. The frequency depends upon the grading of the tumour. Lentigo maligna and melanoma in situ are not regularly followed up, while patients with malignant melanoma need a close follow-up. Breslow's prognostic criteria of less than 1 mm are followed 3-monthly for 3 years, and those with Breslow's prognostic criteria of more than 1 mm are followed 6-monthly for a further 2 years (total 5 years).

Patients should be taught the signs of a nevus becoming malignant. They should see a doctor immediately if any change in the nevus occurs.

Prognosis also depends upon the type of tumour. It is excellent for lentigo maligna, then the superficial spreading, and the acral melanomas. Nodular melanoma has the worst prognosis.

CUTANEOUS T-CELL LYMPHOMA (Mycosis Fungoides)

The name mycosis fungoides is a misnomer as this is not a fungal disease. It is a malignant neoplasm of T cell lymphocytes; the condition is seen mainly in the aged or elderly people, but can occur at any age. It presents as pruritic plaques; these may involute spontaneously or progress to frank nodules and ulceration. The lesions are associated with severe pruritus. Male female ratio is 2 to 3:1.

Histopathology

In the early stages, there is a dense infiltrate of lymphocytes, histiocytes in the superficial dermis. In the infiltrative stage, the mononuclear cells invade the epidermis to produce small microabscesses (Pautrier's abscesses). Mycosis fungoides cell (Sezary cell) is derived by a blast transformation of a lymphocyte, which can be seen under an electron microscope. It is a large cell with a cerebriform nucleus; these are considered pathognomonic for mycosis fungoides.

Clinical Features

The course of the disease may be divided into several stages. In the early stages macules or erythematous patches appear, often with a wrinkled appearance (pseudoatrophy). The common sites of involvement are buttocks, trunk, upper arm and upper thigh. Patches may last for months or years before proceeding to plaque stage, in which eczematous or psoriasiform eruptions occur. Lesions may either regress or develops into nodules. The nodules may arise anywhere on the body, but have a predilection for face and body folds. The nodules may ulcerate and become secondarily infected (Fig. 10).

Mycosis fungoides may also begin as a specific premycotic eruption called poikiloderma atrophicans vasculare; this is characterised clinically by appearance of red patches accompanied by reticulate pigmentation, telangiectasia and atrophy.

Sezary syndrome is a variant of mycosis fungoides in which the T lymphocytes invade the blood stream. It is essentially the leukaemic phase of mycosis fungoides. It is characterised by erythroderma, generalised pruritus, oedema, alopecia, palmoplantar keratoderma, superficial lymphadenopathy and splenomegaly. Sezary syndrome may follow mycosis fungoides or may start *de novo*. There may be a sparing of areas that are frequently folded such as abdomen and axillary area. This sparing is called the "luggage" or "deck chair" sign.

The patient has associated systemic signs such as fever, malaise, weight loss and poor body temperature homeostasis.

Standard for the diagnosis of Sezary syndrome is more than 1000/mm^3 Sezary cells in the peripheral blood.

Variants

- Follicular mycosis fungoides: Malignant T cells are often present in the hair follicle, with deposits of mucin. Hair follicles are destroyed producing alopecia.
- Granulomatous mycosis fungoides: Formation of granulomas in the dermis, with destruction of the elastic tissue, leads to pendulous skin. This is common in the flexures.

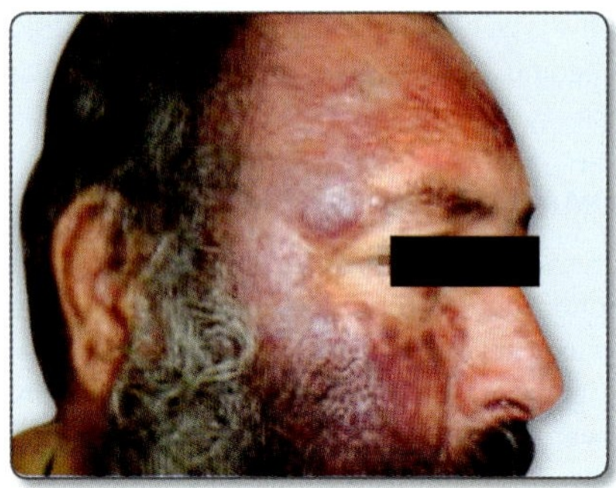

Fig. 10: Mycosis fungoides

- Pagetoid reticulosis: This usually presents as a solitary or few scaly plaques with sharp borders (Woringer-Kolopp type) or the disease may be disseminated and more aggressive (Ketron-Goodman type).
- Pigmented purpura: Sometimes mycosis fungoides may present as pigmented purpura; the lesion should then be differentiated from Schamberg's disease. This is often seen in areas other than the lower leg such as axillae. Lesions larger than 4 cm should be biopsied.

Diagnosis

Mycosis fungoides should be suspected if dermatoses like eczema or psoriais do not respond to treatment. Biopsy might not be specific in the early stages, so repeated biopsies are indicated. Histology, immunophenotype and preferably T cell receptor (TCR) gene analysis should be performed on all tissue samples. Peripheral blood analysis and bone marrow biopsies should be done to diagnose the various variants of T cell lymphoma. In later stages, CT scans would be useful.

Differential Diagnosis

The plaque stage should be differentiated from psoriasis, pityriasis rubra pilaris, lichen planus, parapsoriasis, subacute lupus erythematosus, nummular eczema and seborrhoeic dermatitis. The nodular stage from lepromatous leprosy, generalised leishmaniasis and other lymphomas.

Treatment

Treatment is aimed to control rather than cure the disease. In the early stages the disease may be kept in check by the application of topical steroids; some cases may survive up to 20 years before intensive treatment is required.

In the later stages there are many lines of treatment including PUVA therapy, narrow band UVB, localised radiotherapy, whole body electron beam therapy, topical application of nitrogen mustard and systemic cytotoxic drugs.

Low oral-dose methotrexate, isotretinoin or intramuscular injection of interferon-α is used for recalcitrant cases. Other biological therapies, such as interleukin-12, bexarotene, and fusion proteins such as denileukin diftitox, have also been used.

For Sezary syndrome, chemotherapy is preferred. Extracorporeal photochemotherapy is also found beneficial.

Jean Louis Alibert (1768–1837) is called the father of French Dermatology. He brought fame to the St Louis Hospital as a centre for dermatological training. He was the first to describe keloids and mycosis fungoides. His success was largely stemmed from the fact that in addition to his ceaseless work with both patients and friends, he was a personification of courtesy and kindness.
Sezary and Bouvrain reported a triad of erythroderma, leukaemia with enlarged peripheral lymph nodes, and infiltration with Sezary cells.

PRIMARY CUTANEOUS B-CELL LYMPHOMAS

There are many types of primary B cell lymphomas, such as the follicle cell lymphoma, marginal zone lymphoma and the primary cutaneous diffuse large B cell lymphomas.

Primary cutaneous B cell follicle centre lymphoma is of low-grade malignancy, found predominantly on the head and neck. The tumours appear as nonscaly single or grouped papules, plaques or nodules.

Treatment is by ionising radiation, excision of the solitary lesion, anti-CD20 monoclonal antibody therapy or interferon-α-2. Five-year survival is up to 95%.

Primary cutaneous B cell lymphoma is derived from lymphocytes of the marginal zone of the lymphoid follicle. It usually occurs after the age of 50. The lesions appear as single or multiple, cutaneous or subcutaneous reddish-brown papules and nodules, usually on the trunk. Those that appear on the head and neck or the disseminated form have the worst prognosis.

Treatment is by excision if possible, otherwise ionising radiation or electron beam therapy. Treatment by anti-CD20 monoclonal antibody is also helpful.

Primary cutaneous diffuse large B cell lymphomas are aggressive in nature, occurs predominantly in older women. They are rapidly growing reddish-brown nodules and plaques on the leg, often ulcerated.

This aggressive tumour is treated by polychemotherapy, ionising radiation, anti-CD20 monoclonal antibody, or rituximab. Five-year survival is only 50%.

Kaposi's Sarcoma

Kaposi's sarcoma is a malignant tumour of multifocal origin that manifests primarily as multiple vascular nodules in the skin and other organs. Until recent years, this tumour was rarely seen outside Africa, today it is seen worldwide, and it is one of the manifestations of AIDS.

The cause of Kaposi's sarcoma is multifactorial, involving a genetic predisposition, geographical, and endogenous (probable endocrinal) factors. It is associated with malignant lymphomas and immunological disorders. Two events are responsible for its occurrence; release of angiogenesis factor from a graft-versus-host type of reaction and malignant transfer via an oncogenic virus. Herpes virus 8 is the primary factor in the development of all forms of Kaposi's sarcoma. This also explains the high association of Kaposi's sarcoma with HIV virus.

There is now a general agreement that vascular endothelial cells are the progenitor of Kaposi's sarcoma. The tumour appears in a multicentric fashion; metastatic lesions also develop. The cutaneous distribution is occasionally symmetrical and tends to follow the path of superficial veins.

Clinical Features

There are four major variants of Kaposi's sarcoma are:

- Classic Kaposi's sarcoma (Mediterranean or Jewish origin)
- Endemic Kaposi's sarcoma (African origin)
- Epidemic Kaposi's sarcoma (with AIDS and other immunological disorders)
- Iatrogenic Kaposi's sarcoma (with immunosuppression)

The classical Kaposi's sarcoma begins as reddish-blue black or purplish macules on the feet and ankles, occasionally on the hands, ear or the nose. Nodules develop and by coalescence, large ulcerated fungating or verrucous plaques are formed. Later the legs show a brawny lymphoedema. The disease is unilateral, later becomes bilateral. Lymphadenopathy and visceral involvement may occur (Fig. 11A).

Most aggressive is the African cutaneous Kaposi's sarcoma in which death occurs in a year or two. These are usually seen in the extremities as plaques and nodules; the lesions are locally aggressive, become ulcerative and haemorrhagic, later infiltrate the deeper tissues and bones. There are four subvariants of African Kaposi's sarcoma: nodular, florid, infiltrative and lymphoadenopathic type. In children, Kaposi's sarcoma resembles a lymphoma (lymphoadenopathic type), is usually fatal. The tumour may disseminate with systemic involvement.

Kaposi's sarcoma associated with immunosuppression: This develops in patients with transplant surgery. The tumour is aggressive; lymph nodes and viscera are involved in most cases. Some tumours regressed when immunosuppressive therapy was withdrawn, others responded to radiation and chemotherapy (Fig. 11B).

AIDS-related Kaposi's sarcoma begins as reddish-purple macules; it then rapidly develops to papules, nodules and plaques. Rarely there may be a single cutaneous tumour often on the face. 10% patients have erythema nodosum as the sole manifestation. There is a predilection for the head, neck, and oral mucosa. A fulminant progressive course with nodal and systemic involvement is common.

The disease should not be confused with benign vascular proliferations, histiocytoma or other type of sarcomas.

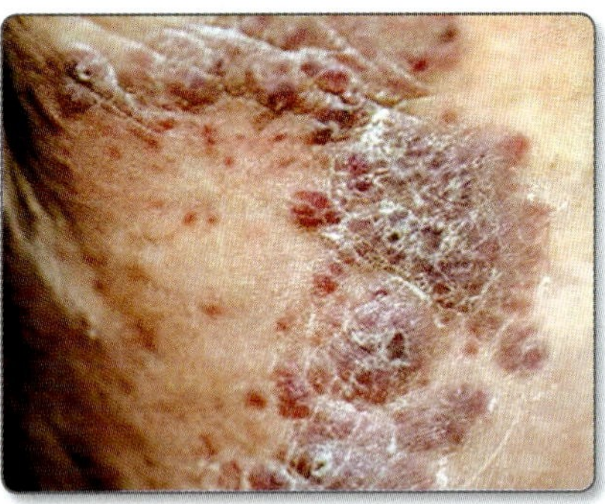

Fig. 11A: Kaposi's sarcoma

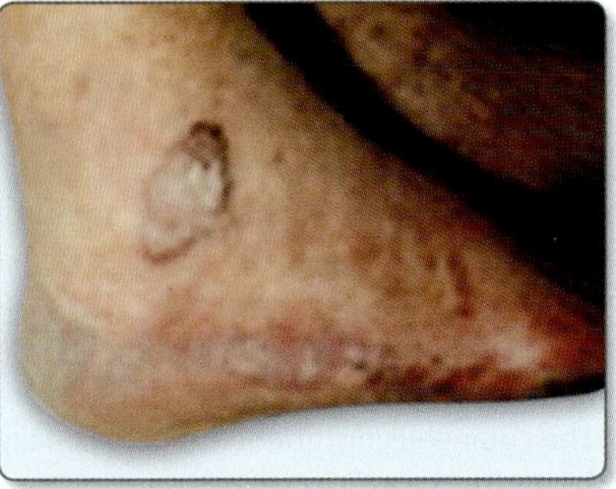

Fig. 11B: Kaposi's sarcoma

Diagnosis

An excisional biopsy is done to confirm the diagnosis. Routine blood parameters and immune status of the patient should be evaluated. HIV infection should be excluded. Depending upon the aggressiveness of the tumour, an abdominal and chest examination should be done including a lymph node sonography.

Treatment

- All types are radiosensitive; local radiotherapy is highly effective. Surgical excision for single tumours and cryotherapy (three treatments at 3-week intervals) are alternatives. Cytotoxic therapy is indicated for rapid progressive disease. The Klein regimen of weekly IV vinblastine 4–6 mg is one of the first line of treatment. Other drugs used are doxorubicin, bleomycin and vincristine.
- AIDS-related Kaposi's sarcoma responds to local radiotherapy, cryosurgery, I/L injections of vinblastine, interleukin or interferon. For systemic disease, highly active anti-retroviral therapy (HAART) is the treatment of choice.

Histopathology

Kaposi's sarcoma has two predominant histological features: the accumulation of spindle cells and the presence of vascular elements. The vascular elements are ectatic capillaries, lymphatics and wide lumen sinuses. In the skin, the tumour cells are found in the middle and lower dermis.

Kaposi was Hebra's successor and son-in-law. He was a man of action and gifted with a brilliant mind. He described many skin disorders, best-known are, Kaposi's sarcoma, Kaposi's varricelliform eruption and xeroderma pigmentosum. He contributed to the existing knowledge of herpes zoster, sarcoidosis, lichen planus and other dermatoses. Kaposi was a master therapist, an excellent teacher and orator with a sparkling temperament.

Paget's Disease of the Nipple

This is due to an extension of an underlying intraductal carcinoma of the breast, extending to the nipple to invade the epidermis. Paget's disease appears as an involuted red scaly eczematous-like patch on the nipple; usually no underlying mass is palpable. Such cases are often treated for eczema, which does not respond. An excisional biopsy should be taken to confirm the diagnosis. Eczema of the nipple is often bilateral and responds to topical steroids. In course of months or years, Paget's disease becomes infiltrated and ulcerated. The nipple may or may not retract. The disease is more common in women, but carries a worse prognosis in men (Fig. 12).

Extramammary Paget's disease commonly involves the anogenital areas. Less common sites are the periumbilical, axillary and the external ear canal.

Histopathology

The disease is characterised by the presence of Paget's cells; these cells are large, round, clear staining with a large nucleus. They appear singly or in small nests between

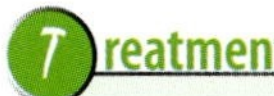

Treatment

This is the same as that of breast carcinoma, mastectomy and removal of the affected axillary glands.

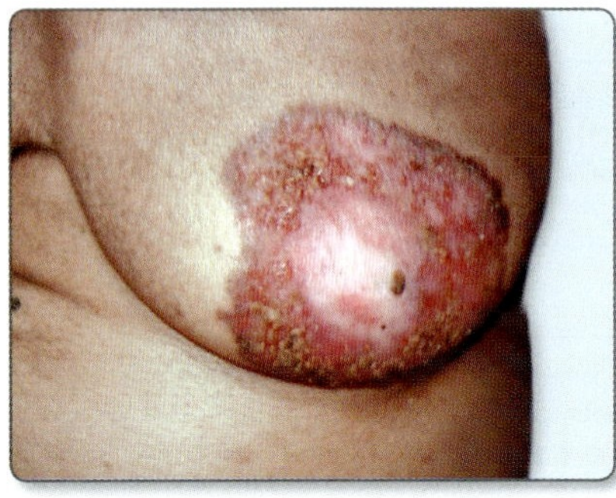

Fig. 12: Paget's disease

the keratinocytes. These cells are positive for carcinoembryonic antigen (CEA). Paget's cells undergoing mitosis are frequent. In the dermis, an inflammatory reaction is often present. Intraductal carcinoma is rarely seen on biopsy.

James Paget (1814–1899) is best known for the eponym Paget's disease of the nipples and Paget's disease of the bones. He discovered trichinella infestation in human muscles. He wrote brilliant essays and gave painstakingly prepared eloquent lectures at St. Bartholomew's Hospital. He had the reputation of being the best surgical diagnostician in Britain.

Merkel Cell Carcinoma

This is an uncommon tumour, usually affecting the elderly, found almost exclusively in the sun-exposed skin. There is a female preponderance. The tumour presents as bluish-red or reddish-brown nodules, often with telangiectasia. It has an aggressive course, grows rapidly, 30–50% metastasize. Immunocytochemical and histochemical investigation show that Merkel cell carcinoma expresses features of neuroendocrine carcinoma. It should be differentiated from a lymphoma, amelanotic melanoma and sweat gland carcinoma. Treatment is by excision.

PREMALIGNANT DERMATOSES

Certain conditions of the skin such as scars, burns, chronic ulcers, long-standing sinuses, and chronic inflammation if left untreated these may become malignant. Some dermatoses such as solar keratosis and leucoplakia may show little evidence of cellular unrest; others such as Bowen's disease may have microscopic features of intraepithelial carcinoma from the beginning, but remain confined by the dermoepidermal junction. A feature common to all is a chronic inflammatory cell infiltrate in the papillary dermis. When the lesion becomes malignant, there is loss of the basement membrane.

Solar (Actinic) Keratosis

These are multiple erythematous scaly lesions that develop on the skin damaged by UVR, commonly seen in persons of skin type 1. The first evidence of solar keratosis is a collection of telangiectatic capillaries, a millimeter or two in diameter; the erythema is followed by the appearance of scales, which are

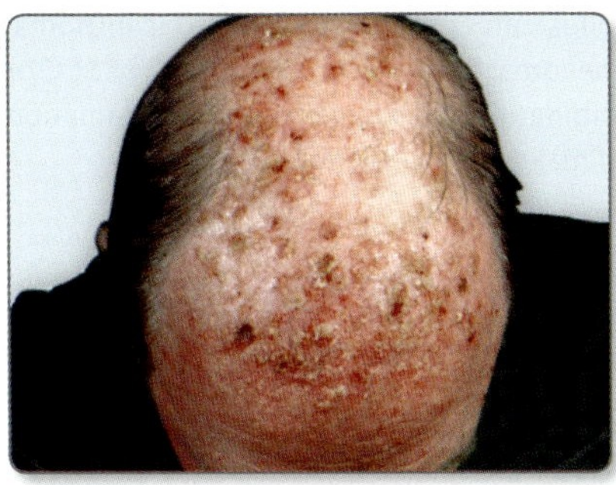

Fig. 13: Solar keratosis

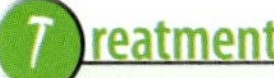

- The patients should be advised to reduce sun exposure
- Avoid sun exposure during mid-day
- Sun screens should be used on exposed skin
- Broad brim hats and protective clothing should be worn
- Cryotherapy
- Topical chemotherapy with 5-fluorouracil for extensive lesions
- Topical immunotherapy with imiquimod cream three times a week for 6 weeks
- Photodynamic therapy
- Excision, if suspicion of malignant change.

yellowish-brown, rough and adherent. It is easier to palpate areas of actinic keratosis as rough areas on the skin than to try and see them. Solar keratosis is usually seen against a background of skin damage such as solar elastosis and dyspigmentation (Fig. 13). The common sites of involvement are the face, arms and hands.

The histology shows epidermal atrophy with dysplastic changes, loss of normal keratinocyte maturation. The pink and blue appearance of the epidermis is characteristic. The hair follicles and eccrine ducts are not involved; they appear blue, while the intervening epidermis appears pink.

The flat keratosis can be mistaken for discoid lupus erythematosus; this is usually bright red in colour and has an easily detachable scale. When the keratosis is pigmented, it may resemble seborrhoeic keratosis, but lacks the granular texture of the lesion. Bowen's disease on the exposed area has more irregular contour and a more erythematous base.

There is usually a period of several years for the transformation of solar keratosis into a SCC. The lesion should be treated in young age.

Cutaneous Horn

It is a premalignant tumour that arises from the keratinocytes. The keratin production is excessive and a hard horn-shaped excrescence is produced resembling an animal horn. The scalp, head and neck areas are the common sites for cutaneous horn. It may arise on normal skin or is superimposed on underlying

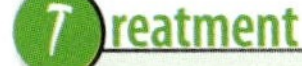

The cutaneous horn should be removed with a currette and the base should be lightly cauterized as these may transform to malignancy.

seborrhoeic keratosis, wart, molluscum contagiosum, keratoacanthoma, epidermal naevus or trichoepithelioma. It may even overly BCC or SCC or premalignant conditions. A combination of induration and inflammation beneath the horn is suggestive of malignant transformation.

Histopathology

There are no atypical cells or loss of polarity, but the granular layer is deficient or absent. In long-standing cases there may be budding from the basal layer signalling transformation into a SCC.

Bowen's Disease

Bowen's disease is an intraepidermal SCC, which has not become invasive. Erythroplasia of Queyrat is Bowen's disease of the glans penis and prepuce. Bowen's disease presents as a reddish-brown scaly raised patch; the patch is non-infiltrative, varies from a few millimeters to many centimeters in diameter, and the lesion is sharply defined. On close examination, a sharply defined border with notches can be seen. As the lesion slowly enlarges, spontaneous cicatrisation may occur in other parts of the lesion. When the growth becomes invasive (Bowen's carcinoma), a nodule is formed that later becomes ulcerative and fungating (Fig. 14). Sun exposure is an important predisposing factor. Formally arsenic was a common cause of Bowen's disease; now HPV is more common.

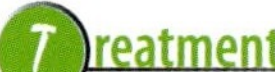

- Surgical excision is the best method of treatment
- Small lesions are treated by electrodesiccation, curettage, cryotherapy in an elderly
- Photodynamic therapy is considered for large lesions on the elderly at sites where healing is poor such as the shins
- Multiple lesions can be treated by 5-fluorouracil, applied twice a day for 4–6 weeks or imiquimod cream 5% daily for up to 16 weeks
- Follow-up of patients is required as recurrences are frequent. Recurrences are due to follicular involvement or due to spread from the lateral margins of the disease.

Bowen's disease can be mistaken for psoriasis, nummular eczema, actinic keratosis, tinea circinata and extramammary Paget's disease.

Histopathology

The epidermis shows hyperkeratosis, parakeratosis, acanthosis and thickening of the rete pegs.

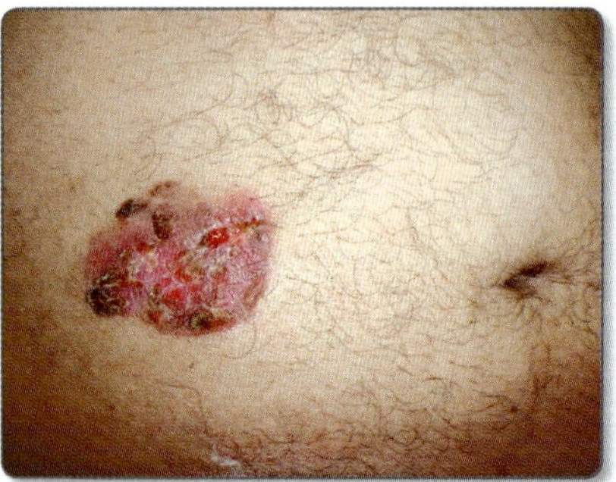

Fig. 14: Bowen's disease with malignant change

John T Bowen (1857–1940)

Bowen was an eminent histopathologist. He was the first to describe the precancerous dermatoses. He also described the epitrichial layer of the epidermis. He was the founder of Boston Dermatological Club.

Leucoplakia

This is a potentially malignant lesion characterised by white patches, mainly on the inner surface of the cheeks, gums and tongue. The cause is unknown but irritation by smoking, eating hot and spicy foods, chewing betel nuts or tobacco and lichen planus are important predisposing factors. The plaque may be small or large but is always well defined. It is first flat but later becomes raised, rough and palpable. Malignant change is represented by vegetating or ulcerative growth. A verrucous lesion, with an admixture of white and red colours, is suggestive of malignancy.

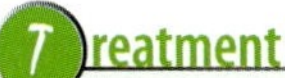

Early lesions respond to avoidance of irritants and topical steroids. Smoking should be forbidden. Persistent lesions should be destroyed by electrosurgery or excised. Vulval leucoplakia develops into carcinoma in half of the cases, which requires vulvectomy.

Leucoplakia may also affect the genitals especially in women; the clitoris and inner surface of the labia are commonly affected. Oral lesions are asymptomatic; genital lesions are pruritic. *Candida* may be superimposed on the lesions of leucoplakia. Soft plaques of *Candida* can easily be removed from the oral mucosa (Fig. 15).

Leucoplakia of the lips closely resembles chronic actinic cheilitis; it is preceded by abnormal dryness of the lips, followed by formation of circumscribed or diffuse keratosis, almost invariably on the lower lips.

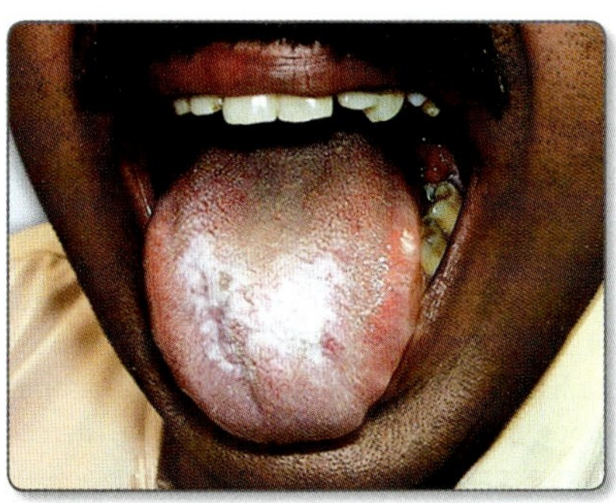

Fig. 15: Leucoplakia

Arsenic Keratosis

This is seen many years after arsenic ingestion. These appear as punctate wart-like keratosis usually affecting the palms and soles. Inflammation, induration and ulceration occur when the lesions become malignant. There may be areas of Bowen's disease at other sites. Multiple BCC develops on the trunk. Diffuse hyperpigmentation interspersed with raindrop like hypopigmented macules is characteristic of arsenic keratosis. Arsenic was given in the past for the treatment of a number of disorders, such as psoriasis, atopic dermatitis, asthma, etc.

Tar Keratosis

The condition is now rare; it was seen in men working with tar and pitch. The lesions appear as plane warts or flat seborrhoeic keratosis on the face and head. Some resemble solar keratosis or even keratoacanthoma. Tar keratosis on the scrotum has a high chance of becoming malignant.

Disseminated Actinic Superficial Porokeratosis

The condition is chiefly seen on the exposed parts of the body of white skin people. The lesions begin as 1–3 mm conical papules, brownish in colour. As these papules enlarge, a slightly raised keratotic ridge develops and spreads out to a diameter of 10 mm or more. The skin within the ring is somewhat atrophic and slightly red. A hypopigmented ring may be seen just outside the ridge. Sweating is absent within the lesion. In a few cases the centre of the lesion becomes inflamed, covered by thick hyperkeratosis; it may become ulcerated. These may become malignant. The lesions respond satisfactorily to freezing with liquid nitrogen.

(Erythroplasia of Queyret and Actinic Cheilitis are described in the chapters 36 and 37)

BENIGN TUMOURS OF THE SKIN

Benign tumours arising from the skin are extremely common and their prevalence increases with increasing age. It is important to diagnose them clinically as many need no other treatment other than reassurance. The common benign tumours are keratin cysts, lipoma, keratoacanthoma, skin tags, histiocytoma, pyogenic granuloma, seborrhoeic keratosis, dermatosis papulosa nigra and chondrodermatitis nodularis helicis.

Benign tumours remain localised at their site of origin. It does not have the capacity to spread to distant sites such as cancers. These tumours increase in size by expansile growth, compressing and possibly distorting the surrounding tissues. Most benign tumours enclose a fibrous capsule around them; this separates them from the surrounding tissue by a zone of compressed connective tissue. A well-marked cleavage exists around these lesions.

Some benign tumours are neither encapsulated nor discretely defined, such as fibroblastoma and vascular benign tumours of the dermis. Occasionally benign tumours may rupture through their capsule to extend pseudopodia into the surrounding tissue. Benign tumours resemble the tissue of origin, there is no anaplasia. They are slow growing, expansile growths.

Epidermoid Cyst

This is a cyst containing keratin and its breakdown products; it is surrounded by a wall of normal epidermis. The epidermoid cyst is thought to arise from the infundibular portion of the hair follicle. These cysts are common affecting young and middle-aged adults. This cyst is situated in the dermis and is attached to the epidermis. A central filled keratin punctum may be seen on the surface of the cyst. The contents of the cyst are cheesy and odorous. The common sites are the face, neck, shoulders and the chest (Fig. 16). These become inflamed and tender from time to time.

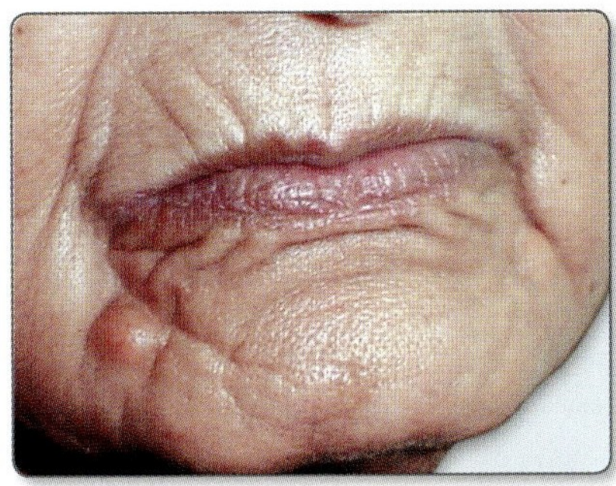

Fig. 16: Epidermoid cyst

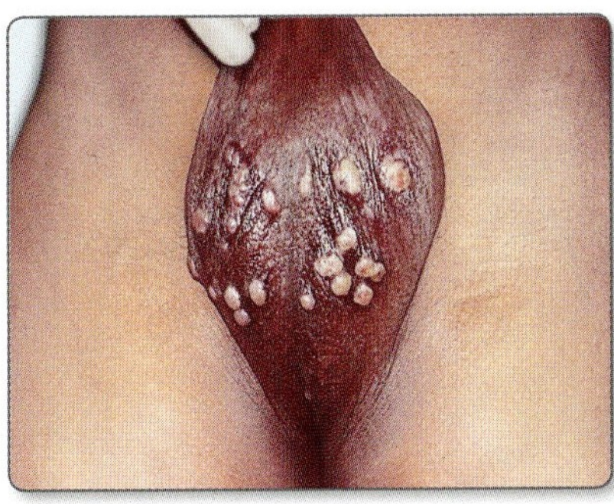

Fig. 17: Scrotal cysts

Variant

Scrotal cysts: These are multiple epidermal cysts on the scrotum; they usually calcify (Fig. 17).

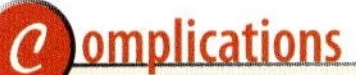

Complications

Infection, rupture, dystrophic calcification; some may become malignant.

Treatment

These cysts should be removed surgically.

Gardener syndrome

This is an autosomal dominant disorder. It is associated with intestinal polyposis, epidermoid cysts, osteomas and congenital hypertrophy of the retinal pigment epithelium. There is a 100% life-time risk of malignancy developing in the colon, if prophylactic treatment is not done.

Epidermoid cyst is often called sebaceous cyst, but it has no association with sebaceous glands. The term should be avoided.

Trichilemmal Cyst

This is also a keratin cyst with a lining resembling the external root sheath of the hair follicle. The granular layer is absent, as opposed to that of the epidermoid cyst, because of trichilemmal keratinisation. These are thought to arise from the isthmus of the hair follicle, the portion between the sebaceous duct and the insertion of the arrector pili muscle. It is usually situated in the scalp; they are firm, smooth, mobile round nodules; large cysts may be

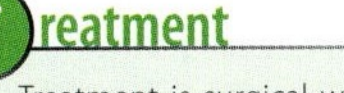

Treatment

Treatment is surgical with total removal of the cyst.

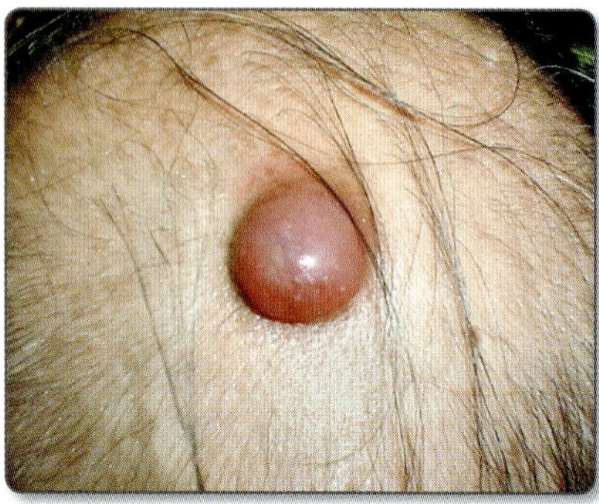

Fig. 18: Trichilemmal cyst

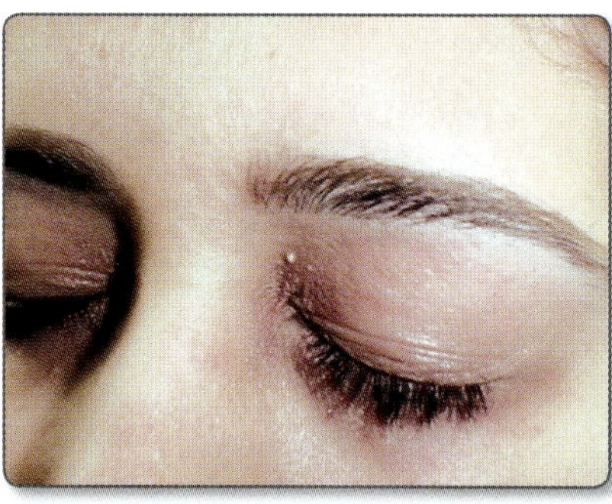

Fig. 19: Milia

lobular. Tenderness occurs when the cyst is inflamed. They do not have a central punctum. The contents are gelatinous and odourless (Fig. 18).

Milia

These are small epidermal keratin cysts which can be primary or secondary. Primary milia are small cysts that arise spontaneously most often on the eyelids or the cheeks. They are derived from the lowest portion of the infundibulum of the vellus hair. Milia are quite common at all ages from infancy onwards. They appear as small white papules; rarely exceed 2 mm in diameter (Fig. 19). Milia on the palate are known as Epstein's pearl. A rare type of primary milia known as milia-en-plaque occurs in middle-aged women; these are grouped milia on an erythematous base, commonly located around the ears.

Secondary milia are retention cysts following injury to the skin. They arise after damage to the skin appendages by radiotherapy, blister formation, sun bathing, burns, dermabrasion, etc.

Milia are treated by excision of the epidermis over the milium with a cutting edge needle or sharp-pointed scalpel and squeezing the contents out. Spontaneous disappearance occurs in milia of infants.

Dermoid Cyst

The dermoid cyst is congenital in origin and occurs chiefly on the lines of cleavage. It may occur in the sublingual region, the external and internal angular dermoid cyst occurs about the eyes; so constant is the dermoid in these positions that it can be diagnosed on sight. These cysts are not attached to the skin and are freely movable. The cyst wall is lined by stratified squamous epithelium containing skin appendages, including lanugo hair. The cyst is the result of sequestration of epidermis in the dermis along the lines of embryonic closure. These cysts should be completely excised. Sometimes a dermoid cyst in the upper eyelid may have a deep extension into the orbit; this should be kept in mind while removing it. It is often called an ovarian teratoma, but the cyst has no relation to ovaries.

Seborrhoeic Keratosis (Senile Wart, Basal Cell Papilloma)

Seborrhoeic keratosis, also called seborrhoeic wart, is not related to seborrhoea. They are masses of basaloid cells arranged in an orderly fashion with overlying hyperkeratosis and increased melanin production. The cause is unknown. They are common in people above the age of 40, seen in both males and females.

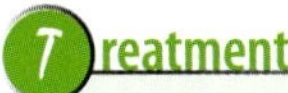

Seborrhoeic keratoses are easily removed by curettage followed by electrodessication, or light freezing with liquid nitrogen. If there is any doubt in its diagnosis, the lesion should be biopsied to exclude a melanoma.

The early lesions are brown or black macules. As the lesions progress, they become elevated plaques with an uneven surface that has a characteristic network of indentation or crypts on its surface, with multiple plugged follicles. Follicular prominence is one of the hallmarks of seborrhoeic keratosis. Seborrhoeic keratosis has an abrupt edge that gives the appearance of plasticine stuck on the surface of the skin (Fig. 20).

Seborrhoeic keratosis can also be flat with a waxy surface and sometimes have small punctate inclusions. The acanthotic type is smooth, dome shaped, and pigmented with horny inclusions. Stucco keratoses are small, pale and usually found on the thigh, legs, or back of the feet. Occasionally they become inflamed; these should then be differentiated from a malignant melanoma.

Sudden appearance of multiple seborrhoeic keratosis is indicative of an internal malignancy, usually of an adenocarcinoma of the stomach (sign of Leser Trelat).

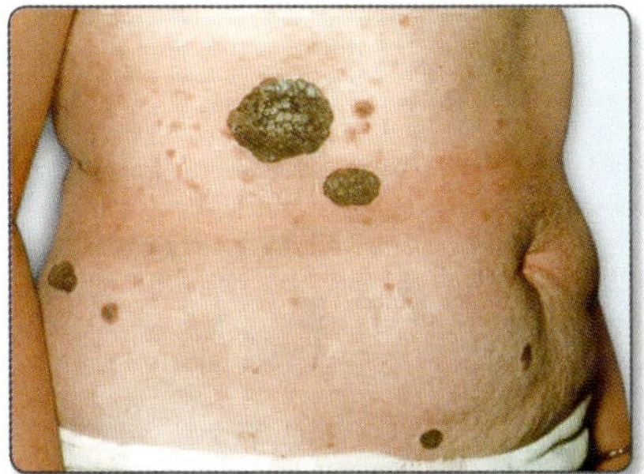

Fig. 20: Seborrhoeic keratosis

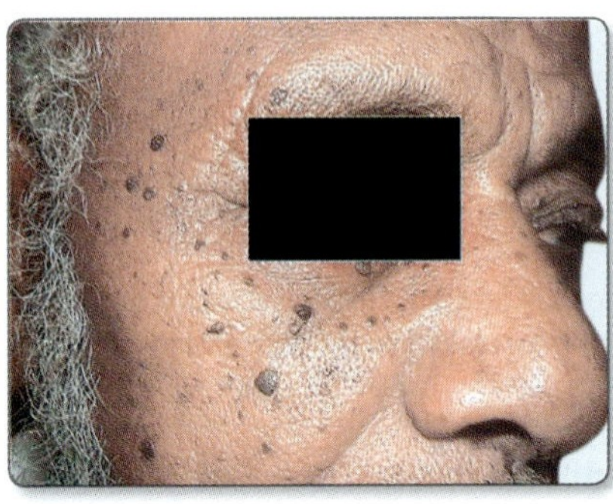

Fig. 21: Dermatosa papulosa nigra

Dermatosis Papulosa Nigra

This is a pigmented papular eruption on the face and neck, commonly seen in black people (Fig. 21). It is a variant of seborrhoeic keratosis; the histology resembles seborrhoeic keratosis. The lesion is probably genetically determined; it is caused by a naevoid developmental defect of the pilosebaceous follicles. The lesions are most numerous on the malar region and on the forehead; they are rare on the lower part of the face and chin. These are easily removed by diathermy or cautery.

Keratoacanthoma

This fascinating lesion looks malignant but acts benign. It is a rapidly growing self-limiting benign growth of unknown cause, located mainly on the exposed parts of the body usually the centre of the face. The rapid growth suggests a viral aetiology, but there is no evidence of any HPV or any other virus involved. Other factors such as UVR, chemical and physical agents have been suggested but again without any evidence.

Histopathology is like that of a low-grade SCC. When properly sectioned, the centre of the lesion shows a crater filled with eosinophilic keratin; sides of the crater are formed by invagination of the epidermis. The cytoplasm has a ground glass appearance.

Clinical Features

The lesion is usually seen on the face of middle-aged people, fair-skinned people are commonly affected. Keratoacanthoma begins as a firm round skin-coloured or reddish papule, which grows rapidly in 6–8 weeks, becomes globular with a central depression filled with keratin plug. Lymph nodes are not enlarged. It then becomes stationary for about 2–6 weeks and finally heals spontaneously in 2–6 months leaving a depressed unsightly scar (Fig. 22). The lesion can evolve into a cutaneous horn.

Keratoacanthoma is usually single; sometimes the lesions can be multiple, in which case an internal malignancy should be excluded. Keratoacanthoma are often associated with immune deficiency. Muir-Torre syndrome, a genodermatosis, is associated with nonpolyposis colonic cancer, with multiple sebaceous tumours and keratoacanthomas. Self-healing tumours of Ferguson-Smith has an autosomal dominant inheritance, patients develop keratoacanthomas during childhood and early adolescence. the lesions are common on the sun-exposed areas, they heal leaving scars. Another variant of multiple keratoacanthoma is generalised eruptive keratoacanthomas of Grzybowski. It is characterised by hundreds to thousands of tiny folllicular keratotic papules all over the body, most severe on the face. Oral and genital mucosa may also be involved.

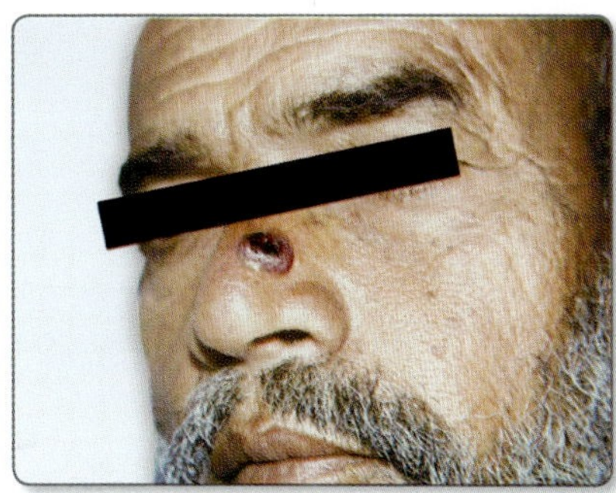

Fig. 22: Keratoacanthoma

Variants

- Giant keratoacanthoma: Sometimes a keratoacanthoma can reach a large size; it may be several centimetres in size
- Keratoacanthoma centrifugum marginatum: In this variant, the keratoacanthoma slowly enlarges with a prominent border. There is slight tendency for regression
- Keratoacanthoma of the nail bed and mucous membrane: These behave like a verrucous SCC.

Treatment

Although keratoacanthoma heals spontaneously, excision biopsy is the treatment of choice for small lesions; large lesions may be curretted and the base is cauterised. Relapses are common; doubtful cases should be treated as SCC. For multiple lesions, methotrexate or acitretin can be tried.

Lipoma

Lipoma is a tumour of the fat cells in the dermis or subcutaneous tissue. They occur most frequently on the trunk, forearm, and axilla. They are soft, single or multiple, small or large, lobulated compressible growths over which the skin becomes dimpled on traction. Lesions on the forehead are often large arising from within or deep to the frontalis muscle. Occasionally there is an angiomatous component (angiolipoma); this type may be tender or spontaneously painful. Another painful lipoma is adiposis dolorosa (Dercum's disease); these are multiple and often occur in menopausal women. Lumbosacral lipomas are congenital; these are often associated with spina bifida. Lipomas should be investigated if they become 10 cm or more in diameter.

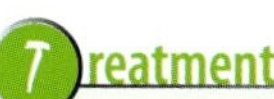

Treatment

Lipomas can be excised for cosmetic reasons.

Pyogenic Granuloma

This small, red and fleshy tumour bleeds profusely on slight trauma. The lesion occurs mostly in children but other age groups are also affected. It is usually formed at the site of injury, cut, scratch or burn. It is composed of newly formed capillaries with fibroblastic proliferation around the vascular tumour. Common sites are periungual in children and gingiva in pregnancy (Fig. 23).

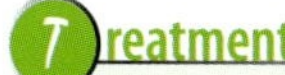

Treatment

Treatment is by excision with cryotherapy or cautery to destroy the granuloma. Pyogenic granuloma can also be treated by shelling out the tumour with a dermal curette and destruction of the base by fulguration or excision.

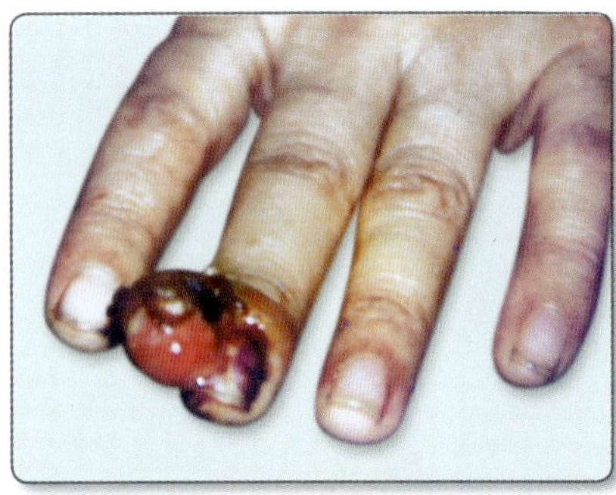

Fig. 23: Pyogenic granuloma

Histiocytoma (Dermatofibroma)

Dermatofibroma is perhaps the most common mesenchymal tumour of the skin. It is also called sclerosing haemangioma; this tumour has various names because of various interpretations on histological findings. It is commonly seen on the lower leg as a reddish-brown or skin-coloured hard papule or nodule which is adherent to the overlying epidermis, it is not attached to the underlying tissue. Lateral compression with the thumb and index finger leads to a dimple-like depression in the overlying skin. This is called the "dimple sign or the Fitzpatrick's sign". These tumours are generally seen in middle-aged adults. The lesions are usually secondary to injury such as insect bites. Multiple dermatofibromas are associated with systemic lupus erythematosus (Fig. 24).

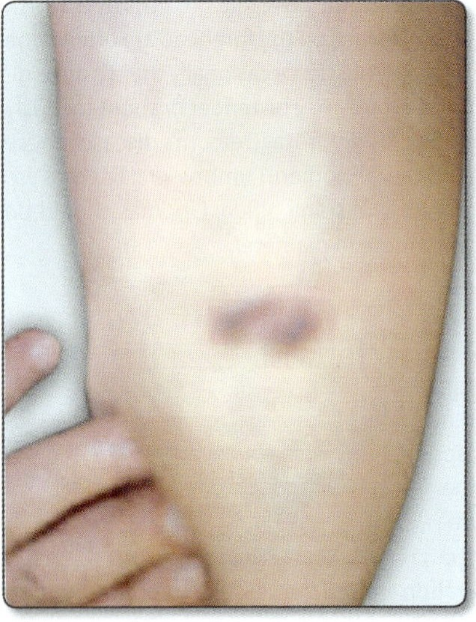

Fig. 24: Dermatofibroma

Histopathology

Fibrous tissue is present in the form of whorls in which fibroblasts and histiocytes are numerous, with collagen in the periphery. There is a great variation in the vascular component, rarely the vascularisation is pronounced; this may suggest a kind of haemangioma. The epidermal changes include acanthosis, increased melanin and hair germs protruding in the dermis. The subcutaneous fat is not involved, except in the cellular variant in which extension into the subcutaneous occurs. Histiocytomas usually do not require any treatment or else they may be excised.

Fibroepithelial Polyp (Skin Tags or Acrochordon)

This is a pedunculated papule consisting of normal epidermis with a loose connective tissue stroma. It is a harmless outpouching of the epidermis and dermis (Fig. 25). Skin tags are common in the elderly, seen in the neck and around the axillary fold. They are common mesenchymal tumours, often multiple, usually 1–4 mm in size, but occasionally 3 cm or more in diameter. It may be a manifestation of aging; they may also be associated with obesity, diabetes mellitus, pregnancy, and some endocrinal disorders. Sometimes they can assume a large size called fibroma pendulans. The larger tumours can become twisted and may undergo infarction. Small lesions are treated with electrodesiccation; larger lesions should be removed by standard or scissor excision.

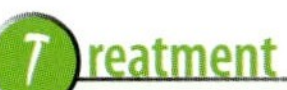

Solitary tumours can be excised. The multiple tumours require plastic surgery. Often leiomyomas occur in the neighborhood of the treated area.

Pain can be relieved by phenoxybenzamine 10 mg, 3–6 times daily with nifedipine 10 mg t.i.d. These relax the smooth muscle fibers.

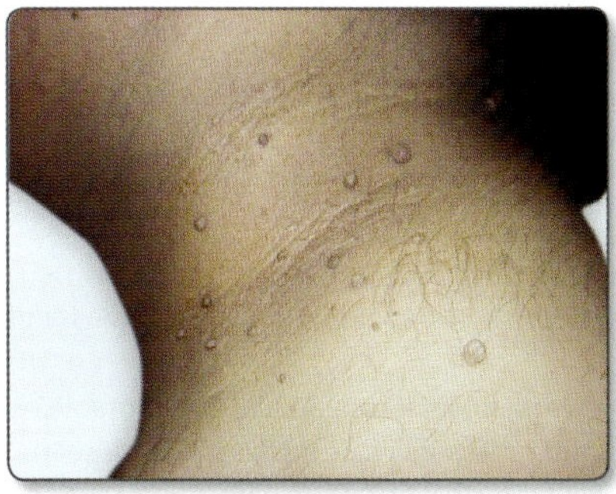

Fig. 25: Skin tags

Tumours of the Smooth Muscles

These tumours develop from the arrector pili muscle, the media of the blood vessels or the smooth muscle of the scrotum, penis, labia majora or the nipple.

Leiomyoma cutis

This develops from the arrector pili muscles; they usually occur in a group as multiple papules of brown colour. They may occur at any age, but are most common in early adult life. The most common site is the extensor surface of the extremities followed by the trunk. The tumours are painful on touch; sometimes even emotional disturbances can cause pain.

Tumours of the other smooth muscles

This may occur on the scrotum (Dartos muscle) at any age; these are usually single. It may also appear on the penis, labia majora and the nipple. Pain is less common than in a leiomyoma.

Angiomyoma

This is a solitary, flesh-coloured tumour; it usually occurs in middle age. It may grow up to 40 mm in diameter. Lower limbs are the most common sites affected. About half of the patients complain of pain.

Tumours of the sweat glands and hair follicles are described in chapters 23 and 24.

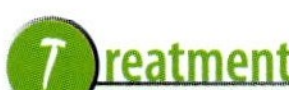

Solitary tumours can be excised, multiple tumours require plastic surgery. Leomyomas often recur adjacent to the treated area.

Pain can be relieved by phenoxybenzamine 10 mg 3-6 times daily with nifedipine 10 mg t.i.d. these relax the smooth muscle fibres.

TUMOURS ASSOCIATED WITH CONGENITAL DISEASES

Neurofibromatosis (von Recklinghausen Disease)

This is an autosomal dominant inherited syndrome, which mainly affects the nervous system, bones, and the skin. Described in 1882, about a century later, Riccardi classified it into seven types:

1. Type 1, which comprises over 85% of cases, is the typical neurofibromatosis with multiple cutaneous neurofibromas; these are derived from the Schwann cells of the peripheral nerves. The three pathognomonic signs are cafe au lait macules, neurofibromas and Lisch nodules of the iris.
2. Type 2 is the central or acoustic neurofibromatosis, characterised by bilateral acoustic neuromas.
3. Type 3 (mixed) having features of both cutaneous neurofibromatosis and acoustic neurofibromas.
4. Type 4 (variant) resemble type 2, but have numerous cutaneous neurofibromas; they are at a greater risk of developing optic gliomas and meningiomas.
5. Type 5 is the segmental neurofibromatosis; it is generally not heritable.
6. Type 6 has no cutaneous neurofibromas, only café au lait spots are seen.
7. Type 7 is the late onset neurofibromatosis. It usually manifests after the age of 20, it is not known whether it is inherited.

Diagnosis and Evaluation

All patients of neurofibromatosis should have an ophthalmic examination, an EEG, CT scan of the skull and orbits, blood pressure and an intelligence test. Yearly evaluation should be done in all cases of neurofibromatosis.

A genetic counselling should be done in patients with neurofibromatosis. There are 50% chances of each child getting the disease.

Clinical Features

Cutaneous neurofibromas are soft, pedunculated or dome-shaped, skin-coloured tumours, widely distributed over the body. Neurofibromas develop in the second decade; these flare at puberty and pregnancy; they continue to develop throughout life. These are soft, nontender skin-coloured tumours, which can invaginate into the underlying dermal defect with a light digital pressure (button-holing) (Fig. 26). The subcutaneous neurofibromas are firm, rubbery, often painful, situated deeply in the dermis.

Plexiform neurofibroma is a diffuse elongated neurofibroma found along the course of a nerve, usually trigeminal or upper cervical nerves (Fig. 27). Large pigmented macules may develop over a plexiform neurofibroma. Pruritus may be severe; this is probably associated with numerous mast cells in the tumour. Plexiform neurofibromas have an increased risk of becoming malignant. Neurofibromas can also be present in the internal organs.

The other cutaneous lesions are cafe au lait macules. These are pigmented macules of more than 5 mm in diameter; six or more of these are diagnostic of neurofibromatosis, freckling in the axillary or inguinal region (Crowe's sign), cutis verticis gyrata and macroglossia may occur. Cafe au lait macules may be present at birth, or develop in the first year.

Lisch nodules (melanocytic hamartomas) are found in the iris. These develop in childhood at about the age of 6 years. The lesions are asymptomatic.

Bony involvement comprise kyphoscoliosis, short stature, macrocephaly, sphenoidal dysplasia, thinning of the cortex of the long bones, psuedoarthrosis of the tibia and atraumatic fractures may occur.

Mental retardation, epilepsy, brain tumours and tumours of the cranial nerves such as optic glioma may occur due to involvement of the central nervous system. Endocrine disorders such as acromegaly, cretinism, hyperthyroidism, myxedema, pheochromocytoma or precocious puberty may be seen.

Treatment

There is no curative treatment. Ketotifen, a mast cell stabiliser, may be beneficial in the treatment of pruritus. There is no treatment of neurofibromas except excision when required. Malignant transformation is seen in 2–5% of neurofibromas.

If juvenile xanthogranuloma is present, always exclude leukaemia in these children.

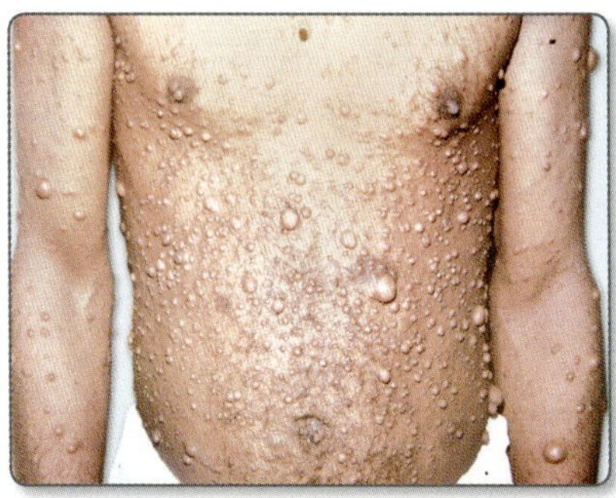

Fig. 26: Neurofibromatosis

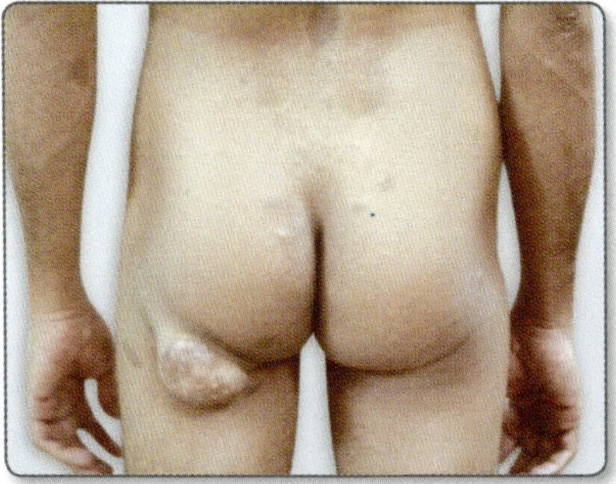

Fig. 27: Plexiform neuroma

Tuberous Sclerosis (Adenoma Sebaceum, Bourneville-Pringle Disease)

This syndrome includes angiofibromata, mental deficiency and epilepsy. Inheritance is autosomal dominant with high penetrance but variable expression. Common cutaneous lesions are ash leaf hypomelanotic macules, facial angiofibromas, periungual fibromas (Koenen's tumours), shagreen patch and forehead fibromatous plaque.

Angiofibromas are characterised by small yellowish-red translucent discrete papules situated on the face; they are principally located on the cheek, nasolabial fold, nose and forehead (Fig. 28). They are present in 90% of patients over the age of 4 years.

The earliest cutaneous sign is the hypomelanotic macules present at birth or early infancy; they are ash leaf or polygonal in shape, present over the limbs or the trunk.

Shagreen patch is an irregularly thickened slightly elevated flesh-coloured plaque consisting of collagen, most commonly situated over the lumbosacral area (Fig. 29).

Koenen tumours are subungual and periungual fibromas; these develop at or after puberty and present as firm flesh coloured growths projecting from the nail folds and beneath the nail plate (Fig. 30).

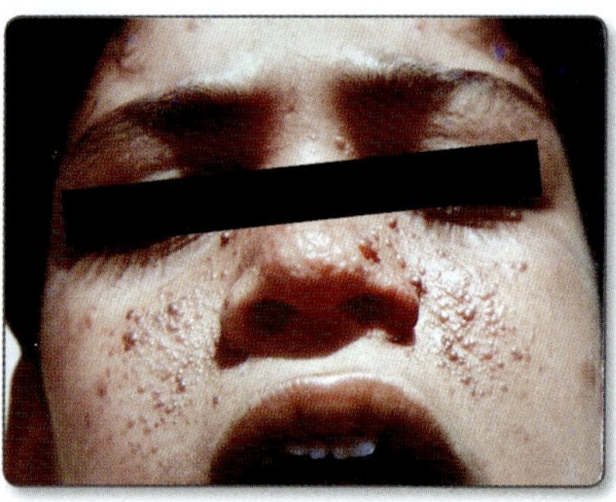

Fig. 28: Tuberous sclerosis: angiofibromas

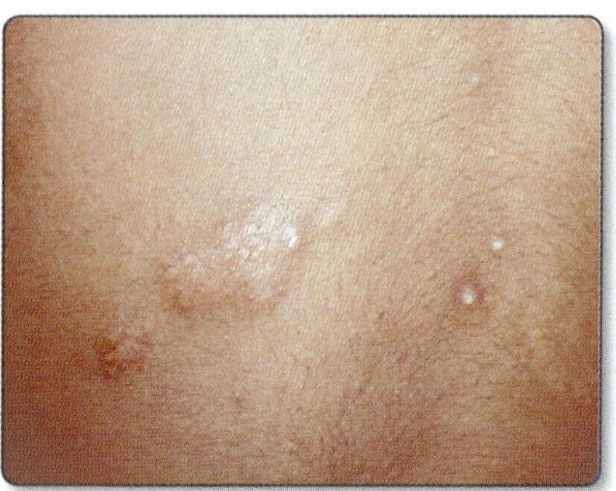

Fig. 29: Shagreen patch

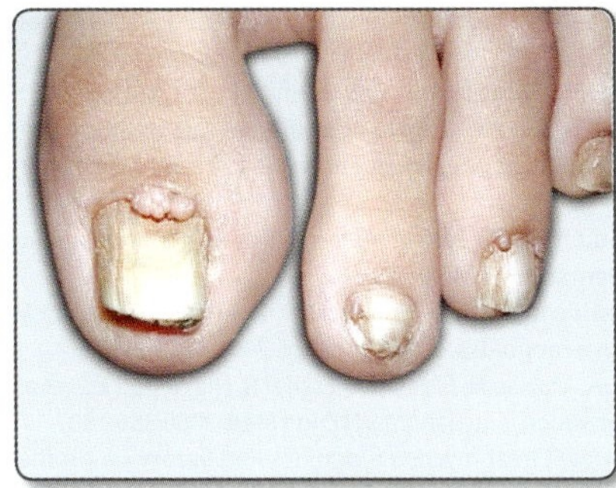

Fig. 30: Koenen tumour

Other tumours in tuberous sclerosis are firm fibromatous plaques on the forehead; fibromatous tumours are occasionally present on the gums and palate.

Mental deficiency is usually seen in early life and epilepsy is variable in severity. About 80% of patients have seizures and nonspecific EEG abnormalities. There may be cerebral calcification; potato-like nodules of glial proliferation characterise the lesions of the central nervous system.

Treatment

There is no specific therapy. Cutaneous tumours can be removed by lasers, but they tend to recur. A neurologist should be consulted; early educational training and guidance for maximum opportunities should be looked into.

Retinal tumours, renal hamartomas and cardiac rhabdomyomas may also occur. About half of the patients have bony abnormalities such as bone cysts and sclerosis. Pits on the enamel of permanent teeth, when more than five, are a marker for tuberous sclerosis. Pulmonary lymphangioleiomyoma may be a forme fruste of tuberous sclerosis.

The prognosis is extremely variable and depends on the severity of clinical manifestations. In severe cases, death may result from epilepsy, infection, cardiac failure or early pulmonary fibrosis.

A child with unexplained seizures should have a Wood's light examination, to search for ash leaf macule, to exclude tuberous sclerosis.

FURTHER READING

1. Ahmed I, Berth-Jones J, Charles-Holmes S, et al. Comparison of cryotherapy with curettage in the treatment of Bowen's disease: a prospective study. Br J Dermatol. 2000;143:759-66.
2. Bernengo M, Novelle M, Quaglino P, Novelli M, et al. Prognostic factors in Sezary syndrome: a multivariate analysis of clinical, haematological and immunological features. Ann Oncol. 1998;9:857-63.
3. Cerroni L, Signoretti S, Hofler G, et al. Primary cutaneous marginal zone b-cell lymphoma: a recently described entity of low-grade cutaneous B- cell lymphoma. Am J Surg Pathol. 1997;21:1307-15.
4. Chor PJ, Santa Cruz DJ. Kaposi's sarcoma in A clinicopathologic review and differential diagnosis. J Cutan Pathol. 1992;19:6-20.
5. Deeths JM, Champman TJ, Dellavalle PR, Zeng C and Aeling L J, et al. Treatment of patch and plaque stage mycosis fungoides with imiquimid imiquimod 5% cream. Amer J Am Acad Dermatol. 2005;52:275-80.

6. Doshi ND, Friedman JA. The new melanoma staging system. Journal of Drugs in Dermatology. 2010;9(8):1026-1029.
7. Gloster HM. Dermatofibrosarcoma protuberans. J Am Acad Dermatol. 1996;35:355-74.
8. Heinzerling L, Dummer R, Kemph W, Sehmid M, Burg G, et al. Intralesional therapy with anti-CD20 monoclonal antibody rituximab in primary cutaneous B- cell lymphoma. Arch Dermatol. 2000;136:374-8.
9. MokenzieMacKenzie-Wood AR, Wood BG. Pyogenic granuloma- like lesions in a patient using topical tretinon. Australas J Dermatol. 1998;39:248-50.
10. Martinez-Gonzalez CM, Veara-Hernando MM, Yebra-Pimentel MT, Del-Pozzo J, Maziara M Fonseca E, et al. Imiquimod in mycosis fungoides. Eur J Dermatol. 2008;18:148-52.
11. Morton LD, Thompson FJ, Cochran JA, Mozillo N, Elashoff R, Essner R, Nieweggg EO, et al. Sentineal-node biopsy or nodal observation in melanoma. N Eng J Med. 2006;355:1307-17.
12. Prince MH, Whittaker S, Hoppe TR. How I treat mycosis fungoides and Sezary syndrome. Blood. 2009;114(20):4337-53.
13. Russel Jones R, Whiltaker S. T-cell receptor gene analysis in the diagnosis of Sezary Syndrome. J Am Acad Dermatol. 1999;41:254-79.
14. Smith JL, Butler JJ. Skin involvement in Hodgkin's disease. Cancer.1980;45:354-61.
15. Sweet RD. The treatment of basal cell carcinoma by curettage. Br J Dermatol. 1963;75: 137-48.

Chapter

28 Naevi and Malformations

INTRODUCTION

Naevi are developmental abnormalities of the skin due to excess or diminution of one or more components of the skin. Naevi are classified according to the predominant cell type, e.g. epidermal naevi, vascular naevi, melanocytic naevi, etc. The most common naevi are the pigmented moles, which occur in 95% of the adults. Some naevi are present at birth (true birthmarks), others do not become apparent until adult life. Naevi may continue to proliferate after birth; some undergo malignant change later in life.

EPIDERMAL NAEVI

These may be present at birth or appear in early infancy or childhood. Occasionally, they may appear for the first time in adult life. There is no sex predominance. It is due to an excessive proliferation of keratinocytes. There are many types of epidermal naevi, but they generally present as dirty grey or brown verrucous papules, present as a localised plaque, or often in a linear morphology. Occasionally they are extensive and affect large areas of the body.

Aetiology

Congenital abnormalities can be caused by genetic or environmental factors. Most of the epidermal naevi reflect genetic mosaicism. They usually appear in linear configuration, originally described by Blaschko. Most of the epidermal naevi having histological features of epidermolytic hyperkeratosis reflect keratin gene mutation. Darier-like epidermal naevus results from mosaicism for the Darier gene. It occurs late in life at about the age of 20 years. The lesions are aggravated by exposure to ultraviolet light (UVL). Similarly, naevoid psoriasis suggests mosaicism for psoriasis. Some naevi are associated with systemic abnormalities such as epidermal naevus syndrome. Organoid naevi feature both epidermal and adnexal structures.

A genetic influence on the development of epidermal naevi is suggested by the occasional reports of the familial occurrences.

Epidermal proliferation and differentiation is largely promoted by the dermis. Epidermal naevi should be removed with the underlying dermis.

Classification of Epidermal Naevi

- Keratinocytic naevi
  - Verrucous epidermal naevus

  - Acantholytic epidermal naevus
  - Inflammatory naevus
- Follicular naevi
  - True hair follicle naevus
  - Comedone naevus
- Sebaceous naevus
- Apocrine naevus
- Eccrine naevus
- Epidermal naevus syndrome

EPIDERMAL KERATINOCYTIC NAEVI

Verrucous Epidermal Naevus (Linear Epidermal Naevus or Linear Epidermal Verrucous Naevus)

These are generally present at birth, or appear within the first few years of life. The individual lesion consists of verrucous papules, brown or dirty grey in colour, arranged in a streak or plaque. Those on the limbs are usually longitudinal, and those on the trunk follow a transverse pattern along the course of the intercostal nerves. They usually do not cross the midline. An epidermal naevus with an extensive distribution is called systemised epidermal naevus. If the lesions are present on one-half of the body, it is termed naevus unius lateris.

The verrucous epidermal naevus usually extends until puberty; they become more verrucous and pigmented. After puberty they remain unchanged, very occasionally they may resolve. Uncommonly benign or malignant tumours may develop in the epidermal naevi. Epidermal naevi may be associated with other cutaneous lesions such as café au lait macules and congenital hypopigmented macules.

The lesions are usually symptomless unless they are present on the nailfold, where they may cause paronychia. In the flexures they may macerate. Megalopinna is reported if the pinna is involved.

Histologically, there is hyperkeratosis, acanthosis and papillomatosis. Five to ten percent of cases show features of epidermolytic hyperkeratosis (Figs 1 and 2).

Differential Diagnosis

Epidermal naevi should be differentiated from the viral warts especially those exhibiting the Koebner's phenomenon. The roughened surface differentiates it from a melanocytic naevus. A linear form of eczema called lichen striatus appears on the limbs of a child that lasts for approximately 18 months and then shows spontaneous resolution.

Treatment

Treatment will depend upon the age of the patient, the location of the naevus and its extent. The prime consideration is complete removal of the naevus with least amount of scarring.

Topical application with salicylic acid, lactic acid, and retinoic acid may help in flattening out the lesion, but this requires persistent application to have any benefit. Systemic acitretin may help epidermolytic naevi.

Surgical treatment should include removal of the epidermis with the underlying dermis to avoid recurrences. Laser removal is often followed by partial recurrence.

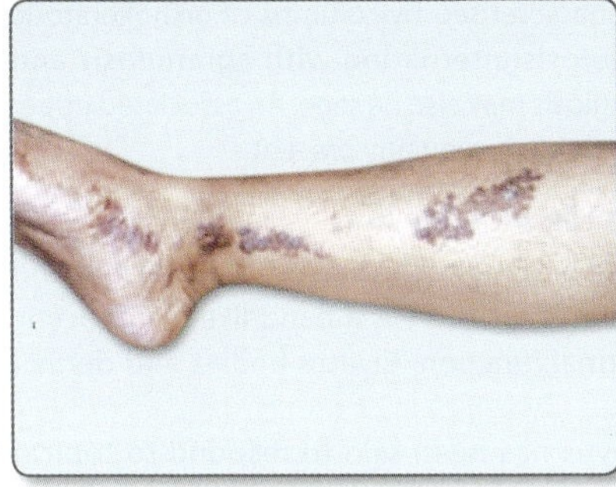

Fig. 1: Linear epidermal naevus

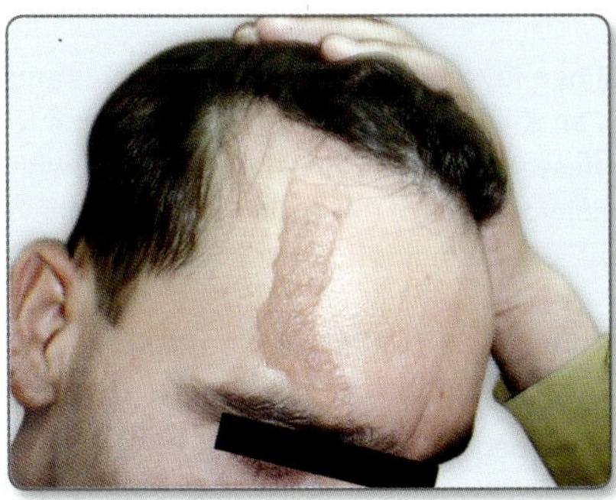

Fig. 2: Epidermal naevus

Acantholytic Naevus

These include Darier-like epidermal naevus and Hailey-Hailey-like epidermal naevus. Darier-like epidermal naevus appears usually late at about the age of 20 years, the lesions are aggravated by sunlight. The lesions resemble those of Darier's disease. Hailey-Hailey-like epidermal naevus is characterised by linear erythematous plaques, which demonstrates vesiculation, erosion and crusting. Histology shows the features of Hailey-Hailey disease. It has a highly characteristic course with periods of spontaneous improvement followed by relapse. It has an early onset.

Inflammatory Epidermal Naevus

These include the inflammatory linear epidermal verrucous nevus, lichenoid epidermal naevus, psoriasiform epidermal naevus and the congenital hemidysplasia ichthyosiform nevus and limb defects (CHILD). All of these show the histological evidence of inflammation.

Inflammatory Linear Epidermal Verrucous Naevus

Previously known as dermatatic epidermal nevus, it usually appears at birth or in the first few years of life. Later onset has been recorded. It usually occurs on the extremities and is pruritic. It is more common in females.

Histopathological picture is characterised by columns of orthokeratotic hyperkeratosis and hypergranulosis alternating with agranulosis and parakeratosis. In some cases, spongiosis may also be seen. An associated upper dermal lymphohistiocytic inflammation is regularly present.

Lichenoid and Psoriasiform Epidermal Naevus

These have the morphological and histological features of lichen planus and psoriasis. In lichenoid epidermal naevus there is a band-like lymphocytic infiltration at the dermo-epidermal junction, Civatte bodies and dermal melanophages are seen.

Psoriasiform epidermal naevus has been said to respond to topical dithranol.

CHILD Naevus

This is an acronym for congenital hemidysplasia, ichthyosiform naevus and limb defects. It is transmitted as an X-linked dominant trait, and lethal to males. CHILD naevus is usually present at birth; it may be associated with bone defects such as scoliosis, and hypoplasia of the phalanges. These naevi are usually refractory to treatment. Oral retinoids may occasionally help.

Pigmented Hairy Epidermal Naevus (Becker's Naevus)

This is a distinct clinical entity; it appears for the first time during adolescence. It is predominantly a disorder of males. It begins as a small area of pigmentation on the shoulder, after a period of a year or two coarse dark hair develop on the naevus. The affected skin becomes thick and rough. Tissue hypoplasia, such as shortening of an arm, and reduced breast development, may underlie Becker's naevus. Spina bifida has been reported.

Histology shows epidermal melanotic hyperproliferation, acanthosis, thickening of the dermis and smooth muscle hyperplasia. Becker's naevus is considered as an organoid naevus, with epidermal and dermal components (Figs 3 and 4).

It should be differentiated from a pigmented naevus, which usually begins at an earlier age or is present at birth. Naevus of Ito has a bluish colour because of its dermal location.

The lesion is usually extensive, treatment is therefore difficult. Lasers and plastic surgery may be considered.

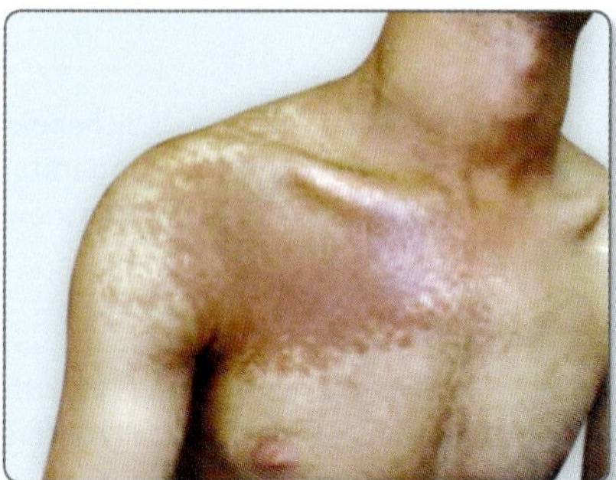

Fig. 3: Becker's naevus (early stage)

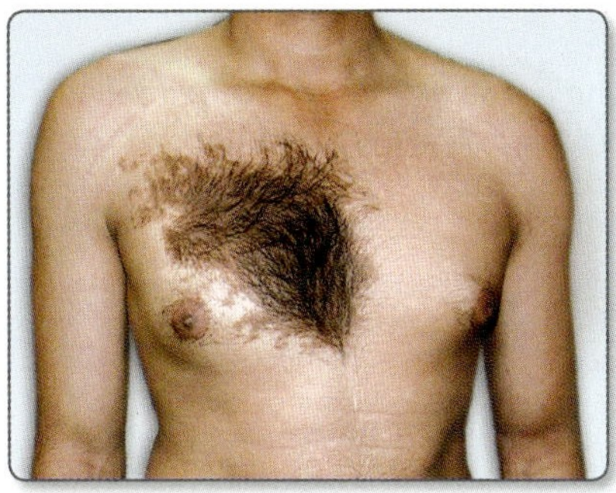

Fig. 4: Becker's naevus (late stage with hair)

FOLLICULAR NAEVI

Naevus Comedonicus

These naevi are said to be of pilosebaceous origin. They arise from normal, abnormal or ectopic pilosebaceous follicles. There is often incomplete development of the terminal hair and sebaceous glands. Occasionally, they are seen on the palms and soles; some regard the naevi on the palms and soles to be of eccrine origin.

Histopathology

Deep invaginations of the epidermis are seen, which are filled with concentric layers of keratin. These generally represent dilated hair follicles, as hair shafts are present in the deeper part of the invagination; the arrector pili muscles are absent.

Clinical Features

The lesion usually appears in early childhood. These are most commonly seen on the face, neck, trunk and upper arm. Palms and soles are rarely affected. They occur in groups and look like black comedones. These comedones represent epidermal pits filled with keratin. The intervening skin is usually normal. The lesions may be arranged in a linear distribution, these are usually unilateral; bilateral cases may occur but these are rare.

If the lesion becomes inflamed, papules, cysts and scarring may occur. Rarely, naevus comedonicus is associated with defects of the central nervous system (CNS), eyes and bones. In such cases, it is a part of the epidermal nevus syndrome.

Differential Diagnosis

The lesions should be differentiated from porokeratotic eccrine, ostial and dermal naevi and dilated pore naevus. Comedones also occur in familial diffuse comedones, familial dyskeratotic comedones, and linear basal cell naevus.

Treatment

Local treatment with salicylic acid, or retinoic acid improves the cosmetic appearance of the naevus. Ideal treatment is the surgical removal, which includes the dermis. It gives better results than shaving or dermabrasion. Oral isotretinoin is also effective.

Inflamed lesions should be treated on lines similar to acne with nodules and cysts.

NAEVUS SEBACEOUS

Naevus sebaceous of Jadassohn is a sharply circumscribed yellowish orange hamartoma varying from a few millimeters to several centimeters in diameter. The hamartoma consists predominantly of sebaceous glands. It is usually present at birth, most frequently on the vertex of the scalp; it may also be present on the face or neck.

Clinical Features

The lesions are usually single but may be multiple. The naevus is alopecic. Following birth, the lesion tends to remain unchanged until puberty. The naevus is under control of androgens, and grows at adolescence when it becomes thicker and verrucous. Rapid enlargement and ulceration of the growth should arouse suspicion of a malignant growth. Occasionally, it may develop into basal cell carcinoma or other adnexal tumours. Such naevi should always be excised. Naevus sebaceous can develop in association with epidermal naevus syndrome; this is more common in patients with multiple or extensive lesions. It is believed that naevus sebaceous, develops from pluripotential cells. They have the capacity to develop into various epithelial tumours.

Histopathology

In early childhood, the sebaceous glands are underdeveloped, and the lesions consist of immature hair structures. In well-developed lesions, there is a well-developed sebaceous component.

Treatment

The naevus sebaceous should be excised because of the chance of developing malignancy at puberty. Although some authors are of the opinion that because the chances of malignancy is low, the naevus should only be removed if there are signs of a malignant change.

ECCRINE NAEVUS

Eccrine naevi are very rare; it may present as an area of hyperhidrosis in a skin coloured linear plaque, or as a solitary pore that discharges mucoid substance. It may sometimes present as violet plaques or nodules; hyperhidrosis may or may not be present. Treatment is by excision.

EPIDERMAL NAEVUS SYNDROME (Schimmelpenning's syndrome, Solomon's syndrome)

Extensive epidermal naevi are associated with other developmental defects especially those of the CNS, skeleton, cardiovascular system, urogenital system and the eye. They occur sporadically, but there are some reports of an autosomal dominant inheritance. These naevi reflect somatic mosaicism with mutation probably occurring at an earlier embryonic stage, leading to involvement of multiple systems.

Cutaneous abnormalities other than multiple epidermal naevi are haemangiomas, café au lait macules, melanocytic naevus, dermatomegaly and cutaneous malignancies. The majority presents as naevus unius lateris.

Dental anomalies such as enamel hypoplasia, malformation of the teeth and hypodontia may occur. Skeletal abnormalities include scoliosis, kyphosis, limb defects and syndactyly. Neurological abnormalities are common in patients with naevi on the head and neck. Mental retardation, seizures and cognitive development delay are the most common findings. Seizures, spastic paresis, posterior fossa abnormalities, enlargement of the lateral ventricles, agenesis of the corpus callosum and cranial nerve palsies may occur.

Ocular abnormalities include involvement of the conjunctiva and eyelid by the naevus interfering with lid closure, may result in trichiasis. The other ocular lesions include colobomas, choristomas (choristoma is a congenital overgrowth of normal tissue in an abnormal situation), micro-ophthalmia, macro-ophthalmia, corneal opacities and cataract.

Benign and malignant changes may occur in the epidermal naevus. Systemic malignancies include nephroblastoma, salivary gland tumours, glioma, carcinoma of the bladder, intrathoracic tumours, etc.

Management

This requires a multi-disciplinary approach including a dermatologist, neurologist, ophthalmologist, paediatrician, plastic surgeon, etc. Extensive epidermal tumours should be thoroughly investigated for the lesions of the CNS, eye and the skeleton. The naevi should be watched for any change towards malignancy. These naevi need a follow-up at regular intervals. Depending upon the findings, further investigations may be required such as electroencephalography, computed sonography, magnetic resonance imaging, intravenous pyelography, X-ray for bones, etc.

VASCULAR NAEVI

These can be infantile angiomas and vascular malformations.

Infantile Angiomas

These naevi are due to proliferation of vascular endothelium; they are seen shortly after birth and regress by 4–7 years. These are the most common naevi of infancy.

Aetiology

Infantile haemangiomas are benign proliferations of vascular elements. Vascularisation of the fetal skin begins during the third month of life, but these do not anastamose with the deeper vessels until late in gestation. Infantile haemangiomas arise when islands of embryonic cutaneous angioblastic tissue fail to establish communication with the deeper channels.

Capillary endothelial cells have a capacity to develop new vessels under certain conditions. This requires the presence of angiogenic factors. It is said that infantile haemangiomas are able to secrete a factor themselves for their proliferation. Certain cells play a "helper" role in endothelial proliferation such as the mast cells. Endogenous steroid hormones play a role in the growth of infantile haemangiomas.

Strawberry Angioma

These are benign proliferations of the vascular endothelium; they usually appear during the first month of life, these naevi have a characteristic phase

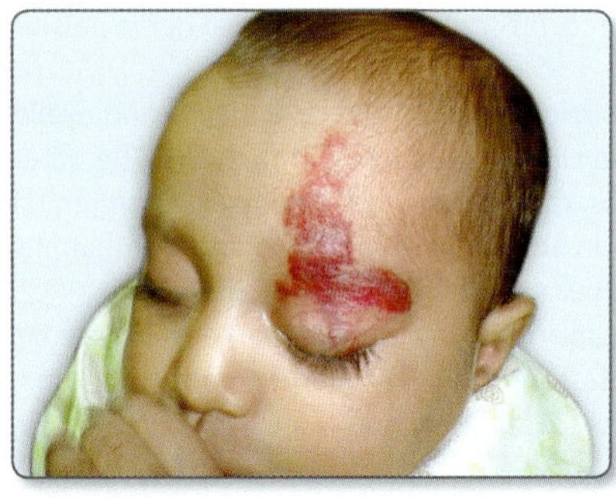

Fig. 5: Haemangioma

of initial growth and later an involution phase. Sixty percent of strawberry angiomas occur on the head and neck, next common site is the trunk. The lesions are dome-shaped dull-red in colour, when involution begins islands of pale pink or white patches appear in the lesion and it starts to flatten. Lesions that are superficial are bright red, and deeper components tend to darken with a bluish hue. These angiomas grow initially for a period of 6–9 months; they remain static for 2–3 years, some resolve completely by the fourth year, and most of them disappear by the seventh birthday. Resolution of an angioma is herald by softening of the lesion and by the appearance of pinkish grey areas in the centre of the surface.

About 50% of children have normal skin after involution; others may have variable atrophy, telangiectasia, or scarring (Fig. 5).

Multiple cutaneous haemangiomas suggest an internal involvement such as haemangiomas of the CNS, liver and gastrointestinal tract. It may be associated with coarctation of the aorta. Genitourinary developmental defects such as imperforate anus, posterior fossa abnormalities such as cerebellar atrophy and arachnoid cysts may also occur.

Complications of the naevi are haemorrhage, infection, ulceration, shunting of large volume of blood from the angioma may lead to high output cardiac failure. Purpura may occur due to consumption of clotting factors within the vascular bed of the angioma and platelet sequestration (Kasabach-Merritt syndrome); it may cause pressure symptoms such as airway obstruction, impairment of vision, interference of feeding due to angiomas in the mouth.

Treatment

In the absence of complications no treatment is required because the haemangioma involutes spontaneously. Intervention is only required when there is severe haemorrhage, cardiac failure, complications due to mechanical obstruction such as difficulty in feeding, respiration, vision, etc. These can be treated with prednisolone 20–40 mg daily for 4–6 weeks; the dose is then gradually tapered over several months. Enlarging haemangiomas may stop growing in 2–3 weeks. Intralesional injections may be effective if systemic steroids fail. Compression bandages may provide temporary relief in reducing the bulk of the tumour. Shrinkage of the tumour may also be brought about by the injection of sclerosing agents such as sodium citrate 30%, glucose 30% and saturated saline, 0.5–5 mL is injected at fortnightly intervals. Pulsed dye lasers have been used to treat ulcerated haemangiomas.

Contd...

Contd...

Interferon-α-2a and 2b are indicated when prednisolone fails to respond, and in cases of life-threatening haemangiomas. It is given subcutaneously in a dose of 3 million U/m^2 daily for 6–12 months. Periodic blood and neurological examinations are required during treatment. Recently, propranolol and other β-blockers have been used successfully for the treatment of infantile angioma.

Special consideration is required when a haemangioma is on the eyelid. Obstruction for even a few weeks may lead to irreversible amblyopia. It is important the eye should be used daily for short periods. The case should be referred to an ophthalmic surgeon.

Embolisation can be used to treat haemongiomas that have not responded to medical treatment. Surgical excision is very rare.

Kasabach-Merritt syndrome

Bleeding in a haemangioma is due to the consumption of clotting factors. This may lead to increased fibrinolysis, which can be detected by the appearance of fibrin degrading products in the circulation. Infantile haemangioma leading to Kasabach-Merritt syndrome are generally deep seated, and often of a large size. The haemorrhage may appear at birth or may appear later. The onset is manifest by increase in size of the tumour, induration and superficial ecchymosis. This may lead to compression of the underlying structures. Internal bleeding may occur in a number of cases.

Treatment is only indicated when there is a threat to patient's life. Corticosteroid injections may be given in a dose of 2–4 mg/kg/day. Fresh plasma and platelet transfusion helps in improving the general condition of the patient. Vincristine and interferon-α-2a have shown response in some cases.

Continuous bandaging may help in some cases. Surgery should be done when adequate control of bleeding has been achieved, otherwise surgical intervention may be catastrophic.

Vascular malformations

Vascular malformations can be arterial, venous, capillary, or mixed. There is a progressive ectatic dilatation of the mature dermal blood vessels with lack of endothelial cell proliferation. They are present at birth and there is no tendency for spontaneous resolution. These malformations grow in proportion to the growth of the child. Initially there is involvement of the superficial blood vessels; later the deeper blood vessels are also involved. The lesions are probably due the weakness of supporting elements of the blood vessel wall.

The lesions on the face occur along the sensory branches of the trigeminal nerve, which suggests that the abnormality may have a neurogenic basis. Sometimes lesions similar to port wine stain occur later in life following trauma, which is probably due to damage to the microvascular nerve supply.

Salmon Patch

This is a pink patch due to dilatation of the blood vessels; it is present in about 50% of newborn infants. The eyelid is the common site, these fade rapidly but those on the nape of the neck (naevus flammeus nuchae) often persist. It has an autosomal dominant inheritance. Nuchal sites appear to be a predilection for other dermatoses such as psoriasis and seborrhoeic dermatitis.

Port Wine Stain (Naevus Flammeus)

This is a naevus on the area supplied by the ophthalmic branch of the trigeminal nerve. It may be present as such or associated with abnormalities of the cerebral blood vessels. In some cases, it may be widespread and may involve as much as half of the body. It is present at birth as small red macules, which enlarge to firm large red patches. These patches are partially or completely blanched by pressure. The surface is smooth, sometimes nodular or warty growths may be present. They persist for life unless treated.

Treatment

As port wine stains occur on the face, they are often a source of psychological trauma to the patient. Cosmetic camouflage creams have been used to cover the disfigurement. Over the years, a number of methods have been used to treat this disorder such as tattooing, excision and grafting, Grenz rays and cryotherapy.

Lasers have been gaining popularity. Lasers used for its treatment include the argon-pumped tunable dye laser, copper vapour laser, and the flash lamp pulse dye laser. The flash lamp tunable dye laser is used for most cases of port wine stain, particularly in the lighter ones seen in children. Adults require more treatments than children. The argon laser is more suitable for adults with deep purplish lesions. Side effects of laser include oedema, bullae, bleeding, pyogenic granuloma, hypopigmentation, hyperpigmentation, and atrophic scarring (Fig. 6).

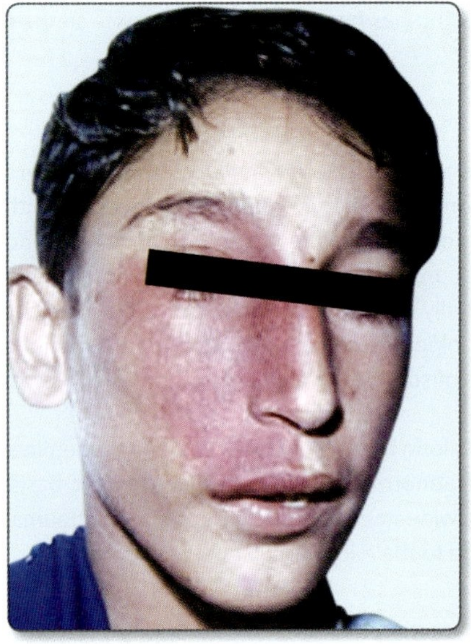

Fig. 6: Port wine stain

Sturge-Weber Syndrome

It is a vascular naevus associated with glaucoma, contralateral Jacksonian epilepsy, paralysis, mental retardation, and retinal detachment. These naevi are persistant, they can be treated by cosmetic camouflage, and pulsed tunable dye laser gives the best result. Results are excellent when treated early in life before they become raised and palpable.

Vascular anomalies occur in any part of the ocular circulation. There may be dilated conjunctival and episcleral vessels, choroidal angiomas may also occur. Glaucoma is present in a number of patients. Choroidal angiomas push the retina forwards producing hyperopia. Degenerative changes of the retina occur later. Glaucoma should always be excluded in a case of port wine stain. An ophthalmic examination is necessary in all cases of Sturge-Weber syndrome.

Klippel-Trenaunay Syndrome

This syndrome is characterised by port wine stain, soft tissue swellings with or without bony overgrowths and associated with arteriovenous fistulae. Most of the lesions are seen on the extremities, these abrupt sharply at the midline. The lesions are patchy; they may extend to the buttocks or the trunk and thoracic region. Varicosities develop when the patient stands and walks. There may be hypoplasia or even atresia of the deep venous system. Augmented arterial blood flow is said to account for bony and soft tissue hypertrophy. The involved limb is usually longer and larger than normal.

Complications include haemorrhage, deep venous thrombosis, pulmonary embolism, and septicaemic episodes (Fig. 7).

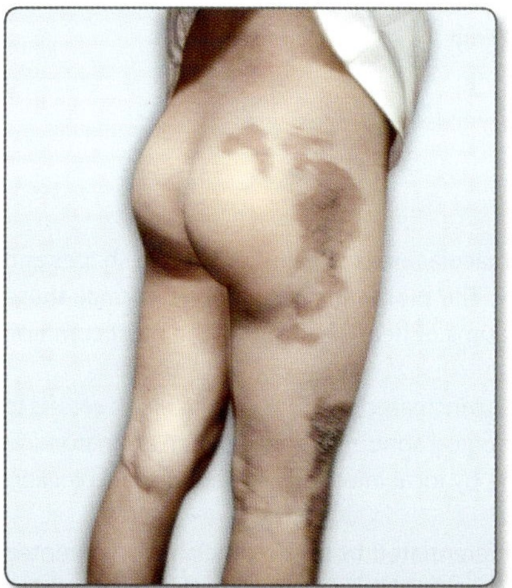

Fig. 7: Klippel-Trenaunay syndrome

The disease should be differentiated from Proteus syndrome; this syndrome comprises an association of asymmetrical overgrowth of almost any part of the body. It is associated with verrucous epidermal naevi, infantile haemangiomas, lipoma-like subcutaneous hamartomas. (The name Proteus is derived after Proteus the man in Greek mythology, who could change his shape at will to avoid capture).

Treatment

Majority of the patients can be helped with an elastic support; this reduces the symptoms of chronic venous insufficiency, decreases the swelling caused by lymphatic stasis and protects the limbs from external trauma.

Treatment is unsatisfactory, clinical evaluation of the patients is done with phlebography, arteriography, roentgenography and radiography before any surgical procedure is carried out. Surgery should be done to correct the inequality of the limbs and to relieve any deep venous obstruction.

VENOUS MALFORMATION

Cavernous haemangiomas are deeper, softer and unlikely to regress spontaneously. These are found mainly on the face, trunk, or extremities. The haemangiomas are usually compressible, because of their slow blood flow, thrombosis may occur. Patients complain of intermittent pain, particularly on awakening in the morning. Thrombosis does not occur in arterial malformations. The overlying skin is bluish in colour. Multiple venous malformations may be familial.

Skeletal abnormalities, such as facial asymmetry and distortion of facial features may occur. Underlying bone hypertrophy can result when cavernous haemangiomas are situated on a limb.

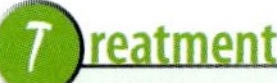

Conservative treatment for cavernous hemangiomas on the limbs consists of elastic support, and low dose aspirin for thrombosis. Sclerotherapy followed by surgery is the best active treatment.

NAEVUS ANEMICUS

The naevus is characterised by macular areas of pallor of varying shapes and size due to reduced blood flow. The pigment production is normal; these areas cannot be made red by trauma or heat. The trunk is the most common site affected.

The condition is probably due to increased sensitivity of the blood vessels to catecholamines. It is a pharmacological abnormality rather than an anatomical one. The pallor can be overcome by local injection of α-adrenergic blockers such as phentolamine.

Naevus anemicus can be differentiated from the other hypopigmented lesions by a diascopic test; the naevus and the surrounding skin become alike on diascopy. Treatment is by camouflage.

BLUE RUBBER BLEB NAEVUS SYNDROME

The syndrome consists of venous malformations in the skin and gastrointestinal tract. Most cases are sporadic; some may have autosomal dominant inheritance. The cutaneous lesions present as compressible, tender blue nodules, present on the trunk and extremities. The gastrointestinal lesions are commonly found in the small intestine, oral and anal mucosa. In some cases, other organs can be affected such as the eye, nasopharynx, brain, meninges, and the heart. Complications include intestinal haemorrhage, volvulus, bowel infarction and rectal prolapse.

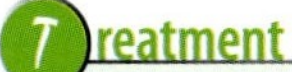

Excision, sclerotherapy, or laser therapy is indicated for the skin lesions. For the intestines cauterisation, sclerotherapy or bowel resection may be necessary.

MAFFUCCI SYNDROME

Maffucci syndrome is a combination of lymphatic-venous malformation and endochondromas. The condition is common on the extremities, 20% of endochondromas may become malignant. The patient is often of short stature. The syndrome should be carefully monitored for any malignant change. Vascular lesions should be treated on a similar line to that of venous malformations.

MELANOCYTIC NAEVI

Melanocytic naevi are the most common naevi, most of these arise during childhood and adolescence. About 1% of new born infants have a melanotic naevus. With advancing age, some naevi may disappear.

Aetiology

The abnormality in the melanocytes and their behaviour is unknown. Melanocytic naevi are common, they are present in about 95% of Caucasians, they should not be considered as an abnormality but as a variation of normal cutaneous reaction.

A hereditary factor has been implicated in some cases, particularly when a large number of naevi are present in successive generations.

A hormonal influence is suggested because a number of these naevi occur at puberty, pregnancy or after taking contraceptive pills.

Exposure to ultraviolet light appears to be an exacerbating factor in the development of melanocytic naevi. Use of sunscreens has shown to decrease the number of new moles in children.

An increase in the number of moles is also been seen in immunosuppression such as AIDS/HIV infection.

There are many hypotheses for the development of melanocytic naevi such as transformation of epidermal melanocytes and migration into the dermis, development from the pigment of the Schwann cells, hamartomatous change, or developing from a defect in the cells of the neural crest.

Types of Melanocytic Naevi

Melanocytic naevi can be epidermal or dermal depending on whether the naevi are derived from the epidermal melanocytes or from the melanocytes derived from the neural crest that have not reached the epidermis, because the cells are arrested in the dermis due to some developmental abnormality.

Melanocytic naevi may be acquired congenital melanocytic naevi.

Acquired Melanocytic Naevi

Acquired melanocytic epidermal naevi begin to appear after the first 6–12 months of life and increase in number until the second or third decade. Acquired melanocytic naevi typically range from 1 mm to 1 cm in diameter and have a round or oval shape with relatively demarcated smooth borders. These have a wide variety of presentations; they may be flat, dome-shaped, or papillomatous. The colour varies from black, shades of brown, skin coloured, or pink. These variations depend upon what stage of their evolution the development stops. Very dark brown or black melanocytic naevi are seldom seen in light coloured people; these colours are more common in dark skin (Fig. 8).

Junctional Naevi

The naevi begin as a proliferation of the melanocytes in the epidermal based layer, at this stage they appear as flat-pigmented macules, brownish-black in colour, round or oval in shape, regular outline and have a sharp border. The size does not exceed 6 mm.

Compound Naevi

In the next phase of development, the proliferating melanocytes migrate into the dermis and form clumps or columns of cells. These naevi that have both junctional and intradermal components are called compound naevi.

These present as small, raised pigmented papules, which have a smooth surface, these often increase in size and pigmentation at puberty, coarse hair may appear.

Intradermal Naevi

The final stage of development occurs when the melanocytes stop proliferating and this naevus becomes entirely intradermal. When the naevus is wholly intradermal, the melanocytes may or may not produce melanin. The

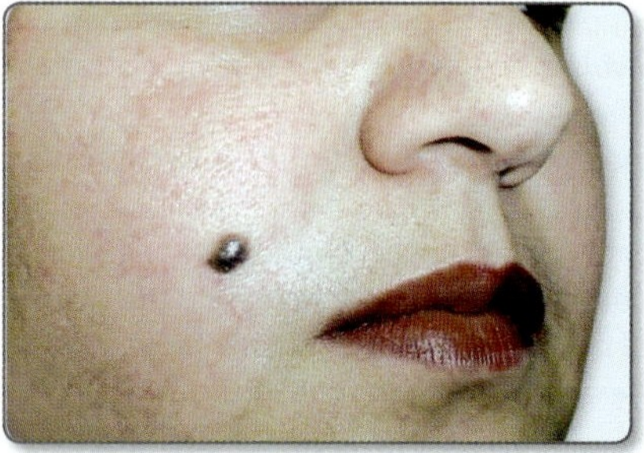

Fig. 8: Acquired melanocytic naevus

intradermal naevus may therefore be pigmented or nonpigmented; it is raised and dome shaped. The higher naevi are darker, deep intradermal naevi are lightly pigmented or skin coloured.

Naevi of the Nail Apparatus

These appear as pigmented streaks of even colour on the nails, extending from the nail matrix to the distal end of the nail. Any extension on the surrounding skin should be considered suspicious for malignancy.

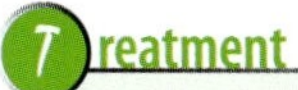

No treatment is required for most melanocytic naevi, apart from cosmetic removal. A nevus, which shows a change in size, color, shape, is inflamed, and the nevus, which has a history of bleeding or itching, should be excised and biopsied to exclude malignant transformation. A nevus, which is at a site of continuous irritation, should also be removed; it could be a site of later malignant change.

Spindle Cell Melanocytic Naevus (Epithelioid Naevus and Reed's Naevus)

The most common presentation is a solitary asymptomatic pink, verrucous or smooth surfaced telangiectatic papule or nodule. A halo of depigmentation is often seen surrounding these naevi. The diameter ranges from several millimetres to several centimetres, an average being about 8 mm. The most common site is the head and neck. Most cases are superficial; some may have a dermal involvement.

On microscopic examination nests of pigmented spindle shaped cells predominate. No cellular atypia is seen, but dermal inflammation can cause confusion with a melanoma. The spindle cells may infiltrate down the eccrine ducts and hair follicles. These cells are large about twice the size of epidermal basal keratinocytes. Mitosis is seen in some of the cells. Eosinophilic granules (Kamino bodies) are seen in 60% of cases.

The naevus should be differentiated from a melanoma and dysplastic naevus. It has a very distinctive star burst pattern on dermoscopy.

Treatment

Complete excision with a clear margin of normal skin.

Naevus Spilus (Speckled Lentiginous Naevus)

Naevus spilus is essentially a lentigo in which naevus cells are sometimes seen. These naevi are large; they can measure up to several centimetres in diameter, which is speckled with dark spots. The naevus is usually oval in shape, the borders are sharply defined. They can appear on any apart of the body. The lesion is benign, no treatment is necessary except for cosmetic reasons.

Congenital Melanocytic Naevus

These are present at birth and may be small (less than 1.5 cm in diameter), medium (1.5–20 cm in diameter) or large (greater than 20 cm in diameter). The giant bathing trunk naevus covers an entire body segment. One percent of all new born babies have a small congenital melanocytic naevus. Giant melanocytic naevi are found 200 times less frequently than the small ones. A striking feature of these naevi, which differentiates it from the acquired naevi, is the increased volume of naevus cells per unit of tissue. The naevus cells infiltrate into the skin appendages, a feature not seen in acquired naevi. The naevus cells can also be found between the collagen bundles and in the vessel wall. Signs of immature skin, young fat cells, cellular collagen and immature sebaceous and sweat glands are other features of congenital melanocytic naevi. Most congenital naevi are hairy, heavily pigmented and have a papillomatous surface. About 5–15% giant cell naevi can become malignant (Fig. 9).

Congenital melanocytic naevi can be junctional, compound or intradermal similar to acquired melanocytic naevi.

The giant congenital naevus (bathing trunk nevus) is extremely rare; it covers a large part of the trunk. There is an increased risk of malignant change in these naevi. These naevi become thick and hairy in childhood; occasionally it may be associated with other congenital abnormalities, such as spina bifida, when it is situated over the spinal column, hypertrophy, or atrophy of the deeper structures when it is on a limb.

Treatment

Treatment depends upon the size and site of the naevus. The reasons for removal are cosmetic and fear of malignant change. Small and medium sized naevi can be excised if required.

Large melanocytic naevi should be removed because of the danger of malignant change. Some authorities believe that dermabrasion should be done in the first week of life to reduce the naevus cell load. An alternative approach is to use the technique of tissue expansion by inserting inflatable balloons under the normal skin, and so create redundant epidermis, which can be used for definite excision and grafting procedure. Patients should be followed yearly; any new nodules that are highly suspicious should be excised.

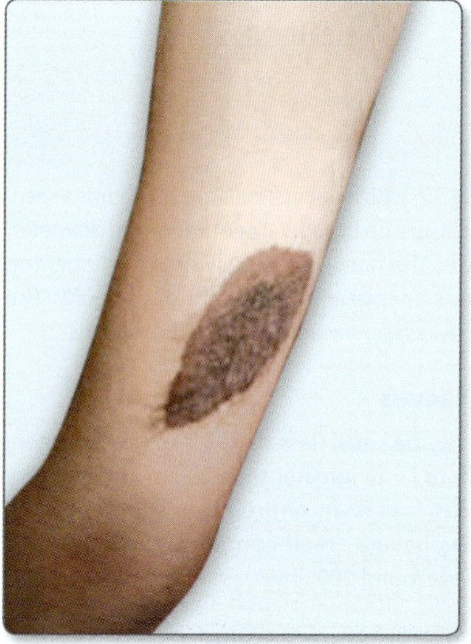

Fig. 9: Congenital melanocytic naevus

Halo Naevus (Sutton's Naevus)

This is a naevus that has a halo of depigmentation around it. This may be seen in childhood or adult life and the naevus gradually disappears after a few months. The area of depigmentation may then repigment. The halo naevus may be found with vitiligo and is thought to be an autoimmune process with antibodies against the melanocytes of the naevus. The lesion is not malignant and no treatment is required.

Blue Naevus

These are dermal proliferation of spindle shaped melanocytes.
Four types are recognised:

1. *Ordinary blue naevus:* This consists of spindle shaped cells with varying degrees of melanin; junctional changes are uncommon. The blue colour is due to the optical effect of dermal melanin. They appear as bluish-grey papules, usually less than 10 mm in diameter, most commonly found on the face or dorsum of the hands and feet.
2. *Cellular blue naevus:* Plump epithelioid cells are present in the deep dermis, often in the subcutaneous fat, sometimes with satellite lesions. Mitosis suggests a malignant change. These appear as bluish-brown or bluish-gray nodules or plaques. Most of these are located on the buttocks or sacrum.
3. *Combined naevus:* This is a combination of blue naevus and a compound naevus. The lesions are bluish-brown or bluish-black in colour, variable in size, they have a smooth or slightly irregular in appearance.
4. *Deep penetrating nevus:* Variant of ordinary blue naevus with junctional component, it extends deep into the dermis, often along adnexal structures, may even involve the subcutaneous fat.

The naevus should be differentiated from malignant melanoma and pigmented dermatofibroma.

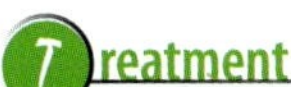

A blue naevus that is stable requires no treatment. Sudden expansion, those larger than 10 mm should be excised along with the subcutaneous fat. Cellular blue naevus should be evaluated because of its malignant potential.

Other Dermal Melanocytic Naevi

These naevi arise from the dermal melanocytes, which have failed to reach the epidermis as opposed to the epidermal melanocytes, which have completed their migration from the neural crest to the basal layer of the epidermis. The most common is the Mongolian spot; this appears as a macular blue grey pigmentation present at birth on the sacral area. The patches are round or oval up to 10 centimetres in diameter. The pigmentation usually disappears by the age of twelve. No treatment is required. A Mongolian spot occurring at extra-sacral location such as hands and feet is called Naevus of Yamamoto.

The other dermal naevi are the naevus of Ota; this is a bluish pigmentation of the sclera and the skin around it. Bilateral naevi of Ota are called naevus of Hori. The naevus of Ito occupies the acromioclavicular region and the upper chest, the blue naevus is found on the extremities. Apart from these, the

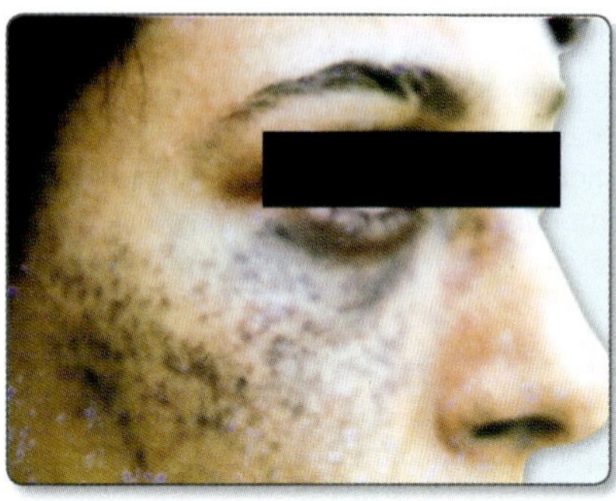

Fig. 10: Naevus of Ota

melanocytic naevi can be combined, i.e. having both a dermal and epidermal component, these naevi are relatively large with irregular borders and are frequently mistaken for a malignant melanoma (Fig. 10).

The blue colour is due to the optical effect of dermal melanin. The longer wavelengths of visible light are absorbed by the dermal melanin. The shorter blue wavelength does not penetrate deeply enough and is reflected back to the observers eye, giving a blue colour to the deeply situated melanin.

ATYPICAL NAEVUS (DYSPLASTIC NAEVUS)

Atypical naevus is larger than the acquired melanocytic naevi and have irregular borders that fade into the surrounding skin. These appear at puberty and continue to grow throughout life. Variations of colour within these lesions are found as well as a degree of inflammation, the diameter varies from 5 mm to 15 mm. Single or multiple lesions may be found in a single patient. These are commonly situated on the upper trunk in males and on the extremities in the females. These naevi show the features of asymmetry, irregular borders, show different shades of colour, diameter greater than 6 mm, and may be elevated (ABCDE rule). Atypical naevi are markers of increased melanoma risk. Atypical naevi are seen in a sporadic or familial setting. In a familial setting particularly in patients who already have one primary malignant melanoma, are at a risk factor for development of a melanoma (Fig. 11).

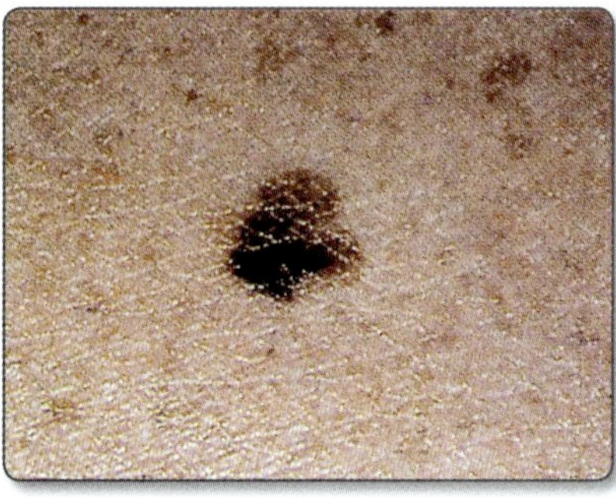

Fig. 11: Dysplastic nevus

Histology

Not all atypical naevi show atypia, but they all show signs of inflammation and fibrosis. Naevus cells are present in the dermis, often associated with impairment of maturation and synthesis of pigment.

The histopathological major and minor criteria for the diagnosis of atypical naevus.

- Major criteria
  1. Basilar proliferation of atypical melanocytes extending to three rete ridges beyond a dermal melanocyte component (if a dermal component is present)
  2. Pattern of intraepidermal melanocyte proliferation, which may be lentiginous or epithelioid
- Minor Criteria
  1. Concentric eosinophilic fibrosis or lamellar fibrosis
  2. Neovascularization
  3. Dermal inflammatory response
  4. Fusion of rete ridges

Diagnosis

These naevi should be differentiated from acquired melanocytic naevi and malignant melanoma. Malignant melanomas are not multiple. First-line blood relatives should be examined for atypical naevi at puberty.

Treatment

Patients showing a few atypical naevi should be excised. Lesions that are difficult to monitor should also be excised. Exposure to sunlight should be avoided.

Those with multiple naevi should have a periodic examination to exclude any suspicious change to melanoma, especially those who have a family history of melanoma. Total body photographs, dermoscopy and patient self-examination are used as adjuvant measures to follow patients with atypical naevi.

DYSPLASTIC NEVUS SYNDROME

The condition is associated with multiple dysplastic naevi and increased risk of malignant melanoma; some pedigrees have increased risk of carcinoma of the pancreas or ocular malignant melanoma. The condition is often familial with autosomal dominant inheritance. A number of genes are associated with familial dysplastic nevus such as CDKN2A (p16) (cyclin-dependent kinase inhibitor) at 9p21 or CDK4.

The condition is associated with multiple dysplastic naevi, often more than 100, most commonly situated on the trunk. There is an increased propensity of these naevi to become malignant. Some melanomas do not arise from the nevus, but from the apparently normal skin.

Complete body examination should be done with regular follow-up at frequent intervals. Total body photographs should be combined with computer-supported dermatoscopic examination. Excision and microscopic examination should be done of large and changing nevus. The patient should be taught self-examination of the naevi; note any change that occurs and to avoid exposure to direct sunlight.

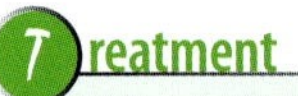

Treatment is similar to that of dysplastic naevus.

SPITZ NAEVI (Juvenile melanoma)

This is a variant of compound naevi; it is commonly seen on the face of young children but can occur at any age. It presents as a slow growing pink or pale brown lesion on the cheek of a child but may be darker in adults. Initially the surface is smooth but later becomes rough and scaly.

Histologically it resembles a compound naevus; however, the cells are larger with abundant eosinophilic cytoplasmic granules (Kamino bodies). The cells may be spindle shaped or epithelioid-like with clusters of giant and multinucleated cells; mitotic figures are seen but these are not numerous. The dermal vessels are dilated and the stroma may be oedematous and infiltrated with lymphocytes. An expert histopathological report is necessary for its diagnosis.

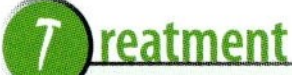

Treatment is by local excision with a wide margin of normal skin to confirm the clinical diagnosis.

Dark pigmented naevi on the acral region, mucosa and nails should be viewed with suspicion irrespective of the skin colour.
Moles exceeding 1 cm in size should suggest a congenital naevus,
Exclude malignancy by the ABCDE rule,
Patients with more than 50 naevi have a fivefold increase of melanoma risk,
Patients with more than 100 naevi have a fivefold increase of melanoma risk.

NAEVUS ACHROMICUS

Areas of depigmentation are present at birth. The lesions may be single or multiple. These may be round in a linear distribution or in whorls. The number of melanocytes in naevus achromic is normal, but there is a defect in the transfer of melanosomes from the melanocytes to the keratinocytes. It should be differentiated from the whorled hypomelanosis of Ito; in this condition there may be associated disorders in the CNS, musculoskeletal defects and the eyes. It should be differentiated from naevus anemicus by diascopy (Fig. 12).

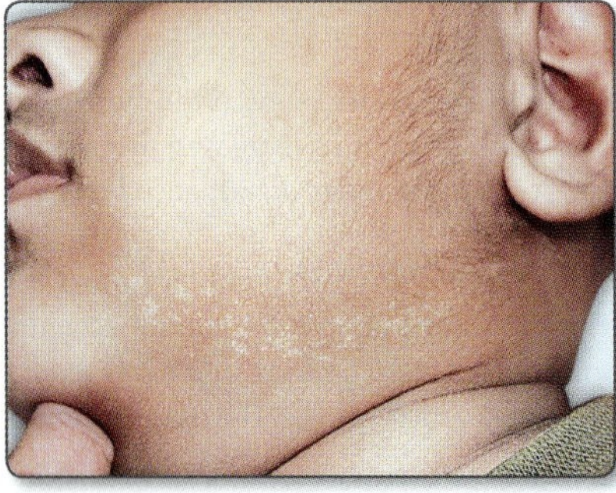

Fig. 12: Achromic naevus

LYMPHATIC MALFORMATIONS

Lymphatic malformations are malformed dilated lymphatic vessels in the skin because the embryonic lymph sacs have not connected correctly with the lymphatic system.

These can present as:

- Lymphangioma circumscriptum
- Cavernous lymphangioma
- Cystic hygroma

Lymphangioma Circumscriptum

Lymphangioma circumscriptum is a microcystic lymphatic malformation. It may be present at any age but is usually noted at birth or appear at childhood. The common sites are the axillary folds, shoulders, neck, proximal parts of a limb, perineum, tongue and the buccal mucous membrane. It presents as a group of deep-seated vesicles-like papules resembling frogspawn. They are yellowish in colour, but some may be pink or red in colour due to the presence of fresh or altered blood. Lymphangiomas rarely involute; they may enlarge or contract according to the changes in the flow of lymphatic fluid, presence of inflammation, or intralesional bleeding. Lymphangioma is often associated with bony hypertrophy especially on the face or extremity (Figs 13 and 14).

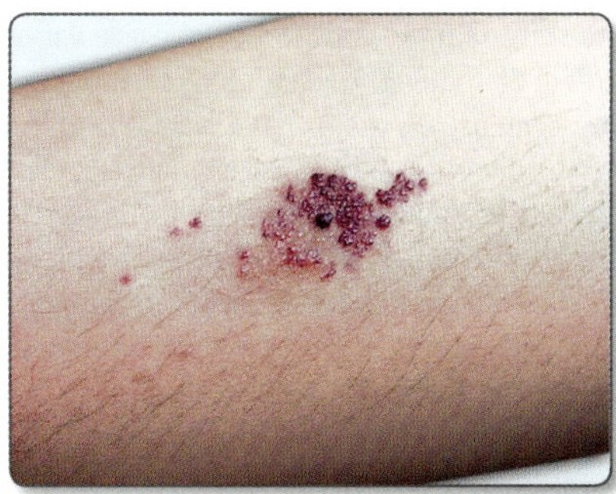

Fig. 13: Lymphangioma circumscriptum

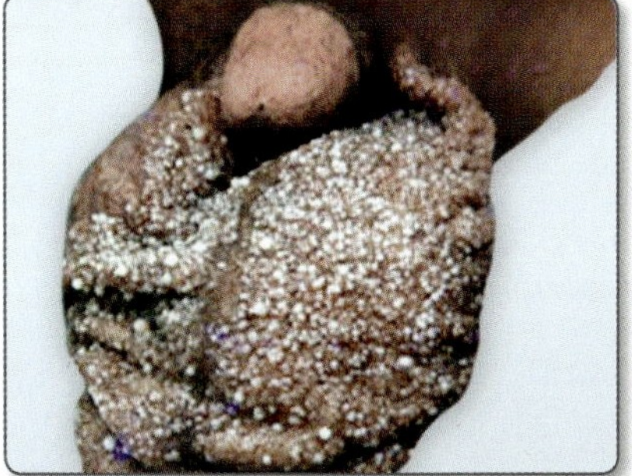

Fig. 14: Lymphangioma circumscriptum of the scrotum

These naevi should be differentiated from molluscum contagiosum. Lymphangioma circumscriptum are compressible with a glass depressor while molluscum is not.

Treatment

Lymphangioma circumscriptum should be removed along with the removal of the subcutaneous tissue or else they may regrow. Small lesions can be treated with laser ablation or cryotherapy.

Cavernous Lymphangioma

Cavernous lymphangioma can affect any site on the body, including the tongue. It presents as a skin coloured, red or bluish rubbery swelling under the skin. Sometimes, it has a period of fast growth in early childhood. Rarely, it may ulcerate. It is distinguished from other vascular naevi by the presence of clear fluid within the lumps and the findings on ultrasound scan.

Cystic Hygroma

These are deep unilocular lymphatic malformations that involve the soft tissues of face and neck, less commonly the axilla or groin.

CONNECTIVE TISSUE NAEVI

Connective tissue naevus is the term used for cutaneous hamartomas comprised primarily of collagen (collagenomas) and elastic (elastomas) tissue, or it may be a combination of these two. These naevi are produced by the fibroblasts. Collagenomas are skin coloured while elastomas may be skin coloured or yellowish. They may be present at birth or appear within the first few years of life. The naevi are soft to firm in consistency; the size varies from a 0.5 cm to several centimetres in diameter. The lesions may be grouped, linear or irregularly distributed. These are usually present as a plaque over the lumbosacral region. Connective tissue naevi can be excised if small (Fig. 15).

Some connective tissue naevi act as cutaneous markers for systemic disease, e.g. shagreen patch in tuberous sclerosis. Multiple connective tissue naevi called dermatofibrosis lenticularis disseminata are composed primarily of elastic tissue; these are cutaneous markers of Buschke-Ollendorff syndrome. This autosomal dominant disorder presents with osteopoikilosis of the bone and connective tissue naevi.

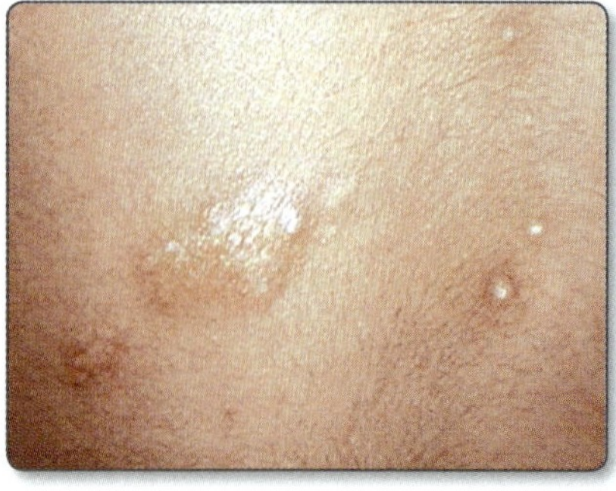

Fig. 15: Connective tissue naevus

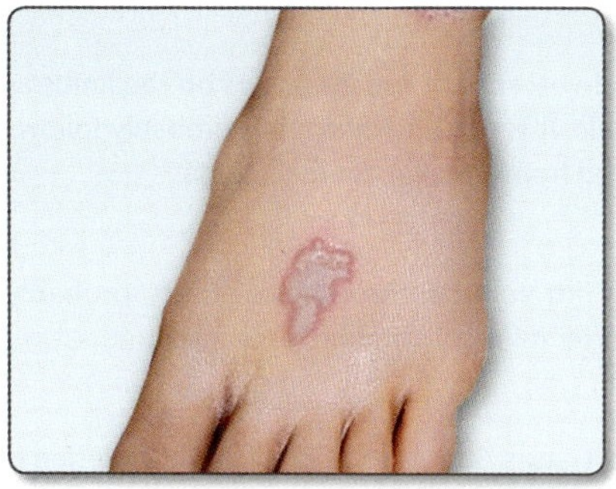

Fig. 16: Angiokeratoma

ANGIOKERATOMAS

Angiokeratoma is the name applied to a number of distinct conditions that share a common clinical presentation; this consists of asymptomatic hyperkeratosis, papillomatosis, acanthosis and superficial dermal vascular ectasia. The following types are recognised:

- Angiokeratoma of Mibelli
- Angiokeratoma circumscriptum
- Angiokeratoma of the scrotum and vulva
- Solitary angiokeratoma
- Angiokeratoma corporis diffusum and fucosidosis (discussed in chapter 31)

Angiokeratoma of Mibelli

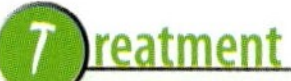

Electrocautery, fulguration and carbon dioxide laser give good results.

This occurs in adolescence often associated with cold intolerance and chilblains. It is an autosomal dominant disorder. The lesions appear as dull red verrucous rounded papules, situated on the dorsum of the fingers, toes, elbows and knees.

Histopathology

Dilated sub-papillary vessels form lacunae; the overlying epidermis is hyperkeratotic with increased thickness of the granular layer.

Angiokeratoma of the Scrotum (Fordyce)

Small red papules with minimal hyperkeratosis are present on the scrotum. Sometimes they may be associated with increased venous pressure in the area, e.g. a varicocele. These angiokeratomas occur in the second to third decade; they become more frequent with increasing age. Similar lesions may be seen in the vulva. Patients complain of pruritus and bleeding. Occasional there is superficial ectasia of the gingiva and oral cavity.

Angiokeratoma Circumscriptum

These are present at birth as a red warty growth. These occur in bands or streaks usually over an extremity.

Solitary Angiokeratoma

This develops in childhood or adolescence. It usually occurs on the limbs as a single bluish-black warty papule. It is not hereditary, but probably follows trauma. It should be differentiated from a malignant melanoma.

Course of Angiokeratomas

All lesions remain static unless intraluminal thrombosis occurs, probably secondary to trauma. Bleeding after minimal irritation is common.

Treatment

No treatment is necessary in most cases. Simple excision of a solitary lesion is curable, diathermy or laser therapy is also helpful. Angiokeratoma of Mibelli responds to cryotherapy. A varicocele if present in angiokeratoma of scrotum should be treated.

FURTHER READING

1. Adams BB, Mutasim DF. Adult onset verrucous epidermal nevus. J Am Acad Dermatol. 1999;41(5 Pt 2):824-6.
2. Ashinoff R, Geronemus RG. Capillary hemangiomas and treatment by the flash lamp-pulsed dye laser. Arch Dermatol. 1991;127(2):202-5.
3. Assmann A, Mandt N, Geilen CC, et al. Buschke-Ollendorff syndrome--differential diagnosis of disseminated connective tissue lesions. Eur J Dermatol. 2001;11(6):576-9.
4. Augustsson A, Stierner U, Suurkula M, et al. Prevalence of common and dysplastic naevi in a Swedish population. Br J Dermatol. 1991;124(2):152-6.
5. Bataille V, Bishop JA, Sasieni P, et al. Risk of cutaneous melanoma in relation to the numbers, type and sites of naevi: a case-controlled study. Br J Cancer. 1996;73(12):1605-11.
6. Cestari TF, Rubim M, Valentini BC. Nevus comedonicus: case report and brief review of the literature. Pediatr Dermatol. 1991;8(4):300-5.
7. Coleman WP, Gately LE, Krementz AB, et al. Nevi, lentigines and melanoma in blacks. Arch Dermatol. 1980;116(5):548-51.
8. DePadova-Elder S, Mols-Kowalczewskii BL, Lambert WC. Multiple connective tissue nevi. Cutis. 1988;42(3):222-4.
9. Donnelly LF, Adams DM, Bisset GS. Vascular malformations and hemangiomas. Am J Roentgenol. 2000;174(3):597-608.
10. Enjolras O, Mulliken JB. Vascular tumors and vascular malformations. Adv Dermatol. 1998;13:375-422.
11. Enjolras O, Mulliken JB. The current management of vascular birthmarks. Pediatr Dermatol. 1993;10(4):311-3.
12. Ezekowitz RA, Mullliken JB, Folkman J. Interferon alfa 2a therapy for the life-threatening haemangioma of infancy. N Engl J Med. 1992;28;326(22):1456-63.
13. Gioglio L, Porta C, Moroni M, et al. Scrotal angiokeratoma (Fordyce): histopathological and ultrastructural findings. Histol Histopathol. 1992;7(1):47-55.
14. Greaves MW, Birkett D, Johnson C. Nevus anemicus: a unique catecholamine dependent nevus. Arch Dermatol. 1970;102(2):172-6.
15. Happle R. Mosaicism in human skin: understanding the patterns and mechanisms. Arch Dermatol. 1993;129(11):1460-70.
16. Harvell JD, Meehan SA, LeBoit PE. Spitz nevi with a halo reaction. A histopathological study in 17 cases. J Cutan Pathol. 1997;24(10):611-9.
17. Kraema KH, Greene MH, Tarone R, et al. Dysplastic nevi and cutaneous melanoma risk. Lancet. 1983;5;2(8358):1076-7.
18. Martinez-Perez D, Fein NA, Boon CM, et al. Not all hemangiomas look like strawberries. Uncommon presentations of the most tumor of infancy. Pediatr Dermatol. 1995;12(1):1-6.
19. Peachey RD, Lim CC, Whimster IW. Lymphangioma of skin. A review of 65 cases. Br J Dermatol. 1970;83(5):519-27.

20. Rogers M, McCrossin I, Commens C. Epidermal nevi and epidermal nevus syndrome. A review of 131 cases. J Am Acad Dermatol. 1989;20(3):476-88.
21. Rogers M. Epidermal nevi and the epidermal nevus syndrome: a review of 233 cases. Pediatr Dermatol. 1992;9(4):342-4.
22. Sahl WJ Jr. Familial nevus sebaceous of Jadassohn. Occurrence in three generations. J Am Acad Dermatol. 1990;22(5 Pt 1):853-4.
23. Smoller BR, Rosen S. Port-wine stains. A disease of altered neural modulation of blood vessels? Arch Dermatol. 1986;122(2):177-9.
24. Tate PR, Hodge SJ, Owen LG. A quantitative study of melanocytes in Becker's nevus. J Cutan Pathol. 1980;7:404.

Chapter

29 Malnutrition and Skin

INTRODUCTION

Malnutrition may be due to improper or inadequate food intake, or it may result from inadequate absorption of food. Certain metabolic abnormalities may also lead to malnutrition. Precise evaluation of food status in chronic malnutrition usually involves deficit of more than a single nutrient.

HYPOVITAMINOSIS A

Vitamin A and its derivatives are required for the normal growth of most cells in the body, especially different types of epithelial cells and transduction of visual images by the retina. It is also responsible for growth and reproduction. Normal amount of vitamin A required for an adult is 5,000 IU daily. Some manifestations of vitamin A deficiency are as follows:

Cutaneous Manifestations

Deficiency of vitamin A in the skin causes proliferation of basal cells, follicular hyperkeratosis and xerosis. Follicular papules are especially seen on the dorsal and lateral aspect of the extremities, called phrynoderma, it later spreads to other parts of the body. The hands and feet are not involved and only rarely are the lesions present on the axillary or anogenital areas.

On the face, the lesions resemble acne because of the presence of comedones, but differ from acne as deficiency of vitamin A is associated with dryness of the skin.

Epithelial metaplasia also occurs in the vagina, urinary tract and testicular epithelium.

Ocular Involvement

Posterior segment of the eye is affected first with impairment of dark adaptation and night blindness. Later the anterior segment of the eye is involved with drying of the cornea, conjunctiva, followed by wrinkling and cloudiness of the cornea known as keratomalacia. Dry silvery plaques appear on the bulbar conjunctiva (Bitot's spots), with follicular hyperkeratosis of the eyelashes.

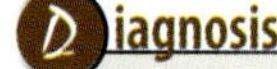

Aided by vitamin A levels in the blood, normally it is over 20 mg/dl.

Treatment

Vitamin A 50,000 IU is recommended daily until symptom resolve and serum vitamin A levels is normalised.

Deficiency of vitamin A also leads to reduced immunity. There is an increased incidence to viral and parasitic infections. The number and function of natural killer cells is also reduced.

HYPERVITAMINOSIS A

Clinically symptoms of hypervitaminosis A resemble those of hypovitaminosis A, most cases of hypervitaminosis A are seen in children. Vitamin A derivatives should be carefully evaluated and monitored when given to children. Children with hypervitaminosis A have anorexia, nausea, and vomiting; there is increasing irritability, limitation of movements and tender swelling of the bones. Roentgenograms reveal hyperostosis affecting several long bones. This is most notable in the middle of the shafts. Alopecia, seborrhoeic dermatitis like skin lesions and fissuring of the corners of the mouth may occur. Papilloedema with pseudotumour cerebri may occur very early, before any other signs appear, apparently due to some idiosyncrasy. It is preceded by headache.

In adults, the premonitory signs are dryness of the lips and anorexia, which may be followed by bone and joint pains, desquamation of the skin, dryness and loss of scalp hair and eyebrows, dystrophy of the nails, and hyperpigmentation of the face and neck resembling chloasma or Riehl's melanosis. Symptoms develop after taking doses in excess of 50,000 IU units daily, taken over months.

Prognosis is good on withdrawal of vitamin A, symptoms subsiding in a few days or weeks.

VITAMIN B COMPLEX

These include a number of vitamins that are important constituents of the enzymes system. These vitamins support and increase the rate of cell metabolism, maintain healthy skin and muscle tone; they also help in the function of nervous tissue and immune system. Since most of these enzymes have closely related functions, lack of one factor can interrupt an entire chain of normal chemical processes and produce diversified clinical manifestations. Diet deficient in one factor of the vitamin B complex series and are frequently poor sources of other vitamin B complex components. Although closely related in function, they vary greatly in chemical composition.

The members of the vitamin B complex series are:

Thiamine (Vitamin B_1)

Thiamine functions as a co-enzyme in carbohydrate metabolism; it is also required for the synthesis of acetylcholine. Its deficiency may result in impaired nerve function, wet (cardiac) and dry (neurological) beriberi. Cutaneous manifestations are limited to oedema, the skin appears waxy, and the tongue is red with burning sensation.

Riboflavin (Vitamin B_2)

Riboflavin deficiency is rarely encountered without other manifestations due to deficiencies of Vitamin B group. Riboflavin forms co-enzymes; this in turn operates as hydrogen carriers in the important oxidative systems of the mitochondria. The deficiency is often seen in children who when weaned from breast milk are not fed on milk. This is common in underdeveloped countries.

Its deficiency is often seen in alcoholics and sometimes in neonates receiving phototherapy for jaundice. The classical findings of the oro-ocular-genital syndrome are present. These include angular stomatitis, nasolabial seborrhoea, blepharitis, cheilitis, atrophic glossitis, magenta red tongue, corneal vascularisation, hyperpigmentation, redness and scaling of the vulva and scrotum.

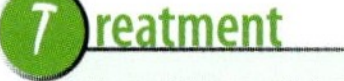

Five milligram of riboflavin daily is required, the response is dramatic.

Pyridoxine (Vitamin B_6)

Pyridoxine acts as a coenzyme in decarboxylation and transamination of amino acids. It is used in the metabolism of cysteine, tryptophan and essential fatty acids. It helps in the conversion of linoleic acid to arachidonic acid.

Pyridoxine deficiency may follow therapy with isonoiazid, hydralazine and penicillamine.

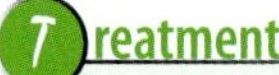

Pyridoxine (10–100 mg) daily may be necessary. Recommended daily allowance is about 2 mg.

Four clinical disturbances due to vitamin B_6 deficiency have been described:

1. Convulsion in infants
2. Peripheral neuritis
3. Dermatitis and
4. Anaemia.

Cutaneous lesions include cheilitis, glossitis, seborrheic dermatitis like lesions around the eyes and nose.

Cyanocobalamin (Vitamin B_{12})

Vitamin B_{12} performs several metabolic functions, and acting as hydrogen acceptor coenzyme. Its most important function is to act as a coenzyme for reducing ribonucleotide to deoxyribonucleotide, a step that is necessary for the replication of genes. It helps in the promotion of growth, RBC formation and maturation. Vitamin B_{12} is essential for neurons and rapidly dividing cells such as the skin cells. Vitamin B_{12} is absorbed through the distal ileum, after binding to gastric intrinsic factor in an acidic pH. Deficiency is seen in pernicious anaemia following gastrectomy.

Glossitis, hyperpigmentation and canities are the main dermatological manifestations. The tongue is bright red and sore, pigmentation is most pronounced in skin flexures, such as those of the fingers, palmar creases and on the knuckles. Pigmented streaks on the nail may be seen.

Folic Acid Deficiency

The most important function of folic acid in the body is the synthesis of purine and thymine, which is required for the formation of deoxyribonucleic acid. Folic acid is converted to folinic acid, which is the biologically active form;

vitamin C is required for its conversion. Therefore, folic acid like vitamin B_{12} is also required for the replication of cellular genes. It is important for the maturation of RBC.

Deficiency of folic acid gives rise to diffuse hyperpigmentation, glossitis, cheilitis and megaloblastic anaemia resembling vitamin B_{12} deficiency. Folic acid deficiency in pregnancy can lead to neural tube defects in the fetus, supplements of folic acid are therefore essential in pregnancy especially in the first trimester.

Biotin B_7 (Vitamin H)

Biotin acts as a coenzyme in decarboxylation and other enzymatic processes. Deficiency can occur by eating raw egg white; avidin in the egg binds biotin and makes it poorly absorbable.

Biotin deficiency results in seborrhoeic dermatitis like lesions, alopecia, conjunctivitis, hyperesthesia, and paraesthesia. Biotin is used in high doses for the treatment of Leiner's disease.

Niacin (Vitamin B_3, Nicotinic Acid)

Niacin functions in the body as coenzymes in the form of nicotinamide adenine dinucleotide (NAD) and nicotinamide adenine dinucleotide phosphate (NADP). These coenzymes act as hydrogen acceptors. When niacin is deficient, the normal rate of dehydrogenation cannot be maintained, and oxidation delivery of energy from the foodstuffs to functional elements cannot occur at normal rates. Niacin is obtained from the diet, it is also synthesised from tryptophan.

In early stages of niacin deficiency, simple physiological changes such as muscular weakness and poor glandular secretions occur, but in severe cases of niacin deficiency actual death of the cells may occur.

Deficiency of niacin results in pellagra (*pellis*, skin; *agra*, rough). This deficiency disease affects all tissues of the body. The classical triad of pellagra include: diarrhoea, dermatitis, and dementia. The most characteristic manifestations are cutaneous, which may develop suddenly or insidiously, sunlight may exacerbate these lesions. The lesions appear as symmetrically developed erythema of the exposed areas. The erythema resembles sunburn. The lesions are sharply demarcated from the healthy tissue around them. The appearance on the hands is known as the pellagrous glove, and similar demarcation is seen on the foot and leg is known as the pellagrous foot and that of the neck is the Casal's necklace. The pellagrous nose is characteristic. There is dull erythema on the bridge of the nose with slight scaling. The scaling gives a powdery appearance. Thickening of skin follows the erythema. After several weeks or months the epidermis desquamates leaving the affected parts deeply pigmented. The eruption has a tendency to be worse in summer months.

In some cases vesicles and bullae develop. The healed part of the skin remains pigmented. The cutaneous lesions are sometimes preceded by the symptoms of the alimentary tract such as stomatitis, glossitis, vomiting and diarrhoea. The tongue is intensely red with swelling of the papillae, ulcerations may even occur. Nervous system signs include depression, disorientation insomnia and delirium.

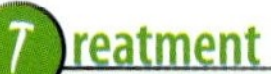

Treatment

Nicotinamide (100 mg) is given four times a day, along with adequate nutrition such as animal proteins, eggs, milk and vegetables.

Pellagra is caused by a deficiency of niacin or its precursor tryptophan. It is often seen in maize eating people. Maize contains a low concentration of niacin. It is also present in people eating jawar, in which the leucine content is high; this alters the tryptophan metabolism. Pellagra-like lesions may also occur in Hartnup disease in which there is a failure in the absorption of tryptophan from the gastrointestinal tract. In carcinoid syndrome, pellagra-like lesions is seen because tryptophan is unable to produce niacin due to the altered metabolism of tryptophan. Some drugs can induce pellagra-like lesions such as isoniazid, 6-mercaptopurine 5-fluorouracil, sulphonamides, anticonvulsive and antidepressive drugs.

No skin changes are seen in deficiency of pantothenic acid—vitamin B_5.

VITAMIN D

Vitamin D is also called the sunshine vitamin as vitamin D is produced in the skin from 7-dehydrocholesterol with the help of ultraviolet light. Deficiency of vitamin D results in tetany and rickets in children and osteomalacia in adults. Rickets can be congenital or acquired. There are two types of vitamin D-dependent rickets (DDR). Type I DDR is due to an inborn error of renal metabolism, it is not associated with skin disease. Type II DDR is genetically determined; it is an autosomal recessive disorder, most often caused by mutations in the vitamin D receptor gene. It is characterised by progressive diffuse alopecia in the first year of life.

Rickets is characterised by craniotabes (thinning of the skull bones), rachitic rosary (costochondral thickening, which looks like a string of rosary beads), pigeon breast (sternum protrusion) and Harrison's groove (depression along the line of diaphragmatic insertion into the rib cage). Osteomalacia resembles osteoporosis.

Acquired vitamin D deficiency is due to decreased exposure to sunlight, poor intake of vitamin D, taking of anticonvulsive drugs, malabsorption, pancreatitis, or biliary disease.

Treatment

Daily administration of 1,500–5,000 units of vitamin D will produce healing in 2–3 weeks. Therapeutic overdose of vitamin D will result in hypercalcaemia and generalised calcinosis. Metastatic calcification may be produced in the skin.

VITAMIN K

Vitamin K is necessary for the synthesis of prothrombin, factor VII, IX and X by the liver, which are important in blood coagulation. Purpura occurs due to vitamin K deficiency. Dicumarol produces hypoprothrombinemia; Salicylic acid is a degradation product of dicumarol also produces hypoprothrombinemia. Large doses of salicylic acid should be avoided in treating cutaneous disorders associated with vitamin K deficiency. Vitamin K is used in the treatment of haemorrhagic disease of the newborn in which prothrombin levels are low.

VITAMIN E (α-tocopherol)

Vitamin E is a fat soluble antioxidant and may be involved in nucleic acid metabolism. It is widely distributed in foods. In animals, its deficiency causes degeneration of the germinal epithelium in testis resulting in male infertility. Lack of vitamin E also causes resorption of the fetus after conception. It increases sperm motility. Vitamin E is often called the "anti-sterility" vitamin.

Various dermatological diseases and conditions have been said to respond to vitamin E. It has an inhibitory effect on hyaluronic acid and a protective effect on cellular membrane. It is an antioxidant, and it may have an anti-wrinkling effect.

It has been suggested that large doses of vitamin E have been shown to reduce the risk of myocardial infarction.

VITAMIN C (Ascorbic acid)

Vitamin C is a strong organic acid; it is required for the growth and repair of tissues in all parts of the body. It is necessary to form collagen, tendons, ligaments and blood vessels. Vitamin C is an antioxidant, a co-factor in many enzymatic reactions. It is used for removing wrinkles, and is used in anti-aging creams. Vitamin C also helps in the formation of hard keratin. It is also reported that vitamin C, in addition to removing free radicals, also increases the capacity of fibroblasts to repair potentially mutagenic DNA, it also stimulates the fibroblasts and promotes their migration to wounded areas.

Vitamin C in small amounts is found in all fruits and vegetables. Increased concentrations are found in citrus fruit, strawberries, tomatoes, green leafy vegetables, cabbage and broccoli. Daily requirement is 80 mg.

Deficiency of vitamin C leads to impaired formation of collagen and ground substance; this leads to symptoms involving the bones, mucous membranes, cartilage and the skin.

The cutaneous changes manifest after several months following the deficiency of vitamin C. These include follicular keratosis with associated hair coiled (corkscrew hair) in the follicle. The lesions are found on the upper arms, back, buttocks and lower extremities. This is followed by perifollicular purpura, particularly on the legs. This is due to the decrease in dermal collagen that provides vascular support. Generalised ecchymosis can occur. There is a delay in wound healing, and a tendency in breaking of old scars. Other manifestations include edema of the lower extremities, swelling and bleeding from the gums. Gingival necrosis may occur.

MINERALS

A number of minerals have nutritional significance. These include calcium, magnesium, potassium, sodium, phosphorus, sulphur and chloride. Iron, cobalt, and iodine are present in the body in important organic complexes. The trace elements fluoride, copper, zinc, manganese, selenium, silicon, boron, nickel, aluminium, arsenic, bromine, molybdenum, and strontium are present in the diet, but their significant functions in the body are not fully understood.

Minerals of dermatological importance are zinc, sulphur, calcium, copper, and selenium.

Zinc

Zinc is an integral part of many enzymes; one of the most important enzyme is carbonic anhydrase present in high concentrations in the RBC. Zinc is also present in the gastrointestinal mucosa, tubules of the kidney and epithelial cells of many glands of the body. Zinc in small quantities is essential for the performance of many reactions relating to carbon dioxide metabolism. Zinc is also a component of lactic dehydrogenase. This is important for the interconversion between pyruvic acid and lactic acid. Zinc is a component of some peptidases, which are used for the digestion of proteins from the gastrointestinal tract.

High concentrations of zinc are present in nuts, shellfish, legumes and green leafy vegetables. Phytate interferes with zinc absorption therefore high fibre content in the diet interferes with the absorption of zinc from the gastrointestinal tract. Zinc deficiency may be inherited (acrodermatitis enteropathica) or acquired.

Acute Zinc Deficiency

The symptoms of acute deficiency include septicemia, photophobia and mental depression. Eczematous changes are seen on the hands, feet, anogenital regions, and around the body orifices. The palmar and finger creases show bullae surrounded by reddish-brown erythema. There is paronychial inflammation, angular stomatitis with sparing of the vermillion border of the lips.

Chronic Zinc Deficiency

The patient is often listless and depressed. Skin lesions are seen at the site of repeated trauma such as: knees, elbows, knuckles, and malleolar region of the ankles. The lesions are thick, well-demarcated brownish in colour. Lichenification and scaling are often present. Seborrhoeic dermatitis-like lesions are often seen on the face. The growth of the hair and nails are slow; there is diffuse thinning of the scalp hair, total alopecia may often result. Beau's lines may be seen on the nails due to the arrest of growth.

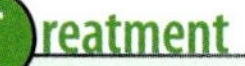

Zinc in a dose of 0.2 mg/kg of the body weight/day is required (10–20 mg/day). In acrodermatitis enteropathica higher doses of 2 mg/kg are given due to poor zinc absorption.

Selenium

Selenium is an integral part of the enzyme glutathione peroxidase. It plays an important role in preventing oxidative damage by endogenous peroxides. The exact role of selenium on the skin is not known. Patients of acne, psoriasis, seborrhoeic dermatitis and dermatitis herpetiformis have low glutathione peroxidase activity than normal subjects. Serum glutathione levels have a prognostic value in the follow-up of malignant melanoma and cutaneous T cell lymphoma. Selenium sulphide shampoos are used in the treatment of seborrhoeic dermatitis.

Selenium perhaps plays a protective role in cardiovascular, cancer and rheumatic diseases.

Sulphur

Sulphur is a vital element for normal functions of the human body. It is an essential component of the amino acids methionine and cysteine, and of chondroitin sulphate, these are involved in keratinization and formation of dermal collagen. When the supply of sulphur containing amino acids is inadequate, less sulphur is available for the nail and hair growth, but skin keratin production is normal. In exfoliative dermatitis, there is excessive loss of sulphur from the scales of the skin. Hair loss in exfoliative dermatitis is due to the diversion of sulphur containing amino acids to skin proteins instead of hair keratin formation.

Trichothiodystrophy is a syndrome in which hair are brittle due to sulphur deficiency. The hair is short and sparse the disease is inherited as an autosomal recessive trait.

Calcium

The human body contains more calcium than any other mineral. It is a key to skeletal muscle and myocardial contraction, neurotransmission and blood coagulation. Calcium-protein complex is important for skin permeability. Calcium is present in the body mainly as calcium phosphate in the bone. Excessive quantities of calcium in the extracellular fluid can cause the heart to stop in systole, and it can also cause mental depression. Low levels of calcium can cause spontaneous discharge of nerve fibres resulting in tetany.

Excessive intake of vitamin D, milk and alkalis containing calcium may result in metastatic deposit of calcium in the skin.

Silicon

Silicon is an essential trace element for the formation and maintenance of connective tissue. It increases the tissue levels of hydroxyproline, one of the key amino acids required for the formation of collagen. Studies have shown improvement in skin roughness, firmness and strength by silicon. Silicon also improves the brittleness of nails and hair.

Manganese

Manganese is present in melanocytes in high concentration. It is necessary for arginase activity in the epidermis. Changes in hair colour and slow growth of hair can occur in patients with manganese deficiency.

ESSENTIAL FATTY ACIDS

Essential fatty acids are those that the body cannot synthesize, and therefore, have to be taken from the diet. Amongst these are linolenic acid and oleic acid. Linolenic acid is the parent molecule of arachidonic acid. The essential fatty acids contribute to the formation of lamellar granules of the stratum corneum.

Deficiency of essential fatty acids can occur in patients who are on prolonged parenteral diet with impaired fat absorption, or those who take skimmed milk as diet substitute. Deficiency can lead to dry, scaly skin, loss of hair and weeping intertriginous eruptions. Periorificial lesions similar to zinc deficiency are also reported. Systemic manifestations include fatty liver, thrombocytopenia, anaemia, impaired wound healing, and increased susceptibility to infection.

Treatment is with essential fatty acid replacement. Linolenic acid (5 g) daily is required to prevent deficiency.

Hydration: Water and the Skin

Water forms a major part of our body, it constitutes about two-thirds of our body weight. Water helps in many body functions such as digestion, absorption, circulation and excretion. In the skin, it helps in its hydration and allows the skin to maintain its elasticity and suppleness. Certain toxins can also be excreted through the pores of the skin. About eight glasses of water are required by the body in a day.

The ground substance of the dermis is made of glycosaminoglycans, which supports the collagen and elastic tissue, it has a remarkable capacity to hold water, and it helps in the passage of nutrients, hormones, and fluid molecules through the dermis. Glycosaminoglycans are attached to a protein core to form proteoglycans. These form enormous hydrated space filling polymers in extracellular matrix. Proteoglycans form healthy and resilient connective tissue.

Glycosaminoglycans and in particular hyaluronic acid and chondroitin sulphate are easily hydrated; they combine with water molecules to form highly viscous fluid. In the skin, this affinity for water molecules helps in removing wrinkles, and sagging of the skin seen with aging. Glycosaminoglycans are used in cosmetic dermatology as fillers for rejuvenating the skin.

High amounts of hyaluronic acid and dermatan sulphate are present in the lesional skin of pseudoxanthoma elasticum. Pseudoxanthoma alters the metabolism of key polysaccharides.

Dry skin causes pruritus; it is a common problem seen in the elderly, in atopic dermatitis, ichthyosis, leprosy, thyroid disorders, chronic renal failure, etc. Moisturisers and increase in water intake are required to keep the skin hydrated.

MARASMUS

Marasmus is derived from a Greek word "*marasmos*" which means wasting. It is a severe form of starvation often seen in developing countries due to economic problems, improper weaning due to ignorance, poor hygiene, etc. Intake of all nutrients is reduced. Protein-calorie malnutrition leads to suppression of growth, loss of weight and emaciation results. The skin is dry, loose and wrinkled due

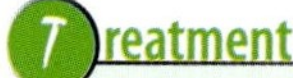

Complete and balanced diet has to be instituted. Skin ulcerations may respond to topical zinc paste or oral zinc in addition to a protein rich diet. Low level of zinc is a predominant feature in marasmus.

to the loss of subcutaneous fat. The sunken and drawn appearance of the face is due to the loss of buccal fat giving the typical monkey facies appearance. Follicular hyperkeratosis may be prominent in adult persons. The hair is thin and sparse, nails are fissured, and cutaneous ulcerations may occur.

KWASHIORKOR

Kwashiorkor is characterised by protein malnutrition that impairs growth, produces changes in the skin and hair; there is edema of the feet and a potbelly prominence. Other deficiencies also co-exist such as zinc deficiency, essential fatty acid deficiency associated with the presence of free radicals and leukotrienes.

The changes in the skin and hair are striking; they vary from reddish-yellow to grey or even white. The hair is dry, scaly, and lustreless; curly hair becomes straight, especially striking is the "flag sign" affecting the long-dark hair. During periods of poor nutrition, the hair is pale, alternating bands of dark and light hair is thus seen, indicating period of good and poor nutrition.

The skin in the early stages is scaly and erythematos, later these patches become hard, scaly, and distinctively elevated; "enamel paint" appearance. Other signs of malnutrition are present as angular stomatitis and glossitis.

Children affected with kwashiorkor have poor development, their height and weight is below normal, and diarrhoea is common. There is oedema of the feet and face due to hypoalbuminemia. The oedema later becomes generalised, subcutaneous fat is lost, and muscles become wasted. The child is irritable, does not smile, and when he does it is a sign of recovery. The child is prone to bacterial and parasitic infection.

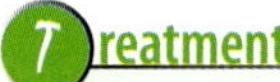

Balanced diet supplements with higher protein and vitamins should be given. Electrolyte levels should be corrected.

PLUMMER-VINSON SYNDROME

Plummer-Vinson syndrome is a combination of microcytic anaemia: dysphagia and glossitis seen mostly in middle-aged women. The anaemia is hypochromic and microcytic due to deficiency of iron, the skin is dry and wrinkled, hair is scanty, and koilonychia is seen in 40–50% of patients; the tongue is smooth and atrophic.

The lips are thin, opening of the mouth is small and inelastic, and difficulty in swallowing is characterised by feeling of food becoming stuck in the throat. Often a radiological examination demonstrates oesophageal stricture at the postcricoid region. The syndrome is precancerous, it can give rise to cancer of the oesophagus and mouth, and often the oesophageal stricture is the site of carcinoma.

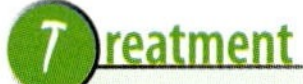

Treatment is by iron therapy and a high vitamin diet.

OBESITY

Obesity is an excess proportion of total body fat. The most common measure of obesity is the body mass index or BMI. A person is considered overweight if BMI is between 25 and 29.9; a person is considered obese if BMI is over 30. Obesity increases the likelihood of various diseases, particularly heart disease, type 2 diabetes, hypertension, stroke, infertility, and osteoarthritis.

Obesity can lead to a number of skin problems such as intertrigo. This is due to friction between the skin surfaces, which leads to secondary bacterial and fungal infection. Striae are common; these are prominent on the arms, thighs, buttocks and abdomen. Skin tags, acanthosis nigricans, and hirsutism are other skin conditions seen in obese patients. It is important that the underlying cause of obesity is removed to eradicate the cutaneous lesions which occur due to obesity.

Control of diet, eating healthy food and exercise are helpful in reducing obesity. Bariatric surgery can reduce the risk of disease in people with severe obesity.

FURTHER READING

1. Berkner KL, Runge KW. The physiology of vitamin K nutriture and vitamin K-dependent protein function in atherosclerosis. *J Throm Haemostat*. 2004;2:2118–32.
2. Bjorntorp P. Obesity. *Lancet*. 1997;350:423–5.
3. Harris SS. Vitamin D and African Americans. *J Nutr*. 2006;136(4):1126–9.
4. Harris SS, Soteriades E, Coolidge JAS, et al. Vitamin D insufficiency and hyperparathyroidism in a low income, multiracial elderly population. *J Clin Endocrinol Met*. 2000;85(11):4125–30.
5. Kiamal S, Thappa DM. Diet in dermatology revisited. *Ind J Dermatol Venereol Leprol*. 2010;76(2):103–15.
6. Natajaran VS, Ravindran S, Krishnaswamy B, et al. High prevalence of nutritional disorders and nutrient deficits in elderly people in a rural community in Tamil Naidu. *J Hong Kong Ger Soc*. 1995;6:40–3.
7. Pence BC, Delver E, Dunn DM. Effects of dietary selenium on UVB-induced skin carcinogenesis and epidermal antioxidant status. *J Inves Dermatol*. 1994;102:759–61.
8. Purba MB, Kouris-Blazos A, Wattanapenpaiboon N, et al. Skin wrinkling: can food make a difference? *J Am Coll Nutr*. 2001;20(1):71–80.
9. Ross EM. Iron deficiency anemia: risks, symptoms and treatment. *Nutr Clin Care*. 2002;5: 220–24.
10. Wahliqvist ML, Savige GS, Lukito W. Nutritional disorders in the elderly. *Med J Aus*. 1995;163:376–81.

Chapter

30 Primary Cutaneous Immunodeficiency

INTRODUCTION

The immune system is divided into two functional components: the innate and the adaptive. Innate immunity is the first-line of defense in the body; it is comprised of phagocytes, these consist of neutrophils, monocytes and macrophages. The adaptive immune system comes into play when there is a breach in the innate system. This system produces a specific reaction to each infectious agent and prevents it from attacking the body when it is introduced later.

INNATE IMMUNITY

This system consists mainly of the phagocytes. Natural killer cells, acute phase proteins and complement also help in innate immunity.

The phagocytes include the fixed macrophages of the reticuloendothelial tissues in the lungs, spleen, liver, lymph nodes and bone marrow. It also consists of the wandering macrophages: the polymorphonuclear leukocytes and monocytes of blood. Eosinophils may be involved in the phagocytosis of the antigen antibody complexes.

Phagocytes

Neutrophils and monocytes attack and destroy invading bacteria and other infectious microorganisms. The neutrophils are mature cells that destroy these organisms, in the circulating blood. Blood monocytes are immature cells that have very little ability to fight against infection. Once they enter the tissues, they change into macrophages, which are extremely capable of combating infection.

The most important function of neutrophils and macrophages is phagocytosis. This it does with the help of acute phase proteins, natural killer cells and complement. Thus, both the innate immune system and adaptive immune system are inter-related. Macrophages when activated are much more powerful phagocytes than neutrophils. They can phagocytise as much as hundred bacteria; they can even phagocytise whole RBC and even malarial parasites. Neutrophils are not capable of phagocytising particles larger than bacteria. Macrophages can also phagocytise necrotic tissue and even dead neutrophils.

Macrophages and neutrophils are stimulated to phagocytosis by cytokines from other cell, particularly the lymphocytes. On stimulation, they produce a number of cytokines and enzymes to kill the invading microorganism. Macrophages also present processed antigens to T and B lymphocytes. Some of the bactericidal substances produced by phagocytes are lysozymes, lactoferrin and hydrogen peroxide.

Natural Killer Lymphocytes

When a cell becomes infected with an invasive microorganism, its surface molecules are altered. These alterations are recognised by the natural killer cells, which engulf the microorganism and kill it. Cells infected with virus produce interferons, which prevent viral replication. Interferons are also released by T lymphocytes.

Acute Phase Proteins

The serum concentration of a number of proteins increases rapidly during infection. The acute phase proteins include C-reactive protein, so called because of its ability to bind to the C-protein of pneumococci. C-reactive proteins provide binding of the complement. It enhances phagocytic phagocytosis, this is known as opsonisation.

Complement

The complement is a group of about twenty proteins in the blood, which interact with one another and with the other components of innate and adaptive immune system. The microorganisms activate the complement system. It stimulates the antigen-antibody complexes via the alternative or classical pathway. The principal activities of the complement system are directed at protection against infection. It has a wide range of biological effects. One of its components C_3 seems to play a role in immunological memory.

The complement helps in the following biological effects:

- Histamine release
- Neutralisation of viruses
- Release of kinins
- Increased vascular permeability
- Leukocyte immobilisation
- Promotion of phagocytosis
- Promotion of fibrinolysis
- Promotion of coagulation.

ADAPTIVE IMMUNITY

Two basic types of adaptive immunity occur in the body: humoral immunity and cell-mediated immunity.

Humoral immunity: The body develops circulating antibodies, which are capable of attacking the invading organism. This is called the humoral immunity and is brought about by B lymphocytes; these change to plasma cells to produce the respective antibodies.

Cell-mediated immunity: The adaptive immunity is achieved through the formation of large number of activated lymphocytes that are specially designed to destroy the foreign agents. This immunity is called the cell-mediated immunity. It is brought about by the T lymphocytes.

The lymphocytes are formed in the bone marrow. Those lymphocytes, which are destined to form activated T lymphocytes first migrate to and are processed by the thymus, for this reason they are called T lymphocytes. They are responsible for cell-mediated immunity.

The other populations of lymphocytes that are destined to form antibodies are processed in the liver during mid-fetal life, and in the bone marrow in late fetal life and after birth. These cells were first discovered in birds, in which the processing occurs in Bursa of Fabricius, were called B lymphocytes.

HUMORAL IMMUNITY

This is carried out by the B lymphocytes. The B cells transform into plasma cells, which produce and secrete antibodies or immunoglobulins. An antibody first binds to the specific antigen and then inactivates them. T helper cells aid both cell-mediated immunity and antibody-mediated immunity.

Immunoglobulins

Immunoglobulins consist of four chains of polypeptides: two short and two long chains. These are parallel to each other, the short lighter chain (L); enclose a pair of large heavy chains (H). All four chains are joined at intervals by sulphydryl bonds. Within the light and heavy chains are two distinct regions. The tip of H and L chains is called the variable region or fragment (V); it contains the specific antigen binding sites (Fab). The variable region is specific for each antigen. The antibody recognises a particular antigen and binds to it. The remainder of the H and L chain is called the constant region or fragment (C, Fc). The constant region is nearly the same in all immunoglobulins of the same class. Its structure serves as a basis of distinguishing the five different types of immunoglobulins. The constant region is also responsible for the particular mediators of the antigen-antibody reaction that occurs, after binding of the antigen to the antibody (Fig. 1). The different types of immunoglobulins are IgG, IgM, IgA, IgD and IgE.

IgG

This accounts for 73% of the total immunoglobulins. It is found in the blood and interstitial tissue. It is the only globulin that crosses the placenta. It plays the major part in the antibody activity of an individual, it neutralises soluble toxin. It has an opsonic effect on bacteria.

It has four subclasses, which have different biological activities. The molecular weight (MW) is 150,000. Normal serum level is 1,000–1,259 mg/100ml.

IgM

It is a predominantly intravascular immunoglobulin. It constitutes 7% of the total immunoglobulin. It is especially effective in activating complement to

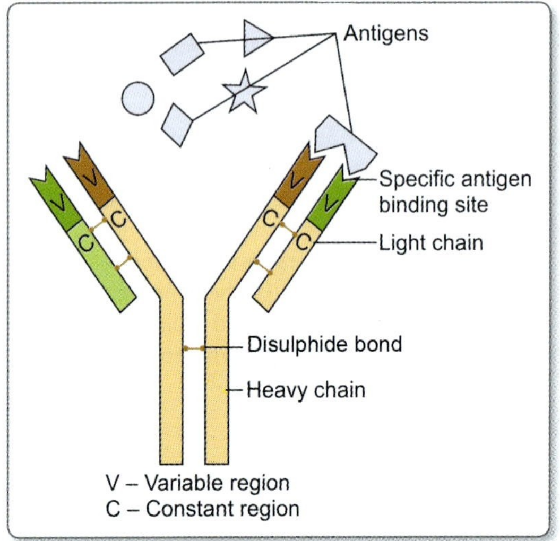

Fig. 1: Structure of an antibody

produce immune lysis of foreign cells. It is more effective than IgG in linking particulate antigen for agglutination and phagocytosis. For an antigenic stimulus, the immediate antibody response is often an IgM antibody, followed some days later by IgG antibody.

Molecular weight is 900,000. Normal serum level is 50–125 mg/100 mL.

IgA

This accounts for 19% of total serum immunoglobulins. It is found in colostrum, saliva, intestinal fluid and respiratory secretions. The major site of IgA synthesis is the lamina propria underlying the mucous membrane throughout the gastrointestinal and respiratory tract. These antibodies are vital in defense of the gut and other mucosal surfaces against microorganisms and toxins. It plays a major role as an antiseptic secreted over the mucous surfaces of the body. Another proposed function of IgA is to mask the antigenic substances absorbed through the mucous membranes and to prevent these substances from causing allergy. There are two subclasses of IgA; the serum level is 150-400 mg/100 mL.

IgD

This immunoglobulin has some properties of IgG; it is found exclusively on the surface of B lymphocytes and may be involved in their regulations. The serum level is 3 mg/100 mL.

IgE

This has a very low serum level. It has distinctive affinity for cell surface and constitutes an integral part of immediate hypersensitivity reactions such as asthma, hay fever etc. They are present on the surface of mast cells and basophils. The physiological function of IgE is obscure; perhaps it plays a part in defense against helminthic infestations. Its serum level is 10–70 µg/100 mL. The amount is too small to be measured by precipitation or agglutination techniques. There are special techniques to measure the amount of IgE in the blood.

Immunological reactions help the body to fight against microorganisms and thus prevent disease. Sometimes, an aberrant reaction occurs, which may cause diseases such as pemphigus, systemic lupus erythematosus. Several types of allergic reactions are recognised.

CLASSIFICATION OF HARMFUL ALLERGIC REACTION

Type 1 (Immediate Hypersensitivity Reaction)

In this reaction, a circulating IgE antibody becomes bound to tissue cells such as mast cells. When the antigen often a foreign protein (pollens, food, insect venom) come in contact with the antibody, it degranulates the mast cell, histamine and other vasoactive amines are discharged from the cell, e.g. anaphylaxis, asthma, urticaria, hay fever, etc.

Type 2 (Cytotoxic Reaction)

In this reaction, the antibody is IgG or IgM, it reacts with an antigen bound to the cell surface. The reaction, which involves the complement, results in damage to the affected cell, e.g. pemphigus, pemphigoid, autoimmune haemolytic aanemia.

Type 3 (Circulating Immune Complexes)

This reaction occurs when the antigen and antibody are present in the circulation in roughly equal proportions. The resulting immune complexes tend to precipitate in small blood vessels. Circulating complement activates an intense inflammatory reaction, e.g. vasculitis, systemic lupus erythematosus.

Type 4 (Delayed Hypersensitivity)

In this reaction, the sensitised lymphocytes react with the antigen deposited at a local site to provoke a slow evolving mixed cellular reaction that involves mainly the T cells. B cells and macrophages may also be activated. The sensitised T lymphocytes release lymphokines, which recruit non-sensitised lymphocytes to the area and bring about an immune response. The tuberculin reaction is a classical type 4 reaction. Most eczema belong to delayed hypersensitivity reaction.

Type 5 (Antibody-Dependent Cell-mediated Toxicity)

This is a mixed form of reaction in which two types of non-immune killer cells (K cells) act in conjunction with antigen and antibodies to damage the target cells. This type of reaction is seen in malignant melanoma.

Type 6 (Granuloma Formation)

Granulomas arise as an inflammatory response to a wide variety of infectious agents and irritant substances. An allergic reaction such as delayed hypersensitivity reaction is associated with granuloma formation. Granulomatous skin diseases include tuberculosis, leprosy, syphilis, sarcoidosis, necrobiosis lipoidica, etc.

CELL-MEDIATED IMMUNITY

Cell-mediated immunity begins with activation of T cells by a particular antigen. Once a T cell is activated, it undergoes proliferation and differentiation into a clone of effector cells. These are a population of identical cells that can recognise the same antigen.

Types of T Cells

There are several different types of T cells: helper T cells, cytotoxic T cells, suppressor T cells, memory T cells and regulatory T cells.

T Helper Cells

T cells that display CD4 develop into T helper cells (T_H). Resting T_H cells recognise antigens belonging to MHC-11 molecules; they are co-stimulated by interleukin-1 secreted by macrophages. These cells are stimulated by antigen presenting cells. On stimulation they start secreting a variety of cytokines. An important cytokine produced by T_H cells is IL-2. T_H cells do not directly destroy the target cells but augment all aspects of the immune respond. There are two main subsets of T_H cells: T_{H1} and $T_{H2.}$ T helper cells enhance the activation and proliferation of T cells, B cells and natural killer cells.

T_{H1} cells rally a cell-mediated (cytotoxic T cell) response, which is appropriate for infections with intracellular microbes such as viruses. T_{H1} response is seen in psoriasis.

T_{H2} cells promote humoral immunity by B cells, and increase eosinophil activity for defense against parasitic worms.T_{H2} response is seen in atopic dermatitis.

Whether a naïve T cell becomes a T_{H1} cell or T_{H2} cell depends on which cytokines are secreted by macrophages, as it presents the antigen to the T cells. Interleukin-12 drives naïve T cell specific to the antigen towards T_{H1} production. Interleukin-4 favours the development of T_{H2} cell. Thus by means of macrophage secretion, the non-specific immune system can influence the whole tenor of specific immune system.

Other sub-classes of T_H cells are also identified such as T_{HF}, which helps B lymphocytes to develop into plasma cells. T_{H17} protect surfaces such as skin, lining of intestines against extracellular bacteria.

Cytotoxic T Cells

T cells that display CD8 develop into cytotoxic T cells, these are also known as killer T cells. Cytotoxic T cells recognise foreign antigens belonging to MHC-1 molecules on the surfaces of body cells infected by viruses, some tumour cells and cells of tissue transplants. In order to be cytolytic they have to be stimulated by IL-2 and other cytokines secreted by T_H cells. Cytotoxic T cells are especially effective against slow growing organisms such as tuberculosis, brucellosis, some viruses, fungi, cancer and transplanted cells. Once activated the cytotoxic T cells directly or indirectly destroy the target cell infected with the antigen.

Suppressor T Cells

These T cells are distinct from T_H and cytotoxic T cells. The nature of the receptors for antigens is not known. They may down-regulate the immune response by producing cytokines such as TNF-β which inhibits proliferation of T cells. Another possibility is that they directly destroy activated lymphocytes. The suppressor cells suppress both B cell antibody production and cytotoxic and helper T cell activity.

Memory T Cells

These cells are programmed to recognise the original invading antigen. If the same antigen invades the body again, thousands of memory cells are able to initiate an initial response swiftly and vigorously.

Regulatory T Cells

T lymphocytes that do not take part in the immune response are known as regulatory T lymphocytes. They modulate the activities of B cells, cytotoxic T cells, macrophages and their own activities.

LABORATORY DIAGNOSIS AND ASSESSMENT OF IMMUNOLOGICAL DISORDERS

Tests for Humoral Immunity

- Circulating autoantibodies and antigens, these are estimated in diseases such as collagen vascular disorders, e.g. ANA.
- Complement levels: Circulating immune complexes usually depress total complement levels. The CH50 measures the overall complement system (CH50 refers to serum complement hemolysis of 50% RBC *in vitro*). Individual levels such as C_3 and C_4 can also be measured.
- Level of circulating immune complexes.
- Indirect measurement by finding low complement levels, or increased levels of complement breakdown products as C_3c and C_3d.
- Labeled Clq binding: Labeled Clq globulin is incubated with test specimen and the amount of radioactivity incorporated in the immune complex is measured.
- Cryoglobulin: Immune complexes tend to precipitate at temperatures below blood temperature. The cryoglobulin in connective tissue diseases are often mixtures of IgM and IgG immune complex.

Tests for Cell-mediated Immunity

E-Rosette Test

Normally about 75% of the circulating lymphocytes are T cell lymphocytes. The E-rosette test uses sheep erythrocytes to bind T cell to form rosettes.

Lymphocyte Transformation

Lymphocytes are incubated in tritiated thymidine. They are grown in culture with and without phytohaemagglutinins. Transformation to lymphoblast is indicated by incorporation of tritiated thymide into the newly synthesised DNA.

Dinitrochlorbenzene Sensitisation

Dinitrochlorbenzene (DNCB) acts as a hapten, in a normal individual with normal functioning T lymphocytes. Skin sensitisation occurs after 10 days.

Inhibition of Leukocyte Migration

Lymphocytes that are immunologically active will when challenged with a ubiquitous antigen release lymphokines, which further inhibit leukocyte migration.

WHEN TO SUSPECT IMMUNODEFICIENCY

Immune deficiency should be suspected when patients have recurrent infections of increased duration, of intense severity and with unusual organisms. There is often inadequate response to treatment. Children have delayed milestones, some show failure to thrive.

Immune deficiency is associated with cutaneous and systemic disorders. Cutaneous abnormalities include infections, alopecia, poor wound healing, atopic dermatitis or seborrhoeic dermatitis like manifestations, petechiae, cutaneous granulomas and lupus like changes.

Systemic manifestations include gastrointestinal, respiratory and urinary tract infections, hepatosplenomegaly, arthritis, lymphadenopathy associated with haematological abnormalities. There is failure to thrive, visceral infections, autoimmune disorders and malignancy.

Immune deficiency should be suspected when an individual has repeated skin infections especially by rarer organisms. The infections are difficult to treat or show a poor response to treatment.

Classification of Immunodeficiency States

- Disorder of Phagocytosis
  - Neutropenia
  - Chronic granulomatous disease (CGD)
  - Chediak-Higashi syndrome
  - Leukocyte adhesion deficiency (LAD)
  - Hyperglobulinaemia E syndrome
- Disorders of Thymus and T lymphocytes
  - Congenital aplasia of thymus (DiGeorge syndrome)
  - Nezelof's syndrome
  - Chronic mucocutaneous candidiasis
- Antibody Deficiency
  - X-linked hypogammaglobulinemia
  - Isolated IgA deficiency
  - Isolated IgM deficiency

- Combined T cell and Antibody Deficiency
  - Wiskott-Aldrich syndrome
  - Ataxia telangiectasia
- Severe Combined Immunodeficiency (SCID)
- Complement Deficiency
  - Leiner's disease.

DISORDERS OF PHAGOCYTOSIS

Disorders of phagocytosis lead to recurrent skin and pulmonary infections, lymphadenopathy, hepatosplenomegaly and ulcerative stomatitis.

Neutropenia

Quantitative deficiency of neutrophils may be primary or secondary. Familial neutropenia may occur at any age; it may be due to either depression of the bone marrow or destruction of neutrophils by autoantibodies. This may be due to drugs, radiation, and infection. There may be recurrent cycles of neutropenia of unknown cause (cyclic neutropenia). Cycles of neutropenia occur at intervals of 21–28 days, and persist for 2–3 days. Oral manifestations include ulcerative gingivitis and mucosal ulcers. Repeated cycles of neutropenia lead to periodontal disease and bone loss.

Treatment

The following methods may be employed in the treatment of neutropenia:

- Supportive therapy with antimicrobials.
- Elimination of the factors responsible for suppression of neutrophils, good nutrition.
- Transfusion of fresh blood or concentrated white blood cells.
- Treat the underlying disease.

Chronic Granulomatous Disease (CGD)

This is an hetrogenous group of X-linked and autosomal recessive disorders, in which 90% of the patients are males. In patients with CGD, the membrane associated nicotinamide adenine dinucleotide phosphate (NADPH) oxidase system fails to produce superoxide and other toxic oxygen metabolites, which are required for bactericidal activity after phagocytosis. There is a pronounced deficiency of degranulation and stimulation of oxidative mechanisms, which accompany phagocytosis. The metabolic abnormality is the basis of nitroblue tetrazolium (NBT) test; it is diagnostic of the disease. Both neutrophils and monocytes are unable to kill ingested bacteria. The disease presents during the first year of life. Prenatal diagnosis can be made by the NBT slide test.

The disease is characterised by persistent and frequently fatal infections, often caused by organisms of low virulence. Recurrent infections involve the long bones, lymphatic tissue, liver, skin and lungs. Cutaneous lesions comprise furunculosis, subcutaneous abscesses, especially around the anal area. Eczematous lesions are present on the scalp,

Treatment

Treatment of the infection should be early, aggressive and prolonged. The disease varies in severity, but is generally fatal in the first five years of life.

behind the ears and face, suppurative lymphadenopathy usually affects the cervical nodes.

The affected tissues show a granulomatous reaction with the formation of microabscesses and draining sinuses.

Chediak-Higashi syndrome

This is a rare autosomal recessive disorder. It is characterised by the presence of giant granules in the leukocytes, melanocytes and many other cells. There is oculocutaneous albinism, neutropenia, the abnormal neutrophils do not phagocytize. The skin is typically fair but areas of pigmentation are seen. Hair shafts have clumped pigmented granules. Infections are common in the skin and the respiratory system. Early death usually occurs due to malignant lymphoma or other forms of cancer.

The albinism is due to defective melanocytes, containing very few or large melanosomes. Ocular hypopigmentation can lead to nystagmus, strabismus and photophobia.

Prenatal diagnosis is done by examining the hair from fetal scalp biopsies, and finding the giant granules in lymphocytes from fetal blood samples.

Treatment

Prompt treatment of infections and bone marrow transplantation. Vitamin C has been found to be helpful in a dose of 200 mg daily in a few cases.

Leukocyte Adhesion Deficiency

In this disorder there is deficiency of cell surface glycoproteins (β_2-integrins) that are responsible for the adherence of leukocytes. This is a rare autosomal recessive disorder. The patients have frequent skin, mucosal and ear infections. Skin infections often present as necrotic abscesses that resemble pyoderma gangrenosum. Cellulitis of the face and perirectal area is common. Gingivitis with periodontal disease may result in loss of teeth. Death often occurs before the child's second birthday, unless a successful bone marrow transplantation is done.

Hyperimmunoglobulinaemia E Syndrome

The disorder is characterised by increased levels of IgE, atopic-like dermatitis, peripheral eosinophilia, recurrent cutaneous and systemic infections and defective neutrophil and monocyte chemotaxis. Cutaneous abscesses are found mainly on the head and neck, pulmonary infections are most frequent. Dental abnormalities include retention of primary teeth, and lack of eruption of secondary teeth.

Job's syndrome is similar to hyperimmunoglobulinaemia E syndrome, but the inflammatory response is less severe; cold abscesses are often found. The syndrome occurs mainly in girls with red hair, freckles, blue eyes and hyperextensible joints.

Treatment is symptomatic with antibiotics. IgG and interferon-γ has been used successfully.

DISORDERS OF THE THYMUS AND T LYMPHOCYTES

The features of T lymphocyte deficiency include recurrent infections with low grade or opportunistic organism. There is a high incidence of malignancy and short life span.

Thymic Hypoplasia (DiGeorge Syndrome)

The syndrome includes congenital absence of the parathyroid glands and thymus; associated with an abnormal aorta. These abnormalities suggest a developmental defect of structures arising from the third and fourth pharyngeal pouches of the brachial arch. Most patients have associated B cell immune deficiency; due to effects of T cells on B cells.

Neonatal tetany is often the first sign of the disease. Aortic and cardiac defects are the most common causes of death. T cell defects are present, cell-mediated immunity is absent or depressed. The lymph nodes display abundant follicles and plasma cell, but there is depletion of lymphocytes in the paracortical areas. Characteristic abnormalities of DiGeorge syndrome include short philtrum, low set ears and hypertelorism. Cutaneous manifestations often present as chronic mucocutaneous candidiasis and increased susceptibility to viral infections. Infants have associated neonatal tetany with hypocalcemia due to aplasia of parathyroid glands. Cardiac abnormalities are frequent such as truncus arteriosus, abnormal aortic arch vessels and septal defects.

Treatment

Transplantation of fetal thymic tissue would appear to be the treatment of choice.

Thymic Dysplasia with Normal Immunoglobulins (Nezelof's Syndrome)

In Nezelof's syndrome, there is a faulty development of the thymus, cell-mediated immunity is lacking, serum inmunoglobulins are normal. Despite the presence of immunoglobulins, antibody production is often low or absent. Onset is in early infancy with repeated fungal, viral and bacterial infections. Patient usually dies from overwhelming viral infections.

DISEASES DUE TO DEFICIENCY OF ANTIBODIES

Deficiency of antibodies include infection with extracellular encapsulated bacteria, chronic sino-pulmonary infection, lymph glands are usually not enlarged. The condition is compatible with survival. A patient can live for many years, unless complicated by autoimmune disease or malignancy.

X-linked Hypogammaglobulinaemia (Bruton's Disease)

This is a rare hereditary immunological disorder of X-linked inheritance. It is due to the failure of maturation of B lymphocytes. The disease becomes apparent after 6 months of age, with the disappearance of maternal antibodies. There is a great susceptibility to Gram-positive pyogenic infection. There is an increased tendency to develop atopic dermatitis, diffuse vasculitis, dermatomyositis, urticaria and viral infections. Parasitic and viral infections are also seen despite normal cell-mediated immunity. Lymphoreticular malignancies may develop.

Cutaneous infections present with recurrent furunculosis and impetigo, prominent around the body orifices. An atopic like eczematous eruption is often seen. Pyoderma gangrenosum and cutaneous granulomas are frequently reported.

IgA, IgM, IgE and IgD are absent from the serum. IgG is present in small amounts. Defect is in the maturation of B cell differentiation.

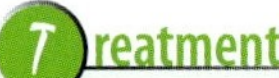

Gamma globulin is helpful but does not control the disease.

Isolated IgA deficiency

The condition is due to a maturation defect of B-lymphocytes as it transforms into an IgA producing plasma cell. The defect is transmitted as autosomal recessive trait. Drugs can also induce the disease such as phenytoin.

Most of the patients are asymptomatic, those who manifest symptoms have repeated infections, and some have collagen vascular disease. There is an increased association of ulcerative colitis and regional ileitis.

Isolated IgM deficiency

This is probably due to a defect of IgM producing plasma cells. Eczematous dermatitis is present in about one fifth of cases. Affected persons are predisposed to severe infections, verrucae occur in great numbers.

COMBINED ANTIBODY AND T-CELL DEFICIENCY

Wiskott-Aldrich syndrome

This is a rare X-linked recessive disorder, seen exclusively in young boys with a triad of chronic eczematous dermatitis, increased susceptibility to infection and thrombocytopenia. There is an intrinsic abnormality of platelets. T cells progressively decline in number and activity.

Spleen and liver are enlarged. Bloody diarrhoea or haemorrhage during the first month of life is the initial clinical manifestation. Decreased humoral immunity leads to severe bacterial and viral infections. Atopic dermatitis like lesion is present in the first year of life. Death usually occurs by the age of six from infection or bleeding.

Ataxia telangiectasia is described in the Chapter 15.

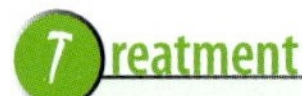

Platelet transfusions, antibiotics and immune globulins are helpful. Splenectomy and bone marrow transplantation are also recommended. Human stem-cell gene therapy has emerged as an innovative therapeutic strategy for the treatment of Wiskott-Aldrich syndrome and other primary immunedeficiency disorders.

SEVERE COMBINED IMMUNODEFICIENCY

Severe combined immunodeficiency (SCID) is a severe disorder associated with combined humoral and cell-mediated deficiency. Most of the cases are seen in boys due to X-linked recessive inheritance. The other types of inheritance are autosomal recessive (Swiss type agammaglobulinemia) and by spontaneous mutation. Patients rarely survive beyond 2 years of age without treatment. Patients have deficiency of CD8, natural killer cells. Although the number of B cells is normal, patients have difficulty in activation of B lymphocytes. There is defect in cytokine production especially IL-2.

Patients with SCID suffer from repeated infection; bacterial, fungal and viral. Mucocutaneous candidiasis is common. Viral infections are often fatal.

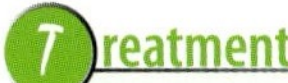

Bone marrow transplantation, IL-2 injections are also helpful.

Hereditary Thymic Dysplasia (Swiss Type Agammaglobulinemia)

Hereditary thymic dysplasia was the first type of SCID discovered in 1950s. It is an inherited autosomal recessive disorder, in which there is a decrease in both T and B lymphocytes. The presumed basic defect is in the lymphopoietic stem cells, which fail to differentiate into lymphoid cells. The thymus is small and so are the lymph nodes, while pulp of the spleen, lamina propria of the gut is devoid of lymphocytes and plasma cells. There is an absence of lymphocytes in the tissues and blood, the tonsils are absent. There are repeated fungal and viral infections; the condition is fatal in early life.

The children with hereditary thymic dysplasia should not be vaccinated, as it may lead to fatal infections.

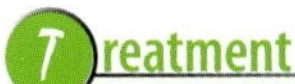

Success has been reported in patients with daily injections of thymosine. This has led to a complete return of lymphocytes, decrease in infections and weight gain.

All newborn infants should be screened for SCID
SCID is also known as the 'Bubble disease'. A boy is said to have survived for 12 years by being kept in a plastic germ free cell.

Complement deficiency (Leiner's disease) is discussed in Chapter 9.

FURTHER READING

1. Blume RS, Wolff SM. The Chediak-Higashi syndrome: study in four patients and review of literature. Medicine. 1972;51(4):247-80.
2. Buztug K, Schmidt M, Schwerzer A, et al. Stem-cell gene therapy for the treatment of Wiskott-Aldrich syndrome. The New Eng J of Med. 2010;(363):1918-27.
3. Figueroa JE and Densen P. Infectious diseases associated with complement deficiencies. Clin Microbiol Rev. 1991;4(3):359-95.
4. Gatti RA, Periman S, Becker-Catana S. Ataxia telangiectasia. Semin Pediatr Neurol Clin. 2003;10(3):173-82.

5. Gherardi R, Beloc L, Mhiri C, et al. The spectrum of vasculitis in Human Immunodeficiency Virus-infected patients: a clinicopathological evaluation. Arthritis Rheum. 1993;36(8):1164-74.
6. Glover MT, Atherton DJ, Levinsky RJ, et al. Syndrome of erythroderma, failure to thrive and diarrhoea in infancy: a manifestation of immune deficiency. Pediatrics. 1988;81(1):66-72.
7. Jemec GB, Moe AT. Topical treatment of skin ulcers in prolidase deficiency. Pediatr Dermatol. 1996;13(1):58-60.
8. Ochs HD, Smith CIE, Puck JM. Primary immunodeficiency diseases: molecular and genetic approach. New York: Oxford University Press, 1999.
9. Rashner AJ, Kinnion C. The Wiskott-Aldrich Syndrome. Clin Exp Immunol. 2000;120(1):2-9.
10. Rosen FS, Cooper MD, Wedgwood RJP, et al. The primary immunodeficiencies (review article). N Eng J Med. 1995;333(7):431-40.

Chapter

31

Cutaneous Manifestations of Systemic Diseases

INTRODUCTION

The skin serves as a window through which the physician can detect internal disease. Therefore, a careful examination can be valuable in diagnosing systemic disease. The principal cutaneous signs are described here; the reader should refer to a general medical text for a detailed study of the systemic disorders. The cutaneous lesions generally require no specific treatment except that of the systemic disorder; therapy for skin lesions is seldom required.

DIABETES MELLITUS

Diabetes mellitus has several cutaneous manifestations; these changes are secondary to the changes in the blood vessels or nerves. Thirty to forty percent of patients with diabetes have cutaneous manifestations.

Vascular Changes

Both small and large blood vessels are involved.

Microangiopathy

This may result in erysipelas like erythema in the legs or feet of an elderly diabetic, cardiac decompensation may be involved.

Rubeosis is a reddening of the face, hand and feet seen in a patient of long-standing diabetes; this is due to the decrease in vascular tone.

Diabetic dermopathy is the most common dermatosis associated with diabetes; microangiopathy and neuropathy are involved. The initial lesion consists of red papules on the shin (shin spots) (Fig. 1); these can also occur on the forearm, thigh, and bony prominences; it heals leaving atrophic brown scars.

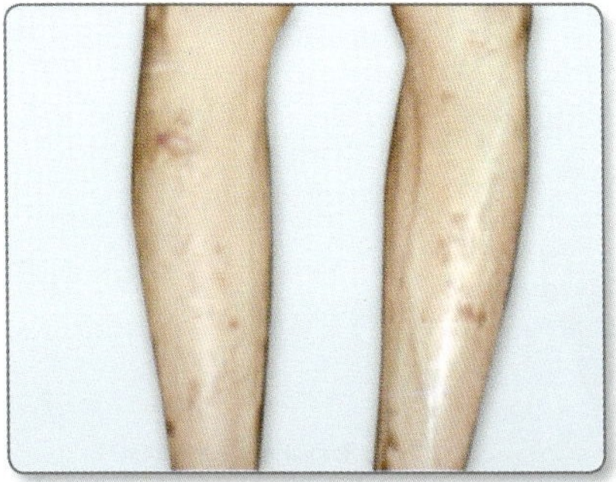

Fig. 1: Diabetic dermopathy

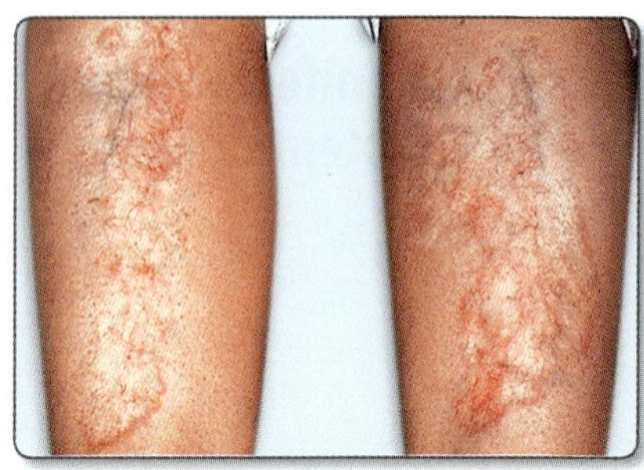

Fig. 2: Necrobiosis lipoidica

Necrobiosis lipoidica diabeticorum consists of discrete reddish papules that develop into waxy reddish plaques with violaceous borders and yellowish atrophic depressed areas in the centre of the plaque, covered with telangiectasia and occasional central ulceration (Fig. 2). These lesions may be single or multiple. The legs (pretibial area) are the most common site of necrobiosis lipoidica diabeticorum, but it may also appear on the forearms or elsewhere on the body. It is usually painless due to damage to nerves; some cases may be extremely painful. Control of diabetes does not alter the course of the lesion.

Necrobiosis lipoidica diabeticorum may precede the onset of frank diabetes. It is a disorder of collagen degeneration with a granulomatous response, thickening of blood vessels and fat degeneration. The cause of the lesion is uncertain, diabetic microangiopathy is the most likely cause. Other theories suggest neuropathy, trauma, inflammatory, or metabolic change. The condition is more common in females.

Macroangiopathy

Cutaneous changes due to large vessel involvement are because of atherosclerosis. The patients complain of intermittent claudication; the skin of the extremities is pale and cool. This may lead to ischaemic gangrenous lesions of the legs and feet (Fig. 3). Nail dystrophy and hair loss may occur.

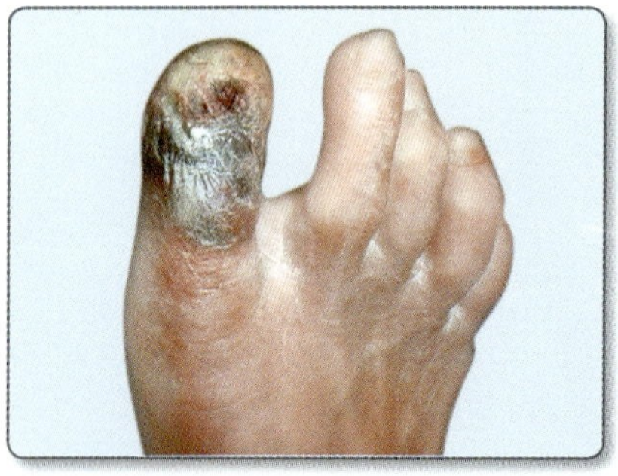

Fig. 3: Diabetic gangrene

Diabetic Neuropathy

This affects the sensory nerves, motor nerves and the autonomic nervous system. Sensory abnormalities include numbness, tingling, aching and burning. Burning feet and restless legs are frequent complaints. Motor neuropathy is characterised by dorsally subluxed digits, distally displaced plantar footpads, depressed metatarsal heads, hammertoes and pes cavus. Autonomic neuropathy may result in decreased or absent sweating of the lower extremities with compensatory sweating of the other areas of the body such as trunk.

Painless slow penetrating ulcers on the sole and at other pressure sites are suggestive of diabetes. A diabetic foot requires special care; it has a multifactorial aetiology. Peripheral neuropathy causes ulcers due to lack of sensations and vascular abnormalities.

Bacterial Infections

Bacterial infections are common in diabetes. The cause is unknown; perhaps it may be due to the decrease in neutrophilic functions. Furuncles, carbuncles and styes are common. Malignant otitis externa due to pseudomonas may progress to osteitis, cranial nerve damage and meningitis. Candidiasis may be a presenting feature of the disease; it may affect the mouth, nail folds, genitals and intertriginous skin areas. Less common but more serious are mucormycosis and clostridial gangrene.

Miscellaneous Disorders

Miscellaneous disorders associated with diabetes are disseminated granuloma annulare, pruritus, vitiligo, lichen planus, eruptive xanthomas, skin tags, Kyrle's disease, acanthosis nigricans, haemochromatosis, and diabetic bullae. Diabetic bullae occur spontaneously on the hands and feet on an uninflamed skin, heal in 2–5 weeks without scarring. Carotenaemia is a yellowish discolouration of the skin, especially of the palms and the soles. The sclera remains white. This is due to the reduced conversion of carotene to vitamin A in the liver.

Stiff thick skin of diabetes (diabetic sclerodactyly) is seen on the skin of hands and fingers, demonstrated by the "prayer sign", in which the fingers and palms cannot be opposed properly.

LIVER DISEASE

The association between the liver and the skin has been known since centuries. Barmaids in New York spotted spider naevi in customers with advanced liver disease. Liver disease is frequently associated with abnormalities of the skin, hair and the nails. As a general rule, the cutaneous findings are non-specific and may even be absent in severe liver disease.

Pigmentary Abnormalities

Jaundice is first visible as a yellowish hue of the sclera and soft palate before it becomes generalised.

The common cutaneous manifestation is pruritus. It is due to the presence of bile salts in the skin, but other liver products may also be involved. There is no indication of the release of histamine and the use of antihistamines is therefore limited; oral cholestyramine 4 g daily in a diet rich in polyunsaturated fatty acids may produce relief. The dose is gradually increased up to 24 g/day in two doses with meals. Rifampicin 150 mg/day, can also be used which can be increased to 600 mg/day. Opiate antagonists such as naltrexone and nalmefene are other options.

Hyperpigmentation is diffuse or it may be localized in the perioral or periorbital region. Pallor is due to anaemia. A diffuse muddy grey pigmentation is seen in cirrhosis of the liver; this is due to basal cell melanin.

Vascular Abnormalities

Urticaria may be due to the presence of circulating immune complexes.

Telangiectasia

Rapid development of multiple spider naevi is seen in chronic liver disease.

Paper Money Skin

Patients with spider angiomata may also show numerous small vessels resembling silk threads in the US paper money; these are scattered in random fashion especially over the face, neck and upper trunk. These may be associated with telangiectatic mats consisting of plaques of telangiectatic vessels.

Bier Spots

Small irregularly shaped hypopigmented patches appear on the arms and legs in patients of hepatic cirrhosis. These are thought to be due to vasoconstriction induced by venous stasis. Bier spots disappear on pressure. Raising the limbs from a dependent position causes the spots to disappear. On cooling the skin of cirrhotic patients, especially on exposure to cold air, these spots appear on the arms and buttocks.

Palmar Erythema

Crimson florid colouration can occur on the palms and fingertips. Palmar erythema is most prominent on the hypothenar eminence.

Bywater's Lesions

The lesions comprise of small painless reddish brown infarcts in the nail fold, with minute digital ulcerations; it may be associated with maculopapular haemorrhagic painful lesions on digital pulp. The changes are due to vasculitis; also seen in rheumatoid arthritis.

Haemorrhagic Manifestations

The cause of bleeding in liver disease depends upon the aetiology of the underlying disorder. It may be due to a failure of absorption of vitamin K in biliary obstruction, failure of production of coagulative factors and abnormal platelet function. The cutaneous haemorrhage may range from petechiae and ecchymosis to haematoma.

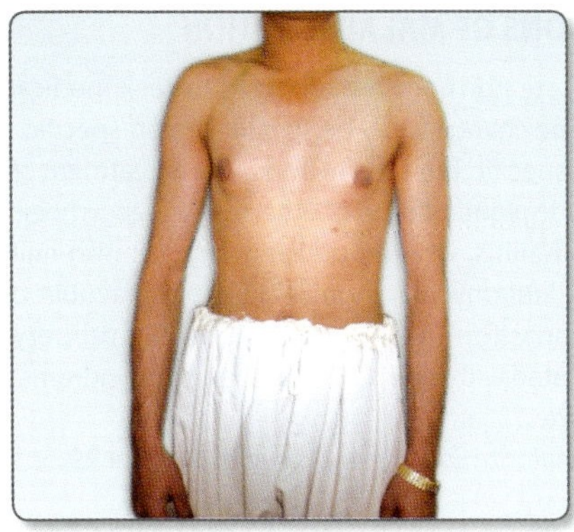

Fig. 4: Gynaecomastia

Hormonal-Induced Changes

Testicular atrophy, gynaecomastia (Fig. 4) and loss of axillary and pubic hair may occur due to the liver being unable to metabolise oestrogens; the level of oestrogen rises. The changes are more common in patients with alcoholic cirrhosis.

Hair and Nails

Severe alopecia indicates associated zinc deficiency. Nail changes include clubbing, white flat nails (leukonychia), striations and white bands. In Wilson's disease, the lunula attains a characteristic azure colour. Terry's nail (half-and-half nails) is characterised by a powdery white discolouration and ground glass opacity of the proximal two-thirds of the nail, the distal one-third is reddish brown in colour due to telangiectasia. The white colour is thought to reflect hyperplasia of connective tissue between the nail and bone.

Miscellaneous Changes

Striae distensae (cutaneous stretch marks) are seen especially on the lower abdomen probably due to hormonal imbalance. Eruptive xanthomas and plain xanthomas may develop on the hands and the fingers. Dilated abdominal veins including caput madusae occur in cirrhosis with portal hypertension. Dupuytren's contracture is associated with stiffness of the finger joints; the patients cannot fully flex or extend the fingers. A genetic factor probably plays a part; associated with disorder of collagen metabolism.

PANCREATIC DISEASE

Cutaneous manifestations of pancreatic disease are rare except jaundice, these are not generally helpful from a diagnostic point of view. Those sometimes found include bruising of the skin around the flanks (Grey Turner's sign) and umbilicus (Cullen's sign) in acute pancreatitis. Other signs include metastatic fat necrosis, panniculitis, thrombophlebitis migrans and xanthomata. Sweat abnormalities as seen in fibrocystic disease are also observed.

CUTANEOUS MANIFESTATIONS OF MALABSORPTION

Twenty percent of patients with steatorrhoea are reported to seek medical attention on account of rashes. The changes may be specific or non-specific.

The majority of these are non-specific, but tend to improve on treatment of steatorrhoea. These changes include pigmentation, haemorrhages, seborrhoeic dermatitis, angular stomatitis, cheilitis, vitamin deficiencies, hair and nail changes (clubbing, koilonychia, leukonychia, monilial infection), acquired ichthyosis, eczematous and psoriasiform rashes, and small blue rubbery nodules on the upper trunk associated with blue rubber bleb naevus syndrome, also known as the Bean's syndrome.

The specific changes due to malnutrition are discussed in Chapter 29.

MISCELLANEOUS DISORDERS OF GASTROINTESTINAL TRACT

Acrodermatitis Enteropathica

This is an autosomal recessive disorder due to a defect in zinc absorption, frequently seen after the infant is weaned off breast milk. It is characterized by diarrhea, dermatitis and alopecia. It presents as erythematous, raw and pustular areas around the mouth, anus, fingers, and toes. Severe diarrhoea is common, and if the condition is not recognised and treated, hair and nails will be shed. Oral zinc supplements bring about dramatic and rapid improvement, and must be continued for many years, possibly for life. A similar condition is seen in patients receiving total parenteral nutrition or elemental diets in which zinc is lacking. The lesions clear rapidly with treatment.

Gluten-Sensitive Enteropathy

Gluten-sensitive enteropathy is common in dermatitis herpetiformis (DH) which is a papulovesicular, intensely pruritic dermatosis with granular deposits of IgA in the dermal papillae. Anti-gluten and anti-gliadin antibodies result in asymptomatic villous atrophy of jejunal mucosa. Several serological abnormalities and diseases have been found to occur more frequently with DH. These include gastric hypoacidity and gastric atrophy associated with anti-gastric parietal cell antibodies, clinical or serological evidence of thyroid disease, IgA nephropathy, and finally increased incidence of lymphomas of the gastrointestinal tract. The incidence of gut lymphoma is significantly reduced if gluten-free diet is introduced early.

Pyoderma Gangrenosum

Pyoderma gangrenosum may precede the development of frank gastrointestinal symptoms in both ulcerative colitis and Crohn's disease. Patients with Crohn's disease also tend to have multiple perianal skin tags, ulcers and fistulae, and occasionally severe oral ulceration. It is also associated with rheumatoid arthritis and Still's disease.

Peutz-Jeghers Syndrome

Peutz-Jeghers syndrome is characterized by lentiginous pigmentation on and around the lips, and polyposis of the gastrointestinal tract, particularly the small bowel. Intussusception may develop, polyps can be premalignant.

Cronkhite-Canada Syndrome

Hyperpigmentation, alopecia, and onychodystrophy are associated with adenomatous polyps in the gastrointestinal tract. Malabsorption occurs; the condition is fatal as there is no effective treatment.

RENAL DISEASE

Cutaneous manifestations of renal disease fall into two categories:

- Hereditary or acquired disorders with renal and cutaneous changes.
- Cutaneous changes due to renal insufficiency, these are usually non-specific.

Dryness of the skin is the most common cutaneous finding in renal disease due to dehydration and use of diuretics (Fig. 5).

Generalised Pruritus

Generalized pruritus is the most common manifestation of chronic renal disease. This may be related to the increase in blood urea, dehydration from the use of diuretics, decrease in the size of the sweat glands, secondary hyperparathyroidism and mast cell hyperplasia. Pruritus is relieved as the general condition of the patient improves. Oral antihistamines are usually ineffective apart from their sedative effect. Emollients are given for the dryness of skin. Oral cholestyramine resin has been reported to decrease pruritus due to absorption of a circulating toxin from the gut. Phototherapy is most successful. Narrow band UVB is widely used. Phototherapy induces the formation of photoproducts which have antipruritic effect by inactivating pruritogenic substances. Topical tacrolimus, opioid antagonists, charcoal (6 g/day), topical capsaicin, thalidomide and IV lidocaine can also be used to treat pruritus. Subtotal parathyroidectomy may be very helpful, but the problem often recurs.

Other Manifestations

Anaemia with resulting pallor is an early sign of renal failure due to decreased haemopoiesis and increased haemolysis. Purpura may occur in the form of

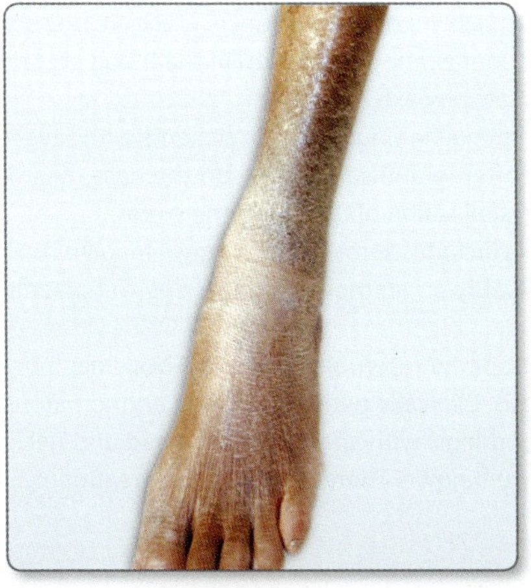

Fig. 5: Xerosis

scattered ecchymosis and petechiae. Purpura due to mild thrombocytopenia may be corrected by dialysis.

Diffuse hyperpigmentation with accentuation in the sun-exposed areas is characteristic of uraemic patients; this is due to retention of chromogens and deposition of melanin due to impaired renal processing of melanocyte-stimulating hormone (MSH).

A yellowish discolouration of the skin can occur due to lipochrome and carotenoids deposition in the dermis and subcutaneous tissue. Elastosis is seen as yellowish atrophic plaques in sun-exposed areas of the body.

A self-limiting bullous dermatosis similar to that of porphyria cutanea tarda is seen in patients undergoing dialysis; this is due to the high levels of uroporphyrins that do not cross the dialysis membrane.

Premature aging of the skin and solar keratosis have been described in renal failure; the patients should avoid excessive UVB therapy for pruritus. Forty percent of the patients undergoing dialysis may develop gynaecomastia. A low phosphorus diet and aluminium hydroxide gel may reverse this.

Kyrle's disease occurs in both diabetes and renal failure; these consist of hyperpigmented papules up to 1 cm in diameter with a keratin plug. The extensor surface of the limbs is commonly affected.

Half-and-half nails have been emphasised as a marker for uraemia. It consists of proximal white and distal end reddish-brown in colour, due to changes in the nail bed. The nail plate is unaffected.

Terry's Nail. The proximal end of the nail is white; it stops 1–2 mm from the distal end of the nail, which is pinkish-brown in colour. This is present in all the nails. It is also associated with cirrhosis of the liver, congestive cardiac failure, and adult-onset diabetes.

Leukonychia is seen in end-stage renal failure.

Hypocalcemia is due to decreased calcitriol production by the kidney. This leads to secondary hyperparathyroidism, which mobilises calcium and phosphorus from the bones in the blood. When these solubility products are exceeded in the blood, metastatic calcification occurs. Cutaneous calcification is uncommon and is seen around the large joints and flexures. These appear as firm papules or plaques, with a chalky-white appearance. These are present around the joints and fingertips. Metastatic calcification in the blood vessels may lead to skin necrosis called calciphylaxis.

Uraemic frost a distinctive terminal finding is seen in patients with severe uraemia. The numerous white-to-tan granules are seen on the nose, beard, arm and neck; they represent crystallisation of urea from the sweat.

Oral manifestation of uraemia includes xerostomia, gingival friability, and ulcerative stomatitis; this is probably an ammoniacal burn due to bacterial decomposition of salivary urea.

Nephrogenic fibrosing dermopathy resembles scleromyxoedema; most cases are seen after haemodialysis. Clinically patients develop erythematous sclerotic plaques on the arms and legs, with sparing of the head and neck. Pruritus is common. The cause is unknown. There is no effective treatment.

RHEUMATOID ARTHRITIS

Several skin changes are seen in the patients of rheumatoid arthritis. These are mainly due to increased deposition of fibrous tissue or those due to vasculitis.

Rheumatic Nodules

Palpable subcutaneous skin coloured nodules occur in 20% of patients of rheumatoid arthritis. It is commonly seen in the ulnar border of the forearms, dorsum of the hands, knees, scapula, sacrum, buttocks, heels, and ears. Nodules are associated with more severe form of the disease. Rheumatic nodules may occur in the sclera which then becomes atrophic and even perforate (scleromalacia perforans), leading to blindness.

Linear Subcutaneous Bands

These are elongated bands 3–5 mm wide and about 10 cm or more in length. These are seen in the axilla extending to the iliac crest.

Histologically the nodules consist of fibrous tissue in which foci of fibrinoid necrosis are scattered. These necrotic areas are surrounded by a palisade of cells mainly fibroblast and histiocytes.

Vascular Lesions

The most characteristic lesions are small infarcts around the nails; these infarcts are transitory, painless, lasting for 2–3 days. Occasionally an infarct may cause grooving of the nail. Digital necrosis similar to that of systemic lupus erythematosus may occur; it may be confused with occupational trauma. Palmar erythema similar to systemic lupus erythematosus is also seen in rheumatoid arthritis.

Small painful purpuric nodules (Bywater lesions) are seen on the pulp of the fingers. Palmar erythema is common. Leg ulcers are seen in 18% of rheumatoid patients due to venous insufficiency, complicated by immobility and postural factors.

The skin may show necrotic arteritis. Haemorrhage occurs without preceding trauma; it may vary in size from small petechiae to large ecchymosis that may ulcerate. Gangrene may result from changes in the digital vessels; sometimes it may involve a large part of the hand and foot in a few days. Bullae of the fingers or toes may occur; occasionally it may spread to involve other areas of the body.

Peripheral sensory and motor neuropathy is due to occlusion of the vasa nervosum. Pyoderma gangrenosum is another complication of rheumatoid arthritis. Pressure sores are common because of immobility. Ridging of the nails may occur; the lunula may be red.

Atrophic Skin in Rheumatoid Arthritis

In patients over the age of 60, the skin over the dorsum of the hands becomes loose, thin, inelastic, and transparent, so that the veins and tendons are easily seen. The change is generalised but is seldom conspicuous except on the hands and the forearms. Histologically the dermis is thinned but shows no distinctive signs.

Rheumatoid Neutrophilic Dermatosis

The lesion is characterised by the appearance of symmetrical erythematous nodules and plaques on the dorsum of the hands, arms, extensor surface of the joints, neck, and the trunk. They are sometimes tender. Histologically there is a dense infiltration of neutrophils in the dermis.

HYPERTHYROIDISM

The classical triad of Grave's disease are enlarged toxic goitre, exophthalmos and acropachy. The skin is moist, warm and smooth. Palmar erythema is frequently seen; the hair is thin and has a downy texture. The skin may be diffusely pigmented; sometimes melasma is also present. Thyroid acropachy is characterised by digital clubbing and diaphysial proliferation of the acral and distal long bones. Pretibial myxoedema is seen on the anterolateral aspects of the shin and is characterised by pink, waxy, yellow or skin coloured plaques, with prominent hair follicles giving a peau d'orange appearance. Localised hypertrichosis in the lesions is often noted. It is treated with intralesional steroids.

HYPOTHYROIDISM

Mild hypothyroidism results in cold hands and feet in the absence of vascular disease, sensitivity to cold weather, lack of sweating, tendency to put on weight, drowsiness in the day, and constipation. Severe hypothyroidism in adults results in myxoedema; this condition is characterised by accumulation of mucopolysaccharides in the dermis. The skin is dry and rough; in some cases ichthyosis may be simulated. The facial skin is puffy, expression is dull and flat, and macroglossia may be present. Diffuse hair loss is common and the outer third of the eyebrow is shed. The hair becomes coarse and brittle. The free edges of the nails break easily.

Cretinism is thyroid deficiency in fetal life. In juvenile hypothyroidism, there is abnormal physical and mental development. The children develop hypertrichosis on the upper back and shoulders.

CUSHING'S SYNDROME

This is usually iatrogenic due to prolonged use or high dose of corticosteroids. The use of steroids should therefore be carefully assessed and monitored. The cutaneous manifestations are similar to those caused by endogenous or iatrogenic hypercortism. The subcutaneous fat is redistributed from the limbs to the trunk, so that the trunk becomes obese with a "buffalo hump", while the limb remains slim. The plethoric "moon face" is pathognomonic of increased circulating glucocorticoids. Thinning of the skin due to collagen loss may result in large purple striae. Cushing's syndrome increases the susceptibility to cutaneous infection especially to candidiasis and tinea versicolor. The skin is fragile, heals poorly, the blood vessels rupture easily; purpura and bruises are common. Osteoporosis and compression fractures of the vertebrae may occur. If the adrenal androgens are also produced in excess then there may be hirsutism, seborrhoea, and acne.

ADDISON'S DISEASE

Addison's disease is manifested in the skin primarily by hyperpigmentation. The skin becomes darker, particularly in the sun-exposed areas, buccal mucosa, lips, nipples, genitalia, and sites of friction such as the knees, elbows, palms and soles. Females lose axillary and pubic hair. Acne improves due to decreased levels of adrenal androgen secretion.

XANTHOMATOSIS (HYPERLIPIDEMIAS)

Xanthomatosis are cutaneous manifestation of hyperlipidemia. The hyperlipidemias are classified into six types based on biochemical, electrophoretic, and ultracentrifugational abnormalities. The types are not absolute. Patients may change from one type to another; more than one type may be present in a patient.

Aetiology

The hyperlipidemias may be primary or secondary to hepatic and pancreatic disorders, diabetes mellitus, myxedema, leukemias, alcoholism, hyperuricemia and dysproteinemia. They may also be drug induced by vitamin A derivatives such as acitretin, isotretinoin, oestrogens and oral prednisolone therapy.
Cutaneous lesions are classified as:

- Xanthelasma
- Xanthoma tuberosum
- Tendinous xanthoma
- Eruptive xanthoma.

Xanthelasma

This is the most common type of xanthoma. It occurs on the eyelids near the inner canthi as soft, yellowish or orange plaques. They may be associated with other types of xanthomas, but are usually present without any other disease. The disorder is seen during middle age. It is common in women who have hepatic or biliary disorders, myxoedema, diabetes and pancreatic disorders, but more than half of the patients are normal. A patient with xanthelasma should be investigated for serum lipids, liver and renal functions, diabetes to exclude any systemic disorder (Fig. 6).

The best method for treatment is surgical removal. Fulguration, trichloroacetic acid cauterisation and carbon dioxide laser vaporization are other methods of treatment. However, removal does not prelude the possibility of other new lesions developing.

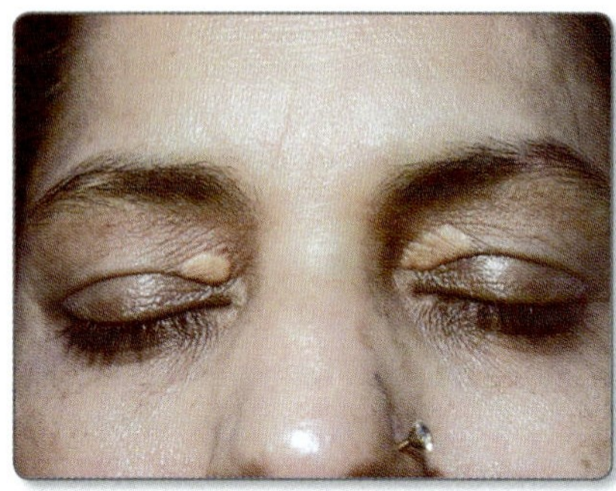

Fig. 6: Xanthelasma

Xanthoma Tuberosum

This begins at any age as flat or elevated yellowish orange or reddish-brown papules; common sites are the knees, elbows, buttocks, and heels. These occur in association with markedly elevated triglycerides. A corneal arcus may be present. It is present in type II-B and type III hyperlipidemia.

Tendinous Xanthomas

These are soft yellowish nodules over the tendons. Tuberous and tendinous xanthomats are present in type II and type III hyperlipidemias.

Eruptive Xanthomas

It consists of small yellowish orange or reddish-brown papules often on an erythematous base; they appear in crops all over the body and mucous membrane, usually found on the extensor surface of the limbs and the buttocks. They are present in type I, IV and V hyperlipidemia (Fig. 7).

Palmar Xanthomas

Palmar xanthomas are characteristic; they are linear yellow xanthomas in the palmar creases. It is present in type III hyperlipidemia.

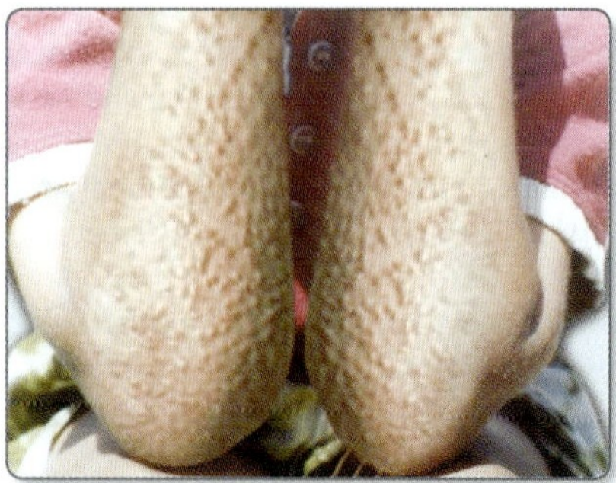

Fig. 7: Eruptive xanthoma

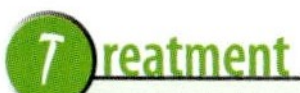

This requires a strict fat-modified diet often in combination with drugs such as statin clofibrate, cholestyramine and nicotinic acid. Xanthomata respond well to lowering of lipid intake.

DISORDERS OF LIPID METABOLISM

These rare diseases are associated with disturbances of lipid metabolism. Some of these are:

Lipoid Proteinosis (Hyalinosis cutis et mucosae)

This is a rare autosomal recessive disorder, characterised by infiltration of hyaline material. The nature of the hyaline material is unknown. There is mutation in the extracellular matrix protein-1 gene. A change is seen in the fibroblasts of patients with lipid proteinosis. Various other cell constituents such as myoepithelial cells, smooth muscle cells and Schwann cells are also held responsible for the production of hyaline material. It often manifests in infancy as hoarseness.

Distinctive histopathological features are extreme dilatation of the blood vessels, thickening of their walls and infiltration of the dermis and subcutaneous tissue by extracellular hyaline deposits.

Cutaneous Lesions

Lipid proteinosis (Fig. 8) develops early in life, mild skin injury and inflammation results in scarring. Early infiltration of the skin results in formation of papules and nodules. These are especially seen in the muzzle area of the face. Beaded papules are present on the upper and lower eyelids; there may be total loss of the eyelashes. Nodules may be present on the elbows, finger joints, axillae and the scrotum. Nodular lesions resemble xanthomas. Patchy alopecia occurs if the scalp is involved.

Mucosal Lesions

Hoarseness develops in infancy; it may progress to complete aphonia, fortunately breathing difficulty is rare. The tongue is wood like and moves

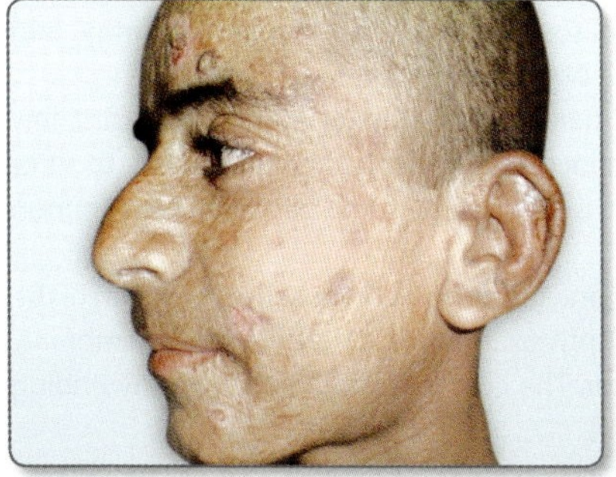

Fig. 8: Lipid proteinosis

with difficulty. It is difficult to protrude the tongue. Yellowish deposits similar to that of the skin are seen in the mucosal lesions.

The rhinecephalon is the cerebral representation when the muzzle area is involved; here taste, smell and correlated reflexes are controlled. Other cerebral manifestations include epilepsy and abnormal behaviour. Calcification of the cerebral lesions is common. Calcification on either side of the sella turcica is said to be pathognomonic of lipid proteinosis.

There is no effective therapy for lipid proteinosis. Dermabrasion and chemical peeling can improve the skin lesions cosmetically. Acitretin may show a clinical response after 2–3 months of therapy. Dissection of the vocal nodules may improve the hoarseness; it is only temporary. Clearance of the laryngeal and skin lesions has been reported with dimethylsulphoxide.

Gaucher's Disease

This is an autosomal recessive disorder due to decrease of beta-glucocerebrosidase. This results in accumulation of glucocerebrosides in the reticuloendothelial (Gaucher's) cells of the liver, spleen, and the bone marrow. Gaucher's cells are large cells with a small nucleus and pale staining cytoplasm; these contain glucocerebrosides within the distended lysosomes.

Clinically there are two types of Gaucher's disease: infantile and adult. The infantile variant begins in infancy and usually ends fatally by the second year of life. The symptoms are mainly neurological and laryngeal. Cutaneous lesions are not seen. The child often dies of acute respiratory infection.

The adult type is more common and it starts insidiously. It is characterised by hepatosplenomegaly, rarefaction of the long bones, pingueculae of the sclera, and bronze discolouration of the skin due to melanin. Deeper pigmentation which extends from the knees to the feet is due to haemosiderin. Initial complaints are of weakness and mild bleeding tendencies. Anaemia and pancytopenia are almost constant findings.

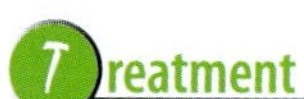

Bone marrow transplantation has halted the neurological progress of the disease. Treatment is symptomatic. X-ray therapy to the long bones may be given for bone pains. Splenectomy is indicated for anemia and thrombocytopenia.

Niemann-Pick Disease

This is an autosomal recessive disorder due to lack of sphingomyelinase. The disease is characterised by hepatosplenomegaly, lymphadenopathy, and accumulation of foam cells in the bone marrow.

The systemic symptoms are manifested by loss of weight in the first few months of life. Muscle weakness increases and the patient is unable to sit or raise his head, as the muscle tone is lost. Deafness and blindness are common features.

The cutaneous changes are characterised by yellowish discolouration of the skin, resembling the lesions of eruptive xanthoma. On the mucous membrane, black macular patches may occur. The course is progressive usually ending fatally in the first three years of life.

No treatment is effective. Bone marrow transplantation has shown good response in a few cases.

DISORDERS OF AMINO ACID METABOLISM

Phenylketonuria (PKU)

Phenylketonuria is an autosomal recessive disorder in which there is deficiency of phenylalanine hydroxylase, the enzyme which catalyses phenylalanine to tyrosine. This leads to accumulation of phenylalanine, phenylpyruvic acid, and their metabolites. Levels of phenylalanine are high in the urine. The reduction in melanin formation is due to reduction of tyrosine; the hair will darken if large amounts of tyrosine are ingested.

Clinical Features

Cutaneous lesions occur predominantly in the Caucasians. The children are usually blue eyed with blonde hairs and fair complexion. The patients are extremely sensitive to light. Fifty percent have eczematous dermatitis similar to atopic dermatitis. Skin lesions may also be sclerodermatous in nature. Induration of the thigh and buttocks are present in infancy. The incidence of pyogenic infection is also increased.

Systemic Manifestations

The affected children are of average birthweight and height. Brain damage due to phenylalanine and its metabolites occur during rapid phase of brain development just before and after birth. Mental retardation, epilepsy and extrapyramidal manifestations occur due to the brain damage.

Diagnosis

Blood phenylalanine levels should be done in the first week of life. Urine tests may be negative in the first few months of life. The presence of phenylpyruvic acid in the urine is demonstrated by a deep green colour when a few drops of ferric chloride are added to it. (Green diapers also occur in histidinemia).

Guthrie test which detects raised blood phenylalanine levels is carried out routinely in most developed countries.

Treatment

A diet low in phenylalanine brings about normal development if begun shortly after birth. The amount of phenylalanine supplied in the diet should be low enough to prevent its accumulation in the blood, but high enough to allow protein synthesis and growth. The diet may be relaxed at 6–8 years, but some restriction of the diet is still essential throughout life.

Alkaptonuria

Alkaptonuria is an autosomal recessive disorder caused by a lack of homogentisic acid oxidase, the enzyme necessary for the catabolism of homogentisic acid to acetoacetic acid and fumaric acid. Large amounts of homogentisic acid are deposited in the fibrous tissue and cartilage; large amounts are also excreted in the urine. In the skin, it gives rise to a distinctive cutaneous pigmentation.

Drugs such as phenol, resorcinol, mepacrine, and perhaps anti-malarials can also cause alkaptonuria. These drugs also inhibit the enzyme homogentisic acid oxidase. An exogenous ochronosis can also occur from hydroquinone containing bleaching creams.

Clinical Features

The clinical sequel of events is first alkaptonuria then ochronosis and lastly arthropathy. The urine is of normal colour but darkens on exposure to air or after the addition of an alkaline solution. Patients observe that both sweat and urine discolour clothing. Dark urine may be the only manifestation for many years.

Cutaneous manifestations occur in the fourth decade. Blue or brown-coloured macules occur; they have a predilection for the ears, nose, fingers, genital region, apices of the axillae, and buccal mucosa. The skin of the vault of the axilla yields black brown sweat on intradermal injection of epinephrine.

Cartilage is a favourite site for the deposition of homogentisic acid. The earliest sign is pigmentation of the sclera (Osler's sign) and cartilage. The cerumen is often black. Internally the larynx, trachea, valves of the heart, oesophagus, and dura mater may be involved.

Arthropathy may involve the vertebral joints first, giving rise to low backache. X-ray shows early calcification of the intervertebral discs and narrowing of the intervertebral spaces with eventual disc collapse. Other joints involved are shoulders and the hips. Limitation of the expansion of the chest may give rise to dyspnoea.

Atherosclerosis is common in old age. Generally, the disease is benign with normal life expectancy.

Diagnosis

The diagnosis is based on the typical urinary discolouration; the dark urine is examined by chromatography. Other causes of dark-coloured urine should be excluded such as melaninuria, porphyria, myoglobinuria, hematuria, and bilirubinuria. Care should also be taken while testing the urine; an incorrect diagnosis of glucosuria can be made with Fehling's solution.

Treatment

Connective tissue damage can be reduced by ascorbic acid that acts as an anti-oxidant; a long-term therapy may be required. Analgesics and physiotherapy are required for arthropathies.

Hartnup Disease

The disease is named after the Hartnup family in which it was first discovered. This is a rare hereditary autosomal recessive metabolic disorder in which there is a failure in the absorption of tryptophan from the small intestine. Large amounts of indoleacetic acid are found in the urine. Failure of absorption of tryptophan results in a deficiency in the synthesis of nicotinamide, resulting in pellagra-like syndrome.

Clinical Features

The onset is usually in childhood. The cutaneous signs precede the neurological manifestations. Erythematous scaly lesions occur mainly in the sun-exposed areas, which flare up on exposure to sunlight. Neurological manifestations include cerebellar ataxia, nystagmus, diplopia and mild tremors of the hands and feet. Mental retardation and psychiatric manifestations are seen only in a few cases. Other abnormalities include fever, diarrhoea and atrophic glossitis.

Treatment

Skin lesions respond to nicotinamide 200 mg/daily; it may also improve ataxia and psychotic behaviour. Symptoms become milder with increasing age.

MUCOPOLYSACCHARIDOSIS

Mucopolysaccharidosis (MPS) are clinically progressive hereditary disorders characterised by accumulation of mucopolysaccharides (glycosaminoglycans) in the various tissues. There are a number of different types of MPS caused by deficiency of a specific lysosomal enzyme, which are normally involved in the degradation of one or more types of mucopolysaccharides. The group of diseases is separated by genetic, clinical, and biochemical characteristics. Hurler's syndrome are the prototype of these disorders. All MPS are autosomal recessive except Hunter's syndrome, which is X-linked recessive.

Clinical Features

Clinical manifestations related to the eye, heart, brain, skeleton, skin and other systems.

Cutaneous Manifestations

This is characterised by thickening of the skin with ridges and grooves. Large brown coarse hair is present over the extremities. Pebbling of the skin over the inferior angle of the scapular is characteristic of Hunter's syndrome; these are firm flesh coloured to white papules and nodules that coalesce. These may also be present on the nape of the neck, lateral aspect of the arm and thigh. In MPS IV, the skin may hang rather loose over the hands. Gargoyle features are characteristic of Hurler's syndrome; the patients have broad saddle shaped nose, thick lips, and large tongue.

Eye changes include clouding of the cornea, glaucoma and pigmentary retinoid degeneration. These changes are seen in all types of MPS. Progressive degeneration of intellect is the cardinal feature of Hurler's and Sanfilippo syndrome. Hydrocephalus is frequent in Hurler's syndrome.

Skeletal changes are referred to as dysostosis simplex. The joints have limited extensibility, particularly of the fingers. Breadth of the hand is greater than the length; the fingers are maintained in a claw-like position. Coxa valga and genu valgum of moderate degree may be present. The combination of claw like hands, large head, grotesque facies, and deformed limbs accounts for the designation "gargoylism". The sella turcica is often elongated, mandibular condyles are concave. The vertebral bodies are short, the anterior and posterior outlines appear concave and the spinous process is directed backward. The humerus is long and thick, the radius and ulna are short and broad.

All MPS fulfil the following criteria:

- The disorders are progressive.
- Multiple organs are affected.
- The stored material is heterogeneous, e.g. both dermatan sulfate and heparan sulfate are found in MPS I and II.
- Cellular inclusions are present, bounded by a single membrane; this stains positively for acid phosphatase.

Prognosis and Treatment

Treatment is unfavourable; patients remain retarded both physically and mentally. Orthopaedic treatment can help the deformities of the bones and spine.

CALCINOSIS CUTIS

Calcium can be deposited in the skin in a number of disorders. These can be broadly classified as:

- Dystrophic calcification
- Idiopathic calcification
- Traumatic calcification
- Metastatic calcification
- Calcinosis circumscripta
- Familial calcification
- Idiopathic calcification of the scrotum.

Dystrophic Calcification

Calcium is deposited in damaged or altered tissue. Calcium deposition can occur in localised morphoea, rheumatoid arthritis, and pseudoxanthoma elasticum. Other cutaneous tumours and diseases that can calcify are epidermal cysts, trichilemmal cysts, dermoid cysts, haemangiomas, keratosis, neurilemmomas, chondromas, lipomas, foreign body granulomas, and inflammatory lesions such as acne cysts.

Idiopathic Calcification

The deposition of calcium in the dermis, subcutaneous tissue and the muscles is unrelated to any recognised tissue injury or metabolic disorders. This can be localised or generalised.

Generalised Idiopathic Calcification

Nodules or plaques are symmetrically distributed over the extremities and less commonly over the trunk. Fingertip lesions are often painful, while at other sites there may be limitation of movements due to stiffening of the skin. The disease is eventually fatal. Painful lesions can be removed surgically. In some cases corticosteroids may be helpful. Low calcium diet should be initiated.

Calcinosis Circumscripta

There are few calcium deposits in the skin. Most of these cases are found in generalised scleroderma and dermatomyositis. Rarely is it idiopathic. These are chiefly found in the upper extremities, fingers, or the wrists.

Traumatic Calcification

This is a rarely reported entity; traumatic calcification has been reported in people working with calcium chloride containing substances. Prolonged contact with ECG paste, sacks of calcium chloride, limewater compresses, coal mine exposure, and exposure to refrigerant calcium chloride are some of the occupations in which calcium deposition in the skin may occur.

Familial Calcification (Tumoral Calcinosis)

This is a rare familial disease of unknown cause. It appears early in life with large subcutaneous masses of calcium overlying the pressure areas and the joints. Skin involvement apart from tumoral masses is extremely rare, but may occur as localised calcinosis cutis. The internal organs are not involved and the serum calcium levels are normal. Surgical excision is the mainstay of therapy, but recurrences are common.

Metastatic Calcification

This rare entity is characterised by metastatic calcification of the skin; there are elevated levels of serum calcium and phosphates. It is often associated with bone destruction, primary hyperparathyroidism, parathyroid neoplasia, hypervitaminosis D, sarcoidosis, excessive intake of milk or alkali, osteomyelitis, bone tumours, Paget's disease of the bone, metastatic carcinoma, etc. It is also seen in chronic renal failure and hyperphosphataemia. Other organs involved in addition to the skin are lungs, kidneys, heart, eyes, and the stomach.

Treatment of the underlying disease is essential. Involution of the skin lesions is reported with a diet containing 430 mg of phosphorous, 30 g of protein and 60 mL of aluminum hydroxide gel. In hypervitaminosis D and milk-alkali syndrome, improvement can occur with withdrawal of vitamin D or milk from the diet.

Idiopathic Calcification of the Scrotum

This is a rare benign disorder of unknown aetiology. The nodules are small, non-tender and firm. Idiopathic calcification of the penis is also reported. This is sometimes associated with Peyronie's disease.

Osteoma Cutis

Bone formation in the skin may be primary or metastatic. Metastatic osteoma cutis occurs most frequently in pilomatricoma. It may also occur in basal cell carcinoma, intradermal naevi, mixed tumours of the skin, scars, scleroderma, dermatomyositis and some inflammatory disorders.

ANGIOKERATOMA WITH SYSTEMIC DISEASE

Fabry's Disease (Angiokeratoma Corporis Diffusum)

This is an X-linked storage disease in which ceramide trihexoside (glucosyl galactosyl glycosyl ceramide) accumulates in the skin and the viscera. It is due to deficiency of alpha galactosidase A, low levels of which are found in

Clinical Features

The disease is manifest in about 6–7 years of life as remittent attacks of fever, limb pains, dysesthesias of the extremities, intermittent proteinuria, haematuria, and abdominal pain resembling acute appendicitis. Most patients have excruciating pain in their hands. Corneal dystrophy is common. Renal colic, ankle oedema may occur. Cardiac disease and renal insufficiency bring death usually in the fifth decade.

Cutaneous lesions are widespread. These are angiokeratomas; the keratosis is less prominent than in the other forms of angiokeratomas. The skin lesions are grouped, almost black, small telangiectatic papules around the umbilicus and pelvis. Similar papules are also seen on the lower extremities, scrotum, penis, lower trunk, axillae, and lips. Hair growth is scanty. Anhidrosis occurs due to impaired vasomotor control. The lesions are symptomless. Similar lesions are also seen in fucosidosis.

the serum, skin, fibroblasts, and amniotic fluid. The deposits of glycolipids are present predominantly in the endothelial cells, fibroblasts, and pericytes of the dermis.

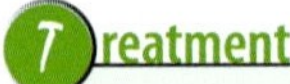

There is no specific treatment. Limb pains may be reduced by phenytoin, carbamazepine either alone or in combination. Infusion of plasma, haemodialysis, and renal transplantation have been tried for symptomatic relief and overall progress.

Fucosidosis

This is a rare autosomal recessive lysosomal disease caused by the deficiency of α-L-fucosidase. It can occur in association with Fabry's disease. Progressive mental and motor deterioration begins in infancy and death occurs by the age of 18–20 years. Numerous empty storage vacuoles are seen in the melanocytes, endothelial cells, sweat glands and fibroblasts, which help it to be differentiated from Fabry's disease.

Motor and mental retardation, visceromegaly, and epilepsy are seen in the first few years of life. The angiokeratomas are more frequent than in Fabry's disease; these may also occur on the tongue.

CUTANEOUS MANIFESTATIONS OF IMMUNOSUPPRESSION

Immunosuppression often results when corticosteroids, cytotoxic therapy, and immunosuppressive drugs are given to transplant patients to suppress the rejection of the graft, or when given for autoimmune disease such as lupus erythematosus, pemphigus, pemphigoid, etc. Most of the published reports relate to kidney transplants. The complications include side effects of the drug such as Cushing's syndrome in corticosteroid therapy, oral ulcers, purpura, and hair loss in cytotoxic therapy. There is an increased susceptibility to infection, increased incidence of malignancy, and drug reactions.

Infections

Viral infections are the most common. Warts occur in 50% of transplant patients; these may be widespread, some may also show a dysplastic or malignant change. Re-activation of the latent varicella-zoster virus occurs; herpes zoster may take a quiescent or fulminant course; chickenpox may be life-threatening. Persistent herpes simplex infection particularly with ulceration of the mouth and perioral skin is frequently encountered.

Furunculosis, impetigo and cellulitis are more common when compared to the general population. Ecthyma gangrenosum with pseudomonas septicaemia may be life-threatening. Long-standing quiescent leprosy and tuberculosis may relapse suddenly.

Candidiasis of the mouth and intertriginous areas of the skin is common. Pityriasis versicolor and Norwegian scabies occur frequently in the immunosuppressed. Invasive Trichophyton rubrum infection may present as subcutaneous nodules.

Neoplasms

Immunosuppression leads to increased incidence of neoplasms of the skin and lymphoreticular system. Cyclosporin induced lymphomas may have a short incubation period. Kaposi's sarcoma is clearly associated with immunosuppressive therapy. The most common cutaneous malignancy of renal transplant patients is squamous cell carcinoma in the sun-exposed area. Solar keratosis, keratoacanthoma and basal cell carcinomas are also seen. Patients should be advised against excessive sun exposure. Dysplastic naevi may become malignant. Malignancy of the anogenital region may be associated with the oncogenic papilloma virus.

CUTANEOUS MANIFESTATIONS OF INTERNAL MALIGNANCY

Changes in the skin can indicate the presence of underlying malignancy in many ways.

Signs of Exposure of the Carcinogen

Brown staining of the fingers due to cigarette smoking is seen in bronchogenic carcinoma. Arsenic, previously used to treat many cutaneous disorders is potentially malignant. Arsenic produces three distinct skin changes: circular brown keratosis of the palms and soles, diffuse pigmentation with raindrop areas of paler normal skin and Bowen's disease on the covered parts of the body. Chronic radiation dermatitis can also lead to malignancy; radiation is used for the treatment of internal malignancy.

Direct Involvement of the Skin by Malignant Cells

Breast cancer cells invade the skin directly to produce the peau d'orange effect due to lymph stasis. An erythematous plaque that resembles erysipelas is sometimes seen. Eczematous eruption of the nipple or perineum is seen in Paget's disease; this is usually unilateral and does not respond to corticosteroid treatment. Skin metastasis is common in terminal cancer but occasionally it may present as a presenting sign. Subcutaneous or dermal nodules are the most frequent manifestations of metastatic carcinoma; the most common site is the scalp or the trunk. Sister Joseph's nodule is a deep subcutaneous nodule around the umbilicus usually due to metastasis from adenocarcinoma of the stomach. Hypernephroma metastasises in the skin as a solitary deposit usually on the scalp.

Miscellaneous Signs of Internal Malignancy

The three most common skin markers of internal malignancy are pallor due to anaemia, pigmentation probably due to ectopic production of melanocytic-stimulating hormone by the malignant cells and generalised pruritus. The latter is particularly common in Hodgkin's disease and may be accompanied by eosinophilia.

The other manifestations include erythroderma, acanthosis nigricans, clubbing, herpes zoster, and dermatomyositis. The rarer manifestations are erythema gyratum repens, acquired hypertrichosis lanuginosa, multiple seborrhoeic warts, acquired ichthyosis, necrolytic migratory erythema, flushing in carcinoid syndrome, bullous pyoderma gangrenosum, paraneoplastic pemphigus, and pemphigoid may occasionally occur in patients with carcinoma.

Secondary Skin Involvement in Lymphoid Neoplasias

The skin involvement occurs in the advanced stage of malignancy. Lesions can be by specific infiltration of neoplastic cells or they are non-specific. The specific infiltrates appear as papules, plaques, nodules or as diffuse infiltration. Non-specific skin lesions are seen in about 30% of patients. These include pruritus, erythroderma, oral ulcers, purpura, pyoderma gangrenosum, Sweet's syndrome, urticaria, hair loss and skin infections.

Genetic Syndromes that Predispose to Malignancy

The best known examples are neurofibromatosis and tuberous sclerosis. Gardner's syndrome is associated with multiple epidermal cysts on the face and the scalp, and bone cysts in the jaw. Peutz-Jeghers syndrome is associated with perioral lentigines and multiple small intestinal polyps. Defects in the immune system allow the malignant cells to evade detection and destruction by the immune system, this is seen in both congenital and acquired immunosuppression, e.g. Wiskott-Aldrich syndrome is associated with eczema and purpura. Other diseases associated with malignancies are xeroderma pigmentosum, Bloom's syndrome, epidermodysplasia verruciformis and albinism.

The sorrow that has no vent makes other organs weep.
(Henry Maudsley)

FURTHER READING

1. Abrams JJ. Normocholesterolemic dysbetalipoproteinemia with xanthomatosis Metabolism. 1979;28(2):113-24.
2. Bello YM, Phillips TJ. Necrobiosis lipoidica: indolent plaque may signal to diabetes. Postgrad Med. 2001;109(3):93-4.
3. Bem J, Bradley EL. Subcutaneous manifestations of acute pancreatitis. Pancreas. 1998;16(4):551-6.
4. Bem J, Bradley EL. Subcutaneous manifestations of severe acute pancreatitis. Pancreas; 1998;16(4):551-6.
5. Boscaro M, Barzon L, Fallo F. Cushing's syndrome. Lancet. 2001;357(9528):783-91.
6. Erikson QL, Faleski EJ, Koops MK, et al. Addison's disease: the potentially life-threatening tan. Cutis. 2000;66(1):72-4.
7. Feingold KR, Elias PM. Endocrine and skin interaction. Cutaneous manifestations of pituitary, disease, thyroid disease, calcium disorders and diabetes. J Am Acad Dermatol. 1987;17(6):921-40.
8. Fisch RO, Tsai MY, Gentry WC. Studies of phenylketonuria with dermatitis. J Am Acad Dermatol. 1981;4(3):284-90.
9. Jabbour SA. Cutaneous manifestations of endocrine disorders: a guide for dermatologists. Am J Clin Dermatol. 2003;4(5):315-31.

10. Jones D, Kay M, Craigen W, et al. Coal-black hyperpigmentation at birth in a child with congenital adrenal hypoplasia. J Am acad Dermatol. 1995;33(2 Pt 2):323-6.
11. Jorizzo JL, Daniels E. Dermatologic conditions reported in patients with rheumatoid arthritis. J Am Acad Dermatol. 1983;8(4):439-57.
12. Kaliyaden F, Dharmanatran AD. Q-switched Nd-YAG laser in the treatment of xanthelasma palpebrarum. J Cut Aesth Surg. 2010;3(2):127-8.
13. Kupers DR, Claes K, Evenepoet P, et al. A prospective proof of the study on the efficacy of tacrolimus ointment on uraemic pruritus; in patients with chronic dialysis therapy. Nephrol Dial Transplant. 2004;19(7):1895-901.
14. Lakhanpal S, Conn DL, Lie JT. Clinical and prognostic significance of vasculitis as an early manifestation of connective tissue diseases syndrome. Ann Intern Med. 1984;101(6):743-8.
15. Li CP, Lee FY, Hwang SJ, et al. Role of substance P in the pathogenesis of spider angioma in patients with non-alcoholic liver disease. J Am Acad Dermatol. 1999;94:502-7.
16. Nambu M, Kaneko K, Lilija T. Biochemical and clinical study of muscle atrophy at thenar and hypothenar eminences in patients with cirrhosis. Liver. 1996;16(1):19-22.
17. Rahbour G, Rehanullah M, Yassin N, et al. Cullen's sign: case report with review of literature. Int J Surg Case Rep. 2012;3(5):143-6.
18. Schaberg DS, Norwood JM. A case study: infections in diabetes mellitus. Diabetes Spectrum. 2002;13(1):37-40.
19. Scoggin RB, Haraln WR. Cutaneous manifestations of hyperlipidemia and uraemia. Postgrad Med. 1967;41:357-8.
20. Seyger MM, van den Hoogen FH, de Mare S, et al. A patient with severe scleroedema diabeticorum: partially responded to low dose methotrexate. Dermatol. 1999;198(2):177-9.
21. Vega GL, Denke MA, Grundy SM. Metabolic basis of primary hypercholesterolemia. Circulation. 1991;84(1):118-28.
22. Worth RL. Calciphylaxis: pathogenesis and therapy. J Cutan Med Surg. 1998;2(4):245-8.

Chapter

32

Systemic Effects of Cutaneous Disease: Erythroderma

ERYTHRODERMA

Erythroderma or exfoliative dermatitis is the name given to inflammation of the skin that covers more than 90% of the skin surface. Exfoliative dermatitis does not generally involve the mucous membrane. Men are more frequently affected, and the mean age of onset is around 50 years (Fig. 1).

Just as the skin is affected by internal disease, the internal organs may be affected by cutaneous disease. In erythroderma, the systemic effects may assume major importance. Before the introduction of steroids, erythroderma was fatal in about one-third of cases. Heart failure and pneumonia were the most common causes of death.

Causes of Erythroderma

Erythroderma can be primary or secondary. Primary erythroderma is often idiopathic. The common secondary causes of erythroderma are drug eruptions, eczema, psoriasis, pemphigus, lymphomas and leukemias. Lichen planus, dermatophytosis, crusted scabies, and hereditary disorders such as congenital ichthyosiform erythroderma and pityriasis rubra pilaris are some other causes of erythroderma.

Papuloerythroderma of Ofuji differs from the ordinary erythroderma; in this papular eruption is predominant. It tends to spare the face and flexures.

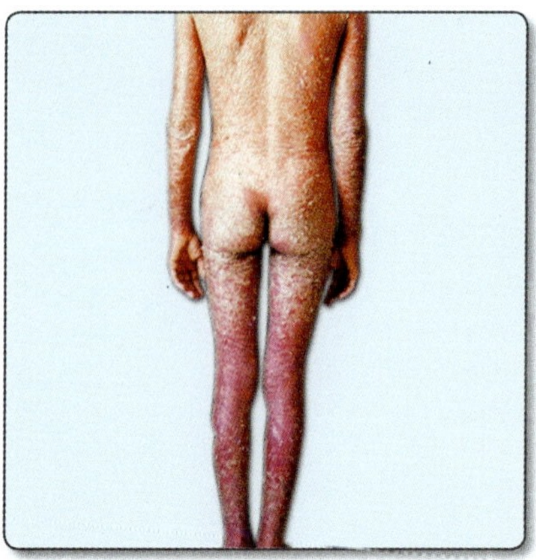

Fig. 1: Erythroderma

The condition is extremely pruritic, blood eosinophils and serum IgE levels are raised.

The drugs most likely to cause erythroderma are nonsteroidal anti-inflammatory drugs (NSAIDs), sulphonamides, thiazides, barbiturates, captopril, furosemide, and cimetidine. The list is continuously increasing.

In children the common causes of erythroderma are bullous and non-bullous ichthyosiform erythroderma, atopic dermatitis, immunodeficiency syndromes, and staphylococcal scalded skin syndrome.

Manifestations Cutaneous

Although the causes of erythroderma are varied, the cutaneous signs are similar in most cases. The skin is erythematous and scaly. The epidermis is thin and shiny. As desquamation progresses the skin becomes dry, scaly and has a greyish hue. If infection is superadded, moist adherent crusts form with a characteristic musky odour.

In chronic erythroderma, lichenification is common, diffuse hair loss occurs, the nails are dry, brittle and ridged. Shoreline nails is characteristic of drug induced erythroderma; there are alternating bands of leuconychia representing the period during which the offending drug was taken. Palmoplantar keratoderma and crusted scaling of the scalp is often associated with chronic erythroderma.

Patchy hypopigmentation and hyperpigmentation, vitiligo, anhidrosis, and xanthomas have been reported after resolution of erythroderma.

Manifestations Systemic

Haemodynamic Effects

In erythroderma, the cutaneous capillary bed is fully dilated and the skin feels hot due to the increased blood flow. There is tachycardia and a collapsing pulse; the cardiac output is also increased. Much of the cardiac output is diverted to the skin, and blood flow to the other organs may be decreased. The plasma volume is increased, and there is often widespread cutaneous oedema due to increased capillary permeability and hypoalbuminaemia.

Thermoregulation

Erythrodermic patients often behave like cold-blooded animals. The inflamed skin may produce a circulatory pyrogen, and the hypothalamic thermostat becomes abnormal so that inappropriate shivering occurs.

Haematological Effects

These include anaemia, leucocytosis and increased erythrocyte sedimentation rate (ESR). Folate and iron deficiency is due to malabsorption. Protein metabolism is also abnormal; plasma albumin is decreased due to hypovolemia, increased capillary permeability and increased protein loss through the bowel and the skin (desquamation). The plasma globulin is often increased, the reason for which is obscure.

Fluid Balance

Thirst and oliguria are common in erythroderma. This positive fluid balance compensates for the increased transepidermal water loss, and plasma loss from the increased capillary permeability.

Intestinal Effects

Erythroderma is associated with malabsorption. There may be a protein losing enteropathy, this dermatogenic enteropathy must be distinguished from the other causes of protein loss from the gastrointestinal tract such as coeliac disease.

Lymphadenopathy

The lymph nodes of the axillae and the groins are usually considerably enlarged in erythroderma from any cause; this may be misdiagnosed as lymphomas. Biopsy shows that the normal architecture is preserved and the lymph nodes contain quantities of lipid and melanin derived from the inflamed skin. This non-specific lymphadenopathy secondary to erythroderma is called "dermatogenic lymphadenopathy".

Miscellaneous Metabolic Effects

Gynecomastia is a common finding in chronic erythroderma; some patients have increased urinary oestrogens. Hyperuricaemia is due to increased cell turnover. Hypocalcaemia and decreased levels of serum iron are due to malabsorption.

Diagnosis

Most information is got from history of the patient. History of previous dermatoses and history of drug intake are important; these often give a clue to the cause of erythroderma. Detail examination of the skin may give a clue to the aetiology of erythroderma, e.g. white reticulate pigmentation of the oral mucosa in lichen planus. Patches of normal skin may be evident in erythroderma due to pityriasis rubra pilaris.

Microscopic examination of an erythrodermic patient is often unsatisfactory to give a diagnosis; most cases give a report of chronic dermatitis, except perhaps mycosis fungoides and Sézary syndrome. Direct immunofluorescence may be helpful in bullous disorders.

Treatment of Erythroderma

Treatment depends upon treating the underlying cause of erythroderma. Acute cases of erythroderma should be hospitalised; chronic cases can be treated in an outpatient department, provided the body has acclimatised to the condition.

The most common cause of erythroderma is reaction to drugs; it is always better to discontinue any suspected offending drug. Cutaneous inflammation is best managed by bland lotions or emollients. Systemic effects may occur with topical application of drugs due to absorption from the skin which occurs more readily because of the inflamed skin.

Systemic steroids should be avoided especially in psoriasis as this may precipitate pustular psoriasis. Systemic steroids may also give rise to the dangers of fluid retention, secondary infection, diabetes, etc. These may be required in severe persistent cases of erythroderma secondary to eczema and drug eruptions. It is best to start with mild-moderate potency steroids, or dose depending upon the cause of erythroderma; these should be tapered rapidly to a maintenance dose. Cyclosporin 4–5 mg/kg/day can be used as an alternative.

Antibiotics should be given in all cases as *Staphylococcus* colonisation may exacerbate erythroderma.

If the patient develops complications of erythroderma, they should be hospitalised and carefully monitored for protein and electrolyte balance, circulatory status, and body temperature surveillance. Rapid cooling and overheating should be avoided. Blood urea, blood electrolytes and fluid balance must be maintained; cardiac failure treated if it develops.

When the erythroderma starts to resolve, the primary treatment of the underlying skin disorder should be initiated.

Course and Prognosis

This depends upon the cause of erythroderma and the age of the patient. Erythroderma due to drugs usually has a good prognosis provided the patient is healthy. Erythroderma due to psoriasis and eczema may continue for months or years, and tend to relapse easily. Prognosis is poor in the elderly due to the associated systemic complications; cutaneous and respiratory infections are common. Pneumonia, heart and kidney failures are the common causes of death.

The three common causes of erythroderma are: drug reactions, atopic dermatitis and psoriasis.

FURTHER READING

1. Freedburg IM, and Baden HP. The metabolic response to exfoliation. J Invest Dermatol. 1962;38:277-84.
2. King LE. Erythroderma: who, what, when, why and how? Arch Dermatol. 1994;130:1545-7.
3. Okoduwa C, Lambert WC, Shwartz RA, et al. Erythroderma: Review of a Potentially Life-threatening Disorder. Indian J Dermatol. 2009;54(1):1-6.
4. Sarkar R. Neonatal and infantile erythroderma: The Red Baby. Indian J Dermatol Venereol Leprol. 2006;31(3):178-81.
5. Wilson DC, Hester JD, King LE. Erythroderma and exfoliative dermatitis. Clin Dermatol. 1993;11:67-72.

Chapter

33

Ages of Man and their Dermatoses

Human life passes through various stages: from neonatal life and infancy, to the school-going child and adolescence, then adult life, with its responsibility of procreation and family, it finally drifts to the wisdom of old age. During these stages changes occur in the skin and other organs. In this chapter, the changes of the skin in the following ages are discussed:

- Neonatal dermatoses
- Changes in pregnancy and menopause
- The ageing skin.

NEONATAL DERMATOLOGY

The neonatal period constitutes the first 4 weeks of extrauterine life. The structure and function of the skin in a neonate are as follows:

The skin of a normal full-term infant has a complete functional stratum corneum with fully developed barrier function. The problems in absorption in a neonate occur because of the greatly increased surface area to the volume. Great care should be taken while applying medications on the skin of a neonate. Aniline dyes, hexachlorophene and related antiseptics, corticosteroids, neomycin, boric acid, resorcinol, benzyl benzoate and salicylic acid should be avoided on the skin of neonates because of the danger of side effects and toxicity.

It has been shown that the oxygen absorption and carbon dioxide excretion through the intact skin are inversely correlated to the gestational age. There is no increase in gas exchange in full-term neonates. Rates in preterm neonates rapidly fall within 2 weeks of birth.

A full complement of normal eccrine sweat glands is present by the 28th week of gestation, but these appear to be functionally immature in neonates before 36 weeks. Response to sweat glands occurs 2 weeks after birth. In neonates born after 36 weeks of gestation, sweat in response to thermal stimulation is present at birth. Such sweating is initially relatively insufficient, as thermoregulatory mechanisms are immature. Care should be taken not to overheat a neonate.

The secretions of the fetal sebaceous glands make a considerable contribution to the vernix caseosa. Sebum secretion rates are high in neonates as compared with the older and preadolescent children. This sebaceous activity reflects maternal androgens transferred through the placenta. Sebaceous activity decreases by the end of first month to the stable level by first year of life.

There is a high incidence of bacterial infections, ease of blister formation, absence of histamine induced urticarial reactions, and immunological incompetence in neonatal skin.

At birth the skin is covered with a whitish greasy film the vernix caseosa. The vernix normally dries rapidly and falls off within a few hours of birth. Its colour may reflect intrauterine disorders, it is golden yellow in haemolytic disease of the newborn and fetal distress. The meconium is greenish when bile salts are present.

The skin of postnatal infants (40 weeks) is dry and cracked soon after birth. Moisturisers are used to soften the skin. The premature infant (born before 37 weeks) is at a greater risk from infection. Their barrier system is not fully developed, and they have even a greater surface area to volume ratio. Local and systemic toxicity can occur from topical application of medicines or even cleansing agents. The skin is very fragile, great care is required while handling these children to avoid injury to the skin. Sweating is reduced; this coupled with loss of subcutaneous fat leads to inadequate temperature regulation.

TRANSIENT NEONATAL DERMATOSES

These dermatoses are common; they often resolve within a month.

Peripheral cyanosis (not involving the mucosa): This is regarded as normal in the first 48 hours or so, it is more prominent in hypothermia.

Erythema neonatorum: This is present in 75% of neonates. A striking generalised erythema is present after birth, which fades spontaneously within 24–48 hours.

Caput succedaneum and cephalohaematoma: Caput succedaneum is subcutaneous oedema present on the presenting part of the scalp in normal delivery. It is due to the shearing forces on the scalp during delivery. It resolves spontaneously in about 7 days.

Cephalohematoma is due to the same cause; it is a fluctuant swelling bound by suture lines. It also resolves spontaneously. If extensive, it can lead to hyperbilirubinaemia.

Harlequin Colour Changes: In about 5% of full-term infants, it is seen that when the baby is on its side the upper half of the body becomes pale and the lower half a deep red colour with a sharp demarcation between the two. If the baby is turned on the other side, the colour reverses. The duration of the attack is between half a minute to twenty minutes; a neonate may have a single attack, or these may recur on several occasions. It appears to have no pathological significance; it is probably due to immaturity of the hypothalamic centre, which is responsible for the control of peripheral vascular tone. If this persists beyond 4 weeks, it may be due to cardiovascular abnormalities associated with hypoxia, which needs investigation.

Marbling of the skin (Cutis marmorata): Newborn infants subject to cooling show distinct marbling of the skin, which disappears on re-warming. This marbling comprises a reticulate blue vascular pattern. This response is physiological and may be seen throughout infancy.

Physiological scaling of the newborn: Superficial cutaneous desquamation occurs in 75% of normal neonates. This usually occurs first around the ankles, it is mostly confined to the hands, and feet; it may gradually spread.

Sucking blisters: One or more solitary blisters may occur occasionally at birth; they are caused by vigorous sucking by the fetus in the uterus.

The scalp hair: The scalp hair is shed synchronously during the 5th month of the fetal life; having regrown enters a telogen phase by about 12 weeks before term. The telogen hair is again shed from the frontal and parietal region and the roots enter the anagen phase from the front and back. At the occipital area, the roots do not enter the anagen phase until term, and therefore a conspicuous alopecia appears at this site.

In some babies there is a synchronous hair loss during the neonatal period resulting in diffuse alopecia of the newborn (Telogen effluvium of the newborn).

Sebaceous hyperplasia: It is due to maternal androgens. This is seen as yellowish papules on the nose, cheeks, upper lip and forehead.

Milia: These are present in neonates; their number varies from few to many. These are 1–3 mm in size; white papules often appear at the site of sebaceous hyperplasia. Larger and single milia are often termed as "pearls"; these disappear by the first week of life.

Epstein's pearls: On the hard palate on either side of the raphe, there may be a temporary accumulation of epithelial cells called "Epstein pearls". Similar retention cysts may be seen on the gums; they disappear within the first few weeks of birth.

Jaundice: It is often present in a newborn child, because the lipid soluble bilirubin (indirect reacting) has to be converted to the water soluble ester glucuronide of bilirubin (direct reacting). This conversion requires an adequate amount of an enzyme, bilirubin glucuronyl transferase; the enzyme is present in small amounts in a newborn infant. This physiological jaundice is visible in the first 2–3 days of life in about two-thirds of infants, and disappears between 5 to 7 days. This is dependent on a rise of serum bilirubin levels, which is due to the breakdown of fetal RBC and transient deficiency of glucuronyl transferase in the liver.

Acne neonatorum: About 50% of neonates develop acneiform eruption on the face. These are hormone mediated due to maternal androgens. They resolve spontaneously; some cases may have to be treated by benzoyl peroxide or erythromycin.

NEONATAL DERMATOSES

These range from transient and benign to serious and life threatening. A history, physical examination, and laboratory findings will help to differentiate these disorders. Recognition of transient disorders will spare a newborn from intensive investigations, potentially harmful medication and prolonged hospitalisation.

Permanent lesions include hair shaft defects, aplasia of skin, keratinising abnormalities (ichthyosis, keratoderma, and pachyonychia), pigmentary abnormalities (albinism), photosensitive disorders (xeroderma pigmentosum), bullous disorders (epidermolysis bullosa, and incontinentia pigmenti), collagen and elastic tissue defects (cutis laxa, and pseudoxanthoma elasticum). These can easily be recognised and are discussed in the corresponding chapters.

The neonatal skin may also reflect systemic abnormalities such as excessive secretion of sodium chloride by the eccrine glands in cystic fibrosis, hyperpigmentation in Addison's disease, abnormalities of the hair in argininosuccinic aciduria. The skin may show changes in systemic diseases such as porphyria and other metabolic disorders, reticuloendotheliosis, various diseases of the connective tissue, etc. All these should be taken into account before concluding whether a skin rash is purely cutaneous, or associated with systemic disease; categorise its severity and treat it accordingly. Staphylococcal scalded skin syndrome, harlequin fetus, and junctional epidermolysis bullosa are some of the serious cutaneous disorders, which need utmost care.

SPECIFIC NEONATAL DERMATOSES

Pustular Erythema Toxicum Neonatorum

This is a benign, self-limiting neonatal eruption seen in about one-third of all full-term newborns. It is seen 24–72 hours after birth; the lesions appear first as erythematous macules, these later change to red or yellowish papules, finally a vesicular or pustular eruption occurs on an erythematous base. They are asymptomatic and evanescent; the individual lesions disappearing in 24–48 hours. Delayed eruption occurring after 10 days has been reported. The sites of predilection are the forehead, face, chest, trunk and extremities. Palms and soles are generally spared.

Giemsa's stain or Wright's stain of the lesional contents demonstrates numerous eosinophils. Bacteria are negative on culture; a biopsy reveals interfollicular, subcorneal pustules with dense accumulation of eosinophils.

Erythema toxicum neonatorum will resolve spontaneously without any side effects the usual duration being less than 1 week. No treatment is necessary.

Miliaria

Miliaria is often seen in the first few weeks of life. It is a transient inflammatory disease that is caused by mechanical obstruction of the sweat ducts. The clinical appearance depends upon the level of obstruction of the duct. Miliaria rubra occurs when swelling and inflammation follow rupture of the sweat duct behind a deeper occlusion. Miliaria rubra may progress to pustular lesions.

Effective management consists in keeping the baby in a cool environment; clothing should be lightweight. Cool soaks provide rapid improvement.

Transient Neonatal Pustular Melanosis

Transient neonatal pustular melanosis (TNPM) is reported to affect 5% of full-term black infants and less than 1% of white newborns. The most common lesion in TNPM is a pigmented macule. The initial lesions are pustules; these rupture leaving brown macules with a collarette of scale; vesicles may be seen occasionally. Lesions are seen primarily on the nape of the neck, forehead, lower back, shins, and under the chin. There are no systemic symptoms. The lesions may persist for several months but usually fade spontaneously within 3–4 weeks.

Giemsa's stain or Wright's stain of lesions in TNPM demonstrates polymorphic neutrophils and occasional eosinophils. Bacteria are absent and cultures are negative.

The lesions are transient and no treatment is required.

Acropustulosis of Infancy

Acropustulosis is a relatively rare disorder; the condition has its onset within the first few months of life, but it can begin shortly after birth.

The lesions begin as red papules that change within 24 hours to vesicles and pustules. These pustules are very pruritic; they last for 7–10 days, and appear in crops every 2–3 weeks. They are found predominantly on the hands and feet, less frequently on the face and scalp.

Gram's stain, Giemsa's stain and Wright's stain of the lesions reveal numerous neutrophils; bacteria are absent. On biopsy, the pustules are seen to be subcorneal.

The disease is self-limiting, it exacerbates and remits over 2–3 years and then resolves completely.

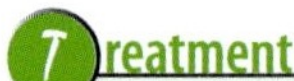

Treatment

Topical steroid therapy may be effective; antihistamines relieve itching in older children; in neonates it is contraindicated due to excessive sedation. Dapsone in a dose of 2 mg/kg/day may be effective.

Eosinophilic Pustular Folliculitis of Infancy

This rare disorder has a male predominance, it can be present at birth. The disorder is characterised by eosinophilic infiltration of hair follicles resulting in pruritic grouped follicular papules and pustules. The lesions appear in a perifollicular pattern on the scalp, hands and feet. They occur in recurrent crops; there is no systemic involvement.

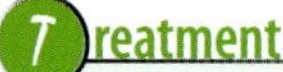

Treatment

Potent topical corticosteroids reduce itching and abort eruption in a number of cases. Sulphones and systemic steroids are used in adults.

Cultures of bacteria are negative. Giemsa's and Wright's stain show numerous eosinophils. Some patients have eosinophilia as well as leukocytosis. The pustules are intraepidermal.

Cradle Cap

The term "cradle cap" is generally applied to conditions in which there are adherent scales on the scalp in infancy. Strictly speaking, it is said to be a form of seborrhoeic dermatitis manifested by patches of greasy scales on the scalp with exudation and crusting. The disease gradually spreads beyond the scalp to the forehead, ears, postauricular region and neck. In extreme cases, greasy dirty crusts with an offensive odour cover the entire scalp.

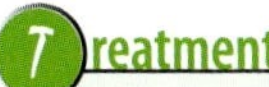

In the neonatal period, the scalp should be regularly oiled with olive oil. In the more refractory cases, water soluble emollients are applied on the scalp twice a day. Salicylic acid should not be used in neonates; it is used for older children as 1% sulphur and 1% salicylic acid preparation.

PANNICULITIS IN NEONATES

Sclerema neonatorum and subcutaneous fat necrosis of the newborn occur in the perinatal period and have a marked different prognosis.

Sclerema Neonatorum

This is often associated with an underlying serious disease such as severe diarrhoea, intestinal obstruction, respiratory distress, convulsions, pneumonitis or shock. It is due to cold exposure with vascular collapse and an increase in saturated fat relative to unsaturated fat; this leads to a diffuse solidification of the tissues. Histopathology shows oedema of fibrous septa surrounding the fat lobules.

The infants are often of low birthweight not necessarily premature. Most of the patients succumb to the concurrent illness, those who survive the sclerema resolves without complications.

Sclerema neonatorum presents as tallow-like indurations, which remain localised to the extremities or buttocks, or spread rapidly to involve most of the body surface. The skin is bound down to the underlying structures and is cold to touch. Palms, soles and genitalia are often spared. Biopsy shows the presence of fibrous bands in the subcutis, cellular infiltration and fat necrosis is absent or minimal. Occasional lipocytes are engorged with fat or replaced with firm needle-shaped crystals.

Treatment

Treatment is supportive and specifically directed at the underlying disease.

Subcutaneous Fat Necrosis

This is a self-limiting disease affecting healthy neonates. The fat of neonates contains more saturated fatty acids; this has a higher melting point than adult fatty acids. Once the temperature of the skin drops below the melting point of fat, crystallisation occurs within the subcutaneous fat cells and a granulomatous reaction ensues.

The lesions present as multiple violaceous firm nodules on the buttocks, shoulders or trunk; these tend to be discrete rather than confluent; liquefaction and calcification are common. A viscous grey material can be aspirated from the lesion. The nodules resolve spontaneously within a period of 6 months. Infrequently hypercalcaemia can occur with associated symptoms such as irritability, vomiting, weight loss and failure to thrive.

On biopsy ruptured fat cells surrounded by a florid inflammatory reaction and necrosis is seen. A few needle-shaped crystals are found within the fat cells and crystallisation of the saturated fat may be detected, but there is no fibrosis in the subcutaneous tissue.

Treatment

No treatment is indicated and under no conditions should the mass be incised. Fluctuant lesions can be aspirated to avoid subsequent scarring. The calcium level should be monitored in these infants: as the skin lesions resolve transient hypercalcaemia can occur and this should be treated.

OEDEMA OF THE NEWBORN

This is a rare disorder of unknown cause seen in weak newborns especially in premature infants. It is characterised by widespread pitting oedema of the extremities and trunk by pallor and lividity of the skin. It is fatal in most cases, those who survive the oedema gradually disappears as the general condition of the infant improves. The condition should be differentiated from sclerema neonatorum and scleredema of Buschke. No specific therapy is known.

Congenital Naevi discussed in chapter 28 and Neonatal Herpes discussed in Chapter 6.

CUTANEOUS CHANGES IN PREGNANCY

Pregnancy (Physiological Changes)

In pregnancy changes occur in the body due to the production of hormones by the pituitary, thyroid, adrenal and ovaries. Hormones are also produced by the placenta such as human chorionic gonadotropin, human placental lactogen as well as oestrogen and progesterone. The impact of these hormones is of importance in certain obstetric conditions, but their action on the skin is not clear.

In pregnancy there is deposition of fat and an increase in tissue fluids resulting in temporary coarsening of the features and an altered appearance. The sebaceous secretions increase perhaps due to progesterone, and the scalp becomes greasy. The scalp hair under the influence of oestrogens often enters a resting phase, moulting tends to occur in a few weeks following delivery.

The increase in pigmentation is mainly due to the increase in melanocyte stimulating hormone (MSH) or oestrogens; this may result in increased freckling and darkening of the areola. It is also responsible for melasma (mask of pregnancy), linea nigra, and darkening of the vulva.

Mild hirsutism is seen during pregnancy; it resolves after delivery. After delivery telogen effluvium may be significant up to 6 months postpartum. Regrowth occurs within a year. Androgenetic alopecia may improve due to increase of oestrogens.

The deeper layers of the skin crack due to stretching by the increase of subcutaneous fat. This causes striae gravidarum which occurs mainly on the abdominal wall, thigh, upper arm and breast. These are permanent, purplish red when originally formed; they become silvery and inconspicuous in later years. Skin tags tend to increase in pregnancy.

Granuloma gravidarum also known as pregnancy tumour is a pyogenic granuloma of oral cavity (particularly the gingiva); it is often associated with pregnancy gingivitis. Glomus tumours may appear or enlarge during pregnancy.

Spider naevi and palmar erythema are common; moles tend to enlarge genital warts and candidiasis gets worse.

Pregnancy may alter the course of a number of skin disorders, such as acne, eczema and psoriasis, and may trigger erythema multiforme.

SPECIFIC DERMATOSES OF PREGNANCY

The specific dermatoses of pregnancy are:

- Pruritus gravidarum
- Pemphigoid gestationis
- Polymorphic eruption of pregnancy
- Prurigo of pregnancy
- Pruritic folliculitis of pregnancy
- Papular dermatitis of pregnancy
- Autoimmune progesterone dermatitis of pregnancy
- Impetigo herpetiformis.

Pruritus Gravidarum (Intrahepatic Cholestasis of Pregnancy)

This is a mild variant of cholestasis of pregnancy; it occurs in 0.02–2.4% of pregnancies. The itching usually begins in the 3rd trimester; it is often localised to the abdomen, although it may be widespread. The patient may be mildly icteric, and liver function is usually abnormal with raised alkaline phosphatase. The condition is associated with fetal mortality and premature delivery. Postpartum hemorrhage may occur.

It is possible that irritation results from abnormal hepatic production of bile acids induced by endogenous oestrogens and progesterones. The itching usually subsides after childbirth, but may recur after subsequent pregnancies, and with the use of contraceptive pills.

Treatment

Pruritus is treated with bland emollients and topical antipruritic therapy such as calamine lotion. Other treatment modalities are antihistamines, ultraviolet B (UVB) and cholestyramine (8–10 g/day in 2–3 divided doses). Ursodeoxycholic acid 15 mg/kg have been used with success in some patients.

Polymorphic Eruption of Pregnancy (Pruritic Urticarial Papules and Plaques of Pregnancy-PUPPP)

The incidence of this eruption is 1 in 240 pregnancies. It begins in the 3rd trimester usually of a first pregnancy, or it may be delayed a few days postpartum. It rarely recurs in subsequent pregnancies. It has been postulated that excess of abdominal distention may act as a trigger for the skin changes.

The patient complains of intense itching. The skin lesions usually begin within the abdominal striae; it then spreads to the chest, buttocks and thigh, face and mucous membranes are spared. The lesions commonly consist of urticarial papules and plaques, vesicles, target and polycyclic erythematous lesions. There is no risk to the child.

The condition is treated with topical calamine lotion, topical steroids, sedatives, antihistamines are often affective. The condition subsides within a few days after delivery.

Prurigo of Pregnancy

This disorder begins between 25 weeks and 30 weeks of gestation. It occurs in 1 in 200 pregnancies, clinically there are multiple excoriated papules over the abdomen and on the extensor surface of the limbs. Many of these patients have atopic diathesis, and their skin condition flares up in pregnancy. The lesions continue throughout pregnancy and in the puerperium. It may occur in subsequent pregnancies. Treatment is symptomatic.

Pruritic Folliculitis of Pregnancy

This disorder begins in the 1st or 2nd trimester of pregnancy and usually resolves within 2 weeks of delivery. Clinically the lesions consist of itchy-red follicular pustules, which may be generalised or limited to the extremities. There is no adverse effect on the mother or fetus.

Papular Dermatitis of Pregnancy

The disease is rare, occurs in 1 in 24,000 pregnancies. The lesion consists of intensely itchy papules with a central crust. Laboratory abnormalities include raised urinary chorionic gonadotrophic hormone and low urinary estriol levels. About 30% fetal abnormality is associated with this eruption.

Autoimmune Progesterone Dermatitis of Pregnancy

Only a few cases has been reported of this eruption. It occurs as acneiform rashes on the extremities and buttocks. A skin sensitivity test is positive for progesterone.

Impetigo Herpetiformis

This is severe form of pustular psoriasis in pregnancy. It has a febrile onset; grouped pustules appear on an erythematous base, which begins in the flexures such as groins, axillae and neck. The lesions are usually annular. There is a high peripheral blood count and hypocalcaemia may be present. The patient is ill with fever, nausea, vomiting and tetany. Mortality rate is high.

The condition resolves with delivery but recurrences can occur with subsequent pregnancies. It may be associated with hyperparathyroidism, or it may lead to hyperparathyroidism. Fetal death may occur due to placental insufficiency.

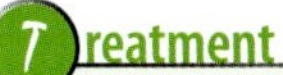

Multidisciplinary management is required with the paediatrician, obstetrician and dermatologist. Systemic corticosteroids 40–60 mg daily are required with supportive care.

Pemphigoid gestationis described in chapter 12.

CUTANEOUS CHANGES AT MENOPAUSE

Menopause literally speaking is the last menstrual period. Climacteric is a transitional phase lasting from 1 year to 5 years, during which the genital organs involute in response to cessation of gonadal activity.

During reproductive years, the ovaries produce oestrogens and progesterone, but at menopause, there are very few follicles left and the levels of ovary-derived oestrogens fall. After menopause, most of the oestrogens are derived from direct peripheral conversion of oestrone and androstenedione. Some oestrone may also arise from the alternative pathway via testosterone and oestradiol.

These hormonal changes are reflected in a number of physiological changes. Breast glandular tissue decreases and fibrous tissue increases. The body of the uterus becomes smaller, its muscles are partly replaced by fibrous tissue, endometrium becomes atrophic, and it retains the capacity to respond to endogenous hormones. The vagina becomes shorter and narrower, the vaginal epithelium atrophies. The vaginal pH increases and infections become more frequent. The external genitalia atrophy with loss of subcutaneous fat.

Skin is a target organ for oestrogens. The concentration of oestrogen receptors in the facial skin is more than on the breast or thigh. Changes in the skin seen at menopause such as dryness, epidermal thinning; loss of dermal elasticity may be due to decreased oestrogen levels. Oestrogen given to postmenopausal women, increases dermal thickness and decreases breakdown of collagen. Hormonal replacement therapy may increase the skin water-holding capacity.

The women become coarser in built and appearance, they develop features suggestive of a mild degree of acromegaly. The shoulders become broader, the waistline is lost and there is a slight growth of hair on the face; axillary and pubic hairs are not shed as these are dependent on adrenal rather than the ovarian androgens. Body hair becomes sparse as a result of senile changes affecting the hair follicles. Increase in weight is common. This may be due to increased appetite because of emotional stress, or it may be because of alteration of metabolism that lowers the nutritional requirements.

SKIN DISORDERS OF MENOPAUSE

Atrophic Vulvovaginitis

This responds to topical estrogens.

Menopausal Flushing

The most distressing complaint of menopause is flushing. There is a sudden feeling of intense heat in the face, neck and chest often accompanied by discomfort and sweating. It lasts for 4–5 minutes. Visible changes are seen in 50% of cases; this consists of blotchy erythema on the face, neck and chest. Some patients develop palpitations and throbbing in the head and neck. Headache, nausea and vomiting may occur. Some physiological changes such as increase in temperature, pulse rate and respiratory rate are also seen.

Flushes may be related with pulsatile release of luteinising hormone due to low circulatory oestrogen levels. This perhaps is not the only mechanism as flushing is also seen after hypophysectomy. It may be due to the alteration of hypothalamic catecholamine levels, and a failure in the normal response of central thermoregulatory centres. Flushing may be produced by encephalin analogue; this is blocked by naloxone infusion.

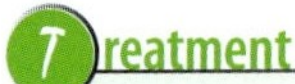

Flushes are treated by oestrogen therapy; it is the most effective treatment for symptomatic hot flushes, other alternatives are a mixture of ergotamine, belladonna alkaloids and phenobarbitone.

Keratoderma Climatericum

This is a thickening of the palms and soles especially around the heels. As it is also seen in men, it is a non-specific effect. It is treated by salicylic acid topically and systemic retinoids orally.

Complications of Hormonal Replacement Therapy

Hormonal replacement therapy (HRT) is used to prevent osteoporosis and cardiovascular diseases. It may increase the chances of carcinoma of the breast and genital tract. Oestrogen therapy may exacerbate chloasma, spider angiomas, darkening of the naevi and acanthosis nigricans. Urticarial and eczematous dermatitis appears in many patients, which subside on cessation of treatment.

THE AGEING SKIN

Ageing is a natural process as we grow; changes appear in the appearance and function of the skin. Ageing of the skin is brought about by both intrinsic (Programmatic theory) and extrinsic (Stochastic theory) changes. The intrinsic changes appear to be engendered in the tissue themselves, and those that are a result of alterations caused by changes in the other organs. Genetic changes may be programmed by the genes or caused by errors in the replication of genetic information in the cells. The ultraviolet radiation is the main cause of extrinsic ageing. Intrinsic ageing is universal and inevitable; extrinsic ageing is neither universal nor inevitable.

Intrinsic Ageing (Programmatic Ageing)

During mitosis the somatic cells cannot replicate the final base pairs of each chromosome, and thus resulting in progressive shortening of each chromosome. Human telomere length shortens by 30% during adulthood. The telomere of fibroblasts is used to detect ageing in premature ageing syndromes. Short telomeres signal cell arrest or apoptosis.

The limited capacity of cells to undergo cell division is called cellular senescence. Senescent cells display short telomeres, irreversible growth arrest, resistance to apoptosis and altered differentiation. Senescence cells show blocking the cells in the G1 phase of the cell cycle. Other genes associated with senescence are those that encode for proteins such as fibronectin and proteases, which are involved in the formation of collagenase and stromelysin. The proteins in the extracellular matrix may be responsible for regulating cellular proliferation and perhaps ageing.

Photoageing (stochastic ageing) is described in chapter 20.

SKIN CHANGES IN THE AGEING SKIN

Dermis

The wrinkling of the skin seen in old age is almost entirely due to changes in the dermis. In young adults the collagen fibers form a rhomboid network; within these collagen bundles lie the elastic fibres. With age the collagen bundles become fragmented and disoriented and the elastic fibres are gradually reduced. In the exposed skin, there is a striking increase of fragmented elastic fibres giving rise to solar elastosis.

Nerves and sensations: Age decreases sensory perception and increases the threshold of pain. This is due to the loss or disorganisation of some sense organs.

There is loss of dermal thickness and reduction of mast cells, and reduction of vasculature surrounding the hair bulbs. Eccrine and apocrine glands may contribute to their gradual atrophy and fibrosis with age. There is a decreased rate of dermal clearance. Senile purpura is due to the lack of support of the vasculature by collagen tissue and reduced perivascular veil cells.

Epidermis

The ageing changes in the skin are difficult to interpret due to the difference in the epidermis in the different regions of the body. There is in general a flattening of the dermal-epidermal junction. This results in a smaller surface contact between the dermis and the epidermis, which means less communication and nutrition transfer, this poor adhesion between the epidermis and dermis results in superficial abrasions, minor trauma and increased prevalence of bullous disorders in the elderly. The permeability of the skin also changes. The capability of the skin to restrict water loss does not change but the skin is more permeable to chemical substances. The chemical substances enter the skin more quickly, but are removed slowly due to changes in the dermal matrix and reduction in vasculature. A change in the nature of corneocyte is also seen especially in the skin of the lower legs; the skin becomes dry and itchy. In females, slight hirsutism occurs as a result of endocrine changes.

Sebaceous and Apocrine Glands

Sebum production is greatest in young adults and then lessens with age. The size of the sebaceous glands increases because the turnover of the cells is slower. Apocrine glands regress with age and produce less odour.

Eccrine Glands

The number of eccrine glands decrease with age and therefore ageing people sweat less with age in response to heat.

Pigmentation

Yellow or brown macules develop on the back of the hands and face. These consist of localised proliferation of melanocytes at the dermoepidermal junction. There is a general darkening of the skin.

Changes in the Hair

Graying usually becomes evident around the age of 50 years. The hair bulb shows abnormalities; they are deficient in tyrosinase. The follicles of white hair may completely lack melanocytes. Changes in the hair follicle vary with the site, e.g. greying starts at the temporal region of the scalp, eyebrows become bushier in males and hair develops along the external auditory meatus. On the scalp, density of the hair decreases, the capacity to produce long hair decreases due to the shortened anagen phase, rather than a decrease in the growth rate. There is an increase of hair follicles in the telogen phase. The diameter of the hair follicle is also reduced.

Androgen-dependent hair of the beard, axilla, pubis and chest reaches a peak in mass and density in the 3–4 decade; it is then followed by a decline. The linear growth of the hair is related to the level of 5 α-dihydrotestosterone (DHT), whereas the density is related to testosterone levels in the plasma.

Nails

The rate of linear nail growth is decreased with age; it is more marked in females than males.

Langerhans Cells and Immune Function

Langerhans cells and T cells are reduced in number, the number of B cells is not affected but their dysfunction is reflected by an increased antigen antibody formation. Elderly skin has a reduced capacity to produce cytokines. There is a decreased intensity of delayed hypersensitivity reactions. The increased risk of photocarcinogenesis and chronic skin infections are some of the consequences of the ageing process.

The buttocks show the most significant site of intrinsic ageing, similar to the exposed areas in extrinsic ageing. A dramatic comparison is that the buttocks of a 60-year-old is as aged as a facial skin of a 20-year-old. This just shows how great the effect of ultraviolet radiation on the skin is.

HISTOLOGICAL FEATURES OF THE AGEING SKIN

Epidermis

Flattened dermal epidermal junction, variable thickness, variable cell size and shape, occasional nuclear atypia, fewer melanocytes, and fewer Langerhans' cells.

Dermis

Reduction in dermal volume with fewer fibroblasts, fewer mast cells, fewer blood vessels, shortened capillary loops, and abnormal nerve endings.

Appendages

These changes include depigmented hair, loss of hair, and fewer glands. Dryness of the skin is one of the most common complaints of the ageing population.

DERMATOSES OF THE ELDERLY

Many dermatoses of the elderly reflect the higher prevalence of systemic diseases such as diabetes mellitus, vascular insufficiency and various neurological syndromes. Some diseases such as cutaneous infections may be due to reduced local skin care. Reduced tolerance to systemic drugs is well documented. Delay in dermal clearance of absorbed substances and possible reduced metabolic capacity may render old age to both beneficial and adverse effects of topical application of drugs.

Skin diseases of old age include pruritus, senile xerosis, asteatotic eczema peripheral leg ulcers, herpes zoster and skin tumours; some benign growths of old age are acrochordon, cherry angiomas, seborrhoeic keratosis, lentigo and sebaceous hyperplasia.

PREMATURE AGEING SYNDROMES

Most of the premature ageing syndromes are inherited and the defect is obvious within the first few years of life. Cutaneous signs of premature ageing include wrinkling, atrophy of the skin, loss of subcutaneous tissue, greying, thinning and loss of hair, dystrophy of the nails, hypopigmentation and hyperpigmentation, sclerosis and ulceration of the skin.

The premature ageing syndromes include:

- The classical inherited syndromes
  - Pangeria
  - Progeria
  - Acrogeria
  - Metageria
- Due to excessive photosensitivity
  - Xeroderma pigmentosum
  - Porphyria
  - Rothmund-Thomson syndrome
  - Cockayne's syndrome
- Due to loss of subcutaneous fat
  - Lawrence-Seip syndrome
  - Leprechaunism
- Miscellaneous ageing disorders
  - Down's syndrome
  - Prolidase deficiency
  - Diabetes mellitus
  - Osteodysplastic geroderma
  - Wiedemann-Rautenstrauchs syndrome
  - Baraitser syndrome

Pangeria (Werner's Syndrome)

This is an autosomal recessive disorder. The ageing process starts at puberty. The disease affects both the skin and the internal organs. Most patients are of short stature; there is microsplanchnia and generalised atheroma. Cataracts develop between the ages of 20 years and 35 years. The incidence of malignancy is high. Death usually occurs in the 4–6 decade, due to myocardial infarction.

The earliest cutaneous change is greying of the hair at the temples, which develops at the age of 14–18 years. This then becomes generalised. There is loss of subcutaneous fat, which is mostly marked in the lower leg, feet, forearms and hands. Face and neck is less affected. The trunk is normal or appears obese. The skin is tense, shiny and adherent; there may be sclerodactyly and acral gangrene. Keratoses develop over the pressure points.

The epidermis is atrophic, the appendages are sparse, the dermis is thickened and the subcutaneous tissue is lost; it is hyalinised.

Progeria (Hutchinson-Gilford Syndrome)

This disorder is due to an autosomal dominant mutation. The onset of the disease is in early childhood. The major changes are seen in the skin, bone and cardiovascular system.

Atrophy of the epidermis and dermis, loss of subcutaneous fat and hyalinisation of dermal collagen characterise the cutaneous changes. The cardiovascular system shows extensive atheromas; fractures occur due to osteoporosis.

The disorder begins in childhood; growth is retarded. The face has typical characteristics with a large cranium, frontal bossing, prominent eyes, sparse hair on the scalp, eyebrows and eyelashes. The lips are thin and the nose beaked.

The skin is taut, shiny and thin in some areas, and wrinkled at other sites. The nails are small thin and dystrophic. Dentition is abnormal, progressive bone resorption leads to fractures and dislocations. Sexual maturation is absent, and intelligence is normal. Death usually occurs in the second decade due to atheromas.

The lack of photosensitivity and absence of large hands and feet should differentiate the disease from Cockayne's syndrome.

Acrogeria (Gottron's Syndrome)

The disorder begins at birth or soon after; acrogeria is an autosomal recessive disease. The ageing changes are localised to the skin; the internal organs are not affected. The skin over the extremities is thin, dry and wrinkled. The cutaneous changes develop soon after birth. The skin bruises easily, poikiloderma and telangiectasia are present. The hair growth is normal. The face has a hollowed appearance due to loss of subcutaneous fat. The nose is beaked and the lips are thin.

The stature is short, but the general health and life expectancy are normal.

Metageria

The condition is very rare; only a few cases are reported. The onset of the disease is at puberty; the patient is tall and thin. There is loss of subcutaneous fat; the facial appearance is characteristic with a beaked nose. Diffuse mottled hyperpigmentation and hypopigmentation develops at puberty. Hair is thin but not in density; the colour is normal. The peripheral circulation is poor. Patients may develop diabetes mellitus in the second decade.

Wiedemann-Rautenstrauch Syndrome

This is an autosomal recessive disorder with marked physical and mental retardation. The onset is in early life; the facies is characterised by frontal bossing, small facial bones, small mouth, low set ears and abnormality of the dentures. The scalp hair is long and sparse. The extremities are thin; hands are large with long fingers and the nails are atrophic.

Diabetes Mellitus

Diabetes may be classified as an ageing syndrome due to changes in the internal organs such as atheromas, development of cataract, and reduced life expectancy. Some patients with insulin-dependent diabetes have tight waxy skin and limited joint motility; life expectancy is reduced due to microvascular damage to the renal and coronary arteries. Poor vision is due to changes in the retinal arteries.

The impaired joint mobility is due to enzymatic digestion of tendon, and collagen in young patients; these changes normally occur in a person 60–65 years of age.

Prolidase Deficiency

It is a rare inborn error of collagen metabolism of autosomal recessive inheritance due to deficiency of prolidase. Skin ulceration and mental retardation characterise the disease. The other cutaneous changes are photosensitivity, telangiectasia, purpura, premature greying of the hair, and lymphoedema. Large amounts of iminodipeptide are excreted in the urine, and proline; hydroxyproline ratio is increased.

Prolidase deficiency is diagnosed by the presence of iminodipeptiduria and prolidase deficiency in the RBC, WBC and cultured fibroblasts.

Baraitser Syndrome

This syndrome is characterised by low birthweight, short stature, mental retardation, multiple pigmented naevi, and a distinctive facial appearance with loss of subcutaneous fat.

Osteodysplastic geroderma

This syndrome manifests in early life; it is characterised by changes in the skin and bones. There is stunting of growth, senile changes in the skin, generalised osteoporosis, multiple fractures and skeletal abnormalities. Skin biopsy shows fragmented elastic fibers.

DIAGNOSIS OF AGEING SYNDROMES

Fibroblasts have a limited life span in culture. This is universally proportional to the age. In all ageing syndromes, there is reduction in fibroblast growth potential. Telomeres are shortened. Enzyme activities of cultured fibroblasts are helpful to study the ageing process. Enzymes of hexose monophosphate shunt have an increased heat labile fraction that is also useful in studying old age.

Enzymes involved in purine metabolism are also altered during ageing in human erythrocytes.

In normal ageing process, there is an increase of insulin binding, and relative insulin resistance is seen in the elderly people.

Other abnormalities include decrease in surface membrane human leukocyte antigen (HLA).

Premature ageing syndromes have multiple features; these are difficult to attribute it to a single enzyme or protein defect. These syndromes may be due to genetic abnormalities, which regulate various metabolic pathways.

METHODS OF IMPROVING THE SKIN IN AGEING

All-trans retinoic acid (tretinoin): Topical administration of tretinoin produces improvement in skin roughness, fine and coarse wrinkling, and mottled pigmentation. The beneficial effects are dose dependent and increase with duration of therapy. Improvement in wrinkling is due to increased collagen deposition in the papillary dermis, and increase in anchoring fibrils. Increased vascularity of the dermis is also well documented. Tretinoin reverses the histological changes associated with ageing.

Alpha-hydroxy acids: These are acids produced from fruits such as glycolic acid from sugar cane, citric acid from citrus fruits, maliec acid from apples. These acids produce subtle changes in the sun-damaged skin such as dyspigmentation and roughness. Fine wrinkling shows improvement when used over time.

Antioxidants: Naturally occurring antioxidants include vitamin A, C and E, β-carotene and bioflavonoid; these are effective when taken orally, but their effects when applied topically are not effective.

Hormone therapy: Both systemic HRT and topical oestrogen therapy are said to improve age-related changes in postmenopausal women. They are said to increase total skin thickness, and dermal collagen. Increased sebaceous gland activity, decreased roughness, and increased hydration of the skin are reported. Oestrogen therapy is said to improve the appearance of skin in elderly women.

In men growth hormone therapy increases skin thickness, which suggests that decrease in growth hormone could also relate to cutaneous ageing.

Moisturisers should be used liberally to moisturise the dry skin.

Peeling, botox and fillers are described in Chapter 44.

Like a candle in a holy place,
So is the beauty of an aged face.

Abraham Lincoln

In the end it is not the years in your life that count.
It is the life in your years.

FURTHER READING

1. Ambros-Rudolphf CM, Mullegger RR, Vaughan-Jones SA, Kerl H et al. The specific dermatoses of pregnancy revisited and reclassified: a retrospective two-center study on 505 patients. J Am Acad Dermatol. 2006;54:395-404.
2. Chamlin SL, McCalmant TH, Cunningham BB, et al. Cutaneous manifestations of hyper- IgE syndrome in children and infants. J Paed. 2002;141:572-5.
3. Ghosh S and Chaudhuri S. Intrahepatic Cholestasis of Pregnancy. A Comprehensive review. Indian J of Dermatol. 2013;58(4):327-31.
4. Gilkes JJH, Sharvill DE, Wellse RS. The premature ageing syndromes. Br J Dermatol. 1974; 91:343-62.
5. Harpin VA, and Rutter N. Barrier properties of the newborn infants skin. J Paed. 1983;102:419-25.
6. Harpin VA, and Rutter N. Sweating in preterm babies. J Paed. 1982;100:614-18.
7. Keitel HG, and Yadav V. Etiology of toxic erythema. Am J Dis Child. 1963;106:306-9.
8. Wahliqvist ML, Savage GS, and Lukito W. Nutritional disorders in the elderly. Med J Aust. 1995;163:376-81.

Chapter

34

Skin and Sports

INTRODUCTION

Since time immemorial sports have played an important role in human life. Today more and more amateurs are turning into professionals; sport has become a primary source of income for many. Most of these professional sportsmen play or practice all year round. They suffer from cutaneous injuries, these injuries vary in players, they are sport-specific. Minor skin injuries become infected, and close physical contact amongst players increases the risk of infectious diseases such as scabies, herpes simplex and fungal infections. Skin-related problems are more common in warm and humid climates. Skin injury like other injuries may result in loss of training time, or the player may be disqualified because of an infectious skin disorder.

Prime function of the skin is to protect the body against mechanical trauma. Stratum corneum acts as a first line of defence against minor penetrating and abrasive injuries. Beneath the stratum corneum and the epidermis, is the dermal connective tissue; it consists of tough collagen and elastic fibres, which protects the body against shearing and indenting forces.

Sport-related skin problems can be studied under the following headings:

- Skin diseases that prevent sports
- Skin diseases that can be transmitted to other players
- Skin injuries due to sports
- Skin diseases aggravated by sports.

SKIN DISEASES THAT PREVENT SPORTS

There are a number of cutaneous disorders that prevent sports. Patients of xeroderma pigmentosa, porphyria, actinic dermatitis and albinism are unable to play in the sunlight due to the damaging effects of ultraviolet radiation. In epidermolysis bullosa, blisters appear at the site of trauma, which prohibit sport. Occasionally, sport can elicit the onset of Weber-Cockayne syndrome or epidermolysis bullosa simplex. Severe palmoplantar keratoderma interferes with playing. In anhidrotic ectodermal dysplasia, hyperpyrexia occurs due to physical exertion. In conditions like Ehlers-Danlos syndrome, pseudoxanthoma elasticum and cutis laxa impaired wound healing prevents sports. Besides these disorders, severity of any disease would prevent active participation in sporting activity.

DISEASES TRANSMITTED TO OTHER PLAYERS

Contact sports like rugby, wrestling, boxing and swimming can transmit infectious disease. Besides the major contagious diseases, importance lies in preventing the spread of minor infectious diseases that are easily overlooked. Players who have infections like herpes simplex, warts, molluscum contagiosum, ringworm infections, tinea versicolor, folliculitis, impetigo, pediculosis and scabies should be prevented from taking part in sports, until the infection is eradicated. Mini epidemics of scabies have occurred in games like cricket, where players stay together for long periods.

Pyogenic skin infections are common amongst players who work in teams. Factors associated with the spread of infection include lack of shower facilities, sharing of a common bath, towels and clothes. Infection with nephritogenic streptococcus has caused an epidemic of glomerulonephritis in a rugby team. Pseudomonas infections often occur in sports associated with water. Infections such as otitis externa, pseudomonas folliculitis, green nails and web space infection have been found in players habitually exposed to water. These are often due to contaminated pools or infected players allowed to take part in water-related games. A number of skin infections can be prevented by good personal hygiene and adequate public health facilities.

There is a growing concern related to blood borne pathogens during contact sport such as rugby and boxing. Minor cuts and abrasions can be portal of entry for hepatitis B and HIV virus.

All players should be screened for any cutaneous infection before competing in sports. Players with a history of herpes should have prophylactic antiviral drugs, such as acyclovir to prevent an outbreak of disease during the playing session. Players who are potential carriers of infection should be treated before participating in games.

CUTANEOUS INJURIES DUE TO SPORT

The cutaneous injuries due to sport can be:

- Injuries due to mechanical trauma
- Injuries due to heat
- Injuries due to cold
- Injuries due to the sun
- Contact dermatitis
- Miscellaneous.

INJURIES DUE TO MECHANICAL TRAUMA

These can be in the form of haemorrhage, corns and callosities, blisters, striae, traction alopecia and acne mechanica.

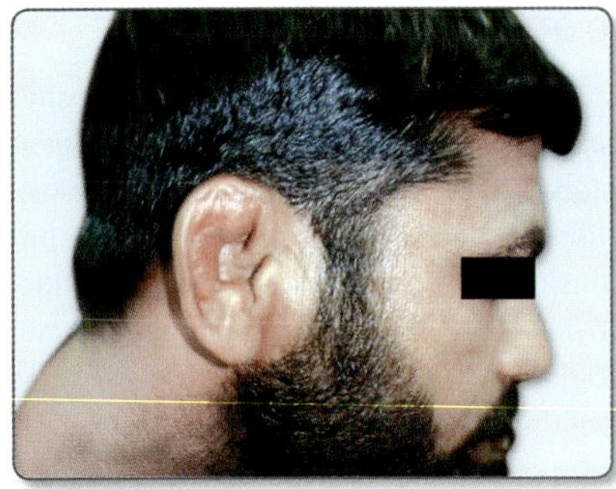

Fig. 1: Cauliflower ear

Haemorrhage

This can occur in the form of cauliflower ear, black heel, black palm, tennis toe and purpura.

Cauliflower Ear

Haemorrhages can occur in any game due to injury. Typical example is the cauliflower ear seen in boxers and wrestlers (Fig. 1). An acute injury can result in the formation of a haematoma, which is characterised by fluctuation and swelling. The chronic cauliflower ear is marked by fibrosis, calcification, new cartilage formation and deformity. This requires a careful reconstruction. A note of interest is that wrestlers who develop cauliflower ear get them bilaterally, and not only on the counter dominant side as seen in boxers.

Black Heel (Calcaneal Petechiae)

This is common in games like tennis, squash, football, volleyball and basketball. Games in which there are sudden abrupt stops and starts, bleeding occur as punctuate haemorrhage in the skin, localised mainly at the periphery of the heel. The condition is due to accumulation of coagulated blood in the superficial dermis and overlying epidermis. It is caused by sudden shearing forces or repeated minor trauma to the skin. The condition can be prevented by well-fitting shoes, by inserting a piece of felt inside the heel of the shoe, wearing thick socks also provides adequate protection to the heel. The condition resolves spontaneously. It should be differentiated from a melanoma to avoid unnecessary surgery. It can easily be distinguished by paring the surface when black dots appear.

Black Palm

It is a condition similar to black heel, seen in the palm of weight lifters.

Tennis Toe

This occurs in games that are similar to those mentioned under black heel. Painful splinter-like haemorrhages in the longest toenail is characteristic of the condition. This is due to the toenail being propelled against the tip of the shoe. In 25% of the population big toe is the longest, in 25% of the population the second toe is the longest, and in the remaining 50% of the population both the big toe and second toe are of equal size. Tennis players also have transverse ridging of the nail plate, some have onycholysis. The condition resolves spontaneously with cessation of activity.

Purpura

This is seen in sports played in extreme cold such as skiing, ice hockey, ice fishing, and mountaineering. Vasoconstriction due to cold is a protective mechanism to prevent loss of heat from the body. With more severe exposure to cold, vasodilatation occurs, this leads to purpura.

Blisters

Blisters occur on the hands of players by holding rackets, bats, and oars in rowing. They occur on the feet from ill-fitting shoes. Blister formation occurs due to accumulation of fluid in the epidermis, resulting from horizontal shearing forces acting on the skin. The blisters develop secondary to prickle cell necrosis. Wearing proper fitting shoes, applying emollients or talc at the site where the shoe rubs against the skin can prevent blister formation. Small blisters heal spontaneously; large blisters can be drained keeping the blister roof intact.

Corns and Callosities

Callosities are circumscribed plaques of hyperkeratosis induced by repeated or prolonged friction. Corns are localised callosities usually on the feet or toes. Corns are painful, after paring a central translucent core that interrupts the normal papillary line pattern, becomes obvious in a corn.

Palmar callus result from batting or any hand gripping activity. Some specific lesions include callus on the first finger of the pitcher's hand. Balls that are without holes gives callus on the right middle and ring finger. Balls with holes give callus on the lateral aspect of the second, third and fifth finger. Martial arts produce callosities on the lateral aspect of the hands from chopping and on both heels from kicks.

Callus can be a pride of many sport veterans, but it may be source of discomfort to others. Corns can be treated by salicylic acid plasters and paring, or by curettage of central core. Callosities require treatment that is more prolonged. Care should be taken to identify poorly fitting shoes, anatomic malformation of the feet and other factors. Referral to a podiatrist or an orthopaedic surgeon may be required in difficult cases.

Striae Distensae

These are seen in gymnasts and weight lifters. It is due to the excessive stretching of the skin. These occur mainly over the anterior shoulders, lower trunk and thighs perpendicular to the direction of skin tension. There is no treatment for striae, but avoidance of extreme tension may prevent some from developing, (Fig. 2).

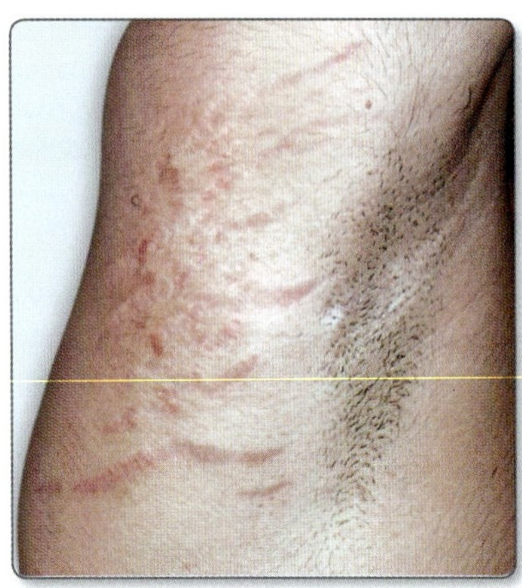

Fig. 2: Striae

Traumatic Alopecia (Balance Beam Alopecia)

This is a pattern of alopecia secondary to physical stress. A typical example in sports is the "balance beam alopecia" seen in gymnasts. It is due to repeated headstands and rollovers performed on a balanced beam. This is a patch of alopecia, which extends from the frontal to the occipital region on either side of the midline.

Acne Mechanica (Footballer's Acne)

Although called footballer's acne, it can occur in any game secondary to chin straps, headbands, wristbands, back pads, shin pads, life jackets and helmets of all kinds. It is due to friction, pressure, and occlusion. Ideal treatment would be removal of the exacerbating items.

HEAT-INDUCED INJURIES

These occur in outdoor summer sports. Heat produces hyperhidrosis, miliaria, heat exhaustion and heat stroke. Hyperhidrosis in a sportsman can be generalised due to heat, or palmoplantar due to emotional stress, which a sportsman often faces due to competitive sports. Generalised hyperhidrosis may cause infections like intertrigo, erythrasma, and pitted keratolysis. It can exacerbate contact dermatitis, fungal and other infections.

Miliaria occurs when the flow of sweat is impeded by the obstruction of the sweat duct. Miliaria profunda is seen almost exclusively in the hot tropical climate after recurrent episodes of miliaria rubra. Patients may develop a state of heat intolerance termed tropical anhidrotic asthenia. The treatment lies in placing the individual in a cool environment. In this setting, the keratinous plug blocking the sweat ducts is shed. Besides this the clothing should be lightweight. Topical treatment is of little benefit but powders and lotions such as calamine lotion may absorb sweat and cause symptomatic relief.

Erythema ab igne

This is seen in sportsmen who apply local heat in the form of hot water bottles and electric heating pads to treat painful muscles and joint. Erythema ab igne (EAI) is characterised by persistent reticulate erythema with hyperpigmentation and telangiectasia. The condition is usually irreversible.

COLD-INDUCED INJURIES

A large number of cold-induced injuries occur in sports like mountaineering, ice hockey, ice fishing, skiing, etc. The common cold injuries are chilblains, frostbite, Raynaud's disease and phenomenon, skier's cheilitis and cold urticaria. Although any physical urticaria can occur in sports, cold urticaria is most common followed by dermographism and heat urticaria. Cold desensitisation was accomplished in a young swimmer who had to abandon championship swimming due to cold urticaria. After one week of programmed cold exposure, he was able to resume swimming and subsequently was symptom free with daily cold showers. Sportsmen playing winter sports should keep themselves warm, and special care should be taken of their hands and feet. Shoes should be water-proof.

Skier's Cheilitis

This results not only from cold, but also from the wind and sun. In severe cases skier's cheilitis can present as atrophy and a polymorphous eruption of the upper lip. Applying lipsticks containing sunscreen can prevent the condition.

INJURIES DUE TO THE SUN

These can be acute in the form of sunburn or suntan, chronic as premature ageing of the skin and malignancy. Most of the damage due to the sun is by ultraviolet B. Ultraviolet A is responsible for most of the photosensitive eruptions. Ultraviolet C is absorbed by the ozone layer, but can cause sunburn; it is a matter of concern in near future, because of the changes in the ozone layer. Ultraviolet light is also reflected from the snow and water, and it passes through the clouds; it is therefore advisable for all sportsmen to use sunscreens to protect themselves from the damaging effects of ultraviolet radiation in both sunny and cloudy days.

CONTACT DERMATITIS

Despite a wide variety of irritants and sensitisers encountered in sports, only a few cause morbidity. Common allergens are rubber and leather found in gloves, shoes, jackets, headbands, chin bands, wristbands, kneepads, swimming equipment, rubber balls, etc. Grip aids, such as resin, beeswax and tincture of benzoin, are sensitising agents. Successful treatment of contact dermatitis is to avoid the use of the offending allergen. As with other skin problems of athletes, it is necessary to minimise or eliminate the effects of heat, humidity, friction, and maceration. The player should be advised to visit a contact dermatitis clinic for follow-up.

MISCELLANEOUS

Swimming

Swimming is a very popular sport, along with its many advantages; cutaneous insults due to swimming are many. Swimmers are prone to dryness, especially during the cold weather. This is due to washing of the skin lipids during swimming, and due to the exposure of chlorine in pools.

It is important to differentiate between of the effects on the skin of chlorinated pool, fresh water, and seawater swimming.

Chlorinated Pools

Irritation of the skin due to chlorine is very common. It is seen especially in people who have a dry skin such as patients of atopic dermatitis, and the elderly. Applying emollients following a shower after swimming is helpful.

Bleaching of the hair is due to chlorine which is a very powerful bleaching agent. This can be prevented by shampooing the hair after swimming.

Green colouration of the hair is seen only in blondes. It is due to the copper tubings and algaecides in the pool. Shampooing the hair after swimming can prevent this.

Swimmer's Ear (Otitis Externa)

This is due to the macerating effects of water and failure to dry the ear after swimming. The organism being most frequently encountered is pseudomonas but streptococci and staphylococci are also found. A combination of polymyxin B, colistin, and neomycin is used typically for treatment, but consultation with an ear, nose and throat surgeon is recommended, as vigilant supervision is required to prevent malignant otitis externa.

Swimming Pool Granuloma

This results from the cutaneous inoculation of *Mycobacterium marinum*. The name swimming pool granuloma was given when 290 cases were traced from the same pool. The infection can also be acquired from fresh water and salt water swimming including home pools. Spontaneous healing occurs within a few months. Recommended treatments are numerous, suggesting that no single treatment is best. Localised lesions can be excised, but those in which the infection has spread can be treated by cotrimoxazole, minocycline hydrochloride, tetracycline, rifampicin and ethambutol.

Salabrasion

This manifests as abraded denuded skin in areas where the swimsuit is tight. It is the result of friction and abrasive action of the salt in water. It is more common by swimming in salt water.

Tinea Pedis

This occurs on the feet of those who swim frequently. Decks around the pool are the source of infection.

Contact Dermatitis

This can occur from swimming suits, goggles, flippers, etc. The main allergens are rubber or elastic in the garments. The use of nylon has decreased the frequency of rubber allergy. Rare causes of dye allergy are also seen.

Aquagenic Urticaria

This is due to pressure of water on the skin while swimming irrespective of its temperature.

Freshwater swimming: This results in "swimmers itch". It is called schistosomal cercarial dermatitis. Ducks or rodents are the definite host; both excrete contaminated ova, which further develop in the snail. These snails release cercaria, which infect man. It involves the area not covered by the swimming suit. Pruritic papules and wheals develop. Sloughing of the cercaria occurs in 3–7 days with spontaneous healing.

Seawater swimming: Sea swimmers meet a large number of unpleasant surprises. These are seen in sports like scuba diving and spear fishing. "Sea bather's eruption" occurs on parts of the body covered by the swimming suit. Erythematous macules, papules and weals develop in a short time after bathing in the sea; these disappear spontaneously in a week's time. Exact cause is unknown, but may be due to the crushing of the spawns of jellyfish and Portuguese man of war under the swimsuit. Showering immediately after coming out of the seawater is the best prophylaxis.

Coelenterates, including jellyfish, Portuguese man-of-war, sea anemone, corals and hydroids, are some example of marine animals which live mostly in ocean water. When skin contact is made with these organisms, a toxin is released through small spicules producing severe local dermatitis as well as fatal systemic reactions. Fortunately, the number of fatalities encountered from these animals is extremely small compared to those due to wasps and bee stings.

Dogger Banks Itch

It is an eczematous dermatitis caused by *Alcyonidium hirsutum*, a seaweed-like animal colony.

Seaweed Dermatitis

It is caused by marine plants; prophylaxis is achieved by refraining from swimming in muddy water, and by taking a shower shortly after swimming.

Hunting

Hunting, like swimming, is a sport of the medieval ages. The hunters are prone to bites by snakes, scorpions, fleas, ticks, mite, etc. Two common infections reported in hunters are sporotrichosis and tularaemia.

Sporotrichosis: This is caused by fungus *Sporothrix schenckii* that grows on decaying vegetable matter. Hunters are infected through trauma by a thorn or splinter. Ulcerated nodules develop at the site of injury followed by appearance of painless nodules along the line of lymphatic vessels. It is treated by saturated solution of potassium iodide. If iodine therapy fails, amphotericin is the treatment of choice.

Tularaemia: Tularaemia is an infection caused by *Francisella tularensis*. The hunter acquires the infection by arthropod bites or by the bite of wild rodents who are reservoirs of infection. An ulcerated nodule develops at the point of inoculation, with regional adenopathy. Systemic symptoms and toxemia may be severe. Gentamicin or streptomycin is the treatment of choice.

Athletics

Athletes are prone to a number of injuries like blisters, corns, callosities, bruises, abrasion, etc. Injuries specific to athletes are "runner's rump", piezogenic pedal papules, and turf toe. Runner's rump is pigmentation due to ecchymosis at the upper end of the gluteal region. The athlete is also prone to get piezogenic pedal papules. These are soft skin coloured papules appearing on the side of the heel, when the subject is standing and disappearing when the weight is taken off the feet. It is due to herniation of fat into the dermis. Turf toe is a painful erythema and oedema of the great toe, it affects athletes who play on artificial turf surfaces.

Jogging

Jogging is gaining popularity worldwide. Millions of people are jogging and running; about 70% of them will at some time sustain a running-related injury. Specific cutaneous manifestation of jogging is the jogger's nipple. It is due to the friction of the nipple from the hard fiber vest. The nipples are painful, fissured and may bleed. Appropriate firm clothing and a petrolatum covering may be useful for protection. Judo jogger's itch is seen with jogging following vigorous judo, but may be a manifestation of dry skin subjected to abnormal physical and climatic trauma. Multiple Beau's lines or periodic shedding of the nails are found in runners. Black heel from cutaneous haemorrhage is also seen in jogger's and marathon runners.

Squash

Being hit by a squash ball is momentarily painful, but results in a characteristic colourful bruise that lasts for several days. The center of the ball is quite pale, while the periphery is at first erythematous and later takes on the colour of a fading bruise.

Lime Burns

Chalk (calcium carbonate) is normally used to line sports fields. But if calcium hydroxide or calcium oxide is used instead, chemical burns can occur. The severity of burns depends upon the time spent on the field, and delay in taking a shower after the game. Second and third degree burns have been recorded. These are found in soccer, football, and rugby players.

SKIN DISEASES AGGRAVATED BY SPORTS

Many pre-existing skin problems can be aggravated by sports. These can be diseases aggravated by heat, cold, stress, and ultraviolet radiation. Frequent bathing may lead to dry skin, especially seen in atopic patients and the elderly. Acne can be aggravated by perspiration, heat and pressure by head bands, chin bands, etc. Almost any type of physical urticaria can occur in sports; treatment of the physical urticaria must be tailored to the clinical type present.

The importance therefore lies not only in diagnosing and treating injuries due to sports, but also to create an awareness of sport injuries, and how to prevent them.

The Love of the Game

The time, the effort, the pain, the passion, the strength, and courage
You sacrifice it all in the game

Happiness, spirit, dreams, success, respect and enthusiasm
You gained it all from the love of the game

FURTHER READING

1. Houston SD, Knox JH. Skin problems related to sports and recreational activities. *Cutis*. 1977;19:487-91.
2. Philpott JA Jr, Woodburne AR, Philpott OS. Swimming pool granuloma. A study of 290 cases. *Arch Dermatol*. 1963;88:158-62.
3. Spoor HJ. Sports identification marks. *Cutis*. 1977;19:453-6.
4. Zaidi Z. Skin and Sports. Specialist. 1991;8(1):71-7.
5. Zinder SM, Basler RSW, Foley J, et al. Athletic Trainers Association Position Statements: Skin Diseases. J of Athletic Training. 2010;45(4):411-28.

Chapter

35

Skin and Psychiatry

INTRODUCTION

Skin and psychiatry have a long association. Skin is the only organ that is visible, it plays a vital role in the overall appearance of the human body, consequently it becomes the matrix for body ego. Skin lesions which are unsightly or disfiguring, such as port-wine stain or congenital melanocytic naevus, have a deleterious effect on the emotional development of a child at an early stage. Facial acne in adolescence leads to poor self-image. In the aging population, especially celebrities, wrinkles and blemishes are a cause of great concern. Stress and anxiety make skin disorders worse. A dermatologist must be familiar with the psychological factors that influence skin disease and dermatology-psychiatry liaison services should be available when necessary.

CLASSIFICATION OF PSYCHOCUTANEOUS DISORDERS

Psychocutaneous disorders can be classified as:

- Primary psychiatric disorders with dermatological symptoms
- Primary cutaneous disorders that are exacerbated by psychophysiological mechanisms

PSYCHIATRIC DISORDERS WITH DERMATOLOGIC SYMPTOMS

These disorders have received little emphasis in the psychodermatological literature; even though they may be associated with suicide and unnecessary surgical procedures. Most of these disorders occur in the context of somatoform, anxiety, factitious, eating or obsessive compulsive disorders.

Dermatitis Artefacta

Dermatitis artefacta (DA) is a psychocutaneous disorder in which the patient inflicts cutaneous damage which the patient typically denies having induced. The condition is more common in women. The lesions are usually within easy reach of the dominant hand and may have bizarre shapes with sharp geometrical or angular borders, or be in the form of burn scars, purpura, blisters, and ulcers. Erythema and edema may be present. Patients may induce these lesions by rubbing, scratching, picking, cutting, punching, sucking, biting or by applying dyes, heat or caustics (Fig. 1). The lesions are difficult to assign to any dermatological disorder. Reported associated conditions include obsessive compulsive disorder, borderline personality disorder, depression, psychosis, and mental retardation. Direct confrontation with the patient should

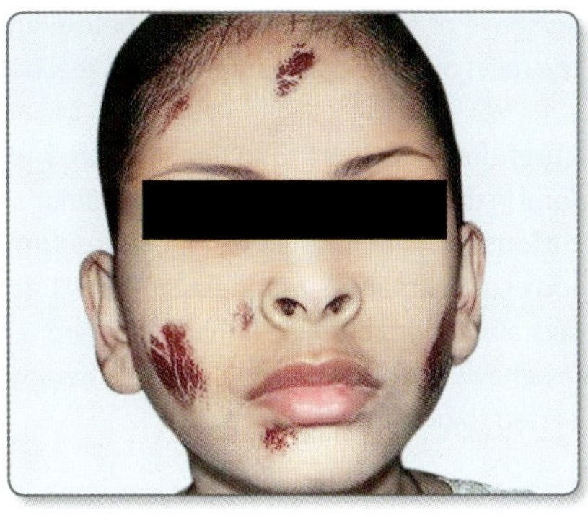

Fig. 1: Dermatitis artefacta

be avoided, and a supportive non-judgmental approach is the mainstay of management. Patients should be seen on an ongoing basis for supervision and support, whether or not lesions remain present.

Delusions of Parasitosis

Delusions are fixed false beliefs that the patients holds with unshakable conviction. Patients believe that organisms infest their bodies; they often present with small bits of excoriated skin and debris that they show as evidence of the infestation. The patients complain of a feeling of insects crawling on their skin, biting or stinging them. Pimozide, 1–10 mg had been the treatment of choice in past; risperidone, trifluoperazine, haloperidol, chlorpromazine and electroconvulsive therapy are among other treatments reported to be useful.

Trichotillomania

Trichotillomania is recurrent pulling out of hair resulting in noticeable hair loss. Scalp is the most common site producing non-scarring alopecia. The patients present with irregular areas of hair loss with broken hair of different length; occasionally follicular haemorrhage can be seen. Hair pull test is normal. Other body areas include eyelashes, eyebrows, and pubic hair. Some patients pull hair at more than one site (Fig. 2). Repeated trauma can result in scarring. The

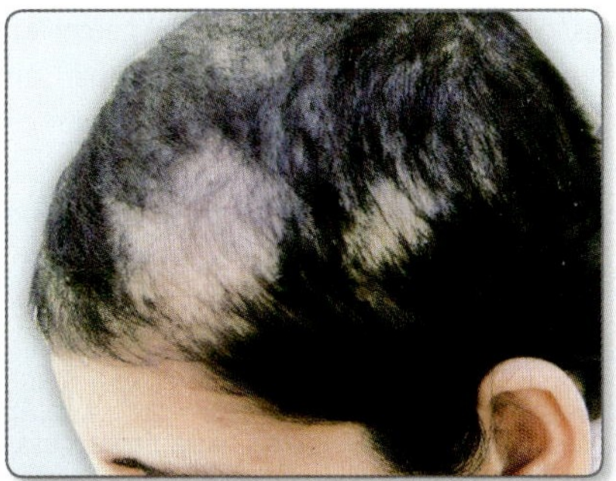

Fig. 2: Trichotillomania

patients experience an increasing sense of tension immediately before an episode of hair pulling; they feel the relief of tension and sometimes a feeling of gratification after hair pulling.

Habit reversal therapy and careful evaluation for anxiety, mood and obsessive symptoms has been helpful in the management of these conditions.

Associated psychiatric conditions may include anxiety, depression, dementia, mental retardation, mood or adjustment disorder, abuse and eating disorder. Fluoxetine, paroxetine, sertraline, clomipramine, lithium, buspirone, risperidone, aripiprazole, cognitive behavioural therapy, habit reversal therapy and hypnotherapy have been reported to be beneficial.

Obsessive-Compulsive Disorders

Cutaneous obsessive-compulsive behaviour includes compulsive pulling of scalp hair, eye brows or eye lash hair, biting of nails, lips, tongue and cheeks, and excessive hand washing. Hand washing is the most common compulsion recorded. It is also called the Lady Macbeth syndrome. It is said that Lady Macbeth would often wash and rub her hands to get rid of the guilt in helping her husband to murder the king of Scotland.

The patients typically have increased level of psychiatric symptomatology compared to age and sex matched controls taken from the general population of dermatology patients. Many patients experience negative stigmatization in their daily life. Selective serotonin re-uptake inhibitors (SSRIs), clomipramine, behaviour modification and habit reversal therapy and psychodynamic psychotherapy have been reported to be effective.

Body Dysmorphic Disorder

This condition is also called dysmorphophobia or dermatological non-disease. This is a psychiatric disorder in which patients of normal appearance is preoccupied with an imagined defect in appearance, or overconcerned about a minor abnormality. These patients are rich in symptoms but poor in signs of organic disease. Self-reported complaints or concerns usually occur in three main areas: face, scalp, and genitals. Facial symptoms include excessive redness, blushing, scarring, large pores, facial hair, and protruding or sunken parts of face. Other symptoms are hair loss, red scrotum, urethral discharge, herpes and AIDS phobia. Strategies to relieve the anxiety due to the perceived defects may include camouflaging the lesions, mirror checking, comparison of defects with the same body parts on others, questioning/re-assurance and seeking advice.

Patients with body image disorders, especially involving the face may be suicidal. Associated comorbidity in dysmorphophobia may include depression, impairment in social and occupational functioning, social phobias, obsessive-compulsive disorder, marital difficulties and substance abuse. Selective serotonin re-uptake inhibitors, clomipramine, haloperidol, and cognitive behavioural therapy have been used in this condition with variable success.

Neurotic Excoriations

In this disorder, patient's produce repetitive, compulsive excoriations of the skin. Unlike patients of dermatitis artefacta, they admit their role in producing the lesions. Repeated excoriations can lead to the development of itch-scratch-cycle. Neurotic excoriations typically present as weeping, crusted or lichenified lesions with postinflammatory hypopigmentation or hyperpigmentation. Psychopathologically, patients with neurotic excoriations have personalities with compulsive and perfectionist traits. Common concurrent psychiatric diagnoses are obsessive compulsive disorder, and other anxiety disorders such as mood disorders, body dysmorphic disorders, substance abuse disorders, eating disorders, compulsive buying, and personality disorders. Phenomenologically, there is an overlap between trichotillomania and pathological skin picking; both conditions are similar in demographics, psychiatric comorbidities, and personality traits. Selective serotonin re-uptake inhibitors, doxepin, clomipramine, naltrexone, pimozide, olanzapine, benzodiazepines, amitriptyline, habit reversal behavioural, therapy and supportive psychotherapy have been used in the treatment.

Psychogenic Pruritus

In this disorder there are cycles of stress leading to pruritus, and pruritus contributing to stress. Psychological stress and comorbid psychiatric conditions may lower the itch threshold, or aggravate itch sensitivity. Stress liberates histamine, vasoactive neuropeptides and mediators of inflammation, while stress-related haemodynamic changes such as variation in skin temperature, blood flow and sweat response, may all contribute to the itch-scratch-itch cycle. Psychogenic pruritus has been noted in patients with depression, anxiety, aggression, obsessional behaviour and alcoholism. The degree of depression may correlate with pruritus severity. Habit reversal training; cognitive behavioural therapy, and antidepressants may be beneficial.

Psychogenic Purpura (Gardner-Diamond Syndrome)

This condition also known as autoerythrocyte sensitisation syndrome is seen primarily in emotionally unstable adult females. These patients present with bizarre painful recurrent bruises on extremities frequently after trauma, surgery, or severe emotional stress. The exact mechanism is unclear; however, hypersensitivity to extravasated red cells, autoimmune mechanism, and increased cutaneous fibrinolytic activity has been implicated in the pathogenesis. These patients may have overt depression, sexual problems, feeling of hostility, obsessive-compulsive behaviour, borderline personality disorder, and factitious dermatitis. The diagnosis can be made in a patient who has atypical history and clinical picture of the syndrome and in whom a skin test with use of the patient's blood reveals a positive reaction.

Atypical Chronic Pain Syndrome

Patients occasionally present to the dermatologist with symptoms such as pain, or dysesthesias on the skin or mucous membranes for which no obvious cause can be found. The patients are anxious, and make the burden of chronic pain difficult to bear. The condition can be further complicated if the patient has been taking analgesics. The comorbid psychological disorders include anxiety, behavioral problems, depression, and personality vulnerabilities. Antidepressants are helpful, but it is best to refer these patients to a multidisciplinary pain clinic for evaluation and treatment.

DERMATOLOGIC DISORDERS THAT ARE EXACERBATED BY PSYCHOPHYSIOLOGICAL MECHANISMS

This category includes patients who have emotional problems as a result of having skin disease. The skin disease in these patients may be more severe than the psychiatric symptoms and even if not life-threatening, it may be considered "life ruining". Symptoms of depression and anxiety, work-related problems, and impaired social interactions are frequently observed. Major depression and social phobia may develop. Suicide has been reported in patients with longstanding debilitating skin diseases, which must be considered when evaluating these patients.

Some of these disorders are chronic eczema, atopic dermatitis, acne, chronic urticaria, alopecia, vitiligo, psoriasis, various ichthyosiform syndromes, rhinophyma, neurofibromas, hyperhidrosis, herpes simplex, warts, and other cosmetically disfiguring cutaneous lesions that have grave effects on psychosocial interactions, self-esteem, and body image.

APPROACH TO PATIENTS WITH PSYCHOCUTANEOUS DISORDERS

Emotional influences can affect the skin through the autonomic nervous system such as sweating, vascular tone, or through the arrector pili function. Emotional influences can also affect the voluntary nervous system such as by rubbing, scratching, and excoriation of the skin, hair, or nail. The teeth can produce cutaneous lesions such as nail biting, knuckle chewing, and cheek biting.

Clinical Findings

The lesions suggesting an emotional basis are persistent, atypically located, bizarre, presence of scratch marks and excoriation, chemical and physical marks such as caused by biting, tearing and pulling out the skin, nail and hair. One should conclude emotionally related dermatoses only after excluding all other possibilities of organic disease.

Clues of Emotionally Disturbed Persons

The patient may be indifferent, over anxious, apathetic, euphoric, reluctant to speak, or talkative, preoccupied, inordinately tidy or unkempt. Personality problems are often present with premenstrual tension, extreme mood swings, chronic indigestion, and children with a history of bedwetting.

Patients response to the disease is also significant, either the patients may be indifferent to the disease, or may show extreme anxiety; the patient may be distressed, non-accepting, unduly questioning, complaining of ill treatment with derogatory remarks.

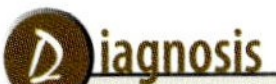

Clinically the diagnosis of emotionally-related dermatoses could only be based on the basis of positive evidence of a relative nature, and never because of conjecture. It should be emphasized that even if personality assessment suggests emotional factors, the possibility of organic dermatoses should be ruled out.

Interestingly stressful life events tend to have little effect on the skin, whereas difficulties in personal relationship play a significant role in emotional dermatoses. Unresolved hostility may be towards a parent, spouse, sibling, and relationship with the employer or a rival for promotion. Envy, jealousy and frustrations are all important factors in producing emotionally-related dermatoses such as lichenification and anogenital pruritus.

Severity Scale of Self-Inflicted Damage

The damage to the skin is in proportion to the degree of emotional disturbance. Blisters and ulcerations produced by heat or chemicals are at one end of the scale, suicide tendencies are at the other end. According to Anderson and Cross, the patient can also be graded in emotional instability by the part of body affected. The face is said to be highly cathectic part of the body followed by the external genitals, trunk, limbs and the hands are the least affected grades in severity.

Role of a Psychiatrist in Dermatology

The concept of liaison psychiatry can be ideally applied in the management of cases where skin disorder is associated with a psychiatric problem. The identification of an emotional problem in these patients should in no way be distracted from applying the standard methods of dermatological treatment. It is often said that "the more or less homespun psychotherapy of the dermatologist is often more efficacious than the more scientifically ordered psychotherapy of the psychiatrist". The simple reason being that the patient has developed a trust and rapport in his dermatologist. The anxieties and fears of the patient can be removed by reassurance, and a sympathetic approach by the dermatologist. In cases with associated gross personality problems and evidence of moderate to severe anxiety, depression or psychotic disorders, psychiatric consultation is invaluable. Management of the patient's mental state is clearly vital in treating these disorders.

FURTHER READING

1. Barsky AJ. Overview of hypochondriasis, bodily complaints and somatic styles. Am J Psychiatry. 1992;140:101-8.
2. Cash TF. The psychology of hair loss and its implications for patient cure. Clin Dermatol. 2001;19:161-6.
3. Jafferany M. Psychodermatology: a guide and understanding. Common psychocutaneous disorders. J Clin Psychol. 2007;9(3):203-13.
4. Kellelt SC, Gawkrodger DJ. The psychological and emotional impact of acne and its effect of treatment with isotretinoin. Br J Dermatol. 1999;149:273-82.
5. Marzuk PM, Tiney H, Tardiff K et al. Increased risk of suicide in persons with AIDS. JAMA. 1988; 259:1333-7.
6. Ross S, Health N. A study of self-mutilation in a community of adolescents. J Youth Adolesc. 2002;31:67-77.

Chapter

36 Diseases of the Oral Cavity

INTRODUCTION

Diseases of the oral cavity are those related to local causes in the oral cavity, or may be a manifestation of cutaneous or systemic disorder. There are number of similarities between oral mucosa and the skin. Like the skin, the major function of the oral cavity is that of protection, it acts as a barrier against environmental factors. The mucosa of the oral cavity is continuous with the skin externally and the mucous membrane of the oropharynx and nasopharynx internally.

The mucous membrane of the oral cavity is divided into masticatory mucosa, lining mucosa, and the specialised mucosa. The masticatory mucosa is present on the gingiva and the anterior hard palate. The lining mucosa comprises the greatest area of the oral mucosa; it includes labial and buccal mucosa, mucosa of the floor of the mouth, ventral surface of the tongue, mucosa of the posterior hard palate, soft palate and uvula. The specialised mucosa is present on the dorsal surface of the tongue.

The mucous membrane on the dorsum of the tongue is divided by a V-shaped groove, the sulcus terminalis into an anterior two-thirds and a posterior-third. The mucous membrane of the anterior two-thirds of the dorsum of the tongue has numerous papillae, which are responsible for taste. These are of three types:

1. Filiform papillae, these are most numerous conical, thread like and arranged in rows.
2. Fungiform papillae, these are numerous small round mushroom-like situated on the tip and lateral surface of the tongue
3. Circumvallate papillae, these are only 7–12 in number, situated just in front of sulcus terminalis.

The normal morphological pattern of the oral integument is not different from that of the cutaneous element. The lining mucosa consists of stratified squamous epithelium overlying a connective tissue stroma, the lamina propria. The stratified squamous epithelium of the lining mucosa is not keratinised; it normally does not have a granular, or a keratinised layer. The masticatory mucosa consists of stratum granulosum, distinct keratohyalin granules, and a stratum corneum.

Melanocytes are also present in the oral mucosa in variable numbers, occurring in groups or in isolation in the basal layer. Local concentration of melanin is common in Negroids especially prominent on the anterior dorsal surface of the tongue and fungiform papillae. Langerhans cells are also present in abundance in the gingival epithelium, dorsum of the tongue, and hard palate. It is less abundant in the lining mucosa. Indeterminate dendritic cells are present in the basal and suprabasal layers.

The lamina propria and the submucosa contain fibroblasts, collagen connective tissue bundles, blood vessels, nerves, sensory receptors, etc. The connective tissue is thrown into folds and finger-like papillae. These are more prominent in the masticatory mucosa providing an increased area of contact between the epithelium and the underlying stroma.

The absence of cornified epithelium, and prominence of vascular network in the underlying connective tissue results in the normal reddish-pink colour of the lining mucosa.

Lesions on the mucous membrane are more difficult to diagnose than that of the skin. There is less contrast of colour, and greater likelihood of alteration in the original appearance because of secondary factors such as maceration from moisture, abrasion from food and teeth. Vesicles and bullae rupture easily to form erosions; grouping and distribution is less distinctive in the mouth than on the skin.

ULCERS OF THE ORAL CAVITY

There are innumerable causes of ulcers in the oral cavity. Some of these are:

Local causes

- Recurrent aphthous stomatitis
- Herpes simplex
- Traumatic such as from teeth biting, dentures, etc.
- Vincent's infection
- Eosinophilic ulcer of the tongue

Cutaneous causes

- Viral: Herpes simplex, herpes zoster, hand, foot and mouth disease
- Pemphigus
- Mucosal pemphigoid
- Behcet's disease
- Reiter's disease

Systemic causes

- Systemic lupus erythematosus
- Syphilis
- Tuberculosis
- Gastrointestinal disorders such as Crohn's disease, gluten sensitive enteropathy
- Erythema multiforme
- Pernicious anaemia
- Takahara's disease
- Cyclical neutropenia.

Recurrent Aphthous Stomatitis

Recurrent aphthous stomatitis (RAS), also known as canker sore, is characterised by recurrent painful ulcers of the oral cavity without evidence of systemic disease. These can be triggered by a number of factors such as emotional stress, nutritional deficiencies, hormonal changes such as menstrual cycle, food allergies, etc.

Classification

- Minor aphthae
- Major aphthae
- Herpetiform ulcers.

Minor Aphthae

These are the most common types of aphthae; they vary in number from one to six, and account for 63% of all RAS patients. These are shallow, round or oval ulcers having a yellowish grey base, a regular border, and a thin discrete erythematous margin. They occur frequently in the lining mucosa especially buccal and labial mucous membrane. They heal in 7–10 days and recur at variable intervals (Fig. 1).

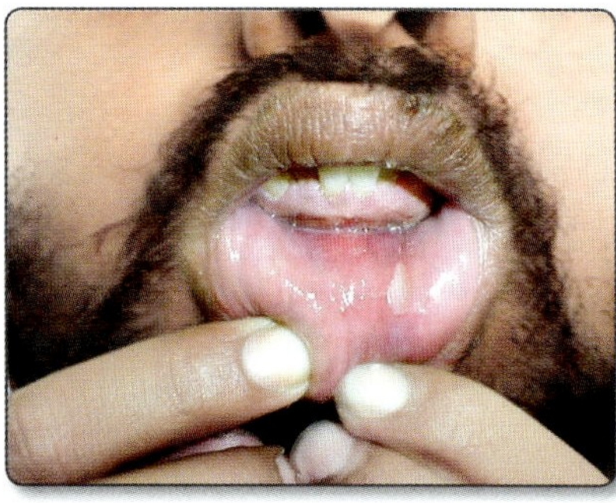

Fig. 1: Aphthous ulcer

Major Aphthae (Sutton's Ulcer)

These ulcers were previously known as "periadenitis aphthae". These ulcers are larger about 10 mm or more in diameter; they are more painful than the minor aphthae. They are found on any part of the oral mucosa including the dorsum of the tongue. They heal slowly and may take up to a month to heal; some may heal with scarring.

Herpetiform Ulcers

These ulcers appear in a slightly older age group with a female preponderance. The ulcers are many, vary in number from 10 to 100, initially small they later coalesce to form large lesions. These ulcers are very painful; they occur very frequently and are virtually continuously present in the oral mucosa.

Many patients report a prodromal period of 24 hours or less prior to the appearance of lesions, in which they have a burning, itching or tingling sensation.

Aetiology

The aetiology of RAS is not clear; a number of factors have been considered for its aetiology. A family history is found in about one-third of patients, and there is a frequency of human leucocyte antigen (HLA)-A2, HLA-B12 and HLA-DR2 supporting a genetic basis for its aetiology.

Infections or immunological mechanisms are felt to be significant causes. *Streptococcus sanguinis* has been found to have an antigenic overlap with the human oral mucosa. This might account for autoantibody and cell-mediated immune factors directed against the oral mucosa. Vasculitis with tumour necrosis factor-α (TNF-α) may also mediate aphthous stomatitis.

Cell-mediated immune response appears to be involved in the pathogenesis of RAS. In the lesion, helper T cells predominate, and there are some natural killer cells. There is evidence for an antibody-dependent cellular cytotoxicity reaction.

Predisposing factors: These include low serum iron, folate or vitamin B_{12}. Stress and anaemia may also precipitate aphthous ulcers. Aphthae are also seen in Behcet's syndrome, Sweet's syndrome, and human immunodeficiency virus (HIV) infection. It may be associated with gastrointestinal diseases such as celiac disease and Crohn's disease.

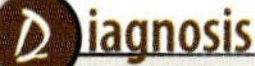

Diagnosis

Diagnosis is mainly clinical; biopsy is only required when some other cause is suspected, and the diagnosis is in doubt.

Treatment

Numerous therapeutic regimens have been tried, but permanent remissions have not been obtained. Therapy is clinically symptomatic and therapeutic.

Topically applied steroids in adhesive base, so that it stays in contact with the oral mucosa, it should be applied 4–5 times a day; it gives good results. Soluble steroid tablets may also help in many cases, when used for rinsing the mouth.

Antihistamine like diphenhydramine held in the mouth 5 minutes prior to meals has a soothing local anaesthetic effect; it is helpful in allaying pain. Local application of gentian violet, cauterisation with 10% silver nitrate may be recommended in intractable cases.

Tetracyclines seem to reduce the duration, size and pain of the ulcer. Tetracycline suspension (250 mg/5 ml) four times a day is swished over the ulcer for 2 minutes before swallowing; this appears to be an effective method for reducing pain and healing time.

Major aphthae have responded to thalidomide 300 mg/day initially, 200 mg/day after 10 days, and 100 mg/day after 2 months. For relapses, the treatment is 100 mg/day for 12 days. Side effects such as teratogenic effects, and neuropathy must be considered before giving thalidomide.

Patients having low levels of folate, iron, or vitamin B_{12} should be given in cases of nutritional deficiency. Oral zinc sulphate is helpful in patients with low levels of serum zinc.

Other therapies of RAS include levamisole, dapsone, and colchicine. These play a role in individual cases but are generally not effective. Thalidomide blocks TNF-α can be used as an alternative treatment. Psychosomatic overlay seen in some patients may require anxiolytic therapy.

The differential features of minor, major and herpetiform aphthous ulcers are shown in Table 1.

Eosinophilic Ulcer of the Mouth

Eosinophilic ulcer may develop anywhere on the tongue. It is a shallow ulcer covered by a pseudomembrane. Histological findings show a predominance of eosinophilic infiltration with some histiocytes and neutrophils. It may respond to cryotherapy with liquid nitrogen.

Table 1: The differential features of minor, major and herpetiform aphthous ulcers

Aphthous ulcer (Minor)	*Aphthous ulcer (Major)*	*Aphthous ulcer herpetiform*
Age of onset		
Childhood and adolescence	Childhood and adolescence	Later onset
Size of ulcer		
< 10 mm	> 10 mm	1–3 mm
Number of ulcers		
< 6	< 6	10–100
Sites affected		
Any site, mainly vestibule, buccal and labial mucosa	Any site, mainly overlying minor salivary glands, lips, soft palate and fauces	Any site, mainly posterior part of oral cavity
Pain		
+	++	+
Duration		
About 10 days	About 1 month	About 10 days, recurs very frequently
Frequency		
80%-most common	10–15%	7–10%-least common
Healing		
No scarring	Scarring present	Scarring may be present

Fusospirochetal Gingivitis (Vincent's Infection)

This is an acute necrotising ulcerative gingivitis. It is thought to be due to the presence of necrotic tissue that provides an anaerobic environment for the infection by fusospirochetal organisms such as *Bacteroides fusiformis*, *Borrelia vincentii* and other organisms. Poor oral hygiene and malnutrition are predisposing factors.

Clinical Features

The disease has a rapid onset characterised by punched out ulcers beginning in the gingiva and may then spread to the lining mucosa; a slight pressure causes bleeding. There is a characteristic foul smelling odour from the mouth.

Treatment

Good oral dental hygiene is necessary. Penicillin, erythromycin, clindamycin or tetracycline with metronidazole for anaerobic organisms. Oral tetracycline mouthwashes with 3% hydrogen peroxide, or chlorhexidine mouth washes several times during the day. A dental consultation is necessary.

Noma (Cancrum Oris)

It is a fusospirochetal gangrenous stomatitis of children with low resistance and malnutrition. There is extensive ulceration of the oral mucosa, which

Treatment

Treat the predisposing factors such as malnutrition. Medical treatment is the same as for Vincent's infection. Reconstructive surgery should only be initiated when complete healing occurs.

rapidly becomes gangrenous. It may extend to the skin above and to the bone below. It often ends fatally.

Behcet's Syndrome

Behcet's syndrome is common in Middle East and East Asia. The syndrome was originally described as a triad of oral aphthae, genital ulcers, and uveitis. It is now recognised as a multisystem disorder involving the skin, eyes, genitourinary tract, gastrointestinal tract, joints, vascular and the central nervous system (CNS). The basic pathological process in Behcet's syndrome is a vasculitis principally involving the veins and venules.

Aetiology

The aetiology is uncertain. Viral, immunological, bacterial, genetic, and ecological causes have been postulated.

Studies show HLA association in Behcet's syndrome. These appear to be geographical in distribution and possibly associated with disease localisation. HLA-B5 may be a marker for ocular disease, HLA-B27 for arthritis and HLA-B12 for mucocutaneous disease. In Turkey, there are a high proportion of HLA-B5 patients.

Histopathology

The early lesions show a leucocytoclastic vasculitis. There is perivascular infiltration chiefly lymphocytic in the older lesions.

Clinical Features

The disease is usually seen in males in the third to fourth decades. The oral lesions are indistinguishable from RAS especially those of minor or herpetiform variants. Only a small percentage have lesions similar to major aphthae. The lesions are very painful.

Genital lesions: The ulceration is similar to those of the mouth. Swelling of the regional lymph nodes and fever may accompany the oral and genital lesions.

Ocular lesions: The disease starts with intense periorbital pain and photophobia. Retinal vasculitis is the chief cause of blindness. Conjunctivitis and iridocyclitis frequently occur. Untreated disease may lead to blindness from optic atrophy, glaucoma, or cataract.

Neurological manifestations: These resemble those of multiple sclerosis, neurosyphilis or systemic pseudobulbar palsy. Steroid therapy is helpful.

Vascular: Large vessel vasculitis associated with pulmonary artery, and aortic aneurysms may occur. Lesions such as thrombophlebitis may be seen in some cases, thrombosis of the superior vena cava may also occur.

Joints: Arthralgia may occur in the form of polyarthritis.

Cutaneous lesions: Venepuncture is followed by pustulation (pathergy); this is said to be characteristic of Behcet's disease. Other skin lesions include folliculitis, acneiform eruptions, vesicles, necrotising vasculitis, and erythema nodosum-like reactions.

Diagnostic Criteria

Major criteria

- Oral aphthae
- Neuro-ocular lesions

- Genital ulcers
- Dermatological lesions.

Minor criteria

- Proteinuria and haematuria
- Thrombophlebitis
- Aneurysm
- Arthralgias.

Diagnosis

The diagnosis is clinical although there are no universally accepted diagnostic criteria: the occurrence of two to three major and one minor criterion are accepted as diagnostic. Screening for organ involvement, and a positive pathergy test suggest diagnosis. Histology will show neutrophilic infiltrate or vasculitis.

Treatment

Response to treatment is poor. For oral and genital lesions, topical or intralesional corticosteroids are effective. Cyclosporin is most effective for uveitis. Colchicine 0.6 mg three times a day (tid) with topical corticosteroid therapy is effective in more severe mucocutaneous disease. Topical tacrolimus may also be considered in resistant cases.

Patients who have severe mucocutaneous lesions and have systemic involvement, a more aggressive therapy is required. Prednisolone with immunosuppressive agents, such as cyclosporin, azathioprine, chlorambucil or cyclophosphamide, is needed.

Other therapies include colchicine 1–1.5 mg daily, dapsone 0.5–2 mg/kg daily, thalidomide 100 mg/day, prednisolone 15–20 mg/day, methotrexate 15–20 mg/week and levamisole.

Subcutaneous injections of 3 million units of interferon α-2A have shown good response to ocular, genital and skin lesions in some studies.

Hulusi Behcet (1889–1948)

Behcet was a Turkish professor of dermatology. He described the clinical triad of recurrent oral and genital ulceration with a relapsing inflammation of the eyes. The disease is frequently seen in Greece, Turkey, Cyprus and other Eastern Mediterranean countries.

Cyclic Neutropenia

It is characterised by a decrease of circulating neutrophils from the blood and dermatological manifestation. At regular intervals (21 days) neutropenia occurs with mouth ulcerations, accompanied by fever, malaise and arthralgia. The oral ulcers are extensive irregular in outline and are covered with a greyish white necrotic slough. In addition cutaneous infections, such as abscess, boils, cellulitis, urticaria and erythema multiforme, are also reported.

The cause of cyclic neutropenia is not known. Nothing is known that will influence the course of the disease. The use of antibiotics during infection helps in recovery. Attention should be paid towards good oral hygiene. Death may occur from pneumonia, sepsis, gangrene or granulocytopenia.

Takahara's Disease (Acatalasemia)

This is a rare recessive inherited disease; the enzyme catalase is deficient in the liver, muscles, bone marrow, erythrocytes, and the skin.

The disease may be mild, moderate or severe depending upon the amount of catalase present. The mild type is characterised by rapidly recurring ulcers. In the moderate type alveolar gangrene develops, teeth fall out spontaneously. In the severe type, there is widespread destruction of the jaw. After puberty all the symptoms heal.

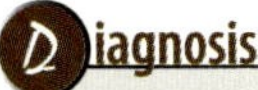

Upon addition of hydrogen peroxide to an acatalase blood, the blood turns blackish brown and does not foam. Normal blood remains bright and foams.

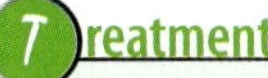

Extraction of the diseased tooth and, use of antibiotics, helps to control the infection.

WHITE LESIONS OF THE ORAL MUCOSA

White lesions in the mouth may be congenital or acquired; these may be benign or malignant. Following are some of the causes:

Local causes

- Congenital white sponge naevus
- Oral florid papillomatosis
- Candidiasis
- Smoker's keratosis
- Leukoplakia
- Actinic cheilitis
- Recurrent aphthous stomatitis
- Herpes simplex
- Fordyce's spots
- Gingival cyst of newborn (Epstein's pearl)
- Submucous fibrosis.

Cutaneous diseases

- Lichen planus
- Pachyonychia congenita
- Dyskeratosis congenita
- Darier's disease.

Systemic diseases

- Syphilis
- Koplik's spots of measles
- Chronic renal failure
- Systemic lupus erythematosus
- HIV infection (white hairy leukoplakia).

White Sponge Naevus

The disease is inherited as an autosomal dominant disorder, oral mucous membrane is commonly involved; vagina and rectum may also be the site of white sponge naevus. It is present at birth, the condition is stable. White overgrowth of the mucous membrane is seen. Histologically, there is acanthosis, vacuolated prickle cells, and acidophilic concentrations in the cytoplasm of the keratinocytes; these are aggregates of tonofilaments. There are no extra-mucosal lesions. There is no treatment, although it has been suggested that antimicrobial therapy clear the lesions.

Oral Florid Papillomatosis

This is a confluent papillomatosis covering the mucous membrane of the oral cavity. The lesion appears as a white mass resembling a cauliflower, overlying the tongue and extending into the nasopharynx. The disease is progressive; it may develop into a squamous cell carcinoma in which metastasis occurs very late or not at all. The histological features are those of papillomatosis, acanthosis without disruption of the basal layer. The condition should be differentiated from leukoplakia. Treatment is by surgical removal.

Fordyce Spots

These are ectopic sebaceous glands present in the lining mucosa of the oral cavity. It may also be present in the glans penis and labia minora. It is a common disorder more obvious in males with a greasy skin. Clinically, it is characterised by pinhead sized yellowish white macules or papules. There is no indication for treatment; the condition is asymptomatic and benign.

Smoker's Patches (Stomatitis Nicotinica)

The condition is due to smoking, especially pipe and cigar. Despite the name, the lesion is not due to nicotine, but due to tar and heat in tobacco smoke.

The lesion is characterized by distinct umbilicated papules on the palate. The ostia of the mucous duct appear as red pinpoints surrounded by milky white umbilicated papules. These are asymptomatic. The intervening mucosa later becomes white and thick with a tendency to desquamate leaving raw beefy areas.

Treatment is abstinence from the use of tobacco.

White Hairy Leukoplakia

Hairy leukoplakia is seen in patients with immune defects such as HIV infection. It is due to infection with Epstein-Barr virus. The lesion is often associated with candidiasis. The site of predilection is the parakeratinised mucosa as that of the lateral margin of the tongue.

Clinically the lesion is characterised by white corrugated or hairy appearance on the lateral surface of the tongue. The condition is asymptomatic.

Hairy leukoplakia needs no treatment; those patients infected with HIV infection tend to improve with zidovudine, acyclovir is also effective.

Submucous Fibrosis

Submucous fibrosis is a disease of the Indian subcontinent confined to people using areca nut and betel leaves. The condition develops insidiously, presenting

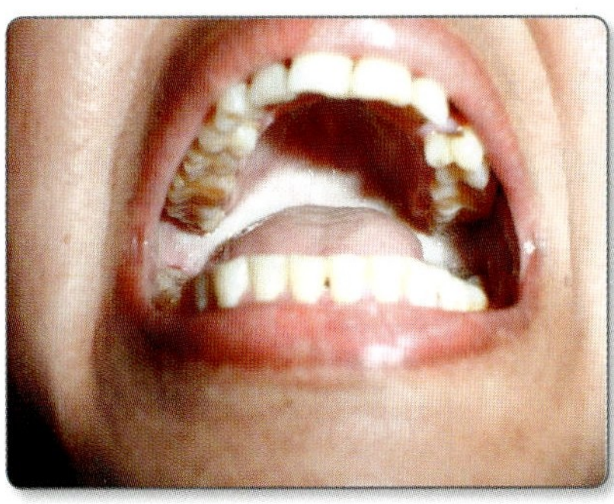

Fig. 2: Submucous fibrosis

as oral dysesthesia, and a nonspecific vesicular stomatitis; later there is fibrosis of the tissue, mainly in the buccal mucosa, lip and palate. When the condition becomes severe, fibrotic bands are seen involving the palatoglossal folds; due to which there is difficulty in opening the mouth and eating. The condition is premalignant and oral cancer can develop in 2–10% of cases (Fig. 2).

Treatment is difficult, intralesional injections of triamcinolone and jaw exercises are required in the early stages. Surgery to relieve the fibrotic bands is done in the later stages. CO_2 laser provides instant relief but not long-term cure. Vitamin A supplements along with zinc and folic acid relieve the chronicity of the lesion.

Lichen Planus

The mucous membrane of the mouth is frequently affected. The lesions are usually located on the inner side of the cheeks; these consist of pinhead sized white papules that form annular lesions, linear patterns, or appear as discrete puncta. More commonly, there is an aggregation of these to form a reticulated or lace-like pattern. Similar lesions occur on the palate, lips and tongue. On the tongue, plaque-like lesions may appear resembling leukoplakia. On the lips, the papules are often seen in an annular form, and there is an adherent scale similar to that of lupus erythematosus. Vesicular and bullous lesions are also observed; these may ulcerate. The ulcers are painful and may undergo malignancy. These lesions need careful follow-up (Figs 3 and 4).

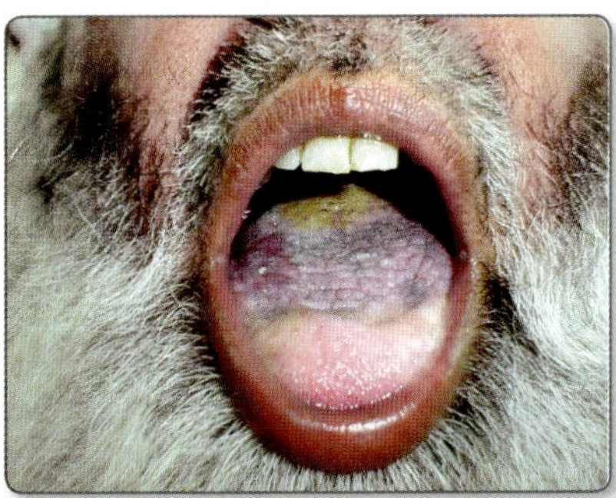

Fig. 3: Lichen planus (tongue)

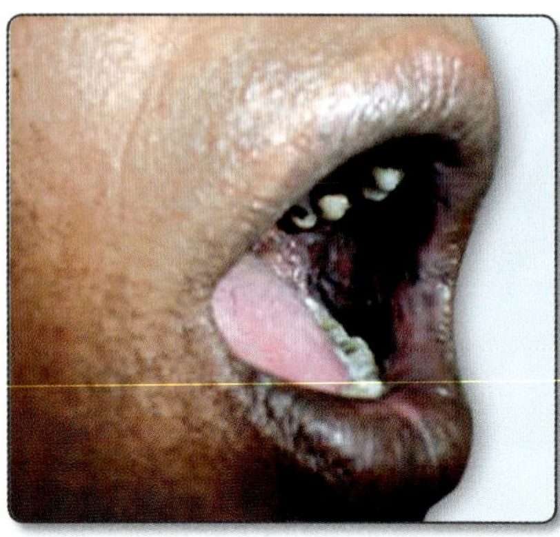

Fig. 4: Lichen planus (oral cavity)

Psoriasis

Oral lesions of psoriasis are unusual. They may give rise to both white and red lesions; they are mostly associated with pustular and exfoliative psoriasis. The lesions appear as demarcated plaques or annular lesions that range in colour from grey to white. Geographical tongue is also seen in pustular and exfoliative psoriasis.

Candidiasis

Candida of the oral cavity (thrush) is usually seen in infants. It appears as greyish white plaques on the tongue and buccal mucosa. It is produced by the growth of *Candida albicans* on the superficial layers of the mucous membrane. The base of the plaque is moist, reddish and macerated; the angles of the mouth may be involved. In adults, candidiasis is due to malnourishment, immunosuppression, AIDS, diabetes and in other debilitating conditions. Oral broad-spectrum antibiotics can also produce oral thrush. In some patients, candidiasis may be the first manifestation of an occult primary masked neutropenia (Fig. 5).

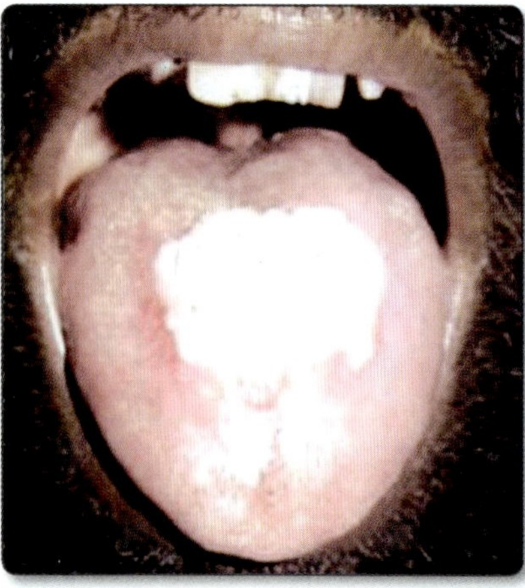

Fig. 5: Thrush

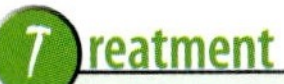

Local application of antifungal medicines such as nystatin in the form of drops or creams often suffices. In AIDS or patients with immunosuppression, systemic antifungal therapy is required.

The condition should be differentiated from curd often seen in the infant's mouth after taking milk; this is loosely attached on the surface of a normal mucous membrane. Diphtheric plaque is grayish and cannot be easily separated from the mucosa. Leukoplakia affects the older age group; it is due to hyperplasia and hypertrophy of the mucosa.

Table 2 shows the difference between oral leukoplakia and oral candidiasis.

Table 2: Difference between oral leukoplakia and oral candidiasis

Candidiasis	*Leukoplakia*
White patch on oral mucosa, which can be rubbed off.	The white patch on oral mucosa cannot be rubbed off.
Age of onset Neonates and young children. In adults it can occur in diabetes, immune-deficiency, severe debilitating diseases, after antibiotics.	Middle age
Yeast infection	Premalignant lesion
Histopathology Dyskeratosis absent	Dyskeratosis present
Yeast on microscopy	Yeast absent
Treatment Antifungal drugs	Excision

Leukoplakia is described in chapter 27.

BLACK/BROWN PIGMENTED LESIONS OF THE ORAL MUCOSA

Local causes

- Tattoos
- Melanocytic naevus
- Lentigines
- Melanoacanthoma
- Malignant melanoma.

Cutaneous disorders

- Incontinentia pigmenti
- Riehl's melanosis.

Systemic disorders

- Drug induced
- Black hairy tongue
- Peutz-Jeghers syndrome
- Albright's syndrome
- Malignant acanthosis nigricans
- Neurofibromatosis.

Melanocytic Naevus

Melanocytic naevi are generally uncommon in the oral mucosa. In mucosal naevi, cellular naevus is the most common, compound naevus and junctional naevus occurs only rarely. Blue naevus may occasionally occur.

Lentigines

Lentigines are due to increase in the number of melanocytes in the basal layer. They appear as hyperpigmented macules in the oral mucosa.

Oral Melanoacanthoma

Oral melanoacanthoma is a simultaneous proliferation of keratinocytes and melanocytes. Most lesions are present on the buccal mucosa. It seems to be a reactive process following trauma, resolves spontaneously in 40% of cases.

Melanoma

Occurs in older persons, it is larger than the benign lesions, irregular in shape, it has a tendency to ulcerate and bleed. A peripheral areola of pigmented spots may be present. Melanoma is most common on the palate and gingiva. The prognosis is poor.

Inflammatory Acquired Oral Pigmentation

This starts as distinct macules, which progress to diffuse oral pigmentation. It may be due to some undefined inflammation, there is slow partial resolution.

Tattoos

This also gives rise to focal hyperpigmentation, usually from fragments of silver amalgam implanted in the gums.

Drug-Induced Hyperpigmentation

Drugs such as antimalarials, cytotoxic drugs, phenothiazine, minocycline, contraceptives, steroids, mephenytoin, heavy metals, some antibiotics and iron therapy produce oral pigmentation.

Antimalarials produce a variety of pigmentation ranging from yellow with mepacrine to bluish black with quinidine. Minocycline produces bluish grey gingival pigmentation caused by staining of the underlying bone. Bismuth and lead produce a pigmented line along the gum margin. Purplish gingival pigmentation may be seen after treatment with gold salts.

Black Hairy Tongue

This represents a benign hyperplasia of the filiform papillae of the tongue. These appear as pigmented hair-like projections that are made up of orthokeratotic and parakeratotic cells.

Black hairy tongue may be associated with several conditions such as excessive smoking, use of oral antibiotics; tetracycline being the most common cause of black hairy tongue. Oral candidiasis on the dorsum of the tongue may sometimes give rise to black pigmentation.

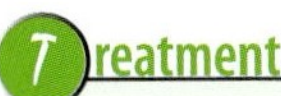

Scrub the projections with a tooth brush, application of isotretinoin may be helpful. Remove the predisposing causes such as smoking and antibiotics. Good oral hygiene should be maintained.

RED LESIONS OF THE ORAL MUCOSA

Congenital and hereditary

- Haemangioma
- Sturge-Weber syndrome
- Maffucci's syndrome
- Hereditary haemorrhagic telangiectasia.

Acquired

- Purpura
- Geographical tongue
- Infections such as scarlet fever
- Deficiency glossitis
- Erythroplakia
- Telangiectases
- Betel leaf stomatitis.

Benign Migratory Glossitis

Geographic tongue (benign migratory glossitis) is a benign condition that occurs in up to 3% of the general population. The patients are often asymptomatic; however, some patients report increased sensitivity to hot and spicy foods. Geographic tongue affects both males and females, it is more prominent in adults than children.

The classic manifestation of geographic tongue is an area of erythema, with atrophy of the filiform papillae of the tongue, surrounded by a serpiginous, white, hyperkeratotic border. The patient often reports spontaneous resolution of the lesion in one area, with the return of normal tongue architecture, only to have another lesion appear in a different location of the tongue.

The aetiology and pathogenesis of geographic tongue is still poorly understood; it may be a manifestation of atopy, psoriasis, stress, and Reiter's syndrome.

No treatment is necessary. Topical tretinoin 0.1% may be helpful.

Betel Leaf Stomatitis

Betel leaf stomatitis, also called the "*pan*" mouth, is a common clinical condition seen in the Indo-Pakistan subcontinent. It is due to the perpetual contact of the oral mucosa with betel leaf (called *pan* in India and Pakistan) coated with slaked lime and catechu (a bark). This is often retained in the mouth for long hours.

Burgundy-coloured, bizarre irregular patches with a somewhat corrugated buccal mucosa may look frightening, though it is often naïve in nature. However, in rare instances a malignant lesion may remain masqueraded underneath. Hence in suspicious cases thorough removal of the red pigmented patch should be undertaken, and careful follow-up is required.

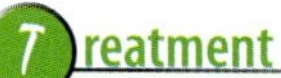

There should be total abstinence from consumption of *pan*, as malignancy may supervene.

Plasma Cell Mucositis

Plasma cell mucositis (PCM) is a rare plasma cell proliferative disorder of the upper aerodigestive tract with an unknown aetiology. PCM affects adult patients at an average age of 50–55 years.

Clinical features are an intensely erythematous mucosa with papillomatous, cobblestone, nodular, or velvety surface changes.

Symptoms include oral pain of long duration, dysphagia, persistent hoarseness, and pharyngitis. The majority of cases have a history of autoimmune or immunologically mediated disease. Stenosis of the respiratory passages has been reported.

The histopathologic features of a dense, submucosal plasma cell infiltrate is not specific and must be differentiated from other reactive and neoplastic conditions.

Diagnosis of PCM depends on clinical pathologic correlations.

Treatment for PCM is not established. Reports have described the use of both topical and systemic corticosteroids, cytotoxic and radiation therapy, and surgical intervention.

TUMOURS OF THE ORAL CAVITY

A number of tumours affect the oral cavity. These may be benign, premalignant and malignant.

Benign growths

- Pyogenic granuloma
- Molluscum contagiosum
- Epulis
- Warts
- Mucous cyst
- Hemangioma
- Lymphangioma
- Fibroma.

Premalignant

- Leukoplakia
- Local epithelial hyperplasia
- Submucous fibrosis.

Malignant

- Squamous cell carcinoma
- Melanoma
- Erythroplakia
- Sarcoma
- Kaposi's sarcoma.

Mucous Cyst

It is frequently seen in dermatological practice. These appear as soft bluish white papules or nodules, most commonly seen on the inner surface of the lower lips, but may also occur on the tongue and buccal mucosa. They are about 2–10 mm in diameter, painless, fluctuant, and tense. Incision releases a sticky straw-coloured fluid, bluish if haemorrhage has occurred (Fig. 6).

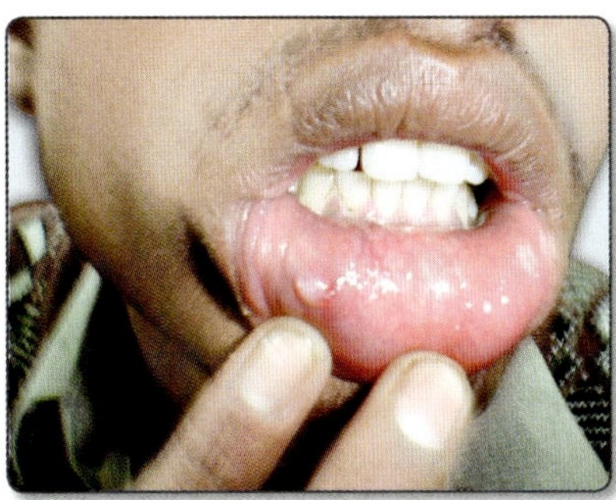

Fig. 6: Mucous cyst

Mucous cyst is caused by rupture of the mucous duct with the extravasation of mucin in the submucosa to produce cystic spaces. Granulation tissue formation is followed by fibrosis.

Treatment is by surgical excision.

Leukoplakia

This is a chronic hypertrophy and hyperkeratosis of the mucous membrane especially of the buccal mucosa and tongue. It usually affects people past the middle age. In the mouth, it is more common in males; on the vulva, females are often affected.

The main causes of buccal leukoplakia are cigarette or pipe smoking, poor oral hygiene, strong alcohol, dental caries, jagged tooth, etc.

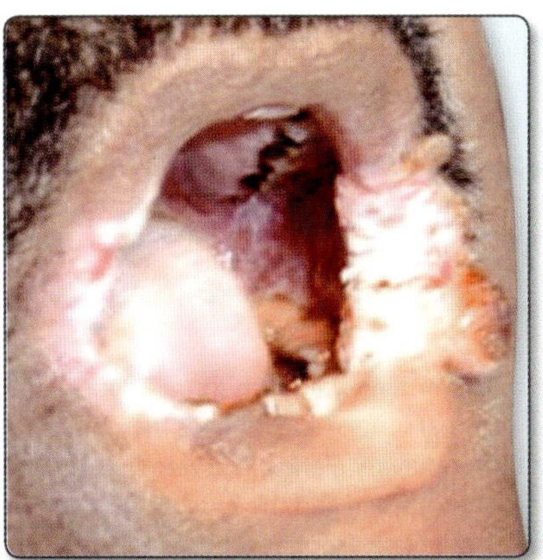

Fig. 7: Leukoplakia with malignant change

Clinical Features

Dry, whitish irregularly shaped but well-defined plaques characterise the lesion. The surface may be smooth or verrucous. It has a typical leathery feel. The condition is premalignant. The white colour may be attributed to an increased epithelial water uptake (moist hyperkeratosis).

Clinically premalignant leukoplakia should be differentiated from the malignant lesion. Induration is often the first marker of malignancy; erosions and ulcerations on the surface are most likely to be precancerous. Carcinoma generally follows anywhere between 1 years and 20 years.

Leukoplakia of the lips is usually secondary to actinic damage (Fig. 7).

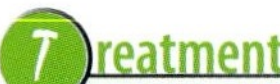

Remove the provocative causes such as smoking. Every case of leukoplakia should be thoroughly examined to exclude malignancy. Fulguration, laser ablation and simple excision are some of the methods to treat leukoplakia. Cryotherapy is also effective.

Erythroplakia

This is a premalignant condition of the oral cavity, it is commonly found in men in the fourth to seventh decade. It is analogous to the Bowen's disease of the skin. The lesions appear as red velvety patches or they may be slightly depressed. The patches vary in size; these are mainly found on the tongue or the cheeks. Erythroplakia may gradually progress to squamous cell carcinoma.

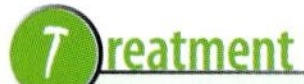

The lesion should be excised with a healthy margin of normal mucosa.

Squamous Cell Carcinoma

Roughly, 85% of the oral tumours are squamous cell carcinoma. This is the most common tumour of the oral cavity. It often occurs on the lower lip, secondary to ultraviolet radiation, or on the anterior two-thirds of the tongue secondary to leukoplakia; it may occur at the site of chronic ulceration or irritation. Regional lymph node metastasis frequently occurs. It appears as a keratinous growth, ulcer or soreness of the lip.

Any exophytic growth that bleeds on touch should be subjected to biopsy. Depending upon the result of biopsy and the grading of cancer, the choice of treatment could be radiation, laser vapourisation, surgical extirpation or chemotherapy. Squamous cell carcinoma secondary to herpes virus responds to acyclovir. The overall prognosis is extremely poor. Prevention from consumption of tobacco, maintenance of good oral hygiene and nutrients are protective measures to be taken.

CHEILITIS

The lips are two fleshy folds of orbicularis oris muscle which surround the orifice of the mouth with the skin on the external surface and mucous membrane on the inner surface. Lips are rich in minor salivary glands. The vermilion zone is the transitional zone between the glabrous skin and the mucous membrane. The epithelium of the vermilion is distinctive as it has a prominent stratum corneum. The oral commissure is the angle where the upper and lower lips meet. The upper lip includes the philtrum or the midline depression extending from the columella of the nose to the superior edge of the vermilion zone.

The common causes of cheilitis are:

- Allergic contact cheilitis
- Actinic cheilitis
- Cheilitis exfoliativa
- Angular cheilitis
- Glandular cheilitis
- Cheilitis granulomatosis
- Plasma cell cheilitis.

Allergic Contact Cheilitis

The vermilion border of the lip is more likely to develop allergic contact cheilitis. It is often secondary to lipsticks, drugs, sunscreens, cigarettes, cosmetics, food, etc. The condition is characterised by dryness, fissuring, oedema, and crusting of the lips.

Treatment is by removing the offending agent and use of topical corticosteroids.

Actinic Cheilitis

The condition is mostly seen in outdoor workers or athletes. The lower lip is involved is almost all cases. The vermillion border being the most commonly affected site, it is analogous to actinic keratosis, but the risk of squamous cell carcinoma is much greater in actinic cheilitis.

Clinical Features

In early stages, the lips are red and edematous, and then they become dry and scaly. In later stages, the lips become thick with small greyish white plaques. Fissuring, erosion and crusting may occur. Ulceration is rare; if it does occur it is a sign of malignancy.

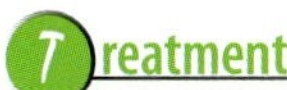

Treatment

Prolonged exposure to sunlight should be avoided. Application of sun blocks, 5% fluorouracil, topical tretinoin or trichloroacetic acid may provide relief in some cases. If malignancy develops, the treatment is vermilionectomy or laser ablation.

Angular Cheilitis

Angular cheilitis (perleche) is inflammation of the angle of the mouth comprising the skin and contiguous labial mucosa. It is commonly seen in old age and children.

In old age, it is due to mechanical factors such as ill-fitting dentures, drooling of the saliva from the angle of the mouth, due to overhanging of the alveolar ridges, which occurs in old age. In females, it could be related to Plummer-Vinson syndrome.

Clinical Features

Angular cheilitis presents as a triangular area of erythema and edema at the angles of the mouth; radiating furrows are seen in severe cases. Recurrent exudation and crusting are common. In some cases, especially those following atopic dermatitis, the angle of the mouth is dry and scaly. Thickening and hyperpigmentation may be combined with radial fissures.

Treatment

It is necessary to remove the underlying cause of disease such as dentures should be corrected; these should be kept out of the mouth in an anticandida and antiseptic solution at night. Improve the nutritional status of the patient. Surgery is only required for the intractable cases to restore the normal commissural anatomy.

Recurrent infection should be treated with topical miconazole cream after meals and at bedtime. Topical polymyxin B or mupirocin is valuable in treating staphylococcal colonization.

In children, especially in underdeveloped countries, angular cheilitis is due to nutritional deficiencies such as that of riboflavin, iron, protein and folic acid.

A high incidence of bacterial and yeast infection is responsible for angular stomatitis especially in people wearing dentures, in diabetic patients and those associated with immunodeficiency. Other causes of angular stomatitis are sinuses at the angle of the mouth, Down's syndrome and Crohn's disease.

Cheilitis Exfoliativa

This is a mild inflammation of the lip; it may be primary or secondary to atopic dermatitis, psoriasis, retinoid therapy, lip licking, actinic exposure, contact dermatitis, etc. The lower lip is usually involved. Most cases occur in young women, a personality disorder with licking and biting of the lips is frequent.

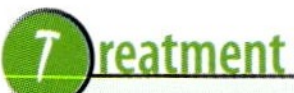

Treatment

Remove the causative agent, topical steroids and zinc are usually helpful.

Glandular Cheilitis

This is an inflammation of the salivary glands of the lips due to chronic exposure to sunlight or lip licking. The lower lips are usually involved.

Clinical Features

The lower lip is the site of predilection. In the early stages, the lip is thickened, pinhead size orifices of the ducts are seen, from which mucous saliva can be expressed. When the lip is palpated between the thumbs and index finger, the enlarged mucous glands feel like pebbles beneath the surface. Mucous exudes freely from these glands to form a gluey film that dries over the lips and causes the lips to stick together at night.

In the more severe form (Volkmann), the lower lip as enlarged, there is pain and tenderness of the lips. There may be deep-seated infection and abscess formation. The condition may become malignant.

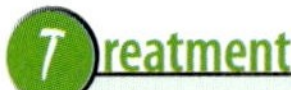

Treatment

Avoid lip licking; protect the lips from sunlight; for enlarged lips, surgery may be required.

Cheilitis Granulomatosis

It is a granulomatous inflammation of both the lips of unknown aetiology giving rise to macrocheilia. Usually the upper lip is involved first; after a lapse of several months, the lower lip is involved. It may be a part of Melkersson-Rosenthal syndrome (Granulomatous cheilitis, facial palsy and fissured tongue). Some cases may represent a localised form of sarcoidosis, ectopic Crohn's disease or orofacial granulomatosis.

The disease has its onset in childhood. The earliest manifestation is the formation of nodules or diffuse swelling of the upper lip then the lower lip; the cheeks may be involved, fissured tongue is seen in 20–40% of patients. There may be a loss of taste and decreased salivary gland secretion. Facial palsy is seen in 30% of cases.

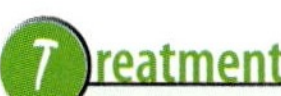

Intralesional injection of triamcinolone 10 mg/mL into the lips may be effective. The injections are to be repeated every 4–6 weeks. Surgical repair of the enlarged lips gives good results. Drugs such as clofazamine, metronidazole may also produce resolution in granulomatous cheilitis.

Plasma Cell Cheilitis

Plasma cell cheilitis is a counterpart of Zoon's plasma cell balanitis. It is characterised by sharply demarcated red plaques with lacquer-like glazing on the lower lips in an elderly patient.

Histologically there is plasma cell infiltration of the lips in a band-like pattern.

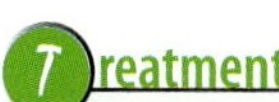

Success has been reported with clobetasol propionate ointment or intradermal injection of triamcinolone. Griseofulvin is also effective.

FURTHER READING

1. Alinovi A, Banoldi D, Pezzarossa E. White sponge nevus: successful treatment with penicillin. Acta Derm Venereol. 1983;63(1):83-5.
2. Barnard NA, Scully C, Eveson JW, et al. Oral cancer development in patients with oral lichen planus. J Oral Pathol Med. 1993;22(9):421-4.
3. Caniff JP, Harvey W, Harris M. Oral submucous fibrosis: its pathogenesis and management. Br Dent J. 1986;160(12):429-34.
4. Fernandez JF, Benito MA, Lizaldez EB, et al. Oral hairy leukoplakia: a histopathologic study of 32 cases. Am J Dermatopathol. 1990;12(6):571-8.
5. Ho KK, Dervan P, O'Loughlin S, et al. Labial melanotic macules. A clinical, histopathological and ultrastructural study. J Am Acad Dermatol. 1993;28(1):33-9.
6. Lim J, Ng SK. Oral tetracycline rinse improves symptoms of white sponge nevus. J Am Acad Dermatol. 1992;26(6):1003-5.
7. Maher R, Lee AJ, Warnakulasuriya KA, et al. Role of acreca nut in the causation of oral submucous fibrosis. A case-control study in Pakistan. J Oral Pathol Med. 1994;23(2):65-9.
8. Pillari R, Balaram P, Reddiar KS. Pathogenesis of submucous fibrosis. Relationship to risk factors associated with oral cancer. Cancer. 1992;69(8):2011-20.
9. Porter S, Scully C. Aphthous stomatitis: an overview of aetiopathogenesis and management. Clin Exp Dermatol. 1991;16(4):235-43.
10. Preeti L, Magesh KT, Rajkumar K and Karthik R. Recurrent Aphthous Stomatitis. J Oral Maxillofac Pathol. 2011;15(3):252-6.
11. Swerlick RA, Cooper PH. Cheilitis glandularis: a re-evaluation. J Am Acad Dermatol. 1984;10(3):466-72.

Chapter 37

Cutaneous Manifestation of Diseases of External Genitalia

INTRODUCTION

The female external genitals comprise the mons pubis, labia majora, labia minora, clitoris, and the vestibule. The vestibule is the area within the labia minora, which contain the urethral meatus, the vaginal orifice and the ducts of the Bartholin glands situated on the posterior part of labia majora. Numerous small mucous glands, and the lesser vestibular glands open on the surface of the vestibule. The greater vestibular glands are homologous to the bulbourethral glands in the male. These are two small round oval bodies reddish-yellow in color situated on each side of the vaginal orifice.

The female urethra is short with the Skene's glandular tubes located at the lower end. The vagina is lined with stratified squamous epithelium; it is rather resistant to gonococcal infection, but is often infected by trichomonas and candidiasis.

The superficial inguinal glands drain the lymphatics of the lower part of the external genitalia, and perineum. The cervix and upper end of the vagina drain into the external iliac nodes. The lower part of the anus drains into the superficial inguinal nodes and the rest of the anal canal into the internal iliac nodes.

SPECIFIC DISORDERS OF FEMALE EXTERNAL GENITALIA

Infections in the vulval region can be purely cutaneous, or purely vaginal, or both. The infection is often complicated by secondary yeast, or bacterial colonization. The vaginal secretions should be examined and cultured in vulval infections. Contact dermatitis by topical therapy often self-administered by patients may further exacerbate the problem. The warm moist environment of the vulva may alter the morphology of lesions such as absence of scales. Vulval scarring can lead to narrowing of the introitus.

Vulval Dystrophies

The term vulval intraepithelial neoplasia (VIN) replaces the previously used terms as: carcinoma *in situ*, Bowen's disease, Bowenoid papulosis, leucoplakia and erythroplasia of Queyrat. Vulvar intraepithelial neoplasia is the presence of abnormal cells in the vulvar skin.

Vulval Intraepithelial Neoplasia

The cause of VIN is unknown; it may be associated with syphilis, granulomatous lesions, herpes simplex, viral infections, obesity, diabetes mellitus, and poor hygiene. Recurrent irritation and radiation to the pelvis may play a part. The role of human 'papillomavirus (HPV) remains uncertain; HPV 16, 18 and 31 have been found to have malignant potential. There is also an association with immune suppression. It may be due to spirochetal infections, malignancy is sometimes associated with Lyme's disease.

Vulvar intraepithelial neoplasia was previously classified as follows:

- VIN I: Mildly abnormal changes in the skin cells (mild dysplasia)
- VIN II: Moderately abnormal changes in the skin cells (moderate dysplasia)
- VIN III: Severely abnormal changes in the skin cells (severe dysplasia).

CLASSIFICATION

The International Society for the Study of Vulvovaginal Diseases (ISSVD) has reclassified VIN. They recommended that the term VIN I, previously used to describe a mild change in the lower epithelial lining, should no longer be used, as these changes have been found to be due to irritation or non-precancerous viral wart infection, and often clear up without treatment. The ISSVD recommended that the term VIN should be used for high grade abnormal squamous lesions (these were previously known as VIN II and VIN III) (Fig. 1).

VIN is now classified as:

1. VIN usual or undifferentiated type.
2. VIN rare or differentiated type
3. VIN rare and unclassified type

VIN 1 can be described by the pathologist as warty, basaloid or mixed VIN. These types of VIN are due to infection with cancer-forming (oncogenic) types of human papillomavirus (HPV) and are more likely to occur in women who smoke.

VIN 2, the 'differentiated' type of VIN is not caused by human papillomavirus and is associated with rapidly growing squamous cell carcinoma. It arises in about 5% of women with lichen sclerosus or lichen planus.

VIN 3-unclassified type, is rare and is of unknown origin.

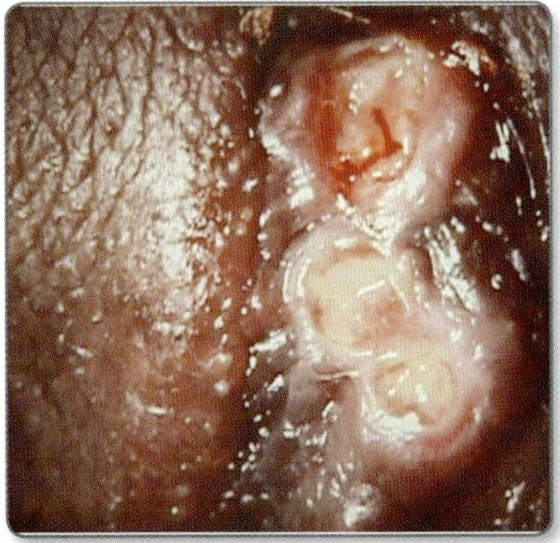

Fig. 1: Vulvar Intraepithelial Neoplasia

Clinical Features

Vulvar intraepithelial neoplasia is commonly seen in the age range of 40–45 years. Most patients complain of pruritus, burning or a severe tingling sensation that can become worse when passing urine; or it may be asymptomatic.

Multicentric or confluent areas of different size, color, and appearance are seen. The areas may be white, brown or red, and ulcerated or warty. Any part of the vulva may be involved, but VIN is most commonly seen in the perineal skin, the preclitoral area, and labia minora. The risk of progression to invasive carcinoma is greater in elderly patients.

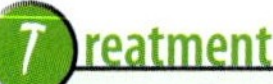

Treatment

Usually all VIN lesions are treated to reduce the risk of developing cancer. The mainstay of treatment is to remove all affected tissue. This may be done with laser ablation, or surgical excision usually under general anesthesia.

Other treatment methods include imiquimod, and 5-fluorouracil creams. These cause severe inflammation, the treatment is also prolonged (several weeks), this is usually not tolerated by all women.

Careful follow-up after treatment is essential as VIN may recur.

Prevention

Immunisation with HPV vaccine has been shown to decrease the risk of VIN as well as cervical cancer.

All vulval disorders such as lichen planus, lichen sclerosus et atrophicus, should be promptly treated to prevent VIN.

Lichen Sclerosus (Lichen Sclerosus et Atrophicus)

Lichen sclerosus was previously called lichen sclerosus et atrophicus. It is also known as hypoplastic dystrophy, kraurosis vulvae, and white spot disease (Fig. 2).

Aetiology

The aetiology is unknown. The cause of lichen sclerosus is not fully understood, it may be autoimmune, genetic, hormonal or an infectious disorder. It was previously thought that the disease occurs only in the elderly, but lichen sclerosus can also occur in younger women due to oestrogen deficiency.

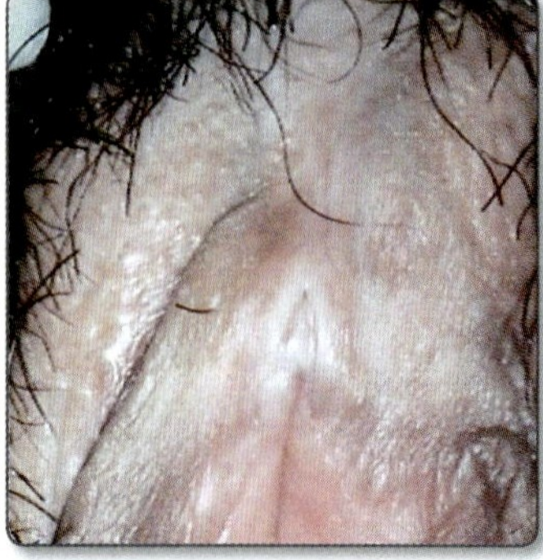

Fig. 2: Lichen sclerosus

Abnormalities of keratin synthesis and androgen abnormalities have been postulated in the pathogenesis of lichen sclerosus.

Lichen sclerosus may be due to IgG antibodies against extracellular matrix; it is associated with autoimmune disorders, anti-thyroid antibodies; antibodies against the gastric parietal cells are found in some cases. It may be associated with alopecia areata, vitiligo, thyrotoxicosis, hypothyroidism, diabetes mellitus, and systemic lupus erythematosus.

Histopathology

Histopathology shows atrophic epidermis, vacuolar degeneration of the basal layer, band-like infiltrate in the superficial dermis, ectatic capillaries, and lymphocytic infiltration. Inflammation and altered fibroblast function in the papillary dermis leads to fibrosis of the upper dermis. The role that hypoxia and ischaemia have in the initial cellular and vascular damage is supported by the finding of increased Glut-1 (Glucose transporter 1) and decreased vascular endothelial growth factor (VEGF) expression in affected skin.

Clinical Features

The disease is ten times more common in women; it usually affects women after the age of 50 years, but it may also occur in pre-pubertal girls. The condition may follow or coexist with lichen simplex, candidiasis, or erosive lichen planus. It may cause no symptoms, or it is extremely pruritic.

The lesion affect the pudendum, either partially or completely as a figure of "8" lesion, encircling the vestibule and involving the clitoris, labia minora, inner aspect of the labia majora, and skin surrounding the anus.

Lichen sclerosus is also known as the white spot disease. In the early stages, there are white flat-topped discrete papules, dark follicular plugs, and an erythematous halo around the papules. The papules gradually flatten, undergo atrophy and become depressed below the surface. Later, the lesions coalesce to form large atrophic patches; itching is usually severe. In course of time, there is considerable hyperpigmentation at the periphery, and the affected skin becomes smooth, wrinkled soft, and white. The classic presentation is of a hypopigmented well-defined plaque with a crinkled or cellophane paper-like texture. Excessive itching may result in thickened hyperkeratotic skin. Long-standing cases produce scarring with resorption of labia minora, and narrowing of the vaginal opening. Lichen sclerosus never affects the vagina. The vulval lesions can lead to the development of squamous cell carcinoma.

Lichen sclerosus when it occurs in girls is at extragenital sites often involutes at puberty; it may be seen occasionally in men causing scarring phimosis.

The disease should be differentiated from guttate morphoea, lichen planus of the atrophic type, VIN, and extramammary Paget's disease.

Treatment

Ultrapotent glucocorticoids are effective in reducing symptoms in a few days. The treatment has to be continued for several months with close monitoring for side effects of steroid application. The disease recurs once treatment is stopped.

Tacrolimus and pimecrolimus have also helped resistant cases of lichen sclerosus.

Two to three percent testosterone ointment gives relief in some cases. It is applied daily until a good response is seen, and then weekly for maintenance. If hypertrophy of the clitoris or hoarseness develops, the treatment should be stopped and then resumed at half strength until symptoms subside.

Carbon dioxide laser, acitretin, and potassium para-aminobenzoate have been used for the treatment of lichen sclerosus.

Plasma Cell Vulvitis

This appears as sharply demarcated erythematous shiny plaques on the vulva. Erosion, haemorrhages, synechiae, and slate to ochre pigmentation may supervene. The epidermis is atrophic; papillary dermis is infiltrated with plasma cells. Topical steroids are helpful and may even be curative.

MALE EXTERNAL GENITALIA

The scrotum is a cutaneous pouch containing the testes and the lower part of the spermatic cord. It is divided into a right and left halves by a ridge or raphe, which is continued forward to the under surface of the penis and backwards to the anus. The skin of the scrotum is thin, brownish in colour, and thrown into folds and rugae. The dartos muscle is a thin layer of unstriped muscle fibres; it is closely united to the skin. The subcutaneous tissue of the scrotum is devoid of fat.

The skin covering the penis is remarkable for its thinness; it is dark in colour. The superficial fascia is devoid of fat; it contains a few fibres of the dartos muscle. The lower part of the penis is the glans, which is covered with skin (prepuce) in uncircumcised men. Coronal sulcus is the constriction behind the glans.

In men, the urethra is divided into prostatic, membranous and spongy urethra. The spongy urethra is the longest and traverses the whole length of the corpus spongiosum. The Cowper's glands are present on both sides of the membranous urethra. The Tyson's glands are proximal to the coronal sulcus and open on both sides of the frenum. The lymphatic vessels of the skin of the external genitalia and perineum drain into the inguinal lymph modes.

SPECIFIC DISORDERS OF MALE EXTERNAL GENITALIA

Balanitis and Balanoposthitis

Balanitis is an inflammation of the glans penis; posthitis is an inflammation of the foreskin. Posthitis does not occur in circumcised men. In young males, the incidence of balanoposthitis is common between the ages of 2 years and 5 years; in children the foreskin is partly or completely nonretractable. The characteristic findings include erythema, pain, discharge, dysuria, bleeding and ulceration of the foreskin. The infecting organisms are usually *Streptococcus haemolyticus* and *Staphylococcus aureus*. In adults, diabetes is often a predisposing factor.

The condition should be differentiated from irritant or allergic contact dermatitis, Reiter's syndrome, and extramammary Paget's disease.

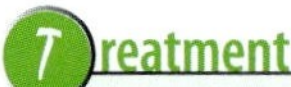

Remove any predisposing cause, antibiotics for the treatment of infection, and the foreskin should be retracted. The sexual partner should also be treated for the elimination of infection.

Balanitis Xerotica Obliterans

The condition occurs after repeated episodes of acute balanitis. The patient presents with complaints of reduced urinary stream, or repeated acute attacks of balanoposthitis. The prepuce is thickened, contracted, and fixed over the glans, which cannot be retracted. The condition is also associated with lichen sclerosus. Potent corticosteroids are effective. Invasive squamous cell carcinoma can occur in long-standing cases.

Lichen Sclerosus

The condition is similar to that of females. The lesion present as ivory white macules and plaques on the glans or inner aspect of the prepuce. The surface is smooth or hyperkeratotic. It may occur around the urethral meatus resulting in stricture of the meatus, and obstruction to the flow of urine. It can develop into squamous cell carcinoma. Patients should be monitored at regular intervals. Potent steroids are very effective in the early stages of the disease.

Plasma Cell Balanitis (Zoon's Balanitis)

This presents as a solitary erythematous plaque on the glans of an uncircumcised usually elderly male. The coronal sulcus and the inner surface of the prepuce may be involved. Histologically, the lesion is benign, and consisting of lozenge-shaped keratinocytes with mild spongiosis. Dermis shows a band-like infiltrate of plasma cells and vascular proliferation. There is poor response to local treatment; circumcision is curable.

Erythroplasia of Queyrat

The condition is characterised by single or multiple well-circumscribed erythematous, velvety plaques on the glans penis of uncircumcised men, usually over the age of 40 years. Symptoms include localised pain, pruritus, and difficulty in retracting the foreskin over the glans. The lesion is similar to Bowen's disease, but this is confined to the penis and perianal areas (Fig. 3). Predisposing factors include poor hygiene, friction, trauma and genital herpes simplex infection. Malignant transformation is common. It is treated by excision, Mohs surgery, carbon dioxide laser ablation or topical application of 5-fluorouracil.

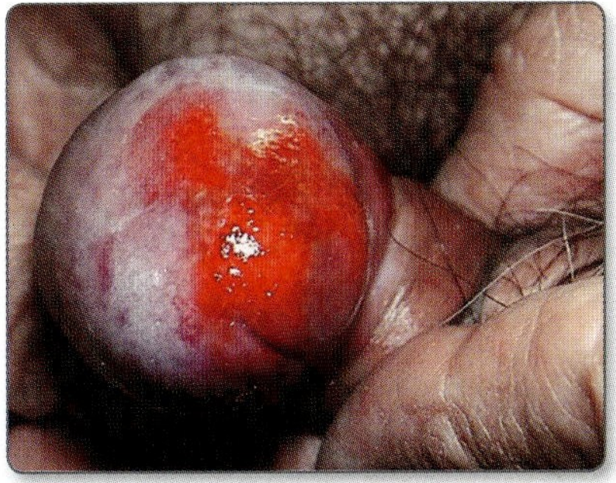

Fig. 3: Erythroplasia of Queyrat

Pearly Penile Papules

These are tiny harmless angiofibromas, which are skin coloured or pearly, situated around the corona (Fig. 4). The condition is symptomless. They can be mistaken for condylomas.

Genital lesions require no therapy. If they occur on the face then can be removed for cosmetic reasons. Recurrences are common.

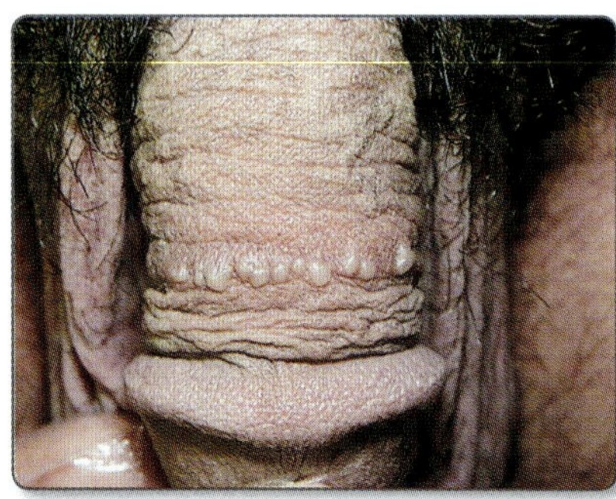

Fig. 4: Pearly penile papules

Peyronie's Disease

This is an idiopathic disorder in which there is excessive fibrosis of the tunica albuginea, the covering sheath of the corpora cavernosa. This fibromatosis may be associated with Dupuytren's contracture and plantar fibromatosis. The fibromatosis leads to distortion, and angulation of the erectile penis. Intralesional injection of corticosteroids in the fibrotic plaque may help some patients. Surgery is often indicated.

Pseudoepitheliomatous, Keratotic and Micaceous Balanitis

This is a rare papulosquamous dermatoses of the glans penis. Clinically a well-demarcated micaceous hyperkeratotic plaque is seen on the glans penis of a circumcised male. The condition is pre-cancerous, and it may develop into an invasive squamous cell carcinoma.

Sexually transmitted diseases are described in chapter 8.

FURTHER READING

1. CM. Lichen sclerosus et atrophicus. BMJ;1987;295:1295-6.
2. Cooper SM, Wojnarowska F. Influence of treatment of erosive lichen planus of the vulva and its prognosis. Arch Dermatol. 2006;142(3):289-94.
3. Edwards L, Hansen RC. Reiter's syndrome of the vulva. Arch Dermatol. 1992;128:811-4.
4. Hart WR. Vulvar intraepithelial neoplasm: historical aspects and current status. Int J Gynaecol Pathol. 2000;20:16-30.
5. Harvood CA, Mortimer PS. Acquired vulval lymphangiomata
6. Heller DS. Report of a new ISSVD classification of VIN. J of Lower Gen Tract Dis. 2007;11(1): 46-7.
7. Kadish AS. Biology of anogenital neoplasm. Cancer Treat Res. 2001;104: 267-86.

8. Kirby B, Whitehurst C, Moore JV, et al. Treatment of lichen planus of the penis with photodynamic therapy. Br J Dermatol. 1999;141:765-6.
9. Meffert JJ, Davis BM, Grimwood RC. Lichen sclerosus. J Am Acad Dermatol. 1995;32:393-416.
10. Neill SM, Ridley CM. Management of anogenital lichen sclerosus. Clin Exp Dermatol. 2001;126:637-43.
11. Porter W, Bunker CB. Treatment of pearly penile pruritic papules with cryosurgery. Br J Dermatol. 2000;142:847-8.
12. Tanebe H, Kishigawa T, Sayama S, et al. A case of giant extramammary Paget's disease of the genital area with squamous-cell carcinoma. Dermatology. 2001;202:249-51.
13. Waugh MA. Balanitis. Dermatol Clin. 1998;16:757-62.

Chapter

38 Miscellaneous Disorders

POIKILODERMA

Poikiloderma is a descriptive term characterised by hyperpigmentation, hypopigmentation, telangiectases and atrophy. It may manifest as a primary disorder, it may be secondary to cutaneous dermatoses, or associated with syndromes, such as Bloom's syndrome and Fanconi's syndrome.

Poikiloderma Vasculare Atrophicans

Poikiloderma vasculare atrophicans (PVA) follows various cutaneous disorders such as mycosis fungoides, large plaque parapsoriasis, dermatomyositis, lupus erythematosus, acrodermatitis chronica atrophicans (ACA), xeroderma pigmentosum, and dyskeratosis congenita. The changes are also seen after radiation (Fig. 1).

The histological findings vary according to the stage of the disease. Early changes show dilatation of the superficial vessels, perivascular round cell infiltration, increase or loss of pigment. Atrophy occurs later, the dermal papillae are flattened, and degenerative changes are seen in both the collagen and elastic tissue. Treatment depends upon the cause.

Hereditary Sclerosing Poikiloderma

This is an autosomal dominant disorder. The skin changes consist of generalised poikiloderma, with hyperkeratotic and sclerotic bands extending across the antecubital spaces, axillary vaults and popliteal fossae. There is sclerosis of the palms and soles, clubbing of the fingers and calcinosis cutis. There is no effective treatment.

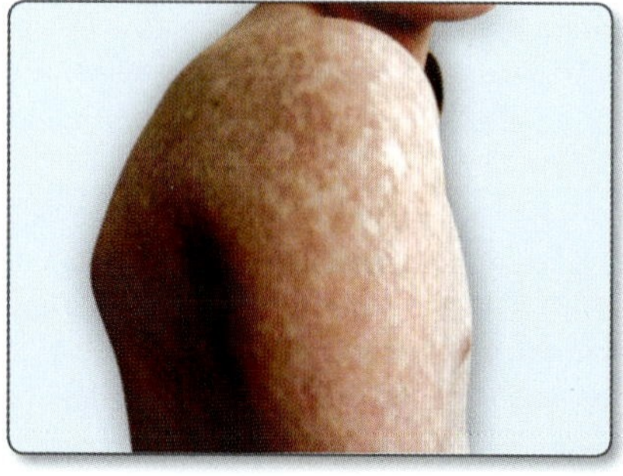

Fig. 1: Poikiloderma vasculare atrophicans

Weary-Kindler Syndrome

This is an autosomal recessive disorder. The disease starts at the age of 1–3 months, it has manifestations of both epidermolysis bullosa and congenital poikiloderma. Vesicopustules occur on the hands and feet often following trauma, which resolve in childhood. Photosensitivity develops early in life, gradual appearance of poikiloderma, which persists until adult life. Keratotic papules develop on the hands, feet, knees, and elbows that persist indefinitely. Early loss of deciduous teeth, severe periodontal bone loss around many permanent teeth, and fragile bleeding gingiva are key features of the syndrome. The defect lies in kindlin-1 a protein found within basal keratinocytes.

Poikiloderma of Civatte

This is a reticulate pigmentation limited to the face, neck and upper part of the chest. The eruption is symmetrical, reddish brown in colour, intermingled with superficial white atrophic spots and telangiectasia (Fig. 2). It is due to photosensitising chemicals in perfumes and other cosmetics. There is no effective treatment, patient should apply sunscreens and avoid exposure to the sun.

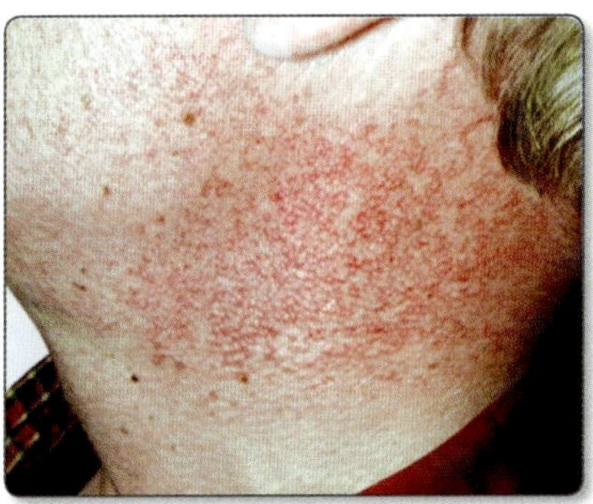

Fig. 2: Poikiloderma of Civatte

ACANTHOSIS NIGRICANS

Acanthosis nigricans is characterised by hyperpigmentation of the axillae, groins, sides of the neck and palms of the hands. The skin becomes thick with pronounced ridging and papillomatosis, which gives the skin a velvety or in severe cases, a warty appearance (Fig. 3). It is believed that acanthosis nigricans is associated with insulin resistance.

Pathogenesis

High concentrations of insulin stimulate deoxyribonucleic acid (DNA) synthesis and cell proliferation in vitro, through the insulin-like growth factor 1 (IGF-1). IGF-1 receptors are present in the keratinocytes, ovaries and in the heart. The insulin receptor has an intrinsic tyrosine kinase activity; this could be responsible for the hyperpigmentation.

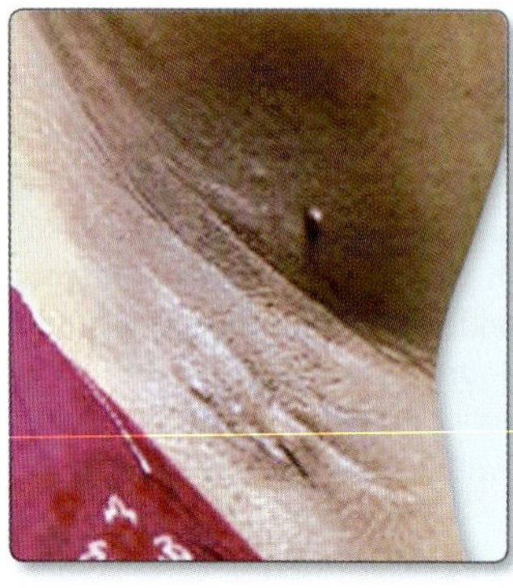

Fig. 3: Acanthosis nigricans

Histopathology

This shows papillomatosis without thickening of the malpighian layer, hyperkeratosis and slight increase in pigmentation of the basal layer.

Classification

Acanthosis nigricans can be:

- Familial
- Benign
- Malignant
- Drug induced
- Naevoid

Familial acanthosis nigricans (true benign acanthosis) is due to an irregular dominant gene. The condition is present at birth or appears during childhood. The lesion becomes worse at puberty and later becomes static or it will regress. It is not associated with any endocrine abnormality.

In benign acanthosis nigricans, the lesions appear secondary to a number of endocrine disorders such as polycystic ovaries, Addison's disease, Cushing's syndrome, hyperandrogenic states, and insulin-resistant diabetes. Acanthosis nigricans is also associated with various syndromes such as Bloom's syndrome, Rud's syndrome and Wilson's disease.

Malignant acanthosis nigricans usually appears at late middle age, it is more severe and more extensive. Thickening of the palms (tripe palms) is frequent, nails may be ridged and brittle, and they may shed. The mucous membrane is involved in 50% of the cases. It is often secondary to carcinoma of the stomach, breast or the lung. Removal of the tumour is associated with regression of clinical signs, but relapses are common.

Pseudoacanthosis nigricans is seen in obese people, often associated with numerous skin tags; histologically, it is indistinguishable from true acanthosis nigricans. This is more common in dark coloured individuals.

Treatment

Removal of the cause may result in moderate improvement of acanthosis nigricans. Pseudoacanthosis nigricans will improve on weight loss. Acitretin has been used in the treatment of hereditary benign acanthosis nigricans.

Drug-induced acanthosis is associated with drugs such as nicotinic acid, fusidic acid, glucocorticoids, stilboestrol, and contraceptive therapy. Triazinate, a folic acid antagonist, is also reported to produce acanthosis nigricans.

Naevoid acanthosis nigricans is uncommon; it is unilateral and is not associated with endocrine abnormalities.

PYODERMA GANGRENOSUM

Pyoderma gangrenosum is an uncommon condition of uncertain aetiology; systemic disease is seen in 50% of cases. This is a destructive, necrotising non-infective ulceration of the skin. It presents as a furuncle like nodule, pustule or haemorrhagic bulla. Pyoderma gangrenosum is often associated with ulcerative colitis, rheumatoid arthritis, leukaemia, myeloma, chronic active hepatitis, lupus erythematosus and Takayasu disease. A number of cases of pyoderma gangrenosum occur without any associated cause; the aetiology remains unknown.

Histopathology

It shows features of a large sterile abscess in which venous and capillary thrombosis, haemorrhage, necrosis and massive cell infiltration are present. Polymorphs are numerous, but epithelioid and giant cells may also be seen.

Clinical Features

It is a rare disorder, occurring mainly in adults. Any area of the body may be involved; thighs, calves, buttocks and face are more prone to develop pyoderma gangrenosum. The typical lesion begins as a small, red, tender nodule or pustule, which breaks down rapidly to form an ulcer. It is surrounded by an erythematous halo. The painful gangrenous ulcer may show satellite violaceous papules, which may break down to fuse with the central ulcer. The ulcer may increase in size to 10 cm or more in size, or it may remain indolent for a long time. The edge of the ulcer is bluish in colour, usually raised and thickened, but sometimes ragged and undermined. It can extend to the underlying fat, fascia and even the muscles. The lesions are sterile on bacterial culture. The ulcer heals forming an atrophic thin flexible scar (Fig. 4).

A rare bullous variant, which remains superficial and maintains an expanding bullous margin, is seen in association with haematological disorders.

Pyoderma gangrenosum displays pathergy: skin trauma, such as biopsy, insect bite can trigger a pustule formation.

Cullen's syndrome a variant of pyoderma gangrenosum includes peristomal pyoderma gangrenosum, and postoperative cutaneous gangrene.

Differential Diagnosis

Severe infections, brown recluse spider bite, artefact, calciphylaxis, coumadin and heparin necrosis.

Course and Prognosis

If pyoderma gangrenosum is related to an underlying disease, then the skin lesions often parallel the course of the illness. If no underlying disease is present, then the course of the disease is very variable. It may persist for years and then the lesion shows spontaneous healing, but new ones develop at other sites. Occasionally the disease will burn out itself after one or two years.

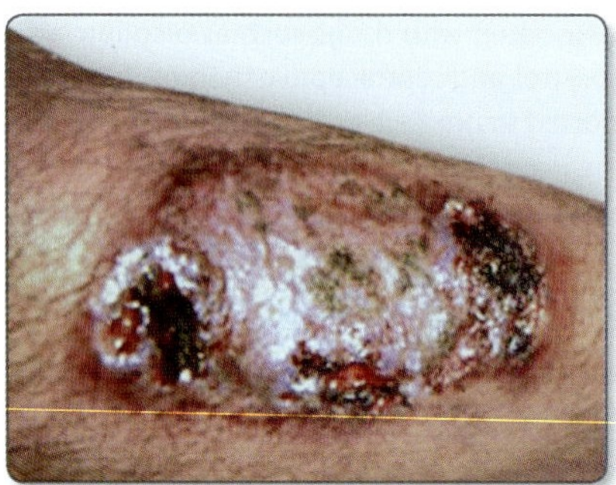

Fig. 4: Pyoderma gangrenosum

Treatment

Treat the underlying disease. Hyperbaric oxygen therapy has been successful in many patients.

Corticosteroids are the mainstay of therapy. High dose of corticosteroids should be given orally in a dose of 1–3 mg/kg of the body weight/day. A pulse therapy with methylprednisolone 1 g/day for 5 days in 150 mL of 5% dextrose infusion is given over an hour.

Cyclosporin is effective, suggesting that T cells may play a part in the pathogenesis. About 5–10 mg/day, which is reduced to half as healing occurs, but the treatment has to be continued for several months.

Treatment with sulphapyridine or salicylazosulphapyridine 0.5 g every 3 hours for 10 days has been helpful. Dapsone and anti-tumour necrosis factor-alpha (anti-TNFα) are also effective.

MALIGNANT ATROPHIC PAPULOSIS

Malignant atrophic papulosis (Degos disease) is a potentially fatal multi-organ vasculopathy. The aetiology is uncertain. The actual physical damage to blood vessels involves impaired fibrinolytic activity, and alterations in platelet function. A genetic influence is seen in most cases. Specifically, it is a progressive, small-size and medium-size arterial occluding disease leading to tissue infarction, and initially involving the skin. Degos disease occurs both in a limited benign, cutaneous form and in a potentially lethal multi-organ, systemic involvement. Lesions in the eyes and central nervous system (CNS) are common. The disease occurs typically in young adults.

Histopathology

There is obliteration of the arterioles and small arteries with proliferation of the intima with subsequent thrombosis. There is dermal necrosis below an area of epidermal atrophy. In the older lesions, there is absence of inflammatory cells; in early lesions, mucin deposits are common.

Clinical Features

The disease is characterised by presence of pale rose coloured papules frequently surrounded by a pink oedematous ring. Later the lesions become umbilicated with a central depression. The center then becomes porcelain white, while the periphery is livid red and telangiectatic, atrophy finally occurs. New lesions appear from time to time, and lesions of different stages can be seen at the same time. Lesions may coalesce to form polycyclic atrophic areas. Degos disease usually does not involve the face, scalp, palms and soles.

Contd...

Contd...

The significance of the condition is that it is associated with endovasculitis of the gut. This is usually lethal. The condition manifests a colicky abdominal pain, vomiting and enteritis. Death is usually due to peritonitis following perforation of the intestines. Occasionally death may also occur following cerebral infarction.

Neurological manifestations comprise hemiparesis, seizures and multiple cranial nerve involvement. Other organs can also be involved such as the lungs, and cardiovascular system. Malignant atrophic papulosis can also be associated with systemic lupus erythematosus and acquired immune deficiency syndrome (AIDS).

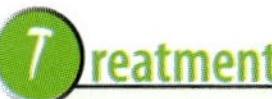

Treatment

The prognosis is poor. Anti-platelet drugs (e.g. aspirin, and dipyridamole) may reduce the number of new lesions in some patients, usually those with only skin involvement. The duration of treatment is about 18–20 months. Anticoagulants have also been used. Pentoxifylline, which facilitates blood flow through the narrowed capillaries by making erythrocytes more flexible, may be helpful.

Eculizumab can effectively treat systemic Degos disease. Corticosteroids are not used; they may even cause gastrointestinal haemorrhage.

SWEET'S SYNDROME (ACUTE FEBRILE NEUTROPHILIC DERMATOSIS)

Tender erythematous plaques, appearing typically on the face, neck and extremities, characterise Sweet's syndrome. The condition is seen typically in middle-aged women; fever and systemic illness accompany the disease.

Pathogenesis

The cause of Sweet's syndrome is unclear. It could be secondary to bacterial or viral infections. Some authors think, it is due to a hypersensitivity reaction to an upper respiratory tract infection. Other associations are internal malignancy and drugs. It can also occur in association with inflammatory disorders such as systemic lupus erythematosus, rheumatoid arthritis or inflammatory bowel disease.

The drugs responsible for Sweet's syndrome are antibiotics, antiepileptics, oral contraceptives, and retinoids; it may also be seen in patients receiving granulocyte colony-stimulating factor (G-CSF).

Clinical Features

The skin lesions are tender red or bluish papules or nodules that coalesce to form irregular plaques. Common sites are the face, arms and neck. Generalised cases may be associated with malignancy. Lesions on the leg resemble panniculitis. Later lesions appear pseudovesicular, because of prominent dermal oedema. The top of the papules occasionally become studded with pustules, resulting from neutrophilic migration. The lesions resolve after weeks or months without scarring (Fig. 5).

The systemic symptoms include fever, headache, arthralgias and generalised malaise. Conjunctivitis and scleritis may occur. Lesions of the oral mucosa should be differentiated from aphthae.

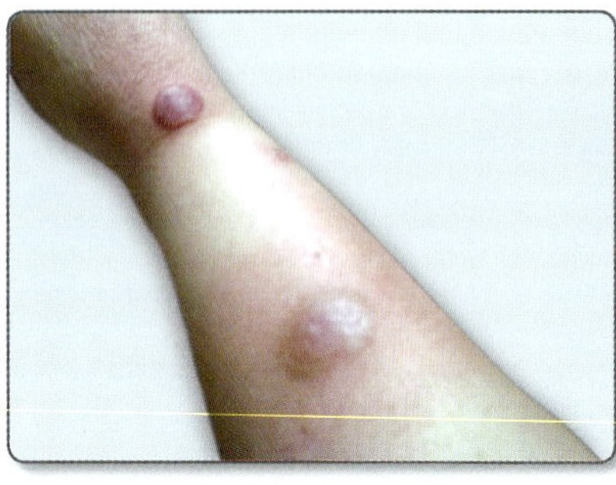

Fig. 5: Sweet's syndrome. Note the vesiculation effect due to dermal oedema

Histopathology

A distinctive band of edema in the papillary dermis, with intense focal infiltration of neutrophils in the upper and mid-dermis, is characteristic of Sweet's syndrome. Varying amounts of fragmentation of the neutrophils occur, with presence of nuclear dust and ingestion of neutrophils by macrophages (bean bag cells). Vasodilatation and minor degree of endothelial swelling is seen in the blood vessels. There is little evidence of acute or chronic vasculitis on light microscopy.

Laboratory Findings

Elevated erythrocyte sedimentation rate (ESR), peripheral leucocytosis and neutrophilia are consistent findings. White blood cells (WBC) counts range from 10,000/mm^3 to 20,000/mm^3.

Treatment

Although systemic symptoms such as fever and leucocytosis suggest a systemic infection, there is no response to antibiotics. Systemic corticosteroids such as prednisolone in a dose of 30–60 mg is given daily and then tapered to 10 mg in 2–3 weeks. A rapid response is also seen with potassium iodide, 100 mg daily for 2 weeks. Recently colchicine 1.5 mg daily for 3 weeks has also produced good results.

Methotrexate, clofazimine and thalidomide are also helpful.

Benign Cutaneous Lymphocytic Infiltration

Lymphocytes may infiltrate the skin in a number of cutaneous disorders such as infections, inflammatory diseases, autoimmune diseases, malignancy, etc. In benign cutaneous lymphocytic infiltration lymphocytes accumulate in the skin without any known cause.

Lymphocytoma Cutis

This is a benign cutaneous infiltration of the skin usually confined to the head and neck. Females are commonly affected.

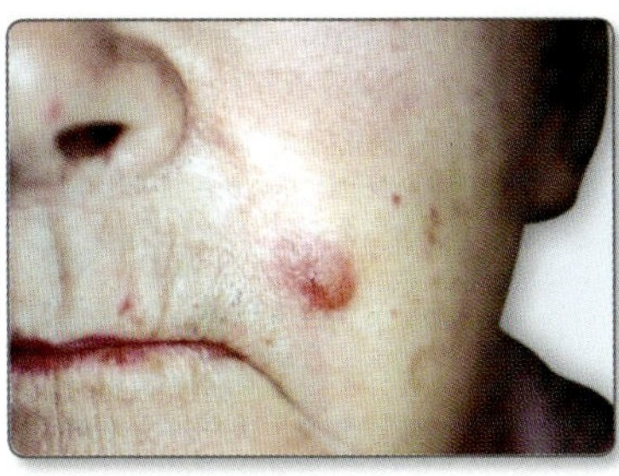

Fig. 6: Lymphocytoma cutis
Source: Dr Ian McColl. Global Skin Atlas

Histopathology

The epidermis is usually normally separated from the dermis by a Grenz zone. The dermis is infiltrated with histiocytes, and lymphocytes arranged in follicles. The blood vessels and appendages are spared. Most of the lymphocytes are B lymphocytes.

Clinical Features

The disease may be localised or generalised. In the localised form, nodules red or purple in colour are seen on the head and neck especially the forehead and ear lobes. A number of cases are also seen on the scalp. There is no internal manifestation (Fig. 6).

In the disseminated form, miliary papules or indurated nodules are found on the face, trunk, and extremities. Progression to lymphoma may occur.

Treatment

There is no specific treatment. Excision, intralesional steroids, antibiotics, antimalarials, radiotherapy, avoidance of sunlight and use sunscreens are helpful.

JESSNER'S LYMPHOCYTIC INFILTRATION

This is a chronic T cell disorder characterised by pink or reddish brown flat discoid plaques. The lesions are usually found on the face, neck, and upper back. Eyelids and zygomas are frequently involved. The condition is seen most frequently in men.

Histopathology

In the dermis, there is intense perivascular infiltration of lymphocytes. There is no follicular arrangement as in lymphocytoma cutis.

Treatment

Treatment is unsatisfactory. Chloroquine, radiotherapy, cryotherapy, corticosteroids and psoralen ultraviolet A (PUVA) have been used in the treatment. Most of the lesions involute after several years.

PSEUDOLYMPHOMAS

This is a persistent lymphocytic infiltration of the skin with T or B lymphocytes. These present as multiple cutaneous nodules often present after systemic therapy with drugs such as β-blockers, amitriptyline, anti-scabietic treatment, insect bites, etc. Histology shows mitotic figures and cellular atypia. The condition is benign. Careful drug history should help in differentiating the condition from a lymphoma. In most cases, pseudolymphoma is a self-limiting condition, once the offending agents are removed.

LYMPHOMATOID PAPULOSIS

There are two types of lymphomatoid papulosis; in type A the atypical cell is the histiocyte, and in type B the proliferating cell is the T helper cell.

Histopathology

The histological appearance of both types of lymphomatoid papulosis is that of malignancy, although the condition is mostly benign. Cell phenotype reveals antigen associated with lymphoma rather than benign inflammation. DNA analysis also supports the view that the condition is a T cell lymphoma. About 10% of cases will eventually develop into a lymphoma which maybe mycosis fungoides, Hodgkin's disease or non-Hodgkin's lymphoma.

Clinical Features

The condition is characterised by self-healing recurrent eruptions of haemorrhagic papules. These heal spontaneously in 6–8 weeks; the lesions are present on the trunk and extremities. The disease is common in middle-aged males. The lesions of lymphomatoid papulosis are in constant activity, with old lesions resolving and new ones developing at the same time. Mild pruritus may occur (Fig. 7).

Treatment

Treatment is often unsatisfactory; PUVA, corticosteroids and methotrexate have been used for the treatment.

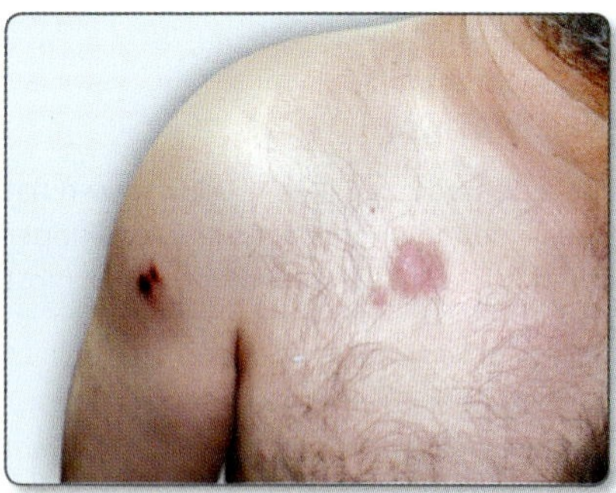

Fig. 7: Lymphomatoid papulosis

GANGRENE OF THE SKIN

Gangrene is death of tissue. It is due to vascular occlusion, it may have a neural association as in diabetes mellitus. Gangrene may be 'moist' which is associated with bacterial invasion and putrefaction, or 'dry' without bacterial decomposition as seen in large vessel occlusion.

Clinical Appearance

The gangrenous part is cold, arterial pulsations are absent. The colour changes due to ischaemia are as follows: initially there is pallor, later there is a dusky grey or purple discolouration due to pooling of blood and finally the colour changes to brownish-black due to disintegration of hemoglobin and formation of iron sulphide.

Dry Gangrene

This is due to arteriosclerosis and takes place over a period of weeks or months. This is seen secondary to arteriosclerosis, polyarteritis nodosa, Raynaud's phenomenon, thromboangiitis obliterans (Buerger's disease), frostbite, etc. If this occurs on an exposed part such as limbs, the part of the extremities dries up before necrosis occurs. The dryness discourages the growth of bacteria and putrefaction does not occur. There is no foul odour. The gangrenous area is dry, wrinkled and black.

Moist Gangrene

This occurs, when at the time of vascular occlusion the area is moist. Putrefaction of tissue proteins takes place and infection sets in, producing a foul smell. This is seen when an artery is suddenly occluded by an embolus or ligature, venous obstruction and arterial occlusion occur together. In diabetes, there is increased likelihood of bacterial infection and so is the case in gangrene of the internal organs.

Wet gangrene of the limb manifests as swelling and discolouration, the epidermis is raised in blebs, and vesicles appear. In gas gangrene, crepitus can be felt on palpation.

A number of bacteria are associated with gangrene, such as Clostridia, β-Haemolytic *Streptococcus*, Pseudomonas, Bacteroides, Fusospirochaetes, *Haemophilus influenzae* and some anaerobic organisms. Gangrene may also be associated with viral infections, such as vaccinia gangrenosum, severe varicella infection and fungal infections such as mucormycosis (Fig. 8).

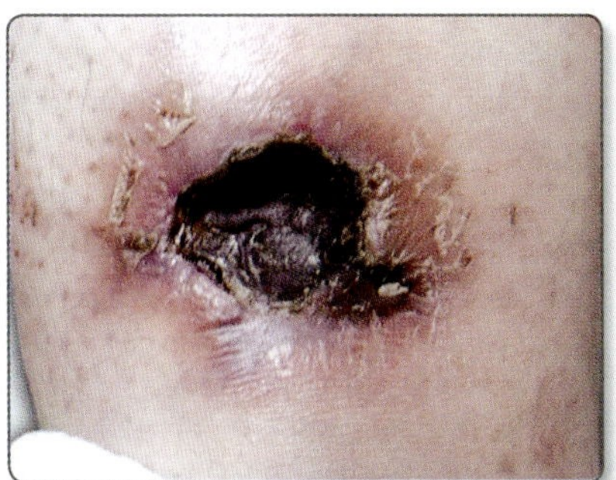

Fig. 8: Gangrene

Gas Gangrene (Clostridial Myonecrosis)

This is usually rare in civilised life. It often results from infections of deep lacerations and wounds of muscle tissue. It may be a complication of compound fracture, bowel surgery, after septic abortions and delivery.

Pain is the first indication of gas gangrene. The patient has an anxious look. Clostridial septicemia is characterised by irritability, dyspnea and tachycardia, which is out of proportion to pyrexia. There is a peculiar sickly-sweet odour from the wound linked to that of decaying apples. The area around the wound is red and swollen. Gas gangrene spreads along the muscle planes. Crepitus is present due to the air entrapped in the tissue.

The causative organisms are *Clostridium perfringens*, *C. oedematicus*, *C. septicum* and *C. histolyticum*. These are thick Gram-positive rods.

Non-Clostridial Gas Gangrene

This is often due to anaerobic streptococcus. It may complicate diabetes mellitus. The onset is delayed for several weeks. The purulent exudate has a foul odour. It can be treated with hyperbaric oxygen. This is of value if immediately administered.

Necrotising Fasciitis

The condition is characterised by necrosis in addition to cellulitis. It has a rapid fulminant course, with the appearance of bullae at the site of an abscess, furuncle or injury. In about 2–4 days, there is a bluish discolouration at the affected site and a gangrenous area is found on the skin. There is extreme apathy and weakness.

Treatment is surgical with wide incisions in the infected area. Initially, high-dose penicillin intravenously or broad-spectrum coverage, switching to culture sensitive antibiotic as soon as possible.

Fournier's Gangrene

This is a malignant dangerous infection of the penis and scrotum due to group A streptococcus associated with enteric bacilli and anaerobes. It is a form of necrotising fasciitis.

Meleney's Gangrene

This is a postoperative synergistic gangrene. It often follows drainage of an abscess or chronic empyema. After a week or two, the drainage site has a carbunculoid appearance, with well-differentiated three zones: an inner gangrenous zone, middle dusky purple and an outer zone of bright red colour. The pain is severe. The gangrene is due to microaerophilic nonhaemolytic *Streptococcus*.

Ecthyma Gangrenosum

This is often seen in debilitated persons as those suffering from leukemia or any terminal malignant disease, severe burns, pancytopenia and chronic terminal systemic illness. The causative organism is *Pseudomonas aeruginosa*.

Clinically, the ecthyma becomes tender or painful, large tense grouped vesicles appear surrounded by a pink or violaceous halo. The vesicles then become haemorrhagic, and they rupture to form ulcers with necrotic black centres. The lesion is usually on the extremities or buttocks.

Treatment is with aminoglycoside and antipseudomonal penicillin such as piperacillin.

Traumatic Gangrene

This is due to direct or indirect trauma. The most common example is the bedsore; it can also be due to the pressure of splints and plasters.

Bedsore

These commonly develop in a patient who is bedridden. Two most important factors in its development are pressure and loss of the trophic influence of nerves. Bedsores develop rapidly in anaemic and malnourished patients. Moisture increases the rate of extension of a bedsore. The common sites for the development of bedsores are the sacrum, greater trochanters and the heel.

TREATMENT OF GANGRENE

After removing the gangrenous area, the aim of treatment is to save the limbs or tissues from amputation if possible. For impending cases of gangrene, improvement of the blood supply can be done by direct arterial surgery or by interruption of the sympathetic nerve supply. These measures are adopted if the arterial supply above the gangrenous area is good. If gangrene is spreading rapidly, amputation has to be carried out to save the patient's life.

General treatment

Treat the underlying cause of gangrene such as vasculitis, diabetes, infections, etc. If no major arterial obstruction is present, the effort is made to save the limbs as far as possible. In severe infections, drainage of the affected area with removal of the slough must be carried out.

Treatment of Bedsores

A foam mattress should be used. Bed sheets should be kept free from wrinkles. Urine and feces should be cleaned immediately. The affected area should be clean and dry. The patient's position should be changed two hourly. A special mattress with honeycomb cavities may help. Alternate cavities are filled with air. These are emptied every few minutes by a motorised pump. In this way, a constant pressure on any area of the skin in prevented.

Occlusive dressings made of various polymers have made a significant contribution to ulcer therapy. These dressings keep the ulcer moist, a factor that helps in epidermal repair, through migration of epithelial cells over the ulcer. Initially, large amounts of exudate forms under the dressing (crust and necrotic debris); these dressings are changed daily; later as the ulcer heals they can be changed at 2–3 days interval.

The infected wound should be treated with an appropriate antibiotic given systemically. Locally the infected wound should be cleaned with an antiseptic.

HISTIOCYTOSIS

Histiocytosis is a group of diseases that are characterised by the accumulation of reactive or neoplastic histiocytes in various tissues. Histiocytes are cells derived from the circulatory monocytes, which have their origin in the bone marrow. The Langerhans cell is an antigen-presenting histiocyte, which has migrated into the epidermis. It has staining reactions for S-100 protein, CD1a, and CD4 as for macrophages. The factors that control the migration of Langerhans cells into the epidermis are poorly understood. A possible immediate precursor of Langerhans cells in the epidermis is the indeterminate cell; this resembles the Langerhans cell but lacks the Birbeck granules. The fate of the Langerhans cells is unknown, it has been reported by some authors that the cells migrate from the skin into the lymphatics as veiled cells, and eventually develop into interdigitating reticulum cell in the para-cortical zone of the regional lymph nodes. If Langerhans cells are cultured, they lose their characteristic phenotype and assume an interdigitating reticulum cell phenotype.

Histiocytes can be broadly divided into two groups of cells: one responsible for phagocytosis and the other as antigen-presenting cells. Langerhans cells are the antigens-presenting histiocytes.

CLASSIFICATION OF HISTIOCYTOSIS

- Class I Langerhans cells histiocytosis
- Class II Histiocytosis of mononuclear phagocytes
- Class III Malignant histiocytic disorders.

Class I Histiocytosis: Langerhans Cell Histiocytosis

In this class of histiocytosis, cells with the phenotype of Langerhans cells accumulate in the various tissues and cause damage. The damage is perhaps due to the presence of cytokines. The condition was previously known as Histiocytosis X, a word coined by Louis Lichtenstein in 1953. He chose the suffix "X" to represent an undetermined cause of disorder. He thought that the suffix "X" has the advantage of brevity and by implication emphasizes the necessity for intensive search for the aetiological agent. We now know that these cells are the Langerhans cells.

The Langerhans cells histiocytosis is characterised by granulomatous proliferation of Langerhans cells. The disease involves the skin, bones, lungs, nervous system and other organs. Several entities have been grouped which have a great deal of overlap. In some cases, only the bones are involved in others there may be involvement of the CNS. Diabetes insipidus may occur which is controlled by vasopressin. Purpura and petechiae are associated with poor prognosis. Lesions on the trunk and scalp may resemble seborrhoeic dermatitis. Eczematous changes are present in the body folds. Nail changes include onycholysis, subungual hyperkeratosis, and onychodystrophy. Oral mucosa may show white plaques or nodular infiltrations. Displaced teeth and loss of alveolar bones are characteristic findings.

The different clinical entities of Langerhans cell histiocytosis are:

Letterer-Siwe Disease

The condition is seen in infants. Lesions are present in the lungs, lymph nodes, liver, spleen and bone marrow. Eighty percent of patients develop cutaneous lesions, which consist of petechiae, crusted papules on the scalp, trunk, groin and face. The treatment consists of a combination of drugs such as vincristine, methotrexate and prednisolone.

Hand-Schuller-Christian Disease

The disease is usually seen in children, but may develop in adults. It is characterised by a triad of exophthalmos, diabetes insipidus and defects in the membranous bones, especially that of the skull. Cystic changes are also seen in other parts of the skeletal system. Cutaneous lesions are present in about one-third of the patients. Most of the lesions resemble seborrhoeic dermatitis, both of the scalp and trunk lesions present as yellowish-brown scaly papules, these may become nodular, it may exudate and crust. Purpura is often found. There is bronze pigmentation of the skin.

Bone involvement is most frequent in the skull. Femur, scapula, ribs mandible, and vertebrae are also often affected. Lesions appear as osteolytic areas that are sharply demarcated; deafness may occur if the mastoid is involved.

Visceral lesions involve the liver, spleen, brain and lungs. Hepatosplenomegaly and enlargement of the lymph nodes may occur. The disease runs a chronic progressive course that ends fatally in 20–50% of cases.

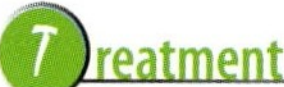

Treatment includes oral prednisolone alone or in combination with vinblastine or methotrexate. Radiation is given to those patients who do not respond to chemotherapy. Bad prognosis includes patients with onset under the age of 6 years, extra-osseous lesions, and multiple organ involvement.

Eosinophilic Granuloma of the Bone (Large Cell Granuloma)

This is the most benign type of Langerhans cells histiocytosis. It is characterised by granulomas in the bone with osteolysis. Cutaneous lesions when present resemble those of Letterer-Siwe disease. Periorificial involvement is characteristic. The course of the disease is benign.

In congenital self-healing reticulohistiocytosis, multiple firm reddish-brown papulonodar lesions are present at birth. These clear spontaneously by 2–3 months of age.

Class II Histiocytosis: Histiocytosis of Mononuclear Phagocytes

These are non-malignant disorders in which the phagocytic histiocytes accumulate in the various tissues, where they may or may not cause symptoms, e.g. dermatofibroma, juvenile xanthogranuloma and multicentric reticulohistiocytosis. They are usually S-100 and CD1a negative. These include a series of nonaggressive, self-healing diseases affecting both children and adults. Some of these are juvenile xanthogranuloma, generalised eruptive histiocytosis, benign cephalic histiocytosis, and sinus histiocytosis with massive lymphadenopathy.

Juvenile Xanthogranuloma

Two clinical forms are distinguished, papular and nodular. The papular form is characterised by numerous yellowish-brown papules, distributed all over the skin. The nodular form may be associated with systemic involvement, juvenile chronic myeloid leukemia has been reported. The cutaneous lesions tend to flatten with time.

Multicentric Reticulohistiocytosis

Multicentric reticulohistiocytosis (MR) is a systemic granulomatosis; the skin and joints predominate the clinical picture. The granulomas consist chiefly of histiocytes of irregular size and shape.

Clinical Features

The disease typically affects the middle-aged women, about two-thirds of the patients first note arthritis, about one-fifth note skin nodules first, and in one-fifth of the cases skin and joint lesions appear simultaneously. About half of the cases eventually develop mucous membrane manifestation.

Cutaneous Changes

The face particularly the nose and the paranasal areas, nails especially the nail folds, ears, forearms, scalp (behind the ears), neck and trunk are involved in descending order of frequency. The lesions are hemispherical nodules of reddish-brown colour; they vary in size from a few millimeters to several centimetres. Ulceration normally does not occur, pruritus may be present. Lesions around the nail fold are said to have a coral bead appearance.

Articular Lesions

There is symmetrical involvement of the interphalangeal joints, knees, shoulders, wrists, hips, ankles, feet, elbows, and vertebral joints in a descending order of frequency. The arthritis is destructive, and severe deformities may result. The fingers may be considerably shortened, but pulled out to their full length, these are called the opera glass hand or telescopic fingers.

Differential Diagnosis

The disease should be differentiated from rheumatoid arthritis, lepromatous leprosy, sarcoidosis, xanthoma disseminatum and gout.

Mucosal Changes

About half of the patients have mucosal lesions; nodules are seen similar to those of the skin.

Lesions may also occur in other tissues and organs, such as muscles, lymph nodes, stomach, eyes, thyroid and salivary glands. Gallium scans are often used as a screening method to assess the extent of the disease.

Treatment

In about one-fourth of patients the disease involutes spontaneously in 6–8 years. No treatment is of consistent value. Alkylating agents such as cyclophosphamide and nitrogen mustard prevent disfiguring arthritis and skin lesions. prednisolone, vinblastine and PUVA have also been helpful.

Class III Histiocytosis: Malignant Histiocytosis

The malignancies comprise monocytic leukemia, malignant histiocytosis, and true histiocytic lymphoma; there is an enormous overlap between the conditions and sometimes it is not possible to differentiate them.

In monocytic leukemia, the malignancy involves the bone marrow and blood. In malignant histiocytosis, there is widespread involvement of the reticulohistiocytic system. In true histiocytic lymphoma, the malignancy arises from the fixed tissue histiocytes and the tumours are localised.

Monocytic leukemia may have secondary cutaneous manifestations which may be specific or non-specific. Malignant histiocytosis usually involves the liver, spleen, lymph nodes, and bone marrow. Cutaneous infiltrations are seen as extranodal extension of the disease and in generalised dissemination.

True Histiocytic Lymphoma

This may be nodal or extranodal. Constitutional symptoms such as fever, malaise, anorexia, and sweating may be present. Extranodal presentation may be cutaneous which usually presents as bluish-red tumours; these attain a large size. One-third of the cases are seen on the thighs or buttocks. Peak incidence is in the 7th decade. Several histological variants are described including myxoid, inflammatory, angiomatoid and giant cell types. The cells stain positively for vimentin.

The prognosis depends on the site; the deeper and more proximally located tumours have a poor prognosis. Angiomatoid variants in younger patients have a poor outlook. The myxoid variety is less prone to metastasis, localised recurrence is common, and metastasis to the lung is a frequent cause of death.

Always biopsy infants who do not respond to treatment of seborrheic dermatitis to exclude histiocytosis

MUCINOSIS

Mucinosis are disorders, characterised by deposition of mucin focally or diffusely in the dermis. Mucins are jelly-like acid mucopolysaccharides of the ground substance produced by the fibroblasts. There are a number of conditions in which mucin deposits are present in the skin, such as in thyroid disease (pretibial myxedema, and scleromyxedema), monoclonal gammopathy and lupus erythematosus. Mucinous infiltration in the skin may be primary or secondary.

Primary mucinosis may be diffuse, focal or follicular. Secondary mucinosis may be found in collagen disorders, Degos syndrome, and eosinophilic-myalgia syndrome; it may accompany mesenchymal renal tumours, lymphomas. Secondary mucinosis may also occur in basal cell carcinoma, tumours of the sweat gland, pyogenic granuloma, and granuloma annulare.

Lichen Myxedematosus (Papular Mucinosis)

This is a disease of adults. The disease may manifest as generalised papules, nodules or annular lesions, or rarely as urticarial nodules and plaques.

Histopathology

Mucinous deposits are found in the middle and deeper layers of the dermis. The deposits can be seen on staining by alcian blue or toluidine blue.

Clinical Features

The disease is seen mostly between the ages of 30–50 years. It is characterised by the formation of small papules over an erythematous and hardened skin. The skin is thickened but is movable over the subcutis. The infiltration is most noticeable on the forehead with accentuation of the folds and creases that form a vertical swelling at the root of the nose. A woody fibrous sclerosis of the skin is characteristic. General health is not affected. Scalp and mucous membranes are not involved.

A paraproteinaemia is always present, which is seen on electrophoresis. The protein is an immunoglobulin G (IgG), which causes proliferation of the fibroblasts. Other laboratory abnormalities are elevation of ESR; eosinophilia in seen is some cases.

Treatment

Melphalan is the treatment of choice; it results in gradual resolution of the skin lesions in about 3 months. Retinoids have also produced good results. Topical betamethasone, photochemotherapy, and electron beam therapy have also been used in the treatment.

Reticular Erythematous Mucinosis (REM Syndrome)

The disease usually affects the middle-aged females. A relationship between reticular erythema and Jessner's lymphocytic infiltration has been suggested.

The disease is characterised by the formation of papules and plaques on the mid-chest and upper back, over a persistent reticular erythema. Deposits of mucin are found between the collagen fibres, there is perivascular and periappendageal lymphocytic infiltration.

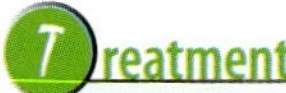

Antimalarial therapy is effective in some cases of REM syndrome.

Follicular Mucinosis

The disease is characterised by the deposition of mucin in the outer root sheath of the hair follicles and sebaceous glands. The lesion is a mucinous plaque, which may be hypopigmented, erythematous and scaly, or eczematous, studded with follicular papules. These are present mainly on the face and neck; dysesthesia to cold is reported in some cases with a resultant misdiagnosis of leprosy. The plaque is alopecic.

Three categories of patients have been identified; younger patients with a few lesions, the disease resolves spontaneously in 2 months to 2 years. The lesion in the older age group are more numerous and widespread, resolution takes place in a number of years. The third group affects still the older age group; it is mostly seen in association with mycosis fungoides. Anaesthesia to cold and touch may occur in many cases.

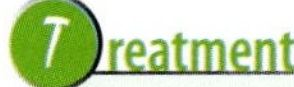

Spontaneous involution may occur. Corticosteroids, dapsone and PUVA have been found to be effective.

A variant common in young girls presents as round or oval clusters of hypopigmented follicular macules on the outer aspect of the arms. Intralesional injection of triamcinolone acetonide permits repigmentation in 3–4 weeks.

Follicular mucinosis may occur in association with reticulosis or lymphomas.

Cutaneous Focal Mucinosis

The condition is seen mostly in childhood as a solitary symptomless nodule or papule. The surface is smooth. Histologically, it may resemble a myxoma, myxoid cyst, or a ganglion. Treatment is by excision.

Myxoid Cyst

This is a focal accumulation of mucin in the dermis present on the dorsal aspect of the distal phalanx or proximal nail folds of the fingers, less often on the toes.

The cysts are 5–7 mm in diameter, opaque, shiny and dome shaped with a smooth surface. On puncture mucin is exuded. The nail often shows a longitudinal groove due to the presence of the cyst.

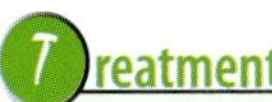

Treatment

Treatment is usually disappointing for the cyst reappears in spite of any method of therapy. The cyst can be punctured, excised or removed by electrofulguration. Splinting of the distal interphalangeal joint for 4–6 weeks interferes with the replenishment of its contents, but the cyst reappears later. Combination of squeezing the gelatinous contents and then freezing with cryotherapy, a method known as Epstein's technique, is also quite successful.

Scleredema, myxedema and pretibial myxedema are described in chapters 11 and 33.

NECROBIOTIC DISORDERS

Necrobiotic lesions exhibit a primary focus of localised damage to the dermis that affects the cells more than the fibres, and it is accompanied by deposits of abnormal substances. These areas of necrobiosis are surrounded by a granulomatous reaction in which loosely arranged histiocytes have a tendency to point towards the centre of the granuloma.

Granuloma annulare, actinic granuloma, necrobiosis lipoidica, rheumatic and rheumatoid nodules belong to the group of necrobiotic disorders. Recently cat scratch disease has also been included in this group of disorders.

Granuloma Annulare

Granuloma annulare is a necrobiotic disorder characterised by focal destructive process in the dermis, which stimulates a histiocytic and granulomatous response resulting in a palisading granuloma. The granuloma is present in the middle and upper dermis; mucin deposition may occur in the foci of altered collagen.

Aetiology

The exact cause is unknown. It may be a delayed hypersensitivity response to unidentified antigens. Cases have been reported following insect bites, trauma,

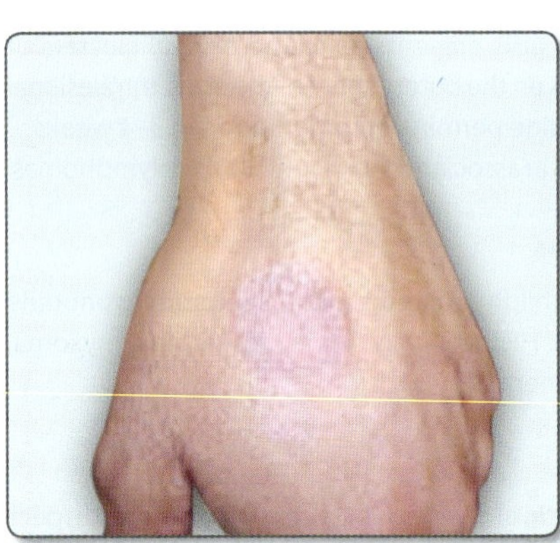

Fig. 9: Granuloma annulare

Clinical Features

Granuloma annulare can be localised, generalised, nodular and perforating.

Localised granuloma annulare: The dorsal surface of the hands, feet and fingers are the common sites affected. The lesion consists of small papules closely set, arranged in form of a ring. These are skin coloured or erythematous. On stretching the skin, the underlying whitish beaded papules are revealed. The lesions enlarge by centrifugal extension. The condition is symptomless. Multiple lesions may occur; the disease does not affect the mucous membrane. Granuloma annulare disappears spontaneously without scarring. Recurrences are common (Fig. 9).

Generalised granuloma annulare: Numerous papules or nodules develop over the trunk and limbs. The lesion may remain discrete or coalesce to form reticulate and circinate patterns. The lesions may be pruritic. It is often associated with diabetes mellitus. The condition is seen in both children and adults.

Nodular granuloma annulare: This is usually seen in children. The scalp, palms, buttocks and legs are commonly involved.

Perforating granuloma annulare: This may be localised or generalised. The papules develop a yellowish centre due to perforation of collagen. On gentle squeezing a clear viscous fluid is discharged, which dries to form a crust.

Differential Diagnosis

The condition should be differentiated from the other annular lesions such as tinea corporis, annular lichen planus, annular psoriasis, erythema annulare centrifugum and annular sarcoidosis. The absence of symptoms, site and biopsy will differentiate granuloma annulare from other disorders.

Treatment

Spontaneous resolution occurs in a number of cases, so no treatment is required. Trauma of biopsy, injection of sterile water and freezing are believed to initiate treatment. Intralesional steroids and dapsone are also helpful. In generalised eruption, systemic steroids are effective. A few studies have also shown response by fumaric acid esters.

gold therapy, sun exposure, PUVA therapy, etc. Generalised granuloma annulare is associated with diabetes mellitus. Epstein-Barr virus and HIV infection raise the possibility of a viral etiology.

Granuloma Multiforme

This is also a necrobiotic granuloma characterized by focal necrobiosis and histiocytic proliferation. The disease is mainly found in Central Africa where leprosy is endemic. The local inhabitants often call the disease "giant ringworm".

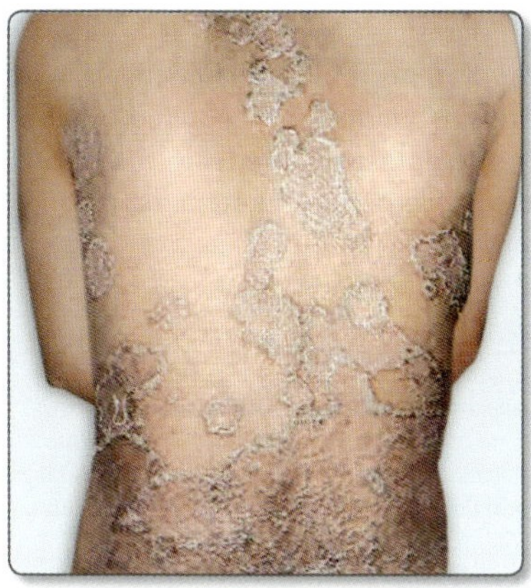

Fig. 10: Granuloma multiforme

Clinical Features

The upper trunk and arms are commonly affected. The initial lesion is a papule, which later becomes annular with raised margins and a slightly depressed centre. The lesions may coalesce to form polycyclic patterns. The condition lasts for months or years. The general health remains unaltered. There is no loss of sensation. The cutaneous nerves are not enlarged (Fig. 10).

There is no known treatment of granuloma multiforme.

The histology resembles granuloma annulare but multinucleated giant cells are present. The aetiology of granuloma multiforme is unknown.

Necrobiotic granulomas of rheumatoid arthritis and necrobiosis lipoidica are described in chapter 31.

PERFORATING DISORDERS

These are a group of disorders in which altered components of the skin are eliminated via the epidermis, a process termed as transepithelial elimination (TEE). In most of these conditions, TEE is secondary to some underlying diseases such as granuloma annulare, chronic renal failure, diabetes mellitus, pseudoxanthoma elasticum, etc. There are four conditions considered as primary or major perforating disorders. These may be due to some defect in the epithelial keratinocytes, hair follicles, collagen or elastic fibres. The primary perforating disorders are:

- Reactive perforating collagenosis
- Elastosis perforans serpiginosa
- Kyrle's disease
- Perforating folliculitis.

Reactive Perforating Collagenosis

This is a rare disorder beginning in early childhood in which traumatically altered collagen is extruded by a process of TEE.

Histopathology

In papillary dermis the collagen bundles, necrobiotic connective tissue, degenerating inflammatory cells are surrounded and engulfed by focal epidermal proliferation. Eventually, the epidermis overlying the papilla atrophies, disruption of the site over the papilla occurs. The abnormal collagen is eliminated via transepithelial migration.

Clinical Features

The disorder begins in early childhood, as tiny papules on the extensor surface of the hands, elbows and knees. These papules increase in size to 5–10 mm over 3–5 weeks, and then become umbilicated with a keratinous plug. In 6–8 weeks, they regress leaving a small scar with altered pigmentation. The lesions are precipitated by superficial trauma; deep trauma may fail to cause them. Lesions have arisen at the site of acne vulgaris (Fig. 11).

Treatment

There is no specific treatment for the formation of new lesions. Improvement has been reported with the topical application of 0.1% tretinoin cream, corticosteroid occlusion and simple emollients. Methotrexate has also been used in some cases.

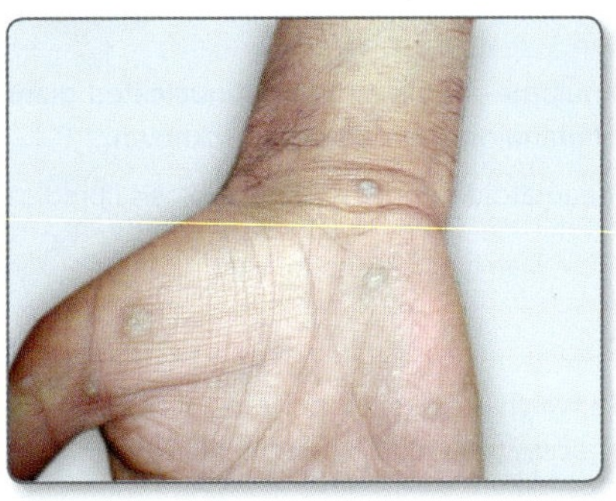

Fig. 11: Perforating collagenosis

Elastosis Perforans Serpiginosa

This is a reactive perforating dermatosis in which altered elastic fibres are extruded through the epidermis.

Histopathology

Altered elastic tissue is found in the upper papillary dermis. This is followed by a reaction of the overlying epidermis that engulfs the elastotic material. The overlying epidermis becomes acanthotic and hyperkeratotic. The papules consist of epidermal horny material in the upper one-third and altered elastic tissue in the lower two-thirds. In the dermis beneath, there is giant cell inflammatory reaction. When the elastic tissue is extruded through the epidermis, there is scarring and warty thickening of the skin.

Clinical Features

The disease usually presents in the third decade, male-female ratio is 4:1. The lesions are usually confined to one anatomic site with predilection in the following order: nape and sides of the neck, upper extremities, face, lower extremities, and trunk. Lesions start as keratotic papules, skin coloured or erythematous arranged in a circular or serpiginos distribution. Satellite lesions may occur. Koebner's phenomenon has been reported. The papules remain small or may enlarge slightly to assume a crateriform appearance with an elevated edge and a central plug. On the other hand, there is an area of atrophic skin surrounded by papules. The lesions may last from 6 months to 5 years.

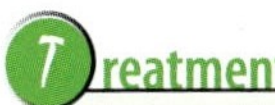

reatment

No successful form of therapy has been found. Removal of the papules by surgery has been advised, it gives reasonable cosmetic results. Oral retinoid therapy has also been used.

Kyrle's Disease

In 1916, Kyrle described this condition as hyperkeratosis follicularis et parafollicularis in cutem penetrans. The disease is due to abnormal keratinisation that forms a keratotic plug. The process of local keratinisation proceeds faster than the adjacent epithelial proliferation. This causes disruption of the epidermis, release of horny material, and a resulting foreign body reaction.

Histopathology

The lesions may be follicular or parafollicular, having an epithelial invagination filled with keratin plug that is partly parakeratotic. Neutrophils and lymphocytic infiltrate are sometimes observed.

Clinical Features

The disease occurs exclusively in adults, between the ages of 20 and 63 years. It may occur anywhere on the body except the palms, soles and mucosa. There is predilection for the lower extremities.

The primary lesion is a skin coloured or greyish papule. The papule then becomes dome shaped with a central keratotic plug. These papules may coalesce to form a plaque. The eruption is asymptomatic; it may sometimes be pruritic (Fig. 12).

reatment

Acitretin and 400 IU of vitamin E may produce improvement after a month of therapy. Flattening of the lesion has resulted from topical retinoic acid.

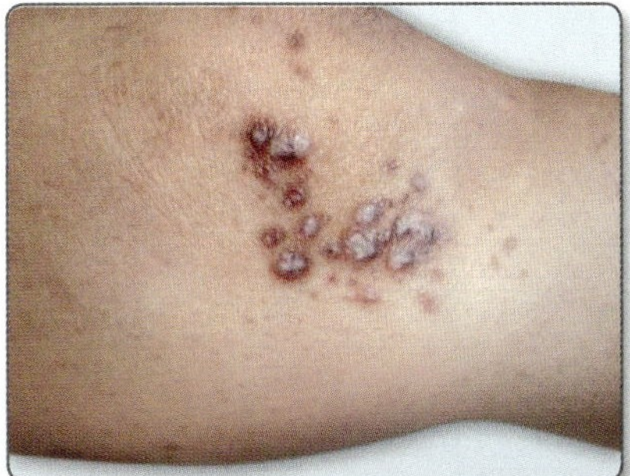

Fig. 12: Kyrle's disease

Perforating Folliculitis

This is a disorder characterised by disruption of the follicular infundibulum.

Histopathology

Widely dilated hair follicles are present within which keratinous debris and degenerated inflammatory debris are found. The follicular epithelium is perforated. Degenerated elastic fibres enter the hair follicle, just above the opening of the sebaceous glands.

Clinical Features

The average age of onset is in the 2–3 decades. Erythematous follicular papules 2–8 mm in diameter are seen on the extensor surface of the upper arm, buttocks or upper thigh. These papules are topped with whitish keratotic plugs. When these are removed, a. bleeding crater is seen.

The disorder may last from several months to several years and may show periods of remission.

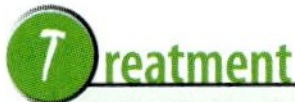reatment

Tropical tretinoin applied twice daily has resulted in complete resolution with atrophic scars.

Piezogenic Papules

Piezogenic papules are due to herniation of subcutaneous fat into the dermis. These painless papules appear on pressure and disappear on removal of force. Piezogenic papules are common, maximum age frequency is 20–30 years. Wrist and ankle joints are subject to repeated physical activity, which probably could be a contributory factor for the fragmentation of elastic fibres in the dermis.

Piezogenic papules occur on the wrist (piezogenic wrist papules) or at the heel (piezogenic pedal papules). Piezogenic pedal papules are examined by making the patient stand while applying pressure at the heel. Piezogenic wrist papules are examined by placing the heels of both palms together and applying pressure (Figs 13 and 14).

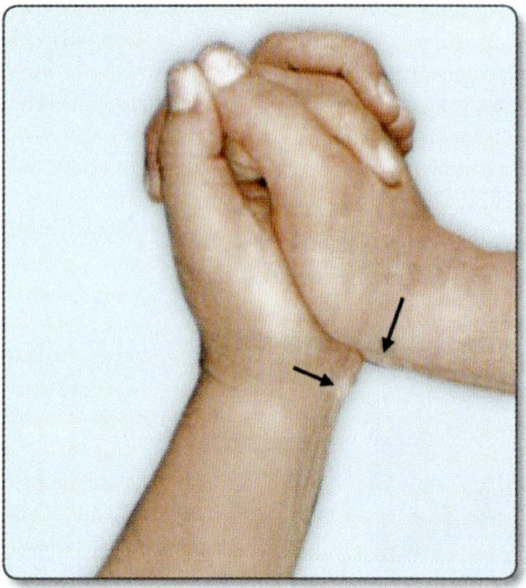

Fig. 13: Piezogenic wrist papules

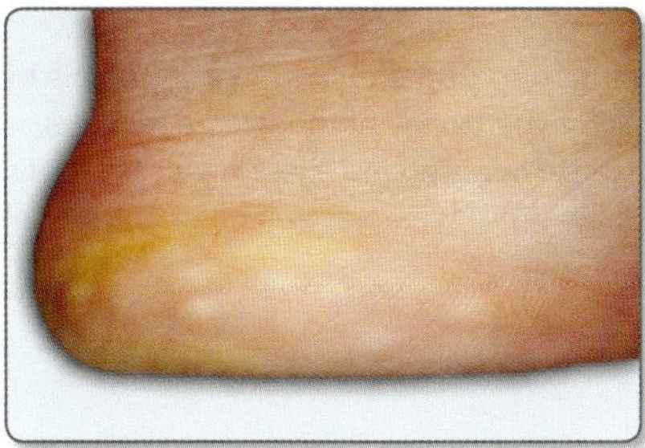

Fig. 14: Piezogenic pedal papules

Papules biopsied on application of pressure show fragmentation of dermal elastic tissue and herniation of subcutaneous fat into the lower dermis.

Painful piezogenic papules are found in only a small number of cases. The painful papules are often associated with latent or inherent defect of connective tissue such as Ehlers-Danlos syndrome.

Piezogenic papules require no treatment. The painful papules are treated by elimination of pressure, heel supports and physiotherapy, and in some cases by surgical removal.

Reiter's Disease

Reiter's disease frequently follows dysentery or non-specific urethritis in HLA B-27 individuals. It is classically defined as a triad of non-gonococcal urethritis, conjunctivitis and arthritis. Its prominent mucocutaneous lesions constitute the clinical tetrad. The skin changes are like psoriasis. The condition may also involve the oral mucosa, cardiovascular and central nervous system.

In the early 19th century, the differentiation of the clinical triad of Reiter's disease from gonococcal infection was difficult. The term keratoderma blennorrhagicum (any excessive discharge of mucus; blennorrhea) was then introduced; it was thought Reiter's disease was a complication of gonococcal infection. Reiter's disease was independently described by Reiter, Feissinger and Leroy during an epidemic of dysentery in the appalling sanitary conditions found in World War I.

Aetiology

Although genetic risk factors and infectious agents have been identified as triggering agents, the mechanism underling the inflammatory process in various tissues is unknown. Lesions of the skin and synovial fluid are sterile. Immunologically-mediated tissue injury is presumed to cause Reiter's disease.

Triggering Infections

The common urogenital infection is *Chlamydia trachomatis*, *Mycoplasma* other organisms are also documented. The most common organisms in the dysenteric cases is *Shigella*, but *Salmonella*, *Yersinia*, *Escherichia coli* and *Mycobacterium phlei* have also been implicated.

Histopathology

The lesion is characterised by infiltration of the epidermis and dermis by neutrophils. There is elongation and hypertrophy of the rete ridges. Intense hyperkeratosis and parakeratosis lead to horny excrescences in the outer layer.

Most penile and oral lesions show similar changes except for absence of hyperkeratosis.

Clinical Features

The disease occurs predominantly in young men, probably the prostate gland serving as a focus for persistent infection. When women are affected, the incomplete form of the disease is more common. The disease is uncommon in children. In children the disease is shorter lived, benign in behaviour and more remittent joint involvement.

The first manifestation is usually urethritis followed by arthritis 10–14 days later. The arthritis is characteristically bilateral; it mainly involves the knees and ankles. This is usually accompanied by conjunctivitis followed shortly by circinate balanitis.

In enteric cases, the dysentery is followed after 10–30 days by urethritis, arthritis and conjunctivitis usually developing within 10 days of each other. Moderate fever is often associated with arthritis.

Urethritis: The features are those of non-gonococcal urethritis. Mild to moderate dysuria with a transient mucopurulent urethral discharge. Prostatitis is often associated, prostate massage is not recommended as it may flare up arthritis. Examination of the morning urine is the only evidence of genital tract inflammation; mucopurulent discharge is noticed on waking. Cystitis and seminal vesiculitis is rare.

Urethritis also occurs in most enteric cases, but it is usually mild and transient.

Ocular manifestations: Non-bacterial conjunctivitis is usually bilateral, mild and evanescent. Anterior uveitis is associated with chronic prostatitis, sacroiliitis and HLA B 27 positivity. It presents as redness, pain and blurred vision. Recurrent uveitis may lead to glaucoma. Keratitis occurs less commonly, recurrent attacks of uveitis may occur.

Arthritis: Joint involvement is non-suppurative, multiple joints of the lower limb are involved, and low backache is common due to the involvement of the sacroiliac joint. Sclerotic patches of bone just above the sacroiliac joint are seen in a number of patients with Reiter's disease, this is not seen in psoriatic arthritis. Para-vertebral ossification is also reported in some cases of Reiter's disease.

Diffuse swellings (sausaging) characterize toe and finger involvement. Usually 4–5 joints are involved especially the knees, ankles, tarsal and metatarsal joints.

Soft tissue inflammation is often associated; it involves the periarticular tissue, adjacent tendon sheaths or bursae. Calcification of the plantar fascia gives rise to calcaneal spur, which is virtually diagnostic of Reiter's disease.

The first attack of arthritis lasts for 1–4 months; recurrent attacks occur in months or may be delayed for decades.

Skin and mucosal lesions: About 36% patients present with skin and mucosal lesions. It usually appears 1–2 months after the onset of arthritis and conjunctivitis. The sole of the foot is always involved; other sites being extensor surface of the legs, dorsal aspect of the toes, feet, hands, fingers, nails and scalp. Occasionally erythroderma may result.

The initial lesions are small vesicles or erythematous macules that coalesce to form irregular scaly plaques, which become hyperkeratotic. The plaques are often psoriasiform with a distinct circular scaly border. Combinations of erythema: crusting, exudation and erosion are often associated. Sometimes the lesions are frankly pustular from the outset, resembling pustular psoriasis.

The most common sites of involvement are the palms and soles, which are densely hyperkeratotic. Isolated lesions are found on the penis, scrotum, trunk, limbs and scalp.

In the uncircumcised male, small superficial ulcers form, which coalesce to give a characteristic circinate distribution known as circinate balanitis. In circumcised males, the lesions evolve to form hard crusts and plaques.

Nails and paronychial involvement is common. Subungual pustules may be seen. Onycholysis is very unusual. Nails may be thick, opaque and ridged. Pitting is absent.

Contd...

Contd...

Oral cavity: The lesions may be transient and are painless. Small vesicles appear; these rapidly rupture to form erosions. Large granular circinate erosions are occasionally seen covered with whitish epithelium resembling leukoplakia.

Other manifestations: The cardiovascular system may be involved; endocarditis, myocarditis and pericarditis are common manifestations. Aortic regurgitation and heart block are seen in 50% of patients. Amyloidosis may occur during the fulminating illness or after a protracted course.

Neurological manifestation occur in 10% of cases. These include peripheral neuritis, optic neuritis and various cranial nerve palsies. Meningoencephalitis is also reported.

The disease is usually self-limiting, resolution occurring within 12 months. Some cases relapse, and become chronic.

Investigation

There is no specific laboratory test for Reiter's disease. The following laboratory and radiological tests may be helpful.

- Overnight urethral secretion for culture may give evidence of genitourinary infection. The smear contains numerous neutrophils. In severe cases, the urethral discharge is purulent. Stool samples may be sent for culture in enteric cases.
- Synovial fluid of the affected joints shows elevation of protein and complement levels. Reiter's cells (macrophages containing ingested neutrophils) may be found. Bacterial culture of the synovial fluid is negative.
- X-ray of the affected joints, calcaneal spur is diagnostic.
- Tissue typing for HLA B-27.
- Examination of the blood: shows anaemia, leukocytosis, thrombocytosis, and elevated ESR.

Differential Diagnosis

Reiter's disease should be differentiated from gonococcal arthritis. The latter does not affect the spine; the cutaneous lesions differ from those of Reiter's disease. Psoriasis, ankylosing spondylitis and Reiter's disease have a common link via HLA B-27 haplotype. Psoriasis usually affects the joints of the hand whereas Reiter's disease mainly affects the lower limbs. Rheumatoid arthritis affects the older age group; it has a dominant upper extremity involvement, rheumatoid factor is positive, subcutaneous nodules may be present (Table 1).

The ocular lesions of Reiter's disease should be distinguished from Behcet's syndrome, which has signs of retinal vasculitis, the lesions are more painful, and the pathergic pustulonecrotic skin lesions appear at the sites of venepuncture.

Treatment

Therapy should be aimed at suppressing articular inflammation and preventing deformities. During the acute phase, bed rest and joint splinting may be necessary. Non-steroidal anti-inflammatory agents, such as indomethacin, and naproxen, are useful. Response to phenylbutazone is often dramatic, but potential haematological toxicity limits its use. Another alternative to the skin and joint involvement is the use of acitretin, especially when the skin lesions are extreme. For chronic arthritis methotrexate and anti-TNF-α agents are helpful.

When triggering infections are present, it should be treated with an appropriate antibiotic. For Chlamydial infections, tetracycline 500 mg is given four times daily for 14 days or until signs of arthritis have cleared. Alternative drugs include minocycline and erythromycin. When the triggering infection is enteric, specific antibiotic therapy is not always indicated; it is treated on its own specific merit.

For cutaneous lesions the topical treatment is on the same lines as psoriasis. In severe cases acitretin is useful.

Eye lesions should be treated with topical corticosteroids; ophthalmic cases should be referred to an ophthalmologist.

Table 1: Differential diagnosis of gonococcal and non-gonococcal urethritis (Reiter's disease)

Gonococcal urethritis	*Non-gonococcal urethritis (Reiter's disease)*
Causative organism *Neisseria gonorrhoea*	*Chlamydia*, *Mycoplasma* or *Salmonella*
Incubation period 3–5 days	7–28 days
Onset Abrupt	Gradual
Urethral discharge Spontaneous and purulent	Not spontaneous and mucopurulent
Burning sensation +++	+
Cutaneous signs Papules and vesicles with a red halo at the extensor surface of extremities	Keratosis of the palms and soles, circinate balanitis. Other skin lesions similar to psoriasis
Cardiac abnormalities Absent	May be present—aortic regurgitation, conduction defects
Eye signs Absent	Present
Arthritis Suppurative, both upper and lower extremities affected. Calcaneal spur negative	Non-suppurative arthritis, lower extremities affected. Calcaneal spur positive
Diagnosis Gram's staining is diagnostic; Gram-negative, intracellular diplococci present, diagnostic	Gram staining is not diagnostic Cervical or urethral smear for chlamydia by direct fluorescent antibody immunoassay Stool culture when bowel symptoms present, usually not conclusive
Treatment Spectinomycin or ceftriaxone	Tetracycline

Course and Prognosis

Arthritis is the most serious and disabling feature of Reiter's disease. In majority of patients, the illness lasts from 3 months to 1 year. Another one-third of patients have a relapsing course, many years separating the attacks. Chronic deforming arthritis is seen in 10–20% of cases. Significant disability results from deformities of the foot, visual loss, or cardiac disease.

Think of Reiter's syndrome when a patient presents with circinate balanitis, keratoderma blenorrhagicum, other psoriasiform lesions on the skin, nail involvement, arthritis of the lower extremities, ocular and oral lesions.

Hans Conrad Reiter (1881–1969)

Reiter described the clinical associations of urethritis, conjunctivitis and arthritis, while in the German army during the First World War. Earlier he had identified the organism of Weil's disease. After the war, he worked with Wassermann and developed a technique for culturing Treponema pallidum. In 1932, Hans Reiter signed the oath allegiance to Hitler and became involved in the infamous studies of eugenics. He was briefly interned in an American prison camp in 1945.

PRURIGO

Prurigo is a term widely used, but it is not well defined. The disease is characterised by a papule, which is dome shaped and topped by a small vesicle. The vesicle soon ruptures due to scratching, as the lesion is very pruritic. Lichenification is often secondary. The term prurigo was originally introduced by Hebra to denote papules induced by scratching.

Aetiology

Prurigo may be caused by sunlight (Hutchinson's summer prurigo), insect bites (papular prurigo), cold (winter prurigo), atopic dermatitis (Besnier's prurigo), pregnancy (prurigo of pregnancy). In many cases, the cause is unknown; it may be due to stress; the disease is often seen in middle-aged women with psychological problems. Whether the lesions are caused by scratching, is highly debatable.

Clinical Features

The initial lesion is the typical prurigo papule topped by a small vesicle. The latter is hardly visible due to scratching. A crusted papule is often visible. The lesion can be acute, subacute or chronic.

Acute Prurigo: This is usually seen after insect bites in both children and adults. It is probably an allergic reaction in sensitised subjects.

Subacute Prurigo (Neurotic Excoriation): This condition often affects middle-aged women. The pathogenesis is unknown; stress appears to be a frequent finding in these women. The typical papule is seldom seen due to excoriation. The lesion usually involves the nape of the neck, scalp and lower extremities; trunk may also be involved. Palms and soles are always spared as the pathology occurs in follicular walls.

Chronic Prurigo: The condition is seen in middle-aged people, more common in women. It may be due to a number of disorders such as ovarian dysfunction, digestive disturbances, focal infection, stress, malignancy such as Hodgkin's disease and polycythaemia.

The lesion usually occurs on the extensor aspect of the limbs, upper trunk, and buttocks. The course is chronic may persist for months or years.

Variants of Prurigo

Nodular Prurigo

This is common in middle-aged women. The lesions consist of intensely itchy nodules on the extensor surface of the legs and forearms.

Clinical Features

The nodules are hard, globular, 1–3 cm in diameter with a warty surface. The early lesions are red which may show an urticarial component. The older lesions are pigmented. Crusting and scaling are present over the recently excoriated lesions.

Pruritus is intense, occurring at intervals and lasting from a few minutes to an hour or two. New nodules develop from time to time. Existing nodules remain for a long time these eventually regress to leave scars (Fig. 15).

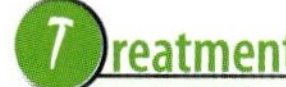

Treatment

Intralesional injection of triamcinolone is helpful. Thalidomide, PUVA and benoxaprofen have also given favorable results.

Thalidomide is given in a dose of 100 mg twice a day; relief is obtained in 2–3 weeks. The treatment should be continued for 3 months. Chronic neuropathy can occur after prolonged use. The drug is contraindicated in pregnancy due to teratogenicity. Cryotherapy is also recommended.

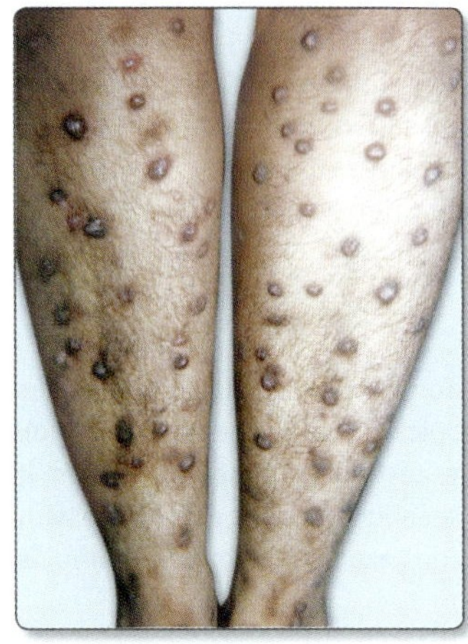

Fig. 15: Nodular Prurigo

Histologically, the lesion resembles lichen simplex chronicus. The hyperkeratosis may be greater, and downward projection of the rete pegs is marked. The dermal infiltrate is dense. Schwann cells are prominent. The neural changes are secondary to the trauma of repeated scratching.

Melanotic Prurigo of Pierini and Borda

This is seen in middle-aged women; it is associated with biliary cirrhosis. The lesions consist of reticulate hyperpigmentation appearing mostly on the trunk. The itching is unbearable.

Prurigo Agria

Prurigo agria is a severe form of chronic dermatitis with secondary infection. The condition is characterised by constantly recurring itchy papules and nodules. It is often associated with atopy.

Prurigo Mitis

The disorder begins in early childhood. The condition is chronic leading to scars, lichenification and eczematisation. The lymph nodes may enlarge; constitutional symptoms are often present. The typical prurigo papule is small, often it is easier to palpate than to see it. The lesions are multiple and symmetrically distributed.

Papular prurigo is discussed in chapter 7.

ATROPHY OF THE SKIN

The term atrophy refers to the diminution in the size of the cell, tissue, organ, or part of the body. Epidermal atrophy is thinning in the number of epidermal cells; the epidermis appears almost transparent, thin and exhibits a fine wrinkling. Skin markings may or may not be retained. Dermal atrophy results from a decrease in papillary or reticular connective tissue; it is usually manifested by depression of the skin. There is often associated loss of hair follicles; telangiectases may be present due to loss of supporting connective tissue. Often epidermal and dermal atrophy may occur in association. If atrophy includes the subcutaneous tissue and the deeper structures, it is then referred to as panatrophy. Cutaneous atrophy may be generalised as in ageing and cutis laxa, or it may be localised. It may be secondary to disease, such as lupus erythematosus, tuberculosis, syphilis, urticaria pigmentosa, leprosy, sarcoidosis, and drugs like penicillamine. It is also seen in normal physiological process such as striae gravidarum; it may be due to drugs such as steroids. It may also be primary without any predisposing factor.

ANETODERMA

This is the localised laxity of the skin with herniation resulting from abnormal elastic tissue. Primary anetoderma maybe of the following types:

- Anetoderma of Jadassohn
- Anetoderma of Schweninger-Buzzi

Anetoderma of Jadassohn

This form of atrophy begins with a preceding inflammation, it begins as an erythematous macular rash, which fades at the centre, and the epidermis becomes wrinkled. In course of time, the lesions become depressed. An examining finger can pass through the depression, which has definite margins. The lesions are commonly seen on the face and the trunk. The aetiology is unknown. No treatment is effective. On histology, there is fragmentation of elastic tissue, which ultimately disappears.

Anetoderma of Schweninger-Buzzi

There is no preceding inflammation in this type of anetoderma. This disease manifests as bluish white or slate coloured bladder-like lesions on which fine telangiectasia are often seen. The tip of the finger can be made to pass through these lesions as in anetoderma of Jadassohn. The trunk is the most common site to be affected. The lesion heals with the formation of soft depressed scars. No treatment is effective (Fig. 16).

Progressive Idiopathic Atrophoderma of Pasini and Pierini

The condition appears to be an atrophic form of morphoea. The lesions are large with sharply defined borders, dropping into a depression without outpouching.

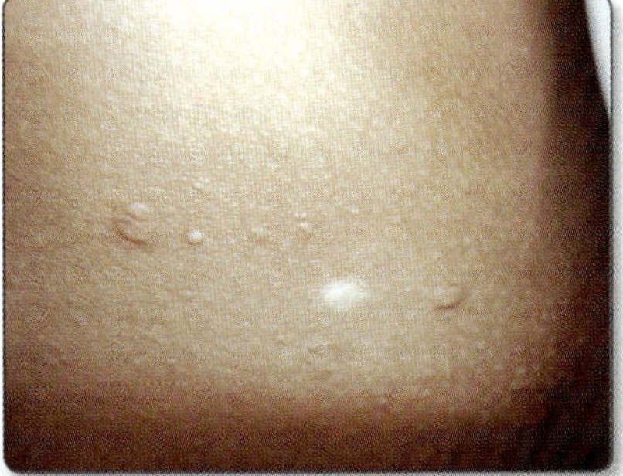

Fig. 16: Anetoderma of Schweninger-Buzzi

The lesions are smooth, slate coloured or violet brown. The trunk especially the back is the most common site affected. On biopsy, elastic tissue is normal, while the collagen tissue is increased. Psoralens have helped a few cases.

Acrodermatitis Chronica Atrophicans

The disease is caused by a *Spirochaete, Borrelia burgdorferi*; it is transmitted to man by the bite of a tick. It is the same organism responsible for Lyme disease. It is said that erythema chronicum migrans represents the early stage of the disease; the late stage is manifested by ACA.

Acrodermatitis chronica atrophicans usually begins as a diffuse or localised erythema on the distal extremities; the underlying dermis is swollen and doughy in consistency. The inflammation spreads favouring the extensor surfaces especially the periarticular areas. After weeks or months, the inflammatory phase is replaced by atrophy, the skin becoming thin and the underlying vessels can easily be seen. The skin can be thrown into fine folds. There is associated loss of sweat glands, sebaceous glands and hair follicles. Hypopigmentation or hyperpigmentation can be seen in the affected areas.

Fibrosis may also occur; this may be seen as ulnar or tibial bands over the respected bones. Localised fibrosis may also occur near the joints. Cutaneous and subcutaneous calcifications, basal and squamous cell carcinoma may develop. Hyperaesthesias, paraesthesias, pain or muscle cramps occur, these are limited to the areas of skin involvement. The underlying bones and muscles may be damaged.

Histologically, there is epidermal and dermal atrophy. The elastic tissue is absent and cutaneous appendages are atrophic.

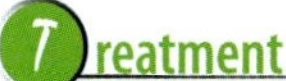

In early stages of the disease, oral antibiotics should be given for a month. Penicillin, tetracyclines and erythromycin are the antibiotics of choice. The improvement occurs gradually. There is no treatment if atrophy has occurred.

Panatrophy

This may be primary or it may be the result of other diseases. In most cases, it is a variant of morphoea; the atrophic areas exhibit a reduced sympathetic response and production of nonesterified fatty acids after stimulation with adrenaline.

Panatrophy of Gowers

This is atrophy without preceding inflammation. In the affected areas, the subcutaneous tissue disappears and the overlying skin appears atrophic. Most cases are seen on the back, buttocks, thigh or upper arm. The atrophy reaches its maximum extent within a few months and then remains stationary.

Sclerotic Panatrophy

This is usually seen after morphoea, but may occur without it. Scar like linear bands may develop along a limb, or encircle the trunk or limbs. The lesions cease to progress after a few months.

CUTIS VERTICIS GYRATA

This is a morphological condition characterised by the presence of folds and furrows in the skin of the scalp, giving a corrugated appearance to the skin. It is due to the overgrowth of the skin in relation to the underlying skull. The folds may number from 2–20; the hair over the folds is of normal growth and black in colour. About one-fourth of the patients exhibit mental retardation and epilepsy. Defects of the cranium and eye may coexist.

Aetiology

The condition may be primary or secondary. Primary cutis verticis gyrata is of autosomal recessive inheritance often lethal to the females. It begins at puberty often associated with epilepsy and cerebral palsy. The intelligence quotient (IQ) is rarely over 35.

Histopathology

The condition is associated with hypertrophy of the epidermis, dermis and neurofibromatous hyperplasia. The nevoid forms are usually melanocytic naevi.

Clinical Features

Primary cutis verticis gyrata begins at puberty; it is usually symmetrical, most prominent at the occipital region. The condition progresses for 5–10 years and then remains stationary. Secondary cutis verticis gyrata is usually localised and asymmetrical depending upon the site of the original pathology (Fig. 17).

Secondary cutis verticis gyrata is associated with developmental abnormalities, localised inflammations, trauma, tumours, naevi and of pachydermoperiostosis. It may also be associated with syphilis, leukemias, acromegaly and mental retardation.

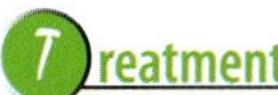

reatment

The treatment is surgical. The condition may not progress after the treatment of the systemic disorder responsible for secondary cutis verticis gyrata.

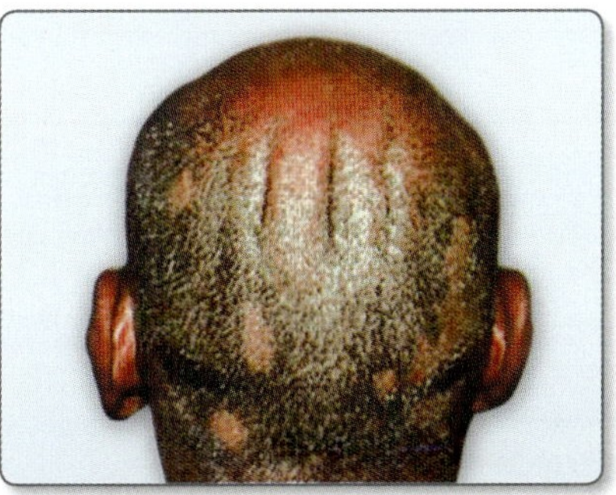

Fig. 17: Cutis verticis gyrata

PACHYDERMOPERIOSTOSIS

The condition is characterised by hypertrophic changes involving predominantly the skin and bones of the extremities. It can be primary or secondary.

Aetiology

Primary Pachydermoperiostosis (Touraine-Solente-Gole Syndrome)

This is an autosomal dominant disorder, it occurs predominantly in men.

Secondary Pachydermoperiostosis

It may be associated with severe pulmonary disease such as adenocarcinoma of the bronchus, bronchiectasis, and carcinoma of the stomach, oesophagus, or thymus. It is also associated with congenital heart disease.

Histopathology

Diaphysis of the tibia, fibula, radius, ulna, and bones of the hand and feet are mainly affected. There is irregular periosteal ossification; this leads to an increase in the circumference of the affected bones, without increasing their length.

The skin shows hypertrophy of the collagen, epidermis and epidermal appendages. There is an increase of acid mucopolysaccharides.

Clinical Features

Primary pachydermoperiostosis begins soon after puberty. It progresses for 5–10 years and then remains unchanged. Skin of the face and scalp is grossly thickened and thrown into folds. The folding of the scalp produces cutis verticis gyrata. The skin of the hands and feet is thickened, but not folded. Sebaceous gland activity is increased on the face and scalp. Hyperhidrosis of the hands and feet may occur. Face and pubic hair are sparse.

Bony changes: The bones of the distal extremities, hands and feet are thickened, producing cylindrical arms and legs. The fingers and toes are clubbed.

Other systemic manifestations: Peptic ulcer and gynaecomastia are present in some patients. Some of the patients may be mentally retarded, working capacity is low.

Secondary Pachydermoperiostosis

This occurs at a later age (30–70 years) predominantly in men. The bony changes are more obvious, often painful. The skin changes are mild. On treating the primary disorder, both skin and bone changes regress.

Differential Diagnosis

The disease should be differentiated from acromegaly, thyroid acropachy. In acromegaly the facial skeleton, jaw and skull are enlarged, visual defects are often found. In thyroid acropachy, there are signs of hyperthyroidism, exophthalmos, and pretibial myxedema.

Treatment

Treat the underlying disease in secondary pachydermoperiostosis.

AINHUM

The word ainhum is derived from the Nagus language of East Africa, meaning "to saw". Ainhum is a painful constricting band around the fifth toe that results in its spontaneous amputation. It is due to abnormal blood supply to the foot. The condition is common in African Negroes who walk barefoot. Trauma precipitates in the development of a groove in the ischaemic toe. This gradually deepens and extends laterally around the toe, until the two ends meet.

Histopathology

Fissuring and hyperkeratosis is followed by fibrosis. The digit distal to the constriction degenerates, leading to its spontaneous amputation.

Clinical Features

The disease often manifests between the ages of 30–50 years. It begins as a painful fissure; this deepens and extends laterally, and the constriction band gradually encircles the toe. The distal end of the toe becomes globular; it is attached to the digit by a thin band of fibrous tissue; this gradually breaks down and the toe is shed. It can be compared to a piece of plastic damaged by repeated flexing.

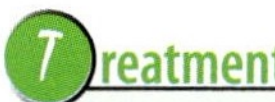

Treatment

Avoid trauma and infection to the foot. If symptoms occur, amputation is indicated. Surgical correction by Z-plasty can produce good results.

PSEUDOAINHUM

Pseudoainhum is more common than ainhum outside Africa. This may be congenital or acquired. Congenital pseudoainhum may be due to amniotic bands or adhesions in utero. It consists of collagen tissue, which penetrates deeply into the subcutis.

Hereditary conditions capable of causing pseudoainhum are hereditary palmoplantar keratoderma, pachyonychia congenita and congenital ectodermal defects.

Acquired pseudoainhum may be associated with infections such as leprosy, injury, systemic sclerosis, neuropathy, syringomyelia, ergot poisoning, palmoplantar keratoderma, fungal infections, psoriasis, yaws, and tumors of the spinal cord. Pseudoainhum can also occur by constriction due to outside forces such as hair or strong thread (factitious).

Pseudoainhum can involve any digit of the feet or hands. Hyperkeratosis is often associated with pseudoainhum. The constricting band in pseudoainhum is more superficial than ainhum. On histopathological examination, the underlying pathology is recognised.

Treatment is similar to ainhum. The underlying associated diseases should be treated aggressively.

RELAPSING POLYCHONDRITIS

The condition can affect any cartilage; it is probably caused by autoimmunity to type 2 collagen. Type 2 collagen is restricted to the cartilage and constitutes to more than 50% of the cartilage protein. Relapsing polychondritis (RP) affects cartilage that lies outside diarthrodial joints; it usually affects the nose, outer ears and trachea.

The ears are the usual target. The overlying skin becomes red, tender and swollen. The disease spares the noncartilaginous portion of the pinna of the ear. The acute inflammation subsides in 1–2 weeks. It is characterised by recurrences which appear after variable periods: from weeks to months. Recurrences lead to auricular chondritis in about 90% patients.

In 25% of cases, the other cartilages may be affected, such as the nose and tracheobronchial tree. Recurrences lead to saddle nose, hoarseness, and respiratory insufficiency.

Less frequently the eyes, cardiovascular system and the inner ear may be affected.

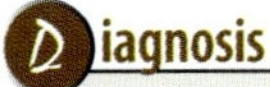

Diagnosis

The clinical picture is characteristic. The only laboratory findings are raised ESR, white blood count is elevated in 50% of patients. Indirect immunofluorescence shows antibodies to type 2 collagen.

Treatment

Mild ear disease responds to low dose steroids or nonsteroidal anti-inflammatory drugs (NSAIDs). Major organ involvement requires high dose steroids in combination with cytotoxic drugs. Dapsone is also helpful. Tracheostomy may be required in some cases.

CUTANEOUS MANIFESTATIONS OF DRUG ABUSE

Drugs are generally taken for medical purposes, but when these are taken to alter the physical and mental functions in a person, it is termed as drug abuse. Any drug abuse can lead to addiction. When such a drug is stopped, withdrawal symptoms are experienced. Most of these drugs are used to produce a state of euphoria and initial wellbeing, without realising the serious effects that it can lead to at the cost of health, family life and economic setbacks. The common age of drug addiction is 15–22 years; peer pressure and a broken family are the common cause of drug abuse.

Drug addiction is an international problem; it affects not only the health of an individual but also the economy of a country. The incidence of drug abuse is increasing; the populations most at risk are the medical and psychiatric patients. All parts of the body are affected by drug abuse, skin being no exception.

The common drugs of abuse are:

- Narcotic analgesics such as heroin
- Stimulants such as amphetamine (ecstasy) and cocaine
- Depressants such as barbiturates, benzodiazepine, and alcohol
- Hallucinogens such as lysergic acid diethylamide (LSD)
- Cannabis such as marijuana, hashish and bhang
- Volatile solvents such as volatile hydrocarbons and petroleum derivatives
- Other drugs such as muscle relaxants, pain killers, antidepressants, antipsychotics, etc.

(Consult a pharmacology book for drug detail).

Clinical Manifestations of Drug Abuse

The clinical manifestation can be cutaneous or systemic. The cutaneous signs range from mild such as skin discolouration to severe such as amputation due to gangrene. The clinical manifestations are due to the pharmacological action of the drug; the withdrawal symptoms by its route of administration.

Cutaneous Manifestations of Drug Abuse

Route of Administration

- Cutaneous signs produced by the administration of drugs by the intravenous route:
  In the West, intravenous route is the most common method of heroin intake; in the Indian subcontinent, it is inhaled. The cutaneous signs due to intravenous administration are:
  - Scarring (needle track scars) and hyperpigmentation at the injection site (Fig. 18)
  - Abscess and necrotic ulceration
  - Fibrosis of the vein
  - Non-pitting oedema of the hands due thrombophlebitis following intravenous injection
  - Keloid formation
  - Tattooing from soot particles on inflamed needles
  - Accidental intra-arterial injection with associated gangrene
  - Necrotising angiitis resembling polyarteritis nodosa
- Cutaneous signs due to subcutaneous route of administration:
  When veins are not accessible, then the subcutaneous route is used to administer drugs; this is known as skin popping. The cutaneous signs are:
  - Skin ulcers
  - Oedema of the hands (Fig. 19)
  - Scars
- Cutaneous signs due to smoking:
  Smoking is the most common method by which charas is used. The cutaneous signs are brown staining of the teeth and nails
- Cutaneous signs due to inhalation of the drug:
  In developing countries such as Pakistan heroin is inhaled. Heroin is put on a foil and heated from below. The fumes that come out are inhaled. About 4–5 persons sit in a group, cover themselves with a large piece of cloth and

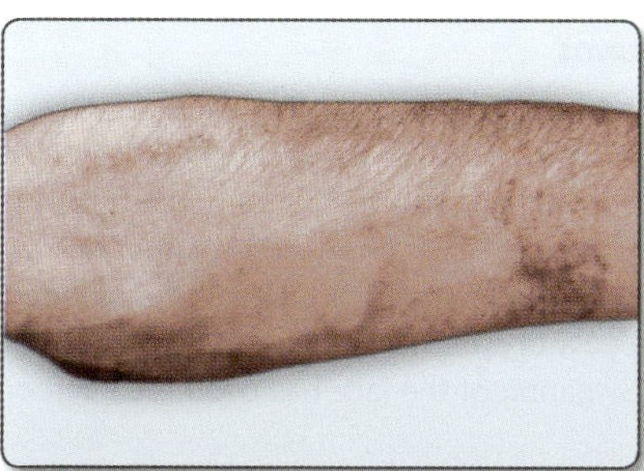

Fig. 18: Needle tracks

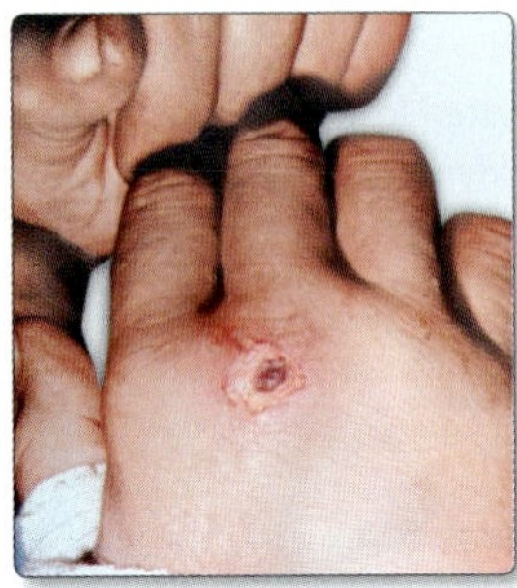

Fig. 19: Subcutaneous route of drug intake—"Skin Popping"

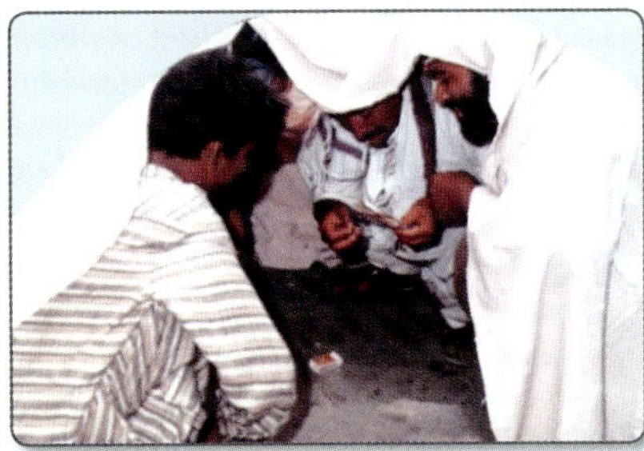

Fig. 20: Inhalation of drugs—"Chasing the Dragon"

inhale the smoke. This method is called "Chasing the Dragon". Cutaneous signs are:

- Pigmentation of the face. The cause of pigmentation is unclear; it may be due to the smoke, sunlight, or due to a cutting agent in the heroin (Fig. 20).

Other Cutaneous Manifestations

These are urticaria, amyloidosis, thermal burns, bizarre macules, bullae, irritant reactions, ulcerations due to cutting agents added to the drug. The cutting agents are also responsible for bacterial and fungal infections and fixed drug reactions. These reactions differ due to different agents added to the main drug. The common cutting agents are quinine, mannite, lactose, and lime juice. Quinine is used for a rush and subjective feeling of acceleration and euphoria. With increase of drug abuse, a number of unusual lesions can be expected due to different cutting agents used. If there is a shortage of one cutting agent, a substitute will be found with unusual reactions.

Cutaneous Signs Due to Pharmacological Action of Drugs and Withdrawal Symptoms

Generalised pruritus is common after the use of heroin; it is due to the release of opioid, and it is relieved by naloxone. Unexplained itching should alert the physician to rule out drug abuse. Pruritus is also seen around the nose and mouth in heroin inhalers.

Piloerection is seen on withdrawal of heroin. Opioids alter the equilibrium point of the hypothalamus heat regulatory mechanism. The body temperature falls giving rise to piloerection. Sweating of the face has been recorded on withdrawal of diazepam.

Systemic Signs of Drug Abuse

These differ according to the different drugs used. The general medical complications include pulmonary infarction, septicaemia, bacterial endocarditis, tetanus, malaria, hepatitis, AIDS and acute fatal reactions. Malnutrition is very common in undeveloped countries, most of the drug abusers have anaemia and other nutritional deficiencies, they are emaciated with reduced muscle mass.

Drug Abuse—Effects on the Family, Society and Nation

Drug abuse not only ruins the health of the individual but also brings the family to shambles in the long run. Often the family of the drug addict become mentally perturbed. Suicide is common in drug addicts. Drug abuse also plays a role in many major social problems such as drugged driving, violence, stress and child abuse.

Motivation and patience are the keys that can help the addict come out of the problem. The cost of treatment is high; it is an economic burden not only on the family but also on the country. Treating a drug addict is the responsibility of the family, society and the health care of the country.

Unexplained itching should alert the physician to rule out drug abuse by heroin in young individuals.

FURTHER READING

1. Aberer E, Breie F, Stanak G, et al. Success and failure in the treatment of acrodermatitis chronica atrophicans. Infection. 1996;24:85-7.
2. Arora K, Hajirmis KA, Sawant S, et al. Perforating disorders of the skin. Ind J Pathol and Microbiol. 2013;56(4):355-8.
3. Beuchnem SA, Rulfi T. Atrophoderma of Pasini and Pierini. J Am Acad Dermatol. 1994;30(3):441-6.
4. Bucsky P, Egeler RM. Malignant Histiocytic disorders in children. Clinical and therapeutic approaches with nostalgic discussion. Hematol Oncol Clin North Am. 1998;12(2):465-71.
5. Callan JP. Pyoderma gangrenosum and related disorders. Dermatol Clin. 1990;7:1249-59.
6. Fisher EA, Desnick RJ, Gordon RE, et al. Fabry disease: an unusual cause of severe coronary disease in a young man. Ann Intern Med. 1992;117(3):221-3.
7. Hodak E, Shamai-Lubovitz O, David M, et al. Primary anetoderma associated with a wide spectrum of autoimmune abnormalities. J Am Acad Dermatol. 1991;25:415-8.
8. Howarth DM, Gilchrist GS, Mullan BP, et al. Langerhans cell histiocytosis. Cancer. 1999;85(10):2278-90.
9. Kuramoto Y, Lizzawa O, Aiba S, et al. Multicentric histiocytosis in a child with sclerosing lesion of the leg. Immunohistopathologic studies and therapeutic trial with systemic cyclosporine. J Am Acad Dermatol. 1989;20:329-35.
10. Langan SM, Groves RW, Card TR, Guiliford MC. Incidence, Mortality and Disease association of Pyoderma gangrenosum in the Unirted Kingdom. J of Inves Dermatol. 2012;132: 2166-70.
11. Lebovits PE, Kouskoukis CE, Weidman AI. Piezogenic pedal papules. Cutis. 1982;29(3):276-7.
12. Meunier L, March Y, Rieyne C, et al. Adult cutaneous Langerhan cell histiocytosis: remission with thalidomide treatment. Br J Dermatol. 1995;132:168.
13. Powell FC, Su WP. Pyoderma gangrenosum: classification and management. J Am Acad Dermatol. 1996;34:(3):395-409.
14. Rapini RP, Herbert AA, Drucker CR, et al. Acquired perforating dermatosis. Evidence for combined transepidermal elimination of both collagen and elastic fibers. Arch Dermatol. 1989;125(8):1074-8.
15. Weary PE, Manley WF, Graham GF. Hereditary acrokeratotic poikiloderma. Arch Dermatol. 1971;103(4):409-22.

Chapter

39 Occupational Dermatoses

INTRODUCTION

Occupational dermatoses are those cutaneous disorders that occur due to work environment, and these disorders will not occur if the individual was not in place of work. Occupational cutaneous disorders are common, and rank second to musculoskeletal injuries which are the most common injuries related to occupation.

The common occupational skin dermatoses are:

- Hand dermatitis
- Contact urticaria
- Infections: bacterial, viral and fungal
- Acne
- Malignancy
- Heat injuries
- Cold injuries
- Vibrating syndrome
- Connective tissue disorders.

OCCUPATIONAL HAND DERMATITIS

From the occupational point of view the hands are the most exposed to chemicals and consequently injuries on the hands are the most common. The vast bulk of hand dermatitis is irritant contact dermatitis (ICD). Common irritants are soaps, detergents, cutting oils and other petroleum products. These injuries are most frequent in nurses and health care workers, beauticians, cooks, gardeners, construction workers and mechanics.

Allergic contact dermatitis (ACD) accounts for about 20% of all cases of hand dermatitis. Common allergens are rubber, fragrance, epoxy resins, chromates, nickel, cobalt, biocides (preservatives) and dyes. These can arise independently or on a background of ICD.

Irritant contact dermatitis can predispose an individual to ACD by epidermal penetration of allergens. Similarly, ACD can also enhance the effect of irritants on the skin. It is often difficult to differentiate between irritant and ACD. Diagnosis is further complicated as often endogenous factors, e.g. atopic eczema, and environmental factors may coexist. Contact urticaria can also gradually progress to hand eczema. The accuracy of diagnosis depends upon the experience, knowledge and skill of the physician. Detailed patch testing and provocation tests may be necessary.

Although contact dermatitis (CD) does not commonly lead to hospital attendance, minor degree of CD is often accepted as a normal hazard to life. The domestic, social and psychological impact on the patient may be considerable. The total economic impact of occupational CD is high. The diagnosis of occupational dermatitis should be accurate, both from the patients perspective and disability payments from the work place.

A detailed history should be taken, such as does the dermatitis improve on vacation, do other workers also suffer from the same dermatosis, is the site of eruption consistent with the exposure, etc. Patch tests help to differentiate ICD from ACD. Always exclude other dermatoses such as psoriasis, lichen planus and tinea manuum. Atopic dermatitis can predispose the individual to CD. A visit to the factory or place of work can help to find out the exact nature of the irritant or allergen.

The treatment is standard including emollients, topical corticosteroids and in severe cases systemic steroids or other immunosuppressive therapy. Protection of hands by gloves and barrier creams as appropriate. In all cases, the patient should be excused from work till recovery.

Assume all cases of hand dermatitis primarily as occupational. Take a detailed history. This allows early intervention and use of protective measures, before serious damage occurs.

CONTACT URTICARIA

This can be immune-mediated contact urticaria (ICU), or non-immune mediated contact urticaria (NICU). The NICU is localised and it is not associated with systemic signs such as, wheezing, rhinorrhoea and syncope. NICU is seen in gardeners due to insects, nettle plants; in cooks due to fish, mustard, preservatives; and in health workers due to local anaesthetics, and tincture of benzoin. ICU is immunoglobulin E (IgE) mediated. People with a history of atopic dermatitis are susceptible. The common substances giving rise to ICU are natural rubber latex, which consists of about 240 different proteins. People with spina bifida have a high incidence of ICU due to natural rubber latex. Other causes of ICU are meat, fish, fragrance, epoxy resins, wood, animal dander, preservatives and disinfectants. ICU is seen in cooks, grocery workers, carpenters, veterinarians and those working with epoxy resins.

INFECTIONS

A number of occupational dermatoses are due to infections. These may be bacterial, fungal or viral.

Bacterial Infections

Any occupation that subjects an individual to minor trauma (like butchers, carpenters, construction workers, etc.) can increase the possibility of resident flora of skin surface, such as *Staphylococcus aureus,* to enter the skin and cause infections like folliculitis, boils, cellulitis, etc. Atopic individuals are more susceptible.

In other cases, bacterial infections from animals can infect people who are in contact with them. Anthrax caused by *Bacillus anthracis* found in horses, sheep, goats and some wild herbivores, people get infected with anthrax who handle these animals such as agricultural workers and meat handlers. The bacteria can cause local skin infection and pulmonary lesions when the spores of anthrax are inhaled. The infection can also be transmitted by animal hides and bones; carpet makers, upholsterers and tanners are subject to infection by them. Erysipeloid is another infection present in many animals such as pigs, poultry and fish; it can affect occupations such as butchers.

Fungal Infections

A range of fungal infections can infect people in different occupations. Superficial fungal infections, such as zoophilic dermatophytosis, can infect butchers, zoo keepers, agricultural workers, farmers and veterinarians.

Candidiasis infects those who are in contact with water for long periods. Chronic paronychia is common in cooks, beauticians, health workers, dish washers and laundry workers. Sporotrichosis is caused by puncture wounds such as thorns or splinters. Sporotrichosis is seen in forest workers, farmers and outdoor workers. Mycetoma is common in farmers who walk barefoot; it is common in underdeveloped countries. A number of deep fungal infections caused by inhalation of the fungal spores can infect the skin by dissemination, e.g. coccidioidomycosis and histoplasmosis.

Viral Infections

Herpes simplex is the most common viral infection transmitted to health care professionals through patients, when localised to the fingers, it is called herpetic whitlow. The same infection when transmitted to wrestlers or rugby players from fellow players is called herpes gladiatorum.

Warts are common in butchers, meat and fish handlers; human papillomavirus 7 has been isolated from these patients.

Orf (ecthyma contagiosum) caused by a pox virus found in sheep and goat; farmers, shepherds and veterinarians are infected.

Milker's nodule, caused by paravaccinia virus, infects the udder of cows. The infection can be transmitted to farmers and veterinarians. Both orf and milker's nodule are self-limiting infections and disappear in 4–6 weeks.

ACNE

Acne is a common disorder of adolescence; it is found in areas rich in sebaceous glands, but when found in other areas, think of acne due to occupational dermatoses. Acne like eruptions can occur in occupations exposed to oil, coal tar and halogenated hydrocarbons. Pitch, tar and cutting oils cause comedonal and pustular acne. Cutting oils cause acne on the thighs or abdomen, areas exposed to the oil. Acne due to coal tar and pitch occurs on the exposed areas, especially the malar areas, white comedones predominate.

Acne due to halogenated hydrocarbons occurs irrespective of the mode of exposure, whether by inhalation, ingestion or direct contact. Chloracne is a sensitive indicator of environmental or occupational exposure to toxic halogenated aromatic hydrocarbons. Exposure may be via military service as seen in soldiers in Vietnam, when exposed to Agent Orange pesticide. Clinically in chloracne the lesions are closed comedones and cysts over the malar areas and retroauricular folds, sparing the nose. Temporal comedones are diagnostic of chloracne. As toxicity increases, the lesions become more widespread. Systemic disease is reported with chloracne such as liver disease, hyperlipidemias and peripheral neuropathies.

MALIGNANCY

A number of occupations can increase the risk of skin cancer. These include occupations with increased exposure to ultraviolet radiation, such as gardeners, farmers, pilots, military personnel, athletes, and X-ray technicians. Exposure to hydrocarbons also increases the risk to cutaneous malignancy as seen in construction workers, iron and steel foundries, tar distillation, and wood impregnation industries. The first known report of occupational skin cancer was of chimney sweeps reported by Percivall Pott in 1775. Skin cancer due to arsenic is common in Bangladesh where arsenic is found in ground water. It is also found in some areas of Taiwan and Argentina where arsenic is found in mining industries. Although the use of arsenic has decreased, it is still associated with glass production and manufacture of semiconductors.

HEAT

Exposure to heat can cause thermal and electrical burns. People exposed to thermal burns are kitchen workers, people working in fast food restaurants, those in contact with liquid metal and tar. Burn injuries have to be carefully evaluated for impairment and disability. Electrical burns result in extensive tissue destruction and fatal cardiac arrhythmias. Burns due to lightning result in characteristic bizarre feather like patterns on the skin.

COLD

Chilblains, frostbite, trench foot and, cold urticaria are seen in occupations exposed to cold such as military personnel, fire fighters, refrigeration workers and people engaged in winter sports.

VIBRATION SYNDROME

Also known as "white fingers" or "dead fingers", occurs due to the vibrating impact of tools such as jackhammers, chain saws and hand grinders. The impact of these tools leads to vasospasm of the vessels of fingers. Symptoms appear after a few months or a few years. These include a feeling of numbness or tingling sensation followed by blanching and stiffening of fingers. Finally weakening of the grip occurs, the condition becomes disabling, leading to job loss. Smoking is an associated risk factor. Improvement in vibrating tools has reduced the incidence of vibration syndrome. The condition is asymmetrical which helps it in differentiating from Raynaud's phenomenon.

CONNECTIVE TISSUE DISORDERS

Raynaud's phenomenon and scleroderma like skin disease is associated with people working with vinyl chloride. The condition is often called "occupational osteolysis". Scleroderma like condition is also seen in photograph developers, people exposed to silica and underground miners. Vibration tools during mining also contribute to the disease.

IMPORTANCE OF OCCUPATIONAL SKIN DISEASES

The diagnosis of occupational dermatoses should be meticulous and precise. The dermatoses can affect the patient economically, psychologically and socially. The heavy burden which the industry has to bear due to disability act is high. The legal issues can be long and drawn out. The cost of occupational dermatitis includes medical care, compensation and disability payment. The loss of income due to lost workdays, and loss of productivity, and the cost of occupational re-training are very high. In a study, it was found that in America the cost of occupational disease ranges from 2.22 million dollars to 1 billion dollars.

DIAGNOSIS OF OCCUPATIONAL SKIN DISEASE

A detailed history, thorough physical examination and comprehensive skin testing is essential in all cases of occupational dermatoses. Diagnosis of occupational dermatoses is a dilemma to the physician, endogenous factors, such as atopic dermatitis, and environmental factors may complicate the diagnosis. Another problem is the accuracy of recall on part of the patient, exposure may have changed over time, past exposure may be over or understated and preventive measures may have been taken after the symptoms occurred. Skin contact with the irritant or allergen is a necessary condition for the diagnosis of occupational dermatitis. The severity of the reaction depends upon the type and intensity of exposure, condition of the epidermal barrier, any endogenous factors associated such as atopic dermatitis, psychological factors, age, gender, etc.

The diagnosis can be further complicated by self-inflicted injury for economic gains. In most cases, the simulators are fully conscious of what they are doing and why, in contrast to those who have a psychiatric problem. There are certain diagnostic criteria to be considered such as the site; it is usually the most easily accessible. The morphology of the lesion; this is often bizarre and irregular. Certain investigations may be required such as histopathological examination, or finding of the extraneous material on the surface of the suspected lesion. It is always best to request a neuropsychiatric consultation.

A complete history and physical examination is required to determine that the lesions are due to place of work. Do the lesions improve on vacations and recur or become worse on return to work? Do the lesions correspond to the working environment? Do other people in the work place have a similar problem are some of the points to be noted in history taking.

The most important irritant is wet work. For industrial work, it is defined if individuals are exposed to liquids longer than 2 hours/day, use occlusive gloves longer than 2 hours/day or washing their hands very often, more than 20 times/day.

Investigation

In occupational dermatology patch testing is of great importance, in order to come to an accurate diagnosis. If the offending agent can be found at comprehensive patch testing (standard allergens and own material), it is of immense value in preventing relapses. The test can be carried out by a dermatologist, who has interest in the field with sufficient experience of patch testing and using materials and products from the patient's work environment. Because of the importance of ACD, a patch test should be done in all cases of CD.

In cases of contact urticaria, a prick test should be performed. A radioallergosorbent test (RAST) is helpful in contact urticaria due to latex. Dimethylglyoxime test for nickel can be done when required.

TREATMENT AND PREVENTION OF OCCUPATIONAL SKIN DISEASE

Treatment of occupational dermatoses is essentially the same as that of non-occupational dermatoses. Importance lies in the prevention and protection from further damage.

Prevention of Occupational Dermatoses

Some skin diseases do not allow a person to work in a particular environment. The list is long only a few are mentioned here:

A person with epidermolysis bullosa should not work at places where trauma is bound to occur, such as labourers, mechanics, carpenters, etc. Patients of anhidrotic ectodermal dysplasia should not be allowed to do jobs which are exposed to heat and temperature. A person with atopic dermatitis should avoid occupations which require constant hand washing such as beauticians, hair dressers, and nurses. Patients with Raynaud's disease or Raynaud's phenomenon should not be exposed to occupations which require working in a cold environment. People with phototoxicity should avoid exposure to ultraviolet light and people with tinea manuum should not work in massage therapy. Job Disability Act helps issues of job placement and accommodation.

Protection and Prevention of Recurrences

Every working place has certain health and safety precautions to be followed. Protection of hands is available at most work places, such as gloves and barrier creams. In some places allergen substitution measures are also provided. Workplace visits by experts also help in making the workplace friendly to the workers.

Protective gloves are widely recommended; they may at times contribute to an exacerbation of the dermatoses. The glove changes the microenvironment, and makes the CD worse. Faulty gloves are even worse. Some people are allergic to rubber or latex gloves. Some chemicals can permeate through the glove. These factors should be taken into consideration before recommending gloves; a follow-up should be done later.

Remove the source of irritation or replacement of harmful exposure, substitute chemicals that are less irritant. Cooperation of the physician, employer, employee, manufacturer, and legislative authorities are required to prevent occupational dermatoses.

Medical Treatment

This does not differ from the treatment offered for other patients visiting the hospital for the same disorder; laying stress upon the prevention of the disorder. This may include protective clothing, gloves, barrier creams, boots, etc. Avoidance of allergens during the active phase of the disease such as rubber gloves in rubber sensitivity.

PROGNOSIS OF OCCUPATIONAL SKIN DISEASE

Prognosis of occupational dermatoses refers to the course of skin disease over a period of time with and without medical treatment. The prognosis of occupational skin disease is poor, it is said that less than half of patients have healed after several years of therapy and follow-up. The prognosis of ACD is worse than that of ICD.

Understanding the course and prognosis of skin disease is important because it enables dermatologists and occupational physicians to predict the course of dermatosis, implement risk management of patients and plan preventive measures.

Bernardino Ramazzini (1633–1714)

An Italian physician is known as the "Father of Occupational Medicine". While still a medical student, his attention was drawn towards the disease of working places. He would visit workplaces, observe workers activities, and discuss their illness.

FURTHER READING

1. Carmichael AJ, Foulds IS. Performing a factory visit. Clin Exp Dermatol. 1993;18(3):208-10.
2. Church R. Prevention of dermatitis and its medico-legal aspects. Br J Dermatol. 1981;105(Suppl 21):85-90.
3. Rudzki E, Rebandel P, Grzywa Z, et al. Occupational dermatitis in veterinarians. Contact Dermatitis. 1982;8(1):72-3.
4. Sasseville D. Occupational Contact Dermatitis. J Allergy Asthma Clin Immunol. 2008;4:59-65.

Chapter

40 Injuries due to Burn

INTRODUCTION

Heat, flame, chemicals, electricity or radiation may cause burn injury to tissues. Burn is injury in which there is transfer of energy into the skin and tissues resulting in disruption of its function. The local response is due to a sudden increase in body surface temperature caused by the dilatation of blood vessels. A further increase in body temperature triggers an inflammatory response.

Around the world millions of people suffer from burns and tens of thousands die from it. Proper treatment requires an understanding not only of local injury but also of bacterial, hematological, nutritional and immunological derangement that occur in burns.

ASSESSMENT OF DAMAGE CAUSED BY BURNS

- Assessment of depth of burns
- Assessment of area of burns.

Assessment of the Depth of the Burn

- First-degree burn: This involves the epidermis only, it is characterized by erythema, pain and swelling. The pain and swelling subside within 48 hours and the superficial epidermis peels off in a few days. New epidermis cover is provided from the underlying basal germinal layer. The skin is unblemished after repair.
- Second-degree burn: This involves the epidermis and the superficial dermis (partial thickness burns). These can be:
  - Superficial partial thickness burns: This involves the epidermis and papillary dermis. Restoration of the skin depends upon the intact epithelial cells within the appendages. Pain, swelling and fluid loss is marked. Blisters are formed; these blisters are thin and rupture easily. The color of the skin is pink, capillary refill is present. These heal in less than 3 weeks (Fig. 1).
  - Deep partial thickness burns: This involves the epidermis and the mid-dermis. The skin is red or pale in color, blisters may or may not form, the blisters are thick, there is no capillary refill, it may or may not be painful. The wound heals in more than 3 weeks, as there are only a few epithelial appendages left to restore the damaged skin. The surviving dermis heals with the formation of ugly hypertrophic scars. Infection will delay healing, converting the injury into a full thickness burn.

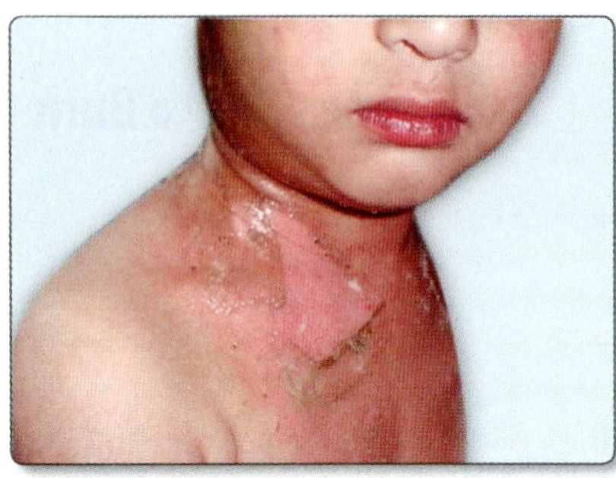

Fig. 1: Superficial burn

- Third-degree burn (full thickness burn): The epidermis and the dermis are destroyed. The destroyed tissue undergoes coagulation necrosis and forms an eschar, which comes off in 2–3 weeks. Fibrosis and ugly contractures are inevitable in these burns.
- Fourth-degree burn: This involves death or injury to the skin, subcutaneous tissue, fat, fascia, muscle or bone.

In children under the age of 5 years and adults over the age of 55 years, the skin is thinner in all areas of the body; therefore, the burns are deeper than the appearance. The anatomic location of the burn is also important in determining the depth of the burn. The skin is thin in areas such as medial thigh, volar surface of the arms, eyelids, ears, perineum, and the scrotum; these also affect the depth of burn injury.

Assessment of the Area of the Burn

Assessment of the area of the burn is important as it indicates the fluid loss and directly affects the fluid resuscitation of the patient. The simplest method is the rule of nine, which divides the body surface into multiples of nine. These are:

Head and neck	9%
Right upper limb	9%
Left upper limb	9%
Front of the chest and abdomen	18%
Back of the chest and abdomen	18%
Right lower limb	18%
Left lower limb	18%
Genitals	1%
Total	100%

CLINICAL ASSESSMENT OF A BURN INJURY

Erythema denotes epidermal damage and blanching on pressure confirms intact dermal capillaries.

Blisters are accumulation of fluid at the junction of the epidermis and dermis and suggest partial thickness damage. The blisters may continue to appear several hours after the injury and are often broken by the time the patient is seen by the doctor.

A dead white appearance indicates full thickness injury, although some may be deep partial burns.

A dry leathery mahogany colored eschar with visible thrombosed veins denotes full dermal thickness burn.

Intracutaneous sensation implies that the epidermal appendages have survived, as they lie in the same level as cutaneous nerve endings in the dermis. Superficial burns thus very painful.

FACTORS TO BE CONSIDERED IN ASSESSING BURN INJURY

- Site of the burn: Burns involving the face, neck, hands, feet and perineum are particularly liable to threaten appearance or function. They require in-patient management.
- Extent of the burn: This can be estimated by the rule of nine; this rule cannot be used in children because of the relatively large size of the head, which accounts for about 20% of the body surface at birth. The lower limbs account for 13% of the body surface. Hypovolemic shock is anticipated if more than 15% of the surface is burnt in an adult or more than 10% in a child.
- Depth of the burn: Superficial burns heal in 3 weeks leaving no scars. Full thickness burns invariably are infected unless excised early.
- Associated respiratory injury: This is extremely common in victims of house fire and is usually due to inhalation of smoke, burning plastic foam upholstery. It is frequently fatal.
- The systemic response occurs when a large area of the body is involved. It may affect the cardiovascular system, kidneys, the gastrointestinal tract, the general metabolism and immunity of the patient. The reduced immunity predisposes the patient to septic complications. In severe burns some 7,000 kcal may be lost daily and weight loss of 0.5 kg/day is not unusual unless steps are taken to prevent it. Hypovolemic shock is anticipated if more than 15% of the surface is burnt in an adult and more than 10% in child. These patients should have intravenous resuscitation. Most of the fluid is lost during the first 48 hours. While replacing the fluid loss, the appropriate type of fluid should be administered in the correct quantity.

SPECIAL TYPES OF BURN

Electrical Burns

These may occur from environmental industries or domestic sources. It may affect multiple organs.

Electrical burns may be high- or low-tension injuries depending upon the amount of voltage of electricity on the body. Low-tensions burns are less than 1,000 volts and high-tension burns are above 1,000 volts. Majority of the domestic burns are of 250 volts alternating current. Damage caused by electrical burns is due to heat caused by the conversion of electrical energy to heat in the body, and partly due to the effect of electric current inducing cell membrane breakdown; a phenomenon known as electroporation.

Burns caused by lightening are very severe; they affect the large part of the body and are deep involving the muscles and bones.

Laser Burns

Laser energy is converted into heat by the body. The effect on the skin depends on the wavelength of the laser and duration of exposure, direction of the beam, and skin color.

Microwave Burn

Microwaves are non-ionizing electromagnetic waves, which generate heat by its effect on the water molecules. Most microwave burns are from contact with steam or hot food. When microwave radiation is absorbed by the body tissues, it can produce heat. This can lead to burns and tissue damage. Sparing of the subcutaneous fat appears to be unique to microwave injury; this is because the radiation is only absorbed by tissues with high water content.

COMPLICATION OF BURNS

Burn wound sepsis: The most important cause of death after massive burn is wound sepsis. The burnt skin being avascular and systemic antibiotics cannot affect bacterial growth. Moreover, host resistance is very low due to reduction in the amount of complement and gamma globulin available, and due to impairment of the activity of neutrophils and monocytes. If local antibiotics are not used, rapid bacterial colonisation will occur. Local antibiotics dissolved in normal saline are distributed deep under the eschar.

Bronchopneumonia and thrombophlebitis frequently occur with massive burns.

There may be some loss of pigmentation in superficial burns, this is temporary. Deep burns are associated with hypertrophic scarring. Malignancy can occur in a burn scar.

Malignancy was first described by Marjolin in 1828. Development of malignancy is characterised by induration, ulceration, appearance of an elevated border or nodule formation.

Smoke inhalation syndrome: If smoke is inhaled in sufficient quantities progressive bronchospasm can develop within 24 hours with expiratory wheezes, tachypnea and respiratory failure.

TREATMENT

Management of a Burn Patient at Home

Chemical Burns

Copious irrigation with water for a minimum of 20 minutes is the key to first aid.

Electrical Burns

The source of current should be switched off and the victim removed from the source of current by non-conductive material.

Burns Due to Fire

Extinguish the fire by rolling the patient on the ground, by water or extinguishing foams or by the application of smothering blanket or coat. The patient should be removed to a smoke-free atmosphere as soon as possible. Mouth-to-mouth respiration is commenced, if necessary. The victim should be placed flat on the ground to avoid flames rising to burn the head and neck with inhalation of smoke and fumes. Clothing continues to burn the body due to heat within it. It should be removed immediately. Cool water is an excellent analgesic and can dissipate heat, but it should be applied with care to prevent hypothermia.

Hospital Management

Minor burns can be treated in an outpatient but moderate and major burns should be hospitalised.

Management consists of tetanus prophylaxis, analgesics and prevention of wound infection. If the patient has had tetanus immunisation during the previous 5 years then tetanus toxin booster dose should be administered. If not anti-tetanus immune globulin, 250 units should be given for passive immunisation and active immunisation started.

In minor burns, sepsis likely to occur due to β-hemolytic streptococcus; therefore, systemic penicillin during the first 72-hour of the burn is necessary. The wound should be dressed, superficial burns are quite painful and an analgesic should be prescribed liberally.

Care of the wound begins at the time of injury and continues until the epithelial cover has been restored. Infection poses the major problem and is the main threat to life once the first 48-hour has passed.

Initial cleaning and debridement: The burn is cleaned meticulously with a mild antiseptic and saline as soon as possible after admission. Staphylococci remain by far the most common infecting organism and *Pseudomonas aeruginosa* remains troublesome in most burn units. Hemolytic streptococci are feared because they can convert a superficial burn into deep burn and can cause severe systemic infection.

Topical antibacterial agents silver sulfadiazine and povidone iodine are valuable local antibacterial agents. These are often used for minor burns. Silver sulfadiazine should be used with cerium nitrate; this produces a calcium-rich layer on the surface of the dermal burn, this minimises infection.

After the initial cleaning, the burn is covered by a layer of sterile paraffin gauze dressing, a layer of cotton gauze swabs, bulky layer of cotton wool and an outer retaining crepe bandage. The bandage is reviewed daily but should be left in place for 8–10 days. If the dressing soaks then it should be changed.

Full-thickness burns need excision and grafting (refer surgical text).

Systemic Treatment

For extensive burns fluid replacement, cardiac monitoring, nutritional care, care of the wound and rehabilitation are necessary (refer surgical text).

REFERRAL TO A BURN UNIT

- Burns greater than 10% of body area
- Electrical burns
- Chemical burns
- Burns on the face, hands, feet, genitalia and major joints
- Circumferential burns of the limbs and chest
- Burns at extreme of age such as the children and elderly
- Burns with pre-existing systemic disorder.

FURTHER READING

1. Baxter CR. Management of burn wounds. Dermatol Clin. 1993;11(4):709-14.
2. Linares HA. From wound to scar. Burns. 1996:22:339-52.

Chapter

41

Fundamentals of Topical Therapy and Some Common Dermatological Preparations

INTRODUCTION

Dermatological therapy may be external or internal. As the skin is easily accessible to the application of topical agents, the external therapy is the easiest mode of treatment. The improvement of the lesion can also be seen by the naked eye.

PRINCIPLES OF TOPICAL THERAPY

- Local therapy should be selected according to the type of eruption, whether it is acute, subacute or chronic, and the site of eruption.
- The more acute the inflammation, the milder should be the treatment.
- Choice of the active ingredient and base depends upon the disease.

As a rule the active ingredient is not given as such but it is diluted in a vehicle or a base to avoid a sensitivity reaction. The base selection depends upon the type of lesion, e.g. acute lesions, which are moist and oozing, respond best to aqueous drying preparations, while chronic scaly lesions are best treated by moisturising and lubricating preparations. It is often said for a skin lesion "if it is dry, wet it; if it is wet, dry it". The local treatment can be in the form of ointments, cream, paste, lotions or solutions depending upon the type of lesion.

The topical preparation should be simple, inexpensive, effective and time tested.

Topical treatment is often the first choice of treatment in dermatological disorders. Systemic therapy is required when the lesions are extensive, not responding to topical therapy or when hard keratin is involved as in treating fungal infections of the hair or nails. Drugs that are used topically do not penetrate the hard keratin.

AMOUNT TO BE DISPENSED

It takes about 30 g of cream to cover the entire body. It takes 10% less ointment than cream and 50% more lotion than cream to cover the same area.

The other method of estimating the amount of medicine to be dispensed is by the fingertip method. The fingertip unit (FTU) is the amount of cream or ointment expressed from a 5-mm diameter nozzle, applied from the distal skin crease to the tip of the patient's index finger. One FTU covers an area of approximately 286 cm^2, (312 cm^2 in males, and 257 cm^2 in females). Approximate FTUs for the face and neck is 2.5, front of the trunk 6.7, back of the trunk 6.8, one arm and forearm 3.3, one hand 1.2, one leg and thigh 5.8, and one foot 1.8 FTU.

PERCUTANEOUS ABSORPTION

Compounds applied topically to the skin pass down along concentration gradients, according to laws governing diffusion of solutes in solvents and their diffusion across membranes. Drugs differ in their physical and chemical properties; this influences the kinetics of their release and absorption. Substances that contain water, alcohol or similar solvents, undergo rapid evaporation. This is recognised as a cooling sensation.

Formulations also mix with the skin surface lipids, and undergo time dependent changes in their composition, which determines the subsequent bioavailability of the active ingredient. Most formulations do not allow the delivery of the compound to the vascular system, because of the high degree of resistance to diffusion within the stratum corneum.

Formulations are designed whether they are to remain on the skin surface, e.g. sunscreens and cosmetics. Whether they have to be delivered to certain skin compartments or whether they have to pass through the dermis for transdermal formulations, such as nitroglycerine, an antianginal drug.

Liposomes as transdelivery systems: These are microspheres comprising a bilayer of lipids that encloses an inner aqueous core. A wide variety of cosmetics contain liposomes. Liposome based formulations are safe and cosmetically well accepted. There is an evidence that liposomes are mildly occlusive, and improve hydration of the stratum corneum. Liposomes based formulations are also said to enhance the penetration of compounds across the skin or to optimise the retention of bioactive compounds in the target tissue.

Reducing the particle size of the active ingredient increases the surface area to volume ratio, allowing for a greater solubility of the drugs in the vehicle. This forms the basis for increased absorption of micro-sized drugs.

Topical drugs that are manufactured are made lipid soluble, so that they penetrate well in the skin. Substances are further added to increase penetration such as dimethyl sulphoxide (DMSO).

Occlusion of the skin by a tight dressing increases the hydration and temperature of the stratum corneum, enhancing drug absorption. To obtain maximum absorption, patients should hydrate the skin by immersion in water for 5 minutes before application of the cream or ointment. Occlusion increases drug delivery by 10–100 times than the amount when not occluded.

Occlusion also leads to adverse side effects of the drug. Corticosteroids lead to atrophy and suppression of the pituitary-hypothalamic axis. Occlusion also promotes infections such as folliculitis, and miliaria.

Presence of hair follicles increases drug delivery. Skin of older individuals is poorly hydrated; they have fewer sweat glands, fewer hair follicles, which impede drug delivery. Penetration of drugs is the greatest from the skin of the scrotum and eyelids followed by the face, back, chest, upper arm and thighs, lower arms and legs, dorsum of the hands and feet. Palmoplantar skin and nails have the least absorption.

Reduced skin barrier function is seen in a number of pathological conditions such as ichthyosis, psoriasis, eczema, etc.; this is due to the structural changes in the stratum corneum. This is partly compensated by the proliferation of keratinocytes.

FREQUENCY OF APPLICATION

Frequency of drug application has little effect on its efficacy. Only once daily application is enough for most topical glucocorticoids. The stratum corneum acts as a reservoir for glucocorticoids. Penetration of nonspecific emollients such as creams and ointments is likely enhanced by more frequent applications.

INGREDIENTS IN TOPICAL PREPARATIONS

Topical preparations consist of vehicles such as ointments, creams, lotions and powder in which the active drug is dissolved or suspended. The term "base" is widely used as a synonym for vehicle.

A vehicle should be non-toxic, non-irritant, non-allergic, chemically stable, bacteriostatic, cosmetically acceptable, and pharmacologically inert. It should be easy to apply and remove. Vehicles contain various substances, such as emulsifying agents, stabilisers, preservatives, antioxidants, thickening agents, emollients and humectants to make the different preparations.

- Emulsifying agents provide stability and homogeneity. They are used to create mixtures containing two immiscible substances. One substance is distributed in small globules throughout the other. Glyceryl monostearate, polyethylene glycol derivatives, sodium lauryl sulphate are such agents.
- The consistency and appearance of creams can be improved by the addition of ethylenediamines, cetyl palmitate and related esters.
- Methylcellulose and gum tragacanth are used as suspending agents in pastes and ointments.
- Preservatives include parabens, benzyl alcohol, sorbic acid and chlorocresol. These are used to increase the shelf-life of the product, and to prevent its decay.
- Lubricants and emollients include fats, oils, waxes, greases (white soft paraffin), cetyl ester wax, etc.
- Penetrating agents include dimethyl sulphoxide (DMSO), propylene glycol, salicylic acid, azone and urea. These have been shown to increase the penetration of the active ingredient. Salicylic acid should be used with great care in children to avoid salicylism.

TOPICAL PREPARATIONS

Lotions

These are suspension of powders in water. Before application, shake the lotion to place the powder in suspension. As the water evaporates, a coating of powder is left on the skin, producing a drying effect. Calamine lotion consists of zinc carbonate coloured with ferrous oxide is soothing, antipruritic and anti-inflammatory. Lotio alba is used for acne.

Tinctures

These are alcoholic or hydroalcoholic solutions, in which the concentration of alcohol is 50%. Tinctures are cool, they dry the skin. Tincture iodine is also used for treating molluscum contagiosum due to its anti-inflammatory effects.

Sprays and Aerosols

They act in a similar way as the solutions and tinctures. They are easy to apply and are cosmetically more acceptable.

Astringents

They are solutions that constitute a combination of alcohol, water and acetone. Astringents contract organic tissue thus lessening secretion, such as silver nitrate, Burrow's solution, potassium permanganate and tincture of benzoin. They are usually applied on the face to obtain a drying cooling effect. They can be irritating.

Paints

These are coloured liquid preparations, either aqueous or alcoholic (tinctures). They are applied on the skin or mucous membranes with a brush. They are cooling, have astringent and antiseptic properties.

Solution

It is a homogenous mixture of one or more substances (solute) dispersed in a sufficient quantity of dissolving medium (solvent), e.g. aluminium acetate, aluminium chloride, silver nitrate, normal saline, formaldehyde, potassium permanganate, Burrow's solution, etc.

Gel

This is a colourless, semisolid, colloidal preparation, which liquefies on application to the skin. Most gels contain water as their main constituent. Gels have the advantage of being colourless and relatively greaseless. They are particularly used for the scalp, as they are not sticky.

Liniment

This is a lotion in an oily/soapy or alcoholic vehicle. These are intended to be rubbed on the skin as a counterirritant or anodyne. It prevents crusting as often seen after the application of lotions. It is therefore possible to change dressings less frequently. The advantage of rapid evaporation and cooling as in lotions is however lost.

Creams

These are semisolid emulsions of oil in water (O/W) (vanishing creams), or water in oil (W/O) (cold creams). In O/W emulsion, the oil droplets are in the discontinuous phase and they are dispersed in the continuous water phase. They also cool inflamed skin by evaporation of the water component. The oily component, which remains on the skin acts as a barrier to the passage of water and helps to protect the skin from external moisture as the nappy rash creams. The oily component may also act as a vehicle for lipid soluble drugs.

Cold creams are water in oil emulsions, in which the water is in the discontinuous phase and oil is in the continuous phase. These are more effective hydrating agents.

Ointments

These generally have no aqueous component. There are three types of ointments; those soluble in water, those that will emulsify in water and those that are insoluble in water.

Paste

These are ointments containing insoluble powders. They may be sufficiently thick to provide physical protection of a healing lesion against abrasion. They are suited for treatment of persistent maceration as diaper dermatitis. They tend to have a drying effect as the paste constitutes about 50% of the powder.

Powders

They increase evaporation and reduce friction. They are often antipruritic and provide a cooling sensation. The common powders used are zinc oxide or zinc stearate, magnesium stearate, talc (magnesium silicate), corn starch, and betonite dioxide.

SOME COMMON DERMATOLOGICAL FORMULAE

Acne

Lotio Alba

Potassium sulphurate	5%
Zinc sulphate	5%
Camphorated water up to	100%

Acne Cream

Acid salicylic	2%
Sulphur	2%
Resorcinol	2%
Aqueous cream up to	100%

Dry Skin

Hydrophilic Ointment

Wool fat	80%
Liquid paraffin	20%

Hydrating Lotion

Glycerine	50%
Aqua rose	50%

Emollient Cream

Liquid paraffin	20%
Glycerine	7%
Emulsifying fat	3%
Chlorbutol	0.5–1%
Water up to	100%

Eczema

Wise's Lotion (Acute Eczema)

Aluminium acetate	15%
Glycerine	20.0%
Talcum powder	25.0%
Zinc oxide	25.0%
Calcium oxide solution	15%

Zinc Liniment (Subacute Eczema)

Zinc oxide	12.5%
Talc	12.5%
Alcohol	12.5%
Glycerine	12.5%
Water	50%

Lassar's Paste (Chronic Eczema)

Acid salicylic	2%
Zinc oxide	24%
Starch	24%
White soft paraffin up to	100%

Fungal Infections

Whitfield's Ointment (for Tinea Infections)

Acid salicylic	3%
Acid benzoic	6%
Emulsifying ointment	100%

Magenta Paint (Castellani's Paint) for Candidiasis

Magenta	0.4 g
Phenol	4 g
Boric acid	0.8 g
Resorcinol	8 g
Acetone	4 mL
Industrial methylated spirit	8.5 mL
Water up to	100 mL

Sodium Thiosulphate Sulphate (for Tinea Versicolor)

Sodium thiosulphate	25%
Water up to	100%

Athletes Foot

Salicylic acid	3%
Benzoic acid	3%
Pyrogallic acid	3%
Thymol iodide	2%
Collodion up to	100%

Hyperhidrosis

Aluminium Lotion

Aluminium chloride	10–25%
Distilled water up to	100%

Aluminium Powder

Aluminium chloride	3%
Salicylic acid	3%
Alum	10%
Talcum powder	84%

Melasma

Depigmenting Cream

Hydroquinone	5%
Retinoic acid	0.1%
Dexamethasone	0.1%
Propylene glycol up to	100%

Azelaic Acid Formula

Hydroquinone	4%
Hydrocortisone	2.5%
Azelaic acid up to	100%

Freckle Peeling Cream

Camphor	2%
Salicylic acid	4%
Bichloride of mercury	0.12%
Alcohol up to	100%

Pruritus

Calamine	15%
Zinc oxide	5%
Glycerine	5%
Water up to	100%

(Menthol 1–2% may be added as an antipruritic)

Schamberg's Lotion

Menthol	0.25%
Phenol	1.00%
Peanut oil	45%
Calcium hydroxide solution	45%
Zinc oxide	8.0%

Psoriasis

Oil of Cade Ointment (Scalp)

Oil of cade	6%
Sulphur	2%
Salicylic acid	2%
Emulsifying ointment up to	100%

Coconut Oil Compound (Body)

Coal tar solution	12%
Sulphur	4%
Salicylic acid	2%
Coconut oil	60%
White soft paraffin	9%
Emulsifying wax	13%

Coal Tar and Zinc Ointment (Body)

Coal tar solution	12%
Zinc oxide	30%
White soft paraffin up to	100%

Dithranol Paste

Dithranol	0.4%
Salicylic acid	2%
Zinc oxide	25%
Starch	25%
White soft paraffin up to	100%

Scabies

Sulphur Ointment

Sulphur	10%
White soft paraffin up to	100%

Benzyl Benzoate Emulsion

Benzyl benzoate	25%
Emulsifying wax/water up to	100%

Warts

Mild Wart Paint

Acid salicylic	2 g
Castor oil	1 mL
Methylated spirit up to	100 mL

Strong Wart Paint

Acid salicylic	16.7%
Acid lactic	16.7%
Flexible collodion up to	100 mL

Topical antibiotics should be avoided as they tend to cause allergic reactions; excessive use may also lead to community based resistant strains of bacteria. Topical anaesthetics also cause allergic reactions.

Silver sulphadiazine may cause reactions in individuals who are sensitive to sulphonamides.

FURTHER READING

1. Gooskens V, Pönnighaus JM, Clayton Y, et al. Treatment of superficial mycosis in the tropics with Whitfields ointment versus clotrimazole. Int J Dermatol. 1994;33(10):738-42.
2. Haroon TS, Jafferani M. Common Dermatological Formulae. Specialist. 3(1):119-122. 1986.
3. Long CC, Finlay AY. The finger-tip unit-a practical measure. Clin Exp Dermatol. 1991;16(6):444-7.
4. Long CC, Mills CM, Finlay AY. A practical guide to topical therapy in children. Br J Dermatol. 1998;138(2):293-6.
5. McClain RW, Yentzer BA, Feldman SR. Comparison of skin concentrations following topical versus oral corticosteroid treatment: reconsidering the treatment of common inflammatory dermatoses. J Drugs Dermatol. 2009;8(12):1076-9.
6. Polano MK, Ponec M. Dependence of corticosteroid penetration on the vehicle. Arch Dermatol. 1976;112(5):675-80.

Chapter

42 Systemic Therapy

INTRODUCTION

The principles of systemic therapy in dermatology are the same as that for general medicine. Systemic drugs are often used for generalised infections, when topical therapy is ineffective, and in treating hair and nail disorders; topical drugs do not penetrate the hard keratin. The common systemic drugs used in dermatology are antihistamines, antifungals, antibiotics, corticosteroids, psoralens, retinoids, antivirals, cytotoxic drugs, antimalarials and the biologics.

CORTICOSTEROIDS

Marion Sulzberger first introduced corticosteroids for dermatological therapy in 1952; since then corticosteroids have been used in the treatment of a number of cutaneous diseases. As corticosteroids are anti-inflammatory, they are often misused.

The daily cortisol production by the human body under normal condition is about 20 mg. Normally only 5% of the circulating cortisol is free; this is the active therapeutic molecule. The remainder is bound to proteins mainly globulin.

Structure of the Steroid Moiety

The structure of a steroid molecule consists of 17 carbon atoms, arranged around a steroid nucleus made of four rings. All steroid molecules consist of the same basic structure, 3 hexanes and a single pentane ring. By convention, these rings are designated A, B, C and D. Individual sites of the molecule are numbered in sequence. Modification of these loci can materially alter and enhance the potency of the individual steroid (Fig. 1).

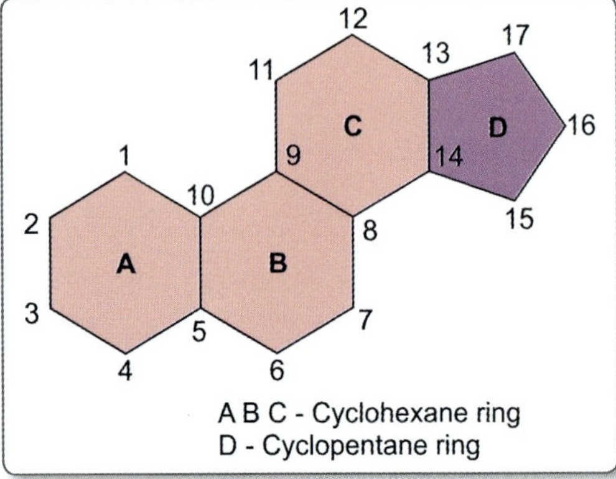

Fig. 1: Steroid molecule

A double bond at C1 and C2 position, increases the effects of hydrocortisone and produces synthetic steroid prednisolone. A fluorine atom at C9 position, not only increases the anti-inflammatory action of the steroid molecule, but also the mineralocorticoid activity. The latter effect can be minimised by various additions; such as addition of an OH group at the 16 α position (triamcinolone), a methyl group at the 16-α-position (dexamethasone), or a methyl group at the 16-β-position (betamethasone).

Esterification of the steroid molecule makes it lipophilic; this is then used for topical application. An acetonide at the C16–C17 position of triamcinolone transforms a relatively inactive topical steroid to a potent topical steroid. An addition of the fluorine atom at the C6 position of the steroid molecule and a 16-α-acetonide ester produces fluocinolone acetonide. Betamethasone valerate is simply a betamethasone with a valerate ester at the C17 position.

Mechanism of Action

Corticosteroids cross the cell membrane, bind to specific receptors in the cytoplasm; this complex is then transported to the nucleus. Here there is an interaction with high affinity binding sites, which results in the formation of new proteins. These proteins are responsible for the various actions produced by the steroids.

When corticosteroids are applied to the skin, the changes produced are: vasoconstriction, reduction of inflammation, immunosuppression and reduction in mitosis.

Effects of Corticosteroids

Metabolic Effects

Corticosteroids stimulate gluconeogenesis. As a result, blood sugar rises, protein is catabolised and insulin is stimulated. Both lipolysis and lipogenesis are stimulated, resulting in redistribution of body fat. There is a net increase of fat deposition in certain areas such as the face (moon face), shoulders and the back (buffalo hump), with reduced fat in the extremities.

Catabolic Effect

Corticosteroids cause muscle protein catabolism. In addition lymphoid tissue, connective tissue, fat and skin undergo wasting under the influence of high concentration of corticosteroid. Catabolic effect can lead to osteoporosis. In children, growth is inhibited.

Immunosuppressive Effect

Corticosteroids suppress T and B cell activity, leading to increased risk of infection due to profound immunosuppression.

Anti-inflammatory Effects

Corticosteroids have a dramatic effect on the distribution and function of leucocytes. They increase the number of neutrophils, decrease the number of lymphocytes, eosinophils, basophils and monocytes. Glucocorticoids also inhibit phospholipase A2, due to steroid-mediated elevation of lipocortin.

This blocks the release of arachidonic acid, the precursor of prostaglandins and leukotrienes.

Mineralocorticoid Effect

Corticosteroids cause sodium retention and potassium excretion. This leads to fluid retention, hypertension and weight gain.

Anti-mitotic Effects

Topical steroids are known to interfere temporarily with epidermal DNA synthesis. This action is important in the treatment of psoriasis. The inhibition of cell division is also responsible for the side effects such as epidermal atrophy.

Vasoconstrictive Effect

This effect is especially useful for ranking the efficacy of topical steroids. Hydrocortisone barely vasoconstricts, fluocinolone acetate produces vasoconstriction 100 times that of hydrocortisone. Betamethasone is 360 times and clobetasol propionate is 1,640 times as potent as hydrocortisone.

Other Effects

Corticosteroid when given in large doses may cause profound behavioural disturbances. Large doses stimulate gastric acid secretion and may lower the resistance to gastric ulcer formation. Long-term corticosteroid therapy may cause severe bone loss, myopathy leads to muscle weakness.

Increased resistance to stress: By raising plasma glucose levels, glucocorticoids provide the body with energy to combat stress, e.g. trauma, flight, etc. Corticosteroids can cause a moderate rise in BP, apparently by enhancing the vasoconstrictive effect of the adrenergic stimuli on the small blood vessels and by salt retention.

Vasoconstriction Bioassay

This test is extremely useful to assess the potency and percutaneous absorption of topical steroids. The degree of blanching at the site of application correlates to the anti-inflammatory potency of corticosteroids. A solution of corticosteroids is applied to the forearms and the area is occluded for 16 hours prior to observation. The assay also measures the penetration and clearance of the steroid.

Classification of Corticosteroids

Based on vasoconstrictor studies, steroids are placed in four classes.

Class I

These are the weakest steroids. 1% hydrocortisone is unlikely to produce side effects. It is not used for treating infections, but it is of choice for treating eczema of the face and flexures.

Class II

These are moderately potent steroids such as fluocinolone acetonide 0.025%, fluocortolone hexanoate 0.1%, triamcinolone acetonide 0.1%. These agents are useful in the treatment of eczema especially atopic eczema in children on areas other than the face, and in the treatment of seborrhoeic eczema in the intertriginous areas.

Class III

These are potent steroids; these include betamethasone valerate 0.1%, fluocinolone acetonide 0.05%, most of these have a fluorine atom in the C9 position. Potent steroids are indicated for more resistant eczema such as seborrhoeic eczema of the trunk, eczema of the hands and feet, lichenified eczema, psoriasis, lichen planus, etc.

Class IV

These are the most potent topical steroids they include clobetasol propionate 0.05%, diflucortolone valerate 0.1% and halcinonide 0.1%. These drugs are used in the treatment of lichen planus, lichen simplex chronicus, localised plaques of discoid lupus erythematosus, vitiligo, alopecia areata. These steroids should be avoided for eczemas except when the disease is localised on the hands and feet. These are potent drugs and the practitioner should be conscious of their long-term usage.

Indications for Corticosteroids in Dermatology

Systemic Indications

- Acute allergic contact dermatitis
- Acute autoimmune connective tissue diseases, such as systemic lupus erythematosus
- Acute anaphylactic reaction
- Chronic immuno-bullous disorders, such as pemphigus and pemphigoid
- Acute generalised exfoliative dermatitis
- Miscellaneous conditions such as severe lichen planus, pyoderma gangrenosum, sarcoidosis, erythema multiforme, and cutaneous T cell lymphoma.

Topical Indications

- Eczema
- Lichen planus
- Psoriasis
- Alopecia areata
- Vitiligo.

Intra-lesional Indications

- Keloids
- Granuloma annulare
- Alopecia areata
- Hypertrophic lichen planus
- Nodular prurigo
- Cystic acne
- Lichen simplex chronicus.

Side Effects of Corticosteroids

These can be studied under the following headings:

- Side effects of systemic steroids
- Side effects of topical steroids
- Side effects of intra-lesional steroid injections.

Systemic Corticosteroids

The side effects produced by the prolonged use of steroids are:

Cushingoid changes: The most common change is the alteration of fat distribution. Buffalo hump, facial and neck fullness, increased supraclavicular and suprasternal fat, gynaecomastia, flattening of the buttocks, and thinning of the extremities.

Suppression of the pituitary-adrenal axis: This occurs by excessive use of potent and moderately potent steroids. The steroids should be given in the morning. This is because the maximum rate of adrenocortisol secretion occurs in the morning; therefore less adrenocortical suppression occurs at this time, while the therapeutic efficacy is maintained.

Purpura or ecchymoses: This is seen especially over the dorsal surface of the forearms in patients over the age of 50 years. It is aggravated by senile purpura.

Steroid acne: Small firm follicular papules on the forehead, cheeks and chest occur. These may persist as long as the corticosteroids are continued even in moderate doses. Steroid acne responds rapidly to tretinoin 0.05%, benzoyl peroxide gel, tetracyclines are also effective.

Striae: These are widely distributed especially over the buttocks, abdomen and thigh.

Gastrointestinal: These include gastritis and peptic ulcer.

Electrolyte imbalance: Changes in electrolytes may lead to hypokalaemia and hypernatraemia.

Metabolic: These include hyperglycaemia and diabetes mellitus. Hypertension occurs due to salt and water retention.

Other side effects. Cataract and glaucoma affect the eye, osteoporosis can result in fractures.

Cutaneous side effects. There may be generalised dryness of the skin, skin becomes thin and fragile, keratosis pilaris and persistent erythema of the skin may occur. Hair loss occurs in half of the patients on corticosteroids. The hair becomes thin and brittle, fractures occur along the hair shaft. There may be increased hair growth on the beard area, arms, and the back with fine vellus hair.

Because of immunosuppression, corticosteroids can flare up latent infections, such as tuberculosis. Always exclude any infection in the body before starting corticosteroids.

Topical Steroid

These can be considered at different levels.

Epidermal effects: Epidermal thinning is associated with a decrease in epidermal kinetic activity. Epidermis becomes atrophic; there is a general flattening of the epidermo-dermal junction. Melanocytes are inhibited and a vitiligo-like condition has been described.

Dermal effects: Collagen synthesis is reduced; this results in the formation of striae. A poor support to the dermal vasculature leads to easy rupture of the blood vessels on trauma, leading to blot haemorrhages, this results in the formation of a stellate scar.

The skin becomes translucent and yellowish, telangiectasia appear. Cutaneous atrophy and telangiectasia are reversible but the striae are permanent.

Vascular effects: Corticosteroids first produce vasoconstriction of the superficial blood vessels, followed by a phase of rebound vasodilatation, which in later stages becomes fixed. As the vasoconstriction wears off, the small blood vessels overdilate, allowing oedema, enhanced inflammation and sometimes pustulation.

Applying the steroids under occlusion enhances the cutaneous changes. When fluorinated corticosteroids are applied on the face perioral dermatitis can occur. Such changes are also seen when 1% hydrocortisone is applied for a long time. Infantile gluteal granuloma is a condition found only in infants who wear napkins. An alteration of the host response to *Candida* under the influence of steroids has been suggested for this condition. When corticosteroids are applied close to the eyes, glaucoma can be a hazard. Allergic contact dermatitis to the steroid molecule can also occur.

Potent corticosteroids can also suppress the pituitary adrenal axis when used extensively for long periods. In children, one should be very careful in using corticosteroids; even hydrocortisone when applied topically can suppress the pituitary adrenal axis.

Prolonged use of potent topical steroids is inadvisable in the following conditions:

- Infancy
- Most facial dermatoses
- Widespread inflammatory disease
- Infected dermatoses unless covered by a simultaneous use of an appropriate antibiotic.

Steroid Injections

The injections may produce subcutaneous atrophy at the site of injection. The patients become aware by noting a depression at the site of injection. It may take as much as 6 months for the lipid to accumulate and fill the gap.

Long-term corticosteroid therapy should be supplemented with antacids to prevent hyperacidity; calcium and vitamin D to prevent osteoporosis.

Corticosteroids are contraindicated in severe infections, gastrointestinal ulcers, osteoporosis, myopathies, glaucoma, psychosis and recurrent thrombosis.

Addison in 1855 described the clinical syndrome resulting from the destructive disease of adrenal glands. Cushing in 1932 described the syndrome of hypercorticism. The preparation of adrenocortical extracts was first accomplished in 1930. In 1948, corticosteroids were used for the treatment of rheumatoid arthritis. Soon therapeutic application was extended to other diseases.

ANTIFUNGALS

At the time of Second World War, only a few local drugs were present for treatment of fungal diseases. In early 1960s, griseofulvin was introduced for the treatment of dermatophytosis. Some of the more recently developed broad-spectrum antifungal drugs are imidazoles, triazole and the allylamines. Most of the superficial fungal infections can be treated with topical medication. Infection of the hair, nails, hyperkeratotic lesions, acute generalised infection and infection resistant to topical treatment require systemic therapy.

Systemic Antifungal Drugs

There are three main families of antifungal drugs: the polyenes, azoles which include the imidazoles and the triazoles, and the allylamines. Other antifungal drugs are griseofulvin and flucytosine.

Polyenes

Nystatin was the first polyene discovered; it was discovered by the New York Research Health Laboratory and named accordingly. The other members of this group are natamycin and amphotericin B.

Nystatin: Nystatin is useful only for candidiasis, intended for cutaneous, vaginal or oral administration. Infection of the nails, hyperkeratinised or crusted lesions do not respond to nystatin. Nystatin is not absorbed from the gastrointestinal tract. It is available in the form of powder, creams, ointment and vaginal tablets. Oral tablets are used to decrease the gastrointestinal colonisation with *Candida* and to prevent the relapse of vaginal candidiasis. It is too toxic for systemic use.

Amphotericin B: Amphotericin B is a naturally occurring polyene macrolide produced by *Streptomyces nodosus*. It is used in the treatment of cutaneous and mucocutaneous candidiasis and almost all deep fungal infections.

Mode of action: Several polyene molecules bind to ergosterol present in the cell membrane of fungal cells, to form pores or channels. This disrupts the membrane function, allowing electrolytes (particularly potassium) and small molecules to leak out from the cell, resulting in cell death.

Amphotericin B is fungicidal; it is effective against a number of fungal infections, such as candidiasis, histoplasmosis, cryptococcosis, coccidioidomycosis, aspergillosis and blastomycosis.

Pharmacokinetics: Amphotericin B is administered by intravenous infusion; the intrathecal route is sometimes used. It is bound to the tissue proteins and is distributed throughout the body. It does not cross the placenta.

It is used in a dose of 0.4–1 mg/kg/day, but toxicity is minimised if there is a build up from a very low dose to full dosage in 3–5 days.

Natamycin is the drug of choice in infection caused by *Fusarium solani*. As it is less irritating for the eyes, it is used in the treatment of fungal keratitis. It penetrates poorly and may not reach deep corneal mycosis.

Side effects: Side effects are anorexia, nausea, vomiting, hypotension, and bronchospasm. Phlebitis is common at the site of infusion. Renal impairment may be severe when amphotericin B is used for systemic mycosis. Renal failure is an absolute contraindication to amphotericin B.

Azoles

These antifungals can be used topically and systemically. These broad-spectrum agents block the synthesis of ergosterol, an essential component of the fungal cell membrane by binding to cytochrome P-450. The azoles block the demethylation of lanosterol to ergosterol; this inhibits the membrane functions by increasing its permeability. They act by damaging the damaging the cell membrane of the fungus, making them leak their intracellular contents. Azoles consist of the following antifungal drugs:

- Imidazoles
- Triazoles
  - Itraconazole
  - Fluconazole
  - Voriconazole
  - Posaconazole

Imidazoles: Clotrimazole and miconazole were the first of the imidazole compounds discovered. Topical compounds include sulconazole, bifonazole, oxiconazole, isoconazole, etc.

Ketoconazole is a broad-spectrum imidazole; it is active against both superficial and deep fungal infections. It is most useful in the treatment of histoplasmosis.

Pharmacokinetics: Ketoconazole is administered orally; it dissolves in the acidic gastric contents and is absorbed via the gastric mucosa. Food and antacids impair absorption. The drug is highly bound to the plasma proteins, penetration into the tissues is limited, and it does not cross the blood-brain barrier. Excretion is primarily via the kidneys.

Adverse effects: Ketoconazole inhibits cytochrome P-450; this enzyme plays an important part in the synthesis of steroid hormones and prostaglandins. Cytochrome P-450 catalyze almost every step in the cascade of cholesterol to the formation of individual hormones. Ketoconazole interacts with each of these enzymes. The interaction with these enzymes includes altered serum levels of steroid hormones.

By inhibiting cytochrome P-450, ketoconazole can potentiate toxicity of cyclosporin, phenytoin sodium and H_1 histamine antagonists such as astemizole. It increases the levels of tolbutamide and warfarin. Rifampicin, an inducer of cytochrome P-450 system can shorten the duration of ketoconazole and other azoles. Drugs that decrease the gastric acidity such as H_2 blockers and antacids can decrease the absorption of ketoconazole.

Triazoles

Triazoles are new group of antifungals similar to imidazoles in both chemical structure and mechanism of action. The triazoles appear less likely to cause hepatotoxicity, they have comparatively little effect on cytochrome P-450. The prototype of triazole class of drugs is terconazole, but because of phototoxicity, its use is limited. The two orally active triazoles are itraconazole and fluconazole.

Itraconazole is active against dermatophytes, *Candida*, *Malasseziz* and against a number of deep fungal infections such as blastomycosis, aspergillosis, coccidioidomycosis and cryptococcosis. It is the treatment of choice for blastomycosis.

The drug is well absorbed from the gastrointestinal tract. It is extensively bound to the plasma proteins, therapeutic concentrations are not attained in the cerebrospinal fluid (CSF). Like ketoconazole, it is extensively metabolised in the liver.

It is normally given in a dose of 100 mg/day for 15 days for tinea corporis. At higher doses, it is possible to use shorter courses, such as 200 mg/day for 1 week in the treatment of tinea corporis. Because it is retained in the nails for long periods, it is used in pulse doses of 200 mg twice daily for 1 week/month for 3–4 months.

Itraconazole may occasionally cause nausea, vomiting, headache, more serious adverse effects such as hepatic reactions and anaphylaxis are extremely rare.

Fluconazole is a broad spectrum antifungal; it is chiefly used in the treatment of oropharyngeal and vaginal candidiasis, cryptococcosis and coccidioidomycosis. It is also shown to be useful in the treatment of blastomycosis and histoplasmosis. A single dose of 150 mg is effective for candidiasis. For dermatophytosis, weekly doses of 150 mg for 2–4 weeks. Similar weekly pulses are also used for onychomycosis. In systemic mycosis, it is the treatment of choice for cryptococcosis.

The drug is administered orally or intravenously. Its absorption is excellent and its absorption does not depend upon gastric acidity. Binding to plasma proteins is minimal. It crosses the CSF barrier and is excreted via the kidney.

Side effects: It is a potent teratogen; this suggests that the other azoles may also be teratogens.

Voriconazole and posaconazole are used to treat serious fungal infections such as invasive aspergillosis, and candidiasis in severely immunocompromised, haematologic malignancies with prolonged neutropenia from chemotherapy.

Allylamines

Allylamines can be used both topically and systemically. Naftifine was the first member of the allylamine series; it can be used only topically. Terbinafine is active both locally and systemically. It is effective against dermatophytes, moulds and dimorphic fungi.

Mode of action: This is a fungicidal antifungal, it acts by inhibiting the fungal ergosterol biosynthesis by specific inhibition of the enzyme squalene epoxidase. Inhibition of squalene epoxidase results in an accumulation of squalene in the cell and a deficiency of ergosterol in the fungal cell membrane. The precise mechanism of the action of squalene is not clear, but it may increase the membrane fluidity leading to disruption of the enzyme function and cell structure.

Allylamines do not inhibit cytochrome P-450; the extent to which allylamines inhibit ergosterol biosynthesis varies between different fungal species. Allylamines are fungicidal to dermatophytes but are fungistatic to *Candida albicans*.

Side effects: There are a few side effects apart from occasional gastrointestinal discomfort. Loss of taste may occur but is reversible. As allylamines do not inhibit cytochrome P-450, it does not interfere in the synthesis of testosterone or steroid hormones like the azole group of drugs. No teratogenic or embryogenic effect was observed in animals.

Griseofulvin

Griseofulvin is fungistatic; it acts only against dermatophytes and is effective only on systemic use. It is not effective on topical application.

Mode of action: It inhibits the formation of the intracellular microtubules within the fungus to disrupt the mitotic spindle and inhibit mitosis. It accumulates in the newly synthesised keratin-containing tissues making them unsuitable for the growth of the fungus. Therapy must be continued until normal tissue replaces the infected tissue, this usually takes weeks to months. In addition to the antimitotic properties, griseofulvin is also anti-inflammatory and anti-chemotactic for neutrophil leucocytes.

Pharmacokinetics: After absorption from the gastrointestinal tract, the drug is concentrated in the stratum corneum within 4–8 hours. Similarly rapid clearance of the drug from the stratum corneum occurs within 42–78 hours after the oral dose. The absorption is more rapid after a fatty meal. Griseofulvin is distributed chiefly to the keratinised tissues; concentration in the other tissues is usually much lower. Griseofulvin induces hepatic cytochrome P-450 activity and can increase the rate of metabolism of a number of drugs, including anticoagulants. Excretion of the drug occurs via the kidneys.

Dose: In adults, the daily dose is 500–1000 mg depending upon the body weight. In children, the dose is 10 mg/kg of the body weight.

Side effects: Toxicity is not generally a clinical problem. The drug potentiates the intoxicating effects of alcohol. Minor effects such as headache, peripheral neuritis, lethargy, mental confusion, vertigo, blurred vision may occur.

Gastrointestinal disturbances such as nausea, vomiting, diarrhoea, flatulence, dry mouth, angular stomatitis may occur. Griseofulvin may cause hepatic toxicity, it is contraindicated in patients with acute intermittent porphyria. Haematological effects such as leukopenia, neutropenia, basophilia and monocytosis occur; this disappears with discontinuation of therapy. Renal effects include albuminuria without evidence of renal insufficiency.

Cutaneous side effects include warm and cold urticaria, photosensitivity, lichen planus, erythema multiforme, vesicular and morbilliform eruptions.

A moderate increase in faecal protoporphyrin has been noted with the drug, when it is used for a long time. Griseofulvin induces hepatic microsomal enzymes; this increases the rate of metabolism of warfarin. The drug may reduce the efficacy of oral contraceptives by a similar mechanism.

Oxford and his coworkers first introduced griseofulvin from Penicillium griseofulvum dierckx in 1939. Because it was ineffective against bacteria, no further attention was paid for sometime. In 1946, Brain and associates found that it produced stunting of fungal hyphae. During the next 10 years, it was used to treat fungal infection in plants and animals. Gentles in 1958 cured mycotic disease of guinea pig by griseofulvin. Soon thereafter the drug was available for general use.

Flucytosine

Flucytosine is a synthetic pyrimidine metabolite, used in combination with amphotericin B for the treatment of systemic mycosis and meningitis caused by cryptococcosis and *candidiasis.*

Mode of action: The drug enters the fungal cell via a cytosine specific permease, an enzyme not found in mammalian cells. Flucytosine is then converted to 5-fluorodeoxyuridylic acid; this false nucleotide inhibits thymidylate synthetase thus depriving the organism of thymidylic acid an essential DNA component. Amphotericin B affects cell permeability thus allowing more of flucytosine to enter the cell.

Pharmacokinetics: Flucytosine is well absorbed by the oral route; it is distributed throughout the body and penetrates well into the CSF.

Side effects: Flucytosine causes reversible neutropenia, thrombocytopenia and occasional bone marrow depression. Reversible hepatic dysfunction and elevation of serum transaminase and alkaline phosphatase may occur. Gastrointestinal symptoms such as anorexia, nausea, vomiting and diarrhoea are common. Severe enterocolitis may occur.

RETINOIDS

Vitamin A is a necessary dietary nutrient, important for growth, vision, reproduction and differentiation of epithelial tissue in all vertebrates. The term vitamin A refers to a group of compounds rather than a single compound. These include preformed vitamin A alcohol-retinol, its aldehyde-retinal, and its acid—transretinoic acid as well as the provitamin—β carotene. Retinoids are naturally occurring and synthetic compounds, with specific biological activities that resemble vitamin A. They are mainly used for disorders of keratinisation.

Mechanism of Action

There are specific receptors of retinol and retinoic acid, the activity of the retinoids is similar to that of steroid hormones. The retinoic acid receptors belong to the family of sterols-thyroid-vitamin D receptors.

These receptors have a more significant effect on differentiation than on inhibition of tumour. The two main receptors are RAR and RXR. There are three different members of RAR (α, β and γ), and RXR (α, β and γ), each encoded by different genes. The human epidermis is mainly regulated by RAR-γ and RXR-α heterodimers.

Effects on differentiation: It has been known for years that vitamin A deficiency results in squamous metaplasia of the epithelial cells and that vitamin A supplement reverses the effect. The functional and structural integrity of the epithelial cells throughout the body is dependent upon an adequate supply of vitamin A. Retinoids enhance the synthesis of some proteins, and reduce the synthesis of others. Retinoic acid is more potent in this respect than retinol.

When there is a deficiency of vitamin A, mature differentiated epithelial cells are replaced by a hyperplastic growth of stratified keratinising epithelium (toad-like skin or phrynoderma). Selected retinoids enhance the differentiation of epithelial cells, stimulate the production of mucus, inhibit keratinisation and inhibit the secretion of sebum. Retinoids are used to treat a variety of keratinizing disorders.

Tumour growth: In experimental animals, deficiency of vitamin A has led to a number of malignancies. Growth of a number of tumours can be reduced by retinoids such as melanoma and non-melanoma skin cancer.

Ageing: The effect of retinoids on the aging skin is complex; it is due to its topical effect. Retinoids show replacement of disorganised collagen fibres, increase in viable epidermal synthesis and a return to its uniform size, electron density of basal and spinous keratinocytes is restored. At least 6 months of treatment is required.

In psoriasis, retinoids lead to a thickening of the granular layer and a normalisation of parakeratosis. It is said to modulate the three main pathological characteristics of psoriasis: keratinocyte hyperproliferation, abnormal keratinocyte differentiation and infiltration of inflammatory cells into the skin.

Isotretinoin

Isotretinoin (13-*cis* retinoic acid), was released in the United States in 1982 for the treatment of severe nodulocystic acne. It decreases the size of the sebaceous glands, alters the keratinisation of the glandular infundibulum, thereby preventing the formation of comedones. The retinoids also inhibit the release of arachidonic acid by the macrophages and in this way contribute to their anti-inflammatory effect.

The other disorders in which isotretinoin is used are Darier's disease, pityriasis rubra pilaris, Gram-negative folliculitis, rosacea, hidradenitis suppurativa, ichthyosis, and steatocystoma multiplex.

Isotretinoin is given in a dose of 0.5–1 mg/kg of body weight.

Etretinate

Etretinate was introduced in 1986 for the treatment of severe psoriasis. This retinoid is replaced by acitretin, which is an active metabolite of etretinate.

The major disadvantage of etretinate is binding to body fat for a period of 2 years, after the course of the drug is completed. For isotretinoin, the period is 1 month.

Etretinate was used for the treatment of psoriasis, ichthyosis, palmoplantar keratoses and malignancies of the skin. It is not a potent sebo-suppressive and is therefore not used in the treatment of acne.

Acitretin

Acitretin is less bound to the body fat than etretinate. The efficacy can be improved by adding ultraviolet A (UVA) and psoralen-UVA (PUVA). It is effective in pustular and erythrodermic psoriasis. In some patients, there is a reverse metabolism to etretinate; therefore the same restriction of 2 years is advised between the end of a course of therapy, and pregnancy to take place.

Bexarotene

Bexarotene is a specific RXR-selective retinoid. It is used mainly for the treatment of mycosis fungoides. Its mechanism of action is similar to other retinoids, but has higher chances of metabolic abnormalities, hypothyroidism and exfoliative dermatitis.

Alitretinoin

Alitretinoin (9-*cis* retinoic acid) acts on both RAR and RXR receptors; it is a pan-retinoid receptor agonist. It was released for use in the United States in 2005. The primary therapeutic potential of alitretinoin appears to be in the treatment of chronic recalcitrant hand eczema. Alitretinoin gel 0.1% is also used for the treatment of AIDS-related cutaneous Kaposi's sarcoma.

Side Effects of Retinoids

A vast majority of patients complain of dryness of the skin, cheilitis, and conjunctival irritation. Hair loss and skin fragility is also common. Headache occurs due to pseudotumour cerebri. Other symptoms include papilloedema, nausea, vomiting and visual disturbances. About 25% of the patients develop hypertriglyceridemia; this is more common in obese patients. Isotretinoin should be discontinued if the triglyceride concentration increases to 500 mg/dl, because of the risk of pancreatitis.

Arthralgia is a common complaint. The risks of premature epiphysial closure and pathological fractures have been observed.

The risk of teratogenicity is an extremely important factor. Major fetal abnormalities, such as hydrocephalus, microcephalus, mental retardation, facial dysmorphea, parathyroid hormone deficiency, micro-ophthalmia, micro-pinna, small or absent external auditory meatus and cardiovascular abnormalities. It may result in premature labour, abortions and stillbirth. Pregnancy is an absolute contraindication to the use of retinoids; the patients should not get pregnant for at least 1 month after isotretinoin and for 2 years after stopping of etretinate therapy.

Less common side effects are alteration of hepatic function, inflammatory bowel disease, decreased night vision and corneal abnormalities. It is important to determine the patient's occupation as this class of drugs should be avoided in airline pilots, rail drivers and long distance lorry drivers due to defective night vision.

Chronic toxicity of retinoids: The most common findings are the bony changes. Demineralisation, thinning of long bones, cortical hyperostosis, periostitis and premature closure of the epiphysis.

Monitoring of Retinoids

The incidence of hypertriglyceridemia is seen 1 in 4 patients on isotretinoin therapy. Pretreatment and follow-up of blood lipids should be obtained under fasting conditions. Tests should be performed on monthly intervals until the lipid response to isotretinoin is established.

Diabetics should have periodic blood sugar determinations during retinoid therapy.

Children receiving retinoids should have periodic bony assessment.

Precautions with Retinoid Therapy

Because of the relationship of retinoids with vitamin A, patients should be advised against taking of vitamin A supplements during retinoid therapy. Tetracycline should not be given with retinoid therapy to avoid pseudotumour cerebri.

Patients should be informed that transient exacerbation of acne might occur during the initial phase of therapy. Patients should refrain from wearing contact lens while on retinoid therapy, due to dryness of the cornea.

All transretinoic acid (ATRA, tretinoin) was the first retinoid to be synthesised. It has no systemic significance. It is used as a topical preparation for disorders of keratinisation such as acne vulgaris, ichthyosis, actinic keratosis, etc. Other topical retinoids are isotretinoin (isomer of tretinoin), adapalene, tazarotene, bexarotene gel and alitretinoin gel.

Night blindness was first described in Egypt around 1500 BC. Hippocrates later suggested eating beef and liver as a cure for the disorder. Clinical and experimental vitamin A deficiencies were first recognised, during the World War I; when it became apparent that xerophthalmia in soldiers was a result of decrease in the contents of butterfat in the diet.

PSORALENS

Psoralens occur naturally in many plants such as citrus fruit, parsley, figs and celery. For therapeutic use, it is available as methoxypsoralen and trimethylpsoralen. The psoralens are furocoumarins; they contain a furan ring fused to a double-ringed coumarin structure.

Mechanism of Action

Psoralens intercalate with DNA in the dark, but do not form covalent bonds. When exposed to light of appropriate wavelength the psoralens form two major types of photoreactants. The first is independent of oxygen and involves formation of adducts with pyrimidine bases, either with one strand or with both strands of DNA. In the second type of reaction, energy is transformed from the psoralens to the oxygen, creating reactive substances such as singlet oxygen or superoxide anion. These substances then mediate the ultimate effects of photochemical reaction.

Psoralens are rapidly absorbed after oral administration; photosensitivity is maximum after 2 hours of ingestion. The drug is metabolised in the liver.

Pharmacological Actions

Psoralens inhibit DNA replication by the formation of photochemical conjugates with nucleic acid.

Psoralens are immunosuppressive; they alter the distribution and function of circulating T lymphocytes and suppress contact hypersensitivity reactions. Psoralens cause depletion of Langerhans cells.

Psoralens increase melanin pigmentation by stimulating mitosis and proliferation of melanocytes, they increase the melanisation of melanosomes, and the transfer of melanin to keratinocytes, and they increase the synthesis and inactivation of tyrosinase. Psoralens are thus useful in the treatment of vitiligo; the action depends upon the presence of functional melanocytes.

Studies on animals also suggest that PUVA suppresses degranulation of mast cells; this explains its use in cutaneous mast cell disease.

Uses of Psoralens

Psoralens are mainly used in the treatment of psoriasis, vitiligo and cutaneous T cell lymphoma. Other conditions in which they can be used are atopic dermatitis, alopecia areata, dyshidrotic eczema, mastocytosis, acute and chronic pityriasis lichenoides, generalized granuloma annulare and pityriasis rubra pilaris.

PUVA can also be used to induce tolerance in some photosensitive disorders such as polymorphic light eruption. PUVA has the advantage of intense and rapid pigment induction at relatively low UVA doses.

Side Effects

Photosensitivity occurs after use of psoralens; pruritus, blistering and painful erythema occur after treatment on exposure to sunlight. This effect can be minimised if the dose of UVA is monitored carefully and the patient avoids exposure to sunlight. Taking the drug with milk can reduce nausea.

Long-term toxic reactions include changes in the skin pigmentation, cataract, increased incidence of skin cancer, particularly squamous and basal cell carcinoma.

Monitoring of Psoralens

The following tests should be done before treatment; the tests should again be repeated after 3, 6 and 12 months of therapy.

- Complete blood test
- Anti-nuclear antibody test
- Liver functions
- Renal functions
- Patients should have an ophthalmic examination before the start of therapy and thereafter yearly.

Before starting psoralen therapy, patients should not sunbathe 24 hours before psoralen ingestion and UVA exposure.

Ultraviolet A absorbing sunglasses should be worn during daylight and 24 hours after psoralen intake. The protective eyewear must be designed to prevent the entry of stray radiation to the eyes. This is to protect the binding of psoralens to the proteins and DNA component of the lens, cataract occurs when the binding occurs.

Patients should avoid sun exposure through the window glass and clouds for at least 8 hours after taking psoralens. Sunscreen should be applied during and after therapy.

During PUVA therapy, eyes and genital areas should be shielded.

Contraindications of Psoralen Therapy

- Patients exhibiting idiosyncratic reactions to psoralen compounds
- Patients with photosensitive disorders
- Patients with cutaneous malignancies
- Patients with absence of lenses, because of significant increase of retinal damage
- Previous history of arsenic poisoning.

The use of psoralens for the treatment of vitiligo dates back to ancient Egyptian and Indian healers. Psoralens are extracts of the plant Ammi majus. In 1974, PUVA therapy came into effect; psoralen administration followed by exposure to UVA, was found to be effective in the treatment of psoriasis.

IMMUNOSUPPRESSIVE AND CYTOTOXIC DRUGS

These drugs are primarily developed for use in oncology. In dermatology, they are used for the treatment of autoimmune disorders such as pemphigus, pemphigoid, systemic lupus erythematosus, histiocytosis and mycosis fungoides.

Some of the drugs used by the dermatologist are:

- Cyclophosphamide
- Methotrexate
- Azathioprine
- 5-Fluorouracil
- Cyclosporin
- Tacrolimus
- Mycophenolate mofetil.

Cyclophosphamide

Cyclophosphamide is an alkylating agent. The effect of the drug is dependent on the alkylation of DNA as the cell enters the S phase of the mitotic cycle. It is well absorbed when taken orally; the drug is activated by hepatic cytochrome P-450-enzyme system. It differs from other alkylating agents because thrombocytopenia is less common. There is more damage to the hair follicles, resulting frequently in alopecia. Acute central nervous system symptoms are not noted. Nausea and vomiting may occur. The drug is not a vesicant and there is no local irritation.

The occurrence of sterile haemorrhagic cystitis is reported in 5–10% of patients. This is due to the chemical irritation produced by reactive metabolites of cyclophosphamide. Its incidence is relieved by the administration of acetyl cysteine. For routine clinical use, ample fluid intake and frequent voiding are recommended. Administration of the drug should be interrupted on occurrence of dysuria and haematuria.

Inappropriate secretion of antidiuretic hormone (ADH) has been observed in patients receiving cyclophosphamide in high doses (above 50 mg/kg). It is important to be aware of the possibility of water intoxication, since these patients are vigorously hydrated.

Dose for dermatological use is 1–3 mg/kg of body weight in 2–3 divided doses. It is used with steroids in the treatment of pemphigus, pemphigoid, Wegener's granulomatosis, systemic lupus erythematosus, polymyositis, mycosis fungoides and histiocytosis.

Methotrexate

Methotrexate is a folic acid antagonist; it binds to dehydrofolic acid reductase and prevents the production of tetrahydrofolic acid, the active coenzyme form of folic acid. It acts on the S phase of the cell cycle. It is also a powerful immunosuppressant, with little anti-inflammatory activity.

Methotrexate is rapidly absorbed from the gastrointestinal tract at doses of less than 25 mg/m^2, larger doses are absorbed incompletely, larger doses are therefore given by the intravenous route. About 35% of methotrexate is bound to the plasma proteins, this may displace phenytoin. Caution should be used if these drugs are used concomitantly. It diffuses poorly in the central nervous system. About 40–50% of the small dose and about 90% of the large dose is excreted unchanged in the urine within 48 hours of administration. A small amount is also excreted in the stools.

Methotrexate is retained in the cells as polyglutamate for long periods, for weeks in the kidney and for months in the liver. There is also evidence of enterohepatic circulation.

Therapeutic Application

Methotrexate is used in the treatment of lymphoblastic leukemia, hydatidiform mole, choriocarcinoma, Burkitt's tumour, and non-Hodgkin's lymphoma. In dermatology, it is used in the treatment of psoriasis, Reiter's disease, pityriasis rubra pilaris, ichthyosiform erythroderma, sarcoidosis, Norwegian scabies and keratoacanthoma. It is effective in pemphigus, pemphigoid and corticosteroid resistant dermatomyositis.

Side Effects

The primary toxic effect of methotrexate is on the bone marrow and intestinal epithelium. The blood cell counts are depressed and there is mucosal ulceration. Such patients may be at risk from spontaneous haemorrhage or life-threatening infection.

The major long-term concern in the use of methotrexate is the development of chronic hepatic toxicity. Major risk appears to be related to the cumulative dose of methotrexate. A cumulative dose of 2,000–4,000 mg of methotrexate is associated with the development of hepatic cirrhosis and fibrosis. Other risk factors appear to be age, obesity and alcohol consumption. Because liver function tests can be normal in the presence of hepatic toxicity, a liver biopsy is indicated in patients who have received more than 1.5 g of methotrexate. Serum level of amino-terminal polypeptide of type III procollagen is a marker for hepatic fibrosis. The other major concern in the long-term use of methotrexate is teratogenicity and pulmonary toxicity. Methotrexate is teratogenic to pregnant women, there is no evidence that methotrexate taken by males or non-pregnant women have any effect on fertility or offspring. Methotrexate occasionally causes oligospermia. This is reversible.

Pulmonary toxicity is related to hypersensitivity syndrome that rapidly reverses on discontinuation of therapy and administration of corticosteroids.

Neurological toxicity is associated with intrathecal administration of the drug. These include subacute meningeal irritation, seizures and encephalopathy. Neurological complications are not reversed by folinic acid (leucovorin).

Additional toxicities include alopecia, dermatitis, nausea, vomiting and diarrhoea. Renal complications are due to the high dose of methotrexate administration.

Folinic acid (leucovorin) is a potent antidote for methotrexate overdose. Leucovorin can be interconverted to other reduced folates and bypass the block in the folate reduction by methotrexate. Folinic acid administered daily in a dose of 5 mg, except on the day methotrexate is taken, can minimize the toxicity of methotrexate. For overdose 25 mg of leucovorin is given by IM injection within the first four hours.

Azathioprine

Azathioprine is a purine analog, derived from 6-mercaptopurine by the addition of an imidazole ring on to sulphur. The major effect occurs on the inhibition of both DNA and RNA synthesis. It is most active in the S phase of the cell cycle.

Azathioprine is a popular immunosuppressive drug; it causes immunosuppression in doses that do not cause significant leucopenia. Its principal use is in the reduction of the steroid dose, required in the induction and maintenance of remission of pemphigus and pemphigoid. Azathioprine is effective in psoriasis, shows some activity in pityriasis rubra pilaris.

Side Effects

Azathioprine causes nausea, vomiting and diarrhoea. Bone marrow depression is the chief toxicity, especially in patients with reduced levels of thiopurine methyltransferase. Hepatic toxicity has been reported.

5-Fluorouracil

5-fluorouracil is a pyrimidine analog; it has a stable fluorine atom in place of a hydrogen atom at the position of the uracil ring. The fluorine interferes with the conversion of deoxyuridylic acid to the thymidylic acid, thus depriving the cell of one of the essential precursors for DNA synthesis.

Pharmacokinetics

Because of severe toxicity to the gastrointestinal tract, 5-fluorouracil is given by the intravenous route or topically administered. The drug penetrates well into all the tissues including the CSF. It is metabolised in the liver largely to carbon dioxide, which is exhaled.

Therapeutic Application

5-fluorouracil is essentially used in the treatment of slow growing solid tumours such as breast, ovary, colon, rectal and gastric tumours. Adjuvant therapy with levamisole improves the survival of patients with colonic cancer.

5-fluorouracil is the most common used cancer therapy in dermatology. Its major use is via the topical application, this admits its use with minimal adverse reactions. 5-fluorouracil is used in the treatment of superficial basal and squamous cell carcinoma, actinic keratosis, kerato-acanthoma, facial warts and lentigo maligna.

Side Effects

These include nausea, vomiting, diarrhoea, alopecia, severe ulceration of the oral and gastrointestinal mucosa and bone marrow suppression. A dermopathy (erythematous desquamation of the palms and soles) called hand-foot syndrome is seen after extended infusion.

Cyclosporin

Cyclosporin belongs to the family of cyclic peptides produced by a ground fungus; *Tolypocladium inflatum* Gams. It is a neutral lipophilic cyclic peptide made of 11 amino acids.

Mode of Action

Cyclosporin suppresses cell-mediated immunity by interfering with the early events involved in the activation of T cells. Its primary target appears to be helper T lymphocytes, with little effect on other aspects of the immune response. The cell cycle of the helper T lymphocytes is blocked in the G_0 or early G_1 phase of the cycle. Because it acts early in the process of T cell activation, it has secondary effects on other cell types that are normally activated by factors produced by the T cells. The production of various lymphokines notably interleukin-2 (IL-2) is therefore inhibited. It may also have some direct effect on DNA synthesis and proliferation of keratinocytes. Unlike other cytotoxic immunosuppressants, therapeutic concentration of cyclosporin does not cause immunosuppression.

Pharmacokinetics

The oral bioavailability of cyclosporin varies from 20% to 50%, peak concentrations of the drug in the plasma is achieved in 3–4 hours. About 60–70% of the drug in whole blood is contained in the erythrocytes; leucocytes contain 10–15% of the circulating cyclosporin. The remainder of the drug circulates largely in association with plasma lipoproteins. It has a half-life of about 6 hours.

Most of the drug is metabolised in the liver and excreted in the bile. Very little appears in the urine. The cyclic peptide structure of the drug is relatively resistant to the attack, but cytochrome P-450 group of enzymes mediate extensive oxidation of the side chains.

Dose

About 2–5 mg/kg/day, increments should not be more than 0.5–1 mg/kg/day at 2–4 week intervals.

Side Effects

The major toxic manifestation of cyclosporin is nephrotoxicity, this occurs in 25–75% of patients treated with the drug. The toxicity is dose related and usually irreversible, nephrotoxicity frequently mandates cessation of the therapy. Plasma concentrations of creatinine and urea are used to guide dosage.

Hypertension (10–15% elevation of blood pressure) is seen in more than 30% of patients receiving cyclosporin. Cyclosporin induces a dose-related rise in arterial blood pressure. Neurological complications are common, seen especially in recipients of hepatic transplant patients. About 50% of patients receiving cyclosporin have elevated transaminase activity or increased concentrations of bilirubin in the plasma. The abnormality usually disappears if the dose is reduced or discontinued.

Hirsutism, gingival hyperplasia is seen in 10–30% of patients who receive cyclosporin, but these reactions rarely affect therapy. Headache, paresthesias, gynaecomastia, conjunctivitis and tinnitus are observed occasionally.

Long-term toxicity includes increased tendency for lymphoma formation.

Drug Interactions

Ketoconazole, erythromycin, amphotericin B increase the blood levels of cyclosporin. Rifampicin, hydantoin, trimethoprim and sulphamethoxazole decrease blood levels of cyclosporin, primarily as a result of induction of hepatic cytochrome P-450 enzyme system. Nonsteroidal anti-inflammatory drugs are seen to increase the nephrotoxicity without changing the blood levels.

Therapeutic Uses

Cyclosporin is used primarily in combination with prednisolone to sustain renal, hepatic and cardiac transplants. Dermatological uses include psoriasis, atopic dermatitis, lichen planus, Behcet's disease, pyoderma gangrenosum, and chronic eczema of the hands. It is also used in pemphigus, pemphigoid, mycosis fungoides, Sezary's syndrome and dermatomyositis.

Mycophenolate Mofetil

Mycophenolate mofetil (MMF) is an ester of mycophenolic acid. Mycophenolic acid was used in the treatment of psoriasis in the early 1970s, but due to its side effects it was discontinued. Its ester mycophenolate mofetil has greater bioavailability and immunosuppressive action. In the body, it is converted to mycophenolic acid; this restrains the proliferation of T and B lymphocytes and reduces the production of cytotoxic T cells. MMF inhibits purine synthesis by inhibiting inosine monophosphate dehydrogenase; the precursor of DNA and RNA synthesis.

It is used as steroid sparing drug when other immunosuppressants cannot be used. It is used in the treatment of autoimmune bullous disorders, atopic dermatitis, psoriasis, pyoderma gangrenosum, graft versus host reaction, etc.

Dose

About 1–2 g/day.

Side Effects

Side effects include nausea, vomiting, leucopenia, anaemia and hepatitis. It should not be given with azathioprine, because azathioprine also blocks purine synthesis by the same pathway. The drug should be monitored frequently for liver functions, blood counts, and haemoglobin levels.

Leflunomide

This inhibits pyrimidine synthesis by inhibiting mitochondrial dihydroorotate dehydrogenase. It also inhibits proliferation of T cells, B cells and polymorphonuclear cells.

The drug is used in the treatment of psoriasis, lichen planus, bullous immune disorders, rheumatoid arthritis and systemic vasculitis.

Dose

The dose is 100 mg/day for 3 days and then 10–25 mg/day. The initial loading dose is more suitable for rheumatoid arthritis; in cutaneous disorders, this form of administration may not be necessary.

Side Effects

Nausea, vomiting, hypersensitivity syndrome, hepatic, and renal toxicity, bone marrow depression, Stevens-Johnson syndrome, and erythroderma.

IMMUNOBIOLOGICS

Immunobiologics are biologically active molecules that have immunological actions. They are specially targeted to initiate or inhibit naturally occurring proteins. The main categories include monoclonal antibodies, fusion proteins and interferons. Monoclonal antibodies can be murine, chimeric, primatised or humanised. These agents play a crucial role in organ transplantation, and in the therapy of autoimmune and inflammatory disorders. Topical immunomodulators are agents that regulate and modify the local immune response of the skin. They are safe therapeutic alternatives for several immune-mediated diseases, such as atopic dermatitis, psoriasis, alopecia areata and vitiligo.

Monoclonal Antibodies

Infliximab

This is a chimeric monoclonal antibody. It inhibits cytokines and tumour necrosis factor-α (TNF-α).

Infliximab is used in psoriasis, rheumatoid arthritis, Behcet's disease, pyoderma gangrenosum, graft versus host disease, toxic epidermolytic necrosis (TEN) and subcutaneous pustular dermatosis.

Dose: About 3–5 mg/kg is given as an intravenous infusion, alone or combined with other immunosuppressants, to decrease the chance of antibody formation. The injection may be repeated every 4–6 weeks as required.

Side effects: Side effects include diarrhoea, headache, upper respiratory tract infections, urinary tract infections, re-activation of tuberculosis and other infections.

Infliximab may produce autoantibody-mediated immune syndrome. Subsequent infusion of infliximab may lead to the development of neutralising antibodies, which may diminish its therapeutic effect, when used in the absence of a concomitant immunosuppressive agent.

Other monoclonal antibodies are basiliximab, daclizumab, and siplizumab. Golimumab is a monoclonal antibody which also inhibits TNF. It is used to treat rheumatoid arthritis, psoriatic arthritis and ankylosing spondylitis.

Efalizumab a humanised monoclonal antibody, was used in moderate-to-severe psoriasis. It inhibited the activation and trafficking of T cells. The drug is now withdrawn because of encephalopathy reported in some patients.

Fusion Proteins

Etanercept

This is a fusion protein that contains soluble TNF-α receptor protein and Fc component of IgG. It inhibits cytokines TNF-α and TNF-β.

Etanercept is used to treat psoriasis, rheumatoid arthritis, cicatricial pemphigoid, and scleroderma. It can be used in combination with methotrexate to treat psoriatic arthritis.

Dose: The dose is 25 mg by subcutaneous injection administered twice weekly. Response to psoriasis is slower than infliximab.

Side effects: Injection site reactions can occur, the drug is otherwise well tolerated.

Etanercept has better safety profile and long remissions rates.

Alefacept

This is a fusion protein combining LFA-3 (CD58) and the constant region (Fc) of human IgG antibody. The LFA component binds to T cells and blocks a co-stimulatory molecule required for activation of antigen processing cells (APC). The Fc segment attracts natural killer cells which cause apoptosis of T cells.

Dose: About 10–15 mg given by intramuscular injection, once weekly for 12 weeks. Effects can be seen after 2 weeks of initiation of therapy, but the peak response is seen in 6–8 weeks after therapy has concluded.

Side effects: Headache, nausea, vomiting and upper respiratory tract infections.

Denileukin Diftitox

This is a fusion toxin that consists of diphtheria toxin and IL-2. It directs cytocidal action of diphtheric toxin, to cells with exposure to IL-2 receptors. Denileukin diftitox should not be administered if the albumin level is below 3 g.

Indication: T cell lymphoma.

Dose: About 9–18 μg/kg/day in an intravenous infusion daily for 5 days, every 3 weeks. Six courses are required to show partial or complete response.

Side effects: Acute hypersensitivity syndrome, flu-like illness, leucopenia, vascular leak syndrome, nausea, vomiting, and cutaneous rashes.

Inhibitors of Interleukin 12 and 23

These include Briakinumab and Ustekinumab. IL-12 and IL-23 are expressed in psoriatic plaques, and inhibitors of these cytokines have shown potential as therapeutic agents for the treatment of psoriasis and psoriatic arthritis.

Human Interferon

These are a family of glycoproteins that are synthesised by leukocytes (IFN-α), fibroblasts (IFN-β), and immune cells (IFN-γ). IFN-α is mainly used for therapeutic purposes. IFN-γ regulates the immune function and inhibits the synthesis of collagen.

Interferons are potent cytokines that possess complex antiviral, immuno-modulating and anti-proliferative effects. Endogenous production and release of interferons occurs in response to viruses especially double stranded RNA viruses. Other inducers of interferons are bacterial endotoxins, certain low-molecular weight compounds and microorganisms capable of intracellular growth.

Mode of Action

When a virus invades a cell, the presence of viral nucleic acid induces cells genetic machinery to produce interferon, which is secreted into the extra-cellular fluid. It warns the healthy cells of the potential viral attack and helps them to resist such an attack. Once released from the virus infected cells, interferons bind with the receptor on the plasma membranes of healthy neighbouring cells and even distant cells, which it reaches via the bloodstream. Here it triggers the production of potential virus blocking enzymes by the host cells. After binding with interferons, these cells synthesize enzymes that will breakdown the viral messenger RNA and inhibit protein synthesis essential for viral replication.

Interferons not only inhibit viral synthesis, but also reinforce other immune activities. They enhance macrophage phagocytic activity and stimulate production of antibodies. It also has anticancer effects.

Pharmacokinetics

Interferons are not absorbed orally, after intramuscular or subcutaneous injections, plasma peak levels appear after 4–8 hours. Initial half-life is about 40 minutes and terminal half-life is about 5 hours. The kidneys excrete negligible amounts.

Side Effects

Influenza-like illness follows systemic administration of alpha interferon. The reaction can be diminished by pretreatment with antipyretics. Bone marrow depression with thrombocytopenia and granulocytopenia is common. Neurotoxicity is characterised by somnolence, confusion and behavioural changes. Renal, hepatic and cardiac toxicity has been reported.

Uses

Interferon is used to treat leukemia, AIDS related Kaposi's sarcoma and condylomata accuminatum. It may be used to treat herpes zoster in immunocompromised patients, herpes keratoconjunctivitis, and hepatitis B virus infection. It is also effective in preventing respiratory infections by rhinovirus, but not by other viruses.

Interferon-α: Intra-lesional injections are administered three times a week for 3 weeks. A second course may be administered at 12–16 weeks.

Interferon-γ is used for the treatment of keloids in a dose of 0.1 mg, intralesionally once a week for 3 weeks. Localised scleroderma/morphea in a dose of 100 μg subcutaneously once a week for 4 weeks. In systemic sclerosis, it is given in a dose of 100 μg subcutaneously three times a week for 4 weeks. Interferon is also used in the treatment of condylomata acuminata, basal cell carcinoma, Bowenoid papulosis, and chronic granulomatous disease.

Key Points

Neutralising antibodies may be formed in response to interferon therapy, but these do not affect their efficacy.

Concomitant use with zidovudine may increase the hepatic complications and bone marrow suppression.

All patients should have a complete blood examination, liver function tests, renal functions, autoimmune profile, hepatitis screen, and chest X-ray to exclude any latent infection or active tuberculosis, before initiating treatment by biologics.

INTRAVENOUS IMMUNOGLOBULIN

Intravenous immunoglobulin are hetrogenous human gamma globulins containing IgG with traces of IgA and IgM. They are safe and effective therapeutic option as immunomodulatory agents in the management of skin disorders, when other immunosuppressive agents cannot be used.

Mechanisms of Action

- Blocks Fc receptors
- Prevents complement-mediated damage
- Inhibits IL-1, IL-6 and TNF-α
- Reduces circulating pathogens and antibodies
- Increases immunoglobulin catabolism.

Uses

Autoimmune bullous disorders, toxic epidermal necrolysis, hypersensitivity syndromes, Kawasaki's disease, graft-versus-host reaction, pyoderma gangrenosum.

Side Effects

The side effects are rare; these are usually self-limiting and may be related to the infusion rate. These include headache, nausea, vomiting, hypersensitivity reactions, acute renal failure, haemolysis and neutropenia.

Key Points

- As IgG is not compatible with normal saline, it has to be diluted with 5% dextrose.
- Serum concentrations are achieved immediately.
- IgG can interact with live virus vaccine, these should not be given for 14 days before and 3 months after IgG infusion.
- Sudden infusion can suppress antibody production, with rebound flare up after discontinuation of therapy. The infusion should be given slowly at the rate of 0.01–0.02 mL/kg/minute, and then slowly increased to a maximum of 0.08 mL/kg/minute.

TOPICAL IMMUNOMODULATORS

These are classified as steroidal and non-steroidal immunomodulatory agents. The non-steroidal immunomodulatory agents are:

- Macrolactams
- Contact sensitizers
- Immunostimulators
- Miscellaneous agents

Macrolactams

These have the structure of a macrolide antibiotic. They inhibit the action of T cells by inhibiting calcineurin. They also inhibit the production of a variety of cytokines including IL-2, IL-3, IL-8, TNF-α and IFN-γ.

Tacrolimus

This is a macrolide antibiotic, its action is similar to cyclosporin. The difference lies in its protein receptor. This protein inhibits calcineurin and the effects produced are similar to cyclosporin. Tacrolimus can be given orally, intravenously or applied locally. In dermatology, the local form is used in the treatment of vitiligo and atopic dermatitis. It does not penetrate the thick skin of psoriasis but can be used in inverse psoriasis.

Topically the side effects include burning, itching, allergic reactions and urticaria. Herpes simplex/zoster and eczema herpeticum are rare complications.

Dose: It is administered as 0.03%, 0.1% ointmemt to be applied twice a day.

Pimecrolimus

This is an ascomycin derivative, and it is a potent calcineurin inhibitor. The indications are similar to tacrolimus. It has a greater safety profile than tacrolimus and can be used in infants as young as 3 months of age.

It is administered as 1% cream to be applied twice a day.

Sirolimus **(***Rapamycin***)**

This is only used for systemic administration and has no topical preparation. It is used in renal transplantation.

Contact Sensitisers

These include dinitrochlorobenzene (DNCB), diphenylcyclopropenone (DPCP) and squaric acid dibutylesters (SADBE).

Dinitrochlorobenzene

Dinitrochlorobenzene modifies the immune response in different ways, either by altering the CD4: CD8 ratios and enhancing the cell-mediated immune response. They are used in the treatment of alopecia areata, warts, and cutaneous malignancies such as Bowen's disease, actinic keratosis, and some basal cell carcinoma.

Dinitrochlorobenzene (DNCB) is mutagenic and should not be administered to women of child bearing age.

Diphenylcyclopropenone/Diphencyprone

The actions are similar to that of DNCB, but it is not mutagenic and has a shorter half-life. It is used in concentrations of 0.1–3% solution in acetone.

Squaric Acid Dibutylesters

The actions are similar to DNCB and diphenylcylopropenone (DPCP); they are not mutagenic and have a shorter half-life than DPCP. It has to be refrigerated.

Immunostimulators

These are stimulators of IFN-γ, inhibits tumour necrosis factor α and a number of cytokines such as IL-1, IL-6, IL-8. Interferons are responsible for antiviral, antitumour and immunoregulatory activities. They stimulate the natural killer cells and enhance migration of Langerhans cells.

Imiquimod is used in the treatment of viral infections such as genital warts, common warts and molluscum contagiosum. It has been used for the treatment of keloids, because it is said to enhance collagenase activity. It is also used in leishmaniasis, some malignant and pre-malignant conditions of the skin. Imiquimod should not be used in children under 18 years.

Dose

Cream (5%) is available to be applied overnight three times a week. Around 6–12 weeks are required to see the response of imiquimod.

Miscellaneous

These include anthralin, calcipotriol, topical BCG vaccine, minoxidil, eflornithine and topical zinc.

Calcipotriol, tacalcitol and calcitriol are vitamin D analogues. They act via vitamin D receptors to regulate cell growth, differentiation and immune response. They are used in psoriasis and other keratinising disorders, morphoea, vitiligo, lichen sclerosus and acanthosis nigricans. They should not be applied if the infected area is more than 35% of the body surface to prevent hypercalcemia. These preparations should not be used on the face or intertriginous areas. Vitamin D_3 derivatives should not be used in patients with disorders of calcium metabolism.

Calcipotriol is available as 50 µg/g cream and ointment, to be applied twice a day. Not used for children under 18 years.

Tacalcitriol is available as 4 µg/g ointment.

Calcitriol has been introduced recently for topical use in psoriasis. It is available as 3 µg/g ointment, it does not smell or stain. It may be more acceptable than tar or dithranol.

Side effects include hypercalcemia, irritation, photosensitivity and allergic contact dermatitis.

ANTIMALARIALS

The antimalarials of dermatological use are the aminoquinolines. These include chloroquine, hydroxychloroquine, amodiaquine and quinacrine.

Mode of Action

The four aminoquinolines have several actions on the biochemical and cellular systems of the body. Some of these actions are:

The interaction with nucleic acid: Aminoquinolines bind to DNA; they inhibit DNA replication and transcription to RNA. This helps in the inhibition of the antinuclear antibody reactions and lupus erythematosus cell phenomenon.

Immunological effects: Aminoquinolines suppress lymphocytes transformation in vitro; they also interfere with complement dependent antigen antibody reaction.

Anti-inflammatory action: Chloroquine has been shown to be a lysosomal inhibitor. It also inhibits hydrolytic enzymes and interferes with prostaglandin synthesis.

Photodermatological properties: Chloroquine absorbs UVA and is bound in the epidermis in high concentrations. However, there is no effect on the minimum erythema dose.

Pharmacodynamics

The aminoquinolines are water-soluble and are readily absorbed from the gastrointestinal tract. The plasma concentration reaches a peak level within 8 hours. Liver, spleen, lungs and adrenals store chloroquine in large amounts. Melanin containing cells have a great affinity for chloroquine. The high intake of chloroquine in the liver may be of importance for the use of this drug in the treatment of porphyria cutanea tarda. The melanin affinity may be the basis for the ocular side effects.

Therapeutic Uses

Malaria and rheumatoid arthritis are the chief indications of aminoquinolines. In dermatology, it is used mainly in the treatment of lupus erythematosus, polymorphous light eruption, porphyria cutanea tarda. Other conditions in which it can be used are sarcoidosis, solar urticaria, scleroderma, lymphatic infiltration of the skin, disseminated granuloma annulare, cutaneous leishmaniasis, epidermolysis bullosa, acrodermatitis chronica atrophicans and lichen sclerosus.

In lupus erythematosus, the full therapeutic effects are seen in a month. Cutaneous symptoms respond better than the systemic involvement. The seriously ill patient with fever, renal damage and haematological abnormalities do not benefit from aminoquinolines. In polymorphous light eruption, the disease is confined to the sun-exposed areas of the skin and the histology shows that immunological factors are involved in the pathogenesis.

Chloroquine has been found to be beneficial in the treatment of porphyria cutanea tarda. The mechanism of action is different from that of lupus erythematosus. There is a high affinity of chloroquine for the liver tissue. Uroporphyrin and chloroquine compete with the same binding site in the liver tissue; chloroquine is able to displace the porphyrins from the tissue. Following the administration of chloroquine, there is a massive excretion of porphyrins in the urine.

Side Effects

Side effects of aminoquinolines are weakness, dyspnea, hypotension, tremor, coma, convulsions and cardiopulmonary arrest. Toxic psychosis, headache and irritability are also seen. All aminoquinolines induce leucopenia within the first few weeks of treatment. Aminoquinolines are teratogenic; they cross the placenta and cause congenital defects such as mental retardation and convulsions in the newborn.

Cutaneous Side Effects

Exacerbation of psoriasis and discolouration of the skin is seen on long-term use. Quinacrine gives a yellowish discolouration after a month of treatment. The other aminoquinolines give a bluish-black pigmentation of the pretibial region, palate, face and nail beds. The pigmentation is reversible over time.

Ocular Side Effects

Ocular side effects are the main disadvantage of amonoquinolines, especially on long-term use. Both chloroquine and hydroxychloroquine give deposits on the cornea. They produce symptoms such as visual halos. Irreversible retinopathy is the most limiting factor for use of aminoquinolines. The retinopathy is dose dependent. The two common views to prevent the side effects are: the accumulated dose of chloroquine should not exceed 200 gram, the other is that the daily dose should not exceed 4.4 mg/kg of the body weight. A daily dose of 250 mg of chloroquine is safe if there is a yearly interruption of therapy for about 2 months. An ophthalmologist should see the patients at regular intervals.

DAPSONE

Dapsone is the drug of choice in the treatment of leprosy and dermatitis herpetiformis.

Pharmacokinetics

After oral administration 80–85% of the drug is absorbed, peak levels are reached in 4–6 hours after a single dose; the half-life of dapsone is from 2–4 days. Its retention in the body is prolonged due to the enterohepatic circulation. Dapsone is excreted via the kidneys.

Dapsone is metabolised in the liver. Two major metabolic pathways are involved, acetylation and hydroxylation. From the clinical standpoint, control of symptoms of leprosy and dermatitis herpetiformis is related to the acetylated metabolite. The hydroxylated form of dapsone is responsible for the methemoglobinemia, haemolysis and Heinz body formation.

Mechanism of Action

Dapsone is a potent oxidant with a notable influence on glutathione. Its bacteriostatic effect is by the interference with folate biosynthetic pathway of bacteria. It also incorporates into lecithin of bacterial cell membrane thereby decreasing phospholipid synthesis.

Various investigations have shown that dapsone inhibits lysosomal activity and interferes with myeloperoxidase-mediated cytotoxic system in neutrophils. Dapsone interferes with the complement activation and deposition. It may also inhibit neutrophils from responding to some chemotactic stimuli.

Interaction with drugs: Probenecid blocks the renal excretion of dapsone; rifampicin increases the rate of dapsone clearance.

Therapeutic Application

Dermatitis herpetiformis, leprosy and erythema elevatum diutinum are particularly affected by dapsone. Other diseases that can be treated by dapsone include chronic bullous diseases such as pemphigus, pemphigoid, linear IgA disease, chronic bullous disease of childhood, subcorneal pustular dermatosis and bullous form of systemic lupus erythematosus. Relapsing polychondritis, acne conglobata, leucocytoclastic vasculitis and granuloma faciale can also be treated by dapsone.

Side Effects

Dapsone therapy produces haemolysis and methemoglobinemia. The hydroxylated metabolite is responsible for these side effects. It can be anticipated that a patient receiving more than 50 mg of dapsone will have some degree of haemolysis, which will be reflected in lowered haemoglobin level. Patients with glucose-6-phosphate dehydrogenase deficiency have a greater decrease of haemoglobin level. Most of the patients tolerate the fall in haemoglobin level well. An increase in reticulocytes will accompany the fall in haemoglobin level. After several months of treatment, the haemoglobin level may rise to almost pre-treatment levels, but the level will usually remain 1 g below the original level.

Methemoglobinemia will also regularly occur in patients treated with dapsone, but it is not a major problem in most patients. The methemoglobinemia is more pronounced at the onset of treatment and it is somewhat dose dependent. Symptoms of methemoglobinemia include weakness, tachycardia, nausea, headache and abdominal pain. These symptoms should be considered when the methemoglobin level is 20% or greater.

Dapsone hypersensitivity may occur after 2–6 weeks of therapy. The clinical features include fever, mononucleosis-like illness, malaise, lymphadenopathy, hepatitis and hypothyroidism. Skin rash may begin as maculopapular rash, may progress on to exfoliative dermatitis. Eosinophils and atypical lymphocytes are present in the peripheral blood.

The other pharmacological effects of dapsone are loss of motor function. It develops during the first two months of therapy. Typically, the distal upper and lower extremities are involved, weakness of the limbs is the most common complaint. Foot drop is a common manifestation. Sensory involvement is rare. Symptoms slowly improve over months to years after stopping the treatment. Hypoalbuminemia, acute psychosis and a potentially fatal mononucleosis-like syndrome is seen in patients with dapsone therapy. Agranulocytosis is also reported.

Monitoring of Dapsone Therapy

Before instituting therapy with sulfones, a full blood count should be obtained. In addition, Asians, Africans and people of the Mediterranean descent should be tested for glucose-6-phosphate dehydrogenase deficiency.

After therapy has begun, leucocyte count with differential and haemoglobin level should be obtained weekly or twice a month during the first 3 months. Thereafter complete blood picture should be obtained every 3–4 months. Liver function tests and renal functions should be obtained before the institution of therapy and periodically thereafter.

Once the disease is under control, the dose of dapsone should be reduced, the patient should use the minimum amount of the drug required. If the dose of the drug has to be altered as in dermatitis herpetiformis, the dose should be gradually increased.

ANTIVIRAL DRUGS

The therapy of viral disease has been more difficult than those of other microorganisms. The virus grows within the cell of the host; the therapeutic agents that act against the virus should be such that they do not affect the host cells. There are only a few of antiviral drugs available. With the spread of AIDS, considerable efforts are being made for the search of new antiviral drugs. Drug resistance may also occur with other antiviral agents, but often there is a modification of viral genome making the drug ineffective to the virus. For the past two centuries live and activated vaccines have been the major weapons against viral infections. Research in antiviral therapy began in the early 1950s, when the search for cancer treatments generated several new compounds capable of inhibiting viral DNA synthesis. One such compound was the pyrimidine analog idoxuridine, which subsequently was approved for the treatment of herpes keratitis.

Acyclovir

Acyclovir is synthetic purine nucleoside analogue; it requires three phosphorylation steps for activation. It is selectively phosphorylated by the herpes virus thymidine kinase to monophosphate derivative. The monophosphate form is subsequently converted to diphosphate and then to acycloguanosine triphosphate (acyclo-GTP) by host cellular enzymes. Acyclo-GTP inhibits herpes virus DNA polymerase, 10–30 times more effectively than it inhibits cellular DNA polymerase.

Pharmacokinetics

Acyclovir is widely distributed throughout the body, however the concentration in the CSF is only one-third to half that of the plasma. Peak plasma levels after intravenous dose of 5 mg/kg of body weight is 10 µg/mL, after an oral dose of 200 mg, it is 1 µg/mL. The elimination half-life of acyclovir is about 2.5 hours in patients with normal renal function. The kidney is the primary route of excretion; dose adjustments are needed in patients with renal insufficiency. Acyclovir is concentrated in mother's milk; it should not be given to nursing mothers.

Antiviral Activity

The drug is active against herpes virus; varicella zoster virus is less sensitive, while Epstein-Barr virus may be inhibited only at high concentrations of the drug. Cytomegalovirus is inhibited at even higher concentrations.

Route of Administration and Dosage

Acyclovir is available as 200 mg capsules. For herpes simplex and genital herpes, 200 mg of acyclovir is given 5 times a day for 7–10 days. For herpes zoster, the dose is 800 mg given 5 times a day for 7–10 days.

For intravenous route, the dose is 5 mg/kg every 8 hours. For encephalitis, the dose is 10 mg/kg every 8 hours. The infusion is given over one hour period.

Oral acyclovir 400 mg every 12 hours or 200 mg every 8 hours is effective for clinical suppression of recurrent genital or labial herpes in patients with frequent outbreaks. Recurrence may resume after discontinuation of suppressive acyclovir therapy.

The ointment should be applied every three waking hours for 7–10 days; care should be taken to prevent autoinoculation.

Side Effects

The toxicity is limited to local irritation and transient burning sensation when applied to the genital region. Intravenous infusion is well tolerated. It is rarely associated with phlebitis, rash, diaphoresis, nausea, haematuria and hypotension. Encephalopathy is reported in 1% of cases.

Oral administration is well tolerated; occasional cases of nausea, vomiting and headache have been reported.

Antiviral Drugs Related to Acyclovir

Ganciclovir

This drug is similar to acyclovir, but differs from it structurally by the addition of a hydroxymethyl group. It inhibits viral DNA synthesis. It is phosphorylated initially to the monophosphate derivative by both viral and cellular kinase, then to diphosphate and triphosphate by the cellular enzymes. The incorporation of the phosphorylated drug to the viral DNA initiates the antiviral activity.

The drug is effective against all herpes virus. It is 100 times more effective against cytomegalovirus than against herpes virus. For the treatment of Epstein-Barr virus an even higher concentration of the drug is required.

Ganciclovir is generally used for the treatment of cytomegalovirus infection. Side effects include nephrotoxicity, metabolic disturbances, hypokalemia and hypocalcemia.

Valacyclovir

Valacyclovir is the valine ester of acyclovir. Valacyclovir is used to treat herpes zoster, varicella zoster, genital herpes and herpes labialis. For the treatment of herpes zoster, the dose is 1 g three times a day for 7 days.

Famciclovir

The drug is well absorbed after oral administration, given in a dose of 250–500 mg, three times daily. The incidence of post-herpetic neuralgia is low after its use.

Penciclovir

This is used in the treatment of severe herpes simplex infection. Because of its toxicity, it is given less frequently than acyclovir.

Zidovudine (Azidothymidine)

The drug is a synthetic thymidine analog. It was first synthesised in search for an anti-cancer drug; about a decade later, it was found to be an antiviral drug.

Mechanism of Action

Zidovudine is first phosphorylated by cellular enzymes to the corresponding deoxynucleoside triphosphate derivative. In this form, the drug inhibits the viral RNA-dependent DNA polymerase (reverse transcriptase). Its antiviral selectivity is due to the greater affinity for viral reverse transcriptase than for human DNA polymerase.

Acyclovir and interferon enhance the antiviral activity of zidovudine, but thymidine and ribavirin antagonize it.

Antiviral Activity

Zidovudine is an active agent against HIV-1 and other mammalian retroviruses. The quality of life is enhanced and the incidence of opportunistic infections is reduced considerably. Zidovudine also inhibits virus associated with T cell leukemia. It is less active against HIV-2 virus. It inhibits Epstein-Barr virus in high concentrations, but has no action against herpes simplex or varicella-zoster virus.

Route of Administration and Dosage

Zidovudine is available as 100 mg capsules for oral administration. The dose is 200 mg every 4 hourly. There is no preparation available for its parental use.

Side Effects

The main side effects are anaemia and neutropenia seen in about 45% of treated patients. The risk is directly related to the number of CD4 lymphocytes and granulocytes present at the time of therapy. Anaemia may occur as early as 2–4 weeks after starting therapy and neutropenia after 6–8 months. Haematological monitoring should be performed at 2 weekly intervals.

Other side effects include headache, nausea, vomiting and myalgia. Progressive pigmentation may occur in Afro-Caribbean patients. Severe neurotoxicity may manifest as seizures and Wernicke's encephalopathy. Seizures may occur as soon as 48 hours after initiation of therapy. Wernicke's encephalopathy may be delayed for 6–17 months. Zidovudine causes chromosomal abnormalities in cultured human lymphocytes; the teratogenicity of the drug is not adequately evaluated.

Other Retroviral Agents

Foscarnet

This is an inorganic phosphate analog. It inhibits viral DNA polymerase and reverse transcriptase. It is active against herpes virus, cytomegalic virus and HIV virus at concentrations of 3 µg/mL. Foscarnet is given by the intravenous route. Foscarnet enters the macrophages and inhibits the replication of HIV within these cells. Foscarnet is eliminated by the kidneys and small amounts accumulate in the bones.

Side effects: The most common untoward effect is reduced renal function. The drug increases both fluid intake and urine output. Other side effects include nausea, vomiting, fatigue and headache. Anaemia is common but neutropenia does not occur. Tremor, hypocalcemia and seizures may occur. Genital ulceration of the penis and the vulva has been reported.

Uses: It is used to treat herpes simplex resistant to acyclovir, cytomegalic virus infection and AIDS in combination with zidovudine.

Zalcitabine and Stavudine

Zalcitabine is a deoxynucleotide and stavudine is a thymidine analogue. Both of these antiviral agents are used to treat zidovudine resistant AIDS infection. It is used to treat patients with very low CD4 counts.

Side effects: Zalcitabine causes severe neuropathy, pancreatitis, rashes and hepatitis. Stavudine causes painful neuropathy.

Idoxuridine

The first antiviral compound demonstrated to be clinically effective was idoxuridine. Idoxuridine is a thymidine analog. The activity of idoxuridine is limited to the DNA viruses such as herpes simplex, poxvirus. Epithelial infections respond best, the results are less favourable when the stroma is involved. It is not given systemically due to hepatic and bone marrow toxicity. The topical form is only used. The primary clinical use of idoxuridine is in the treatment of herpes simplex keratitis. The drug is instilled into the conjunctival sac every hour during the day and every 2 hours during the night until improvement occur. It is then instilled every 2 hours during the day and every 4 hours during the night. Therapy is continued for 3–5 days after healing is complete.

Vidarabine

This is an adenosine analog; it acts by inhibiting viral DNA polymerase. It acts both topically and systemically. It is used to treat herpes virus encephalitis and varicella zoster infection in immunocompromised persons. Its use is now replaced by acyclovir. It is given in a dose of 15 mg/kg of body weight. As it is slightly soluble in water, large volumes of fluids are required to dissolve the compound (e.g. about 2.5 liters). The drug is given by intravenous route at a constant rate over 12–24 hours period for 10 days.

Antiviral Activity

Vidarabine is used in the treatment of herpes simplex encephalitis but acyclovir is superior. In herpes zoster of immunocompromised patients, vidarabine reduces the formation of new vesicles; it also accelerates the clearance of virus from the cells and vesicles, reduces pain, decreases the risk of dissemination and pain of post-herpetic neuralgia. Vidarabine applied locally is as effective as idoxuridine in herpes simplex infection.

Side Effects

These include weakness, thrombophlebitis at the site of drug administration, hypokalemia, inappropriate secretion of antidiuretic hormone. Side effects of the central nervous system include tremors, ataxia and psychosis. Thrombocytopenia, leucopenia and megaloblastic anemia are also recorded.

RIBAVIRIN

Ribavirin is a purine nucleoside analog that inhibits the replication in vitro of RNA and DNA viruses including myxovirus, paramyxovirus, influenza virus, etc. It is mainly used to treat pneumonias and respiratory infections. Patients with AIDS virus may show transient improvement when treated with ribavirin.

Amantadine and Rimantadine are mainly used to treat influenza virus.

PROMISE OF THE FUTURE: GENE THERAPY

Gene therapy is a genetic modification of cells to prevent, alleviate or cure disease. Using modern techniques, it is possible to identify and clone genes, alter DNA or RNA in the laboratory and produce large amounts of this modified nucleic acid. This recombinant nucleic acid coding for a gene will hopefully have a therapeutic effect.

The gene delivery for therapeutic purposes is usually in the form of a modified virus called a vector; it must pass from the plasma and nuclear membranes to be incorporated into the chromosomes. There are two ways of delivering genes in patients; in vivo and ex vivo.

- *In vivo*: Injection of a vector containing the therapeutic gene, directly into the patient, e.g. into a malignant tumour.
- *Ex vivo*: Method is taking the cells from the patient, e.g. stem cells from the marrow, treat them with the vector followed by re-injection of the genetically altered cells into the patient.

Vectors for Gene Therapy

A vector should be safe, efficient, selective and should cause persistent expression of the therapeutic gene. These can be viruses or non-viral vectors.

Viral Vectors

Viruses take over the metabolic machinery of the cell: they invade, and fuse with the host nucleic acid. On entering the cells of the host, the virus can produce undesirable results. Vectors are modified to render them non-pathogenic. Viruses are therefore used in ex vivo attempts for therapy. The viruses commonly used for gene therapy are the retrovirus and the adenovirus.

The retrovirus is incorporated in the host DNA and therefore its action is more persistent. Adenovirus vectors are popular because of the high transgene expression. They transfer genes to the nucleus of the host cell; but are not inserted into the host genome, and so do not produce lasting effects.

Other viral vectors are the herpes virus, disabled version of HIV virus, adeno-associated virus.

Non-Viral Vectors

Non-viral vectors are the liposomes, plasmid DNA and microspheres. These are much less efficient than viruses, and attempts are underway to improve this by incorporating various viral signal proteins in their outer coat.

Control of Gene Expression

Once the gene is introduced into the host, then it should be able to get the desired selective target, i.e. the gene expression should be controlled. It is not easy to transfer the gene selectively to the desired target cells. Gene transfer has been found to be effective in animals but the action on human beings is still experimental. One promising approach is the tetracycline inducible expression.

Problems Facing Viral Vectors

Although the viruses are modified, and made non-pathogenic, they may still acquire virulence during use.

Viral proteins that are immunogenic may produce an inflammatory response.

Viruses with mechanisms that regulate the cell cycle, could result in mutations and malignancy.

Therapeutic Application of Gene Therapy

Approximately half of the gene therapy is on cancer. They are also used to treat single gene defects such as cystic fibrosis and haemoglobinopathies.

An attempt is also made to treat diseases in which there is no genetic factor associated. The gene for endothelial growth factor is being used to stimulate the growth of new blood vessels around blockages in atherosclerotic arteries; some studies have shown encouraging results.

A deficient protein, such as insulin, factor VII, erythropoietin, can be grown in vivo and can be of help in treating diseases such as diabetes, haemophilia or chronic failure.

The first investigators to recognise the clinical potential of microorganisms as therapeutic agents were Pasteur and Joubert who recorded their observation in 1877. They noted that anthrax bacillus grows rapidly when inoculated into sterile urine, but failed to grow when bacteria were introduced into the urine. They commented on the fact that life destroys life.

The modern era of chemotherapy started with the clinical use of sulphonamides in 1936. The golden age of antimicrobial therapy began with the production of penicillin in 1941.

FURTHER READING

1. Castelo-Soccio L, Voorhees ASV. Long-term efficacy of biologics in dermatology. Dermatol Ther. 2009;22:22-33.
2. Crawford F, Young P, Godfrey C, et al. Oral treatment of onychomycosis: a systematic review. Arch Dermatol. 2002;138:811-6.
3. Daneshmend TK. The neurotoxicity of dapsone: adverse drug reactions. Acute Poison Rev.1984;3:53-8.
4. Groustein BN. The mechanism of action of methotrexate. Rheum Dis Clin North Am. 1997;23:739-55.
5. Grant SM, Clissold SP. Itraconazole. Drugs. 1989;37:310-44.
6. Gupta AK, Gollfarb MT, Ellis CN, et al. Side effects, profile of acitretin therapy in psoriasis. J Am Acad Dermatol. 1989;20:1088-93.
7. Lipsky JJ. Mycophenolate mofetil. Lancet. 1996;348:1357-9.
8. Mortel MR, Emer J. Prospective new biologic therapies for psoriasis and psoriatic arthritis. JDD. 2010;9(8):952-62.
9. Opravil M, Hirshel B, Lazzarin A, et al. A randomized trial of simplified maintenance therapy with abecavir, lamivudine and zidovudine in human immune deficiency virus infection. J Infec Dis. 2002;185(9):1251-60.
10. Powell HR, Ekert H. Methotrexate induced congenital malformations. Med J Aust. 1971;2:1076-7.
11. Vinod KV, Arun K, Dutta TK. Dapsone hypersensitivity syndrome: A rare life-threatening complication of dapsone. J Pharmacol Pharmcother. 2013;(2):158-60.
12. Yawalker SJ, Vischer W. Lamprene (clofazimine) in leprosy. Leprosy Rev. 1979;50:135-44.

Chapter

43

Cutaneous Drug Reactions

INTRODUCTION

Cutaneous drug reactions are common, they account for about 14% of skin disorders in admitted patients. The severity ranges from very mild to life-threatening conditions, such as toxic epidermal necrolysis (TEN).

CLASSIFICATION OF DRUG REACTIONS

- Nonimmunological adverse reactions: These are predictable reactions such as those caused by overdose, e.g. taking of sleeping pills in suicide, side effects, e.g. sedation by antihistamines, diarrhoea from antibiotics due to change of intestinal flora, drug interactions, most of these occur in drugs which are metabolised by cytochrome P450 enzymes.
- A number of drug reactions occur due to direct activation of mast cells (pseudo-allergic reaction). These are unpredictable.
- Immunological adverse reactions: These are unpredictable; they are mediated via the immune responses of the body. The immunological reactions are:
  - Type I, immunoglobulin E (IgE) mediated drug reactions
  - Type II, cytotoxic reactions
  - Type III, arthus or immune complex-mediated reactions
  - Type IV, Delayed hypersensitivity or cell-mediated.
- In some patients with hypersensitivity syndromes, there is increased sensitivity to reactive products produced by drugs resulting in Stevens-Johnson syndrome and TEN. The immune system may target the native drug or its metabolites.

Reactivation of herpes 6 virus appears to be common in drug hypersensitivity syndromes

- Idiopathic: The pathogenesis of most drug reactions is not known, although the clinical features of most drug reactions are consistent with immune-mediated diseases.

A number of acquired factors can also alter the risk of drug reactions in a patient, such as viral infections and internal malignancy. Drug reactions can also occur when the drugs are metabolised by the body and they produce toxic or reactive products. The reactive products are rapidly detoxified by the body. Drug-drug interaction can also increase the risk of cutaneous drug reactions. Old age, delays the onset of drug reactions, mortality rate is higher in these patients, who should be carefully monitored.

APPROACH TO DIAGNOSIS OF DRUG REACTIONS

To assess the likelihood that a given agent is responsible for changes in the skin or mucous membranes, a good history is important. However, the patient's notion of a drug may be surprisingly variable; laxatives, hypnotics, and simple analgesics are often regarded as part of a normal diet. The most common drugs responsible for drug reactions are *Betalactam* (β lactam) antibiotics, nonsteroidal anti-inflammatory drugs (NSAIDs), aspirin, barbiturates, sulphonamides and phenolphthalein.

The following points should be noted while taking a history of drug reaction.

- Previous experience with the drug, including the frequency of eruptions associated with the drugs administration and the pattern of morphologic reactions.
- The timing of events: A drug taken for the first time, will not elicit an allergic reaction within the first four days. Re-exposure, cross-reaction, or pseudo-allergic reaction all occur almost instantaneously such as anaphylaxis.
- The drug dose; important in overdose reaction.
- Signs and symptoms of mucous membrane and systemic involvement.
- Does the patient have known contact allergy to para-compounds: This would explain a reaction to sulphonamides, oral hypoglycemic drugs, local anaesthetics and, thiazide diuretics. Similarly, ethyl diamine sensitivity would explain sensitivity to theophylline compounds.
- Family history of drug reaction: Every individual has a unique array of enzymes that may influence how they react to drugs. Some enzymes relating to drug metabolism may have a genetic basis.
- Does the patient have any concomitant illness? Human immunodeficiency virus (HIV), internal malignancy can exacerbate drug reactions.
- Age of the patient: In an elderly patient drug reaction takes time, but has high morbidity.

SKIN LESIONS IN DRUG REACTION

The most common type of drug reactions are the maculopapular eruptions (40%), urticaria and angioedema (37%), fixed drug eruption (6%), EM/TEN (5%), and all other reactions (0–3%). Most drug eruptions have their first manifestations on the skin; this can serve as a warning sign for the more severe reactions.

Maculopapular Eruptions

This is the most common drug reaction. The reaction starts within 1 week of starting the therapy and resolves within 7–14 days. Lesions begin on the trunk, and then spread in a symmetrical manner. The rash appears as small erythematous macules and papules, which become confluent and form red plaques, with variable involvement of mucous membranes, palms and soles. The lesions may be scarlatiniform, rubelliform, morbilliform or a profuse eruption of small papules. The dermis and epidermis are involved. It may be accompanied by fever, pruritus and eosinophilia. This is synonymous with **D**rug **R**eaction, with **E**osinophila and **S**ystemic **S**ymptoms (DRESS syndrome). If administration of the drug is continued exfoliative dermatitis may occur. The most commonly implicated drugs are ampicillin, amoxicillin, aminoglycosides, phenylbutazone, barbiturates, benzodiazepines, phenytoin, carbamazepine, gold and piroxicam.

The reaction should be differentiated from viral exanthems, pityriasis rosea, collagen vascular disease and guttate psoriasis.

Urticarial Reactions and Angioedema

Urticaria is an immediate hypersensitivity reaction characterised by pruritic wheals, dermal vasodilation and oedema (the epidermis is not involved). Individual urticarial lesions rarely last more than 24 hours.

Angioedema (involvement of dermal and subcutaneous tissue) when severe can impair respiration, which may lead to life threatening anaphylaxis. The angioedema is frequently unilateral and non-pruritic. The most common drug responsible for angioedema is angiotensin-converting-enzyme (ACE) inhibitors.

Urticarial reactions are IgE-mediated hypersensitivity (type 1) reaction; urticaria usually occurs within 36 hours after drug administration but can occur within minutes. Direct stimulation of the masts cells may also give rise to similar reactions (pseudoallergic reaction).

Aspirin, penicillin and blood products are the most frequent causes of urticarial reactions. However, urticaria can be caused by other drugs, such as morphine, codeine, angiotensin-converting enzyme inhibitors, animal sera, dextran, cephalosporins, benzoates, hydantoin, toxoids, quinidine, radiocontrast media and the yellow dye tartrazine. Urticaria may accompany serum sickness reactions (type III) or systemic anaphylaxis.

Serum sickness like rash is defined by the presence of fever, arthralgia, an urticarial rash, 1–2 weeks after ingestion of the drug. Lymphadenopathy and eosinophilia may also be present. In contrast to true serum sickness, hypocomplementemia, immune complexes, vasculitis and renal lesions are absent.

Fixed Drug Eruption (FDE)

This is a unique form of drug reaction that produces a reaction at the same site, each time the drug is taken. The lesions are most common on the genitals, face, palms and soles, and mucous membrane. Typically the lesions are 5–10 cm in diameter, often solitary, multiple lesions can also occur. The lesions appear as erythematous plaques or bullae, the blisters then erode, crusting is followed by hyperpigmentation, violaceous or brown in colour (Figs 1 and 2). The lesions are preceded by itching and burning. Fixed drug eruption (FDE) is uncommon in children.

On re-exposure of the drug, the rash usually appears within 30 minutes to 8 hours, at the same site. Some patients may demonstrate a refractory period of weeks to months during which the offending drug does not activate the lesion.

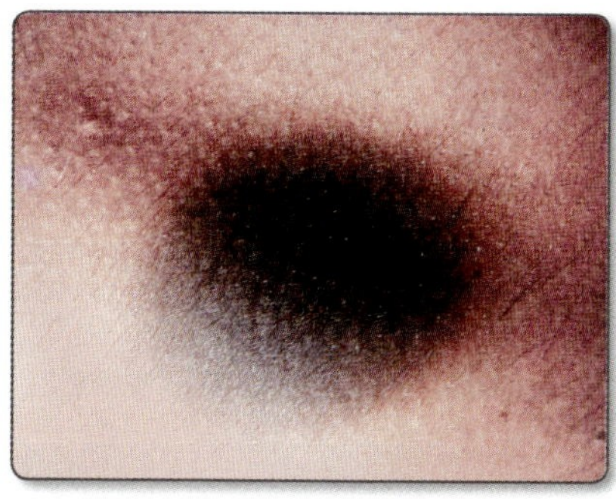

Fig. 1: Fixed drug eruption

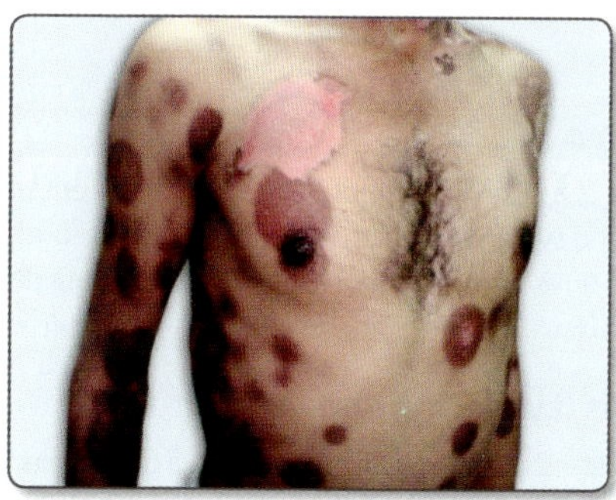

Fig. 2: Fixed drug eruption—generalised

The histology is similar to that of erythema multiforme, with hydropic degeneration of the basal cells, pigmentary incontinence and lymphocytes at the dermoepidermal junction, degeneration of the epithelium with dyskeratosis. There is also evidence of chronic injury, such as acanthosis, hypergranulosis and hyperkeratosis. Eosinophils and neutrophils are also present. T memory lymphocytes are present in the lesional skin, which is said to contribute to immunological memory.

Sulphonamides, aspirin, ibuprofen, tetracyclines, metamizole, hyoscine butylbromide, barbiturates, chlordiazepoxide, dapsone, phenazone, phenolphthalein, quinine, benzodiazepines, systemic antifungal drugs and paracetamol have also been implicated.

Non-pigmented fixed drug reactions have been documented with pseudoephedrine.

SEVERE SKIN REACTIONS

Erythema Multiforme

Erythema multiforme (EM) is an acute, self-limiting inflammatory disorder of the skin, the mucous membrane is rarely involved. Most cases follow herpes simplex, the lesions are present on the distal extremities with the typical target lesion (Fig. 3). EM following drug intake is mostly present on the trunk characterised by macular, papular and urticarial lesions. Distinctive iris 'bull's-

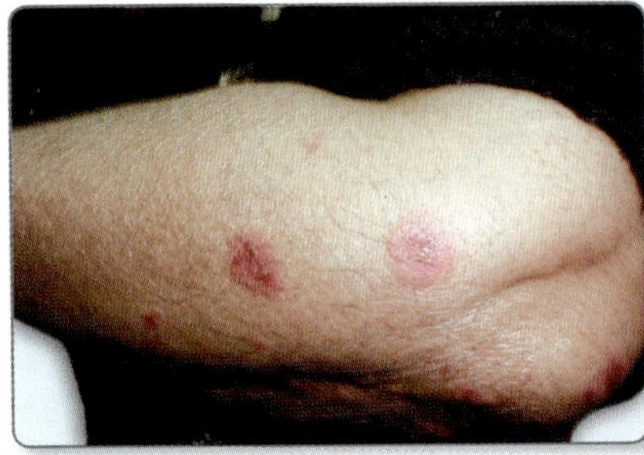

Fig. 3: Erythema multiforme: note the target lesion

eye' or target lesions are seldom found. The skin involvement is usually less than 2%. The lesions if not diagnosed early can lead to more serious Stevens-Johnson syndrome.

Stevens-Johnson Syndrome

Stevens-Johnson syndrome (SJS) is a combination of EM and involvement of mucous membranes, with fever and systemic signs and symptoms. The mouth is involved in all cases, eyes in 70–90%, and genitals in 60–70% cases. The skin involvement is usually less than 10%.

Toxic Epidermal Necrolysis (Lyell Syndrome)

Drug-induced TEN is a potentially life-threatening disorder. There is generalised loss of skin and mucosa. Patients present with a diffusely red, tender skin. Skin involvement is greater than 30%. Skin often comes off in sheets; there is possible loss of hair and nails. Due to the extensive loss of skin, there is fluid and electrolyte imbalance, impairment of temperature regulation and chances of secondary bacterial infection. Disturbance of fluid and electrolytes leads to multiple organ involvement. The condition is fatal in 10–30% of cases. Granulocytopenia for more than 5 days is an unfavourable sign. Gentle lateral pressure on the skin results in epidermal separation, and the formation of erosions (Nikolsky's sign) (Fig. 4).

There is diffuse full thickness epidermal necrosis, with little dermal change. In contrast to staphylococcal scalded skin syndrome, where there is a loss of stratum corneum only.

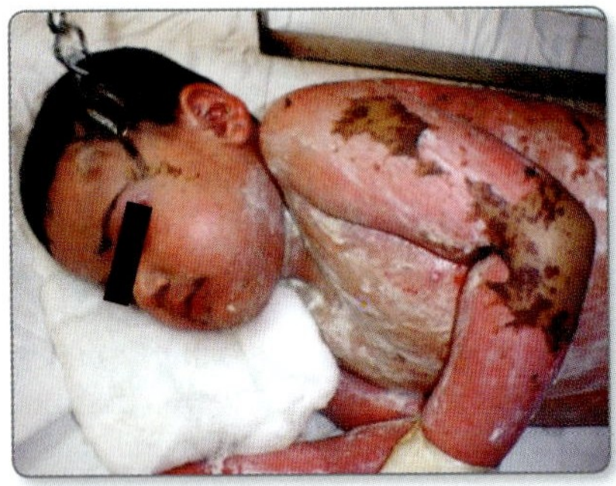

Fig. 4: Toxic epidermal necrolysis

Drugs Causing EM, SJS and TEN

The common drugs are sulphamethoxazole/trimethoprim, sulphonamides, NSAIDs, aminopenicillins, quinolones, cephalosporins, phenytoin, barbiturates, carbamazepine, allopurinol, and valproic acid.

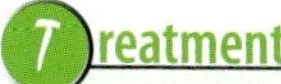

Treatment

All cases of TEN should be treated in a burns ward or intensive therapy unit ward. Careful attention should be given to the fluid and electrolyte replacement, antiseptics for the skin and systemic antibiotic should be prescribed. Intravenous immunoglobulins should be used in severe cases. Ophthalmic monitoring is essential to prevent scarring and blindness.

The use of corticosteroids is controversial, because of the increased risk of secondary bacterial infection, which is one of the major cause of death in TEN.

UNCOMMON REACTIONS

Lichenoid Drug Eruption

Lichen planus like drug reaction is a pruritic eruption, which closely mimics idiopathic lichen planus. It tends to be extensive and even develops into exfoliative dermatitis. β-blockers, captopril, thiazides, gold, bismuth, antimalarials, quinidine, chlorpropamide, penicillamine, carbamazepine, ethambutol, furosemide, isonicotinylhydrazine (INH), methyldopa, phenothiazines, phenylbutazone have been implicated.

Bullous Drug Eruption

Bullae at pressure sites may be seen after overdosage with barbiturates, methadone, meprobamate, imipramine, nitrazepam and glutethimide. Fixed drug eruption and drug-induced vasculitis may have a bullous component and drug-induced TEN is associated with widespread blistering. Phototoxic bullae may be induced by high doses of furosemide, nalidixic acid and non-steroidal anti-inflammatory agents. Pemphigus, pemphigoid, linear IgA disease, cutaneous porphyria, and acquired epidermolysis bullosa can be drug induced.

Drug-Induced Pemphigus

In drug-induced pemphigus, circulating autoantibodies directed against epidermal intercellular substance are not regularly found. The reaction usually regresses within weeks of cessation of therapy, but may persist for years. Penicillamine, captopril, rifampicin, penicillin, ampicillin, and piroxicam are established rare causes of drug-induced pemphigus.

Photosensitisation

Photosensitivity reactions spare the upper eyelids, submental and retroauricular areas. Common photosensitising drugs are amiodarone, chlorpromazine, nalidixic acid, psoralens, sulphonamides (especially cotrimoxazole), tetracyclines (especially demeclocycline) and thiazides.

Exfoliative Dermatitis

Erythroderma can follow the use of some common drugs, such as barbiturates, NSAIDs, captopril, carbamazepine, furosemide, sulphonamides and cimetidine. Because of the large area of skin involved, patients suffer from impaired temperature control, loss of proteins and water loss. With good supportive care, the prognosis is good and complete recovery occurs on withdrawing the drug.

Pigmentation

Pigmentary changes induced by drugs are often insidious, slowly progressive and may be dose related. Colour changes may be a result of direct deposition of a drug or its metabolites in the skin (e.g. minocycline), stimulation of melanocytes (e.g. silver in argyria) or deposition of other pigments, such as iron. Sun exposure may accentuate pigmentary changes. Oral contraceptives, minocycline, antimalarials (chloroquine and mepacrine), chlorpromazine, amiodarone, gold and clofazimine are associated with pigmentation.

Hypertrichosis

The drugs commonly responsible for hypertrichosis are minoxidil, cyclosporin, phenytoin, and androgens. Less common causes include corticosteroids, streptomycin, diazoxide, pencillamine and psoralens.

Purpura

Non-blanching-raised purple papules and plaques are the clinical manifestation of cutaneous vasculitis. Drugs are one of the many causes of cutaneous vasculitis; among those implicated are thiazides, sulphonamides, hydantoin, and non-steroidal anti-inflammatory drugs. The kidneys, central nervous system, joints or other organs may be involved in addition to the skin (Fig. 5).

Allergic Contact Dermatitis

The drugs commonly responsible are antihistamines, local anaesthetics, antibiotics, such as neomycin, penicillin, tetracyclines and sulphonamides.

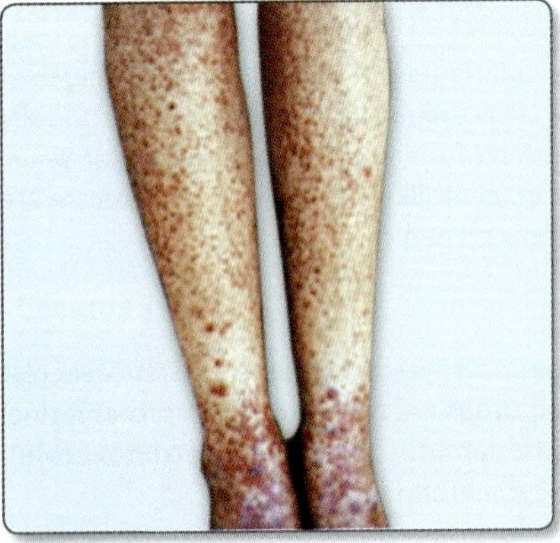

Fig. 5: Purpura

It causes a type 1V hypersensitivity reaction. These medications should be avoided, or used cautiously when used topically.

Systemic Lupus Erythematosus Like Syndrome

Approximately 5% cases of systemic lupus erythematosus (SLE) are drug induced and a number of drugs may exacerbate SLE. Commonly implicated drugs are acetabutalol, chlorpromazine, clonidine, griseofulvin, hydantoin, hydralazine, INH, β-blockers and procainamide.

Erythema Nodosum

Tender, red subcutaneous nodules present on the legs. Sulphonamides, oral contraceptives, a variety of analgesics, antipyretics and anti-infectious agents have been implicated.

Serum Sickness

Serum sickness develops 1–3 weeks after exposure, it is a combination of urticarial, morbilliform or purpuric skin lesions and inflammation of other organs, commonly the liver, joints and kidneys. Fever, arthralgia, lymphadenopathy are common manifestations. Penicillin, streptokinase, halothane, various vaccines and phenytoin have been implicated.

Acute Generalised Exanthematous Pustulosis

Small non-follicular pustules on an erythematous base, often accompanied by fever, are sometimes seen after treatment with drugs, such as penicillin and macrolide antibiotics. Onset is usually abrupt seen within 24 hours after the drug exposure. Patch testing is positive in 80% of cases.

Acral Erythema

A number of cytotoxic drugs, such as 5-fluorouracil, doxorubicin, methotrexate and cytabarine cause painful symmetrical erythema of the palms and soles. These appear days to weeks after initiation of therapy. The side effects is self-limiting and not a contraindication to further therapy.

Diagnosis

History taking is the most important tool in diagnosing drug reactions. A complete list of drug intake should be taken, has the patient had any previous drug reactions. The time period between the drug intake and the reaction gives a clue to the type of reaction. Allergic drug reactions do not occur immediately. Re-exposure to the drug, and pseudo-allergic reactions occur immediately. Many chemotherapeutic agents that inhibit cell division produce dose-related alopecia and mucositis. Any current disease, such as AIDS predisposes to infections, mononucleosis has a high incidence of reaction to ampicillin. Always examine the oral mucosa and see for signs of systemic involvement to assess the severity of drug reaction.

Biopsy

Skin biopsy can sometimes be helpful in diagnosing drug reactions. In TEN, examination of a frozen section of skin biopsy of a patient with sudden onset of generalised blistering shows a deeper epidermal split when the reaction is caused by a drug, the split is higher in staphylococcal infections. In pigmentary alterations, biopsies with appropriate stains can differentiate hyperpigmentation

Contd...

Contd...

due to the deposition of melanin, iron or a drug. Photoallergic and phototoxic reactions also have characteristic histopathological findings. Immunofluorescent examination of a skin biopsy can differentiate SLE from a photosensitivity eruption, a primary blistering disease, such as pemphigoid from a blistering drug reaction. Drug reactions, such as erythema multiforme, erythema nodosom, iododermas and bromodermas and lichen planus also have characteristic histological features.

Drug Allergy Tests

Patch, prick, scratch and intracutaneous tests can all be used, but these should be used carefully. Prick test is used when type 1 reaction has occurred. Patch test is used when a drug has caused type 1V reaction. Severe acute and delayed reactions are possible in such tests, drug allergy tests should be done in a hospital, where resuscitation measures are available. Never re-challenge a drug that has caused severe reactions.

Specific IgE levels can be measured for penicillin allergy, specific IgG and IgM are useful for immune-mediated thrombocytopenia and purpura. Coombs test is useful for drug-induced haemolysis. Complement levels and immune complex assays may be helpful in evaluating vasculitis and serum sickness.

Radioallergosorbent (RAST) test, measures IgE antibodies against specific allergens, has been used to detect immediate hypersensitivity to penicillin and other drugs.

Investigation

Laboratory examinations are not often helpful in the diagnosis and treatment of drug-induced cutaneous reactions. Mild leukocytosis may occur with widespread eruptions, but this finding does not help the clinician to determine whether the condition is due to drugs or infection. Eosinophilia is not a specific indicator of drug allergy. In toxic drug eruptions, measurements of drug levels in the serum and tissues may provide further evidence of the drug intake.

Treatment

The first step in the treatment of a drug reaction is to identify and withdraw the responsible agents. Treatment depends upon the type and severity of the eruption. Simple urticaria can be treated with an oral antihistamine. Morbilliform eruptions can be treated symptomatically with oral antihistamines, topical antipruritic lotions, such as calamine lotion or calamine cream with 1–2% menthol and anti-pruritic baths.

Patients with bronchospasm or signs of anaphylaxis may require emergency treatment with subcutaneous adrenaline 0.5 ml of 1 in 1,000 solution given slowly in 2–3 minutes, as well as parenteral corticosteroids and antihistamines.

Eruptions with prominent oropharyngeal mucous membrane involvement, such as Stevens-Johnson syndrome may require careful monitoring, local analgesia and special diet or even intravenous alimentation. In widespread blistering eruptions; the patient must be monitored for secondary infection and fluid and electrolyte imbalance.

Systemic steroids may be of value in some cases, such as severe exfoliative dermatitis or Stevens-Johnson syndrome. An initial dose of parenteral hydrocortisone is followed by oral prednisolone 1 mg/kg body weight and withdrawn over a period of 7–10 days. Cases of TEN should be treated in a burn unit.

PREVENTION

Most cutaneous reactions are idiosyncratic and serious complications are rare. Patients should not take the same drug again.

Patients with hypersensitivity and severe reactions should wear a bracelet, indicating the nature of reaction they had and the drug used. Genetics also plays a part in cutaneous drug reactions, the first degree relatives are at increased risk over the general populations in getting these reactions. This is especially important in SJS and TEN.

FURTHER READING

1. Clesham GJ, Terry HJ, Jalihal S, et al. Serum sickness and purpura following intravenous streptokinase. J R Soc Med. 1992;85(10):638-9.
2. Grattan CE. Aspirin sensitivity and urticaria. Clin Exp Dermatol. 2003;28(2):123-7
3. Kalish RS. Drug eruption: a review of clinical and immunological features. Adv Dermatol. 1991;6:221-37.
4. Knowles SR, Uetrecht J, Sheer NH. Idiosyncratic drug reactions: the reactive metabolic syndromWe. Lancet. 2000;356(9241):1587-91.
5. Korkij W, Soltani K. Fixed drug eruption: a brief review. Arch Dermatol. 1984;120(4):520-4.
6. Mitchell AA. Teratogens and the dermatologist: new knowledge, responsibility and opportunities. Arch Dermatol. 1991;127(3):399-401.
7. Ozkaya-Bayazin E, Akar U. Fixed drug eruption induced by trimethoprim-sulphamethoxazole: evidence for a link to HLA 30, B-13 Cw6 haplotype. J Am Acad Dermatol. 2001;45(5):712-7.
8. Pellicano R, Ciavarrrrella G, Lomuto M, et al. Genetic susceptibility to fixed drug eruption: evidence to a link to HLA- B22. J Am Acad Dermatol. 1994;30(1):52-4.
9. Porteous DM, Berger TG. Severe drug reactions (Stevens-Johnson syndrome and TEN) in Human Immunodeficiency virus infection. Arch Dermatol. 1991;127 (5):740-1.
10. Routledge PA, O'Mahony MS, Woodhouse KW. Adverse drug reactions in elderly patients. Br J Clin Pharmacol. 2004;57(2):121-6.
11. Shipley D, Omerod AD. Drug-induced urticaria. Recognition and Treatment. Am J Clin Dermatol. 2001;2(3):151-8.
12. Skog E, Gudjonsson H. On the allergic origin of the Jarisch-Herxheimer reaction. Acta Derm Venereol (Stockh). 1966;46(2):136-43.
13. Stern RS, Wintroub BU. Adverse drug reactions: reporting and evaluating cutaneous reactions. Adv Dermatol. 1987;2:3-17
14. Sullivan JR, Sheri NH. The drug hypersensitivity syndrome. What is the pathogenesis? Arch Dermatol. 2001;137(3):357-64.
15. Wintroub BU, Stern R. Cutaneous drug reactions. J Invest Dermatol. 1995;105 (Suppl):S95-8.

Chapter

44

Physical Modalities in Cutaneous Therapy

INTRODUCTION

Dermatological treatment has always included the performance of surgical procedures. Skin is uniquely available for diagnostic procedures as well as for the application of therapeutic agents. A dermatological physician can carry out simple surgical procedures. The larger and complicated ones require the services of a dermatological surgeon.

Before carrying out any surgical procedure, make sure that a written consent is taken from the patient, the patient is not suffering from any bleeding disorder, he is not sensitive to local anaesthetizing agents. Make sure to inform the patient of all the possible risks of surgery beforehand, such as risk of thrombosis if immobilisation is anticipated, risk of recurrence in tumour surgery, risk of structures likely to be damaged, risk of scarring if there is a history of keloids etc. Risks of anaesthesia, wound infection, injury to nerve, lymphatic, etc. should be included in a leaflet, which should be given to the patient at least 24 hours before surgery. Resuscitative measures should be available at hand, particularly for anaphylaxis. For electrosurgical procedures make sure that the patient does not have a pacemaker, as ventricular fibrillations may develop even if the patient is close to a diathermy machine.

Skin is prepared as for any surgical procedure by reducing the extensive bacterial flora present on the skin by antiseptics, hair in the surgical area should be clipped. Local anaesthesia topical or intralesional applied as needed. The surgical staff should be protected against any possible viral infections such as hepatitis B or C and HIV infection, by wearing masks, surgical gloves, and protective eyewear. The risk of cutaneous infection after skin surgery is low. Precautions are needed if the patient is immunosuppressed. For surgery around the lips prophylactic anti-herpes medication is indicated to prevent a relapse of herpes labialis.

Povidone iodine and chlorhexidine are commonly used antiseptics for the skin. Povidone iodine should be avoided around the eyes and the ears. Povidone iodine is toxic to the cornea and the tympanic membrane.

BIOPSY

Punch Biopsy

The biopsy punch is a metal cylinder of diameters ranging from 2 mm to 10 mm. In most cases a punch with a diameter of 3–4 mm is used. It has a sharp cutting edge attached to a handle. Hold the skin taut in the direction of the lines of least tension (Langer's line), the punch is then pushed into the skin with a twisting movement, until a pop is felt, indicating that the subcutaneous fat is reached. By applying gentle pressure on both sides of the defect, the tissue is elevated; the base cut with scissors, the biopsied specimen is then put in a formalin solution. Avoid using forceps, as it damages the tissue which is then not suitable for microscopic examination. The wound is usually left to heal without suturing. Hemostasis is achieved by cauterisation or by a styptic solution.

A punch biopsy is usually required for small superficial lesions of the skin. It cannot be used for deeper lesions, for these lesions, an incisional biopsy is required. For scalp lesions, usually a larger size punch is required so that an appropriate number of follicles can be examined. Punches can also be used for hair transplants. The procedure is simple and quick.

Elliptical Surgical Biopsy

This is one of the most widely used methods of skin biopsy. Small biopsy specimens should be totally excised, a biopsy of a larger lesion should be at right angle through the margin to include the normal adjacent skin. The long axis of the wound should follow the lines of Langer.

Indications

- Lesions deep in the subcutaneous tissue
- Vesico-bullous lesions
- Lesions suspected of malignancy
- Lesions continuous with an important structure, e.g. ears, lips, eyelids nose.

Guidelines for Elliptical Incisions

- The direction of the incision should be along the Langer's lines
- The incision is marked on the skin with alcoholic soluble dyes such as gentian violet
- The length to breadth ratio should be approximately 3.5:1
- Local anaesthesia should be a field block, or 1–2 cm lateral to the perimeter of the excisional site
- Scalpel blades of size No 15 should be used for excision
- Haemostasis is achieved by electrocautery
- Absorbable sutures should be applied for subcutaneous tissue
- The knots are buried to prevent suture elimination through the epidermis (Small wounds do not require subcutaneous sutures)
- Skin is closed with non-absorbable sutures
- Postoperative care involves gentle cleaning with hydrogen peroxide, followed by applications of an antibacterial cream. Non-adherent tape may be used as a dressing
- The timing of the suture removal depends upon the anatomic site and wound tension.
- Sutures on the face are removed after 5 days, while those on the back may remain for 2 weeks.

CURETTAGE

The dermal curette has been used for the removal of a variety of epidermal lesions, e.g. milia, warts, seborrhoeic keratosis and molluscum contagiosum.

The curette does not easily cut through the normal epidermis; curettage is only possible if the material being scraped off is frailer than the surrounding skin or where there is a natural cleavage plane between the lesion and the surrounding normal skin.

Curette is held with one hand while the other hand stabilises the skin. The "Potato Peeler method" is used to remove the lesion. The consistency of the normal dermis is felt as a gritty sensation by the curette, which defines the necessary depth of the excision. With experience one can feel the difference between the lesional tissue and the normal firmer dermis. Haemostasis is achieved by light electrodesiccation. Appropriate size of the curette is also important. Too small a curette may cause severe fragmentations of the specimen. Too large a curette may cause unnecessary damage to the normal tissue and will miss the small extension of the tumour growth into the deeper dermis.

Curettage is contraindicated in the periorbital, periauricular, perilabial, genital and perianal areas. While curetting care should be taken that the curette does not penetrate through the dermis into the fatty layer.

Conditions Suitable for Curettage

- For curettage the lesion should be more fragile than the surrounding skin
- There should be a natural cleavage plane between the lesion and the surrounding skin
- Adjacent skin should not tear easily
- On mobile areas first fulgurate or incise the margin, to obtain a plane of cleavage
- Curettage is used when histology is not an essential characteristic

Contraindications

- Malignancy
- Undiagnosed lesions
- On previous operated sites

SHAVE EXCISION

This technique is best suited for pedunculated, papular or exophytic lesions. The method can also be used for macular or indurated lesions using a deep or rolled shave.

Lesions treated by shave biopsy are seborrhoeic keratosis, intradermal naevi, skin tags, and filiform warts. Small pedunculated lesions do not require a local anaesthesia. The distal end of the lesion is grasped with a fine tooth forceps, it is gently elevated and the base of the lesion is then cut with curved iris scissors. Haemostasis is then controlled with pressure, or styptic solution.

For larger lesions local anaesthesia is required, the shave excision is performed with a No. 15 blade, larger lesions may require No. 10 blade.

After giving the local anaesthesia the lesion is stabilised by pinching the lesion between the thumb and index finger of the left hand. The lesion is then incised by placing the edge of the blade parallel to the skin surface; the excision is performed by one or more sweeping strokes.

The disadvantage of shave excision is that the whole lesion is seldom removed especially when large. There are high chances of recurrence of the lesion.

ELECTROCAUTERY

Electrocautery is a simple process of heating tissues with electricity. The procedure is often used to stop bleeding and to remove unwanted and harmful tissues. A small probe with an electric current flowing through it is used to burn or destroy a tissue. A grounding part is placed on the body, usually the thighs, to protect the body from the harmful effects of electricity. The tip of the probes is of different sizes, depending on the purpose for which the electrocautery is used. Because of the risk of virus transmission, a different clean probe should be used for each patient.

Electrocautery is generally used for small superficial lesions, such as skin tags, molluscum contagiosum, dermatosis papulosa nigra and warts. It is also used to stop bleeding during surgical procedures.

ELECTROLYSIS

One of the first indications of electrosurgery in dermatology was the use of direct current to destroy hair follicles. In this technique heat is actually not a factor. A chemical reaction occurs at the electrode tip, with the evolution of sodium hydroxide at the hair root. When the direct current passes through the electrode tip, the sodium hydroxide produced is responsible for hair destruction.

This is a safe technique with minimal pain and risk of scarring. It is a very slow method, requiring a minute or two for the destruction of each hair. Electrolysis has the advantage over laser, that it can be used for both pigmented and white hair.

THERMOLYSIS

This is a form of diathermy in which high frequency current causes heat in the follicle resulting in tissue destruction. This is more painful and more likely to cause scarring if not properly used. However, it is very fast 100–200 hair may be treated in half an hour session. For this reason, it has replaced electrolysis.

IONTOPHORESIS

This is a method by which ions of soluble salts are introduced into the skin for therapeutic purposes. Basically, it is the process of increasing the penetration of electrically charged drugs into the surface tissues by galvanic current. The systemic side effects of the drug are significantly decreased

Iontophoresis is a method of treating hyperhidrosis of the hands and feet. In this method, a direct current of low voltage can be used to introduce ionised drugs into the skin. Even tap water can be used for the purpose. The electric current and ionised drugs selectively damages and blocks the sweat ducts.

During iontophoresis, patient sits with hands or feet, or both, immersed in shallow trays filled with water for a short period of time (20–40 minutes) while the device sends a mild electrical current through the water. The process is repeated every other day for 5 to 10 days or until sweating is reduced to a comfortable level. Once the desired dryness has been achieved, patients are switched to a maintenance schedule, ranging from once per week to once every four weeks, depending on the individual response. To maintain dryness, iontophoresis must be repeated as soon as sweating begins to return.

MOHS SURGERY

Mohs pioneering work began in late 1930; it is removal of accessible form of cancer under microscopic control. In this method of surgery, the neoplastic tissue is excised, fixed carefully, and marked. Sections of the tissue are cut, examined microscopically; the process is repeated until all the cancer tissue is removed. The method is time consuming, but the success rate is high. This is usually in the range of 99% for primary basal cell carcinoma, and 96% for recurrent lesions. Today instead of using fixed tissue technique frozen tissue technique is used. Mohs surgery provides high cure rates, with minimum damage to the surrounding tissues.

A similar technique is used in Germany (Tubinger Torte). Torte's method of histological control of the entire margin of the incision, by an ingenious plan taking a small peripheral ring of tissue, while Mohs surgery depends upon flattening the excision, and taking sections from the entire base.

Indications

- Mohs surgery is indicated for recurrent basal cell carcinomas, and for cutaneous cancers, when other treatment methods have failed.
- Large or deeply invasive carcinomas
- It is done on the "H Zone" of the face (the naso-labial fold, nasal alae, periorbital region, and periauricular areas), the region where electrosurgery and radiation cannot be done due to complications
- In morphoeic and sclerosing basal cell carcinoma

CRYOSURGERY

The medical use of cold dates back to 2500 BC, it was used by Egyptians to treat inflammation and injuries. Later Hippocrates described its anaesthetic effect. The earliest freezing agent used in the treatment of skin disease was salt ice mixture (-20°C) with Arnott as its pioneer in 1851. Today liquid nitrogen is the most commonly used cryogen, throughout the world, it is efficient, inexpensive and non-combustible. Cryosurgery is used to treat a number of cutaneous disorders; as it also offers partial anaesthesia, a number of lesions can be treated at one time.

Cryogens are easy to apply, require no local anaesthesia, usually leaving no scars after re-epithelialisation. The lower the boiling point of the agent, the more efficient are its freezing capabilities. The boiling point of Freon 12 is -29.8°C, solid CO_2 is -78.5°C, liquid nitrous oxide is -89.5°C, and liquid nitrogen is -195.6°C.

Indications

The most common indications for cryosurgery are warts and actinic keratosis. The other lesions that can be treated by cryosurgery are seborrhoeic keratosis, dermatofibroma, small hemangiomas, granuloma annulare, lentigines, keloids, lentigo maligna, and superficial basal cell carcinoma in the elderly. The patient should be warned about the pain, blister formation and slow healing. This should be specially specified while treating plantar warts.

Contraindications

These include conditions in which there is an abnormal reaction to cold such as cryoglobulinaemia, cryofibrinogenaemia, Raynaud's disease and cold urticaria.

Mechanism of Cell Death by Cryosurgery

- Mechanical damage to cells by intracellular and extracellular ice formation
- Osmotic change related to dehydration of cells and increased concentration of electrolytes
- Denaturing of lipid protein complexes in the cell membrane
- Vascular stasis with resulting necrosis of the tissue.

Histological Changes

Changes are evident within 30 minutes of freezing characterised by pyknotic nuclei, oedema, and coarsely granular and often vacuolated cytoplasm. Within an hour after cryosurgery dermal vascular damage is seen. The cellular infiltrate consists mainly of polymorph leukocytes. Resolution begins within 3 days and healing occurs without scarring.

Melanocytes are more susceptible to damage by cold than keratinocytes; mild hypopigmentation is sometimes seen in areas previously frozen with liquid nitrogen. Fibroblast and stromal structures are less sensitive to the effects of cryosurgery; this may be an important factor in the lack of scarring of superficial lesions.

Clinical Signs after Cryosurgery

A stinging burning pain accompanies freezing, peak effects occur during thawing and for about 2 hours after thawing is over. Freezing on the hands, feet, lips, ears and eyelids is more painful than elsewhere.

Within minutes of thawing a triple response with redness, wheal and a surrounding flare will develop. Intense oedema or blister formation occurs at the dermo-epidermal junction, about 3–6 hours later, this flattens in 2–3 days and sloughs in 2–4 weeks. Re-epithelialisation is seen within 72 hours of superficial freezing, infection is therefore rare.

Cryosurgery may produce nerve damage; special care should therefore be taken where nerves are superficial as the side of the fingers.

Side Effects and Complications

Side effects are common, but transient. The expected side effects are oedema, vesicles, bullae, weeping and crust formation. Scarring can occur if excessive freezing is done. Hypopigmentation is common after freezing, especially in dark skin types, fair skin people are better candidates for cryosurgery. Peripheral hyperpigmentation may be seen on the back and legs. Sensory loss and digital neuropathy has been reported after treating warts on the fingers. Alopecia may occur if the freezing time exceeds 20 seconds on the scalp. Pyogenic granulomas have been reported after treating actinic keratosis or basal cell carcinoma. Headache and or pain around the eyes can occur after treatment of lesions on the forehead.

Liquid Nitrogen

This is the most widely used cryogen. It has a temperature of -196°C. It can be used by a spray method or contact probe. Length of exposure depends upon the thickness of the lesion. Actinic keratosis requires 5–10 seconds. Warts are frozen until the entire lesion and a tiny peripheral rim of white appears.

Liquid nitrogen will rarely cause normal thermos bottles to explode; air ventilation must always be present in all storage apparatus. Quartz size thermos bottles are used to store liquid nitrogen for a few days. Air vent is necessary to prevent explosion.

Carbon Dioxide

The Joule-Thomson refrigeration principle makes snow or dry ice. There are two methods of making this:

- Sparkle method
- Via a chamois leather bag

The chamois leather technique is more commonly used. A chamois leather bag is fitted tightly over the nozzle of a cylinder of carbon dioxide gas. This collects the solid carbon dioxide snow that is formed by the expansion of the gas. The carbon dioxide snow is then put in plastic funnel tubes. These tubes come in varying sizes. The size that correlates with the lesion is used. The snow is held firmly over the lesion, until a spreading ring of white frozen skin appears around the lesion. Time required for the treatment of warts is 1–2 minutes, 5–20 seconds for haemangiomas, 60–150 seconds for deeper tumours.

Carbon dioxide is used as solid stick storage for 2–3 days if possible in a foam container. It can be ground and mixed with acetone in the form of slush, which is then applied with cotton tipped applicator as in acne therapy.

Nitrous Oxide

The gas is easily accessible because of its extensive use in anaesthesia. It is usually applied with cryoprobes.

LASERS

Lasers are an acronym for **L**ight **A**mplification by **S**timulated **E**mission of **R**adiation. Maiman first introduced laser in 1960, Leon Goldman pioneered its dermatological use.

Ordinary light tends to scatter instead of travelling in a straight line, these rays therefore cannot travel very far and tend to become weak in intensity due to the loss and scattering of energy after travelling some distance.

Lasers are electromagnetic waves. Laser machines are energy funnels that emit an electromagnetic energy, which is of a single wavelength (monochromatic), and does not scatter, but travels in the same direction without any change of frequency.

The laser machine consists of an electromagnetic energy source of high output, which is pumped into a laser medium that gives energy which is, monochromatic (of uniform wavelength), collimative (all the light exiting from the laser machine are parallel and will not diffuse over distance) and coherent (all the laser light is in phase and focussed to very small areas). Optical containing mirrors in the laser machine convert the energy into a beam of light as it is emitted. The laser light lies in the infrared and visible light of the electromagnetic spectrum. The laser delivers a non-ionising radiation that destroys the tissue bloodlessly, killing microorganisms in the process and produces a wound that tends to heal with minimum fibrosis. The laser light may be delivered in a continuous stream or by short pulses.

The first cutaneous lasers used continuous beams of laser light, which even when used by expert hands could cause a buildup of thermal energy that diffused to the non-targeted adjacent skin. This led to undesirable adverse effects. Most of the currently used lasers take advantage of the Anderson and Parish's theory of selective photothermolysis, thus minimising the undesired collateral thermal damage. This theory states that selective heating of a target chromophore is achieved when the laser wavelength is preferentially absorbed by the chromophore, the energy of the laser is high enough to damage the chromophore, and the pulse duration of the laser energy is shorter than the thermal relaxation of the target (time it takes for the target to cool by 50% of its peak temperature after the irradiation). The majority of lasers used today work on this principle and attempt to limit the duration of laser lights impingement on tissue. Lasers also have systems to cool the epidermis to prevent collateral damage to the epidermal structures from laser light intended to target deeper structures.

All the cutaneous laser systems in current use target structures in the epidermis or dermis. Most adverse effects and complications of laser treatment can be predicted by understanding that they are mainly due to collateral damage of normal adjacent skin structures. Lasers should only be operated by those who are experienced and trained in the field of laser therapy.

Precautions While Using Lasers

- Environmental protection. There should be ventilation exhaust systems and prevention of spectral reflectance
- Specific eye protection. Eyes should always be protected by safety goggles
- The surrounded skin should be shielded to prevent burning
- Protective gloves must be worn by the operator

A small area of skin should be tested before using laser therapy. It is done to see for the therapeutic efficacy of the laser on the given tissue, and predict the cosmetic result. A watch period of 4 months is recommended for proper evaluation.

Uses of Lasers

Lasers are used to treat a number of dermatological disorders. They are:

Vascular Lesions

Some lasers have special affinity for haemoglobin; these lasers are used to treat capillary malformation such as port-wine stain, angiomas and telangiectasias.

Pigmented Lesions

Melanin can be selectively targeted with ultra-short, high-energy pulse laser. These lasers are used to treat congenital melanocytic nevus, freckles and lentigines.

Hair Removal

Lasers are very popular for removing unwanted hair. Hair removal depends upon the high level of energy in the laser light to be taken up by the melanin pigment within the hair, which converts this energy into heat, destroying not only the hair, but the matrix and hair bulb. The energy generated to the hair follicle is conducted down the base of the follicle more readily in the anagen phase of the cycle. In the telogen phase the energy generated has to cross a gap to reach the future hair producing region. That is why laser-assisted hair removal occurs when the hair is in the anagen growing phase. Several cycles of treatment are required, the spacing between treatments depend upon the area being treated. Lasers do not affect the white hair, they are used only for pigmented hair.

Lasers used for hair removal are the alexandrite, diode and Nd:Yag and long-pulsed ruby laser.

Tattoos

Implanted dermal pigment can be removed by fragmenting the pigment: which allows its removal by phagocytosis, or by producing a burn that heals by secondary intention.

Cutaneous Disorders

Lasers vaporise the body cells and cause cell death. They are used for the treatment of keloids, seborrhoeic keratosis, epidermal naevi, superficial basal cell carcinoma, warts, condylomas and rhinophyma.

Resurfacing

Carbon dioxide and Er:YAG lasers are used to treat extensive areas of skin damage such as photoaging or scarring by acne.

Miscellaneous

Lasers are also used for diagnostic laser imaging and spectroscopy. A near-infrared confocal microscope provides histology like images of human skin. Imaging is painless and takes only a few minutes.

Types of Lasers

Lasers as already said are named after the laser medium used. These lasers act selectively on the different molecules in the skin called chromophores. Lasers are thus selected according to the chromophore on which they act on.

Carbon dioxide Laser

This laser is used for a variety of dermatological lesions. It emits radiation at 10,600 nm in the infrared region of the electromagnetic spectrum. The water in the tissue absorbs this wavelength of light, and this absorption is not dependent on any particular cell of the skin. As the water absorbs energy, the temperature rises vaporising the tissue. The amount of tissue damage depends upon the amount of time the laser impacts on the target tissue, and to the energy setting.

It is used for the treatment of warts, xanthelasma, leucoplakia, tattoos, resurfacing, mucous cysts, superficial basal cell carcinoma, premalignant lesions of the lips and rhinophyma.

The main precaution with carbon dioxide laser is smoke evacuation. During procedure, the laser generates large amounts of smoke that may harbour viral particles. Carbon dioxide laser may also burn any cloth or paper that it comes in contact, therefore appropriate fire precautions must be observed. Eyewear must be used to protect the eyes from injury.

Argon Laser

The argon laser emits 6 wavelengths of light, 80% of it lies within the bands of 488 nm (blue) to 514.5 nm (green). These wavelengths correspond to large absorption peak of oxyhaemoglobin, but melanin also gets absorbed in this range. In clinical application while the dermal vascular region is targeted, melanin in the epidermis also gets heated and causes epidermal damage. Destruction of deeper tissues may result in scarring. For this reason it has been replaced by new and more selected lasers.

Argon laser is not advised for use in children because of the greater risk of scarring. Argon lasers are useful for vascular lesions with large diameter vessels such as venous lakes of the lips and hypertrophied vascular nodules found in the mature port-wine stains.

Pulsed Dye Lasers

The lasers that are pulsed use a variety of techniques to generate laser light. The most common pulsed dye laser uses a flash lamp to energise the laser. The dye is fluorescent; rhodamine is often used as the active medium. This generates a wavelength of 500–700 nm. The vascular pulsed dye lasers use either 577 nm or 585 nm as the preferred wavelength, corresponding to a small peak in the oxyemoglobin absorption spectrum that does not have any competition for melanin.

Pulsed dye lasers are used for treating thin lightly coloured port-wine stains especially those of children. They are also used for treating facial telangiectasia, cherry angiomas, less commonly used for poikiloderma of Civatte and even warts. Damage to the surrounding tissue is very slight and there is virtually no surface damage. Pain is so slight that as a rule no anaesthesia is required. The risk of scarring and pigmentation is very slight.

Pulsed dye lasers are not used to treat thick vascular lesions because the short pulse duration, it is virtually insufficient to target these vessels without increase of power to a level that could lead to generalised damage and scarring.

These lasers are not used to treat venous lesions, as there is significant post-operative purpura that takes 7–10 days to resolve. These lasers are expensive to purchase, operate and maintain.

Krypton Laser

These are continuous mode thermal lasers. The wavelength emitted by krypton laser is 520 nm (green) and 568 nm (yellow). 520 nm is used in epidermal lesions and 568 nm for treatment of thick vascular lesions as that of adult port-wine stain. The biggest problem with krypton laser is the heating of the surface due to scattering of light. It is recommended to cool the skin prior to and during the procedure. The cost is low.

Copper Vapour Laser

These are continuous wave thermal lasers that use electrical energy, to heat metallic copper in a neon gas so that the metal vaporises. The copper generates two wavelengths of 511 nm (green) and 578 nm (yellow). A simple filter is present to emit one or other wavelength of light. The green light is used to treat pigmented lesions, the yellow light for vascular lesions.

Although copper vapour laser is a continuous wave thermal laser, it operates on the concept of selective photothermolysis. The 578 nm of light is absorbed selectively by the oxyhaemoglobin within small vessels.

The major advantage of copper vapour laser is the lack of post-operative purpura, and the larger diameter of the deeper vessels that can be treated. As copper vapour lasers have effective pulse duration of 10 m/second, the surrounding tissue damage is more than the pulsed dye laser, leading to scarring and pigmentation.

Ruby Laser

The ruby laser has an active medium of aluminium oxide that has been chromium doped. This means that the aluminium atoms have been replaced with the chromium atoms. The laser emits a wavelength of 694 nm that is in the red visible light spectrum. The red light is well absorbed by the black, blue and green tattoo pigments. The main disadvantage of ruby laser is that it is absorbed by the melanin in the epidermis and may lead to hyperpigmentation.

Nd:YAG Laser

The Nd:YAG (neodymium-doped yttrium aluminium garnet) laser utilises yttrium-aluminium-garnet crystal in which neodymium has been dispersed. The wavelength of light emitted is 1,064 nm that is in the infrared spectrum of the electromagnetic waves. Nd:YAG lasers are deeply penetrating and cause extensive tissue damage. The Q-Switched Nd:YAG laser has a short pulse in the range of 5–10 nanoseconds. This laser is useful for treating tattoos.

Alexandrite Laser

Alexandrite is a chrysoberyl crystal that has been chromium doped. There are several types of alexandrite laser, which delivers light with a wavelength of 755 nm. Alexandrite laser operates on the concept of selective photothermolysis using an optico-acoustic pulse to fragment the tattoo particles. It is used for the treatment of blue, black and green tattoos. It is also used to treat epidermal and dermal pigmentation. The cost is high.

Erbium-Yag Laser

This has two wave lengths, 2,940 nm (invisible) and 635 nm (red). The longer wave length is used for acne scarring and laser resurfacing. The shorter wavelength is used for epidermal lesions such as solar lentigenes and superficial basal cell carcinoma.

Diode Laser

Diode laser is a semiconductor laser. It produces laser beam in the wave length of 800 nm. It is most popularly used for removal of black /brown hair. Innovative devices with cooling mechanisms give better results with less scarring. Diode lasers have been found to work well on dark skin. In dark skin long pulsed diode laser is preferred.

Diode laser in long pulsed mode is also used for treatment of leg veins. A diode laser of 1,450 nm can be used treat acne scars and wrinkles.

Excimer Laser

This laser uses a combination of a noble gas such as argon, krypton or xenon, and a reactive gas such as fluorine or chlorine. Under appropriate conditions of electrical stimulation and high pressure, a pseudo-molecule called excimer is created, which can only exist in an energised state, and can give rise to laser light in the ultraviolet range. Excimer molecules are also used as a source of spontaneous ultraviolet light. These lasers have cleared psoriasis faster than conventional phototherapy

It is thus seen that various lasers are used in dermatology. To say which is the "Best laser" is a question that has no answer; different lasers are used for different purposes. The effect of laser treatment also depends upon the individuals, their colour and skin type. Each laser is best suited for the type of lesion to be treated and the colour of the patient.

Types of Laser and their Uses

Multiple uses

- CO_2 laser (10600 nm)
- Er:YAG laser (2940 nm)

Vascular lesions

- Pulsed dye laser (585/595 nm)
- Frequency-doubled Nd:YAG (KTP) laser (532 nm)
- Nd:YAG laser (1064 nm)

Pigmented lesions

- Q-switched ruby laser (694 nm)
- Q-switched alexandrite laser (755 nm)
- Q-switched frequency-doubled Nd:YAG laser (532 nm)
- Q-switched Nd:YAG laser (1064 nm)

Hair removal

- Long-pulsed ruby laser (694 nm)
- Long-pulsed alexandrite laser (755 nm)
- Long-pulsed diode laser (810 nm)
- Long-pulsed Nd:YAG laser (1064 nm)

Tattoos

- Q-Switched Ruby laser
- Q-Switched Alexandrite laser
- Q-Switched Nd:YAG laser

The depth of penetration is proportional to the wavelength of the laser. Longer wavelength lasers have a greater penetration.

Laser radiation is absorbed by melanin, other chromophores and water, which are damaged by thermal injury.

INTENSE PULSED LIGHT

Intense pulsed light (IPL) covers a wide spectrum of light ranging from 515 nm to 1,200 nm, with pulses of 2–20 ms, which is transmitted through a small, smooth, transparent hand piece which is gently placed over the skin. Cut-off filters in the hand piece change the wavelength range allowing it to be optimised for different applications and skin types.

Intense pulsed light systems produce light with many wavelengths, unlike lasers which produce light of just one wavelength. The light emitted by IPL is absorbed by chromophores in the skin cells and converted to heat, which impacts the targeted tissue.

Intense pulsed light is mainly used for hair removal (it has a larger field size than a laser), vascular and pigmented lesions.

PHOTODYNAMIC THERAPY (PDT)

This includes the therapeutic combination of photosensitiser administered to the patient and its activation by light. The photosensitisers such as aminolevulinic acid (ALA) or its methyl ester methyl aminolevulinic acid is applied topically on the inflamed tissue which is then activated by concentrated light sources. The emission spectrum of the light source should correspond to the activation spectrum of the sensitiser.

5-aminolevulinic acid applied to the skin is metabolised by the epidermal cells to protoporphyrin IX; which is sensitive to a broad range of light starting at Soret band and through the red region of the visible spectrum. The photochemical reaction between protoporphyrin 1X and absorbed photons produces singlet oxygen along with other reactive oxygen combinations and free radicals. The direct effect of these molecules causes localised membrane damage to cellular and mitochondrial membranes. The photosensitivity is lost in 24 hours; another advantage is that there is no systemic accumulation.

PDT has been used in actinic keratosis, photoaging, acne vulgaris, Bowen's disease, BCC, etc.

COSMETIC DERMATOLOGY

Study of cosmetic dermatology is beyond the scope of this book. Very briefly, the following procedures will be discussed.

Peeling

Peeling with chemical and physical modalities has been a successful treatment for acne scars and pigmentation for many years. Peeling for acne is not much used today as in the past, not because it is ineffective but because more effective treatments have developed. Peels can be superficial, medium or deep. Superficial peels extend up to the epidermis or papillary dermis, mid-depth peels extends up to the upper reticular dermis and the deep peels to the mid-reticular dermis. Mid-depth and deep peels are done by a cosmetic surgeon.

Superficial peels are used to improve the blemishes of the skin. Medium depth peels are used for removing acne and superficial scars. The deep depth peels are used to remove rhytids around the lips and deeper scars.

Superficial Peels

Superficial peels are usually done by beauticians. They are used to treat mild sun damage, light crosshatch wrinkling, muddy, and irregular pigmentation. Repeated every 4–6 months light peels reduce the visibility of acne scars. The wound depth is not below the papillary dermis. These peels contain α-hydroxy acids, such as glycolic acid, malic acid, lactic acid, citric acid or tartaric acid. Glycolic acid is most commonly used in superficial peels, it can be used in concentrations ranging from 10% to 70%. Other superficial peels are Coomb's formula, Jessner's solution (mixture of salicylic acid and lactic acid in ethanol). 10–15% trichloroacetic acid (TCA) will affect only the epidermis, 35% TCA can penetrate up to the papillary dermis.

Method: Face is prepared with washing and degreasing. With superficial peels there is no risk of cardiotoxicity and therefore they can be applied over the whole face in one sitting. The only limiting factor is slight discomfort.

Low-concentration peels are applied 2–3 times on the skin, with a five minute interval between each until a light frost is produced. The peels are applied with cotton balls, gauze squares or cotton tipped applicator. During the first 30–60 seconds, the skin burns so cool compresses or a fan nearby is helpful. A crust is formed after the peel; this is thin and comes of easily. The wound is superficial and heals completely. Patients with a dry skin and fair complexion are the best subjects.

The superficial peels have to be repeated frequently for effectiveness. These can be used on all skin types, and on all body areas.

Side effects: Hyperpigmentation or hypopigmentation may occur; it gradually fades off in 1–3 months.

Prolonged erythema and increased sensitivity to light may occur after a peel.

Contraindications to Chemical Peels: Chemical peels should not be done if the person cannot resist excessive exposure to sunlight, they have active herpes simplex, there is a tendency to keloid formation, and if isotretinoin has been used in the year before.

Medium Depth Peels

These peels remove the skin up to the level of upper reticular dermis. If done well, the skin regenerates without scarring. Medium depth peels usually contain a mixture of 35% TCA and Jessner's solution, 35% TCA and glycolic acid or 50% TCA alone. The preparation is the same as for superficial peels. Oral herpes simplex prophylaxis should be started 2 days before the peel, and continued for at least 5 days afterwards. A pronounced redness is seen 15 minutes after the peel. The redness may persist for about 2 weeks after the peel. These can be repeated every 3–12 months depending upon the skin damage.

Obaji Blue Peel

The Obaji Blue Peel was introduced by *Dr Zein Obaji*. It can be used on all skin types. A blue base is added to the TCA peel. The peel is performed in one to four steps, depending upon the condition of the skin. A slight stinging sensation is felt as each layer is approached. The change in the colour of the dye indicates the level of peel. Each coat of the peel penetrates deeper into the skin; the blue shade of the peel darkens. The blue colour remains for 12–24 hours, and the skin heals in about 10 days. It causes less erythema and inflammation than dermabrasion or lasers.

Deep peels

These peels remove the skin up to the level of mid-reticular dermis. Deep peels contain phenol. Phenol causes immediate coagulation of epidermal proteins. Phenol is used in combination with croton oil, tap water and hexachlorophene. The peel is very painful; it is performed under regional nerve block anaesthesia. In order to reduce phenol toxicity (cardiac arrhythmias) hydration with Ringers solution before, during and after the peel is required. Deep and medium peels may cause hypopigmentation; they are not suitable for dark skin. Oral antibiotics and herpes prophylaxis are given preoperatively.

Deep peels cannot be used on dark skin; the skin remains red and tender for about 3 weeks after the peel. It should only be done by a plastic surgeon. Laser resurfacing has largely replaced deep peels.

Dermabrasion

Dermabrasion was first used as a levelling procedure for smallpox scars. It was performed by Kromayer in 1905. He introduced the concept that freezing the skin makes it rigid and injury above a certain depth does not leave a scar. Dermabrasion is a controlled skin wound, which can be achieved in many ways. There are several dermabrasion systems.

Levels of Dermabrasion

It is possible to visualise the approximate depth of dermabrasion by observing the anatomic changes in the skin as it is removed. These observations are best seen when using a diamond fraise, because it bites less than a wire brush and less freezing is required. In the human facial skin, the following levels are observed:

Level-1 is reached when there is a change to lighter colour, indicating that the epidermis with its melanocytes have been removed. In addition, the tiny blood vessels of the sub-epidermal plexus become visible.

Level-2 is seen when the vessels disappear and small yellow dots just begin to appear. These yellow dots are the most superficial edges of the sebaceous glands, just visible through a few bands of collagen. This indicates that most of the papillary dermis has been removed.

Level-3 is reached when larger and more numerous yellow dots are seen indicating that the middle of the sebaceous glands has been reached; this is essentially the mid-dermis.

Level-4 is when the yellow dots become larger and less in number or disappear, this indicates that the compact dermis is revealed, and rope like bands of collagen is seen.

Level-5, this level is reached when yellow globules of fat appear, indicating the subcutaneous tissue. Ideally this plane should never be reached.

These levels are best appreciated with experience.

Method

The patient is first sedated with diazepam. The skin is cleaned; ears, nostrils and, the eyes are protected. The area to be abraded is frozen, and then abraded to the required depth. Abrading brushes or diamond fraises are used for the abrasion. Bleeding occurs for 10–15 minutes after the abrasion which can be treated by pressure and application of paraffin gauze. These are removed after 24 hours. The crust separates in 7–10 days. Healing is usually complete by 3 weeks. The patient is instructed to avoid exposure to sunlight for 6–8 weeks in order to reduce the incidence of hyperpigmentation.

Complications

- Scarring: this is the most serious complication; it probably indicates a wound in deep compact dermis or subcutaneous tissue. Scars can appear from 6 weeks to 3 months post-treatment
- Hyperpigmentation
- Infection following dermabrasion is rare, herpes simplex infection can be devastating and, acyclovir should be given to those at risk
- Persistent erythema

Microdermabrasion

Microdermabrasion is used by beauticians to remove the stratum corneum and the epidermis. Aluminium oxide or sodium chloride microcrystals are used for the purpose. The microcrystals circulate through a high speed circulator; the waste is collected in a container. The depth of abrasion is controlled by pressure setting on the machine. After a number of treatments, there is thickening of the epidermis, an increase of collagen and elastic fibres. The skin has a smoother contour. This method is used for treating mild blemishes and early photodamage of the skin.

FILLING AGENTS

Battle against ageing has been going on since time immemorial; various methods have been used to fight against damage caused to the skin by ultraviolet light. Filling agents, such as hyaluronic acid, collagen, silicon, microlipoinjection and fibril are yet other armamentarium to the fight against old age.

These implants are injected in a depressed lesion, it should be placed high in the dermis because of migration that naturally takes place. The amount of the filling agent should be carefully adjusted. Overfilling the dermis will cause extrusion below the dermis or into the dermo-epidermal junction, the former is wasteful and the latter will bead up and look like a milium. Care should also be taken that the implant is not injected into the subcutaneous tissue.

It is also necessary to consider the lesion being treated. Deep acne scars should be over corrected so that they may end up with enough implant after the fluids are absorbed. Fine creases need only micro-droplets of the implant. Massage immediately after the injection will help to soothe irregularities to a limited degree.

Indications

- Scars. Acne scars, post- traumatic, post- viral scars, etc. Injections are best suitable for soft, gradual and depressed scars. Fibrotic and sharp walled scars do better with surgical treatment
- Creases, furrows, smile lines, and crow's feet
- There is a large podiatric experience of implants under the corns of feet
- Filling agents have also helped in chondrodermatitis nodularis chronica helicis, if surgery cannot be performed
- Lips can also be made more full with filling agents.

Methods of Injecting a Collagen Implant

Observation is the best way to learn how to inject implants. Most wrinkles and soft scars are significantly altered when a patient moves from a vertical to a horizontal position. Forehead creases are treated best with the patient in a supine position, for all other locations on the face the patient should sit or be upright.

The scar after cleaning is first stabilised between the thumb and index finger of the non-dominant hand. A Zyderm syringe is used to inject the implant. The needle enters 3–5 mm from the scar edge; it is advanced until the tip of the needle enters the scar, which is detected by increased resistance of the scar. The tip is advanced towards the opposite end of the scar, with injection of the implant on withdrawal of the needle.

For small diameter scars, the needle is injected perpendicular to the skin at the centre of the scar. The implant will flow evenly in all directions.

Linear scars are filled by multiple punctures starting at one end and advancing as far as the implant will flow easily. Soft scars fill easily; fibrotic scars may take several treatments.

Complications

- Allergic reaction
- Intermittent swelling
- Mechanical complications such as injecting too much or too little implant, or injecting the implant too high or too low in the skin. Too much implant may result in tissue necrosis. If a dermal arteriole is included, it may lead to ischaemia and necrosis. Vision loss has occurred while injecting collagen in the glabellar region
- Itching, burning and infections have been reported

BOTOX INJECTIONS

Botulinum toxin was first discovered during the Napoleonic wars. It was found to cause food poisoning after eating sausages. The word botulism comes from Latin word "botulus", meaning sausage. A German physician Justinus Kerner gave the full description of food borne botulism in 1820. The interest for therapeutic purposes began in 1949. Much later it was found that patients who were treated for strabismus showed improvement in their wrinkles after the use of botulinum toxin.

Botulinum neurotoxin (BTX) is produced by Gram-negative, anerobic bacteria *Clostridium botulinum*. Eight types of neurotoxin exist, these are A, B, C1, C2, D, E, F and G. Botulinum toxin A (Botox) is the toxin commonly used for the treatment of wrinkles. Botulinum toxin B BTX-B (myobloc, dysport) has a faster onset of action but its duration is shorter, and is more painful than BTX-A. The toxin acts by paralysing the muscles by chemical denervation. Neurotransmission at the neuromuscular junction involves the release of acetylcholine from the presynaptic nerve terminals.

Botulinum toxin-A acts on the wrinkles caused by hyperactive muscles, it does not act on wrinkles caused by loss of collagen and elastic tissue, nor will it act on wrinkles caused by gravity. Selection of the patients is therefore important. Knowledge of the muscles of facial expression and interaction between these muscles is an important prerequisite for botulinum toxin injection.

Botox acts best on wrinkles on the upper part of the face, in particular the crow's feet, glabellar lines and wrinkles on the forehead. Botox injected on the lower half of the face can result in an asymmetrical smile, inability to eat and speak properly, due to impairment of the muscles of mastication. Improvement is seen within a few days following the injection; the maximum effect is seen between 1–2 weeks. The effects of botox injections last for 2–6 months.

Side effects include bruising, haematoma formation, ptosis of the eyelid, double vision, "Mephisto brow" and an expressionless face.

Botox is contraindicated if there is sensitisation to botox injection, diseases of neuromuscular junction such as myasthenia gravis, drugs that interfere with neurotransmission, such as aminoglycosides, penicillamine, quinine, calcium-channel blockers and local infection at the injection site. Patients who are psychologically unstable or those who have unrealistic expectations should also be excluded from treatment.

FURTHER READING

1. Ahmed I, Berth-Jones J, Charles-Holmes S et al. Comparison of cryotherapy with curettage in the treatment of Bowen's disease: a prospective study. Br J Dermatol. 2000;143(4):759-66.
2. Alster TS, Lewis AB. Dermatologic laser surgery. Dermatol Surg. 1996;22(9):797-805.
3. Berneburg M, Rocken M, Benedix F. Phototherapy and Narrowband UVB. Acata Derm Venereol. 2005;85(2):98-108.
4. Campos VB, Dierickx CC, Farinelli WA, et al. Hair removal with 800 nm pulsed diode laser. J Am Acad Dermatol. 2000;43(3):442-7.
5. Colver GB, Cherry GW, Dawber RP, et al. Tattoo removal using infra-red coagulation. Br J Dermatol. 1985;112(4):481-5.
6. Conning DM, Hayes MJ. The dermal toxicity of phenol: an investigation of the most effective first-aid measures. Br J Ind Med. 1970;27(2):155-9.
7. Dierickx C, Alora MB, Dover JS. A clinical overview of hair removal using lasers and light sources. Dermatol Clin. 1999;17(2):357-66.
8. Fitzpatrick RE. Maximizing benefits and minimizing risks with CO_2 laser resurfacing. Dermatol Clin. 2002;20(1):77-86.
9. Goldman L, Dreffer R, Rockwell RJ Jr, et al. Treatment of port wine marks by an argon laser J Dermatol Surg. 1976;2(5):385-8.
10. Greenbaum SS, Koull EA, Watnick K. Comparison of CO_2 Laser and electrosurgery in the treatment of rhinophyma. J Am Acad Dermatol. 1988;18(2 Pt 1):363-8.
11. Jackson R. Basic principles of electrosurgery: a review. Can J Surg. 1970;13(4):354-61.
12. Kantor GR, Wheel and RG, Bailin PL, et al. Treatment of earlobe keloids with carbon dioxide laser excision: a report of 16 cases . J Dermatol Surg Oncol. 1985;11(11):1063-7.
13. Klein AW. Skin filling. Collagen and other injectables of the skin.. Dermatol Clin. 2001;19(3):491-508, ix.
14. Mosley H, Ferguson J. Photochemotherapy: a reappraisal of its use in dermatology. Drugs. 1989;38:822-37
15. Phillips TJ, Gerstein AD, Lordan V. A randomized controlled trial of hydrocolloid dressing in the treatment of hypertrophic scars and keloids. Dermatol Surg. 1996;22(9):775-8.
16. Rapaport MJ, Vinnik C, Zarem H. Injectable silicon: cause of facial nodules, cellulitis, ulceration, and migration. Aesthetic Plast Surg. 1996;20(3):267-76.
17. Ridge MD, Wright V. The directional effects of skin: a bioengineering study of skin with particular reference to Langer's Lines. J Invest Dermatol. 1966;46(4):341-6.
18. Sebben JE. Electrosurgery and cardiac pacemakers. J Am Acad Dermatol. 1983;9(3):457-63.
19. Sheehan MP, Atherton DJ, Norris P, et al. Oral psoralen photochemotherapy in severe childhood atopic eczema: an update. Br J Dermatol. 1993;129:431-6.
20. Spicer MS, Goldberg DJ. Lasers in dermatology. J Am Acad Dermatol. 1996;34(1):1-25.
21. Stegman SJ, Tromoviteh TA. Suturing techniques for dermatological surgery. J Dermatol Surg Oncol. 1978;4:63-8
22. Swanson NA. Mohs surgery. Technique, indications, applications, and the future. Arch Dermatol. 1983;119(9):761-73.
23. Sweet RD. The treatment of basal cell carcinoma by curettage. Br J Dermatol. 1963; 75:137-48.
24. Vano -Galvan S, Jean P. Complications of nonphysician-supervised laser hair removal. Can Fam Physician. 2009;55(1):50-2.

Chapter

45

Radiotherapy in Dermatology

INTRODUCTION

Radiotherapy or radiation therapy describes the use of ionising X-ray for the treatment of mainly malignant tumours but occasionally also benign diseases. Since its infancy, radiotherapy has been closely associated with dermatology. Following the discovery of X-ray in 1895, it was discovered that radiation exposure produced cutaneous reactions, manifesting as erythema, dermatitis and ulceration. Prior to our current understanding of the biological effects of X-ray, radiotherapy was commonly used in a variety of dermatological conditions with both beneficial and detrimental effects. Currently, radiation is selectively used due to its potential genotoxic and carcinogenic side-effects. Radiation therapy is generally indicated in cases in whom surgery is not the preferred option (better cosmetic results or medically unfit). Radiotherapy use is avoided in younger patients and contraindicated in pregnant individuals.

Types of Ionising Radiation used in Dermatology

X-ray (photon) energies are measured in kilovolts (kV) or megavolts (MV). The higher the energy, the more penetrating the X-ray, although MV X-ray tends to produce a skin-sparing effect. Early X-ray machines were capable of generating radiation at about 150 kV, but more powerful 8 MV generators were developed in the 1950s (called linear accelerator or linacs). Although there is diminishing use of kV X-ray due to newer MV linacs, most radiotherapy treatment centres still use low voltage X-ray units due to low cost and convenient treatment delivery techniques. Kilovoltage therapy can be grouped into these categories: Grenz rays (10–20 kV), contact therapy (40–50 kV) that treat up to 2-mm depth, superficial therapy (50–150 kV) treatment up to 5-mm depth, and orthovoltage therapy (200–500 kV). Grenz rays have a very low penetrating power that is limited to the dermis and were previously used to treat superficial lesions (1–2 mm) with the aim of exerting an anti-inflammatory effect (reported to reduce Langerhans cell numbers). In addition to using X-ray, it is also possible to use high energy mega electron volts or MeV electron beams for treating superficial lesions because the majority of the dose is deposited near the surface. As a general rule, superficial X-ray is used to treat lesions within 5-mm depth, less than 4 cm across and away from cartilage and bone. Electron beams are more appropriate for treating depths greater than 5 mm, and wider than 4 cm across, but avoiding eyes (lateral scatter of beam) and air spaces (dose in homogeneity).

Radiation Dose

The gray (Gy) is the SI unit of absorbed dose of ionising radiation. One gray is defined as one joule ionising energy absorbed by 1 kg of matter (usually tissue). The gray replaced the previous unit termed the rad (radiation absorbed dose). The conversion is easy; 1 Gy equals 100 rads or 100 centigray (cGy).

For a given treatment, a radiotherapist will prescribe a total dose, delivered in smaller "fractions" (usually daily), over a defined time. Due to the geometrical variation across tumours, it is unrealistic to expect the whole target area to receive a homogenous dose; to counteract this radiotherapists prescribe a dose range across the target volume that is defined by strict criteria, although the prescription point is fixed. Typical fractionation regimens for curative treatments include 55 Gy in 20 fractions over 4 weeks. The radiotherapist also has to select the most appropriate beam type (kV versus MV energy) or photon versus electron beams. It is usually difficult to repeat a curative radiotherapy treatment as the dose is limited by the toxicity to surrounding normal tissues. In the context of treating benign conditions, the aim is to use the lowest and most effective radiotherapy dose, in order to minimise any long-term toxicity.

Mechanism of Action

The purpose of radiation treatment is to deliver high energy electromagnetic radiation to a defined target (usually cancerous cells) with the required biological effect, through DNA damage, resulting in cell death. Direct or indirect ionisation of the atoms contained within the DNA are responsible for converting high energy radiation into biological effects. Indirect ionisation is mediated through the ionisation of water generating free radicals. These highly reactive hydroxyl radicals damage cellular DNA. Radiotherapy takes advantage of the differential DNA repair ability in cancer cells and the normal tissues. Normal tissues have a more competent repair process compared with cancer cells that are more likely to suffer cell death following formation of a DNA double strand break. This therapeutic window is used in maximising tumour cell death with minimal normal tissue toxicity.

Direct DNA damage is caused by charged particles interacting and causing ionisation of atoms within DNA leading to free radical formation, unlike indirect DNA free radical formation in nearby water molecules. Radiation mediating damage through direct effects has little role in the dermatological setting.

Radiosensitivity

Radiosensitivity is the term used to describe the relative susceptibility of cells to the damaging effects of ionising radiation. According to classical radiobiological principles, cellular sensitivity to radiation is mediated by several factors. Cells are thought to be more sensitive to radiation in the mitotic phase of the cell cycle. Cells that are dividing rapidly are metabolically active and undifferentiated are more prone to radiation-induced damage. Hypoxic tumour cells are relatively protected from the formation of damaging free radicals, although this is reversible through the various methods available for the re-oxygenation of tumours. As outlined above, tumour cells are thought to have an impaired repair capacity in comparison to non-cancerous cells. By delivering the radiation in regular smaller doses, this allows normal tissues to repair DNA damage following irradiation, but inadequate repair time for cancer cells.

Treatment Regimens

The dose of radiotherapy will be tailored to the tumour histology and size, site (surrounding normal tissue may limit total dose), and patient's co-morbidities. Each case must take into account factors such as those highlighted above. Generally speaking the aim is to deliver a curative dose with minimal toxicity to the surrounding normal tissue in the safest and (where appropriate) convenient manner. Most treatment regimens prefer to deliver the treatment by dividing the dose into fractions.

Fractionated radiotherapy is used, providing better sparing of the unaffected skin and tissues. Basal cell carcinoma and squamous cell carcinoma are generally treated with a total of 55 Gy, delivered over 20-treatment sessions. Other treatment regimens include 45 Gy in 10 fractions (lesions smaller than 4 cm), or 60 Gy in 30 fractions (lesions greater than 4 cm at sites of poor radiation tolerance). Studies treating patients with lentigo maligna have reported successful outcomes with doses between 35 Gy and 100 Gy using orthovoltage treatments. Lymphomas are very radiosensitive requiring much lower doses of between 5 Gy and 15 Gy.

Postradiation Changes in the Skin

One of the main concerns regarding radiotherapy use relates to the development of both acute and late radiation-induced side effects to normal tissues. The effects of radiation treatment on normal tissues has been traditionally divided into early (acute) effects that occur within a few weeks of commencing treatment, and late responses where clinical symptoms may manifest themselves over months to years. Tissues that have a rapid cellular turnover and renewal are more prone to an acute response. In addition, damage to the tissue vasculature and connective tissue can also lead to secondary parenchymal death and late effects.

Acute radiation responses occur mainly in tissues where there has been death of critical cell populations such as the basal skin layer. Although these effects occur within 3 months of the initiation of radiotherapy, there is rapid tissue repopulation regenerating the parenchymal cell population thereby not limiting the treatment delivery. The early changes reflect injury, apoptosis and reproductive failure in the basal layer and hair matrix cells. Epidermal cell replacement occurs in 3–5 weeks after radiation. Langerhans cells are relatively radioresistant.

Radiation-induced cell death in normal tissues is thought to occur when the cells attempt to divide and undergo mitosis. Hence, the acute response will occur on a timescale similar to the normal cell turnover. Acute reactions tend to be relatively insensitive to changes in the radiation dose per fraction but are sensitive to the time over which radiation is delivered.

The exact acute effects are dependent upon multiple factors, including age, sex, site of exposure, and radiation dose. Late radiotherapy tissue responses are observed in organs whose parenchymal cells divide slowly and do not express mitotic death until they divide. Late responses usually limit the dose of radiation that can be safely delivered to a patient during a course of radiotherapy. The pathogenesis is linked to the formation of tissue fibrosis that can occur in many different tissue types, and several years after radiation delivery. Radiation-induced fibrosis appears to be mediated through the release of inflammatory cytokines, particularly transforming growth factor-beta (TGF-β), that can stimulate fibroblast proliferation and collagen production. Late toxicity is more sensitive to changes in the radiation dose per fraction and less sensitive to the overall treatment time. Within 2–3 weeks following exposure to high doses of fractionated radiation, acute erythema, (dry and moist) desquamation, and epilation occur. Ulceration is not a common feature, but re-epithelialization commences about 3 weeks following completing of radiotherapy.

Chronic postradiation changes result from injury to dermal structures, particularly the vascular and connective tissue, leading to atrophy of the skin. Progressive postradiation changes are cytokine mediated. In addition to the skin, changes are also seen in the hair. Changes are first seen in the highly proliferative anagen hair matrix. Radiation induces hair dysplasia, and reduced hair length and hair growth rate. Low-dose radiation can also have an effect upon melanin formation, inducing cutaneous hyperpigmentation after minimal inflammation. Pigmentation is directly related to dose rate and total dose. It is characterised by an increase in the number of melanocytes, with increased tyrosinase activity, and by enhanced melanin transfer to the epidermal cells. Higher radiation doses destroy melanocytes with resultant hypopigmentation. Similar changes may occur in anagen hair follicles. At higher doses, hair melanocytes are more susceptible to radiation destruction than epidermal melanocytes.

Indications for Radiation

The application of radiotherapy has been reduced greatly due to newer and advanced methods of treatments such as Mohs surgery and photodynamic therapy. Dermatological radiotherapy still has a place in the treatment of large and complicated tumours.

The most common cutaneous tumours treated with radiotherapy include basal cell and squamous cell carcinomas. Although lesions are amenable to surgical excision, there are indications where radiotherapy should be the preferred option. Older patients, with large superficial lesions, multiple tumours are commonly treated with ionising radiation. Other indications for radiotherapy include patients with multiple lesions, those refusing surgery, or lesions in an area where surgery would cause loss of function or would leave a cosmetic defect. Radiotherapy is also indicated postoperatively in cases with incomplete excision or perineural invasion.

Surgery is best avoided in tumours of the lower eyelid, medial and lateral canthus, nasolabial folds where adequate surgical clearance would be difficult without significant cosmetic deformity. Sites of previous burns and scarring are best avoided for treatment with radiotherapy. Mycosis fungoides is a cutaneous tumour that can either be treated focally (limited

Table 1: Indications of radiation therapy

Malignant tumors	*Benign conditions*
Superficial basal cell carcinoma in a difficult surgical site.	Keloids are the only benign condition which can be considered for radiotherapy
Some cases of squamous-cell carcinoma, lymphoma and Kaposi's sarcoma (outlined above)	
Malignant melanoma is usually not irradiated, except some cases of in situ lentigo maligna	
Merkel cell tumor by excision and radiotherapy	
As palliative therapy for inoperable tumors	
Electron beam therapy for mycosis fungoides	

plaque stage) or more generally using total skin irradiation, giving control in cases of up to 90%.

Recently low dose radiotherapy has been used in the treatment of hidradenitis suppurativa in which all other treatment modalities have failed. As radiation is mutagenic a very careful selection of patients is necessary.

Surgery is the preferred option in younger patients, with small lesions, sites involving relatively radioresistant areas (bone, cartilage, tendon, or joints), uncertain histology, or recurrence postradiotherapy. Areas that poorly tolerate radiation due to relative vascular insufficiency include the dorsum of the hand, digits, or the shin (Table 1).

Side Effects of Radiotherapy and Skin Care

There are four recognised stages of a skin reaction; erythema, dry desquamation, moist desquamation and (rarely) necrosis. Erythema is the initial change, characterised by pink or red skin within the radiotherapy treatment field. The patient may experience pruritus in addition to vesicles or occasionally bullae formation. Dry desquamation is characterised by dry, flaky superficial skin loss which can be seen following erythema (especially in the neck and skin folds). Moist desquamation is characterised by the loss of the epidermis resulting in exudate formation. The exposed surface appears raw, may bleed and is usually seen in the skin folds and areas subject to friction, particularly in patients receiving radiotherapy for head and neck cancers. Necrosis occurs if skin tolerance is exceeded such that the basal cells are killed. It is now uncommon as radiotherapists have more advanced treatment techniques and a better understanding of skin tolerance.

The aims of skin care include prevention, early detection and prompt treatment. General advice includes wearing loose natural fibres, avoiding tight clothing (can cause a shearing force and increase friction), and to minimise any scratching of the area. Hygiene advice includes the use of mild unscented soap, air drying after washing, and avoidance of wet shaving in the treatment area. Emollient creams are used daily to the treatment site (not within 1 hour before treatment). Hydrocolloid dressings provide good symptomatic relief in patients with a moist desquamation skin reaction. Mild steroid creams can be used for problematic itching unresponsive to other measures.

Radioprotectants are currently being evaluated in an attempt to minimise normal tissue toxicity. Misoprostol is a prostaglandin E analogue that may play a role in the future to reduce radiation induced normal tissue toxicity. Following radiotherapy for dermatological malignancies, patients are followed to detect local relapses, and to monitor for signs of late toxicity and radiation-induced cancers (rare).

There is no effective treatment for radiation dermatitis; protection of unaffected areas is of prime importance.

Wilhelm C Roentgen (1872–1919) a physicist discovered the Roentgen rays in 1895. He died of cancer of the intestine. It is not known if the cancer was due to ionising radiations; as all scientific documents were destroyed after his death according to his will. Roentgen received the Nobel Prize for physics in 1901.

FURTHER READING

1. Fuks A, Bagshaw MA. Total skin electron beam treatment of mycosis fungoides. Radiology. 1971;100:145-50.
2. Harwood AR. Conventional radiotherapy in the treatment of lentigo maligna and lentigo maligna melanoma. J Am Acad Dermatol. 1982;6:310-6.
3. James WD, Odom RB. Late subcutaneous fibrosis, following megavoltage radiotherapy. J Am Acad Dermatol. 1980;3:616-8.
4. Kurban AK, Farah FS. Effects of X-irradiation on the skin. Acta Derm Venereol (Stockh) 1969;49:64-71.
5. Lo TCM, Seckel BR, Salzman FA, et al. Single-dose electron beam radiation in the treatment and prevention of keloids and hypertrophic scars. J Radiother Oncol. 1990;19:267-72.
6. Okazki M, Kikuchi I. Radiodermatitis: an analysis of 43 cases. J Dermatol. 1986;13:356-65.
7. Shah N. Hidradenitis Suppurative: A Treatment Challenge. Am Fam Physician. 2005;72(8): 1547-52.
8. Trombetta M, Werts ED and Parda D. The role of radiotherapy in the treatment of hidradenitis suppurativa: Case report and review of literature. Derm Online Journal. UC Davis. 2010; 16(2):16.

Appendix 1 Generalised Eruptions

PAPULOSQUAMOUS LESIONS

Psoriasis, lichen planus, drug eruptions, mycosis fungoides, pityriasis rubra pilaris, Darier's disease, pityriasis lichenoides chronica, parapsoriasis, syphilis (secondary stage).

VESICULOBULLOUS LESIONS

Pemphigus, pemphigoid, dermatitis herpetiformis, linear IgA dermatosis, epidermolysis bullosa, bullous ichthyosiform erythroderma, bullous disease of childhood, acrodermatitis enteropathica, impetigo herpetiformis, eczema herpeticum, bullous drug eruption, bullous systemic lupus erythematosus, bullous lichen planus.

PAPULONODULAR LESIONS

Lepromatous leprosy, diffuse cutaneous leishmaniasis, mycosis fungoides, drug eruptions, neurofibromatosis, generalised xanthomas, generalised granuloma annulare, generalised Kaposi's sarcoma, sarcoidosis, lymphomas, yaws (secondary stage), generalised eruptive histiocytosis, progressive nodular histiocytosis.

ERYTHRODERMA

Eczema, psoriasis, drug eruptions, ichthyosiform erythroderma, Sezary's syndrome, generalised urticaria, pemphigus, pemphigoid, transient erythema of the newborn, TEN (toxic epidermal necrolysis), SSSS (staphylococcal scalded skin syndrome), toxic shock syndrome.

GENERALISED HYPERPIGMENTATION

Genetic, gross malnutrition, deficiency of vitamin B_{12}, deficiency of riboflavin, carbon baby, dyskeratosis congenita (mottled/reticulate hyperpigmentation), chronic renal failure, chronic liver disease, Addison's disease, Gaucher's disease (yellowish-brown), generalised lentigines.

GENERALISED HYPOPIGMENTATION

Albinism, generalised vitiligo, incontinentia pigmenti achromians, selenium deficiency, phenylketonuria, Chediak-Higashi syndrome, Cross syndrome, Luna moon children, Tietz syndrome.

GENERALISED INFILTRATIONS

Scleroderma, scleredema, Myxedema, scleromyxedema, mucopolysaccharidosis, diffuse infiltrating carcinoma, generalised hyaline fibromatosis, acromegaly, Winchester syndrome, lichen myxedematosus, congenital hyalinosis, diffuse cutaneous mastocytosis, infantile restrictive dermopathy, drugs (bleomycin, penicillamine, cocaine), occupational (vinyl chloride, aromatic hydrocarbons, aliphatic hydrocarbons, epoxy resins).

RASH AND FEVER

Measles, scarlet fever, roseola, typhoid fever, rubella, infectious mononucleosis, serum sickness, allergic vasculitis, rheumatic fever, hypersensitivity syndromes, chickenpox, pityriasis lichenoides acuta, erythema multiforme, Rocky Mountain spotted fever, rickettsial pox.

Appendix 2 Hair Disorders

ALOPECIA

Generalised Hair Loss (Non-Cicatricial)

Telogen effluvium, anagen effluvium, alopecia areata-totalis/universalis, androgenetic alopecia (advanced), premature ageing, malnutrition, zinc deficiency, systemic lupus erythematosus, chronic liver disease, post-encephalitis, hypothalamic disorders, damage to the brain stem, syringomyelia, chronic liver disease, anhidrotic ectodermal dysplasia, oral contraceptives, hypothyroidism, hypopituitary states, hypoparathyroidism, diabetes mellitus, secondary syphilis, crash dieting, acute infections, post-febrile, post-puerperium, post-surgical, chronic debilitating diseases, hypothyroidism, endocrinopathies, drugs such as retinoids, anti-convulsants, anti-coagulants anti-thyroid, lithium, indomethacin and heavy metals.

Localised Hair Loss (Non-Cicatricial)

Alopecia areata, tinea capitis, trichotillomania, traction alopecia, folliculitis impetigo, androgenetic alopecia (early stage), dermal dysplasia, anhidrotic ectodermal dysplasia, congenital triangular alopecia, dyskeratosis congenita, Cockayne's syndrome.

Cicatricial Alopecia

Kerion, favus, CDLE, severe bacterial infections such as carbuncles, lichen planus, folliculitis decalvans, naevus sebaceous, herpes zoster, necrobiosis lipoidica, tumours of the scalp, leishmaniasis, pseudopelade, chronic radiation, post-surgical, post-traumatic, burns, acne keloidalis, dissecting cellulitis of the scalp, sarcoidosis, Darier's disease, epidermolysis bullosa, epidermal naevus, Conradi's syndrome, pachyonychia congenita, congenital aplasia of the skin, follicular mucinosis.

HYPERTRICHOSIS

Hypertrichosis Lanuginosa

Congenital, acquired hypertrichosis lanuginosa may be secondary to malignancies of the gastrointestinal tract, bronchus, urinary bladder or the breast.

Hypertrichosis of Vellus Hair

Generalised hypertrichosis: Malnutrition, anorexia nervosa, acrodynia, Hurler's syndrome, Winchester's syndrome, trisomy 18, secondary to drugs such as minoxidil, benoxaprofen, cortisone, cyclosporine, streptomycin, diphenylhydantoin, penicillamine, psoralen.

Localised hypertrichosis: Becker's naevus: on the shoulder or pectoral area, hypothyroidism- back or extensor of limbs, hyperthyroidism: over the plaque of pretibial myxedema, secondary to plucking, dermatomyositis: forearms, legs, temples, plaster of Paris-over the occlusion, secondary to surgical wounds, traumatic sites of epidermolysis bullosa, spina bifida.

Appendix

3 Face

LESIONS ON THE BUTTERFLY AREA OF THE FACE

Systemic lupus erythematosus, rosacea, seborrheic dermatitis, erysipelas, pemphigus erythematosus, photosensitive eruptions, pellagra, carcinoid syndrome, Hartnup's disease, Bloom's syndrome, Rothmund-Thomson syndrome, erythema infectiosum.

MELASMA

Familial, post-pregnancy, drugs such as oestrogens, progesterone, phenytoin, chlorpromazine, amiodarone; Riehl's melanosis, phototoxicity, pigmentation after the use of hydroquinone.

PERIORBITAL PIGMENTATION

Racial, familial, post-traumatic, postinflammatory, chemicals such as mercury, silver and gold, drugs such as minocycline, psoralens, cosmetics, porphyria cutanea tarda, dehydration, exhaustion, chronic illness such as kidney failure, hepatic failure, purpuric plaques of systemic amyloidosis, ochronosis, naevus of Ota.

PERIORBITAL OEDEMA

Cutaneous causes: Angioedema, contact dermatitis, periorbital cellulitis, lymphoedema of rosacea, dermatomyositis, necrotising fasciitis.

Systemic causes: Glomerulonephritis, hypoalbuminemia, cardiac failure, superior vena caval obstruction, thyroid disease, scarlet fever, Chaga's disease.

PERIORAL LESIONS

Angular stomatitis, herpes simplex, perioral dermatitis, contact dermatitis, acrodermatitis enteropathica, South American leishmaniasis, yaws.

FLUSHING

Menopause, rosacea, carcinoid syndrome, pheochromocytoma, mastocytosis, chemicals (alcohol, nicotinamide, prostaglandin D_2, organic nitrates), drugs (calcium channel blockers, disulfiram, cyclosporin, vancomycin), food intolerance, blushing (emotional).

PHOTOSENSITIVE ERUPTIONS

Sunburn, photosensitive eczema, chronic actinic dermatitis, polymorphic light eruption, actinic keratosis, actinic lichen planus, actinic prurigo, rosacea, lupus erythematosus, scleroderma, dermatomyositis, Bloom's syndrome, Cockayne's syndrome, Rothmund-Thompson's syndrome, xeroderma pigmentosum, porphyrias, pellagra, carcinoid syndrome, Hartnup's disease, photosensitive drug eruptions, phototoxicity by chemicals and plants.

LOSS OF OUTER THIRD OF EYEBROWS

Leprosy, myxedema, anhidrotic ectodermal dysplasia, ulerythema oophryogenes, lymphoreticulosis, trichotillomania, sometimes seen in normal elderly patients.

Appendix 4 Upper and Lower Limb

ELBOWS AND KNEES

Papules and plaques: Psoriasis, lichen spinulosus, chronic zinc deficiency, xanthoma tuberosum, pityriasis rubra pilaris (juvenile), follicular ichthyosis, erythema elevatum diutinum, keratosis circumscripta, epidermal dysplasia verruciformis.

Vesicular and bullous lesions: Dermatitis herpetiformis, epidermolysis bullosa.

JUXTA-ARTICULAR NODULES

Xanthoma, rheumatoid arthritis, calcinosis, cutis, synovial cyst, multicentric reticulohistiocytosis, juvenile hyaline fibromatosis, erythema elevatum diutinum intra-joint pathology.

PALMOPLANTAR KERATOSES

Contact dermatitis, fungal infection, psoriasis, lichen planus, pityriasis rubra pilaris, Darier's disease, dyskeratosis congenita, ichthyosis, hereditary palmoplantar keratosis.

NODULES ON THE LEG

Panniculitis—erythema nodosum, Weber Christian disease, Rothmann Makai syndrome, pancreatic panniculitis

Vascular—erythema induratum, polyarteritis nodosa, erythema nodosum migrans, nodular vasculitis,

Tumours—histiocytoma, lymphoma, squamous cell carcinoma, malignant melanoma, Kaposi's sarcoma, basal cell carcinoma, clear cell acanthoma.

Miscellaneous—prurigo, lichen amyloidosis, Majocchi's granuloma.

Leg ulcers described in chapter 18.

Pigmented purpuras described in chapter 19.

Appendix 5

Flexures

Intertrigo
Tinea cruris
Candidiasis
Contact dermatitis
Seborrhoeic dermatitis
Hidradenitis suppurativa
Erythrasma
Inverse psoriasis
Pemphigus vegetans
Hailey-Hailey disease
Fox-Fordyce disease
Acanthosis nigricans
Scrofuloderma
Trichomycosis axillaries
Necrolytic migratory erythema
Extramammary Paget's disease

Appendix 6

Lesions Differentiated by Colour

BLUE LESIONS

Melanocytic—Pigmented lesions with melanocytes in the dermis such as Mongolian spot, naevus of Ota, naevus of Ito, blue naevus.

Vascular—Venous lesions such as cavernous haemangioma, blue rubber bleb nevus.

Miscellaneous—Hidrocystoma, Kaposi's sarcoma (bluish purple), sarcoidosis (bluish-red).

Blue skin colour. Cyanosis.

YELLOW LESIONS

Lipid abnormalities—Xanthomas, xanthelasma, lipid dystrophies,

Elastic tissue abnormalities—Solar elastosis, pseudoxanthoma elasticum,

Sebaceous gland abnormalities—Sebaceous gland hyperplasia, naevus sebaceous, Fox Fordyce spots, sebaceous gland tumours,

Miscellaneous: Necrobiosis lipoidica, epidermal keratin cysts, all pustular lesions,

Yellow skin colour—Jaundice, carotenemia (sclera normal colour), severe anemia.

BROWN LESIONS

Melanocytic abnormalities: Melanoma, melanocytic naevi, pigmented basal cell carcinoma, freckles, lentigenes, café-au-lait patches
Seborrhoeic keratosis

Miscellaneous: Telon noir, dermatosis papulosa nigra, histiofibroma, acanthosis nigricans.

TRANSLUCENT/PEARLY

Molluscum contagiosum, syringoma, apocrine/eccrine hidrocystoma, trichoepithelioma, basal cell carcinoma.

Appendix 7

Lesions Differentiated by Appearance and Texture

Keratotic—Verruca vulgaris, angiokeratoma, tuberculosis verrucosa cutis, chromoblastomycosis

Cystic—Epidermal cyst, dermoid cyst, milia, steatocystoma multiplex

Indented: Molluscum contagiosum, giant comedones, keratoacanthoma, sebaceous hyperplasia, cutaneous penicilliosis

Soft—Lipoma, connective tissue nevus, angiolipoma, neurofibromatosis

Hard—Osteoma cutis, calcinosis cutis, exostosis, chondroma, pilomatricoma.

Appendix 8 Vascular Reactions

Transient erythemas. Urticaria, dermographism, erythema marginatum, flushing syndromes.

Persistent erythemas (livedo pattern). Livedo vasculitis, livedo reticularis, anti phospholipid syndrome, cholesterol emboli, polyarteritis nodosa and other large vessel vasculitis, erythema infectiosum, erythema ab igne, poikiloderma, cutis marmorata telangiectatica.

Persistent erythemas (gyrate, serpiginous and annular pattern). Erythema annulare centrifugum, erythema gyratum repens, erythema chronicum migrans, subacute cutaneous lupus erythematosus.

(*Differentiate from other annular lesions such as granuloma annulare, annular sarcoid, annular psoriasis, ringworm infections, etc.*)

Persistent erythemas (telangiectatic pattern). Essential telangiectasia, unilateral naevoid telangiectasia, telangiectasia of collagen vascular disease, telangiectasia macularis eruptiva perstans, ataxia telangiectasia, radiodermatitis, poikilodermatous conditions.

Persistent erythemas (diffuse). Toxic epidermal necrolysis (early stage), toxic shock syndrome, staphylococcal scalded skin syndrome, scarlet fever, viral exanthems (measles, rubella, roseola), hypersensitivity syndromes.

Appendix 9

Nail Disorders

KOILONYCHIA

Physiological in neonates and infancy, iron deficiency, old age (peripheral arterial disease), soft nail (occupational), Plummer-Vinson syndrome, ectodermal dysplasia, nail patella syndrome, trichothiodystrophy, carpal tunnel syndrome, traumatic (nail of rickshaw drivers), contact with oils, alopecia areata, Darier's disease, Raynaud's phenomenon.

ONYCHOLYSIS

Cutaneous causes: Psoriasis, drugs (bleomycin, minocycline, PUVA, quinine, doxycycline, captopril), alopecia areata, atopic dermatitis, Reiter's disease, actinic reticulosis, mycosis fungoides, hyperhidrosis, histiocytosis, shell nail syndrome, trauma, hereditary, cosmetics, bacterial fungal and viral infections, chemicals-prolonged immersion in water, acids and alkalis, microwave injury, partial hereditary onycholysis, yellow nail syndrome.

Systemic causes: Systemic lupus erythematosus, hyperthyroidism, pregnancy, syphilis, iron deficiency anaemia, carcinoma of the lung, pellagra.

PITTING

Psoriasis, alopecia areata, atopic dermatitis, following severe illness, trauma, contact dermatitis, pityriasis rosea, sarcoidosis, lichen planus, median nail dystrophy, parakeratosis pustulosa, paronychia.

THICKENING

Onychomycosis, psoriasis, aspergillosis, Reiter's disease, onychogryphosis in old age, contact dermatitis, ichthyosis, Norwegian scabies, pachyonychia congenita, pachydermoperiostosis, yellow nail syndrome, hyperuricemia, pityriasis rubra pilaris, Bazex acrokeratosis neoplastica, arsenic keratosis, radiation dermatitis.

THINNING

Lichen planus, iron deficiency anemia, peripheral vascular disease, Darier's disease, familial, congenital, epidermolysis bullosa.

PTERYGIUM FORMATION

Dorsal—lichen planus, congenital, bullous dermatosis, Stevens-Johnson syndrome, graft-versus-host reaction, onychotillomania, radiation dermatitis, Raynaud's phenomenon.

Ventral—congenital, familial, idiopathic, peripheral neuropathy, Raynaud's disease, trauma, scleroderma, chronic disseminated lupus erythematosus, causalgia of the median nerve.

ATROPHY

Vasculitis, lichen planus, ten nail dystrophy.

SHEDDING OF THE NAIL

Trauma, alopecia areata universalis, severe local inflammation (acute paronychia, Kawasaki's disease), severe systemic upset, drugs (PUVA, cytotoxic, retinoids, tetracycline), radiation dermatitis, pemphigus and other bullous dermatosis, Stevens-Johnson syndrome, Lyell's disease, yellow nail syndrome, hypoparathyroidism, acrodermatitis enteropathica, keratosis punctata.

LONGITUDINAL GROOVES

Old age, physiological, Darier's disease, onychorrhexis, myxoid cyst (wide deep longitudinal groove), lichen planus, chronic injury, trachyonychia, Raynaud's phenomenon, lichen striatus, median nail dystrophy.

TRANSVERSE LINES

Beaus lines (high fever, myocardial infarction, measles, Stevens-Johnsons syndrome, Lyell's disease), Mee's lines, Muehrcke's line, contact dermatitis, psoriasis (patterned pitting), physiological (newborn babies), menstrual irregularities, local inflammation, zinc deficiency, overzealous nail manicuring, chronic paronychia, Kawasaki's disease, acrodermatitis enteropathica, hypoparathyroidism, syphilis.

HAEMORRHAGE

Congestive cardiac failure, collagen vascular disease, psoriasis, eczema, rheumatoid arthritis, rheumatic fever, amyloidosis, cirrhosis of the liver, Behcet's disease, Darier's disease, high altitudes, hypoparathyroidism, pityriasis rubra pilaris, scurvy, septicemia, trichinosis, vasculitis, thyrotoxicosis, Raynaud's disease, idiopathic.

Appendix 10 Miscellaneous

ANNULAR LESIONS

Infections: Ringworm infection, annular lupus vulgaris, tuberculoid leprosy,

Infiltrations: Granuloma annulare, granuloma multiforme, Jessner's lymphatic infiltration.

Inflammation: Annular psoriasis, annular lichen planus, subacute lupus erythematosus, annular sarcoidosis, pityriasis rosea,

Erythemas: Erythema annulare centrifugum, erythema chronicum migrans, erythema multiforme, erythema marginatum rheumaticum,

Miscellaneous: Purpura annularis of Majocchi, subcorneal pustular dermatosis, porokeratosis, urticaria, intracellular IgA dermatosis.

LINEAR LESIONS

Along Blaschko's line: Linear epidermal naevus,

Koebner's phenomenon: Psoriasis, warts, molluscum contagiosum

Inflammation: Linear morphoea

Dermatomal: Herpes zoster, segmental vitiligo,
Linear contact dermatitis, e.g. rhus dermatitis

Linear purpura: Vibices

Lymphatic spread: Leishmaniasis, sprotrichosis, atypical mycobacterial infections, tularaemia, glanders, North American blastomycosis, nocardosis, lymphangitis

Venous spread: Superficial thrombophlebitis

Arterial spread: Temporal arteritis, polyarteritis nodosa

Miscellaneous: Lichen striatus, larva migrans, scratch marks, striae.

GROUPED LESIONS

Herpes simplex, herpes zoster, dermatitis herpetiformis, pemphigus herpetiformis, lymphangioma, leiomyoma, lichen spinulosus, lichen scrofulosorum, epidermolysis bullosa herpetiformis.

COMEDONES

Acne vulgaris, naevus comedonicus, hidradenitis suppurativa, senile comedones, Favre-Racouchot syndrome, autoimmune progesterone dermatitis, basal cell naevus syndrome, steatocystoma multiplex.

STERILE PUSTULAR DERMATOSES

Palmoplantar pustular dermatosis, pustular psoriasis, subcorneal pustular dermatosis, erythema toxicum neonatorum, transient neonatal pustular dermatosis, acropustulosis, impetigo herpetiformis, intraepidermal IgA dermatosis, blind loop syndrome, eosinophilic pustular folliculitis, Behcet's disease, pyoderma gangrenosum.

DISEASES ASSOCIATED WITH EOSINOPHILIA

Eosinophilic folliculitis, eosinophilic fasciitis, Well's syndrome, angiolymphoid hyperplasia with eosinophilia, Kimura's disease, hypereosinophilic syndrome, pemphigoid eosinophilia, transient neonatal toxaemia, granuloma faciale, Churg-Strauss syndrome.

NEUTROPHILIC DERMATOSES

Sweets syndrome, Behcet's disease, pyoderma gangrenosum, rheumatoid neutrophilic dermatitis, linear IgA disease, dermatitis herpetiformis, leukocytoclastic vasculitis, erythema elevatum diutinum, dermatitis associated with inflammatory bowel disease, reactions to granulocyte colony-stimulating factor (GCSF).

STIFF SKIN SYNDROME

Scleroderma, scleredema, Winchester syndrome, eosinophilic fasciitis, lichen myxomatosis, congenital hyalinosis, infantile restrictive dermopathy, congenital facial dystrophy, drugs (bleomycin, penicillamine, cocaine), occupational (vinyl chloride disease, aromatic hydrocarbons, aliphatic hydrocarbons, epoxy resins).

ULCERS AT THE SITE OF INJURY

Epidermolysis bullosa (Congenital and acquired) prolidase deficiency, Weary-Kindler syndrome, laryngo-onycho-cutaneous syndrome (Shabbir syndrome), Bart's syndrome.

CUTANEOUS DISEASES ASSOCIATED WITH MALIGNANCY

Congenital disorders: Xeroderma pigmentosum, Cowden's syndrome, Gardner's syndrome. Peutz-Jeghers syndrome, multiple mucosal neuroma syndrome, Muir-Torre syndrome, Howell-Evans syndrome, Gorlin's sundrome, familial atypical multiple melanoma, Carney's syndrome, tumours associated with immunodeficiency.

Acquired disorders: Bazex syndrome, Cronkhite-Canada syndrome, hypertrichosis lanuginosa, malignant acanthosis nigricans, erythema gyratum repens, sign of Leser-Trelat, paraneoplastic pemphigus.

MACROGLOSSIA

Amyloidosis, angioedema, myxedema, acanthosis nigricans, mucopolysaccharidosis, lipidosis, acromegaly, Down's syndrome, haemangioma.

GINGIVAL HYPERPLASIA

Pregnancy, scurvy, drugs (cyclosporine, nifedipine, dilantin, verapamil, hydantoin derivatives), hereditary fibromatosis and hypertrichosis syndrome, inflammatory periodontal disease.

CAFE AU LAIT MACULES

Neurofibromatosis, tuberous sclerosis, Albright syndrome, Bloom syndrome, Wiskott-Aldrich syndrome, Gaucher disease, epidermal naevus syndrome, ataxia telangiectasia, < 3 in 10–15% of normal individuals.

Bibliography

1. Ahsan I. Textbook of Surgery, 2nd Edition. Amsterdam. Harwood Academic Publishers; 1997.
2. Arndt KA. Manual of Dermatological Therapeutics, 7th Edition. Philadelphia. Lippincot. William and Wilkin; 2007.
3. Baran R, Dawber PR, Tosti A, et al. A Text Atlas of Nail Disorders. Techniques in Investigation and Diagnosis, 3rd Edition. New York. Martin Duntz Publication; 2003.
4. Bondi EE, Jegasothy BV, Lazarus GS. Dermatology. Diagnosis and Therapy, 1st Edition. Appleton and Lange Publication; 1991.
5. Brown RG and Burns T. Lecture notes on Dermatology. Diagnosis and Therapy, 3rd Edition. Massachusetts. Blackwell Publishing Ltd; 2002.
6. Brunton LL, Chabner BA and Knollman BC (eds). Goodman and Gilman's The Pharmacological Basis of Therapeutics. 12th Edition. New York. McGraw Hill Publication; 2011.
7. Burns T, Breathnach S, Cox N, Griffiths C (eds). Rook's Textbook of Dermatology, 8th Edition. Oxford. Wiley-Blackwell Publication; 2010.
8. Burton JL. Essentials of Dermatology, 3rd Edition. Edinburgh. Churchill Livingstone Publication; 1990.
9. Crissey JT, Parish LC, Holubar K. Historical atlas of Dermatology and Dermatologists. Washington DC. The Parthenon Publishing Group; 2002.
10. Cunliffe WJ. Acne. 1st Edition. Published by Martin Dunitz. London. Reprint 1993.
11. Davidson's Principle and Practice of Medicine. Edited by Walker BR, Colledge NR, Ralston SH and Penman I. 22nd Edition. London. Churchill Livingstone Publication; 2014.
12. Dawber R and Neste DV. Hair and Scalp Disorders. Common Presenting Signs. Differential Diagnosis, 2nd Edition. Oxford. Blackwell Science Publication; 2004.
13. Doughlas G. A History of Medicine. London. Thomas Nelson and Sons; 1960.
14. Fenella LF, Wojnaewska TT, Shahrad P. Illustrated Encyclopaedia of Dermatology, 1st Edition. MTP Press Ltd; 1981.
15. Fitzpatricks JE and Morelli JG. Dermatology: Secrets Plus. 4th Edition. Philadelphia. Elsevier Mosby Publication; 2011.
16. Fleischer BA, Feldman RA, Katz SA, et al. Twenty Common Problems in Dermatology. Toronto. McGraw Hill Publication; 2000.
17. Gawkrodger DJ and Ardern-Jones MR. Dermatology: An Illustrated Colour Text. 5th Edition. Edinburgh. Churchill Livingstone Publication; 2012.

18. Goldsmith LA,. Katz SI,. Gilchrest BA,. Paller AS, Leffell DJ, Wolff K (eds). Fitzpatrick's Dermatology in General Medicine. 8th Edition. New York . McGraw Hill Publication; 2012.
19. Graham-Brown R and Burns T. Lecture notes: Dermatology. 10th Edition. Oxford. Wiley- Blackwell Publication; 2011.
20. Gulhrie DA. A History of Medicine. London. Thomas Nelson and Sons; 1960.
21. Guyton AC and Hall JC. Guyton and Hall. Textbook of Medical Physiology, 12th edition. Philadelphia. Elsevier/Saunders; 2010.
22. Habif PT. Clinical Dermatology. 5th Edition. Toronto. Mosby Elsevier Publication; 2009.
23. Hughes E and Onselen JV. Dermatological Nursing. A Practical Guide. London. Churchill Livingstone Publication; 2003.
24. Hunter JAA, Weller R, Savin J, Dahl M. Clinical Dermatology. 4th Edition. Oxford. Wiley-Blackwell Publication; 2013.
25. Kane SK, Lio PA, Stratigos AJ, et al. Colour Atlas of Pediatric Dermatology. 2nd Edition. Toronto. McGraw Hill Publication; 2009.
26. Kanerva L, Elsner P, Wahlberg JE, et al. Condensed Handbook of Occupational Therapy. Berlin. Springer- Verlag; 2004.
27. Kerdel A Francisco, Romanelli P, et al. Dermatologic Therapeutics. Singapore. McGraw Hill Publication. International Edition; 2005.
28. Khopkar U, Pande S and Nischal KC. Handbook of Dermatological Drug Therapy. New Dehli. Elsevier; 2007.
29. Kliegman RM, Santon B, St. Geme J, Schor N, Behrman RE (eds). Nelson Textbook of Pediatrics, 19th Edition. Philadelphia. Elsevier Saunders Publication; 2011.
30. Lebwohl MG, Heymann WR, Berth-Jones J, et al. Treatment of Skin Diseases. Comprehensive Therapeutic Srategies, 3rd Edition. China. Mosby/ Elsevier Publication; 2009.
31. Lebwohl MG. Difficult Diagnosis in Dermatology. New York. Churchill Livingstone Publication; 1988.
32. Lever's Histopathology of the Skin. Editor-in-Chief Elder DE, Associate editors: Elenitas R, Johnson BL, Murphy GF, and Xu G. 10th Edition. Philadelphia. Lipponcot Williams and Wilkins Publication; 2009.
33. Lewis P. An Illustrated History of Medicine. Middlesex. Hamlyn; 1968.
34. Mackie R. Clinical Dermatology, 5th Edition. Oxford. Oxford University Press; 2003.
35. Mackie R. Eczema and Dermatitis. How to cope with inflamed Skin, 1st Edition. Prentice Hall Canada Inc; 1983.
36. Magner LN. A History of Medicne, 2nd Edition. Singapore. Taylor and Francis; 2005.
37. Marks JG, Miller JJ. Marks: Lookingbill and Marks. Principles of Dermatology. 5th Edition. London. Saunder Elsevier Publication; 2013.
38. Marks R and Leyden JL. Dermatologic Therapy in Current Practice. London. Martin Dunitz Ltd; 2002.
39. Mckeown T, Rosen G, Brotherston J, et al. Medical History and Medical Care. London. Oxford University Press; 1971.

40. Mehregan AH and Hashimoto K. Pinkus Guide to Dermatohistopathology, 5th Edition. New York. Appleton and Lange Publication; 1991.
41. Menne T and Maibach IH. Hand Eczema. Florida. CRC Press; 1994.
42. Sehgal VN and Jain S. Textbook of Clinical Dermatology, 4th Edition. Jaypee Brothers Medical Publishers Ltd; 2004.
43. Sherwood L. Human Physiology. From Cells to System, 7th Edition. Washington. Thoson/Brook/Cole; 2007.
44. Siegerist HE. Great Doctors. A Biographical History of Medicine. New York. Books for Libraries Press; 1971.
45. Sterry W, Raus R, Burgdorf W. Thieme Clinical Companions- Dermatology, 5th Edition. Printed by Saurabh Printers. New Dehli. International Edition; 2007.
46. Strandring S. Grays Anatomy. The Anatomical Basis of Clinical Practice, 39th Edition. London. Elsevier/Churchill Livingstone Publication; 2005.
47. William D James, Timothy G Berger, Dirk M Elston. Andrews Diseases of the Skin, 11th Edition. Philadelphia. Elsevier/Saunders; 2011.
48. Zaidi Z, Lanigan S. Dermatology in Clinical Practice. London. Springer-Verlog Ltd; 2010.

Index

Page numbers followed by *t* refer to table and *f* refer to figure

A

Acantholysis 56, 334
Acantholytic bullous disorders 335, 342, 342*t*, 343
Acantholytic naevus 607
Acanthosis 56
  nigricans 745, 746*f*
  true 56
Acatalasemia 723
Achenbach's syndrome 416
Achromic naevus 624*f*
Acitretin 269, 816
Acne 484
  adolescent 484
  conglobata 486
  excoriee 485
  fulminans 486
  infantile 485
  inversa 504
  keloidalis 537*f*
    nuchae 536
  mechanica 704
  neonatorum 684
  occlusive 486
  occupational 486
  postadolescent 484
  vulgaris 480, 484*f*, 485*f*
Acquired hypertrichosis lanuginosa 511
Acquired ichthyosis 302, 302*f*
Acquired idiopathic photodermatoses 447
Acquired immune deficiency syndrome (AIDS) 208, 210, 429, 749
Acquired lipodystrophy 565
Acquired melanocytic naevi 618, 618*f*
Acquired palmoplantar keratodermas 283
Acquired patchy pigmentations 429
Acquired toxoplasmosis 169
Acral chronic discoid lupus erythematosus 308
Acral erythema 847
Acral melanoma 578*f*
Acremonium recifei 129
Acrochordon 599
Acrocyanosis 464, 467
Acrodermatitis
  chronica atrophicans 744, 774
  continua 262*f*
  enteropathica 359, 360*f*, 361, 660
Acrogeria 697
Acrokeratosis verruciformis 287
Acrosclerosis 321
Actinic cheilitis 446, 733
Actinic elastosis 446
Actinic granuloma 446
Actinic keratosis 446, 588
Actinic lichen planus 277*f*
Actinic prurigo 448
Actinomadura madurae 129
Actinomyces israelii 90
Actinomyces naeslundii 91
Actinomyces viscosus 91
Actinomycosis 90, 90*f*
Acute arsenic dermatitis 226
Acute eczema 217, 219
Acute intermittent porphyria 453, 451
Acute paronychia 550*f*
Acute zinc deficiency 636
Acyclovir 834
Addison's disease 665
Adenoides cysticum 537
Adenoma sebaceum 602
Adermatoglyphia 431
Adiposis dolorosa 563
Adrenocorticotropic hormone 435, 513
Aerobic diphtheroids 58
African trypanosomiasis 168
Ageing skin 692
Ageing syndrome, premature 695
Agminate folliculitis 112
AIDS, cutaneous manifestations of 210
    systemic manifestations of 212
Airborne allergens 237
Albinism 434*f*, 685
Albright's syndrome 428
Alcyonidium hirsutum 194, 707
Alefacept 825
Alexandrite laser 861
Alezzandrini's syndrome 438
Alitretinoin 816
Alkaptonuria 669
Allergic contact cheilitis 733

Allergic contact dermatitis 221, 223*t*, 782, 846
Allergic vasculitis 374
Allylamines 812
Alopecia areata 523, 525*f*
Alopecia cicatricial 528
Alopecia non-cicatricial 518
Alpha-hydroxy acids 699
Amelanotic melanoma 579
American trypanosomiasis 168
Amino acid metabolism, disorders of 669
Aminolevulinic acid 457
Amphotericin B 810
Amyloidosis 368, 370, 413
Anagen effluvium 527
Anaphylactoid purpura 412
Androgenetic alopecia 509, 518, 519, 521, 522*f*
Androgens
  action of 514
Androstenedione 512
Anetoderma 773
Angioedema 404
Angiokeratoma 627, 627*f*, 628
  circumscriptum 627
  corporis diffusum 673
  with systemic disease 673
Angiolipoma 597
Angioma serpiginosum 393, 394*f*
Angiomyoma 600
Angiotensin converting-enzyme 842
Angular cheilitis 733
Anhidrosis 499
Anhidrotic ectodermal dysplasia 503, 503*f*
Anicteric leptospirosis 102
Animal scabies 188
Annular elastolytic granuloma 446
Annular erythemas 385
Annular psoriasis 259*f*
Anthralin 266
  therapy, routine 267
Anthrax 87
Antibody
  deficiency of 651
  dependent cell-mediated toxicity 645
  positive vasculitis 381
  structure of 644*f*
Antidiuretic hormone 22, 820
Antifungal drugs, systemic 810
Antigen processing cells 256
Antihistamines 237
Anti-hypercholesterolemic drug 531
Anti-neutrophilic cytoplasmic antibody 374, 379
Anti-nuclear antibody 509
Antioxidants 699
Antiretroviral therapy 214
Anti-streptolysin O 59
Antiviral drugs 833, 835
Aphthous ulcer 718*f*, 720*t*
  difference between aphthous ulcers 720*t*
Apocrine bromhidrosis 506
Apocrine chromhidrosis 506
Apocrine gland 24, 45, 694
  diseases of 504
Apocrine hidrocystoma 507
Apoeccrine glands 23
Aquagenic urticaria 402, 707
Argon laser 859
Arodynia 226
Arsenic keratosis 226, 591
Arsenical melanosis 226
Arsenism 226
Arterial and venous ulcer, difference between 422*t*
Arterial ulcer 421, 421*f*
Arthritis mutilans 262
Arthropods 176
Ascorbic acid 635
Ashy dermatosis 391, 391*f*
Aspergillosis 135
Asteatosis 462
Asteatotic eczema 249, 249*f*
Asymmetrical hyperhidrosis 497
Ataxia telangiectasia 394
Athletes foot 114, 801
Atopic dermatitis 220, 234*f*, 235*f*
Atrophic LP 277
Atrophic skin 663
Atrophic vulvovaginitis 692
Atrophie blanche 418
Atrophoderma vermiculatum 290
Atrophy skin 55, 447
Atypical chronic pain syndrome 713
Atypical mycobacteria 77
  classification of 78
Atypical naevus 622
Auspitz sign 52
Autoerythrocyte sensitisation 415
Autoimmune progesterone dermatitis of pregnancy 690
Autoimmune urticaria 403
Autologous serum skin test 403
Axial arthritis 262
Axillae, hyperhidrosis of 496
Azathioprine 821
Azelaic acid formula 801
Azidothymidine 835
Azoles 811

B

Bacillary angiomatosis 94, 212
Bacillus fusiformis 423
Bacterial flora, normal 58
Bacterial infections 58
Balance beam alopecia 704
Balanitis 127, 740
  xerotica obliterans 741
Balanoposthitis 740
Balneophototherapy 268
Bamboo hair 533
Bancroftian filariasis 172
Baraitser syndrome 698
Barbiturates 412
Barraquer-Simons syndrome 564
Bartonella 93
  henselae 93, 94, 212
  quintana 93, 94, 212
Bartonellosis 93
Basal cell
  carcinoma 567, 568, 570*f*
    multiple 573*f*
    pigmented 570, 571*f*
  damage 334
  papilloma 595
Basement membrane 21*f*
  complex 20
  development of 44
Basidiobolus haptosporus 131
Basosquamous cell acanthoma 290
Bathing trunk nevus 620
Bayonet hair 535
Bazex's syndrome 573
Bazin disease 559
Beau's lines 544
Becker's naevus 608, 608*f*, 609*f*, 878
Bedbugs 182
Bedsore 755
  treatment of 755
Bees and wasps 182
Behcet's disease 719, 721, 825
Benign cutaneous lymphocytic infiltration 750
Benign migratory glossitis 729
Benign mucosal pemphigoid 346
Benzyl benzoate emulsion 802
Betel leaf stomatitis 729
Bier spots 658
Biliary cirrhosis 426
Biopsy skin 850
Biotin B7 633
Birthmarks 1, 605
Bitot's spots 630
Black and white comedones 484*f*
Black diccolouration nail 549
Black dot 112
Black hairy tongue 728
Black heel 702
Black palm 702
Black piedra 123
Black widow spider 190
Blaschko's line 41, 888
Blennorrhea 767
Bleomycin 156
Blepharophyma 492
Bloch-Sulzberger syndrome 428
Blood vessels
  and lymphatic system, diseases of 373
Bloom's syndrome 458, 676
Blue naevus 621
Blue rubber bleb naevus syndrome 617
Blue skin colour 883
Body dysmorphic disorder 712
Boeck's disease 363
Bone, eosinophilic granuloma of 757
Borderline lepromatous leprosy 81
Borderline leprosy 81, 82*f*, 85
Borderline tuberculoid leprosy 81
Borrelia afzelii 100
Borrelia burgdorferi 100
Borrelia garinii 100
Borrelia vincenti 423
Borrelial lymphocytoma 101
Borreliosis 100
Botox injections 867
Botulinum neurotoxin 867
Bourneville-Pringle disease 602
Bowen's carcinoma 590
Bowen's disease 590*f*
Bowenoid papulosis 156, 157*f*
Brachioradialis pruritus 474
Brazilian pemphigus 337
Breslow's thickness 581
Brittle nails 552
Bromocriptine 518
Bronze diabetes 426
Brucellosis 97
Bruton's disease 651
Bubonic plague 96
Bulla spreading sign 52, 339
Bullous disorders 334
Bullous drug eruption 845
Bullous ichthyosiform erythroderma 301, 301*f*
Bullous ichthyosis erythroderma 303*t*
Bullous impetigo 60
Bullous LP 278
Burkholderia mallei 95

Burkholderia pseudomallei 95
Burn
complications of 792
depth of 789, 791
extent of 791
full thickness 790
injury 790
second-degree 789
site of 791
third-degree 790
types of 791
wound sepsis 792
Burrow of scabies, 185f, 186
scraping 51
Buruli's ulcer 78
Bywater's lesions 658, 663

C

Cafe au lait macules 890
Calcaneal petechiae 702
Calcinosis 321
circumscripta 672
cutis 672
tumoral 672
Calymatobacterium granulomatis 206
Candida albicans 124, 726
Cancrum oris 720
Candidiasis 114, 123, 125, 135, 264, 726, 727t
Canities, premature 530
Capillaritis of unknown origin 413
Caput succedaneum 683
Carbon dioxide laser 856
Carbuncle 62, 63f
Carcinogen, signs of exposure of 675
Carcinoid syndrome 476
Cardiovascular syphilis 200
Castellani's paint 800
Cat scratch disease 93
Catagen 28
Cauliflower ear 702, 702f
Cavernous lymphangioma 626
Cell cycle 16, 17
Cell mediated immunity 643, 646
tests for 647
Cells of epidermis 18
Cellular blue naevus 621
Cellulitis 65, 66f
Centipedes 191
Central itch 469
Cephalohaematoma 683
Cestodes 175
Chancroid 206
Chanchroid differentiating table with other STDs 209t
Chediak-Higashi syndrome 434, 650
Cheilitis 732
exfoliativa 734
granulomatosis 735
Chemical burns 792
Chemical peels 864
Cheyletiella mites 189
Chickenpox 141, 141f
Chilblain 463, 463f
CHILD naevus 608
Childhood dermatomyositis 318
Childhood linear IgA disease 354
Chlamydia
psittaci 104
trachomatis 205, 207, 767
Chloasma 426, 429
Chlorinated pools 706
Chloroquine 449
Chlorpromazine 412
Cholinergic urticaria 401
Chromium dermatitis 224
Chromoblastomycosis 131
Chromomycosis 131
Chromonychia 549
Chronic actinic dermatitis 448
Chronic arsenism 226
Chronic discoid lupus erythematosus 56, 308, 309f, 463
Chronic eczema 218, 218f, 219, 800
Chronic granulomatous disease 648, 649
Chronic hand eczema 251f
Chronic mucocutaneous candidiasis 127
Chronic paronychia 550f
Chronic urticaria, management of 403
Chronic zinc deficiency 636
Churg-Strauss syndrome 382
Cicatrical alopecia, classification of 528
Cicatricial alopecia 528, 877
Cicatricial pemphigoid 346
Cimetidine 155
Cimex lectularius 182
Ciprofloxacin 449
Circumscript scleroderma 320
Clark's prognostic criteria 581
Closed comedones 482
Clostridial myonecrosis 754
Clostridium perfringens 754
Clothing dermatitis 225
Clubbing of nails 544
Coagulation disorders 411
Coagulation screen 410
Coccidioidomycosis 133

Cockayne's syndrome 458, 697
Cold erythema 465
Cold haemolysis 465, 467
Cold induced injuries 705
Cold panniculitis 465
Cold urticaria 402, 465
Collagen 33
and elastic tissue, hereditary disorders of 328
biosynthesis of 34
disorders 413
Collagenomas 626
Collodion baby 304, 304*f*
Combined antiandrogen oestrogen therapy 489
Combined antibody and T-cell deficiency 652
Comedones 55, 482, 483, 490
Common contact eczemas 223
Compound naevi 618
Condylomata acuminata 155*f*
Condylomata lata 197*f*, 202*t*
Congenital deafness 438
Congenital diseases, tumours with 600
Congenital erythropoietic porphyria 451
Congenital hypertrichosis lanuginosa 511
Congenital ichthyosiform erythroderma 301
Congenital melanocytic naevus 619, 620*f*
Congenital nail disorders 554
Congenital palmoplantar keratodermas 282
Congenital rubella syndrome 160
Congenital syphilis 202
Congenital toxoplasmosis 169
Connective tissue disorders 307, 786
Connective tissue naevi 626, 626*f*
Conradi's syndrome 305
Contact dermatitis 114, 220-222, 705, 707, 783
Contact purpura 413
Contact sensitisers 829
Contact urticaria 783
Copper vapour laser 860
Coral cuts 193
Corn 286, 286*f*
and warts differentiating table 287*t*
Corticosteroids 804
classification of 806
effects on the skin 805
indications 807
mechanism of action 805
side effects 808
Corynebacteria
aerobic 88
anaerobic 88
Corynebacterium diphtheriae 424
Corynebacterium hofmannii 88
Corynebacterium minutissimum 88
Corynebacterium pyogenes 88
Corynebacterium tenuis 89
Cosmetic dermatology 863
Coxsackie virus 158
Cradle cap 687
CREST syndrome 321
Crohn's disease 660, 717
Cronkhite-Canada syndrome 661
Cryofibrinogenaemia 465, 467
Cryoglobulin 466
Cryoglobulinaemia 465, 466
Cryoproteinaemia 412
Cryptococcus neoformans 134
Cullen's sign 659
Cushing's syndrome 664
Cutaneous actinomycosis 91
Cutaneous amoebiasis 163, 370, 371
Cutaneous B-cell lymphomas, primary 585
Cutaneous drug reactions 840
Cutaneous focal mucinosis 761
Cutaneous granuloma faciale 379
Cutaneous horn 589
Cutaneous immunodeficiency, primary 641
Cutaneous sport injuries 701
Cutaneous leishmaniasis 164
Cutaneous mastocytosis 405
Cutaneous nerves 38
Cutaneous pityriasis lichenoides 378
Cutaneous T-cell lymphoma 583
Cutaneous vasculature 37
Cutaneous vasculitis 374, 422
Cutis laxa 329, 685
Cutis marmorata 462, 683
telangiectatica congenita 395
Cutis rhomboidalis nuchae 446
Cutis verticis gyrata 775, 775*f*
Cyanocobalamin 632
Cyclic neutropenia 649, 722
Cyclophosphamide 819
Cyclosporin 269, 822
Cylindromas 501, 501
Cyst 54
Cystic hygroma 626
Cytochrome 451
Cytokines 472
Cytomegalovirus 146, 212
Cytotoxic reaction 645
Cytotoxic T cell 646

D

Dapsone 832
Darier's disease 296, 297*f*, 342, 547
Darier's sign 405
Darling's disease 132
Dartos muscle, tumour 600
Deep partial thickness burns 789
Deep peels 864
Degos disease 748
Degos syndrome 292
Dehydroepiandrosterone sulphate 512
Dehydrotestosterone 512
Dehydroxyphenylalanine 18
Delayed pressure urticaria 402
Demodex folliculorum 188, 491
Demodiciosis 188
Denileukin diftitox 826
Deoxyribonucleic acid 443, 745
Dercum's disease 563, 597
Dermabrasion, levels of 865
Dermal epidermal junction 20
Dermal melanocytic naevi 621
Dermatitis artefacta 423
Dermatitis herpetiformis 348, 350*f*, 351*f*
Dermatofibroma 598, 598*f*
Dermatology, radiotherapy in 869
Dermatomyositis 316, 317*f*
Dermatopathia pigmentosa reticularis 431, 432*f*
Dermatophagoides 188
Dermatophilus congolensis 498
Dermatophytes 51
Dermatophytide 109
Dermatophytoses 107
Dermatosa papulosa nigra 596*f*
Dermatoscopy 51, 510
Dermatoses occupational 782
Dermatosis papulosa nigra 749
Dermis 32
  and subcutaneous tissue, development of 43
  cellular components of 37
  muscles of 39
Dermo-epidermal junction 334
Dermographism 400
Dermoid cyst 594
Dermoscopy 580
Desmoplastic melanoma 579
Desmoplastic neutrotropic melanoma 579
Desmosomes 15, 15*f*
Devil's pinches 416
Diabetes mellitus 413, 476, 655, 697
Diabetic dermopathy 655*f*
Diabetic gangrene 656*f*
Diabetic neuropathy 657
Diaper candidiasis 127
Diaper dermatitis 229
Diascopy 51
Didanosine 214
Diffuse cutaneous leishmaniasis 166
Diffuse cutaneous mastocytosis 406
Diffuse systemic sclerosis 321
DiGeorge syndrome 651
Dihydrotestosterone 480
Dimethylsulphoxide 371, 796, 797
Dimple sign 52
Dinitrochlorobenzene 526, 648
Diode laser 861
Diphencyprone 156, 526
Diphenylcyclopropenone 829
Diphtheria 90
Diphtheritic desert sore 424
Direct fluorescent antibody test 196
Direct immunofluorescence 339, 345, 350
Directly observed therapy (DOT) 76
Discoid eczema 243*f*
Disseminated actinic superficial porokeratosis 592
Disseminated intravascular coagulation 408, 410
Disseminated superficial actinic porokeratosis 295
Distal interphalangeal arthritis 262
Dithranol paste 266, 802
DNA microassays 53
Dogger bank itch 194, 707
Dowling-Degos disease 431
Dracunculiasis 174
Dracunculus medinensis 174
Drug
  abuse 779, 781
  allergy tests 848
  reactions, classification of 840
Dry gangrene 753
Dry skin 799
Dyes, classification of 539
Dyschromatosis 432
Dyskeratosis 56
  congenita 431
Dysplastic nevus 622, 622*f*
  syndrome 623
Dysproteinemic purpura 412
Dystrophic calcification 672
Dystrophic epidermolysis bullosa 357
  differentiating table with other epidermolysis bullosa disorders 358*t*

E

Ecchymosis 808
Eccrine glands 22, 45, 694
  diseases of 496
Eccrine naevus 610
Eccrine poroma 502, 502*f*
Eccrine spiradenoma 502
Echo virus 159
Ecthyma 64, 65*f*
  gangrenosum 92, 754
Ectopic apocrine glands 506
Ectothrix infection 111
Eczema 216
  clinical features and histology 217
  endogenous 230
  exogenous 220
  pathogenesis 216
  treatment 219
Eczematoid like purpura 414
Eczematous drug eruptions 250
Ehlers-Danlos syndrome 330
Eicosanoids 472
Elastin 36
Elastorrhexis systemised 329
Elastosis perforans serpiginosa 764
Electrical burns 791, 792
Electrolyte imbalance 808
Electromyography 318
Elliptical incisions 851
Elliptical surgical biopsy 851
Emollient cream 800
Endemic syphilis 104
Endemic treponematoses 103
Endemic typhus 98
Endogenous eczema 230
Endogenous photosensitisation 450
Endothrix infection 111
Enterobacter alcaligenes 59
Enterovirus 158
Enzyme-linked immunosorbent assay
  (ELISA) 140, 213, 340
Eosinophilic granulomatosis 382
Eosinophilic pustular folliculitis 211, 686
Epidemic typhus 98
Epidermal appendages 22
Epidermal cell necrosis 334
Epidermal naevi 605, 607*f*
  classification of 605
Epidermal proliferation, control of 17
Epidermis 11, 12*f*
  development of 42
  layers of 12
Epidermodysplasia verruciformis 157
Epidermoid cyst 592, 593*f*
Epidermolysis bullosa 355, 359, 685
  acquisita 353, 354
  dystrophica 357*f*
  simplex 355, 356*f*, 358*t*
Epidermolytic hyperkeratosis 56, 301, 359
Epidermophyton 107
Epithelioid naevus 619
Epithelioma cuniculatum 575
Epithelioma of Pinkus, premalignant 573
Epstein's pearls 684, 723
Epstein-barr virus 146, 211
Erbium-YAG laser 861
E-rosette test 647
Eruptions, photosensitive 880
Eruptive xanthoma 666, 666*f*
Erysipelas 65
Erysipelothrix rhusiopathiae 88
Erythemas 383
  annulare centrifugum 385
  chronicum migrans 100, 385, 386*f*
  dyschromicum perstans 391
  elevatum diutinum 377, 378*f*
  gyratum repens 386
  induratum 75, 558, 559*f*
  infectiosum 161
  marginatum rheumaticum 387
  multiforme 387, 388, 389*f*, 843, 844
  neonatorum 683
  nodosum 558, 559*f*, 560*t*, 847
    leprosum 85
  palmare 384
Erythrasma 89*f*
Erythrocyanosis 464
Erythroderma 678, 678*f*, 875
  causes of 678
  desquamatum 241
  treatment of 680
Erythrodermic psoriasis 259
Erythrokeratoderma en cocardes 292
Erythrokeratolysis 292
Erythroplakia 732
Erythropoietic
  protoporphyria 451, 452
  hepatitic and hepatoerythropoietic
  porphyria, difference 455*t*
Esophageal dysmotility 321
Essential fatty acids 637
Etanercept 825
Ethynodiol diacetate 485
Etretinate 815
Eumelanin 425
Excimer laser 861
Exfoliative dermatitis 846
Exogenous eczema 220
Exogenous photosensitisation 449
Exophiala jeanselmei 129

External genitalia 736
disorders of
female 736
male 740
Eythema nodosum 75

F

Fabry's disease 673
Facial oedema, solid 487
Factitious ulcer 423
Famciclovir 835
Familial calcification 672
Fanconi's syndrome 427, 744
Favre-Racouchot syndrome 446
Favus 111, 112, 113*f*
Felty's syndrome 423
Female pattern hair loss 511
Ferriman-Gallwey scoring system 514
Fibreglass dermatitis 225
Fibroepithelial polyp 599
Filaggrin 231
Filariasis 172, 173*f*
Filiform wart 154*f*
First-degree burn 789
Fishing pool granuloma 78
Fissure 55
Fitzpatrick skin types 425
Fixed drug eruption 842, 843*f*
Flare sign 418
Fleas 181
Flexural candidiasis 126*f*
Flexural psoriasis 259
Flies 182
Fluconazole 119
Flucytosine 814
Fluorescent treponema test 198
Flutamide 518
Fogo salvagem 337
Folic acid deficiency 632
Follicular atrophoderma 573
Follicular keratoses 288
Follicular lichen planus 277
Follicular mucinosis 760
Follicular mycosis fungoides 583
Follicular naevi 609
Follicular occlusion triad 530
Folliculitis 61, 62*f*
decalvans 529
Food and food additives 399
Foot and mouth disease 159
Footballer's acne 704
Footwear dermatitis 223
Fordyce spots 724
Forelock, white 438
Fournier's gangrene 754
Fourth-degree burn 790
Fox-Fordyce disease 506
Francisella tularensis 95, 708
Freckle 427, 427*f*
peeling cream 801
Free-androgen index 513
Freshwater swimming 707
Frey's syndrome 497
Frostbite 464
Frostnip 464
Fucosidosis 674
Fumaric acid esters 270
Fungal infection 106
classification of 106
Furosemide 412, 449
Furuncles 63*f*
Furunculosis 62
Fusion proteins 825
Fusospirochetal gingivitis 720

G

Galli-Galli disease 431
Gamma-aminobutyric acid 145
Ganciclovir 835
Gangrene 753*f*
treatment of 755
Gardener syndrome 593, 676
Gardner-Diamond syndrome 713
Gas gangrene 754
Gasterophilus 170
Gaucher's cells 668
Gaucher's disease 668
Gene expression, control of 838
Gene therapy 837
therapeutic application of 839
vectors for 838
Genital herpes simplex 138
Genital lesions 721
Genital mycoplasma 105
Genital warts 155*f*
Geokerman regime 266
German measles 160
Giant porokeratosis 296
Giardia lamblia 213
Giemsa's stain 685, 686
Gingival hyperplasia 890
Glandular cheilitis 734
Glandular fever 147
Glomus tumour 554
Glucosyl galactosyl glycosyl ceramide 673
Gluten-free diet 352

Gluten-sensitive enteropathy 660
Glycosaminoglycans 36, 671
Gnathophyma 492
Gnathostoma spinigerum 171
Gnathostomiasis 171
Gonadotrophic-releasing hormone agonists 518
Gonococcal and non-gonococcal urethritis 770*t*
Gonococcal urethritis 770*t*
Gonorrhoea 204, 205*f*
Gorlin's sign 330
Gottron's papule 318*f*
Gottron's syndrome 292, 697
Gram-negative bacteria 92
Gram-negative folliculitis 487
Gram-negative rosacea 493
Granstein cells 20
Granulocyte colony-stimulating factor 749, 889
Granuloma annulare 761, 762*f*
Granuloma formation 487, 645
Granuloma inguinale 206, 207*f*, 209*t*
Granuloma multiforme 762, 763*f*
Granulomatous mycosis fungoides 583
Granulomatous rosacea 492
Granulomatous vasculitis 374, 379
Gravitational purpura 415
Green nail syndrome 92
Grey Turner's sign 659
Greying of hair, causes of 531
Griseofulvin 118, 119, 449, 813
Gunther's disease 451
Gustatory sweating 23, 496
Guttate psoriasis 259, 259*f*
Gynaecomastia 659*f*

H

Haemangioma 612*f*
Haemophilia A 412
Haemophilia B 412
Haemophilus ducreyi 206
Haemophilus influenzae 753
Hailey-Hailey disease 342, 343
Hair 25, 44
  bleaching of 540
  bulb test 433
  cast 535
  changes 197
  colour 514
  cosmetics 539
  cyclic activity of 28
  discolouration, causes of 531
  disorders 509, 877
  dyes 228
  follicle
    longitudinal section 26*f*
    transverse section 26*f*
    tumorus of 537
  hardening of 541
  loss 877
    pattern of 520
  pluck evaluation 29
  pull test 510
  removal 541, 858
  shaft
    abnormalities of 531
    disorders 532*f*
  softening of 540
  sprays 228
  straighteners 228
  structural defects of 531
  types of 28
  waving of 540
Hairy epidermal naevus, pigmented 608
Hairy leukoplakia, white 723, 724
Halecium beani 194
Halecium dermatitis 194
Half-and-half nails 545
Halo naevus 621
Hamilton's classification 520
Hand dermatitis, occupational 782
Hand eczema 251, 252
  severity of 253
Hand, foot and mouth disease 159
Hands and feet, hyperhidrosis of 496
Hand-Schuller-Christian disease 757
Harlequin colour changes 683
Harlequin foetus 304*f*
Harmful allergic reaction, classification of 645
Hartnup disease 670, 879
Harvest mites 189
Heat
  induced injuries 704
  regulation 46
Helicobacter pylori 491
Heme, synthesis of 452*f*
Hemochromatosis 413
Henoch-Schonlein purpura 412
Hepatic porphyrias 453
Hepatoerythropoietic porphyria 454
Hereditary angioedema 404
Hereditary coproporphyria 454
Hereditary diffuse pigmentation 427
Hereditary patchy pigmentations 427
Hereditary sclerosing poikiloderma 744

Hereditary spherocytosis 423
Hermansky-Pudlak syndrome 434
Herpangina 158
Herpes gestationis 347
Herpes gladiatorum 138
Herpes simplex 138, 139*f*, 209*t*
Herpes zoster 142, 143*f*
Herpetic whitlow 138
Herpetiform pemphigoid 345
Herpetiform ulcers 718
Heterochromia 438
Hidradenitis suppurativa 504, 505*f*
  and scrofuloderma 505*t*
Highly active antiretroviral therapy 214, 565, 587
Hippocratic nails 545
Hirsutism 512, 512*f*, 514
  evaluation of 516
Histamine 471
Histiocytic lymphoma, true 759
Histiocytoma 598
Histiocytosis 756
  classification of 756
Histoplasma capsulatum 132
Histoplasmosis 132
Hormonal replacement therapy, complications of 692
Hortaea werneckii 123
Hot tub dermatitis 93
House dust mite 188
Human bite 192
Human herpes virus 147, 148
Human immunodeficiency virus (HIV) 208, 719
Human interferon 826
Human leukocyte antigen 698
Human papillomavirus 172, 737
Humoral immunity 642, 643
  tests for 647
Hunter's syndrome 671
Hutchinson's summer prurigo 771
Hutchinson-Gilford syndrome 696
Hyalinosis cutis et mucosae 667
Hyaluronic acid 36
Hydrating lotion 799
Hydration 638
Hydroa vacciniforme 448
Hyperglobinaemia 412
Hyperhidrosis 496, 801
Hyperimmunoglobulinaemia E syndrome 650
Hyperkeratosis 56, 282
Hyperlipidemias 665
Hyperostosis 496
Hyperpigmentation 426, 427, 430, 431, 447, 744, 875
Hypersensitivity syndromes 392
Hypertensive ischaemic ulcer 422, 422*f*
Hyperthyroidism 664
Hypertrichosis 511, 846, 877, 878
  lanuginosa 877
Hypertrophic lichen planus 276, 277*f*
Hypervitaminosis A 631
Hypoderma bovis 170
Hypohidrosis 431, 496
Hypomelanosis 433
Hypomelanotic macules 438
Hyponychium 32
Hypopigmentation 432, 435, 875
Hypopituitarism 435
Hypostatic eczema 244, 245*f*
Hypovitaminosis A 288, 630
Ichthyosis 298, 685
  bullous 301
  lamella 299
  non-bullous 301
  rare ichthyosiform disorders 304
  X-linked 299
  vulgaris 298

I

Icteric leptospirosis 102
Idiopathic calcification 672
Idiopathic guttate hypomelanosis 439, 439*f*
Idiopathic hirsutism 516
Idiopathic thrombocytopaenia 411
Idoxuridine 836
Imiquimod 156
Immune complexes 645
Immune mediated contact urticaria 783
Immunodeficiency states, classification of 648
Immunofluorescence 51
Immunoglobulin 643
Immunomodulators, topical 828
Immunorestorative therapy 214
Impetigo 59
  bullous 60*f*
  herpetiformis 690
  non-bullous 60*f*
In situ hybridisation 53
Incontinentia pigmenti 428, 685
  achromians 439
Indeterminate cells 20
Indeterminate leprosy 82, 84
Indirect immunofluorescence 340, 345

Indomethacin 412
Infancy, acropustulosis of 686
Infantile angiomas 611
Infantile atopic dermatitis 242*t*
Infantile seborrhoeic dermatitis 242*t*
Infected scabies 186*f*
Infectious mononucleosis 147, 467
Infective eczema 230
Inflammation, production of 483
Inflammatory acquired oral pigmentation 728
Inflammatory epidermal naevus 607
Inflammatory linear epidermal verrucous naevus 607
Inflammatory melanoma 579
Infliximab 824
Ingrown toe nail 551, 551*f*
Injecting collagen implant, methods of 866
Injection abscess 79
Innate immunity 641
Insect bites 474
Insect venom 645
Insecticides 227
Intense pulsed light 862
Intercellular IgA pemphigus 343
Interdigital candidiasis 126*f*
Internal malignancy 675
Intertrigo 114, 498, 498*f*
Intradermal naevi 618
Intrahepatic cholestasis of pregnancy 689
Intrinsic scarring 41
Inverse pityriasis versicolor 122
Inverse psoriasis 259
Iontophoresis 853
Irregular beading of hair 532
Irritant contact dermatitis 220, 223*t*, 782
Isolated IgA deficiency 652
Isolated IgM deficiency 652
Isoniazid 412
Isonicotinylhydrazine 845
Isotretinoin 815
Itch
  mediators of 470
  receptors 469
  types of 469
Itchy folliculitis 211
Ito, hypomelanosis of 439
Itraconazole 119

J

Jadassohn, anetoderma of 773
Jarisch-Herxheimer reaction 201
Jaundice 684
Jelly fish dermatitis 192
Jessner's lymphocytic infiltration 751
Junctional epidermolysis bullosa 356, 358*t*
Junctional naevi 618
Juvenile hyaline fibromatosis 331, 332*f*
Juvenile melanoma 624
Juvenile plantar dermatosis 250
Juvenile xanthogranuloma 758
Juxta-articular nodules 881
Kala-azar 167
Kamino bodies 619, 624
Kaposi's sarcoma 148, 210, 585, 586*f*
Kaposi's varicelliform eruption 235
Kasabach-Merritt syndrome 410, 612, 613
Kawasaki's disease 392
Keloids 325, 327
Keratin 11
Keratinase 498
Keratinisation
  congenital disorders of 296
  physiology of 16
Keratinocytes 11, 12
Keratitis, ichthyosis and deafness (KID) syndrome 305
Keratoacanthoma 596, 597*f*
Keratoderma 685
  climatericum 692
Keratoelastoidosis marginalis 283, 284*f*
Keratolysis, pitted 498, 498*f*
Keratolytic drugs 488
Keratosis circumscripta 289
Keratosis follicularis spinulosa decalvans 290
Keratosis lichenoides chronica 282
Keratosis pilaris 289, 289*f*
  atrophicans 289
Keratosis rubra pilaris faciei atrophicans 290
Keratosquamous disorders 290
Kerion 112, 113*f*
Ketoconazole 119
Ketoprofen 450
Kitamura disease 431
Klebsiella granulomatis 206
Klebsiella rhinoscleromatis 97
Klippel-Trenaunay syndrome 615, 615*f*
Knuckle pads 327, 328*f*
Koebner's phenomenon 56, 151*f*, 888
Koenen's tumours 602, 603*f*
Koilonychia 544, 886
Koplik's spots of measles 723
Krypton laser 860
Kussmaul-Maier disease 376
Kwashiorkor 639
Kyrle's disease 765, 765*f*

L

Lactobacillus fermentum 238
Lamellar ichthyosis 299, 303*t*, 303*t*
Lamivudine 214
Langer's line 851
Langerhans cells 19
 and immune function 694
 histiocytosis 756
Lanugo hair 28
Large cell granuloma 757
Large plaque parapsoriasis 293
Larva currens 171
Larva migrans 170, 170*f*, 171
Lasers 156, 268, 541, 857
 burns 792
 precautions while using 858
 types of 859
 uses of 858
Lassar's paste 800
Late congenital syphilis 203
Latent syphilis 199
Latrodectus mactans 190
Lawrence-Seip syndrome 564
Lefluonomide 271, 824
Leg ulcers 417, 423
 classification of 417
 difference with arterial ulcers 422*t*
 in tropics 423
Leiner's disease 241, 653
Leiomyoma cutis 599
Leishman-Donovan bodies 164, 166
Leishmania 164
 aethopica 164, 165
 brazeliensis 166
 infantum 164, 165
 major 164
 tropica 164, 165
Leishmaniasis 164
 major 165*f*
 mucocutaneous 167
 recidivans 165,166*f*, 167
 tropica 165*f*
 visceral 167
Lentigines 429, 728
Lentigo maligna melanoma 578*f*
Lepra reactions 85
 treatment of 86
Lepromatous leprosy 79, 81*f*, 84
Lepromatous, borderline and tuberculoid leprosy, differentiation between 80*t*
Leprosy 79, 435
 cardinal signs of 86
 early signs of 86
 neurological manifestations of 83
 types of 79
Leptospiral infection 102
Leptospirosis, treatment of 103
Letterer-Siwe disease 757
Leucocytoclastic vasculitis 375*f*
Leukocyte adhesion deficiency 648, 650
Leukocyte migration, inhibition of 648
Leukonychia 549, 659
Leukoplakia 591, 591*f*, 727*t*, 731
Leukotriene
 inhibitors of 271
 receptor antagonists 404
Levonorgestrel 485
Libman-Sack's endocarditis 313
Lichen amyloidosis 369, 370*f*
Lichen aureus 414
Lichen myxedematosus 759
Lichen nitidus 280, 281*f*
Lichen panus 276*f*
Lichen planopilaris 277
Lichen planus 264, 274, 276*f*, 278, 546, 725, 725*f*, 726*f*
 actinicus 277
 erosive 276*f*
 like eruptions 278
 pemphigoides 345
 pigmentosus 278
 variants of 276
Lichen sclerosus 738, 738*f*, 741
Lichen scrofulosorum 75
Lichen simplex chronicus 247, 264
Lichen spinulosis 288, 288*f*, 289*f*
Lichen striatus 281
Lichenification 57
Lichenoid and psoriasiform epidermal naevus 608
Lichenoid drug eruption 845
Lime burns 708
Linear epidermal naevus 607*f*
Linear epidermal verrucous naevus 606
Linear IgA disease 352
Linear lesions 888
Linear purpura 888
Linear subcutaneous bands 663
Lipid metabolism, disorders of 667
Lipid proteinosis 667*f*
Lipodermatosclerosis 418, 419, 419*f*
Lipodystrophy 563, 564
 Dunnigan type of 564
 partial 563
Lipoid proteinosis 667
Lipoma 597
Lips, lichen planus of 276*f*

Liquid nitrogen 856
Livedo pattern 885
Livedo racemosa 422
Liver diseases 413, 657
Lizard bite 192
Lobomycosis 131
Lotio alba 799
Louis-bar syndrome 394
Loxoceles 189, 190
Lupus anticoagulant syndrome 315
Lupus erythematosus 307, 312*f*
  like syndrome, systemic 847
  systemic 118, 308, 311, 373, 463, 493
Lupus miliaris disseminatus faciei 488
Lupus profundus 310, 310*f*
Lupus tumidus 310
Lupus vulgaris 72, 72*f*
Luteinising hormone 509
Lyell syndrome 390, 844
Lyme disease 100, 385
Lymphangioma circumscriptum 625, 625*f*
Lymphangitis 67
Lymphatic circulation 38
Lymphatic filariasis 172
Lymphatic malformations 625
Lymphatic system, disorders of 396
Lymphocytic vasculitis 374, 378
Lymphocytoma cutis 750, 751*f*
Lymphoedema 396, 419
Lymphogranuloma venereum 207, 209*t*
Lymphomatoid papulosis 752, 752*f*
Lysergic acid diethylamide 778

M

Macroglossia 890
Macrolactams 828
Macular amyloidosis 369, 369*f*
Maculopapular eruption 197*f*, 841
Madura foot 128, 129*f*
Madurella grisea 129
Maffucci syndrome 617
Magnetic resonance imaging 66
Majocchi's disease 415
Majocchi's granuloma 110, 111*f*, 881
Major aphthae 718
Malabsorption 426, 660
Malassezia folliculitis 122, 123*f*
Malassezia furfur 120, 121, 239, 482
Male external genitalia 740
Malignant atrophic papulosis 748
Malignant cells 675
Malignant histiocytosis 759
Malignant melanoma 577
Malignant tumors 554, 873*t*
Malnutrition 413, 630
Malpigian layer 13
Marasmus 638
Marfran's syndrome 331
Marjolin's ulcer 420
Martorell's ulcer 422
Mastocytosis 405
  systemic 406
Measles, mumps and rubella 161*t*
Median nail dystrophy 552
Mediterranean fever 99
Mee's lines 545
Meige syndrome 397
Melanin 18, 443
  synthesis of 19*f*
Melanocyte 18, 443
  stimulating hormone 435, 662, 688
Melanocytic naevi 617, 728
  types of 618
Melanoma 728
Melasma 429, 429*f*, 801, 879
Meleney's gangrene 754
Melioidosis 95
Melkersson-Rosenthal syndrome 735
Melzack and Wall, gate control theory of 470
Memory T cells 647
Mendes de costa syndrome 292
Meningococcal infection 93
Menkes kinky hair syndrome 536
Menopause 691
Mental retardation 428
Mental sweating 23
Mercaptoamines 435
Mercaptobenzothiazole 224
Mercury poisoning 226
Merkel cell 20
  carcinoma 588
Metageria 697
Metallic dyes 539
Methicillin-resistant *staphylococcus aureus* 59
Methotrexate 269, 820
Methoxypsoralen 267
Metophyma 492
Mibelli, angiokeratoma of 627
Micaceous balanitis 742
Microangiopathy 655
Micrococcus sedentarius 498
Microdermabrasion 866
Microscopic polyangiitis 381
Microsporum 107
Microwave burn 792

Milia 594*f*, 684
Miliaria 499, 506, 685
 crystallina 499, 499*f*
 profunda 499
 rubra 499, 500*f*
Milk spots 485
Milker's nodule 151
Millipedes 191
Minimal erythema dose 460
Minor aphthae 718
Mixed connective tissue disease 324
Mohs surgery 854
Moist gangrene 753
Molecular weight 643
Molluscum contagiosum 149, 151*f*
 virus 149
Monilethrix 532
Monoclonal antibodies 824
Mononuclear phagocytes 757
Morbilliform erythema 384
Morbilliform rash 385*f*
Morphea 319, 320, 320*f*
Mosquitoes 183
Mouth, eosinophilic ulcer of 719
M-protein 497
Mucinosis 759
Mucocutaneous leishmaniasis 167
Mucopolysaccharidosis 671
Mucormycosis 135
Mucosal IgA deficiency 232
Mucosal melanoma 579
Mucosal warts 154
Mucous cyst 731, 731*f*
Mucuna pruriens 471
Muehrcke's lines 545
Multicentric reticulohistiocytosis 758
Muscles, tumours of smooth 599, 600
Mycetoma 128
Mycobacteria 70
 classification of 70
Mycobacterium chelonei 79
Mycobacterium leprae 79
Mycobacterium marunim 78, 706
Mycobacterium tuberculosis 70
Mycobacterium phlei 767
Mycophenolate mofetil 270, 823
Mycoplasma 104
 pneumoniae 104, 467
Mycoses, systemic 132
Mycosis fungoides 583
Myeloma 412
Myiasis 180
Myositis-specific antibody 319
Myxoid cyst 554, 761
Myxovirus 159

N

N-acetyl-4-s-cysteaminylphenol 430
Naegeli-Franceschetti-Jadassohn syndrome 431
Naevi 605
 connective tissue 626
 epidermal 605
 lymphatic 626
 melanocytic 617
 vascular 611
Naevoid BCC syndrome 572, 573*f*
Naevus achromicus 624
Naevus anemicus 616
Naevus araneus 395
Naevus comedonicus 609
Naevus depigmentosus 439
Naevus flammeus 614
 nuchae 614
Naevus of Ota 622*f*
Naevus sebaceous 610
Naevus spilus 619
Nail 29, 45, 694
 bed 31
 changes in systemic disease 544
 disorders 544, 886
 eczema 547*f*
 fold, diseases of 550
 lacquers 228
 lichen planus 546*f*
 matrix 31
 patella syndrome 554
 plate 30
  abnormalities of 552
 psoriasis 260*f*, 546*f*
  and onychomycosis, difference between 548*t*
  onycholysis 260*f*
  pitting 260*f*
 shedding of 887
 syndrome, yellow 555
Nalidixic acid 449
Napkin candidiasis 127
Narrowband UVB 267
Natural killer lymphocytes 642
Necrobiosis 57
 lipoidica 656*f*
Necrobiotic disorders 761
Necrolytic migratory erythema 386, 387*f*
Necrotising fasciitis 68*f*, 67, 754
Needle track 779*f*
 scars 779
Neisseria gonorrhoeae 204
Nekam's disease 282

Neodymium-doped yttrium aluminium garnet (ND:YAG) 861
Neonatal dermatology 682
Neonatal dermatoses, specific 685
Neonatal herpes simplex 139
Neonatal lupus erythematosus 316
Nerves and lymphatics skin 44
Netherton's syndrome 305
Neural pathways of itching 470
Neurofibromatosis 600, 601*f*
Neuromelanin 425
Neuropeptide 233, 471
Neurosyphilis 200
  treatment of 201
Neurotic excoriations 713
Neutropenia 649
Neutrophilic dermatoses 889
Neutrophilic vasculitis 373, 374
Newborn, scaling of 684
Nezelof's syndrome 651
Niacin 633
Nickel dermatitis 224, 224*f*
Nicole-Novy-McNeal medium 166
Nicotinamide adenine dinucleotide 633
  phosphate 633, 649
Nicotinic acid 633
Niemann-Pick disease 668
Nikolsky's sign 52, 339, 844
Nitroblue tetrazolium 649
Nitrogen mustard 412
Nitrous oxide 857
Nocardia asteroides 129
Nocardiosis 91
Nodular amyloidosis 369
Nodular elastoidosis 446
Nodular fat necrosis 561
Nodular melanoma, variants of 579
Nodular prurigo 771, 772*f*
Nodular scabies 186
Nodules 54
  on leg 881
Nodulocystic BCC 569
Noma 720
Non-bullous impetigo 60
Non-cicatricial alopecia 519
  causes of 518
Non-clostridial gas gangrene 754
Non-gonococcal urethritis 205, 770*t*
Non-immune mediated contact urticaria 783
Non-nucleoside reverse transcriptase inhibitors 214
Non-steroidal anti-inflammatory drugs (NSAIDs) 68, 213, 450, 486, 679, 778, 841
Non-viral vectors 838
North American blastomycosis 133
Norwegian scabies 187, 188*f*
Nose, fibrous papule of 328
Notalgia paraesthetica 474
Nucleoside reverse transcriptase inhibitors 214
Nystatin 810

O

Oatmeal baths 478
Obaji blue peel 864
Obesity 514, 640
Obsessive-compulsive disorders 712
Ocular rosacea 491, 492
Oedema of newborn 688
Ohara's disease 95
Oil of cade ointment 802
Ointments 799
Oldfield's syndrome 495
Oligoarthritis 262
Onchocerca volvulus 173
Onchocerciasis 173
Onychogryphosis 553, 553*f*
Onycholysis 552, 886
Onychomycosis 117, 117*f*, 120, 547, 548*f*
Opioid peptides 471
Opportunistic fungal infection 134
Oral candidiasis 125, 727*t*
Oral cavity
  diseases of 716
  tumours of 730
Oral contraceptives 558
Oral florid papillomatosis 724
Oral hairy leukoplakia 211
Oral leukoplakia 727*t*
Oral lichen planus 280
Oral melanoacanthoma 728
Oral mucosa, white lesions of 723
Oral ulcers, pemphigus 338*f*
Ordinary blue naevus 621
Organic dyes
  synthetic 540
  temporary 540
Ornithosis 104
Orofacial herpes simplex 138
Oroya fever 94
Osler's sign 670
Osler-Rendu-Weber disease 394
Osteodysplastic geroderma 698
Osteoma cutis 673
Otitis externa 93, 706
Otophyma 492

P

Pachydermoperiostosis 776
primary 776
secondary 776
Pachyonychia 685
congenita 555
Paget's disease 588*f*
of nipple 587
Pagetoid reticulosis 584
Painful bruising syndrome 415
Palmar erythema 658
Palmar keratoderma 282*f*
Palmar xanthomas 666
Palmoplantar hyperkeratosis 282, 282*f*
Palpable purpura 374
Panatrophy of Gowers 774
Pancreatic disease 659
Pangeria 696
Panniculitis 558, 881
in neonates 687
Paper money skin 658
Papillon-Lefevre syndrome 283, 283*f*
Papular acrodermatitis of childhood 161
Papular dermatitis of pregnancy 690
Papular lesions 365*f*
Papular mucinosis 759
Papular urticaria 180, 407
Papules and plaques of pregnancy 690
Papulo-necrotic tuberculid 75
Papulosquamous disorders 255
Papulosquamous lesions 875
Para-aminobenzoic acid 459
Paracoccidioides brasiliensis 133
Paracoccidioidomycosis 133
Parakeratosis 56
Paramyxovirus 159
Paraneoplastic dermatomyositis 318
Paraneoplastic pemphigus 337
Paraphenylenediamine 225, 228, 540
Parapsoriasis 292
Parasitic infestation 163
Parasitosis, delusions of 711
Paronychia 550
Paroxysmal cold haemoglobinuria 467
PASI score, calculations of 264
Pautrier's abscesses 583
Pearly penile papules 742, 742*f*
Pediculus capitis 177, 178
Pediculus corporis 177, 178
Pediculus humanis 177
Pediculus pubis 177
Peeling skin syndrome 292
Pemphigoid 344, 345, 345*f*, 353*t*
gestationis 347
nodularis 344
variants of 344
vegetans 345
Pemphigus 342, 343, 353*t*
erythematosus 337, 339*f*, 342*t*
foliaceus 337, 339*f*, 342*t*
herpetiformis 337
vegetans 337, 338f, 342*t*
vulgaris 338*f*, 342*t*
Penciclovir 835
Penicillin 412, 558
Penicilliosis 134
Penicillium marneffei 134
Percutaneous absorption 796
Perforating collagenosis 763, 764*f*
Perforating disorders 763
Perforating folliculitis 766
Perfumes 229
Periadenitis aphthae 718
Perifolliculitis capitis abscedens et suffodiens 529
Periodic acid-Schiff stain 108, 369, 569
Perioral dermatitis 494, 494*f*
Perioral lesions 879
Periorbital oedema 879
Periorbital pigmentation 431*f*, 879
Periorificial lentigines 428
Peripheral cyanosis 683,
Periungal telangiectasia 313*f*
Periungual erythema 545
Persistent light reactors 450
Personality traits in atopic dermatitis 234
Peutz-Jeghers disease 428
Peyronie's disease 742
Phaeoannellomyces werneckii 123
Phaeohyphomycosis 132
Phagedaenic ulcer, chronic 423
Phagocytes 641
Phagocytosis, disorders of 649
Pharmacodynamics 830
Phenols 435
Phenothiazine 449
Phenylketonuria 435, 669
Pheomelanin 425
Phlebotomy 454
Phosphodiesterase 233
Phospholipase C-activation 233
Photoallergic eruptions 450
Photoallergic reactions 449
Photocarcinogenesis 444
Photochemotherapy 407
Photodynamic therapy 862
Photo-onycholysis 450
Photosensitive eruption, sites of 442

Phototoxic reactions 449
Phrynoderma 288
Phycomycosis 131
Picorna virus 158
Piebaldism 438
Piedra black 123
white 123
difference between black and white piedra 124*t*
Piedraia hortae 123
Piezogenic papules 766
Piezogenic pedal papules 767*f*
Piezogenic wrist papules 766*f*
Pigmentary abnormalities 657
of hair 530
Pigmentation
diseases of 425
lines of 41
physiology of 426
Pigmented purpuric dermatoses, treatment of 415
Pili annulati 533
Pili torti 533
Pilomatricoma 538
Pilosebaceous abnormalities 447
Pimecrolimus 829
Pinta 103, 435
Pioneer dermatologists 4
Piroxicam 450
Pits on hand and feet 296, 573
Pituitary adrenal axis, suppression of 808
Pityriasis alba 248, 248*f*, 435
Pityriasis amiantacea 535, 536*f*
Pityriasis lichenoides
chronica 264, 379
et varioliformis acuta 378
Pityriasis rosea 264, 290, 291, 291*f*
Pityriasis rotunda 292
Pityriasis rubra pilaris 264, 297
Pityriasis versicolor 108, 114, 120, 121*f*, 122, 435
Pityrosporum orbiculare 120
ovale 120
Plague 96
Plantar lichen planus 276*f*
Plant-associated dermatitis 227
Plaque parapsoriasis small, large 293
Plasma cell
balanitis 741
cheilitis 735
mucositis 730
vulvitis 740
Plasma viral load 214
Platelet activating factor 472
Platelet count 409
Platyhelminths 175
PLEVA 378
Plexiform neuroma 601
Plummer-Vinson syndrome 639
Pneumonic plague 96
Pohl-Pinkus constriction 535
Poikiloderma 744
congenitale 459
of civatte 745, 745*f*
vasculare atrophicans 744, 744*f*
Poikilodermic changes 447
Poliosis 438, 531, 645
Polyangiitis 382
Polyarteritis nodosa 376, 377*f*
Polyenes 810
Polymerase chain reaction 53, 213
Polymorphous light eruption 447
Polyneuropathy 497
Polypoid melanoma 579
Pompholyx 245, 246*f*
Porokeratosis 294, 295*f*
of Mibelli 295
plantaris palmaris et disseminata 295
striata 296
Porphyria 450
cutanea tarda 453
treatment of 454
Port wine stain 614, 614*f*
Portuguese man-of-war 192
Positive polymerase chain reaction 75
Postherpetic neuralgia, treatment of 145
Postinflammatory hypopigmentation 435
Postinflammatory pigmentation 429
Postmenopausal pruritus 476
Powders 799
Poxvirus 148
Pregnancy, dermatoses of 689
Pretibial fever 102
Prickly heat 499
Primary systemic amyloidosis 370
Progeria 696
Prolidase deficiency 698
Prophylaxis of postherpetic neuralgia 144
Propionibacterium
acnes 482
granulosum 482
Prostaglandins 472
Protease inhibitors 214
Proteoglycans 21
Prothrombin and partial thromboplastin time 410
Protozoal infestation 163
Proximal nailfold 31
Prurigo 771

agria 772
mitis 772
nodularis 474
of Hutchinson 448
of pregnancy 690
variants of 771
Pruritic folliculitis of pregnancy 690
Pruritic papular eruption 211
Pruritus 469, 474, 661, 801
causes 472
gate control 470
in drug abuse 780
in atopic dermatitis 236
in elderly 695
hiemalis 462
vulvae 474
of undetermined origin 476
ani 474
scalp 474
gravidarum 689
treatment 478
Pseudo colloid milium 446
Pseudoacanthosis 56
Pseudoainhum 777
Pseudoatrophy 583
Pseudofolliculitis 536
barbae 537f
Pseudolymphomas 751
Pseudomonas 59, 92
Pseudomonas mallei 95
pseudomallei 95
Pseudomonas folliculitis 93
Pseudomonilethrix 532
Pseudopelade of Brocq 528
Pseudoxanthoma elasticum 328, 329f, 685
Psittacosis 104
Psoralen 817
monitoring of 818
plus UVA radiation 267
therapy 819
uses of 818
Psoriasiform syphilid 264
Psoriasis 211, 255, 264, 271, 546, 726, 802
aetiology 255
pathogenesis 257
guttate 259
inverse 259
erythrodermic 259
unstable 259
vulgaris 258, 259f
pustular 262, 262f
arthritis 260, 261f
nail 260, 260f
scalp 260, 260f
concomitant diseases 263
method of measuring severity of 264
treatment 265
Psoriatic area and severity index 264
Psoriatic arthritis 260, 261f
treatment of 272
Psychiatric disorders with dermatologic symptoms 710
Psychiatrist in dermatology, role of 715
Psychocutaneous disorders 714
classification of 710
Psychogenic pruritus 476, 713
Pterygium 552
Pulsed dye lasers 859
Punch biopsy 850
Punctate keratosis: 283
Purpura 408, 411f, 422, 447, 467, 703, 808, 846, 846f
annularis telangiectodes 415
of dermatological interest 412
of Doucas 414
of Kapetanakis 414
pigmented 584
simplex 415
systemic causes of 410
Purpuric dermatosis, pigmented 413
Purpuric disorders 415
Pustular erythema toxicum neonatorum 685
Pustular psoriasis 262, 263f
treatment of 272
Pustules 54
PUVA 407
therapy 429
Pyemotes mites 189
Pyoderma faciale 487
Pyoderma gangrenosum 660, 747, 748f
Pyogenic granuloma 487, 597, 598f
Pyridoxine 632

Q

Q. fever 99
Q-switched ruby 430
Queyrat, erythroplasia of 741, 741f
Quincke's oedema 404
Quinidine 412
Quinine 412

R

Racial and ethnic characteristics 41
Radiation therapy 873t
Radioallergosorbent test 233
Radiosensitivity 870
Radiotherapy and skin care, side effects of 873

Rapamycin 829
Rapid plasma reaginic test 198
Rare ichthyosiform disorders 304
Rash and fever 876
Rat-bite fever 97
Raynaud's disease 466
Raynaud's phenomenon 321, 465, 465*f*, 466, 467
Recessive dystrophic epidermolysis bullosa types of 358
Recurrent aphthous stomatitis 717
Recurrent ingrown nail 551
Red lesions of oral mucosa 729
Reed's naevus 619
Refsum's syndrome 304
Regimen of antituberculous therapy 77
Regimen treatment, in radiotherapy 871
Regular beading of hair 532
Regulatory T cells 647
Reiter's disease 767, 770*t*
Relapsing fever 100
Relapsing polychondritis 777, 778
Renal disease 213, 413, 661
Renal disorders 475
Reptiles 191
Reshaping hair 541
Resident flora 58
Resurfacing 859
Reticular erythematous mucinosis 760
Reticular hyperpigmentation 430
Reticular pigmentation 430, 431
Reticulate white streaks 276*f*
Reticulated pigmented anomaly of flexures 431
Retiform parapsoriasis 294
Retinoid therapy
  precautions with 817
  systemic 489
Retinoids 155, 449, 814
  chronic toxicity of 817
  monitoring of 817
  side effects of 816
Retroviral agents 836
Reverse transcriptase inhibitors 214
Rheumatic nodules 663
Rheumatoid arthritis 663
Rheumatoid like polyarthritis 262
Rheumatoid neutrophilic dermatosis 664
Rhino virus 159
Rhinoscleroma 97
Ribavirin 837
Riboflavin 631
Ribonucleic acid 443
Rickettsia 98
  akari 189
  prowazekii 98, 179
  typhi 98
Rickettsial infections, treatment of 100
Rickettsial pox 99
Rifampicin 412
Ringworm infections, management of 118
Ritter's disease 393
Roaccutane 489
Rocky mountain spotted fever 99
Rodent ulcer 569
Rosacea 491, 492*f*
  conglobata 493
  fulminans 493
Rosenbach, erysipeloid of 88
Roseola infantum 148
Rotation of treatment, psoriasis 273
Rothman-Makai syndrome 561
Rothmund-Thomson syndrome 459
Rowell's syndrome 310
Rubber dermatitis 223
Rubella 160
Ruby laser 860
Rud's syndrome 305
Rusters 496

S

Sabra dermatitis 227
Salabrasion 706
Salmon patch 613
SAPHO syndrome 486
Sarcoidosis 363, 365*f*, 412
Sarcoptes scabiei 183
Scabies 183, 802
  burrow 51, 186*f*
  hypersensitivity 186*f*
  in infants 184
  incognito 184
  Norwegian 187
  pathogenesis 184
Scalp psoriasis, treatment of 272
Scar 55
Scarlatiniform erythema 384
Scarlatiniform rash 384*f*
Scarring alopecia 530*f*
Schamberg's disease 413, 414*f*
Schamberg's lotion 802
Schimmelpenning's syndrome 610
Schistosoma haematobium 176
Schistosoma intercalatum 176
Schistosoma japonicum 176
Schistosoma mansoni 175, 176
Schweninger-Buzzi, anetoderma of 773, 773*f*

Sclerema neonatorum 687
Sclerodactyly 321
Scleroderma 319, 322*f*
Sclerosing panniculitis 563
Sclerosis 55
Sclerotic panatrophy 774
Scorpions 189
Scrofuloderma 73, 73*f*
Scrotal cysts 593, 593*f*
Scrotum
 angiokeratoma of 627
 idiopathic calcification of 673
 lymphangioma circumscriptum of 625*f*
Scrub typhus 99
Scurvy 413
Seawater swimming 707
Seaweed dermatitis 193, 707
Sebaceous adenoma 495
Sebaceous carcinoma 495
Sebaceous glands 24, 45
 tumours of 495
Sebaceous
 hyperplasia 684
 sweat and apocrine glands, disorders of 480
Seborrhoeic dermatitis 239, 240*f*, 264
 in infants 241
Seborrhoeic eczema 211
Seborrhoeic keratosis 595, 595*f*
Sebum secretion 481
Selective serotonin reuptake inhibitors 476, 712
Selenium 636
Self-inflicted damage, severity scale of 715
Semi-permanent organic dyes 540
Senear-Usher syndrome 335, 337
Senile comedones 447
Senile purpura 413
Senile wart 595
Sensory functions 46
Sensory nerve receptors 39*f*
Septicaemic plague 96
Serum sickness 847
Severe combined immunodeficiency 649, 653
Severe erythema multiforme 389
Sex hormone-binding globulin 513
Sexually transmitted diseases 195
Sezary cell 583
Shabbir syndrome 359
Shagreen patch 602*f*
Shampoos 119
Shave excision 852
Sheep pox 151
Shoe dermatitis 223*f*
Short contact therapy 267
SICCA syndrome 325
Sickle cell anaemia 423
Sildenafil 466
Silicon 637
Silvery white scales 259*f*
Sirolimus 829
Sjögren's syndrome 325
Sjögren-Larsson syndrome 305
Skier's cheilitis 705
Skin
 development 42
 ethnic characteristics 41
 fragility 353,355,361,745
 functions 46
 lines 40
 structure 10
 types 10
 writing 400
 and ageing 692
 and menopause 691
 and neonatal dermatoses 683
 and pregnancy dermatoses 688
 and occupational dermatoses 786
 and psychiatry 710
 and sports 700
 and ultraviolet radiation 441
Smoker's patches 724
Sneddon Wilkinson disease 343
Solar keratosis 588, 589*f*
Solar radiation on skin 445
Solar urticaria 402, 448
Solitary angiokeratoma 628
Solitary mastocytosma 406
Solitary trichoepithelioma 538
Solomon's syndrome 610
Solvent 798
Soret band 451, 454
South American blastomycosis 133
Sparganosis 175
Spastic paralysis 428
Speckled lentiginous naevus 619
Spider telangiectases 395
Spirillum minor 97, 98
Spirochaetes 100
Spirometra mansonoides 175
Spitz naevi 624
Sponge naevus, white 723
Sponges 193
Spongiosis 57, 334
Sporadic typhus 98
Sporothrix schenckii 130, 707
Sporotrichosis 130, 707
Spun glass hair 534
Squamous cell carcinoma 156, 567, 574, 575*f*, 732

Squaric acid dibutylester 156, 829
Standard erythema dose 442
Staphylococcal scalded skin syndrome 68, 393
Staphylococcus aureus 59, 61, 62, 63, 64, 65, 68, 69, 211, 233, 237, 252, 529, 550
Staphylococcus epidermidis 58, 59, 482
Stavudine 836
Steatocystoma 495
  multiplex 495
  simplex 495
Stein-Leventhal syndrome 515
Sterile pustular dermatoses 889
Stevens-Johnson syndrome 389, 844
Stiff skin syndrome 889
Stomatitis nicotinica 724
Stratum corneum 14
Stratum granulosum 14
Stratum lucidum 15
Stratum malpighii 13
Stratum spinosum 13
Strawberry angioma 611
Streptobacillus moniliformis 97, 98
Streptococcus haemolyticus 59
Streptococcus pneumoniae 59
Streptococcus pyogenes 59, 64, 65
Streptococcus sanguinis 719
Streptococcus viridans 59
Streptomyces pelletieri 129
Streptomyces somaliensis 129
Striae distensae 703
Striate palmoplantar keratoderma 283
Strongyloides stercoralis 171
Sturge-Weber syndrome 615
Subacute eczema 217, 217*f*, 219
Subacute lupus erythematosus 308, 311
Subcutaneous fat
  diseases of 557
  necrosis 687
Subcutaneous mycoses 128
Subcutaneous tissue 39
Subcutaneous zygomycosis 131
Subepidermal bullous disorders 352
Submucous fibrosis 724, 725*f*
Subungual exostosis 554
Sucking blisters 684
Sulphonamides 412, 449, 558
Sulphur ointment 802
Sunlight, spectrum of 441*f*
Sunscreens 228, 459
Superficial BCC 570
Superficial burn 790*f*
Superficial mycoses 107, 108
Superficial peels 863
Superficial spreading melanoma 578*f*
Suppressor T cells 647
Sutton's naevus 621
Sutton's ulcer 718
Sweat glands
  anatomy 22
  congenital disorders of 503
  diseases of 495
  tumours of 500
Sweet's syndrome 719, 750*f*
Swimmer's ear 706
Swimming pool granuloma 706
Swiss type agammaglobulinemia 653
Sycosis barbae 64, 64*f*
Syncope 448
Synovitis 486
Synthesis of collagen 34*f*
Syphilis 195, 209*t*
  primary stage 196
  secondary stage 197
  latent syphilis 199
  tertiary syphilis 199
  treatment 200
  congenital 202
  treatment 203
Syringomas 500, 501*f*
Systemic amyloidosis, primary 370
Systemic disease 655

T

T cell, types of 646
Tacrolimus 266, 828
Taenia solium 175
Takahara's disease 723
Takayasu's arteritis 380
Tar 266
  baths 478
  keratosis 592
Target lesion 56
Tattoos 728, 858
Tazarotene 266
Telangiectasia 55, 321, 393, 447, 658
  macularis eruptiva perstans 406
  primary 393
  secondary 393
Telogen effluvium 527
  causes of 527
Temporal arteritis 380
Tendinous xanthomas 666
Tennis toe 702
Tension lines 40
Terbinafine 119
Terminal hair 28

Terry's nails 545
Tertiary syphilis 199, 200
Testing for plant allergies 227
Testosterone 512
  levels in male and females 514*t*
Thalassaemia 423
Thermal sweating 23
Thermolysis 853
Thermoregulation 679
Thiamine 631
Thiazides 412
Thiols 435
Thrombocytopaenia 411
Thrush 125*f*, 726*f*
Thymic hypoplasia 651
Thymic stromal lymphopoietin 232
Thymus, disorders of 651
Thyroid disorders 475
Ticks 190
  borne typhus 99
Tinctures 798
Tinea barbae 116, 116*f*
Tinea capitis 111, 119
  black dot 112f
  grey patch 112*f*
  favus 112
  kerion 112
Tinea corporis 109, 109*f*, 119
  generalised 110*f*
  variants of 109
Tinea cruris 113, 114*f*, 119, 264
Tinea faciei 116, 117*f*
Tinea imbricata 109, 110*f*
Tinea infections 800
Tinea inguinalis 113
Tinea manuum 115, 116*f*
Tinea nigra 123
Tinea pedis 114, 115*f*, 120, 706
  interdigital 115*f*
Tinea unguium 117, 120
Toll-like receptors 483
Topical preparations 488
Topical therapy, principles of 795
Touraine-Solente-Gole syndrome 776
Toxic epidermal necrolysis 390, 840, 844, 844*f*
Toxic erythemas 392
Toxic shock syndrome 69, 393
Toxoplasma gondii 169
Toxoplasmosis 169
  and pregnancy 169
Transepidermal water loss 236
Transepithelial elimination 763
Transient acantholytic dermatosis 342
Transient bacterial flora 59
Transient neonatal dermatoses 683
Transient neonatal pustular melanosis 686
Traumatic alopecia 704
Traumatic calcification 672
Traumatic gangrene 755
Trematodes 176
Trench fever 93
Trench foot 465
Treponema
  carateum 103
  endemicum 104
  pallidum 103, 195
  pertenue 103, 423
Treponema hemagglutination test 198
Triazoles 812
Trichilemmal cyst 593, 594*f*
Trichloracetic acid 153
Trichoepithelioma 537, 538*f*
Trichogram 510
Trichomonas vaginalis 205, 206, 474
Trichomycosis axillaris 89
Trichonodosis 534
Trichophyton 107
Trichoptilosis 534
Trichorrhexis invaginata 533
Trichorrhexis nodosa 533
Trichoscan 510
Trichosporon asahii 123
Trichosporon beigelii 123
Trichosporosis 123
Trichostasis spinulosa 534
Trichothiodystrophy 536
Trichotillomania 711, 711*f*
Tricyclic antidepressants 449
Trinitrotoluene 531
Triradiate scars 446
Trombidiasis 189
Tropical ulcer 423, 424*f*
Trypanosoma brucei 168
Trypanosoma cruzi 168
Trypanosomiasis 168
Tryptophan 443
Tsutsugamushi fever 99
Tuberculids 74
Tuberculoid leprosy 81, 82*f*, 85
Tuberculosis 70, 72, 75
  classification 71
  diagnosis 75
  cutis orificialis 74
  treatment 76
  verrucosa cutis 73 74*f*
Tuberculous chancre 74
Tuberculous gumma 74

Tuberous sclerosis 602, 602*f*
Tularaemia 95, 708
Tumour necrosis factor-α 257, 271
Tumour necrosis factor-β 492
Tungiasis 181
Turban tumour 501
Tyrosinase albinism negative 433
Tyrosinase albinism positive 433
Tyrosine 443
Tzanck's test 51, 339

U

Ulcers 55
  of oral cavity 717
  site of injury 353, 355, 361, 745
  of leg 417
Ulerythema ophryogenes 290
Ultraviolet light 266, 335, 441, 447, 475, 479, 605
Ultraviolet radiation 18, 441, 568
  spectrum of 442*f*
Unclassified eczema 250
Uncombable hair syndrome 534
Uncommon drug reactions 845
Ureaplasma urealyticum 205
Urocanic acid 443
Urticaria 399, 401*f*, 422, 467
  approach 403
  pathogenesis 400
  classification 400
  autoimmune 403
  pigmentosa 405
  papular 407, 180
  pathogenesis 400
  treatment 404
Urticarial vasculitis 402

V

Vaccination 142, 237
Valacyclovir 835
Vanishing creams 798
Varicella 141
  zoster immunoglobulin 146
  zoster infection, prevention of 146
Variegate porphyria 451, 453
Vascular endothelial growth factor 257
Vasculitis 373
  miscellaneous 381
  systemic 374
Vasoactive intestinal peptide 471
Vasoconstriction bioassay 806
Vasoconstrictive effect 806
Vegetable dyes 539
Veldt sore 424
Vellus hair 28
  hypertrichosis of 511, 878
Venereal disease research laboratory 122, 198
Venomous animals 191
Venomous fishes 192
Venous malformation 616
Venous ulcers 417, 418*f*
  complications of 419
  treatment of 420
Verruca 152
  vulgaris 154*f*
Verrucous melanoma 579
Verruga peruana 94
Vesicle 54
Vesiculobullous lesions 875
Vibration syndrome 785
Vibratory urticaria 402
Vibrio vulnificus 68
Vidarabine 837
Vincent's infection 720
Viral infections 136
Viral vectors 838
Visceral larva migrans 171
Visceral leishmaniasis 167
Vitamin
  B complex 631
  B1 631
  B12 632
  B2 631
  B3 633
  B6 632
  C 635
  D 634
    production 445
    synthesis of 47
  D3 derivatives, topical 265
  E 635
  K 634
Vitiligo 435, 436*f*
  pathogenesis 435
  treatment 437
  segmental 438*f*
Vogt-Koyanagi-Harada syndrome 438
von Recklinghausen disease 600
Vulval dystrophies 736
Vulval intraepithelial neoplasia 736, 737*f*
Vulvovaginitis 127

W

Waardenburg's syndrome 438

Warts 152
  types 153
  treatment 153
  mucosal 154
  treatment resistant warts 155
Warty tuberculosis 73
Waves, permanent 228
Weary-Kindler syndrome 361, 745
Weber-Christian disease 560
Weber-Cockayne syndrome 700
Wegener's granulomatosis 374, 379
Weil's disease 102
Werner's syndrome 696
White blood cells 270, 750
White nail 549
White hair, darkening of 531
Whitfield's ointment 800
Whitmore's disease 95
Wiedemann-Rautenstrauch syndrome 697
Wise's lotion 800
Wiskott-Aldrich syndrome 652
Wood's lamp examination 108
Woolly hair 534
Woringer-Kolopp disease 584
Wright's stain 685, 686
Wuchereria bancrofti 172

X

Xanthelasma 665, 666*f*
Xanthoma tuberosum 666
Xanthomatosis 665
Xeroderma 211
  pigmentosum 457, 685
Xerosis 661*f*
X-linked ichthyosis 299, 303*t*

Y

Yaws 103, 423
Yeast 106, 121, 124
Yellow nails 549
Yellow nail syndrome 555
Yersinia pestis 96

Z

Zalcitabine 214, 836
Zidovudine 214, 835
Zinc 636
  deficiency of 360, 420
  liniment 800
Zinsser-Cole-Engman syndrome 431
Zoon's balanitis plasma cell 735
Zygomycosis 131

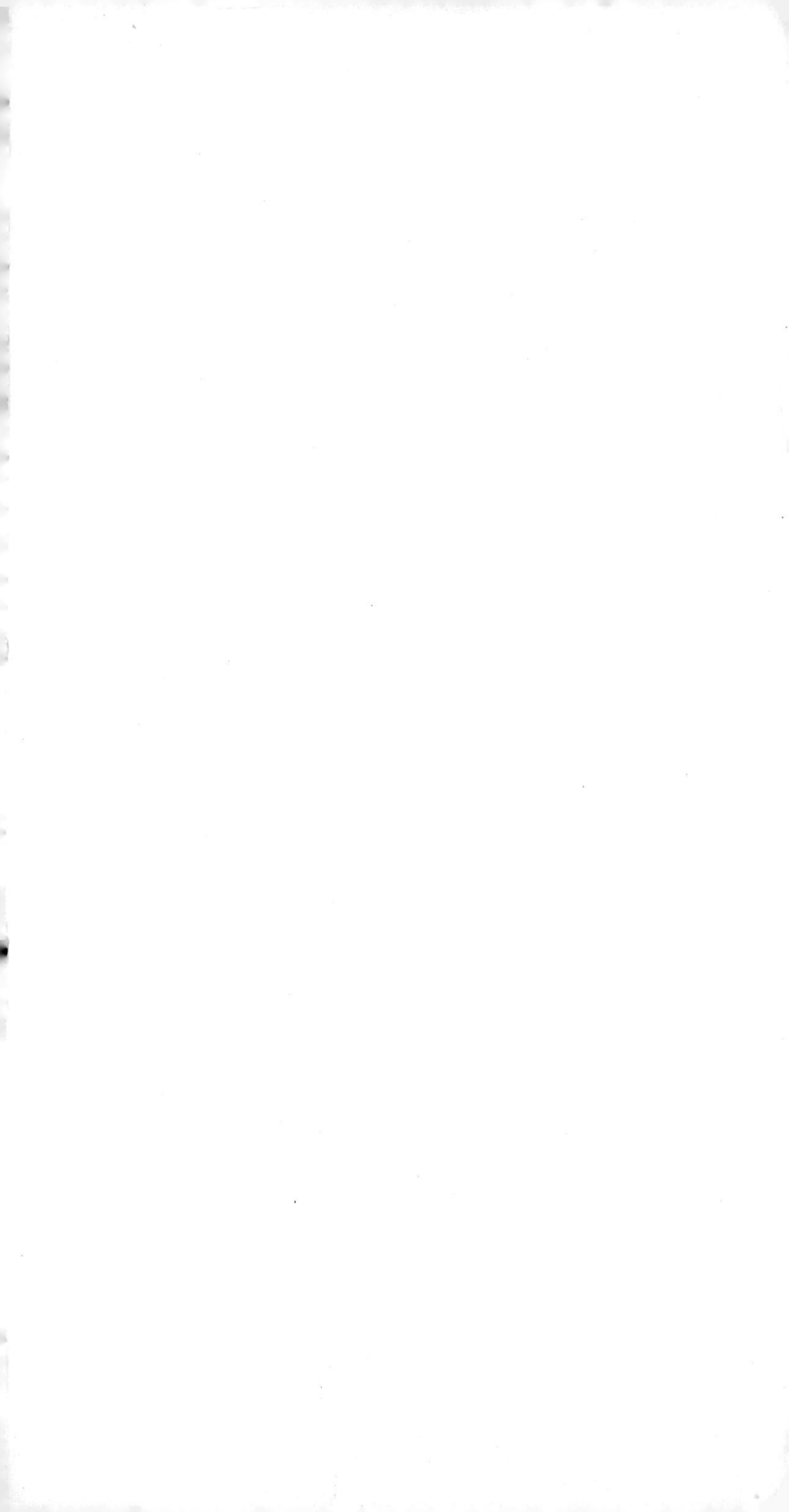